SOURCES AND EFFECTS OF IONIZING RADIATION

United Nations Scientific Committee on the Effects of Atomic Radiation

UNSCEAR 1993 Report to the General Assembly, with Scientific Annexes

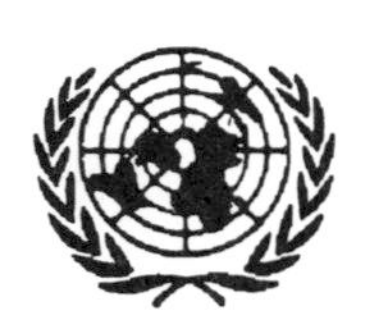

UNITED NATIONS
New York, 1993

NOTE

The report of the Committee without its annexes appears as Official Records of the General Assembly, Forty-eighth Session, Supplement No. 46 (A/48/46).

The designation employed and the presentation of material in this publication do not imply the expression of any opinion whatsoever on the part of the Secretariat of the United Nations concerning the legal status of any country, territory, city or area, or of its authorities, or concerning the delimitation of its frontiers or boundaries.

The country names used in this document are, in most cases, those that were in use at the time the data were collected or the text prepared. In other cases, however, the names have been updated, where this was possible and appropriate, to reflect political changes.

UNITED NATIONS PUBLICATION
Sales No. E.94.IX.2
ISBN 92-1-142200-0

CONTENTS

Report of the United Nations Scientific Committee on the Effects of Atomic Radiation to the General Assembly

CONTENTS

INTRODUCTION

1. The United Nations Scientific Committee on the Effects of Atomic Radiation (UNSCEAR)[a] presents to the General Assembly,[b] and thereby to the scientific and world community, its latest evaluations of the sources of ionizing radiation and the effects of exposures. This is the eleventh in a series of reports issued by the Committee since it began its work in 1955. The major aims of the Committee's work are to assess the consequences to human health of a wide range of doses of ionizing radiation and to estimate the dose to people all over the world from natural and man-made radiation sources.

2. The present report and its scientific annexes were prepared between the thirty-eighth and the forty-second sessions of the Committee. The material of the report was developed at annual sessions of the Committee, based on working papers prepared by the secretariat that were modified and amended from one session to the next to reflect the Committee's views. The Report is based mainly on data provided by the Member States until the end of 1989. More recent information has been used in the interpretation of these data.

3. The following members of the Committee served as Chairman, Vice-chairman and Rapporteur, respectively, at the sessions: thirty-eighth and thirty-ninth sessions: K. Lokan (Australia), J. Maisin (Belgium) and E. Létourneau (Canada); fortieth and forty-first sessions: J. Maisin (Belgium), E. Létourneau (Canada) and L. Pinillos Ashton (Peru); forty-second session: E. Létourneau (Canada), L. Pinillos Ashton (Peru) and G. Bengtsson (Sweden). The names of experts who attended the thirty-eighth to the forty-second sessions of the Committee as members of national delegations are listed in Appendix I.

4. In approving the present Report, and assuming therefore full responsibility for its content, the Committee wishes to acknowledge the help and advice of a group of consultants. These consultants, appointed by the Secretary-General, helped in the preparation of the text and scientific annexes. Their names are given in Appendix II. They were responsible for the preliminary reviews and evaluation of the technical information received by the Committee or available in the open scientific literature, on which rest the final deliberations of the Committee.

5. The sessions of the Committee held during the period under review were attended by representatives of the United Nations Environment Programme (UNEP), the World Health Organization (WHO), the International Atomic Energy Agency (IAEA), the International Commission on Radiological Protection (ICRP) and the International Commission on Radiation Units and Measurements (ICRU). The Committee wishes to acknowledge their contributions to the discussions.

6. In the present Report, the Committee summarizes the main conclusions of the scientific annexes. These results build on previous UNSCEAR Reports and take account of the scientific information that has since become available. A major historical review of the Committee's work including the evolution of concepts and evaluations, was included in the UNSCEAR 1988 Report. The present Report includes a general introduction to the biological effects of ionizing radiation, based on present understanding (Chapter I). In order to quantify the biological effects of radiation and to define the exposures that cause them, it is necessary to

---

[a] The United Nations Scientific Committee on the Effects of Atomic Radiation was established by the General Assembly at its tenth session, in 1955. Its terms of reference are set out in resolution 913 (X) of 3 December 1955. The Committee was originally composed of the following Member States: Argentina, Australia, Belgium, Brazil, Canada, Czechoslovakia, Egypt, France, India, Japan, Mexico, Sweden, Union of Soviet Socialist Republics, United Kingdom of Great Britain and Northern Ireland and the United States of America. The membership was subsequently enlarged by the General Assembly in its resolution 3154 C (XXVIII) of 14 December 1973 to include the Federal Republic of Germany, Indonesia, Peru, Poland and the Sudan. By resolution 41/62 B of 3 December 1986, the General Assembly increased the membership of the Committee to a maximum of 21 members and invited China to become a member.

[b] For the previous substantive Reports of UNSCEAR to the General Assembly, see *Official Records of the General Assembly, Thirteenth Session, Supplement No. 17* (A/3838); *ibid., Seventeenth Session, Supplement No. 16* (A/5216); *ibid., Nineteenth Session, Supplement No. 14* (A/5814); *ibid., Twenty-first Session, Supplement No. 14* (A/6314 and Corr.1); *ibid., Twenty-fourth Session, Supplement No. 13* (A/7613 and Corr.1); *ibid., Twenty-seventh Session, Supplement No. 25* (A/8725 and Corr.1); *ibid., Thirty-second Session, Supplement No. 40* (A/32/40); *ibid., Thirty-seventh Session, Supplement No. 45* (A/37/45); *ibid., Forty-first Session, Supplement No. 16* (A/41/16); and *ibid., Forty-third Session, Supplement No. 45* (A/43/45). These documents are referred to as the 1958, 1962, 1964, 1966, 1969, 1972, 1977, 1982, 1986 and 1988 Reports, respectively. The 1972 Report with scientific annexes was published as *Ionizing Radiation: Levels and Effects, Volume I: Levels* and *Volume II: Effects* (United Nations publication, Sales No. E.72.IX.17 and 18). The 1977 Report with scientific annexes was published as *Sources and Effects of Ionizing Radiation* (United Nations publication, Sales No. E.77.IX.1). The 1982 Report with scientific annexes was published as *Ionizing Radiation: Sources and Biological Effects* (United Nations publication, Sales No. E.82.IX.8). The 1986 Report with scientific annexes was published as *Genetic and Somatic Effects of Ionizing Radiation* (United Nations publication, Sales No. E.86.IX.9). The 1988 Report with annexes was published as *Sources, Effects and Risks of Ionizing Radiation* (United Nations publication, Sales No. E.88.IX.7).

understand the radiation quantities and units. These are discussed in Chapter II, Section A of the Report.

7. The consequences of exposures to radiation are assessed (Chapter II, Section B) by making combined use of the results of radiobiological research and the results of epidemiological studies of exposed human populations. The various sources of human radiation exposures are summarized and evaluated in Chapter III. The doses are estimated from information in the published literature, supplemented by data provided by many of the Member States of the United Nations. Those who make use of the Reports of the Committee often have to take account of the way in which people perceive the risks associated with ionizing radiation. These perceptions depend on various personal and societal factors and interactions. The principal features of radiation risk perception are discussed in Chapter IV. A brief summary and some indication of perspectives are given in Chapter V.

8. The Committee is aware of the wide readership of the Report to the General Assembly and its scientific annexes. Individuals and members of Governments in countries throughout the world are concerned about the possible hazards of radiation. Scientists and medical specialists are interested in the data compilations in the Reports of the Committee and in the methodologies presented for radiation assessments. In carrying out its work, the Committee applies its scientific judgement to the material that it reviews and takes care to retain an independent and neutral position in reaching its conclusions. The results of its work are presented for the general reader in the main text of the Report to the General Assembly. The supporting scientific annexes are written in a format and a language that are essentially aimed at the specialist.

9. Following established practice, only the main text of the Report is submitted to the General Assembly. The full Report, including the scientific annexes, will be issued as a United Nations sales publication. This practice is intended to achieve a wider distribution of the findings for the benefit of the international scientific community. The Committee wishes to draw the attention of the General Assembly to the fact that the main text of the Report is presented separately from its scientific annexes simply for the sake of convenience. It should be understood that the scientific data contained in the annexes are important because they form the basis for the conclusions of the Report.

I. BIOLOGICAL EFFECTS OF IONIZING RADIATION

10. The process of ionization changes atoms and molecules. In cells, some of the initial changes may have both short- and long-term consequences. If cellular damage does occur, and is not adequately repaired, it may prevent the cell from surviving or reproducing, or it may result in a viable, but modified, cell. The two outcomes have profoundly different implications for the organism as a whole.

11. The function of most organs and tissues of the body is unaffected by the loss of small numbers of cells, or sometimes even of substantial numbers. However, if the number of cells lost in a tissue is large enough and the cells are important enough, there will be observable harm, reflected in a loss of tissue function. The probability of causing such harm is zero at small doses of radiation, but above some level of dose (the threshold) it increases steeply to unity (100%). Above the threshold, the severity of the harm also increases with dose. This type of effect is called deterministic, because it is sure to occur if the dose is large enough. If the loss of cells can be compensated by repopulation, the effect will be relatively short-lived. If the doses are caused by an identified event, it will usually be possible to identify the affected individuals. Some deterministic effects have characteristics that distinguish them from similar effects due to other causes, which may help to identify the affected individuals. The occurrence of an initiating event has sometimes been detected by the unexpected appearance of deterministic effects.

12. The outcome is very different if the irradiated cell is modified rather than killed. It may then be able to produce a clone of modified daughter cells. Within the body there are several highly effective defence mechanisms, but it is not realistic to expect these to be totally effective at all times. Thus the clone of cells produced by a modified but viable somatic cell may cause, after a prolonged and variable delay called the latency period, a malignant condition, a cancer. The probability, but not the severity, of the cancer increases with dose. This kind of effect is called stochastic, which means "of a random or statistical nature". If the damage occurs in a cell whose function is to transmit genetic information to later generations, the effects, which may be of many different kinds and severity, will be expressed in the progeny of the exposed person. This type of stochastic effect is called a hereditary effect. Even if the doses are known, the

excess cases of cancer or hereditary disorders can be detected only in a statistical way: the affected individuals cannot be identified. More details are given in later paragraphs.

13. Exposures to radiation are of concern to the Committee mainly in so far as they produce changes in the spectrum of risks to which mankind is subject. It therefore continues to be a major part of the Committee's work to review and interpret data that provide an improved understanding of the quantitative relationships between radiation exposure and effects on health. Except as a result of serious accidents and the unwanted but inevitable irradiation of healthy tissues in radiotherapy, the doses incurred by man are not so large as to produce deterministic effects. Although the Committee continues to take an interest in deterministic effects (one of the annexes to the present Report is concerned with deterministic effects in children), most of its biological work in recent years has been concerned with stochastic effects in human beings.

14. The most relevant sources of information on the biological effects of radiation are those obtained directly from studies of human population groups exposed to known and different amounts of radiation. The comparative study of the health of such groups is known as epidemiology. This is a scientific discipline requiring both medical and mathematical skills. It is discussed further in Section I.B. In addition, a great deal of information about the mechanisms of damage and the relationships between dose and the probability of deleterious effects in man can be inferred from biological research on isolated cells grown *in vitro* and on animals. Studies of this kind allow links to be established between the damage done to cells and the eventual effects in tissues or in the whole organism. It is difficult to make quantitative predictions of the risks to humans from non-human data, but when human data are lacking, animal data may have to be used directly.

15. The main practical interest in the risks of radiation lies in the region of lower doses and dose rates that are experienced in radiation work or in other situations of everyday life. As it happens, however, the strongest epidemiological information comes from situations involving higher doses and dose rates. Some studies at doses of more direct interest, e.g. on radiation workers in the nuclear industry and people exposed to radon in houses, are now under way.

16. It is important to realize that epidemiological studies do not have to be based on an understanding of the biological mechanisms of cancer. However, their interpretation is greatly improved if they are supported by biological information leading to convincing biological models. These can provide a conceptual basis for interpreting the results of epidemiology, essentially by suggesting dose-response relationships, the parameters of which can be fitted to the observed epidemiological results. The information provided by experimental biology is also supplemented by biophysical knowledge of the initial deposition of energy from radiation in the exposed tissues. The theoretical and experimental results are thus combined to obtain a quantitative relationship between dose and the probability of occurrence of the relevant cancer.

A. RADIOBIOLOGY

1. The target for radiation action

17. Deoxyribonucleic acid (DNA), the genetic material of the cells, is the most important target for radiation action. There is compelling evidence from *in vitro* cellular research that the deleterious effects of radiation derive mainly from the damage it causes in cellular DNA.

18. DNA is present in the chromosomes, which are basic components of the cell nucleus. Before every somatic cell division, chromosomes are duplicated so that each daughter cell receives an identical set of chromosomes. Each mammalian species is characterized by a particular and constant chromosome number, size and morphology.

19. To explain the mechanisms by which ionizing radiation damages cells it is necessary to provide a simplified description of the function of the DNA molecule. Although the maintenance of the overall chromosome structure is crucial for several processes involving DNA, it is the DNA polymer itself that is the source of the information that passes from a cell to its descendants. The information is encoded in a linear sequence of alternating molecular structures called base-pairs. These pairs form links between the strands of the double-stranded backbone of the DNA polymer.

20. The base-pair code in DNA is arranged in groups, each providing the basic unit of cellular information and heredity, the gene. In a mammalian cell, it is likely that there are approximately 100,000 genes, each of which depends for its correct function on maintaining a constant base-pair sequence in the DNA. Changes in these sequences, by base-pair substitution, loss or addition, can change the gene function. Such changes are termed genetic mutations.

21. The DNA is known to be damaged by radiation. Two mechanisms are involved: (a) direct effects of ionization in the DNA structure and (b) indirect effects

due to the production of active chemical radicals in the vicinity of the DNA and the diffusion of these radicals to the DNA, where they induce chemical changes. Both direct and indirect effects are of a probabilistic nature, with their probabilities of occurrence increasing with the radiation dose and the volume of the target. There are many other causes of damage to DNA, including errors in replication when cells divide.

22. Damage to the DNA, including radiation damage, is subject to very efficient repair mechanisms mediated by enzyme actions. If the damage to the DNA within a gene is confined to one strand, the repair mechanisms can make use of the information provided by the complementary bases in the other strand. Repair is then highly probable, but as in any complex system, it is not always error-free. Sometimes, however, both strands may be damaged at the same location in the gene. Repair is then more difficult, and genetic code changes or losses are more likely.

23. A track of radiation consists of a series of separate events, each involving a localized deposition of energy. If this deposition is in the immediate vicinity of DNA and is large enough, molecular damage may occur in the DNA bases or in the backbone strands. The nature and likelihood of the biological damage caused by this DNA damage depends on the density of the energy deposition along the tracks that intersect the DNA and also on the complex interplay between the damage and the repair enzymes of the cell. For sparsely ionizing radiations, such as x rays, the net effect of these processes is such that the dose-effect relationship for most stochastic effects is curvilinear. Densely ionizing radiations, such as alpha particles and the protons produced by neutrons, are more effective in producing stochastic effects and the dose-effect relationships are more likely to be linear.

24. In addition to these effects at a single point in the DNA, the presence of a number of ion pairs scattered through the nucleus may cause cellular changes that complicate the simple response pattern described above.

25. Irrespective of the detail of the biological mechanism, the probability that radiation will induce specific changes in the genetic code of cells by single tracks and the additional interaction of multiple tracks, may be expressed as the sum of two terms, one proportional to dose and the other proportional to the square of dose. At low doses with any dose rate and at high doses with low dose rate, only the term proportional to dose is effective. At high doses with high dose rate, both terms are relevant. With densely ionizing radiation, e.g. alpha particles, there are fewer, but denser, tracks per unit dose, and each track is more likely to produce damage that is not successfully repaired, so the relationship is more likely to be proportional to dose at all doses and dose rates.

26. When human tissues are exposed to radiation, various changes in the cell genetic code (mutations) are induced randomly, with probabilities depending on dose as already discussed. For any given change, the expected number of changed cells is the product of the probability and the number of cells at risk. These cells at risk are considered to be the stem cells of tissues, namely the cells that maintain the tissues by division, compensating for cells that mature, differentiate and eventually die, in what is called the cell reproduction cycle.

2. Effects of induced changes in the cell genetic code

27. Some changes in the genetic code are incompatible with the sustained reproduction of the cell, resulting in the death of the cell progeny. Unless many cells are killed, this is usually of no consequence for the tissues and organs because of the large number of cells in the tissue and the very substantial redundancy they provide in the functional capability of the tissue.

28. Cell killing by radiation can be quantitatively studied in cell cultures *in vitro* to gain information on the shape of the dose-response relationship. Radiation accidents and experiments *in vivo* with animals show that high doses can deplete the tissues sufficiently to cause functional failure. In turn, deterministic effects in some tissues, such as the vascular and connective tissues, cause secondary damage in other tissues.

29. Other types of change in the genetic code result in viable, but modified, cells. Some of these cells may belong to gonadal cell lines (ova or sperm) and would express the change as hereditary effects. Others would remain in the exposed tissues, being potential causes of somatic effects. In both cases, the effects are stochastic, governed by the probabilistic nature of the induction of changes in the cell genetic code.

(a) Deterministic effects

30. While individual cell killing is a stochastic effect, organ and tissue failures require the killing of large numbers of cells and therefore have thresholds of dose. Cell depletion is a dynamic process operating in competition with the proliferation of unaffected cells. Tissue failures are therefore dependent on both dose and dose rate. Although the changes in individual

cells are stochastic, the changes in a large number of cells result in a deterministic outcome. These effects are therefore called deterministic.

31. Because the proportion of cells killed depends on dose, the severity of the deterministic effect also depends on dose. If people of varying susceptibility are exposed to radiation, the threshold in a given tissue for deterministic effects of sufficient severity to be observable will be reached at smaller doses in the more sensitive individuals. As the dose increases, more individuals will incur the observable effect, up to a dose above which the whole group shows the effect.

32. Examples of deterministic effects are the induction of temporary and permanent sterility in the testes and ovaries; depression of the effectiveness of the blood forming system, leading to a decrease in the number of blood cells; skin reddening, desquamation and blistering, possibly leading to a loss of skin surface; induction of opacities in the lens and visual impairment (cataract); and inflammation processes that may occur in any organ. Some effects are indirect in that they are the result of deterministic effects on other tissues. For example, radiation that leads to the inflammation and eventual fibrosis of blood vessels may result in damage to the tissues served by those blood vessels.

33. A special case of deterministic effect is the radiation syndrome resulting from acute, whole-body irradiation. If the dose is high enough, death may result from severe cell depletion and inflammation in one or more vital organs in the body (blood-forming organs, the gastro-intestinal tract and the central nervous system, in decreasing order of sensitivity).

34. During organ development *in utero*, deterministic radiation effects are most pronounced at the time when the relevant tissue is being formed. The killing of even a few, but essential, cells may result in malformations because those cells will not have progeny. One important effect of exposure to radiation *in utero* is a dose-related increase in mental impairment, up to and including severe mental retardation.

35. The induction of mental retardation is thought to be the result of the impaired proliferation, differentiation, migration and connection of neural cells at the time when the relevant tissue (brain cortex) is being structured, namely the 8-15 week period after conception in humans. The number of neural cells that are misconnected depends on dose. If, as a first approximation, the magnitude of the mental impairment is taken to be proportional to this number, it would be expected that standard indices of the cognitive functions, e.g. the intelligence quotient (IQ), would reflect this dose dependency.

36. In population groups, the IQ has an approximately normal (Gaussian) distribution, conventionally taken to have a central value of 100. Since the average IQ score decreases as radiation dose increases, apparently without an increase in the amplitude of the spread (standard deviation), the decrease in the values of IQ can be described as a uniform shift of the IQ curve to the left (to lower values). If a pathological condition is defined as a condition in which the IQ of an individual is below a stipulated value, such a shift would increase the number of individuals with the pathological condition. This fact is important for the interpretation of the epidemiologically observed mental retardation induced by radiation, discussed in Section II.B.1.

(b) Cancer induction

37. There is compelling evidence that most, if not all, cancers originate from damage to single cells. Cancer initiation involves a loss of regulation of growth, reproduction and development in somatic stem cells, i.e. the loss of control over the cell reproduction cycle and differentiation processes. Point mutations and chromosomal damage play roles in the initiation of neoplasia. Initiation can result from the inactivation of tumour suppressor genes, some of which play a central role in the control of the cell cycle. Although cells may have undergone initiating changes, they will not express their properties until they are stimulated ("promoted") to reproduce by chemicals, hormones etc. in their environment. The promoting agents may be independent of the initiation agent.

38. Single changes in the cell genetic code are usually insufficient to result in a fully transformed cell capable of leading to a cancer; a series of several mutations (perhaps two to seven) is required. In spontaneous cancers, these mutations will have occurred randomly during life. Thus, even after initial cell transformation and promotion, further mutations are needed, and may well be available, to complete the clonal transition from pre-neoplasia to overt cancer. The whole process is called multi-stage carcinogenesis.

39. It is possible that radiation acts at several stages in multi-stage carcinogenesis, but its principal role seems to be in the initial conversion of normal stem cells to an initiated, pre-neoplastic state. The action of radiation is only one of many processes influencing the development of cancer, so the age at which a radiation-induced cancer is expressed is not likely to be very different from that of cancers arising spontaneously. In some circumstances, however, later stages may be affected by radiation, thus changing the times at which cancers appear.

40. Cancer initiation provides the target cells with some degree of proliferative or selective advantage, which is expressed after adequate promotion. The advantage may be a shorter reproduction time than that of normal cells or a blocking of normal cell differentiation. On the other hand, the very few transformed cells are immersed in a very much larger number of normal cells, and their pre-neoplastic properties can be constrained by their neighbours. An escape from these constraints is a crucial feature of the neoplastic process.

41. Even with their proliferative advantage, transformed cells and their progeny can be eliminated by the random process comprising reproduction, terminal differentiation and death that is at a steady state in mature tissues. The probability of elimination depends on the number of transformed cells and the degree to which they have become autonomous. At least one cell must lead to a clone of modified cells for a cancer to develop. The probability of this occurring is related to dose by the same type of dose relationship (linear or linear-quadratic) as discussed for heritable mutations in the cell. This broadly supports the contention that randomly induced cellular events are responsible for cancer induction.

42. Many animal experiments confirm the predicted shape of the dose-response relationship. It should be mentioned that, at higher doses, cell killing is substantial, competing with cell transformation and causing the dose-response curve to bend downwards. In particular, the following points should be stressed:

(a) unless the single cell origin of most cancers is thought to be unlikely, no low-dose threshold is to be expected;
(b) if radiation acts primarily as an initiating event, providing one among several required mutations, multiplicative models of risk projection in time can be expected to be more realistic than additive models. (See also Section II.B.2).

43. There are problems in assessing the risks of cancer for exposures at low doses and low dose rates, since most human data are available only at high doses and high dose rates. The approach commonly used in risk assessment is to fit a linear dose-response relationship to the data, a procedure that is usually considered to give an upper limit to the risk at low doses. This is because the quadratic term will increase the response at high doses with high dose rates, forcing an increase in the slope of the fitted straight line. From radiobiological considerations, it is then possible to assess the value of the factor by which the slope of the fitted curve should be reduced to give an estimate of the linear component of the linear-quadratic relationship. Direct information on humans exposed at low doses is beginning to emerge and will increasingly provide a check on estimates derived from data at high doses.

44. Novel systems to study cell transformation *in vitro* and cellular and molecular studies with these systems and with animal neoplasms appear to be potentially very productive sources of information about the mechanisms of cancer induction. Modern cellular and molecular studies may make it possible to differentiate between radiation-induced cancer and other cancers. If samples of tumours from radiation-exposed human groups were to be systematically stored, they would then be a very important resource for future studies on oncogenic mechanisms and for the establishment of causality between cancer in the population and physical or chemical carcinogens in the environment.

(c) Hereditary effects

45. If the change in the genetic code occurs in the germ cells, i.e. the egg or sperm or the cells that produce them, the effect is transmitted and may become manifest as hereditary disorders in the descendants of the exposed individuals. Experimental studies on plants and animals show that such changes may range from trivial to severe, causing gross loss of function, anatomical disorders and premature death.

46. Any non-lethal damage to DNA in germ cells can, in principle, be transmitted to subsequent generations. Hereditary disorders in humans vary widely in their severity. Dominant mutations, i.e. changes in the genetic code that produce a clinical effect when inherited from only one parent, can lead to genetic disorders in the first generation progeny. Some of these disorders are very harmful to the affected individual and affect length of life and the likelihood of having offspring. Some dominant mutations can be passed silently through several generations and then suddenly cause their effects. This can occur if the gene is moderated by other genes or is imprinted, i.e. if the expression of the gene is dependent on the sex of the parent from whom it was inherited.

47. Recessive mutations are changes in the genetic code that produce a clinical effect only when two copies of the defective gene have been inherited, normally one from each parent. They produce little effect in the first few generations, as most offspring will inherit the defective gene from only one parent, and carriers are usually not affected. However, recessive mutations may accumulate in the gene pool of the population, as each carrier passes the mutation on to many offspring. As the probability that both parents carry the mutation increases, so too does the risk that a child will inherit two copies of the defective gene and will suffer deleterious effects of the mutation.

48. Two points about recessive mutations are important. A recessive mutation often has some effect, albeit slight, even when only a single copy has been inherited, so it may result in some reproductive disadvantage. Also, recessive mutations introduced into the genetic pool are subject to processes that tend to eliminate them: random elimination, called drift, and selection based on reproductive disadvantage. For this reason, newly induced recessive mutations in the genetic pool cause a finite total damage over the generations of descendants.

49. A third, and frequent, type of deleterious change is due to the interaction of several genetic and environmental factors; these are known as multifactorial disorders. A general increase in mutations would be expected to increase the incidence of multifactorial disorders. The magnitude of such an increase is at present unclear but is likely to be small.

B. EPIDEMIOLOGY

50. Epidemiological studies, when interpreted with the aid of biological knowledge, provide the basis for assessing the consequences of radiation exposures. There are also many qualitative studies that confirm that radiation at high enough doses can induce cancer in most of the tissues and organs of the body. There are, however, several significant exceptions. At present, the three principal sources of quantitative information on stochastic effects of radiation in man are the epidemiological studies on the survivors of the nuclear weapon explosions at Hiroshima and Nagasaki, on patients exposed to radiation for diagnostic and therapeutic procedures and on some groups of workers exposed to radiation or radioactive substances at work. As this Section will show, there is little hope that differences in exposures to natural sources (excluding radon) will be able to provide quantitative information on stochastic effects, but some occurrences of high radon levels or substantial environmental contamination from accidents may well allow further relevant study groups to be identified.

51. Epidemiology is concerned with establishing patterns in the occurrence of diseases, associating these patterns with likely causes and then quantifying the associations. The process is one of observation and inference. Epidemiological studies are inherently observational in nature: they are arranged by circumstances rather than as a result of experimental design. Choices can be made of the groups to be studied and of the methods of analyzing the data, but there is seldom an opportunity to modify the conditions of the study population or the distribution of the causes under investigation. In this way, epidemiology differs sharply from experimental science.

52. Three different types of epidemiological study have been reviewed by the Committee: cohort studies, case-control studies and geographical correlation studies. In cohort studies, a group of individuals, the cohort, is selected on the basis of their exposure to the agent of interest, without prior reference to the disease under study, e.g. cancer. The group is then followed forward in time to record the mortality from or the incidence of relevant diseases. The exposure of the members of the cohort to the suspected causative agent is estimated either from contemporary measurements, as in occupational exposure, or by retrospective studies. It is then possible, by standard epidemiological techniques, to compare the incidence of disease or mortality rates following different levels of exposure.

53. If all the members of the cohort have been exposed and there is not a wide enough range of exposures to provide several groups with different levels of exposure, it is necessary to compare the experience of the cohort with that of a control cohort of individuals with substantially lower exposures. Ideally, the two cohorts should be very similar in characteristics that might influence the incidence of or mortality from the disease under study. Otherwise, these characteristics may act as confounding factors, distorting the observed relationship between disease and exposure. Even within a cohort, there may be potentially confounding factors between the groups with different levels of exposure. When information is available on the values of these factors for the individuals in the cohorts, it may be possible to allow for them. The two obvious factors in the case of cancer, age and sex, always have to be allowed for. More subtle factors, such as diet, social status and hereditary predisposition, may remain and may be difficult to quantify or even to identify.

54. One important cohort study is the Life Span Study of the survivors of the atomic bombings of Hiroshima and Nagasaki. This is based on a large cohort of all ages and both sexes with a very wide range of exposures. About 60% of the original cohort are still alive, so the present conclusions are still based on incomplete data, especially for those exposed in youth, but it remains the most substantial cohort study used by the Committee.

55. In the second type of study, the case-control study, the aim is to ascertain all the cases of the disease in a defined population, e.g. those living in a specified area during a specified period, and then to select for each case one or more control individuals without the disease but drawn from the same population as the case. The cases and controls can then be compared to see if there are significant differences in the exposures. As with cohort studies,

care has to be taken to avoid the effects of confounding factors. This can be done either by matching the controls to the cases for factors such as age and sex or by using statistical techniques in the analysis.

56. Because only the cases and the matched controls have to be investigated, case-control studies can give significant results with smaller study groups than are needed for cohort studies. Case-control studies are therefore useful where the collection of data on the individual exposures requires detailed and extensive fieldwork, making cohort studies impossible or prohibitively expensive. Case-control studies are particularly useful in examining the effects of exposure to radon in dwellings on the risk of lung cancer. In this work, it is important to allow for smoking habits, for which historical data are usually either lacking or unreliable in cohort studies. The necessary data can be sought in case-control studies.

57. The third type of study is the geographical correlation study. These studies are usually the easiest to conduct but are the most difficult to interpret and the most prone to error. In a geographical correlation study, two or more groups of people in different locations are selected on the basis of a difference in long-term exposure to radiation, usually radiation from natural sources. Health statistics for the groups are then compared to identify any relevant differences. This technique takes account of the difference in the average exposure between the groups but ignores the distribution of exposures within the groups, about which information is rarely available. If any important confounding factors, such as age, diet or exposure to pollution, are not randomly distributed between the groups, false conclusions are likely to be reached. Geographical correlation studies have not yet been of much value to the Committee, largely because it is difficult to find groups with a large and accurately known difference in exposure but a small difference in confounding factors.

58. To provide meaningful results, all types of epidemiological study need careful design, execution and interpretation. Moreover, studies that expect a small absolute increase in the incidence of diseases that already exist naturally, such as cancer, must be large if they are to provide statistically significant information. There are two main limitations in epidemiological studies: one, statistical, gives rise to random errors; the other, demographic, gives rise to systematic errors.

59. In many countries, the lifetime probability of dying of cancer is about 20%. If two populations are being compared to detect with confidence the effect of a higher radiation dose in one of them, it is necessary to obtain a difference between them that is statistically significant. To detect an increase in mortality from, say, 20% to 22%, each of the populations would have to number at least 5,000. If the groups were followed to extinction, about 1,000 cancer deaths would be observed in the unexposed group and about 1,100 in the exposed group. The 90% confidence limits on the difference would be about 0-200, just significant. With current estimates of risk, such an increase would result from a lifetime whole-body dose of about 0.4 Sv. This corresponds to an increase by a factor of 5 in the typical lifetime dose from natural sources other than radon (0.001 Sv per year) for the whole 70-year life of the exposed group (0.001 Sv per year × 70 years × 5).

60. The second limitation results from the need to match the study and control groups for any confounding factors that influence the incidence of cancer. Unless the study and control groups are drawn from a single homogeneous population, it is rarely possible to match the groups, or to make allowance for the differences, with sufficient accuracy to detect with confidence a small increase in cancer mortality. Any inadequacy in the matching of the control and study groups may give a bias that cannot be reduced merely by expanding the size of the groups.

61. It is this likelihood of bias that imposes severe limitations on the power of geographical correlation studies of mortality in geographically separated groups such as those used in studies of the effects of exposures to different levels of natural background radiation. It emphasizes the importance of cohort studies, in which a single population can be subdivided into groups with different levels of exposure. There may still be confounding factors that differ from group to group, but they are likely to be fewer in number than between geographically separated groups. Populations that can be subdivided according to exposure include the Life Span Study group in Hiroshima and Nagasaki, groups of patients undergoing radiotherapy and some occupational groups. Because of these limitations it is important to assess the feasibility of any epidemiological study before committing resources.

62. Much of the quantitative information available from the studies on these populations is limited to fairly high doses and dose rates. Estimates of the risks at smaller doses can be obtained only by extrapolation downwards from the results at high doses. The range of this extrapolation is not large, because the small doses of interest are superimposed on the inescapable doses due to natural radiation sources.

63. In the UNSCEAR 1988 Report, the Committee reviewed in detail the high-dose information from epidemiological studies, with an emphasis on the data

from Hiroshima and Nagasaki. It is too soon to repeat a comprehensive review of the Japanese data, but it has been possible to take account of the additional data now available and to reassess the previous conclusions. A substantial study of different methods of interpreting the data has been undertaken. In particular, an examination has been made of available models for projecting risk to give estimates of the lifetime probability of death caused by exposure to radiation. The Committee has also made use of other studies, particulary some recently published data on the effects of occupational exposure at moderate to low doses. These data supplement the results from the Life Span Study but do not yet have the statistical power to add much to the quantitative estimates of risk. The epidemiological studies do not provide significant data for radiation risks in the low-dose range. The extrapolation to the low-dose range has to be validated by experimental biological studies. Therefore the Committee has linked the epidemiological studies with a comprehensive review of the mechanisms of human carcinogenesis and the effects of dose and dose rate on radiation responses. The overall result is to confirm the risk estimates of the UNSCEAR 1988 Report.

64. A great deal of work has been done worldwide on epidemiological studies, but the accumulation of quantitative information is necessarily slow. For example, more than half the study group in Hiroshima and Nagasaki is still alive, and the observed excess of cancer deaths, about 350 to date, is rising slowly. The Committee has concentrated its time and resources on extensive scientific discussions on the implications of the available studies and has not prepared an Annex on epidemiology for publication at this time. The Committee's conclusions are summarized in Section II.B.2 of this Report.

II. QUANTITATIVE ESTIMATES OF RADIATION EFFECTS

A. QUANTITIES AND UNITS

65. A specific set of quantities is needed to describe and quantify radiation and its biological effects. Details of radiation quantities and units and an explanation of the derivations and variations in the use of these concepts were presented in the UNSCEAR 1988 Report. The Committee's use of quantities and units corresponds to accepted international practice.

1. Dosimetric quantities

66. Radionuclides are characterized by unstable configurations of the nucleus of the atom. They decay in spontaneous nuclear transitions and in so doing emit radiation. The characteristic rate of decay of each radionuclide is described by its half-life, the time in which spontaneous transitions will have occurred in one half of the atoms. The rate at which transitions occur in a quantity of a radionuclide is termed the activity, the unit for which is the becquerel (Bq). If a quantity of a radionuclide has an activity of 1 Bq, the transitions are occurring at a rate of one per second.

67. One of the basic quantities used to quantify the interaction of radiation with material is the absorbed dose. This is the energy imparted to a small element of material divided by the mass of that element. The unit of absorbed dose is the joule per kilogram, called for this purpose the gray (Gy). For most purposes, the Committee uses the average absorbed dose in a tissue or whole organism rather than the absorbed dose at a point. Most radiation exposures cause different absorbed doses in different parts of the human body. Absorbed doses from different types of radiation have different biological effectiveness, and the organs and tissues in the body have different sensitivities.

68. For the same absorbed dose, densely ionizing radiations such as alpha particles are more effective in causing biological effects, especially stochastic effects, than are sparsely ionizing radiations such as gamma rays, x rays or electrons (beta particles). It is useful to combine the absorbed doses from different types of radiation to provide a further quantity called the equivalent dose. The equivalent dose in a human tissue or organ is the absorbed dose weighted by a radiation weighting factor that ranges from unity for sparsely ionizing radiation to 20 for alpha particles.

69. The various organs and tissues in the body differ in their response to exposure to radiation. To allow for this, a further quantity, the effective dose, is used. The equivalent dose in each tissue or organ is multiplied by a tissue weighting factor, and the sum of these products over the whole body is the called the effective dose. The effective dose is an indicator of the total detriment due to stochastic effects in the exposed individual and his or her descendants. Since both the radiation weighting factor and the tissue weighting factor are dimensionless quantities, the dimensions of

the equivalent dose and the effective dose are the same as the dimensions of the absorbed dose, and the unit is the same, the joule per kilogram. However, to ensure a clear distinction between the absorbed dose and its weighted analogues, it has been agreed that the unit of equivalent dose and of effective dose should have the special name sievert (Sv).

70. Changes in the radiation and tissue weighting factors in 1990 complicate the comparisons between new and earlier estimates of dose. In general, the Committee has not attempted to reevaluate old data in terms of the new quantities, because the changes are usually small. Where reevaluations have been made, this is indicated in the text.

71. Absorbed dose, equivalent dose and effective dose all apply to individuals or to average individuals. The Committee also uses the collective effective dose, which is the average dose to an exposed population or group multiplied by the number of people in the group. This quantity is defined for a specified source or for a specified unit of a practice. It may refer to the total of the future doses committed by that source or unit of practice, as for instance, the collective effective dose committed by atmospheric nuclear explosions or by one year of medical exposures. If the probability of late effects is proportional to effective dose at low doses, which is probably the case, the collective effective dose is an indicator of the total attributable harm to be expected in that group and its descendants. If the individual doses making up a collective dose cover a wide range of values and extend over very long periods of time, it is more informative to subdivide the collective dose into blocks covering more restricted ranges of individual dose and time. The unit of collective effective dose is the man sievert (man Sv).

72. Some events, especially those involving a release of radioactive materials to the environment, may give rise to exposures extending in time, sometimes for many generations. In these situations, the collective dose is still a useful quantity, provided it is made clear that the collective dose is that committed by the relevant source or unit of practice. To give an indication of the dose committed to a typical, but hypothetical, individual now and in the future, the Committee uses the quantity dose commitment. This is the integral over infinite time (or for a specified period) of the average, per caput, dose rate to a specified population, often the world population, resulting from the event. The dose referred to is almost always the effective dose. The dose commitment has been particularly useful in assessing the long-term consequences of events occurring within a limited time, such as a series of atmospheric nuclear explosions. The unit of effective dose commitment is the sievert.

2. Risk and detriment

73. The Committee has also needed to adopt a consistent method of describing quantitatively the probability and severity of stochastic effects of an exposure to radiation. The term risk has been widely used in this context, but without adequate consistency. It is sometimes used to mean the probability of an undesirable outcome, but at other times to mean a combination of the probability and the severity of the outcome. For this reason, the Committee has tried to avoid the use of the term risk, except in well-established formulations such as "excess relative risk" and "multiplicative risk projection model".

74. One important concept for the Committee is the probability of fatal cancer resulting from an increment of exposure to radiation. The annual probability varies with time after exposure, and the most useful summarizing expression is the probability over the whole of life of dying prematurely as the result of the extra exposure. This is not a simple concept because the total lifetime probability of death is always unity. Any additional exposure to a hazard causing an increase in the probability of death from one cause reduces life expectancy and the probability of death due to all the other causes.

75. For the Committee's purposes, the most appropriate quantity for expressing the lifetime risk of death due to exposure to radiation is the risk of exposure-induced death, sometimes called the lifetime probability of attributable cancer. This quantity takes account of the fact that other causes of death may intervene before the risk of death due to an exposure to radiation can be expressed.

76. Since the effect of the additional exposure is to decrease life expectancy rather than to increase the probability of death, the attributable probability is not an adequate indicator of the effect of an exposure. When summarizing the detriment per unit exposure, the Committee has therefore also used the average period of life lost should an attributable cancer death occur. The combination of this period and the attributable lifetime probability is a measure of the average loss of life expectancy. All these quantities can be used to assess the consequences of a single or continued exposure resulting in a known dose. If the exposures are limited to a range in which the dose-response relationship is approximately linear, the quantities can also be expressed per unit dose. When the relationship is clearly non-linear, the quantities can be specified at a stated dose, usually at an effective dose of 1 Sv.

77. A more complex approach to detriment has been used for protection purposes by the International Commission on Radiological Protection (ICRP). This

approach takes account of the attributable probability of fatal cancer in different organs, of the additional detriment from non-fatal cancer and hereditary disorders and of the different latency periods for cancers of different kinds. All these features are included in the selection of the weighting factors for converting equivalent dose into effective dose.

78. The coefficient linking the probability of fatal cancer to the effective dose is thus a function of the age and sex distribution of the exposed population and of any ethnic variations. Nevertheless, the Committee has found it adequate to use the nominal values adopted by ICRP for most of its own purposes, recognizing that these are necessarily approximate, especially in the case of the medical exposure of patients.

B. EFFECTS IN MAN

79. The effects of radiation, outlined in Chapter I, Section A, can be classified as deterministic or stochastic on the one hand and somatic or hereditary on the other. All deterministic effects are somatic, that is, they occur in the exposed individual, while stochastic effects can be either somatic (for example, radiation-induced cancer) or hereditary.

80. Deterministic effects were quite frequent in the early days of radiation use. In the period between the discovery of x rays and the early 1930s, when protective measures began to be used, more than a hundred radiologists died of deterministic effects. In addition, there were many cases of anaemia and skin damage. After protective measures were instituted, deterministic effects became progressively less frequent, and they are now seen only in the case of accidents or as a side effect of medical radiation therapy.

81. Cancer induction has been detected and quantified by epidemiology in several exposed groups of people. It appears to be the only stochastic somatic effect of radiation. Hereditary effects of radiation have not yet been epidemiologically identified in humans, but there can be no doubt about their existence. They can be recognized in all the forms of animal and plant life in which they have been sought, other than man. The lack of epidemiological evidence is due to the long time between generations and the large number of people required for statistical detection.

1. Deterministic effects

82. Tissues vary in their deterministic response to radiation. Among the most sensitive tissues are the ovary, the testis, the lens of the eye and the bone marrow. The threshold for temporary sterility in the male for a single short exposure is about 0.15 Gy, while for prolonged exposures the threshold dose rate is about 0.4 Gy per year. The corresponding values for permanent sterility are in the range 3.5-6 Gy (acute exposures) and 2 Gy per year (chronic exposures). In women, the threshold dose rate for permanent sterility is in the range 2.5-6 Gy for an acute exposure, with women approaching the menopause being more sensitive. For exposures continuing over many years, the threshold dose rate is about 0.2 Gy per year. These thresholds, like all thresholds for deterministic effects, apply to persons in a normal state of health. For individuals who are already close to exhibiting the effect from other causes, the threshold will be lower. Even in the extreme case where the effect is already present, there will still be a threshold representing the radiation dose needed to produce an observable change in the individual's condition.

83. The threshold for lens opacities sufficient to result, after some delay, in vision impairment is 2-10 Gy for sparsely ionizing radiation (and about 1-2 Gy for densely ionizing radiation) in acute exposures. The threshold dose rate is not well known for long-term chronic exposures, but it is likely to exceed 0.15 Gy per year for sparsely ionizing radiation.

84. For acute exposures of whole bone marrow, the threshold dose for clinically significant depression of blood formation is about 0.5 Gy. The corresponding threshold dose rate for long-term exposure is somewhat above 0.4 Gy per year. Bone-marrow failure is an important component of the radiation syndrome that follows whole-body exposures. An acute whole-body dose of between 3 and 5 Gy causes death in 50% of the exposed population group in the absence of specific medical treatment.

85. In the case of skin exposures, the threshold for erythema and dry desquamation is in the range 3-5 Gy, with symptoms appearing about three weeks after exposure. Moist desquamation occurs after about 20 Gy, with blistering appearing about one month after the exposure. Tissue necrosis, appearing after three weeks, occurs after more than 50 Gy.

(a) Effects on the developing brain

86. Only two conspicuous effects on brain growth and development have emerged from the studies at Hiroshima and Nagasaki. There are some cases of severe mental retardation and some of small head size without apparent mental retardation. Additionally, some groups among those exposed *in utero* have shown lower than average intelligence scores and poor performance in school.

87. An excess of severe mental retardation was observed in some children exposed to radiation *in utero* at Hiroshima and Nagasaki. While no mental retardation was observed in cases where exposure occurred before 8 weeks after conception, a sensitive period was identified, 8-15 weeks, followed by a substantially less sensitive period of 16-25 weeks from conception.

88. As discussed in Chapter I, Section A.2(a), the mechanism of mental retardation induction is thought to be the production of a dose-dependent lack of functional connections of neurons in the brain cortex. This lack of connections causes a downward shift (shift to the left) of the IQ distribution, the value of which is estimated to be about 30 IQ points per sievert, for exposures in the period between 8 and 15 weeks.

89. Normal IQ distributions have a stipulated average value of 100 IQ points and a standard deviation of about 15 IQ points. The region to the left of two standard deviations from the average, i.e. values less than 70 IQ points, corresponds to the clinical designation of severe mental retardation. The radiation-induced shift, for a dose of 1 Sv, would result in severe mental retardation in about 40% of the exposed individuals.

90. However, bearing in mind the shape of the Gaussian distribution, the fraction of extra cases caused by the shift induced by a small dose would be substantially less than that calculated directly from a linear relationship of 40% per sievert (about one order of magnitude less). The dose required to cause an IQ shift large enough to make an otherwise normal individual severely mentally retarded would be high (in the region of 1 Sv or more), while the dose required to bring an individual who without radiation exposure would have a low IQ into the category of severely retarded, by crossing the borderline, might be a few tenths of a sievert.

(b) Effects in children

91. During childhood, when tissues are actively growing, radiation-induced deterministic effects will often have a more severe impact than they would during adulthood. Examples of deterministic damage resulting from radiation exposure in childhood include effects on growth and development, organ dysfunction, hormonal deficiencies and their sequelae and effects on cognitive functions. Most of the information comes from patients who have received radiotherapy and is derived by new analytical methods and by continued careful monitoring. The Committee has reviewed this information to identify the nature of the effects in various tissues and the magnitude of the doses causing these effects.

92. Many factors complicate the study of the dose-effect relationship. These include the underlying disease and the modality of the treatment, which often includes surgery and chemotherapy in addition to the radiotherapy. For these reasons, the estimates of threshold doses in healthy children are still qualified by substantial uncertainties. Only general indications of levels can be provided. Unless otherwise stated, the doses are from fractionated exposures.

93. The effects of radiation on the testis and the ovary are dependent on both age and dose. Testicular function can be compromised at doses of 0.5 Gy. At doses of 10 Gy, gonadal failure occurs in most irradiated boys. In girls, a small proportion show amenorrhea following doses of 0.5 Gy, the proportion increasing to about 70% at doses of 3 Gy. Infertility occurs in about 30% of cases following doses of 4 Gy. A dose of 20 Gy results in permanent infertility in all cases.

94. Many other organs are damaged by doses in the range 10-20 Gy. In contrast, thyroid damage may occur at doses as low as about 1 Gy. Several effects have been shown in the brain, including atrophy of the cortex, after a single dose of 10 Gy or an accumulated dose of 18 Gy delivered in about 10 fractions. The endocrine system is affected by radiation, showing clearly impaired secretion of growth hormones at fractionated doses totalling 18 Gy. Thyroid doses in the region of 1 Gy, protracted over two weeks, resulted in hypothyroidism in patients treated by cranial radiotherapy. Cataracts and impairment of breast development have been seen at 2 Gy.

95. Deterministic effects in several other organs have been identified and quantified. Reduced total lung capacity has been shown at doses of 8 Gy and restrictive lung changes at doses of 11 Gy. Five exposures per week over six weeks require a total dose of more than 12 Gy to produce liver damage, and protracted doses of about 12 Gy are sufficient to produce kidney damage. Radiation nephritis has been reported at 14 Gy. A dose exceeding 20 Gy is required to stop bone formation, with partial effects following doses in the range 10-20 Gy and no effects below 10 Gy. Damage to the heart muscle leading to clinical failure is seen after a dose of about 40 Gy.

2. Radiation-induced cancer

96. Mechanistic models for the induction of cancer by radiation can be formulated from radiobiological information: these models suggest the choice of the dose-response function. Human epidemiology provides the data to be interpreted using such models, which are particularly important in the extrapolation of the

data to the low dose region, where epidemiological data are lacking or extremely imprecise.

97. Since the period of observation of an exposed population sample rarely extends to a full lifetime, it is usually necessary to project the frequency of cancer induction noted during the period of observation to the lifetime of the exposed population, in order to obtain the full lifetime risk. Two principal models have been used for this purpose, one the absolute, or additive, projection model and the other the relative, or multiplicative, model.

98. The simple absolute (additive) model assumes a constant (dose-related) excess of induced cancer throughout life, unrelated to the age-dependent spontaneous rate of cancer. The simple relative (multiplicative) model, assumes that the rate of induced cancers will increase with age as a constant multiple (dose-related) of the spontaneous cancer rate. Both models may be extended to replace the constant values by functions of age at exposure and of time since exposure.

99. The simple additive model is no longer seen to be consistent with most epidemiological observations, and radiobiological information seems to favour the multiplicative model. It should be noted, however, that neither of the simple models fits all the information; for example, the multiplicative model has difficulties with the case of exposure of young children, and neither of the simple projection models is consistent with the data for leukaemia or bone cancer.

100. Three projection models for solid cancers have been examined by the Committee. The first is the simple model with a constant excess risk factor. The second and third use a decreasing factor for times more than 45 years after exposure. Although the leukaemia risk is not yet fully expressed in the Japanese survivors, the residual risk is now sufficiently small to make the use of different projection models unnecessary.

101. The two models with decreasing relative risk factors reduce the estimates of lifetime risk following a single exposure by a factor of about 2 for exposure in the first decade of life and by a factor of 1.5 in the second decade, with only a small effect for older ages at exposure. Because the reduction in probability occurs at older ages, these models show slightly larger loss of life per attributable cancer than does the simple model.

102. An important element in the assessment of the radiation risks of cancer at low doses is the reduction factor used to modify the direct linear (non-threshold) fit to the high-dose and high-dose-rate epidemiological data in order to estimate the slope of the linear component of the linear-quadratic function. From basic radiobiological information, animal studies, and data relevant to cancer induction in man, this factor is now estimated, with substantial uncertainty, to be about 2 for the dose range providing most of the epidemiological data. The epidemiology results do not exclude this value, but except for leukaemia, they do not support it.

103. In the UNSCEAR 1988 Report, the Committee derived risk coefficients (risk per unit dose) for high-dose and high-dose-rate situations for various tissues. For the purpose of this Report, it is sufficient to deal with the total risk of cancer mortality when the whole body is exposed.

104. In recent years, epidemiological studies have been reported on occupationally exposed persons, on population groups living in areas having different levels of background radiation and on people exposed by the release of radioactive materials to their environment. For such studies to provide useful quantitative information on the consequences of exposure to radiation, they must be of a substantial size and must be extended over long periods. Historically, only the studies of radon-related lung cancer in miners have been able to provide quantitative relationships, and these are specific to radon. At present, the most promising studies of general application are those of workers exposed to several kinds of radiation in the course of their work. These studies are now beginning to show positive results.

105. The statistical power of these studies is still low, but it will increase with time as the data accumulate. The results are consistent with those from studies at high doses and high dose rates and provide no indication that the current assessments underestimate the risks.

106. The data now indicate with reasonable certainty that the cancer risks associated with high doses of sparsely ionizing radiation are about three times greater than they were estimated to be a decade ago. The 1988 estimate of probability of lifetime fatal cancers using the preferred multiplicative risk projection model was 11 10^{-2} per Sv for the exposed populations at Hiroshima and Nagasaki, of whom more than half in the epidemiological study are still alive. The Committee's estimates relate only to the Japanese population represented by the Life Span Study cohort. These studies are continuing, but there is as yet insufficient information to suggest a change in the risk estimates.

107. The Committee discussed the factor by which risk estimates derived from studies at high doses should be reduced when used to derive estimates for

low doses. No single figure can be quoted, but is clear that the factor is small. The data from the Japanese studies suggest a value not exceeding 2. If a factor of 2 is used, a value of 5 10^{-2} per Sv is obtained for the lifetime probability of radiation-induced fatal cancers in a nominal population of all ages. A smaller average value of about 4 10^{-2} per Sv would be obtained for a working population (aged between 18 and 64 years) exposed during their working lives. The Committee suggests that a reduction factor should be applied for all doses below 0.2 Gy and for higher doses when the dose rate is less than 6 mGy per hour averaged over a few hours.

3. Hereditary effects

108. Epidemiology has not detected hereditary effects of radiation in humans with a statistically significant degree of confidence. The risk estimate based on animals is so small that it would have been surprising to find a statistically significant effect in the end-points studied in Hiroshima and Nagasaki. Nevertheless, there can be no doubt of the existence of hereditary effects in man. Risk estimation therefore rests on genetic experimentation with a wide range of organisms and on cellular studies, with limited support from the negative human findings.

109. Two considerably different methods of estimating genetic risk have been used by the Committee. One is the doubling dose (or indirect) method. This assessment excluded the multifactorial disorders. For a reproductive population, a risk value of 1.2 10^{-2} per Sv was given for all generations after exposure or, expressing the same risk in a different way, a risk of 1.2 10^{-2} per generation for a continued exposure of 1 Sv per generation. The corresponding risk in the first two generations after exposure was estimated to be 0.3 10^{-2} per Sv in the reproductive segment of the population.

110. The Committee's other method of assessing genetic risk is the so-called direct method. It applies to clinically important disorders expressed in first-generation offspring of exposed parents. The estimate of risk was 0.2-0.4 10^{-2} per Sv in the reproductive part of the population. It is reassuring that the two different methods of genetic risk assessment give reasonably similar estimates.

111. There are many diseases and disorders of complex, multifactorial aetiology. In addition, there are a number of newly recognized, non-traditional, mechanisms of transmitting hereditary disease. The effect of radiation upon the incidence of these multifactorial and non-traditionally transmitted diseases is highly speculative, but may be slight. More research is needed to make it possible to derive risk estimates for all of the mechanisms that could cause diseases in the offspring of exposed individuals.

III. SOURCES OF RADIATION EXPOSURE

A. BASIS FOR COMPARISONS

112. The radiation to which the human population is exposed comes from very diverse sources. Some of these sources are natural features of the environment. Others are the result of human activities. The radiation from natural sources includes cosmic radiation, external radiation from radionuclides in the earth's crust and internal radiation from radionuclides inhaled or ingested and retained in the body. The magnitude of these natural exposures depends on geographical location and on some human activities. Height above sea level affects the dose rate from cosmic radiation; radiation from the ground depends on the local geology; and the dose from radon, which seeps from the ground into houses, depends on local geology and on the construction and ventilation of houses. The exposures due to cosmic rays, terrestrial gamma rays and ingestion vary only slightly with time, so they can be regarded as the basic background exposure to natural sources.

113. Man-made sources of radiation include x-ray equipment, particle accelerators and nuclear reactors used in the generation of nuclear energy, in research and in the production of radionuclides that are then used in medicine, research and industrial operations. Past testing in the atmosphere of nuclear devices still contributes to worldwide exposures. Occupational exposure, i.e. the exposure of workers, is widespread but involves groups of limited size.

114. Some sources of exposure, e.g. natural sources, can be viewed as continuing at a constant level. Others, e.g. medical examinations and treatments and the generation of nuclear power, continue over long periods, not necessarily at a constant level. Still others, e.g. test explosions in the atmosphere and accidents, are discrete events or discrete series of events. Sources that release radioactive materials to the environment deliver their doses over prolonged periods, so that the resulting annual doses do not provide a satisfactory measure of their total impact.

115. Given these complexities, there is no satisfactory single way of presenting the resultant dose to man. However, there is some advantage in attempting a compromise presentation that allows all the sources to be seen on a common basis, while preserving a more selective presentation for the details of the exposure from each type of source. One method is to present the average annual doses from various sources up to the present time. This type of presentation demonstrates the historical significance of the sources to date but gives no indication of any future dose already committed. The Committee has partially avoided this difficulty by using the dose commitment, which takes account of future doses committed by the source. However, neither the dose commitment to date nor the collective dose committed to date provides an adequate representation of the doses from practices that are likely to be continued into the future. For this, some system of forecasting is needed.

116. The approach to be used in this Report to compare radiation exposures from various sources consists of presenting the collective dose to the world population received or committed (a) from the end of 1945 to the end of 1992 (47 years) for discrete events and (b) for a period of 50 years at the current rate of practice or exposure for all other sources, including natural sources. This approach assumes that the current rate of practice is reasonably typical of a period of 50 years, 25 years before and after the present. It is likely that this assumption overestimates the future doses from practices that are not rapidly expanding, because improved techniques and standards of protection will reduce the doses per unit of practice. No assumption is needed for discrete events.

117. This Chapter summarizes the Committee's evaluation of exposures of the public and workers to radiation from the various sources. The detailed information is to be found in the Annexes to this Report.

B. LEVELS OF EXPOSURE

1. Exposures from natural sources

118. The worldwide average annual effective dose from natural sources is estimated to be 2.4 mSv, of which about 1.1 mSv is due to the basic background radiation and 1.3 mSv is due to exposure to radon. The cosmic ray dose rate depends on height above sea level and on latitude: annual doses in areas of high exposure (locations at the higher elevations) are about five times the average. The terrestrial gamma-ray dose rate depends on local geology, with a high level typically being about 10 times the average. The dose to a few communities living near some types of mineral sand may be up to about 100 times the average. The dose from radon decay products depends on local geology and housing construction and use, with the dose in some regions being about 10 times the average. Local geology and the type and ventilation of some houses may combine to give dose rates from radon decay products of several hundred times the average.

119. Table 1 shows typical average annual effective doses in adults from the principal natural sources. With the accumulation of further data and minor changes in the methods of assessment, the estimate of the annual total has been almost constant: 2.0 mSv in the UNSCEAR 1982 Report, 2.4 mSv in the UNSCEAR 1988 Report and 2.4 mSv in Table 1.

120. The typical annual effective dose of 2.4 mSv from natural sources results in an annual collective dose to the world population of 5.3 billion people of about 13 million man Sv.

Table 1
Annual effective doses to adults from natural sources

Source of exposure	*Annual effective dose (mSv)*	
	Typical	*Elevated* [a]
Cosmic rays	0.39	2.0
Terrestrial gamma rays	0.46	4.3
Radionuclides in the body (except radon)	0.23	0.6
Radon and its decay products	1.3	10
Total (rounded)	2.4	-

[a] The elevated values are representative of large regions. Even higher values occur locally.

2. Medical exposures

121. Wide use is made of radiation in diagnostic examinations and in treatments. Of these, diagnosis is by far the more common. Most people are familiar with x-ray examinations of the chest, back, extremities and gastro-intestinal tract and dental x rays, as these are the examinations most frequently performed. The provision of medical radiation services is, however, very uneven in the world, with most of the procedures being carried out in industrialized countries, which contain only one quarter of the world's population.

122. Based on a correlation between the numbers of medical x-ray equipment and examinations and the number of physicians in countries, the Committee has evaluated medical radiation exposures for four levels of health care in the world, from level I in industrialized countries to level IV in the least developed countries. This broad classification is useful, but it sometimes conceals substantial variations within countries.

123. As health care improves, countries move between health-care levels. Thus, the number of people living in the different categories of countries changes with time. Between 1977 and 1990, the greatest change was an increase of population in level II countries from about 1.5 billion to about 2.6 billion. The estimates for 1990 show level I at 1.35 billion, level II at 2.63 billion, level III at 0.85 billion, and level IV at 0.46 billion.

124. Representative estimates of examination frequencies and doses per examination have been obtained from a worldwide survey conducted by the Committee. For countries of health-care level I, the annual frequency of medical (i.e. non-dental) x-ray examinations was 890 per 1,000 population. For levels II, III and IV, the frequencies per 1,000 were 120, 70 and 9. The number of examinations is closely proportional to the number of physicians. In each level, there are differences within and between countries, with most countries lying within a factor of about 3 from the mean of the health-care level. The spread is wider in countries at the lower health-care levels.

125. The doses per examination are generally low, but there is a wide range both within and between countries. The data from level II, and more particularly from levels III and IV, are very limited but show no obvious differences from level I data. Despite the low doses per examination, the magnitude of the practice makes the diagnostic use of x rays the dominant source of medical radiation exposures. Nevertheless, doses from the use of radiopharmaceuticals and from therapeutic treatments have also been evaluated.

126. Patient doses are expressed in terms of effective dose. This permits comparisons between time periods, countries, health-care levels, medical procedures, and sources of exposure. However, patients differ from the population at large in age- and sex-distribution and in life expectancy, so the nominal fatality coefficients discussed in Chapter II, Section A, are only very approximate.

127. When considering the implications of the dose to patients, it is important not to lose sight of the associated benefits. Reducing an individual dose in diagnosis will decrease the detriment to the patient, but it may also decrease the amount or quality of the diagnostic information. In therapy, too small a dose may completely eliminate the benefit of the treatment. In screening studies, the benefit of early detection of a condition must take account of the consequent opportunity for improved management of the individual case, because detection alone is not necessarily beneficial. Collective dose can be a misleading basis on which to make judgements. In many countries, an increase in collective dose would signal an increase in the availability of health care and a net increase in benefit.

128. Information on the mean annual effective dose per patient from x-ray diagnosis is available from 26 counties, of which 21 were in level I, 4 in level II, and 1 in level III. In countries of level I, there has been a widespread downwards trend in the dose per patient for most types of examination. The notable exception is in computed tomography, where the doses have tended to increase. In the countries for which data are available, the values of the annual effective dose per patient are mainly within the range 0.5-2.0 mSv. For individual examinations, values may fall outside this range, being lower for examinations of the extremities and skull and higher for examinations of the gastro-intestinal tract.

129. The annual effective dose per caput is available from 21 countries in level I, 5 in level II, and 2 in level III. The values in level I show a range of 0.3-2.2 mSv. It is not easy to make reliable estimates for countries in the lower levels of health care. However, for levels II and III, the range seems to be about 0.02-0.2 mSv. The population-weighted average for level I is 1.0 mSv, the same as reported in 1988. The average for the world is 0.3 mSv. One cause of uncertainty in these values is the use of fluoroscopy. This procedure results in much higher doses than those from radiography, and its prevalence is both uncertain and changing with time.

130. The diagnostic use of radiopharmaceuticals has stabilized in countries of level I but is probably increasing in countries of levels II-IV. There have

been significant changes of technique in this field. The use of long-lived nuclides in developing countries results in a higher dose per examination than in countries where short-lived alternatives are available. In particular, the use of iodine-131 has decreased sharply, although it still contributes substantially to the collective dose in industrialized countries. The annual effective dose per caput is still only about 10% of that attributable to the diagnostic use of x rays. For countries of level I, the annual effective dose per caput is about 0.09 mSv. For countries of lower health-care levels, it is an order of magnitude less. Worldwide, the annual effective dose per caput from diagnostic nuclear medicine is 0.03 mSv.

131. The estimated annual effective dose per caput from all diagnostic uses of radiation is 1.1 mSv in countries of health-care level I and about 0.3 mSv averaged over the whole world. The annual collective effective dose worldwide from diagnostic medical exposures is about 1.8 10^6 man Sv. This is the largest exposure from man-made sources or practices and is equal to about one seventh of the annual collective dose to the world's population from natural sources of radiation.

132. The dose to individual patients undergoing radiotherapy is very much higher than in diagnosis, but the number of patients is smaller. There are difficulties in defining an appropriate quantity for expressing dose outside the target organ. The Committee has used a quantity analogous to effective dose, but ignoring the dose to the target tissue. For most practical purposes, this quantity may be considered the same as the effective dose.

133. With this simplification, the worldwide annual total collective effective dose from therapy is about 1.5 10^6 man Sv, about the same as that from diagnosis. The comparison of doses in diagnosis and therapy may not, however, correctly reflect the relative detriment. The difference in age distributions does not appear to be marked, but the subsequent expectation of life is likely to be less for the therapy patients. This gives less time for late effects to develop and thus reduces the relative detriment.

134. Exposures from medical radiation usage can be expected to increase as populations age and become urbanized and as health-care services spread throughout the world. There are also, however, trends towards lower doses per examination and the substitution of alternative techniques, such as imaging by magnetic resonance and ultrasound. There will be great differences in the trends in countries of different levels of health care.

3. Exposures from nuclear explosions and from the production of nuclear weapons

135. Nuclear explosions in the atmosphere were carried out at several locations, mostly in the northern hemisphere, between 1945 and 1980. The periods of most active testing were 1952-1958 and 1961-1962. In all, 520 tests were carried out, with a total fission and fusion yield of 545 Mt.

136. Since the Treaty Banning Nuclear Weapon Tests in the Atmosphere, in Outer Space and Under Water, Signed at Moscow, on 5 August 1963, almost all nuclear test explosions have been conducted underground. Some of the gaseous fission products were unintentionally vented during a few underground tests, but the available data are insufficient to allow an assessment of the resultant dose commitment. The total explosive yield of the underground tests is estimated to have been 90 Mt, much smaller than that of the earlier atmospheric tests. Furthermore, although the underground debris remains a potential source of human exposure, mainly locally, most of it will be contained. The earlier atmospheric tests therefore remain the principal source of worldwide exposure due to weapons testing.

137. The total collective effective dose committed by weapons testing to date is about 3 10^7 man Sv. Of this, about 7 10^6 man Sv will have been delivered by the year 2200. The rest, due to the long-lived carbon-14, will be delivered over the next 10,000 years or so. Another way of expressing these findings is to use the integral over time of the average dose rate to the world population, the dose commitment. The dose commitment to the year 2200 from atmospheric testing is about 1.4 mSv; over all time, it is 3.7 mSv. Both figures are of the same order of magnitude as the effective dose from a single year of exposure to natural sources. The fraction of the dose commitment delivered by 2200 (38%) is not the same as the fraction of the corresponding collective dose (23%) because the world population is expected to rise from 3.2 billion at the time of the main weapon testing programmes to a constant 10 billion for most of the 10,000 years.

138. These global estimates include a contribution from the doses to people close to the sites used for atmospheric tests. Although this contribution is small in global terms, some local doses have been substantial. The thyroid doses to children near the Nevada test site in the United States may have been as much as 1 Gy. Similar, but somewhat larger, thyroid doses were incurred between 1949 and 1962 in settlements bordering the Semipalatinsk test site in the former USSR. Some doses near the Pacific test site in the United States were also high, largely because the wind

changed direction after one thermonuclear test. Ground contamination near Maralinga, Australia, the site of British nuclear tests, has been sufficient to restrict subsequent access. Without further decontamination, unrestricted continuous occupancy might cause annual effective doses of several millisieverts in two areas, with values up to 500 mSv in small areas immediately adjacent to the test sites. The local and regional collective effective dose from the whole test series was about 700 man Sv.

139. The operations needed to produce the world supply of nuclear weapons are also a source of exposure. The processes start with the mining and milling of uranium. The uranium is then enriched, either to a high degree for weapon components or slightly for use in reactors producing plutonium and tritium. The scale of these activities is not publicly available and has to be assessed indirectly. The resultant dose commitments are then estimated by applying dose per unit release factors from nuclear power production, for which more data are freely available. The local and regional collective effective dose to the public committed by these operations is estimated to be about 1,000 man Sv. The global collective dose will be larger by a factor of between 10 and 100. Even if the total collective dose is taken to be 10^5 man Sv, it is a small fraction of the collective effective dose committed by the test programmes.

140. As in the case of testing, some local doses have been substantial. The doses near the plutonium production plant at Hanford, Washington, United States, are currently being evaluated. Preliminary results suggest that thyroid doses might have been as high as 10 Gy in some years in the 1940s. The release to the environment of the wastes from the processing of irradiated fuel at the Soviet military plant near Kyshtym, in the Ural mountains, resulted in cumulative effective doses of about 1 Sv at some riverside locations up to 30 km from the site over a few years in the early 1950s.

4. Exposures from nuclear power production

141. The generation of electrical energy in nuclear power stations has continued to increase since the beginning of the practice in the 1950s, although now the rate of increase is less than that for electrical energy generation by other means. In 1989, the electrical energy generated by nuclear reactors was 212 GW a, 17% of the world's electrical energy generated in that year. The total electrical energy generated by reactors from the 1950s until 1990 was slightly less than 2,000 GW a.

142. As in previous UNSCEAR Reports, the collective effective dose committed by the generation of 1 GW a of electrical energy by nuclear sources has been estimated for the whole of the fuel cycle from mining and milling, through enrichment, fuel fabrication and reactor operation, to fuel reprocessing and waste disposal. No specific allowance has yet been made for decommissioning, partly because of the limited experience available to date and partly because it is already clear that the contribution is likely to be small.

143. Detailed information was obtained on the releases of radionuclides to the environment during routine operations from most of the major nuclear power installations in the world. From this information, the Committee has assessed normalized releases per unit of electrical energy generated. The collective effective doses committed per unit energy generated were then estimated with the help of the generalized environmental models developed by the Committee in previous UNSCEAR Reports. Separate estimates were made for the normalized components resulting from local and regional exposures and from exposures to globally dispersed radionuclides. The main contributions are shown in Table 2. These committed collective doses were truncated at 10,000 years because of the great uncertainties in making predictions over longer periods.

144. The value of 3 man Sv $(GW\ a)^{-1}$ for the normalized local and regional collective dose committed per unit of energy generated is slightly smaller than the value estimated in previous Reports. The main reductions have been in reactor operation and reprocessing, with some increase in the estimates for mining and milling. The current value is therefore not representative of the entire period of nuclear power production, the normalized dose in the earlier part of the period being somewhat higher than the average. The total collective dose committed by effluents released from the nuclear fuel cycle up to the end of 1989 is estimated to be slightly more than 10,000 man Sv. The collective dose committed by globally dispersed radionuclides and by solid waste disposal is uncertain, since it depends on future waste manage ment practices and the evolution of the world's population over the next 10,000 years. Using the estimate of 200 man Sv $(GW\ a)^{-1}$ shown in Table 2, the total nuclear power generated, 2,000 GW a, is estimated to have committed a collective effective dose of 400,000 man Sv.

145. If the current rate of generation and the normalized values of Table 2 are representative of the 50-year period centred on the present, the 50-year collective effective dose from nuclear power generation is about 2 10^6 man Sv.

Table 2
Normalized collective doses to the public from nuclear power production

Source	*Collective effective dose committed per unit energy generated [man Sv (GW a)$^{-1}$]*
Local and regional component	
Mining, milling, and tailings	1.5
Fuel fabrication	0.003
Reactor operation	1.3
Reprocessing	0.25
Transportation	0.1
Total (rounded)	3
Global component (including solid waste disposal)	
Mine and mill tailings (releases over 10,000 years)	150
Reactor operation waste disposal	0.5
Globally dispersed radionuclides mainly from reprocessing and solid waste disposal	50
Total (rounded)	200

146. The doses to individuals from the generation of electrical energy differ very widely, even for people near similar plants. Some estimates of the maximum doses have been made for realistic model sites. For the principal types of power plants, the annual effective doses to the most highly exposed members of the public range from 1 to 20 μSv. The corresponding annual figures for large fuel reprocessing plants are 200-500 μSv.

5. Exposures of the public from major accidents

147. As in all human activities, there are accidents at work. The exposure of patients to radiation for diagnostic or therapeutic reasons is also subject to failures of equipment or procedures. The doses resulting from minor mishaps at work are included in the routine monitoring results. Some accidents, both occupational and medical, have serious consequences for the individuals involved. Such accidents are fairly frequent (perhaps a few hundred each year worldwide), but the probability that any given member of the public will be involved is very small. This Section deals only with the major accidents affecting members of the public.

148. The production and subsequent transport of nuclear weapons have resulted in several accidents. The transport accidents caused local contamination by plutonium. The collective dose committed by these accidents is small. In one accident, at Palomares, Spain, the highest committed effective dose was about 200 mSv. Other accidents on land and the loss of nuclear weapons at sea have caused negligible doses to people.

149. The two most serious accidents in nuclear weapons production were at Kyshtym in the southern Ural mountains of the Soviet Union in September 1957 and at the Windscale plant at Sellafield in the United Kingdom in October of the same year.

150. The Kyshtym accident was a chemical explosion following a failure of the cooling system in a storage tank of high-activity waste fission products. The principal fission products released were isotopes of cerium, zirconium, niobium and strontium. The doses were due to fission products deposited on the ground and strontium entering the food chain. The collective dose was shared about equally between those who were evacuated from the area of high contamination (about 10,000 people) and those who remained in the less contaminated areas (about 260,000 people). The total collective dose over 30 years was estimated to be about 2,500 man Sv. The highest individual doses were to people evacuated within a few days of the accident. The average effective dose for this group of 1,150 people was about 500 mSv.

151. The Windscale accident was a fire in the natural uranium and graphite core of an air-cooled reactor primarily intended for the production of military plutonium. The principal materials released were isotopes of xenon, iodine, caesium and polonium. The most important route of intake was the ingestion of milk, which was controlled in the area near the accident. Further away, the uncontrolled consumption of milk and inhalation were significant sources of exposure, with iodine-131 and polonium-210 being the two most important nuclides. The total collective effective dose in Europe, including the United Kingdom, was about

2,000 man Sv. The highest individual doses were to the thyroids of children living near the site. These ranged up to about 100 mGy.

152. There have been several accidents that have damaged nuclear power reactors, of which the accident at Three Mile Island in the United States and Chernobyl in the Soviet Union were the most important. The Three Mile Island accident caused serious damage to the core of the reactor, but almost all the fission products were retained by the containment system. The resulting collective effective dose was not more than about 40 man Sv. The doses to individual members of the public were low, the highest dose having been slightly less than 1 mSv.

153. The Chernobyl accident was discussed in detail in the UNSCEAR 1988 Report. The explosion and subsequent graphite fire released a substantial fraction of the core inventory and caused a distribution of effective doses in the northern hemisphere, mainly in the Soviet Union and Europe. The collective effective dose committed by the accident is estimated to have been about 600,000 man Sv. The doses to individuals varied widely, with a few people in the evacuated group receiving effective doses approaching 0.5 Sv. The average annual effective dose in the strict control zones surrounding the evacuation area fell from about 40 mSv in the year following the accident to less than 10 mSv in each of the years up to 1989.

154. An international review of the situation in the zones around the evacuation area was conducted in 1990. The project corroborated the estimated doses and found that the health of the population at that time was comparable to that of the population in nearby uncontaminated settlements.

155. Sealed sources used for industrial or medical purposes are occasionally lost or damaged and members of the public injured. Four severe accidents of this kind have occurred since 1982. In Mexico, in 1983, an unlicensed teletherapy source containing cobalt-60 was sold as scrap metal. Apart from the widespread contamination of steel products in Mexico and the United States, about 1,000 people were exposed to substantial levels of radiation, with effective doses up to about 250 mSv. About 80 people received higher doses, up to 3 Sv, with seven with doses in the range 3-7 Sv. There were no deaths.

156. In Morocco, in 1984, eight members of one family died after they found and kept at home a sealed industrial radiography source containing iridium-192. The effective doses were in the range 8-25 Sv. In Goiania, Brazil, in 1987, a caesium-137 teletherapy source was removed from its housing and broken up. Severe doses were received from direct radiation and from the localized contamination. Doses to individuals ranged up to 5 Sv. Fifty-four people were hospitalized and four died. In Shanxi Province, China, in 1992, a cobalt-60 source was lost and picked up by a man. Three persons in the family died of overexposure. In 1993, an accident occurred at a plant near Tomsk in the Russian Federation. The information on this accident has not yet been fully assessed, but it appears that the exposures were very low and that few members of the public were involved.

6. Occupational exposures

157. Occupational radiation exposures are incurred by several categories of workers who work with radioactive materials or are exposed at work to man-made or natural radiation sources. The Committee has conducted a survey of countries worldwide to obtain information that would allow comprehensive review of occupational radiation exposures.

158. Many workers in occupations involving exposure to radiation sources or radioactive material are individually monitored. One major exception is the large workforce exposed to enhanced levels of radiation from natural sources, e.g. in parts of the extractive industries. The main reason for monitoring radiation exposures in the workplace is to provide a basis for controlling the exposures and for ensuring compliance with regulatory requirements and managerial policies. Both of these requirements go beyond the simple compliance with dose limits, and may include requirements to achieve and demonstrate the optimization of protection. Inevitably, the design and interpretation of monitoring programmes reflect local needs. There are advantages in extending these objectives to permit comparisons between different operations, if this can be done without too much difficulty. Such extensions would greatly assist the Committee in its compilations and comparisons of data.

159. For most workers involved with radiation sources or radioactive materials, the main sources of exposure are those external to the body. The doses due to internal sources are usually insignificant, apart from those due to the radon naturally present in all workplaces. Furthermore, it is much easier to monitor for external exposures than for internal ones. As a result, many workers are monitored for external exposures, even when their doses are expected to be low, but monitoring for internal exposure is carried out only when it is really needed. However, some areas of occupational exposure may not be adequately monitored. The extent and reporting of the occupational exposure in medical work is thought to be good in large medical installations, but it is likely to be less satisfactory in small installations.

160. It is not possible to make direct measurements of the effective dose to workers. In most monitoring for external exposure, the results from small personal monitoring devices are usually taken to be an adequate measure of the effective dose. The doses from internal sources are estimated from a number of measurements, including the amount of radioactive material excreted or retained in the body, and the concentration of radioactive substances in the air of the workplace. The estimates depend on models of the time distribution of the intakes and of the transfer and retention processes in the body. Substantial uncertainties are inevitable.

161. There is some difficulty in presenting information about the typical individual dose to workers because policies for issuing monitoring devices differ. In particular, the widespread issue of monitoring devices to workers whose exposures are likely to be low artificially decreases the average recorded exposure of the exposed workforce. The Committee has made some use of the mean dose per measurably exposed worker, thus avoiding the distortion introduced by those who are monitored but receive trivial doses. Not all countries provide information in a form that allows this quantity to be estimated, so it cannot be used in the overall summary of data. For some purposes, the collective dose is a more satisfactory quantity, being little affected by the inclusion of large numbers of individually trivial doses.

162. There are wide variations between occupations in the recorded annual doses to monitored workers and also between countries for the same occupation. The detailed information from the Committee's review has allowed comparisons to be made between five-year periods from 1975 to 1989. This summary concentrates on the most recent quinquennium and comments on the trends over the previous periods. The worldwide average annual doses to monitored workers and the associated collective doses for 1985-1989 are summarized in Table 3.

Table 3
Annual worldwide occupational exposures to monitored workers, 1985-1989

Occupational category	*Annual collective effective dose* [a] *(man Sv)*	*Annual average effective dose per monitored worker (mSv)*
	Nuclear fuel cycle	
Mining	1200	4.4
Milling	120	6.3
Enrichment	0.4	0.08
Fuel fabrication	22	0.8
Reactor operation	1100	2.5
Reprocessing	36	3.0
Research	100	0.8
Total (rounded)	2500	2.9
	Other occupations	
Industrial applications	510	0.9
Defence activities	250	0.7
Medical applications	1000	0.5
Total (rounded)	1800	0.6
	All occupations	
Grand total (rounded)	4300	1.1

[a] Doses due to adventitious exposures to natural sources are not included. The annual collective dose from these natural sources is estimated to be about 8,600 man Sv, with the main contribution coming from underground, non-uranium mining. About half of this contribution comes from coal mining.

163. Workers in occupations involving adventitious exposure to natural sources, such as non-uranium mining, are not usually monitored and their doses are excluded from the figures in Table 3. The principal occupations in this category are in aviation and mineral extraction industries. The annual effective dose to aircrew is typically between 2 and 3 mSv, with higher values in some supersonic aircraft. In the extractive industries, the annual effective doses are typically in the range 1-2 mSv in coal mines and 1-10 mSv in other mines. The annual occupational collective dose to these workers is estimated to be 8,600 man Sv. This estimate is, however, quite uncertain because of the limited monitoring data for these workers.

164. The estimates summarized in Table 3 differ in some respects from those in earlier Reports. These changes are due mainly to the improved database now available. The largest change is in the estimates of the doses from medical applications, much of which is due to radiation of low penetrating power. The personal dosimeters worn on the surface of the body then overestimate the effective dose, especially if, as is common, there is some partial shielding of the body by installed shields and protective aprons. The present estimate of collective dose is lower by a factor of 5 than the previous one and may still be too high by a factor of 2.

165. In the nuclear industry, the average annual collective dose has not varied substantially in the last 15 years, notwithstanding increases in electrical energy generated during this period by over a factor of 3 and in the number of workers by a factor of 2. The collective effective dose per unit electrical energy generated declined by 50% and the average individual dose by 30%. Average individual doses are highest for workers in mining and milling operations. Reductions in individual doses to reactor workers come from a combination of improved operating practices and modifications to plants in the mid-1980s. Further improvements can be expected as new plants are commissioned.

166. There has been a decrease by a factor of about 2 in both individual and collective doses in general industry. Since the number of monitored workers has changed only slightly, this represents an overall improvement. In the defence industries, both collective and individual doses have decreased, mainly due to improvements in the operation and maintenance of nuclear-powered vessels.

167. When allowance is made for the overestimation in earlier Reports, the occupational exposures in medicine show no trend in collective dose. There has been a reduction in the average individual dose, partly explained by an increase in the number of monitored workers.

168. It is rare for workers to be seriously exposed to radiation as the result of accidents. Minor incidents that cause unexpected, but not directly injurious, exposures are more frequent, but the policy for reporting these differs widely from place to place. The Committee has received information concerning about 100 accidents causing fatalities or having the potential to cause deterministic injuries in the workforce in the period since 1975. The list is almost certainly incomplete. The accident at Chernobyl was by far the most serious, causing 28 deaths from radiation-related causes. The doses to about 200 workers were high enough to cause clinical deterministic effects. Three deaths due to radiation in other accidents have been reported. Accidents involving the public were discussed in the previous Section.

169. The collective dose due to exposures in minor accidents is included in the routine reports of occupational exposure. That due to serious accidents is not easy to estimate but is certainly small compared with the total occupational collective doses. One component of collective dose that has not yet been reported with other occupational exposures is that due to the emergency work undertaken to contain the damaged reactor at Chernobyl. This was not an accidental exposure, although it was the direct result of an accident. Some 247,000 workers were involved. The average dose from external exposure was estimated to be 0.12 Sv, giving a collective dose of about 30,000 man Sv. The doses from internal exposure varied during the work, but were mainly in the region of 10% of those from external exposure.

7. Summary of current information

170. Typical collective effective doses committed by 50 years of practice for all the significant sources of exposure and by discrete events since the end of 1945 are shown in Table 4. The bases for the values in this table are given in the earlier parts of this Section, which in turn summarize the detailed evaluations given in the Annexes to this Report.

171. Table 4 shows the relative importance of radiation sources in terms of the resulting collective doses. By far the largest source of exposure is the sum of natural sources. The whole world population is exposed to cosmic rays and radiation from naturally occurring radioisotopes of potassium, uranium, radium, radon, thorium etc. in soil, water, food and the body. The next most significant radiation source is the medical use of x rays and radiopharmaceuticals in various diagnostic examinations and treatments. The doses from both diagnosis and treatment have been included in Table 4, although they are not strictly comparable in terms of the resulting detriment.

172. Exposures from the atmospheric testing of nuclear weapons have diminished. There have been no further tests since the last one in 1980. Only small contributions to the collective dose are made by the generation of electrical energy by nuclear reactors, accidental events, and various occupational exposures, but these contributions are nevertheless important from the point of view of the radiation protection of individuals.

173. Apart from the doses from natural sources, the variation of individual doses over time and from place to place makes it impossible to summarize individual doses coherently. However, some indications can be provided.

174. The average annual effective dose from natural sources is 2.4 mSv, with elevated values commonly up to 10 or 20 mSv. Medical procedures in developed countries result in an annual effective dose to the average person between 1 and 2 mSv, of which about two thirds comes from diagnostic radiology. Average annual doses to individuals in the mid-1970s from atmospheric weapon tests were reported in the UNSCEAR 1977 Report. By that time, most of the short-lived nuclides had decayed. The annual effective doses were about 5 μSv. Annual effective doses at the time of maximum testing were probably between 100 and 200 μSv in the northern hemisphere. Annual effective doses to the most highly exposed people near nuclear power installations are in the range 1-200 μSv. Occupational annual effective doses to monitored workers are commonly in the range 1-10 mSv.

Table 4
Collective dose committed to the world population by a 50-year period of operation for continuing practices or by single events from 1945 to 1992

Source	*Basis of commitment*	*Collective effective dose (million man Sv)*
Natural sources	Current rate for 50 years	650
Medical exposure	Current rate for 50 years	
Diagnosis		90
Treatment		75
Atmospheric nuclear weapons tests	Completed practice	30
Nuclear power	Total practice to date	0.4
	Current rate for 50 years	2
Severe accidents	Events to date	0.6
Occupational exposure	Current rate for 50 years	
Medical		0.05
Nuclear power		0.12
Industrial uses		0.03
Defence activities		0.01
Non-uranium mining		0.4
Total (all occupations)		0.6

IV. THE PERCEPTION OF RADIATION RISKS

175. The word "risk" has several different meanings. It is often used descriptively to indicate the possibility of loss or danger, as in "the risks of hang-gliding". In technical contexts it is used quantitatively, but without any general agreement on its definition. Sometimes it is used to mean the probability of a defined adverse outcome, but it is also widely used as a combination of that probability and some measure of the severity of the outcome. These different meanings cause confusion among specialists but probably have little influence on the attitude of the general public. To the public, risk is largely descriptive or qualitative. Some risks are seen as worse than others partly because the outcome is thought to be more likely and partly because the outcome, if it occurs, is less welcome. There is little or no attempt to make a formal separation between these aspects or to combine them in anything more than an intuitive sense. Many factors influence the public's view of a risk. These include its source, its nature, the extent to which it is a familiar part of life, the degree of choice and control thought to be available to the individual, the confidence in the originator and regulator of the risk, and many others. Inevitably, any quantified discussion of risks involves both scientific and social judgements.

176. Against this background, there is no reason to expect the public attitude towards a risk to be the same as the attitude of those who estimate risks quantitatively, assess their importance and manage them. The task of the Committee is to provide quantitative estimates of the risk associated with ionizing radiation. The effects of exposure have been expressed in terms of the probability of their occurrence, the years of life lost in the case of fatal consequences and the severity of non-fatal consequences. The Committee is not con-

cerned with making judgments about the relative importance of different kinds of risk to society or with the management of risks. It therefore aims to present its findings in a neutral way and has thought it desirable to take some account of the probable differences in the way its conclusions will be perceived by non-specialist readers.

177. The most important conclusion is that there is no uniformity of evaluation, comparison or acceptance of risks across individuals or societies. Considerable progress has been made, mainly in the last 20 years, in establishing a structured presentation of the factors that influence perceptions and in grouping them into classes. Some of the factors relate to the personal characteristics and experience of an individual, others are associated with the characteristics of the society in which the individual lives. Much depends on the individual's awareness of the source and character of the risks in question.

178. In all occupations and activities involving radiation, the quantification of and the perception of risks have been recognized as important issues. A major difficulty in managing risks has been to satisfy the concerns of individuals, communities and society. The basic approach in risk management has been to justify activities or practices by the benefits provided and to do all that is reasonable to reduce the risks. Views on the extent to which this approach has succeeded depend heavily on the perceptions of the viewer.

179. There are major difficulties in communicating information about radiation to the public. Even in countries that are highly developed technologically, many people do not know what radiation is, even in simple terms. Most of those who do know something about it associate it with accidents, weapons, fallout and cancer. Very few associate radiation and medical diagnosis or are aware of the normal background exposure to natural sources of radiation.

180. The Committee recognizes that many factors outside its remit influence the way in which its findings are viewed. Public concern about the levels and effects of radiation is more influenced by the perceived merits and social implications of the source of radiation than by the magnitude of the resulting exposures and risks. Nevertheless, the Committee recognizes its obligation to evaluate radiation exposures and to provide estimates of radiation risks that are soundly based, consistent and unbiased. The information must be trustworthy and clearly communicated if it is to contribute to achieving positive decisions for the whole of society.

V. SUMMARY AND PERSPECTIVES

A. LEVELS OF EXPOSURE

181. The Committee's estimates of the levels of exposure throughout the world are improving as the provision of data improves. As a very broad generalization, it can be concluded that improved procedures are decreasing the exposure per unit of practice by an amount that is sufficient to offset increases in the level of the practices.

182. Some sources of exposure continue at a constant level. Some continue over long periods, not necessarily at a constant level. Others are discrete events, or discrete series of events such as weapons tests. Sources that release radioactive materials to the environment deliver their doses over prolonged periods, so that the resulting annual doses do not provide a satisfactory measure of their total impact.

183. This Report presents the collective dose to the world population received or committed from the end of 1945 to the end of 1992 (47 years) for discrete events and for a period of 50 years at the current rate of practice or exposure for all other sources. The results were shown in Table 4.

B. BIOLOGICAL EFFECTS

184. The Committee's interest in the biological effects of radiation is mainly concentrated on the effects of low doses. These effects have a low probability of occurring but are serious when they do occur. Statistical limitations prevent epidemiological studies from providing direct estimates of risk at low doses, making it necessary to rely on radiobiology to provide a basis for interpreting the results of epidemiology. The combination of epidemiology and radiobiology, particularly at the molecular and cellular levels, is a useful tool for elucidating the consequences of low doses of radiation.

185. One of the most rapidly developing fields of work is concerned with the mechanisms of cancer induction as a result of changes in the molecular structure of DNA. Although rapid progress is also being made in the study of hereditary disorders, quantitative estimates of hereditary risk must still be derived from animal studies. Even the substantial exposures at Hiroshima and Nagasaki have not made it possible to obtain quantitative estimates of hereditary risks with a sufficient degree of confidence.

186. Despite the rapid progress in radiobiology and the increasing amount of data from epidemiology, the Committee has not yet found it necessary to make any substantial changes in its risk estimates.

C. PERSPECTIVES

187. The Committee's estimates of radiation exposure and its estimates of the risk of exposure indicate that radiation is a weak carcinogen. About 4% of the deaths due to cancer can be attributed to ionizing radiation, most of which comes from natural sources that are not susceptible to control by man. Nevertheless, it is widely (but wrongly) believed that all the cancer deaths at Hiroshima and Nagasaki are the result of the atomic bombings. The studies in the two cities have included virtually all the heavily exposed individuals and have shown that, of 3,350 cancer deaths, only about 350 could be attributed to radiation exposure from the atomic bombings.

188. One way of providing a perspective on the implications of man-made radiation sources is to compare the resulting doses with those from natural sources. This is easy to do from a global point of view, which deals with total (or average) worldwide exposures. The collective doses were presented in Table 4. However, many man-made sources expose only limited groups of people. The following paragraph attempts to distinguish between these situations.

189. On a global basis, one year of medical practice at the present rate is equivalent to about 90 days of exposure to natural sources, but individual doses from medical procedures vary from zero (for persons who were not examined or treated) to many thousands of times that received annually from natural sources (for patients undergoing radiotherapy). Most of the doses committed by one year of current operations of the nuclear fuel cycle are widely distributed and correspond to about 1 day of exposure to natural sources. Excluding severe accidents, the doses to the most highly exposed individuals do not exceed, and rarely approach, doses from natural sources. Occupational exposure, viewed globally, corresponds to about 8 hours of exposure to natural sources. However, occupational exposure is confined to a small proportion of those who work. For this limited group, the exposures are similar to those from natural sources. For small subgroups, occupational exposures are about five times those from natural sources. The collective dose committed over 10,000 years by atmospheric nuclear testing is fairly uniformly distributed and corresponds to about 2.3 years exposure to natural sources. This figure represents the whole programme of tests and is not comparable with the figures for a single year of practice. Only one accident in a civilian nuclear power installation, that at Chernobyl, has resulted in doses to members of the public greater than those resulting from the exposure in one year to natural sources. On a global basis, this accident corresponded to about 20 days exposure to natural sources. These findings are summarized in Table 5.

Table 5
Exposures to man-made sources expressed as equivalent periods of exposure to natural sources

Source	*Basis*	*Equivalent period of exposure to natural sources*
Medical exposures	One year of practice at the current rate	90 days
Nuclear weapons tests	Completed practice	2.3 years
Nuclear power	Total practice to date One year of practice at the current rate	10 days 1 day
Severe accidents	Events to date	20 days
Occupational exposures	One year of practice at the current rate	8 hours

Appendix I

MEMBERS OF NATIONAL DELEGATIONS ATTENDING THE THIRTY-EIGHTH TO FORTY-SECOND SESSIONS

ARGENTINA	D. Beninson (Representative), E. d'Amato, C. Arias, D. Cancio, A. Curti, E. Palacios
AUSTRALIA	K.H. Lokan (Representative)
BELGIUM	J. Maisin (Representative), R. Kirchmann, H.P. Leenhouts, P.H.M. Lohman, K. Sankaranarayanan, D. Smeesters
BRAZIL	E. Penna Franca (Representative), J. Landmann-Lipsztein
CANADA	E.G. Létourneau (Representative), A. Arsenault, D.R. Champ, R.M. Chatterjee, P.J. Duport, V. Elaguppilai, N.E. Gentner, B.C. Lentle, D.K. Myers
CHINA	Li Deping (Representative), Liu Hongxiang (Representative), Wei Lüxin (Representative), Leng Ruiping, Pan Zhiqiang, Tao Zufan, Wu Dechang
EGYPT	M.F. Ahmed (Representative), F.H. Hammad (Representative), F. Mohamed (Representative), H.M. Roushdy (Representative), S.E. Hashish
FRANCE	P. Pellerin (Representative), E. Cardis, R. Coulon, H. Dutrillaux, A. Flury-Hérard, H. Jammet, J. Lafuma, G. Lemaire, R. Masse
GERMANY [a]	A. Kaul (Representative), W. Burkart, U.H. Ehling, W. Jacobi, A.M. Kellerer, F.E. Stieve, C. Streffer
INDIA	D.V. Gopinath (Representative), U. Madhvanath (Representative), N.K. Notani (Representative)
INDONESIA	S. Soekarno (Representative), S. Wiryosimin (Representative), K. Wiharto
JAPAN	H. Matsudaira (Representative), Y. Hosoda, T. Iwasaki, A. Kasai, S. Kumazawa, T. Matsuzaki, K. Nishizawa, H. Noguchi, K. Sato, K. Shinohara, S. Yano
MEXICO	E. Araico Salazar (Representative)
PERU	L.V. Pinillos Ashton (Representative)
POLAND	Z. Jaworowski (Representative), J. Jankowski, J. Liniecki, O. Rosiek, S. Sterlinski, I. Szumiel
RUSSIAN FEDERATION [b]	L.A. Ilyin (Representative), R. Alexakhin, R.M. Barhoudarov, Y. Buldakov, V. Bebeshko, N.A. Dolgova, A. Guskowa, D.F. Khokhlova, Y. Kholina, E. Komarov, O. Pavlovski, G.N. Romanov
SLOVAKIA [c]	M. Klímek (Representative)
SUDAN	O.I. Elamin (Representative), A. Hidayatalla (Representative)
SWEDEN	G. Bengtsson (Representative), L.-E. Holm, J.O. Snihs, L. Sjöberg
UNITED KINGDOM OF GREAT BRITAIN AND NORTHERN IRELAND	J. Dunster (Representative), R.H. Clarke, J. Denekamp, Sir Richard Doll
UNITED STATES OF AMERICA	F.A. Mettler (Representative), L.R. Anspaugh, J.D. Boice, C.W. Edington, J.H. Harley, N.H. Harley, C. Meinhold, P.B. Selby, W.K. Sinclair, E.W. Webster, H.O. Wyckoff

[a] At the thirty-eighth and thirty-ninth sessions: Federal Republic of Germany.
[b] At the thirty-eighth, thirty-ninth and fortieth sessions: Union of Soviet Socialist Republics.
[c] At the thirty-eighth, thirty-ninth, fortieth and forty-first sessions: Czechoslovakia.

Appendix II

SCIENTIFIC STAFF AND CONSULTANTS COOPERATING WITH THE COMMITTEE IN THE PREPARATION OF THIS REPORT

D. Beninson
B.G. Bennett
A. Bouville
R. Cox
J. Dunster
D. Goodhead
L.E. de Geer
J. Hall
L.E. Holm
G.N. Kelly
M. O'Riordan
W.J. Schull
P. Selby
J.W. Stather
J. Valentin
F. Vogel

Scientific Annexes

ANNEX A

Exposures from natural sources of radiation

CONTENTS

INTRODUCTION

1. Natural ionizing radiation arises in outer space, where cosmic rays are formed, and in and on the earth, where radionuclides normally present in soil, air, water, food and the body undergo radioactive decay. Penetrating radiations and radioactive materials pervade the natural environment. The main types of radiation are gamma rays, alpha and beta particles, neutrons and muons. Human exposure occurs by irradiation from sources outside the body (external exposure) and upon the decay of radionuclides taken into the body through ingestion and inhalation (internal exposure). The assessment of radiation doses in humans from natural sources is important because natural ionizing radiation is the largest contributor to the collective effective dose received by the world's population. In this Annex, the expressions "natural radiation" and "natural radiation background" are often used to refer to "natural sources of ionizing radiation".

2. Some of the contributions to the total exposure from the natural radiation background are quite constant in space and time and practically independent of human practices and activities. This is true, for example, of the doses received from the ingestion of ^{40}K, a long-lived radioisotope of an element that is homeostatically controlled, and also of doses from the inhalation and ingestion of cosmogenic radionuclides, which are relatively homogeneously distributed at the surface of the globe.

3. Other contributions depend strongly on human activities and practices and are therefore widely variable. In particular, the doses from indoor inhalation of short-lived decay products of radon gas are influenced by local geology and by building design, as well as by the choice of building materials and of ventilation systems. Also, concentrations of the short-lived decay products are, as a rule, higher indoors than outdoors. Therefore, people who reside somewhat above the ground surface in apartment blocks or who mostly stay outdoors in the open air are likely to incur far less exposure to radon than those who occupy single dwellings or who spend most of their time in enclosed spaces.

4. Intermediate types of exposure are those that are neither widely variable nor relatively constant at the surface of the globe. Examples are (a) external doses from cosmic rays, which vary with altitude and, to a much lesser extent, with latitude, and (b) external doses from radiation of terrestrial origin (that is, the radionuclides present in the crust of the earth and in building materials), which are affected by location and accommodation.

5. Doses from the inhalation of radon in dwellings are much greater than those from all other components of natural radiation. The main cause of high concentrations of radon in dwellings is the influx of the gas from the subjacent earth; high doses are caused by geological circumstances modified by the manner in which a dwelling is built and used. Since increasing attention is being devoted worldwide to both the radiological and the epidemiological aspects of this topic, considerable emphasis is placed in this Annex on exposure to radon and its decay products in air.

6. Since the publication of the UNSCEAR 1988 Report [U1], further information on radiation exposures from natural sources, especially with regard to radon and its short-lived decay products, has become available. This Annex updates the evaluation of exposures presented in the UNSCEAR 1988 Report [U1]. The additions and modifications present a broader view of average radiation exposures worldwide and of the range of levels experienced in particular locations. The procedures for estimating the tissue doses from inhalation of radon short-lived decay products are under continuing review and the International Commission on Radiological Protection (ICRP) has assigned new radiation- and tissue-weighting factors to define the effective dose [I6]. Despite these changes, the overall assessment of dose from natural sources of radiation is similar.

7. Radiation exposures from extra-terrestrial sources (cosmic rays and cosmogenic radionuclides) and from terrestrial sources (^{40}K, ^{87}Rb and radionuclides of the uranium and thorium series) may be said to form the basic natural radiation background because of the relative constancy of exposure. These exposures are discussed in Chapters I and II in this Annex. Among the terrestrial radionuclides, the radon isotopes in the uranium and thorium decay series play an important role because of the magnitude of the doses they deliver and because of the variability of those doses. The radon isotopes are given special consideration in Chapter III. Exposures related to the extraction and processing of earth materials are considered in Chapter IV, with the exception of the extraction and processing of uranium, which is part of the nuclear fuel cycle and is dealt with in Annex B, "Exposures from man-made sources of radiation".

8. The exposures assessed in this Annex are those to members of the public. They include the exposures outdoors and indoors in normal circumstances both at home and at work. The additional exposures that people receive at work because they are exposed to man-made radiation sources or to elevated levels of natural radiation caused by their work are discussed in Annex D, "Occupational radiation exposures".

I. COSMIC RADIATION

A. COSMIC RAYS

1. The radiation environment

9. Space is permeated by ionizing radiation. The radiation consists of various charged particles of various origins and energies. All are of concern in space travel, and some by creating secondary particles, lead to human exposure during air travel and on earth, with decreasing intensity from the highest altitudes down to sea level. In this Chapter, emphasis is placed on the everyday circumstances of exposure, and brief reference is made to exposure in space.

10. Radiations in space may be classified according to origin as trapped particle radiation, galactic cosmic radiation or solar particle radiation [A1, C1, F1, N1, S1]. Trapped radiation consists mainly of electrons and protons held in orbits around the earth by its magnetic field. Galactic cosmic radiation consists mainly of protons with some helium and heavier ions. Solar particle radiation has similar composition. These three classes are described in turn.

11. Trapped protons and electrons are in two zones or radiation belts, one within and one outside of 2.8 earth radii at the equator, with greater intensities and energies in the outer zone. There are appreciable temporal variations in intensities; energies of electrons reach several megaelectronvolts (MeV) and energies of protons reach a few hundred MeV. Trapped protons are more important than electrons for manned missions in low earth orbit. Although particles trapped in radiation belts can present a radiation hazard for space travellers, they do not result in any radiation dose at ground level.

12. Galactic cosmic rays are created outside the solar system; they are generally believed to be produced and accelerated as a consequence of stellar flares, supernova explosions, pulsar acceleration or the explosion of galactic nuclei [O9]. There is, however, no generally accepted theory of their generation and acceleration. Cosmic rays in our galaxy have a mean residence time of about 200 million years, being contained by the magnetic field of interstellar space [O9]. Energies of the cosmic-ray particles are mostly between 10^2 and 10^5 MeV, but they can reach much higher values [S1]. The spectrum is affected by changes in the magnetic fields within the solar system, caused by solar activity, with maximum intensity at periods of low activity and vice versa. Of the heavy ions, called HZE particles (high atomic number and energy), that are components of the cosmic-ray flux, iron is the most significant for exposure because of its relative abundance and high atomic number [L1]. Galactic cosmic rays are also affected by the geomagnetic field near the earth, which prevents some

particles from reaching the atmosphere but is progressively less effective in doing so from the geomagnetic equator to the poles. This class of space radiation is the most significant for exposure on earth and in aircraft.

13. When the primary particles from space, mainly protons, enter the atmosphere, those with high energy interact with nuclei present in the air (nitrogen, oxygen, argon) to produce neutrons, protons, muons, pions and kaons, in addition to a variety of reaction products, some of the more important of which, from the dosimetric point of view, are ^{3}H, ^{7}Be and ^{22}Na. These high-energy reactions are called spallation reactions. Many of the secondary particles have sufficient energy to initiate whole sequences of further nuclear reactions with nuclei present in the air. A cascade process is the result [I2]. The properties of some of the more important cosmic-ray particles are listed in Table 1 [E6, U5].

14. The nucleonic components, protons and neutrons, are mainly produced in the upper layers of the atmosphere. The protons are formed mainly in spallation reactions, while neutrons are produced both by spallation reactions and by the so-called evaporation of neutrons due to low-energy (p,n) reactions. Neutrons lose energy by elastic collisions and, when thermalized, are captured by ^{14}N to form ^{14}C. Because nucleons rapidly lose energy through ionization and nuclear collisions, the nucleonic flux density is considerably attenuated in the lower part of the atmosphere and accounts only for a few per cent of the dose rate at sea level [U5]. The neutron spectrum covers a wide energy range in the lower atmosphere, from thermal to 100 MeV and more, but the high-energy neutrons are most significant because of their high fluence to equivalent dose conversion coefficients.

15. Pions and kaons have short lives and essentially decay in the atmosphere before reaching ground level. The electromagnetic cascade is initiated from photons produced in the decay of neutral pions. These photons create electron-positron pairs and Compton electrons, which in turn produce additional photons by bremsstrahlung and positron-electron annihilation. As the number of shower particles increases, their average energy decreases. Finally, the majority of electrons will drop to energies where collision losses dominate and the cascade will die out [I2]. Except in the lower layers of the atmosphere, electrons are main sources of ionization [U5]. On the other hand, muons, which have a small cross-section for interaction with atomic nuclei and a mean life of 2.2 μs before decay, penetrate into the lower layers of the atmosphere and are the main constituent of cosmic rays at sea level [U5]. Most muons occur in the energy range 0.2-20 GeV, with a median value of 2 GeV [N2].

16. Solar particle radiation, as the name implies, comes from the sun. Particles of very low energy are generated continuously, but more energetic particles are emitted more copiously during magnetic disturbances. Large emissions associated with flares, called solar particle events, occur occasionally during the active period of the 11-year solar cycle [H1]. Energies are usually between 1 and 100 MeV but can be an order of magnitude higher. Such events are important in low earth orbit, but anomalously large solar particle events, which occur about once a decade, may be of vital importance for manned missions beyond the magnetosphere. Although the fluence rate of solar particles over several years exceeds the fluence rate of galactic particles, solar particles are less significant for radiation exposure in the atmosphere, because most have insufficient energy to penetrate the earth's magnetic field. The emission of solar particle radiation follows the 11-year solar cycle, reaching a maximum during increased solar activity and a minimum during the period of the quiet sun. Because the less energetic galactic cosmic-ray particles are deflected away from the solar system by the magnetic irregularities transported by the solar particle radiation, an 11-year modulation of the galactic cosmic-ray flux density at the earth is produced, the cosmic-ray flux density being lowest during times of maximum solar activity and vice versa (Figure I).

2. Factors affecting dose

17. To estimate human doses from cosmic rays, it is necessary to consider the effects of altitude, latitude and shielding.

(a) Altitude

18. The absorbed dose rates in air from the directly ionizing and indirectly ionizing (neutron) components of cosmic ray are shown in Figure I as a function of altitude at a geomagnetic latitude of 50° N. These results are based on numerous measurements on the ground and aboard aircraft, which were compiled in the UNSCEAR 1977 Report [U4]. During periods of maximum solar activity, dose rates of the ionizing component are reduced about 10% at 10 km altitude and to a lesser degree at sea level.

19. The dose rates from neutrons, the dominant indirectly ionizing component, are much less than those due to the ionizing component, but they increase more rapidly with altitude, peaking at 10-20 km. The variations during the solar cycle are greater, with decreases in the dose rates of a few tens of per cent at an altitude of 10 km during solar maxima and to a lesser degree at sea level.

20. The values of the production rate of cosmic ray ions at sea level reported after 1960 for mid- and

high-latitudes show relatively good agreement, with a cluster of values around 2.1 cm^{-3} s^{-1} and extremes at 1.9 and 2.6 cm^{-3} s^{-1} [U3]. Since 1977, the Committee has consistently adopted a value of 2.1 cm^{-3} s^{-1} for the purposes of computing the absorbed dose rate from the directly ionizing component. Assuming that each ion pair in moist air requires 33.7 eV to be produced, the absorbed dose rate in air is 32 nGy h^{-1} at sea level at mid- and high-latitudes. Since the dose is delivered mainly by muons, for which the radiation weighting factor is unity [I6], this numerical value may also be taken for the equivalent dose rate in the open.

21. The cosmic-ray neutron flux density at sea level is small and difficult to measure, mainly because the neutron energy spectrum extends over a very wide range, from fractions of eV to tens of GeV. At 50° N latitude, the neutron flux density is about 0.008 cm^{-2} s^{-1} at sea level [H2, H12]. A range of estimates of equivalent dose rates from 1.4 to 3.3 nSv h^{-1} were reported in the UNSCEAR 1988 Report [U1] for different computational geometries and exposures. The lowest values are found for low latitudes (24° N) [N23], suggesting the presence of a substantial latitude effect, even at sea level. In the UNSCEAR 1988 Report, the average effective dose equivalent rate was taken to be 2.4 nSv h^{-1}. Changes to the radiation-weighting factor were recommended by the ICRP in 1991 [I6]. Considering the neutron energy spectrum, those changes lead to an increase of about 50% of the effective dose rate from neutrons [H20]. The average effective dose rate from cosmic-ray neutrons at sea level is, therefore, estimated to be 3.6 nSv h^{-1}.

(b) Latitude

22. Lower-energy charged particles are deflected back into space by the earth's magnetic field. This effect is latitude-dependent, so that a greater flux of low-energy protons reaches the top of the atmosphere at the poles than in equatorial regions. Thus, the ionization produced in the atmosphere is also latitude-dependent. This latitude effect increases with altitude; at sea level, the cosmic-ray absorbed dose rate from the directly ionizing component gradually declines to 90% of its high-latitude value between 40° and the geomagnetic equator [T11]. For example, the cosmic-ray absorbed dose rate in air has been found to be 27-31 nGy h^{-1} at Hong Kong (latitude 22.3° N) [T11] and 28 nGy h^{-1} at Shenzen, China (latitude 22.6° N) [Y1]. These figures are to be compared to the value of 32 nGy h^{-1} observed at high- and mid-latitudes.

(c) Shielding

23. Ordinary buildings such as houses and offices provide some shielding against the directly ionizing component of cosmic rays, but data are still scarce; the magnitude of the effect depends on the structure and composition of the buildings. Limited measurements and calculations, summarized in the UNSCEAR 1988 Report [U1] and elsewhere [N2], give shielding factors from 0.96 for small wooden houses to 0.42 for substantial concrete buildings. Calculations for muons yield dose reductions ranging from 10% to 30% compared to the value in a reference room, when the parameters affecting exposure (size of building, thickness of structural elements, proximity to other buildings) are varied within reason [F2]. Without more information on shielding and on the nature of buildings, the same universal shielding factor of 0.8 is retained as before [U1]. It is recognized, however, that there may be 25% uncertainty associated with this value.

24. Information on the shielding effect of ordinary buildings on the neutrons in cosmic rays is more limited than for muons, although the broad spectrum must be affected to some degree, with virtually no attenuation by a shingle roof, for instance, and an order of magnitude attenuation by a substantial concrete element [N3]. In this Annex, no account has been taken of the shielding effect of the neutron component.

3. Exposures

(a) Ground level

25. With the conventional indoor occupancy factor of 0.8, that is, the fraction of time persons are deemed, on the average, to be indoors at home and at work [U1], the annual effective dose from the directly ionizing component of cosmic rays is estimated to be 240 μSv at sea level. Since the shielding effect is ignored for the neutron component of cosmic rays, an occupancy adjustment is not needed. The annual effective dose from the neutron component of cosmic rays is approximately 30 μSv at sea level. The uncertainty in this estimate is, clearly, appreciable.

26. To estimate the population-weighted annual effective dose from cosmic rays at ground-level, account needs to be taken of the variation of the effective dose rate with altitude and of the distribution of the world's population with altitude. Analytical expressions have been developed for the general relationship between annual dose and altitude for both the directly and indirectly ionizing components [B1]:

$$\dot{E}_I(z) = \dot{E}_I(0)[a_I \exp(-\alpha_I z) + b_I \exp(\beta_I z)] \quad (1)$$

where $\dot{E}_I$ is the effective dose rate in μSv a^{-1} for the directly ionizing component; $\dot{E}_I(0)$ is the reference value at sea level, 240 μSv a^{-1}; z is the altitude in km; $a_I = 0.21$; $\alpha_I = 1.6$ km^{-1}; $b_I = 0.80$; $\beta_I = 0.45$ km^{-1}.

$$\dot{E}_N(z) = \dot{E}_N(0)\exp(\alpha_N z) \qquad (2)$$

$$\dot{E}_N(z) = \dot{E}_N(0)[b_N \exp(\beta_N z)] \qquad (3)$$

with equation (2) applying for z < 2 km and equation (3) applying for z > 2 km, where $\dot{E}_N$ is the effective dose rate in μSv a^{-1} for the indirectly ionizing component from neutrons and $\dot{E}_N(0)$ = 30 μSv a^{-1}; α_N = 1.0 km^{-1}; b_N = 2.0; and β_N = 0.70 km^{-1}. These equations may be applied to estimate doses from cosmic rays at habitable elevations around the world. They include an allowance for shielding, as described above.

27. The distribution of the world population by altitude and urbanization has been analysed [B1], with some simplifying assumptions. When the foregoing equations are applied and the two components summed, the distribution of collective effective dose with altitude is obtained. The annual value of the average effective dose worldwide is estimated to be 380 μSv, with the directly ionizing and indirectly ionizing components contributing 300 μSv and 80 μSv, respectively. The global value of the collective effective dose is about 2 10^6 man Sv, some 90% of which occurs in the northern hemisphere by virtue of the population distribution. Somewhat less than one fifth of the collective dose is attributable to China, when account is taken of both population and elevation [H13, N22].

28. Since human habitations are mostly at lower altitudes, about one half of the collective dose is received by the two thirds of the world population that lives below 0.5 km. The one fiftieth (approximately) of the population living above 3 km receives a disproportionate one tenth of the collective dose. Table 2 lists average annual doses from cosmic rays with the separate contributions of the directly and indirectly ionizing components indicated. In high altitude cities the increasing importance of neutrons with elevation is evident. There is considerable variability in total dose. The annual value in La Paz, for example, is five times the global average. In round terms, annual values of the effective dose from cosmic rays range from 270 to 2,000 μSv, with a population-weighted mean of 380 μSv.

(b) Air travel

29. Flight pattern and duration are the principal determinants of cosmic-ray doses to aircrew and passengers. Modern commercial aircraft have optimum operating altitudes near 13 km, but flight paths are assigned according to use and safety requirements, and adequate data do not seem to be available for flight patterns [W1]. In the UNSCEAR 1988 Report [U1], a representative operating altitude of 8 km was assumed, because of the predominance of short-travel flights, with an average speed of 600 km h^{-1}. Alternative assumptions are also made; for example, an altitude of 9 km and a speed of 650 km h^{-1} were used for an assessment in the United Kingdom [H3], and an altitude of 7 km is indicated for flights by United States carriers lasting less than an hour and 11 km for longer flights [O9]. Computational codes have been developed to allow calculating radiation levels throughout the atmosphere (see, e.g. [O9]), and additional measurement experience is being acquired (see, e.g. [N12, R8, S30]). For a given altitude, dose rates for flights over the poles are substantially greater than those for flights over equatorial regions.

30. An international digest of air traffic statistics is published routinely [I3]. Data for 1989 show that 1.8 10^{12} passenger-kilometres were flown in that year, which translates into 3 10^9 passenger-hours aloft. With an effective dose rate of 2.8 μSv h^{-1} at 8 km, calculated using equations (1) and (3), the collective effective dose from global air travel is about 10,000 man Sv for the year. Worldwide, the annual value of the per caput effective dose due to air travel is, therefore, about 2 μSv; in North America it is around 10 μSv. These values are small in comparison to the estimated annual per caput effective dose at ground level of 380 μSv.

31. A limited number of supersonic airplanes operate commercially and cruise at about 15 km. Doses on board are routinely determined with monitoring equipment. Effective dose-equivalent rates are generally around 10 μSv h^{-1}, with a maximum around 40 μSv h^{-1} [U1]. In two years from July 1987, the overall average on six French airplanes was 12 μSv h^{-1}, with monthly values up to 18 μSv h^{-1} [S11]; in 1990, the average was 11 μSv h^{-1} and the annual dose to aircrew was about 3 mSv [M16]. During 1990, the average dose rate for about 2,000 flights by British airplanes was 9 μSv h^{-1}, with a maximum value of 44 μSv h^{-1} [D4]. The equivalent dose rates so far reported in this paragraph do not take into account the changes in the radiation weighting factors for neutrons that were recommended by ICRP in 1991 [I6]. The effective dose rates, estimated with the new radiation weighting factors for the neutron component, are higher than the numerical values reported above by about 30%. The monitoring equipment serves to warn of solar flares so that the airplanes can be brought to lower altitudes. This is a very small sector of the commercial air transport industry.

B. COSMOGENIC RADIONUCLIDES

32. Cosmic rays produce a range of radionuclides in the atmosphere, biosphere and lithosphere by a variety of nuclear reactions. The four most important radionuclides in terms of dose are ^{3}H, ^{7}Be, ^{14}C and ^{22}Na, and the most important mechanism of human exposure is ingestion.

33. The most significant of the four radionuclides considered is ^{14}C. The assessment of its contribution to the dose from natural sources is useful for the derivation of doses from man-made environmental releases of ^{14}C. The annual natural production of ^{14}C is 1 PBq and the specific activity of ^{14}C is 230 Bq per kg of carbon, leading to an annual effective dose of 12 μSv [U4]. The spatial variability of the dose from ^{14}C is not radiologically significant.

34. Annual effective doses to adults from the ingestion of ^{3}H, ^{7}Be and ^{22}Na in food and water have been derived from estimated average annual intakes [N2, U3, U4], applying standard coefficients for dose per unit intake [I4, N5] and assuming an equilibrium situation. The annual effective doses obtained for those three radionuclides are much smaller than that for ^{14}C. The annual intakes and effective doses for the four cosmogenic radionuclides are summarized in Table 3.

C. SUMMARY

35. Cosmic rays, which originate in space, and solar particles enter the earth's atmosphere and begin a cascade of secondary interactions and decays. The resultant ionization is a function of both altitude and latitude. The ionizing component of cosmic rays produces, on average, an absorbed dose rate in air of 32 nGy h^{-1} at sea level in the mid-latitudes, corresponding to an effective dose rate of 32 nSv h^{-1}. The neutron component of cosmic rays results in an effective dose rate of 3.6 nSv h^{-1}. The intensities of both components increase with altitude, more so for the neutron component.

36. Taking into account shielding by buildings for the ionizing component and the distribution of world population with altitude, the population-weighted average annual effective dose from cosmic rays is 380 μSv. The effective dose rate received during a commercial flight is about 3 μSv h^{-1}; the per caput annual effective dose for the world population due to air travel is 2 μSv.

37. Exposures to cosmogenic radionuclides, produced by cosmic ray interactions in the atmosphere, result primarily from ingestion and are relatively uniform throughout the world. The radionuclides include ^{3}H, ^{7}Be, ^{14}C and ^{22}Na. The annual effective dose from ^{14}C is 12 μSv. Exposure from the other radionuclides is negligible.

II. TERRESTRIAL RADIATION

38. Only nuclides with half-lives comparable with the age of the earth (or decay products, whose concentrations are governed by them) exist in terrestrial materials. In terms of dose, the principal primordial radionuclides are ^{40}K (half-life: 1.28 10^{9} a), ^{232}Th (half-life: 1.41 10^{10} a) and ^{238}U (half-life: 4.47 10^{9} a). Of secondary importance are ^{87}Rb (half-life: 4.7 10^{10} a) and ^{235}U (half-life: 7.04 10^{8} a). The thorium and uranium radionuclides head series of several radionuclides, many of which contribute to human exposure. The decay series headed by ^{238}U and ^{232}Th were illustrated in the UNSCEAR 1988 Report [U1]; the radionuclides in the series headed by ^{235}U are less important from a dosimetric point of view. There may be some local departure from secular radioactive equilibrium in the series because of physicochemical processes in the earth, such as leaching and emanation. The mass ratio of natural ^{235}U to ^{238}U is about 0.0073 and the activity ratio 0.046. A slight degree of spontaneous fission occurs in the uranium series. Both ^{40}K and ^{87}Rb undergo beta decay to stable species.

39. Natural radionuclides are also present to varying degrees in the air, in water, in organic materials and in living organisms. Human beings are therefore exposed to external and internal irradiation by gamma rays, beta particles and alpha particles with a range of energies. The main circumstances of external and internal exposures are considered in this Chapter. Separate consideration is given in Chapter III to the inhalation of the radon isotopes in the uranium and thorium series.

A. EXTERNAL EXPOSURE

1. Outdoors

40. Exposure to gamma rays from natural radionuclides occurs outdoors and indoors. Surveys by direct measurements of dose rates have been conducted during the last few decades in many countries. They are summarized in Table 4 and illustrated in Figure II. For the doses outdoors three

fifths of the population of the world is represented. National averages range from 24 to 160 nGy h^{-1}. The population-weighted average is 57 nGy h^{-1}. This is little different from the value of 55 nGy h^{-1} estimated in the UNSCEAR 1988 Report [U1].

41. In the open, much human exposure occurs over paved surfaces, but some also occurs over soil; it is determined by the activity per unit mass of the principal radionuclides in the superficial layer. Large surveys of natural radionuclides in surface soils were carried out in the United States [M1] and in China [N22]; the results are presented in Table 5. Samples were taken from fallow land. Variability is quite marked. Similar mean values for uranium and radium are reported for the United States and China, but the mean values for thorium and potassium are somewhat higher in China than in the United States, and the distributions are wider.

42. In the UNSCEAR 1988 Report, the average concentrations of ^{238}U and ^{232}Th in soil were taken to be 25 Bq kg^{-1} for each radionuclide. Although it is difficult to estimate average concentrations for the wide distributions presented in Table 5, it seems that 40 Bq kg^{-1} would be a better estimate of the average concentration of ^{238}U and ^{232}Th in soil. Data on the concentrations of naturally occurring radionuclides in various types of soils in the Nordic countries, presented in Table 6, are in agreement with the revised estimate.

43. The dose rates per unit activity concentrations of radionuclides have been calculated; for example, Monte Carlo calculations give the kerma in air for terrestrial gamma rays [P2, S12]. Since the mass energy transfer and absorption coefficients for air are not notably different in the energy range of interest here, these coefficients may be deemed compatible with those for absorbed dose rate in air used in the UNSCEAR 1988 Report [U1, B3]. When these dose factors, which are included in Table 5, are applied to the radionuclide concentrations in soil, the average dose rates in air are 72 and 55 nGy h^{-1} in China and the United States, respectively. According to Table 4, the population-weighted average absorbed dose in air for China was 62 nGy h^{-1} and that for all countries reporting survey results 57 nGy h^{-1}. Since human habitations are mostly in areas of sedimentary geology and since radionuclide concentrations in bedrock and overburden are similar in such circumstances [W2], the values from Table 5 in the narrower range, 10-200 nGy h^{-1}, may be considered to be broadly typical for the world population. Areas of high activity are discussed later.

44. The water content of the soil and snow cover can affect absorbed dose rates in air. On the whole, increasing water content and snow cover reduce dose, but these are second-order phenomena [D3, F3, G2] when averaged over a year in temperate zones with moderate precipitation. In extreme climates with heavy snow cover, however, the reduction may be as much as 20% [S5, S35]. The addition of phosphate fertilizer, discussed in Section IV.C, may cause a second-order increase in dose rate [P3].

45. Areas of markedly high absorbed dose rates in air around the world are associated with thorium-bearing and uranium-bearing materials. Mineral sands containing monazite are prime examples of the former. Absorbed dose rates in air from gamma rays near separated monazite may reach 10^5 nGy h^{-1} depending on geometry [M6]. It is not surprising, therefore, that dose rates over sands can be remarkable. Two such areas are well known: on the Arabian Sea coast of Kerala in India, where dose rates in air range from 200 to 4,000 nGy h^{-1} [S6, S7] and on the Atlantic coast of Espírito Santo in Brazil, where dose rates in air range from 100 to 4,000 nGy h^{-1} approximately [P4]. Radiation exposures due to mining and milling of mineral sands are discussed in Section IV.D.

46. Other areas of high background radiation have also been identified. On the Nile Delta, dose rates in air are estimated to range from 20 to 400 nGy h^{-1} [E2] and on the Ganges Delta from 260 to 440 nGy h^{-1} [M7]. Dose rates in air of up to 12,000 nGy h^{-1} have been reported over thorium-bearing carbonatite in an area near Mombasa on the coast of Kenya [P6]. An area of volcanic intrusives in Minas Gerais, Brazil, with mixed thorium and uranium mineralization, has dose rates in air roughly from 100 to 3,500 nGy h^{-1} [P17]. Ramsar, on the Caspian Sea in Iran, has dose rates up to 30,000 nGy h^{-1} because of thorium and uranium deposition by hot springs in travertine [S33]. Many granite areas have elevated natural radiation levels [M2, W10]. Localized dose rates in air around 100,000 nGy h^{-1} have been found over uraniferous rocks in Sweden [S8]. Dose rates associated with uraniferous phosphate deposits are appreciably lower; on the phosphate lands of Florida, they range from 30 to 100 nGy h^{-1} [N2].

2. Indoors

47. During the last decade, several surveys have been made of the dose rate in air from terrestrial gamma rays inside dwellings. The results are included in Table 4. Over a third of the world population is represented. The surveys are not quite as complete as outdoor investigations. National averages range from 20 to 190 nGy h^{-1} with a population-weighted average of all the data being about 80 nGy h^{-1}. This value is somewhat higher than 70 nGy h^{-1}, selected in the

UNSCEAR 1988 Report [U1] as representative for indoor exposure worldwide.

48. In comparing the indoor and outdoor averages, it is seen that the overall effect of surrounding building materials is to increase the dose rate 40%-50%. As indicated in Table 4 and illustrated in Figure III, the ratio of indoor to outdoor dose rates varies from 0.8 to 2.0. In only two countries, Iceland and the United States, are average absorbed dose rates indoors judged to be less than outdoors. This ratio is sensitive to the structural properties of dwellings (materials, thicknesses and dispositions) and is of limited utility for estimating exposures in particular cases from outdoor data. However, the relatively narrow range of the indoor-outdoor ratio reflects the fact that building materials are usually of local origin and that their radionuclide concentrations are similar to those in local soil. The building materials act as sources of radiation and also as shields against outdoor radiation. In wooden and lightweight houses, the source effect is negligible and the walls are an inefficient shield with respect to the outdoor sources of radiation, so that the absorbed dose rate in air could be expected to be somewhat lower indoors than outdoors. In contrast, in massive houses made of brick, concrete or stone, the gamma rays emitted outdoors are efficiently absorbed by the walls, and the indoor absorbed dose rate depends mainly on the activity concentrations of natural radionuclides in the building materials. Under these circumstances, the indoor absorbed dose rate is generally higher as the result of the change in source geometry, with the indoor-outdoor ratio of absorbed dose rates in air between 1 and 2.

49. There is considerable uncertainty in estimates of indoor dose rates. It is clear that the dose rates in masonry dwellings are appreciably higher than in wooden ones, as explained in the previous paragraph. For improved estimates of doses, it would be necessary to have data for representative housing stock around the world. Data for houses in warm climates are underrepresented in Table 4; these may be constructed very differently from houses in cold climates. It is expected that the percentage of houses that are largely made of wood and other lightweight materials is greater in warm climates than in cold climates, so that for the same average absorbed dose rate in air outdoors, the average absorbed dose rate in air indoors would be lower in warm climates than in cold climates. This needs to be confirmed by measurements. Such an important source of human exposure should be quantified more extensively.

50. The dose rates in masonry dwelling are determined by the characteristics of the masonry materials: 30 g cm^{-2} of masonry, for example, provides 90% of the gamma rays from an infinitely thick source [N2]. If construction materials with elevated concentrations of natural radionuclides are used, dose rates in air indoors will be elevated accordingly. Some measurements have been made of dose rates in relation to building materials. Measurements in Sweden gave values of about 230 nGy h^{-1}, on average, in houses with outside walls made of lightweight concrete, some of which contained uraniferous alum shale [M9, M27]. Measurements in former Czechoslovakia gave values approaching 1,000 nGy h^{-1} in houses with outside walls containing uraniferous coal slag [T3]. Measurements in a granite region of the United Kingdom, where some of the houses are made of local stone, gave 100 nGy h^{-1} [W3]. Estimates for houses made with mud blocks in Jamaica reach 200 nGy h^{-1} [P18]. It is useful, therefore, to calculate the effect of using building materials with different activity characteristics.

51. In round terms, the activities per unit mass of ^{40}K, ^{226}Ra and ^{232}Th in building materials A_K, A_{Ra}, and A_{Th} are typically 500, 50 and 50 Bq kg^{-1}, respectively [N10]. If the dose coefficients given in Table 5 are applied, it is possible to construct an activity utilization index that facilitates the calculation of dose rates in air from different combinations of the three radionuclides in building materials. This may then be weighted for the mass proportion of the building materials in a house. The activity utilization index is given by the expression

$$\left(\frac{C_K}{A_K} f_K + \frac{C_{Ra}}{A_{Ra}} f_{Ra} + \frac{C_{Th}}{A_{Th}} f_{Th}\right) w_m \qquad (4)$$

where C_K, C_{Ra} and C_{Th} are actual values of the activities per unit mass of ^{40}K, ^{226}Ra and ^{232}Th in the building materials considered (Bq kg^{-1}); f_K, f_{Ra} and f_{Th} are the fractional contributions to the dose rate in air from the standard or typical concentrations of these radionuclides; and w_m is the fractional usage of the building materials in the dwelling with the activity characteristic. For full utilization of typical masonry, the activity utilization index is unity by definition and is deemed to imply a dose rate of 80 nGy h^{-1}. In Table 7, illustrative examples are given of the use of the activity utilization index.

52. To estimate the effect of using atypical materials, it is necessary to determine the fractional utilization by mass, identify the associated dose rate and then subtract the corresponding dose rate for typical masonry. Thus, 0.5 utilization of granite would increase the dose rate by 70 – 40 = 30 nGy h^{-1} and 0.5 utilization of alum shale would increase it by 390 – 40 = 350 nGy h^{-1}. One quarter utilization of

phosphogypsum would cause an increase of 50 nGy h^{-1}, but a similar fraction of natural gypsum would lead to a decrease of 15 nGy h^{-1}. Because of the simple irradiation geometry and rounded parameter values, this approach is only very approximate, but there is some experimental confirmation [E3], and it does describe the circumstances mentioned earlier.

53. In Kerala, some of the more radioactive stretches of sand have concentrations of ^{40}K, ^{226}Ra and ^{232}Th of 100, 1,000 and 7,000 Bq kg^{-1}, respectively [L6], which would lead, according to the foregoing formulation, to 5,000 nGy h^{-1} in dwellings, since structures there provide little shielding against gamma rays from the ground. Measured dose rates in air in an earlier survey approached 4,000 nGy h^{-1}, with an arithmetic mean around 700 nGy h^{-1} for the population on the segment of the coast with the most radioactive sand [S6]. Large-scale surface mining and subsequent refilling with monazite-free tailings have, however, reduced the external radiation fields substantially, e.g. at some locations from 4,000 nGy h^{-1} to 300 nGy h^{-1}, and improvements in socio-economic conditions have resulted in structural modifications of the hutments, which have reduced indoor external radiation exposures by a factor of 3 [P6].

54. Some of the short-lived decay products of ^{222}Rn, always present in air, emit gamma rays. A semi-empirical analysis for a single-family house yielded an absorbed dose rate in air of 0.01 nGy h^{-1} per unit activity concentration of radon progeny at equilibrium expressed as Bq m^{-3} [M10]. For 20 Bq m^{-3}, a representative activity concentration indoors, the dose rate would be about 0.2 nGy h^{-1}, which is relatively trivial in relation to direct gamma rays from the building materials and the dose to human lungs from alpha particles emitted by the other radon progeny. Another semi-empirical estimate for gamma rays from radon progeny outdoors yielded an increment of 0.5% per Bq m^{-3} over the fluence rate of photons directly from the earth [N11]. For an equilibrium equivalent concentration outdoors of 8 Bq m^{-3}, this implies a dose rate increment of 2 nGy h^{-1}, that is, a few per cent of the prevailing dose rate from the earth. Monte Carlo calculations [F12] substantiate these estimates.

3. Dose

55. In the UNSCEAR 1988 Report [U1], a coefficient of 0.7 Sv Gy^{-1} was used to convert absorbed dose in air to effective dose equivalent. This refers to adults and is based on an analysis in the UNSCEAR 1982 Report [U3] of experimental and calculational data on environmental exposure to gamma rays. A more recent assessment [P19, S12] provides coefficients for exposure to terrestrial gamma rays not only for adults but also for children and infants. Reference data are given in Table 8. The overall value is not altered appreciably by weighting for the typical radionuclide composition of soil. These results were derived from Monte Carlo calculations for mathematical phantoms, those for adults being based on ICRP Reference Man [I5] and those for the younger persons on computed tomographic data for patients. In round terms, therefore, the conversion coefficient of 0.7 Sv Gy^{-1} still seems to be suitable for adults [U1]. Because of the circumstance of irradiation, it seems unlikely that the conversion coefficient to effective dose would differ appreciably from this value.

56. The assumption has been made in previous UNSCEAR Reports [U1, U3, U4] that the indoor occupancy factor is 0.8, implying that 20% of time is spent outdoors, on average, around the world. There is no way at present of validating this assumption, but the indications are that 0.8 is low for industrialized countries in temperate climates, where an appreciable fraction of time is spent indoors in structures other than the home [N2, W3], and high for agricultural countries in warm climates, where a substantial fraction of time is spent out of doors even at night [E5]. As more information becomes available, it may be possible to refine the estimate of the occupancy factor, but at present there is no basis for changing the conventional value.

57. With values for the conversion coefficient to effective dose (0.7 Sv Gy^{-1}) and the occupancy factor (0.8), it is possible to combine outdoor (57 nGy h^{-1}) and indoor (80 nGy h^{-1}) exposures to terrestrial gamma rays to estimate the average effective dose. The arithmetic annual mean worldwide, weighted for population, is 0.46 mSv, somewhat higher than the value for cosmic rays (0.38 mSv), the other component of external exposure to natural radiation sources. For children and infants, the values are about 10% and 30% higher.

58. It is of interest to present some national estimates of average annual effective dose from terrestrial gamma rays. This is done in Table 9. The underlying assumption in each case that the effective dose equivalent and the effective dose are numerically the same for this circumstance. The values range from 0.23 to 0.65 mSv, with a median value of 0.40 mSv. The population-weighted value for these 13 countries is 0.45 mSv, in agreement with the result quoted in the previous paragraph.

59. To complete the consideration of the external component of natural background exposure, the doses

from external irradiation by environmental beta particles should be mentioned, although these mainly affect the superficial tissues of the body. Calculations for soil show that the absorbed dose rate in air from beta particles is similar at the surface of the ground to that for gamma rays, but that it drops to 20% of the latter at 1 m above the surface [O4]. Furthermore, the dose throughout the organs of the body generally is about two orders of magnitude less than the dose to the skin. Similar circumstances exist indoors. The absorbed dose rate from airborne beta emitters is comparable to that from surface emission indoors and about an order of magnitude less outdoors. If these relationships are applied to the average values for the absorbed dose rates from gamma rays outdoors and indoors, the annual absorbed dose to the skin from beta particles is estimated to be about 0.2 mGy overall. The contribution to dose from beta particles from the surfaces of particular materials, such as the mineral sands in Kerala, would be much more [S7].

B. INTERNAL EXPOSURE

60. After cosmic rays and terrestrial gamma rays, the third element of basic background exposure is that from long-lived natural radionuclides in the human body, which arises from inhalation and ingestion. Potassium-40 and the uranium and thorium series radionuclides are treated separately. Radon is considered in Chapter III.

61. Data on ^{40}K in the human body are well established, mainly from direct measurements of persons of various ages [I5, U5] but also from the analysis of post-mortem specimens [F13]. At the age of 30 years, approximately the median for industrialized countries [U11], the body content of potassium is about 0.18%, at 10 years about 0.2%, and is assumed to be the same at 1 year, these being the averages for the sexes. Potassium is under homeostatic control in the body, although there are disease states that affect the level. The isotopic abundance of ^{40}K is 1.18 10^{-4}. With an average specific activity of 55 Bq kg^{-1} of body weight and a rounded conversion coefficient of 3 μSv a^{-1} per Bq kg^{-1} [N2], the annual effective dose equivalent from ^{40}K in the body is 165 μSv for adults, most of the dose being delivered by beta particles. The value for children is 185 μSv.

62. Doses from radionuclides in the uranium and thorium series, on the other hand, reflect intake to the body with diet and air. In previous UNSCEAR Reports [U1, U3, U4, U5], doses were estimated from measured activities in tissues and appropriate dosimetric coefficients, but intake data were also provided. In this Annex, intake data are translated to committed effective doses for adults and also for children and infants, so as to indicate the effect of intake with age. Although the determination of dose from concentrations in tissue is more direct, the data on intake provide a good secondary indication.

63. A reference food consumption profile is presented in Table 10. This is based on the normalized average consumption rate adopted by WHO [W4], derived from the food balance sheets compiled by the Food and Agriculture Organization (FAO) [F4]. These estimates refer to raw, unprepared products with no account taken of losses in distribution and utilization; consequently, average values are usually overestimates. Data on food consumption by age are usually obtained from nutritional studies, but because the information is rather limited, relative rather than absolute values are best inferred [V2]. In Table 10, therefore, the average values [W4] are adopted for adults, and the consumption rates for children and infants are taken to be two thirds and one third of the adult values, except for milk products, which are higher than unity [V2]. Intakes of water, both directly and in beverages, are based on reference ICRP water balance data [I5]. The tabulated values are compatible with other assessments [C4, N13, U1]. There are, of course, departures from the reference consumption: the Chinese diet, for example, is low in milk, the African diet in leafy vegetables [W4] and the Indian diet in meat [R11]. Cereal consumption, on the other hand, is much the same in all types of diet. The nominal nature of the data in Table 10 and the resulting uncertainties in the dose estimates must be stressed. Reference ICRP breathing rates [I5] are also given in Table 10.

64. The next step is to establish reference activity concentrations in dietary materials and air. The values for food and water in Table 11 rely heavily on data for northern temperate latitudes [F5, L5, N2, P5, P20, S13, S14, S44] and are compatible with data in the UNSCEAR 1988 Report [U1]; fish, for which data are scarce and disparate, includes a 10% admixture of invertebrates [C5, J7]. All food values are for wet weight. Reference concentrations in air in Table 11 are from the same sources [F5, L5, N2, U1] and are deemed to apply outdoors and indoors.

65. Information on effective dose per unit intake of activity of naturally occurring radionuclides by adults is given in Table 12 [I4]; it is based on the biokinetic models of ICRP. It is assumed in this Annex that the doses per unit activity intake for natural radionuclides are not age-dependent.

66. Average age-weighted annual intakes by ingestion and associated effective doses have been estimated using the fractional distribution of adults, children and infants of 0.65, 0.3 and 0.05, respectively; the results are presented in Table 13. The intake values are generally similar to those in the UNSCEAR 1988 Report [U1], although the ^{210}Po value is

somewhat higher, mainly because fish and, in particular, invertebrates were included. The dominant radionuclides are ^{210}Pb and ^{210}Po. There is a scarcity of environmental data for ^{231}Pa and ^{227}Ac [K10, V7], but if they were present to the same degree as ^{235}U, the overall effective dose would be increased by approximately 1%. Along the same line, the intake of ^{228}Th has been assumed to be equal to that of ^{232}Th. In fact, the intake of ^{228}Th should be greater, because of some ingrowth of that radionuclide in foodstuffs following the decay of ^{228}Ra [L11]; this ingrowth, which is difficult to quantify, would result in an increase in the overall effective dose of less than 2%.

67. Table 13 includes analogous information for inhalation. The values are similar to those in the UNSCEAR 1988 Report [U1]. The dominant radionuclide is ^{210}Pb. It may be noted that smoking 10 cigarettes a day would double the intake of ^{210}Po [N2]. The decay products of ^{235}U would, once more, add about 1%.

68. The doses from reference annual intakes of the long-lived series radionuclides can be compared to the annual doses re-estimated from the UNSCEAR 1988 Report [U1] with the new ICRP tissue weighting factors [I6]. For uranium and thorium series radionuclides, the effective doses are 62 μSv committed from annual intake and 130 μSv annually from average body content. For ^{40}K the same doses are 170 and 180 μSv, respectively. The total effective doses are 230 μSv by intake and 310 μSv by body content. The results are fairly consistent and support the validity of the intake estimation method. The advantages of this method over that based on post-mortem analyses are that there are more data on activities in foodstuffs than in human tissues and that it facilitates the estimation of doses from high intakes of activity in unusual circumstances. It is recognized, however, that there are large uncertainties in the values of the dose coefficients, mainly owing to uncertainties in the values of the gut absorption fractions (also called f_1) for many radionuclides. These uncertainties may arise for a variety of reasons, including the chemical nature of the radionuclide ingested, biological variability in humans and extrapolation from animal data when human data are sparse. It would be desirable to carry out more post-mortem analyses of tissues to determine natural radionuclide concentrations, as such analyses would allow a more direct assessment of the absorbed doses.

69. The variability of activity concentrations in foods is clearly shown in Table 14, where selected information on elevated levels is presented. The reference values can be exceeded by orders of magnitude. In the volcanic area of Minas Gerais, Brazil [A4, A8, L10, V3] and in the mineral sands area of Kerala, India [L6], there is evidence of excess activity in milk, meat and grain, leafy vegetables, roots and fruits. In the granitic area of Guandong, China, excess activity has been reported in foodstuffs such as rice and radishes [Z1]. Mention might also be made of the elevated levels of ^{210}Po in yerba maté, a plant used to make a beverage in South America [C15]. For radiological significance, however, the most pronounced increase over reference levels occurs in the Arctic and sub-Arctic regions, where ^{210}Pb and ^{210}Po accumulate in flesh of reindeer and caribou [H7, P7], an important part of the diet of the inhabitants of those regions. Reindeer and caribou feed on lichens, which accumulate these radionuclides from the atmosphere. If the annual consumption of reindeer and caribou meat is taken into account [K3], it is possible to evaluate the effective dose from this intake. Assuming the reference intakes for other foods and water apply, the overall dose from ingestion is estimated to be about 300 μSv for adults. This is one example of a community exposed under unusual circumstances.

70. Selected information on elevated levels of activity concentrations in potable waters is shown in Table 15 with values for some bottled mineral waters and ground waters. These elevated levels are to be compared with the reference levels presented in Table 11. As with foods, reference values are exceeded by orders of magnitude. Bottled waters in Brazil include some from areas of high natural radiation levels [P8]. The results for France [M19, P5, P9, R12, R13, R14, S11] represent all the principal sources of mineral waters in that country. Commercially available waters were widely sampled in Germany [B12, G4, G5]. The selection of Portuguese waters was broadly representative [B6]. An extensive survey in Sweden of public and private water supplies [K4] yielded high levels of ^{226}Ra in some wells with an average of 45 mBq kg^{-1} in water from deep-bored wells. In Finland, remarkably high concentrations have been discovered in wells drilled in bedrock throughout the south of the country near Helsinki [S15]. If allowance is made for the extra dose from these waters with otherwise reference intakes, the overall value of the committed effective dose becomes 550 μSv for annual intakes by adults. This is another example of a community with unusual circumstances of exposure.

C. SUMMARY

71. Natural radionuclides of significance in soil, air, water and living organisms include ^{40}K and the isotopes of the ^{238}U and ^{232}Th decay chains. Exposures occur by external irradiation and from internal irradiation following ingestion or inhalation of the radionuclides.

72. The dose rate in air outdoors from terrestrial gamma rays in normal circumstances is around 57 nGy h^{-1}. National averages range from 24 to 160 nGy h^{-1}. Soil and survey data yield similar values. Communities living on mineral sands may well be exposed at two orders of magnitude more. The gamma-ray dose rate indoors is estimated to be 80 nGy h^{-1}, the population-weighted mean of measured values worldwide, and the range of reported national averages is 20-190 nGy h^{-1}. These results are in accordance with values inferred from outdoor measurements and the concentrations of radionuclides in building materials. Applying a coefficient of 0.7 Sv Gy^{-1} to convert absorbed dose rate in air to effective dose and using an indoor occupancy factor of 0.8, the world-wide average annual effective dose from external exposure to terrestrial radionuclides is 0.46 mSv.

73. Effective doses resulting from intake of natural radionuclides in air, food and water may be determined from measured concentrations in the body or estimated from concentrations in intake materials. The worldwide average committed dose from annual intakes is estimated to be 0.23 mSv, of which 0.17 mSv is from ^{40}K and 0.06 mSv from radionuclides of the ^{238}U and ^{232}Th series. Variations in exposures occur from variations in the latter component. Communities receiving higher effective doses include consumers of reindeer meat (average annual effective dose: 0.3 mSv) and consumers of deep well water in some locations (average annual effective dose: 0.5 mSv). Little information exists on the variability of dose from the inhalation of long-lived activity in air, but inhalation is dominated by radon isotopes and their short-lived decay products, which are the subject of the next Chapter.

III. RADON

74. Exposure to radon is the most significant element of human irradiation by natural sources. It is distinguished from the other three elements of basic background because exposure varies markedly in ordinary circumstances and because high exposures may be avoided with comparative ease. The most important mechanism of exposure is the inhalation of the short-lived decay products of the principal isotope, ^{222}Rn, with indoor air. Concentrations of ^{222}Rn and its progeny are usually higher in indoor air than in outdoor air; exceptions are in tropical areas, where ^{222}Rn concentrations in well-ventilated dwellings are essentially the same as in outdoor air.

75. There are three natural isotopes of the radioactive element radon: ^{219}Rn (actinon) in the ^{235}U series; ^{220}Rn (thoron) in the ^{232}Th series; ^{222}Rn (radon) in the ^{238}U series. Because of the low activity concentrations of ^{235}U and the short half-life of ^{219}Rn, this isotope is not significant for human exposure. Because of its short half-life, ^{220}Rn is of concern only where the concentration of ^{232}Th is high. Owing to its relatively long half-life, ^{222}Rn is the most significant isotope, and there is much information on it. Table 16 gives the alpha decay properties of ^{220}Rn and ^{222}Rn and their short-lived decay products [B7, M11].

76. Radon is a noble gas with slight ability to form compounds under laboratory conditions [S16]. The density of radon is 9.73 g l^{-1} at 0° C [W5]. There is very little radon in air, typically about one atom per 10^{18} atoms of air indoors, and so it does not stratify. Its solubility in water at 0° C is 510 cm^3 l^{-1} decreasing to 220 cm^3 l^{-1} at 25° C and 130 cm^3 l^{-1} at 50° C.

A. SOURCES AND MOVEMENT

1. Production in terrestrial materials

77. The production of ^{220}Rn and ^{222}Rn in terrestrial materials depends on the activity concentrations of ^{228}Ra and ^{226}Ra present. Indicative values for these radium isotopes in soils may be inferred from Table 5. Some values for rocks, taken from extensive analyses [C14, W6], are given in Tables 17 and 18. On average, granites are high in radium, basalts are low and sedimentary and metamorphosed rocks have intermediate values. In the main, the results are fairly consistent with the soil values, although exceptional values of ^{226}Ra do occur in some detrital sedimentary rocks [A5].

78. Earth materials may be envisaged as a porous matrix through which fluids can move. To be free to do so, radon must first emanate from the mineral substance into the pore space. This is brought about mainly by the recoil of radon atoms on formation, with a typical range of 20-70 nm in minerals, and by molecular diffusion [T4]. Emanation is thought to be amplified by the superficial disposition of radon precursors and the damage caused by radioactive decay. The fraction of radon formed that enters the pores has variously been called the emanating power, the ratio, the coefficient and the fraction. Values of the emanation fraction, as it is called here, for various earth and building materials are given in Table 19. The results relate to ^{222}Rn and are supported by other studies of soils [B13, M20, M21]. Relatively little

information exists for ^{220}Rn, but similar values would be expected because of the physical processes involved.

79. Moisture and temperature affect radon emanation. The presence of water increases the probability that the recoils will terminate in the pores rather than the matrix and that more radon will therefore be available for movement [T4], but this trend is later reversed as the water content grows. Increasing temperature also increases emanation, probably because of reduced adsorption, but the mechanism and magnitude of this effect are not as well understood or quantified [S18]. Of the two, the moisture effect is the more significant.

2. Diffusion

80. The movement of radon in porous material is brought about by concentration and pressure gradients; the mechanisms of movement are molecular diffusion and forced advection [N14]. Both are modified by radioactive decay. Consideration here is limited to the movement of radon from the ground into the open atmosphere and from the ground and building elements into confined spaces such as dwellings. Attention is first given to diffusion.

81. If earth is regarded as a porous mass of homogeneous material semi-infinite in extent, the flux density of radon at the surface J_D (Bq m^{-2} s^{-1}) is given [U1] by the expression

$$J_D = C_{Ra} \lambda_{Rn} f \rho [D_e / (\lambda_{Rn} \varepsilon)]^{0.5} \quad (5)$$

where C_{Ra} is the activity concentration of ^{226}Ra in earth material (Bq kg^{-1}); λ_{Rn} is the decay constant of ^{222}Rn (2.1 10^{-6} s^{-1}); f is the emanation fraction for earth material; ρ is the density of earth material (kg m^{-3}); D_e is the effective diffusion coefficient for earth material (m^2 s^{-1}); and ε is the porosity of the earth material. The first four parameters in the equation comprise the volumetric production rate of radon (Bq m^{-3} s^{-1}); the expression in brackets is the diffusion length.

82. If a building element, such as a wall or floor, is similarly regarded as a semi-infinite slab of porous material, the flux density of radon from one side is given [U1] by the expression

$$J_D = C_{Ra} \lambda_{Rn} f \rho [D_e / (\lambda_{Rn} \varepsilon)]^{0.5} \tanh d [D_e / (\lambda_{Rn} \varepsilon)]^{-0.5} \quad (6)$$

where d is the half-thickness (in metres) of the element and the other symbols refer to the same parameters as in equation (5), but where the values are for the building material rather than the earth material. The two equations are the same apart from the hyperbolic term, which takes into account the finite thickness of the slab and has a value less than unity.

83. Since diffusion dominates over advection as the mechanism by which radon enters the atmosphere from the surface of the earth [N14], it is possible to calculate the flux density by using appropriate values for the parameters in equation (5). Values of C_{Ra} are in Table 5 and values of f, D_e and ε in Table 19. Representative values are C_{Ra} = 40 Bq kg^{-1}; f = 0.2; D_e = 5 10^{-7} m^2 s^{-1}; ε = 0.25. The value of ρ is about 1,600 kg m^{-3}, and λ_{Rn} = 2.1 10^{-6} s^{-1}. These yield an estimate for J_D of 0.026 Bq m^{-2} s^{-1}, somewhat higher than the weighted value of 0.016 Bq m^{-2} s^{-1} from measurements over various soils [W7] but quite close to the average value of 0.022 Bq m^{-2} s^{-1} estimated for Australia [S36] and compatible with the indications for sedimentary areas of France [R15]. It must be noted, however, that the calculated value of J_D is critically dependent on the value adopted for C_{Ra} and that the measured value is critically dependent on the weighting procedure for soil type. The volumetric production rate, given by the first part of the equation, is about 0.027 Bq m^{-3} s^{-1}.

84. For building elements, the flux density due to diffusion may be calculated by substituting the appropriate values in equation (6). Such values of C_{Ra}, f, D_e and ε are in Tables 7 and 19: C_{Ra} = 50 Bq kg^{-1}; f = 0.1; D_e = 1 10^{-8} m^2 s^{-1}; ε = 0.15. As before, λ_{Rn} = 2.1 10^{-6} s^{-1}, and the value of ρ is taken to be 1,600 kg m^{-3}; for elements 0.2 m thick, d is 0.1 m. These yield an estimate for J_D of 0.0015 Bq m^{-2} s^{-1} and a volumetric production rate of 0.017 Bq m^{-3} s^{-1}. Whereas the production rate is comparable to the volumetric value for earth material, the flux density from a building material element is about an order of magnitude less. Volumetric production rates for radon inferred from measurements on laboratory specimens of ordinary concrete are in accordance with the calculated value, but the rates for natural gypsum and ordinary clay bricks are lower than estimated [C6, J2, T5, U1]. Most measurements of radon flux density have been made on laboratory specimens of building materials; since these have a much higher surface-to-volume ratio than building elements, the results underestimate the flux density in practical circumstances [C6]. Some measurements on sections of building elements do, however, give results that are fairly compatible with the calculations for ordinary concrete and ordinary clay bricks but appreciably lower for natural gypsum [B9, P10, S20].

85. As in the UNSCEAR 1988 Report [U1], a model building is defined so as to illustrate the relative importance of the various sources of radon indoors. A

simple masonry structure is envisaged with a volume, V, of 250 m^3 and a surface area, S_B, of 450 m^2. The characteristics broadly reflect construction in temperate climates. An air exchange rate of 1 h^{-1} is postulated. The rate U of radon entry from the building elements (Bq m^{-3} h^{-1}) is given by the expression

$$U = (3.6\ 10^3\ S_B J_D)/V \qquad (7)$$

where J_D is defined in equation (6). The resulting value of U is almost 10 Bq m^{-3} h^{-1}. Without a masonry floor, the rate of entry by diffusion from bare earth would be about 37 Bq m^{-3} h^{-1}, this being calculated by substituting the surface area of the floor, S_E = 100 m^2, for S_B and 0.026 Bq m^{-2} s^{-1} for J_D in equation (7). An intact concrete floor 0.2 m thick would, however, reduce the rate of entry by a factor of about 14 [C7, U1] to 2.6 Bq m^{-3} h^{-1}, which is comparable to the contribution from such a floor element.

86. It should be recognized that floors are unlikely to be intact and that holes and cracks greatly facilitate the entry of radon. The effect of cracks has been modelled in a mathematical sense for a stylized pattern of penetrations through a floor element [D6, L8]. With an array of 1 cm wide cracks every 1 m through a 0.2 m thick floor and a diffusion coefficient of 5 10^{-7} m^2 s^{-1} for the underlying earth, the rate of entry by diffusion is about 20% of that from bare earth [D6], implying 7.5 Bq m^{-3} h^{-1}, which in turn implies a flux density, averaged over the whole floor, of 0.0052 Bq m^{-2} s^{-1}. In the reference building, therefore, 1% discontinuity in the floor permits 20% diffusion from the earth.

3. Advection

87. Attention is now turned to the forced advection (also frequently called convection) of radon from the earth into a building. This is caused by the slightly negative pressure differences (underpressure) that usually exist between the indoor and outdoor atmospheres. Two mechanisms are mainly responsible, wind blowing on the building and heating inside the building [N15]. Other mechanisms, such as changes in barometric pressure and negative pressure caused by mechanical ventilation, may also be significant [N14].

88. Wind creates a negative pressure drop across the shell of a building. The magnitude of the drop is determined by the configuration of the building and varies with the square of the windspeed; in a light breeze, it may be a few pascals [N14]. Outdoor air is therefore drawn inwards through gaps in the shell or through the subjacent earth with radon entrained. The rapidity with which a pressure drop is transmitted depends on the permeability of the ground and can vary from seconds for sand to weeks for clay [N14].

89. Heat also creates a pressure drop across the shell of the building with the gradient towards the higher temperature. This phenomenon, usually called the stack effect, also draws air through and under the shell. The drop is proportional to the temperature differences [F7]; for 20° C, it also amounts to a few pascals. In severe climates, however, it would be much more and in tropical climates much less. The overall effect of both mechanisms is assumed to create a pressure difference, Δp, of about 5 Pa [R4].

90. If a masonry floor is intact, advection from the earth cannot take place. The presence of cracks in the element allows advection, however, and a mathematical model has been used to determine the influx of radon [D7]. As with diffusion through cracks [D6], the finite difference method is used to solve numerically the steady-state transport equation for advection. Apart from Δp, the parameter of prime importance is the permeability, k, of the subjacent earth material, which varies in value through several orders of magnitude from a low of 10^{-16} m^2 for fine clay to a high of 10^{-8} m^2 for coarse gravel [N14].

91. Application of the model to a floor element with an array, as before, of 1 cm wide cracks every 1 m, yields ratios between the advective and diffusive influxes for a range of permeabilities [W8]. These ratios vary from about unity at lower permeabilities to an order of magnitude greater when k is about 10^{-10} m^2 and then decline towards unity again at higher permeabilities. Extension of the model to a bare earth floor yields estimates of influx for lower and intermediate permeabilities, but the method breaks down at higher permeabilities. When these results are applied to the model building for an underpressure of 5 Pa, they give the flux densities in Table 20, which are averaged over the whole area of the floor. They should be compared to the diffusive flux densities of 0.0052 Bq m^{-2} s^{-1} for the cracked floor and 0.026 Bq m^{-2} s^{-1} for the bare earth estimated earlier. Values of the flux density similar to those shown in this Table would be obtained for similar values of the product kΔp within the underpressure range 1-10 Pa [D7].

92. Radon entry rates by advection are calculated from equation (7) by again substituting S_E = 100 m^2 for S_B and by replacing the diffusive flux density by the advective values in Table 20. The outcome is also shown in Table 20. Entry rates vary from zero for an impermeable floor element, through 10 Bq m^{-3} h^{-1} for a cracked floor on earth material of low permeability, to 274 Bq m^{-3} h^{-1} for a bare floor of fairly high permeability. The decline in rates at the higher

permeabilities is due to the depletion of radon in the earth near the walls of the building by the passage of fresh air [D7, W8]. If an intermediate permeability of 10^{-11} m^2 for sandy-silty earth material is deemed to be typical and accordant with the diffusion coefficient adopted earlier, it becomes clear from the Table and from the earlier paragraphs that advection is likely to dominate over diffusion as a source of radon in buildings under common circumstances.

93. It is possible to estimate an upper value of the entry rate by advection from the earth in a simple manner if the fraction ϕ is known of the air exchange rate for the building that takes place through the earth. It is given by the expression

$$U = \phi \lambda_v [(C_{Ra} f \rho)/\varepsilon] \quad (8)$$

where λ_v is the air exchange rate (1 h^{-1}) and the other symbols represent the same quantities as before with the same values. The terms in brackets refer to the radon concentration in equilibrium with radium at depth in the earth; their conjoint value is about 5 10^4 Bq m^{-3}. A value of 0.02% for ϕ would yield an entry rate of 10 Bq m^{-3} h^{-1} for the model building and thus match the contribution by diffusion from the building elements. Values of ϕ two orders of magnitude greater may be realized [S21] for solid floors on the earth, sometimes called slab on grade. This simple analysis does not, however, take into account the depletion of radon near the surface of the earth.

94. It must be stressed that entry by advection is quite dependent on the configuration of the floor and that any estimate of an illustrative value is quite uncertain. Even for the simple slab on grade of the model building, structural details and the nature of the underfill make estimating difficult. For suspended floors, entry is severely influenced by the degree to which the living space is decoupled from the earth. For buildings with basements, the difficulty is compounded by the extensive area of contact between the structural elements and the backfill or earth. Much still remains to be done to clarify these issues [G10, H15, M22, N16, R4], and it must be realized that reliable estimates of indoor radon concentrations are best obtained from measurements of radon in air.

4. Infiltration

95. Fresh air enters a building through open doors, windows and ventilators and through inadvertent gaps in the superficial shell. Although the term infiltration properly refers to the passage of air through small openings, it is used here to describe the overall degree of direct exchange between outdoor and indoor air. Outside air brings with it radon, usually at a low concentration.

96. Concentrations of radon outdoors are determined by the flux density from the earth and by dispersion in the atmosphere; both are affected by meteorological conditions. There are pronounced diurnal variations, mainly because of changes in atmospheric stability, and pronounced seasonal variations, mainly because of changes in patterns of air mass circulation. Water masses such as lakes and oceans make a negligible contribution to the atmospheric inventory of radon [N17]. On the basis of exhalation data, NCRP [N2] estimated the average outdoor concentration over continents to be 8 Bq m^{-3}. Hourly measurements over several years at an inland and a coastal site in the United States yielded average values of 8 and 4 Bq m^{-3} [F8], respectively, but successive quarterly measurements with integrating devices nationwide at 50 sites gave 15 Bq m^{-3} [H16]. Year-long measurements with integrating detectors throughout the United Kingdom gave a population-weighted average of 4 Bq m^{-3} [W3]. Integrating devices deployed in an urban area of Japan also yielded a year-long average of about 4 Bq m^{-3}, with seasonal variations from 2.6 to 6.1 Bq m^{-3} [M23]. Summertime measurements across Canada gave 11 Bq m^{-3} in the eastern provinces and 56 Bq m^{-3} in the prairie provinces, which were particularly dry and where the levels were reduced by a factor of 5 in the following summer [G11]. Protracted measurements in France showed 60 Bq m^{-3} in sedimentary regions, with marked temporal and spatial variations throughout the country [R15]. Whereas a tentative estimate of 5 Bq m^{-3} was made for the population-weighted parameter worldwide in the UNSCEAR 1988 Report [U1], the developing evidence, especially for continental as opposed to island air, suggests that it is probably closer to 10 Bq m^{-3}.

97. With a direct air exchange rate, λ_v, of 1 h^{-1} and an outdoor concentration, χ, of 10 Bq m^{-3}, the rate of entry of radon to the reference building by infiltration is the product of the two values, 10 Bq m^{-3} h^{-1}.

5. Transfer from water and natural gas

98. As noted earlier, radon is soluble in water. It follows that water supplies bring radon indoors and that some de-emanation of the water occurs, thus contributing to the radon entry rate, sometimes to an appreciable degree. Concentrations of radon in water vary markedly. Supplies may be classified broadly as surface water, groundwater or well water. As shown in Table 21, radon concentrations in these classes differ by an order of magnitude, and utilization also varies considerably [N18, O5]. Surface waters with the

least radon but the greatest variability in concentration [H5, H6, N15] are used the most. The weighted average of the radon concentrations for the reference set of supplies is somewhat above 10,000 Bq m^{-3} but not unlike the estimate for the United States [C8]. In the UNSCEAR 1988 Report [U1], a reference value of 1,000 Bq m^{-3} was adopted, but it was noted that countries such as Finland and Sweden had population-weighted averages of over 30,000 Bq m^{-3} [K4, S15]. Comprehensive surveys of well water from southern Finland yielded a median concentration of 210,000 Bq m^{-3} and isolated values approaching 50 MBq m^{-3} [J8]. It is assumed in this Annex that the worldwide average concentration of radon in water is 10,000 Bq m^{-3}.

99. Radon is slowly removed from still water by molecular diffusion, but agitation and heating cause water to de-emanate rapidly and transfer the gas to the indoor air. The transfer factor for buildings, defined as the ratio of the concentrations of radon in water and air, has been determined both experimentally and analytically. Values are distributed log-normally, but the average is about 10^4. For 10,000 Bq m^{-3} in water, this implies 1 Bq m^{-3} in air; for an air exchange rate of 1 h^{-1}, this implies a radon entry rate of 1 Bq m^{-3} h^{-1} to the model building.

100. In the interest of completeness, natural gas is mentioned as a potential source of radon. It contains various concentrations of the radioactive species, determined mainly by the geology of the gas field and the delay in transmission to the user. When it is burned indoors, the radon is released. In the UNSCEAR 1988 Report [U1], an entry rate of 0.3 Bq m^{-3} h^{-1} to the model building was deemed appropriate. This estimate still seems to remain valid.

6. Entry rates

(a) Radon

101. Radon entry rates for the model building are summarized in Table 22, and the relative importance of the various sources of radon in a temperate climate is illustrated. It will be recognized from the preceding text that the selection of illustrative values is rather arbitrary, since it depends on the values chosen for the parameters that determine the significance of the various mechanisms of entry. Nevertheless, the overall entry rate is not greatly at variance with that inferred from radon measurements in many buildings in temperate climates. With a contribution of over 50%, mostly from forced advection through discontinuities in the floor, radon entry from the subjacent earth dominates over all other sources. Diffusion from the building elements is also important, as is the infiltration of outdoor air, but the other sources are relatively unimportant. Table 22 focuses attention on the importance of advection in such typical circumstances; the text emphasizes its importance in atypical circumstances where high radon levels occur indoors. In tall blocks of dwellings, however, the earth contribution would virtually disappear the overall entry rate would at least be halved, and the percentages would be altered accordingly.

102. If a building with dimensions similar to those of the model but of non-masonry construction is envisaged for a tropical climate, it is possible to estimate the entry rate of radon by crudely adjusting the data in Table 22. Diffusion from building elements virtually disappears, but diffusion from the subjacent earth may contribute 37 Bq m^{-3} h^{-1} because board floors would not appreciably impede the ingress of radon. Advection from the earth may also disappear with calm air, balanced temperature and high ventilation. On the other hand, the contribution from infiltration would increase twofold, to 20 Bq m^{-3} h^{-1}, with a direct air exchange rate of 2 h^{-1}. The other mechanisms would remain unimportant. Overall, therefore, the entry rate of radon under such conditions should not be much different from that in Table 22, although the individual percentages would change.

(b) Thoron

103. There is less information on entry rates of thoron into buildings. Since the precursors of ^{220}Rn and ^{222}Rn have about equal activities in earth and building materials (see Tables 5, 6, 17 and 18), the rates at which the two isotopes are produced are also about equal. It is usually assumed that the emanation fraction is the same for each.

104. By definition, the diffusion coefficient is the same for both isotopes, so the diffusive flux density in terms of activity is proportional to the square root of the decay constants (0.0126 s^{-1} for thoron and 2.1 10^{-6} s^{-1} for radon) implying a value 77 times higher for thoron. The measured values for thoron, about 1 Bq m^{-2} s^{-1} from earth materials and 0.05 Bq m^{-2} s^{-1} from building materials [D11, F6, N19, S19, S36, U3], reflect this ratio, although there is considerable variability in the value.

105. As for advection, the flux density should, in principle, be the same for both isotopes in materials with the same permeability, if all the atoms produced are forced to the surface [N19]. Overall, the rate of entry of thoron into a building with unfinished walls and floors is likely to appreciably exceed that of radon. However, owing to its short half-life of 55 seconds, only the superficial layers of walls and floors contribute to the rate of entry of thoron into a

building, so that covering the floors and walls with plastic materials, tiles or paint is likely to reduce the rate of entry of thoron by at least an order of magnitude. This effect was indirectly demonstrated in Japan, where indoor measurements generally detected high concentrations of thoron (up to 400 Bq m^{-3}) near unfinished soil walls, but no thoron near walls covered by plastic or by paint [D2].

106. From the relatively few measurements of thoron outdoors [N19, S23, U3] it would appear that activity concentrations of thoron at or very near the surface of the earth exceed those of radon. As altitude increases, however, the situation reverses because of the disparity in decay constants. A representative value of 10 Bq m^{-3} might be chosen for head height, which is the same as the value adopted earlier for radon. With a direct exchange rate between outdoor and indoor air of 1 h^{-1}, the rate of entry to the model building by infiltration is also about 10 Bq m^{-3} h^{-1}.

107. The average rate of entry of thoron to a building from all mechanisms is crudely estimated in this Annex to be similar to that of radon, i.e. about 50 Bq m^{-3} h^{-1}. This estimate is highly uncertain.

B. EXPOSURE

1. Indoor concentrations

(a) Radon

108. It is possible to estimate the activity concentration χ (Bq m^{-3}) for the model building from the expression

$$\chi = U/(\lambda_v + \lambda_{Rn}) \qquad (9)$$

where the symbols refer to quantities defined previously. With U (the radon entry rate) = 49 Bq m^{-3} h^{-1} (Table 22), λ_v = 1 h^{-1} and λ_{Rn} = 0.00756 h^{-1}, the value of χ is 48.6 Bq m^{-3}. In round terms, therefore, one would generally expect radon gas concentrations of about 50 Bq m^{-3} in masonry buildings in temperate climates and 30 Bq m^{-3} in tropical timber buildings. With thoron, however, the decay constant of 45.4 h^{-1}, rather than the air exchange rate, determines the concentration: for U = 50 Bq m^{-3} h^{-1}, χ = 1 Bq m^{-3} of thoron gas. It should be noted that the indoor radon and thoron concentrations calculated from equation 9 represent averages throughout the building. Because of its short half-life, thoron does not become uniformly distributed. Strong gradients of thoron concentration have been predicted and observed according to distance from the wall [D2, D9, K15]. In any case, because of the large uncertainties in the estimation of the rate of entry of thoron into buildings, it is not recommended to use equation 9 to predict the indoor thoron concentration; it is better to rely on direct measurements of indoor concentrations, discussed in Section III.B.1.b.

109. It is now appropriate to compare expectation with observation. Although most large surveys are of radon gas concentration, χ_{Rn}, some surveys have been conducted of the decay products. The parameter of interest in the latter case is the equilibrium equivalent concentration (EEC) of radon χ_{Eq}, and the two quantities are related through the equilibrium factor F, defined by the expression

$$F = \chi_{Eq}/\chi_{Rn} \qquad (10)$$

where χ_{Eq} is $0.105\chi_1 + 0.515\chi_2 + 0.380\chi_3$. The symbols χ_1, χ_2 and χ_3 represent the activity concentrations of ^{218}Po, ^{214}Pb and ^{214}Bi; the constants are the fractional contributions of each decay product to the total potential alpha energy from the decay of unit activity of the gas [I7]. By analogy, the equilibrium equivalent concentration of thoron is 0.913 χ_1 + 0.087 χ_2, where χ_1 and χ_2 now represent the activity concentrations of ^{212}Pb and ^{212}Bi.

110. Many surveys have been made during the last decade of radon concentrations in dwellings. An extensive compilation was included in the UNSCEAR 1988 Report [U1]; it is updated here by the information in Table 23. Data are now available for 35 countries representing almost two thirds of the world population. The list is not comprehensive; some scattered observations for other countries are omitted, and summary results for a few countries with advanced radon programmes may not have been available. The purpose here is not to record all such data, but to select information that is representative of the various countries. The distribution of the survey data of Table 23 is illustrated in Figure IV.

111. Whereas early surveys were based on discrete sampling of radon decay products, usually called grab sampling, because it lasted a matter of minutes, surveys of substance are now made by sampling radon gas for extended periods of time, several days for charcoal detectors and several months for track etch detectors. Mass surveys of radon decay products are not feasible because the equipment and human resources required to conduct them would be very costly.

112. A satisfactory national survey might be defined as one in which measurements of adequate quality are made throughout a year in the living and sleeping rooms of a stratified sample of at least 1 in 10,000 of the housing stock. Not many surveys meet these criteria. Some are not large enough; many are made in the rooms with the highest radon levels; some are

biased to areas of the country with high radon concentrations; most do not follow a statistical design. As a result, any estimate of a representative or typical world value is quite uncertain. Distributions of radon concentrations are usually reported as being log-normal, although departures are sometimes seen. Arithmetic means are frequently cited or may be calculated from the geometric mean and standard deviation. Extreme values are often given.

113. Owing to the large populations of China and India, the results for these countries weigh heavily in the estimation of a worldwide radon concentration. Definitive national surveys have not yet been conducted, but the population-weighted mean of somewhat disparate and developing data for China [C10, R5, U1, Z2] is about 20 Bq m^{-3} [P21]. Exploratory data for India [S37], pending the completion of a national survey, suggest an arithmetic mean of 57 Bq m^{-3}, with lower values in cities such as Bombay [M12] and higher values in cities such as Nagpur [S24] and an equilibrium factor approaching 0.4 [S25]. A national residential radon survey [M24, O10, U12] recently completed in the United States yielded an arithmetic mean of 46 Bq m^{-3}, which is consistent with the outcome of a structured survey in the state of New York [P11].

114. Results from several studies in southern Europe have become available. Generally radon values are lower than in northern Europe: for example, only 3.2% of the 244 Spanish dwellings investigated in Madrid and Barcelona exceeded 200 Bq m^{-3} [G1]; only about 20% were above 100 Bq m^{-3} in a Turkish survey of 400 houses in Istanbul [K14]; and about 5% of Portuguese dwellings had average radon concentrations in excess of 200 Bq m^{-3} [F14]. However, in Italy the use of natural building materials (tuffs, pozzuolana) with elevated ^{238}U activity concentrations ranging up to 400 Bq kg^{-1} can result in elevated indoor radon levels in the areas concerned (arithmetic average: 93 Bq m^{-3} [B16]). Frequently, seasonal changes are seen to have a pronounced effect on indoor radon concentrations in southern climates, with winter values up to 80% higher than corresponding summer values [B16, G1].

115. Little information is available for large parts of Africa and for tropical regions in the Americas, Asia and Oceania. For well-ventilated buildings, indoor and outdoor radon concentrations should be essentially equal; thus, indoor radon levels should be lower in tropical areas than in temperate areas if the outdoor radon concentrations are similar [M12, S25]. The limited results available for Egypt and Thailand [C23, H18] show that, for well-ventilated buildings in tropical areas, indoor radon concentrations are approximately equal to those measured outdoors; furthermore, a gradual increase in the ratio of indoor-to-outdoor radon concentration from low latitudes (23° N) to temperate latitudes (40° N) has been observed in China [P21]. However, Figure V, where the average indoor radon concentrations from Table 23 are plotted against the latitude of the countries or the main population centres, shows a considerable scatter, as well as some average indoor radon concentrations at high latitudes that are similar to those at low latitudes.

116. The different results of radon concentrations with latitude may be due to local geology, atmospheric conditions or building design. Local geology and atmospheric conditions may result in outdoor radon levels that are high in low latitudes and low in high latitudes. For example, the average outdoor radon concentration measured in Bangkok [C23] is 40 Bq m^{-3}, while that in the United Kingdom is 4 Bq m^{-3} [W3]. Such a difference alters the indoor-to-outdoor concentration ratio for most dwellings. Also, the sharply contrasted rainy and dry seasons in tropical areas may influence the annual average of the indoor radon concentration in a manner that is not clearly understood. Finally, the design of traditional sub-Saharan houses explains the relatively high radon concentrations in that region [O6].

117. In the UNSCEAR 1988 Report [U1], a population-weighted value of 40 Bq m^{-3} was adopted for the arithmetic mean worldwide. This value still appears to be representative. Given the gross uncertainty in this value and the climatic complications, the degree of agreement with the estimate for the model building is probably more coincidental than conclusive. It is clear that additional research and measurements are needed in tropical areas in order to estimate more accurately the worldwide average of indoor radon concentration. It is hoped that more data from countries at low latitudes will become available from a radon survey programme that is being initiated by IAEA [S22].

118. Because of the trend away from the measurement of radon decay products, there is no new information of substance on the value of the equilibrium factor F indoors; it is taken, as before, to be 0.4 [U1]. The position is much the same for outdoor air; the previous value of 0.8 is also adopted here. In terms of equilibrium equivalent concentration, therefore, the worldwide values of the arithmetic mean, population-weighted, are about 16 Bq m^{-3} indoors and 8 Bq m^{-3} outdoors.

119. For the major surveys in temperate climates, the value of the geometric standard deviation is typically 2.5. This may be somewhat high for tropical climates, but any adjustment would be arbitrary, and so it is considered to be generally valid. The arithmetic mean of the radon gas concentration is 40 Bq m^{-3}, and the

geometric mean is about 26 Bq m^{-3}. The corresponding values of the equilibrium equivalent concentration are 16 Bq m^{-3} indoors (arithmetic mean) and 10 Bq m^{-3} (geometric mean). Estimates of the 98th percentiles are 200 Bq m^{-3} for the radon gas concentration and 80 Bq m^{-3} for the equilibrium equivalent concentration. It can thus be suggested that about 2% of dwellings worldwide may have concentrations in excess of these values. Further, about 0.02% of dwellings may be in excess of 800 Bq m^{-3}. Concentrations far in excess of 800 Bq m^{-3} are, however, frequently reported in the literature; values more than an order of magnitude greater are sometimes encountered, which may reflect the possibility of positive divergence from a log-normal distribution at higher concentrations [N20]. Competent authorities who have considered the effects of human exposure to radon in homes are generally agreed on the desirability of taking action at concentrations exceeding 400 Bq m^{-3} [O8]; worldwide, a few homes in a thousand probably exceed that level. Remedial measures in those houses will reduce the number of persons exposed to high doses from the inhalation of radon progeny but it will not change significantly the average levels.

(b) Thoron

120. Limited information on thoron concentrations has been reported since the publication of the UNSCEAR 1988 Report [U1]. A representative value of 10 Bq m^{-3} was adopted earlier for thoron gas in outdoor air. Equilibrium equivalent concentrations of about 0.1 Bq m^{-3} have been adopted elsewhere [N2, N19, N20], somewhat lower than the previous value of 0.2 Bq m^{-3} [U1]. Estimates of the gas concentration indoors point to around 3 Bq m^{-3} [N20, S23], and limited surveys of the equilibrium equivalent concentration [C16, D8, G9, M14, M25, N19, P21, R1, S23, T7, W3], taken together, indicate about 0.3 Bq m^{-3}, again somewhat lower than the previous value of 0.5 Bq m^{-3} [U1]. There is considerable uncertainty in these figures, pointing to a need for systematic measurements.

(c) Average concentrations

121. The foregoing estimates of the concentrations of radon and thoron in outdoor and indoor air are summarized in Table 24. Both the gas and equilibrium equivalent values are given. They are intended to represent the population-weighted arithmetic means worldwide, but it is necessary to bear in mind that considerable uncertainty attaches to them, mainly because of the general paucity of data for thoron and some geographical bias in the origins of the radon data. They are, nevertheless, robust and round enough to allow calculating the radiation doses from inhalation for the gas and decay products.

2. Dose

(a) Inhalation

122. Exposure to radon, thoron and their progeny comes mainly from the inhalation of the decay products of radon and thoron, which deposit inhomogeneously within the human respiratory tract and irradiate the bronchial epithelium. Compared with the lung dose from inhaled decay products, the dose contribution from the inhaled radon (or thoron) gas itself, which is soluble in body fluids and tissues, is small under normal conditions of exposure. The two contributions to the annual effective dose are considered in turn.

123. Conversion coefficients relating average annual concentrations to effective dose equivalent were presented in the UNSCEAR 1988 Report [U1] for radon and thoron progeny. These were based mainly on a comprehensive report on lung dosimetry published in 1983 [N21] and other earlier analyses [I7, J3]. Parallel and later developments were recognized, however, that pointed to the need for a re-evaluation of the radon dosimetry [J4, N17, V4].

124. Dose to lung tissues depends, among other things, on the fraction f_p of the total potential alpha energy associated with the mixture of decay products not attached to the ambient aerosol [N21]; as the value of f_p increases, so does the dose. Values from 0.04 to about 0.20 have been found in several dwellings in the United Kingdom [J5, S27]. A similar range was determined in several Norwegian dwellings [S28]. For a Japanese dwelling, however, the range was 0.031 to 0.064, with an arithmetic mean of 0.043 [K6], reflecting perhaps the different lifestyle [H8]. In Germany, the arithmetic mean for many rooms without additional aerosol sources was 0.096, whereas for a few with cigarette smoke it was 0.006 and for outside air, about 0.02 [R9]. A study in a test dwelling in Germany yielded values around 0.1, but ranging below 0.01 as a result of smoking [R10]. A review of these and other data leads to a value of around 0.1 [P16]. Further results reveal 0.077 [H21] and 0.20 [S46] for single-family dwellings and 0.086 as an average for five dwellings [T13]. Such values may be contrasted with those from 0.02 to 0.03, adopted previously for dosimetric purposes [I8, N21, U1]; they appear to be about three times greater indoors, the implication being that the equivalent dose to the bronchial epithelium might be somewhat larger than previously estimated [J11].

125. The rate of attachment of radon decay products to the ambient aerosol increases as the aerosol concentration increases [P12]. With other aerosol conditions constant, therefore, a higher aerosol

concentration means a lower value of f_p and a lower dose. In dwellings, the aerosol concentration generally increases as the infiltration rate of outside air decreases, with the result that the values of f_p and dose also decrease. For a given concentration of gas at a fixed value of f_p, the dose increases as the value of the equilibrium factor F increases; the value of F, however, increases with decreasing infiltration rate. The effects of f_p and F on dose, with other aerosol conditions constant, are therefore counterbalanced.

126. Concurrent measurements of f_p and F [J5, P13, R9, R10, S28] demonstrate that values of f_p are negatively correlated with values of F. Concurrent measurements of decay product concentrations, infiltration rates and size distributions of ambient aerosols in rooms [V4, V5] and the use of a room model [P14] to estimate the value of the unattached fraction also substantiated the inverse relationship between f_p and F [P16]. Further calculations of doses to lung tissues with two reference dosimetry models [N21] showed that the gas concentration was an adequate indicator of effective dose equivalent; a conversion coefficient of around 50 μSv a^{-1} per Bq m^{-3} of radon gas was deemed appropriate [V5]. A similar conclusion had been reached in an earlier assessment [J5] and was supported by a later analysis [H9]. On the other hand, a more recent assessment indicates that the coefficient may be around 25 μSv a^{-1} per Bq m^{-3} [J10]. Given the preponderance of radon gas measurements as opposed to decay product measurements in surveys of dwellings, there is some merit and much convenience in applying such a conversion coefficient directly to the results, but unanimity is lacking on the most appropriate value to use.

127. The dosimetry of radon and decay products is under review to account for the introduction of the new ICRP recommendations [I6] and to develop a new dosimetric model for the respiratory tract [B2]. Dosimetrists are considering new physical information on the indoor aerosol, new insights into the regional sensitivity of the respiratory tract and the new tissue weighting factors.

128. For the purposes of this Annex, it seems reasonable to keep the dose coefficients that were adopted in the UNSCEAR 1988 Report. In that Report, an indoor exposure to radon at a concentration of 40 Bq m^{-3} was estimated to correspond to an annual effective dose equivalent of 1.0 mSv as a result of the irradiation of tissues of the respiratory tract by the radon progeny. This is numerically equivalent to an effective dose coefficient of 25 μSv a^{-1} per Bq m^{-3} of radon gas for indoor exposure, assuming an occupancy factor of 0.8 (7,000 hours spent indoors in a year), or to 3.6 nSv per Bq h m^{-3} of radon gas.

129. When the effective dose coefficient is expressed in terms of equilibrium equivalent concentration (EEC) of radon, the result is slightly different from that adopted in the UNSCEAR 1988 Report, because the EEC of radon is estimated in this Annex to be 16 Bq m^{-3} instead of 15 Bq m^{-3}, as in the earlier Report, the radon gas concentrations being the same. Expressed in terms of the EEC of radon, the effective dose coefficient is found to be $3.6 \times 40 \div 16 = 9$ nSv per Bq h m^{-3} for EEC of radon instead of 10 nSv per Bq h m^{-3}, as in the UNSCEAR 1988 Report. The value 9 nSv per Bq h m^{-3} for EEC of radon is also used in this Annex to estimate effective doses resulting from the inhalation of radon progeny outdoors.

130. It is convenient at this point to consider the doses from the inhalation of radon gas in somewhat more detail. Since the gas is soluble in body fluids and tissues, it is transported throughout the body. Doses are delivered from the decay of the gas itself and the short-lived decay products. Equivalent dose rates to some tissues of interest from constant inhalation of the gases at concentrations of 1 Bq m^{-3} are 1.2 nSv h^{-1} in fat, 0.75 nSv h^{-1} in lungs and 0.094 nSv h^{-1} in bone marrow from radon and 0.004 nSv h^{-1} in fat, 0.58 nSv h^{-1} in lungs and 0.039 nSv h^{-1} in bone marrow from thoron [J3]. The effective dose rates are 0.17 nSv h^{-1} from radon and 0.11 nSv h^{-1} from thoron. The resulting annual effective doses per unit concentration in air are 1.5 μSv per Bq m^{-3} of radon and 0.96 μSv per Bq m^{-3} of thoron. These values are supported by a more recent assessment [P15]. The relatively high dose rate from radon in fatty tissue is due to the high solubility of radon. In an earlier investigation [H10], the distinction was made between fatty and normal marrow; the ratio of the dose rates was about 5. From these dose coefficients it may be estimated that the equivalent dose to the marrow from the worldwide average value of radon and thoron is about 0.03 mSv a^{-1}, an order of magnitude less than the equivalent dose from cosmic rays.

131. The dose coefficients corresponding to the inhalation of the thoron progeny are taken to be the same as those adopted in the UNSCEAR 1988 Report, namely 10 nSv per Bq h m^{-3} for outdoor exposure and 32 nSv per Bq h m^{-3} for indoor exposure.

132. The effective dose coefficients related to the inhalation of radon gas, thoron gas, radon progeny and thoron progeny are summarized in Table 24. Annual effective doses corresponding to the worldwide average concentrations are estimated from those effective dose coefficients, assuming average occupancy factors of 0.2 for outdoors and 0.8 for indoors; the results are included in Table 24. The average annual effective dose from inhalation of radon and its progeny is estimated to be 1200 μSv, while the dose from thoron and its progeny is about 70 μSv.

(b) Ingestion

133. When internal exposures were considered in Section II.B, the dose from the ingestion of radon in water was not included. These doses are estimated here. Application of a modified ICRP model to the ingestion of radon in water [K7] leads to a value of 10^{-8} Sv Bq^{-1} for the committed effective dose per unit intake, with virtually all of the dose coming from the gas rather than the decay products. Doses to children and infants, scaled from body masses, are 2 10^{-8} Sv Bq^{-1} and 7 10^{-8} Sv Bq^{-1}, respectively. Since radon is readily lost from water by heating and bottling, the consumption of interest here is that of water directly from the tap. Annual intakes by adults and children are about 50 l and 75 l, with 100 l by infants when scaled by metabolic rate [I5]. The estimate for adults is supported by other statistics [H11]. For the reference concentration of 10,000 Bq m^{-3} adopted earlier, the annual effective doses are 5 μSv to adults, 15 μSv to children and 70 μSv to infants. Assuming that a representative population consists of 5% infants, 30% children and 65% adults, the population-weighted average annual effective dose from ingestion of radon is about 10 μSv, which is small in comparison to doses from the inhalation of radon or thoron progeny. However, persons who consume deep well waters with the reference concentration of 10^5 Bq m^{-3} will incur doses an order of magnitude greater. This gives an indication of the range experienced by communities with atypical supplies.

C. SUMMARY

134. Radon and its decay products make the most significant contribution to exposures from natural radiation. In particular, levels indoors can build up following entry from subjacent soil, building materials and the infiltration of outdoor air. Extensive national surveys have been conducted to determine both typical and extreme levels in houses.

135. The population-weighted average radon concentration is 40 Bq m^{-3} indoors. Most of the data are from temperate regions. Average levels outdoors are 10 Bq m^{-3} in continental areas and somewhat less in coastal regions. Levels indoors in tropical regions should be comparable to outdoor levels in consideration of construction materials and probable ventilation, but more data are needed to substantiate this. The equilibrium factors to determine equilibrium equivalent concentrations (EEC) are taken to be 0.4 for indoor exposure and 0.8 for outdoor exposure. The population-weighted average EEC radon concentra-tions are therefore estimated to be 16 Bq m^{-3} indoors and 8 Bq m^{-3} outdoors.

136. The dosimetry of radon and its decay products is at present under review, and uncertainty prevails about a conversion coefficient suitable for deriving the effective dose from the concentration. In this Annex, the effective dose coefficient that was adopted in the UNSCEAR 1988 Report for inhalation of radon progeny has been kept; in numerical terms, the effective dose from 1 Bq h m^{-3} radon EEC is estimated to be 9 nSv for both indoor and outdoor exposures. The average annual effective dose from the inhalation of radon progeny outdoors is estimated to be 8 Bq m^{-3} (EEC) × 9 nSv h^{-1} per Bq m^{-3} (EEC) × 0.2 (occupancy) × 8760 h a^{-1} = 0.13 mSv. For radon indoors, it is 16 Bq m^{-3} (EEC) × 9 nSv h^{-1} per Bq m^{-3} (EEC) × 0.8 × 8760 h a^{-1} = 1.0 mSv. The dose from inhaled radon that becomes dissolved in tissues is estimated to be [(10 Bq m^{-3} × 0.2) + (40 Bq m^{-3} x 0.8)] × 1.5 μSv a^{-1} per Bq m^{-3} = 0.051 mSv. Thus, the total estimated average annual effective dose is 1.2 mSv. The corresponding annual effective dose from inhalation of thoron and its decay products is 0.07 mSv. An additional annual effective dose to adults of 0.005 mSv is estimated to result from ingestion of radon.

IV. EXTRACTIVE INDUSTRIES

137. The extraction and processing of earth materials affect exposure to natural radiation of the general public when these earth materials, or their industrial products or by-products, contain above-average concentrations of natural radionuclides. The earth materials that are considered in this Annex exclude uranium, which is discussed in Annex B, "Exposures from man-made sources of radiation". In the industrial processes associated with the extraction and processing of earth materials, the hazard from radiation is generally small compared to that from other chemical substances, so radiation is not systematically monitored. The assessment of such exposures is based on sketchy information derived from isolated surveys. This Chapter reviews the information available on radiation exposures from four types of activity: (a) combustion of coal; (b) other energy production from fossil fuels; (c) use of phosphate rock; and (d) mining and milling of mineral sands. Except for the Section on mining and milling of mineral sands, this Chapter essentially summarizes the review presented in the UNSCEAR 1988 Report [U1], as very little new

information has since been published. Collective effective doses committed from atmospheric discharges of radioactive materials are estimated using the crude models described in the UNSCEAR 1982 Report [U3].

138. In order to allow their comparison with the doses from natural radiation background, the annual per caput effective doses resulting from the extraction and processing of earth materials have been estimated. In doing so, crude assumptions have been made about the dynamics of the dose rate and the duration of the practice considered. It is emphasized that all estimates of dose resulting from the extraction and processing of earth materials are fraught with large uncertainties.

A. ENERGY PRODUCTION FROM COAL

139. The world production of coal, expressed in coal equivalent for energy purposes, was 3.1 x 10^{12} kg in 1985, the main producers being China, the republics of the former Soviet Union and the United States [U13]. A large fraction of the coal extracted from the earth is burned in electric power stations; about 3 x 10^9 kg of coal is required to produce 1 GW a of electrical energy. In the UNSCEAR 1982 Report [U3], the Committee estimated the average concentrations of ^{40}K, ^{238}U and ^{232}Th in coal to be 50, 20, 20 Bq kg^{-1}, respectively, based on the analysis of coal samples from 15 countries, and noted that the concentrations varied by more than two orders of magnitude. The results of an extensive survey of coal from China, which produces 20% of the world's total, point to concentrations that are appreciably higher: 104, 36 and 30 Bq kg^{-1} for ^{40}K, ^{238}U and ^{232}Th, respectively [P22]. The higher concentrations of natural radionuclides in coal from China do not result in substantial increases in the worldwide averages, which are little more than educated guesses, but they do allow a better assessment of the doses due to the uses of coal in China. Radiation exposures occur throughout the fuel cycle, which consists of coal mining, the use of coal and the use of fuel ash.

1. Coal mining

140. Members of the public are exposed to the radon present in the exhaust air of coal mines. Since there are currently no measured data on the emission of radon from coal mines, the Committee, in the UNSCEAR 1988 Report [U1], used two different, very crude approaches to estimating the annual releases of radon from coal mining all over the world; the figures obtained were 30 and 800 TBq, leading to collective effective doses per year of practice of 0.5 and 10 man Sv, respectively. Dividing by the world population of 5.3 10^9 yields an annual per caput effective dose of 0.1-2 nSv.

2. Use of coal

141. There are vast differences in the relative use of coal in various countries. In the OECD countries, which account for about one third of the world's coal production, 68% of the coal produced is burned in electric power stations, 30% in coke ovens and other industrial operations and 2% in dwellings [U13]. In China, 25% of the coal produced is burned in electric power stations, 59% in other industries and 16% in dwellings [P23]. Assuming that the usage distribution of coal in China is representative of the distribution in countries that are not members of the OECD, the average worldwide usage of coal is as follows: about 40% is burned in electric power stations, 10% in dwellings and 50% in other industries. When coal is burnt, the naturally occurring radionuclides are redistributed from underground into the biosphere. The resultant doses from burning coal in power stations and in dwellings are considered below. There is not enough information on the releases of radionuclides from burning coal in other industries to assess this use of coal.

(a) Coal-fired power plants

142. Coal is burned in furnaces operating at up to 1,700° C in order to produce electrical energy. In the combustion process, most of the mineral matter in the coal is fused into a vitrified ash. A portion of the heavier ash, together with incompletely burned organic matter, drops to the bottom of the furnace as bottom ash or slag. The lighter fly ash, however, is carried through the boiler, together with the hot flue gases and any volatilized mineral compounds, to the stack, where, depending on the efficiency of emission control devices, most is collected while the rest (escaping fly ash) is released to the atmosphere. Owing mainly to the elimination of the organic content of the coal, there is approximately an order of magnitude enhancement of the concentrations from coal to ash. Consequently, the natural radionuclide concentrations in ash and slag from coal-fired power stations are significantly higher than the corresponding concentrations in the earth's crust. Arithmetic averages of the reported concentrations in escaping fly ash are 265 Bq kg^{-1} for ^{40}K, 200 Bq kg^{-1} for ^{238}U, 240 Bq kg^{-1} for ^{226}Ra, 930 Bq kg^{-1} for ^{210}Pb, 1,700 Bq kg^{-1} for ^{210}Po, 70 Bq kg^{-1} for ^{232}Th, 110 Bq kg^{-1} for ^{228}Th and 130 Bq kg^{-1} for ^{228}Ra ([U3], Annex C, paragraph 11).

143. The amounts of natural radionuclides discharged to the atmosphere from a power plant depend on a number of factors such as the concentrations in coal,

the ash content of the coal, the temperature of combustion, the partitioning between bottom ash and fly ash and the efficiency of the emission control device. In the UNSCEAR 1988 Report [U1], the Committee estimated the amounts of radioactive materials discharged to the atmosphere for typical old and modern plants. The resulting normalized collective effective doses were 6 and 0.5 man Sv $(GW\ a)^{-1}$ for typical old and modern plants, respectively. Data from China indicate that because of higher-than-average concentrations of natural radionuclides in coal, relatively low filter efficiencies (90%) and high population densities around the plants, the normalized collective effective doses arising from atmospheric releases of radioactive materials from plants there is approximately 50 man Sv $(GW\ a)^{-1}$ [P22]. Assuming that, worldwide, one third of the electrical energy produced by coal-fired power plants is from modern plants, with another third from old plants and the remaining third from plants with characteristics similar to those in China, the average normalized collective effective dose is 20 man Sv $(GW\ a)^{-1}$.

144. According to the dose assessment methodology used in the UNSCEAR 1988 Report, about 70% of the effective dose resulting from atmospheric releases of natural radionuclides from old plants is due to the inhalation of long-lived radionuclides as the cloud passes. The remainder of the effective dose is due to external irradiation from radionuclides deposited on the ground and to the ingestion of foodstuffs contaminated by radionuclides deposited on the ground. It is assumed that the deposited activity becomes unavailable to the vegetation, with a mean life of 100 years for all the natural long-lived radionuclides. On the whole, the effective dose per unit release is delivered at a rate that decreases slowly over a century or so.

145. Assuming that (a) $3\ 10^{12}$ kg of coal is produced in a year; (b) 40% of the coal production is burned in electric power stations; and (c) $3\ 10^{9}$ kg of coal is required to produce 1 GW a of electrical energy, the annual electrical energy produced by burning coal worldwide is 400 GW a. The collective effective dose per year of practice is therefore estimated to be 20 man Sv $(GW\ a)^{-1} \times 400$ GW a = 8,000 man Sv.

146. Crude assumptions are necessary to derive the annual per caput effective dose from the collective effective dose per year of practice. If it is assumed that similar amounts of radioactive materials have been released into the atmosphere by coal-fired power plants year after year for the last century or so, then the collective effective dose per year of practice would be approximately equal to the annual collective effective dose. In fact, coal has been used for about a century to produce electrical energy, but information is lacking regarding the magnitude of the environmental releases during that time. Given the large uncertainty associated with the estimate of the collective effective dose per year of practice, it is assumed in this Annex that the annual collective effective dose has the same numerical value as the collective effective dose per year of practice. The annual per caput effective dose is obtained by dividing the annual collective effective dose (8,000 man Sv) by the current world population ($5.3\ 10^{9}$); the result is about 2 μSv.

(b) Domestic use

147. Another significant use of coal is for domestic cooking and heating. No information has been found in the literature on the environmental discharges of natural radionuclides from this source. The use of coal for cooking or heating in private houses may, however, be estimated to result in high collective doses since chimneys are not equipped with ash removal systems and the population densities around sources of emission are generally high.

148. Assuming that the concentrations in smoke are equal to those in coal and that 3.5% of the coal is emitted as smoke, the annual worldwide atmospheric releases caused by the domestic burning of coal are estimated to be 0.7 TBq of ^{40}K and 0.3 TBq of each of the radionuclides of the ^{238}U and ^{232}Th series (radon and thoron excepted); these figures become 20 times greater if it is assumed that the concentrations in smoke are equal to those in ash and that the coal burned has a 5% ash content. Taking the average population densities around the houses to be $10^{3}\ km^{-2}$ leads to collective effective doses committed from yearly worldwide use of coal in the range of 2,000-40,000 man Sv. This estimate is highly uncertain, as it is not supported by any discharge or environmental data.

149. It is assumed that the annual collective effective dose to the world's population is in the same range as the collective effective dose per year of practice (2,000-40,000 man Sv). It follows that the annual per caput effective dose attributable to the use of coal for domestic cooking and heating would be 0.4-8 μSv.

3. Use of fuel ash

150. Large quantities of coal ash (fly ash and bottom ash combined) are produced each year throughout the world. In the UNSCEAR 1988 Report [U1], the Committee estimated that about 280 million tonnes of coal ash are produced annually in coal-fired power stations. Coal ash is used in a variety of applications, the largest of which is the manufacture of cement and concrete. It is also used as a road stabilizer, as road

fill, in asphalt mix and as fertilizer. Data on the various uses of coal ash in several countries have been reported [G8]. About 5% of the total ash production from coal-burning power stations is used for the construction of dwellings; this represents an annual usage of 14 million tonnes.

151. From the radiological point of view, the use of coal ash in building materials, which may affect indoor doses from external irradiation and the inhalation of radon decay products, is the most significant. With respect to external irradiation, the Committee estimated in the UNSCEAR 1988 Report, on the basis of measurements made by Stranden [S47], that the use of concrete containing fly ash for constructing dwellings would result in additional annual effective doses of 70 μSv and 30 μSv in concrete and wooden houses, respectively. Taking the amount of fly ash concrete to be 1.3 tonnes in a wooden house and 4 tonnes in a concrete building and assuming that an average of four persons live in each house and that the lifetime of the house is 50 years, the collective effective dose arising from external irradiation attributable to the annual use of fly ash for constructing the dwellings is estimated to be about 50,000 man Sv.

152. The annual collective effective dose to the world's population depends on the number of dwellings built with concrete containing coal ash during the last 50 years. Assuming that the practice of building dwellings with concrete containing coal ash began 25 years ago and that 14 million tonnes of coal ash have been used each year for that purpose, the annual collective effective dose to the world's population from external irradiation from that source is half the collective effective dose per year of practice, or 25,000 man Sv. The corresponding annual per caput effective dose is 5 μSv.

153. There are conflicting views on the impact of the use of fly ash on the dose from inhalation of radon decay products. According to some investigators, the indoor dose should be higher in a house with fly ash concrete than in a house built with ordinary concrete [B4, S45]; according to other investigators [S47], the indoor dose should be lower, while another group concluded that there should not be any significant change [U14, V9]. In this Annex, as in the UNSCEAR 1988 Report, it is assumed that the use of fly ash in building materials does not result in any additional dose due to the inhalation of radon decay products.

B. OTHER ENERGY PRODUCTION

154. In addition to the use of coal in power plants to generate electrical energy, other minerals, including oil, peat and natural gas, as well as geothermally heated water, are also used for this purpose. The natural radionuclides in these materials, the amounts released and the resultant doses are considered in this Section.

1. Oil

155. Oil has a large number of fuel applications, the most important being for road transport vehicles, for the generation of electrical energy and for domestic heating. Approximately 3×10^{12} kg of crude petroleum is produced in the world annually. In power plants, about 2×10^{9} kg of oil is needed to produce 1 GW a of electrical energy. As the ash content of oil is very low, oil-fired power plants are usually not equipped with efficient ash removal systems. On the basis of limited measurements, the Committee in the UNSCEAR 1988 Report estimated that the amounts of radioactive materials discharged from oil-fired power plants are similar to those from coal-fired power plants fitted with efficient aerosol control devices; the resulting collective effective dose is about 0.5 man Sv $(GW\ a)^{-1}$. About half of the effective dose results from inhalation during passage of the cloud and the other half from external and internal irradiation from deposited activity. Assuming that 15% of the worldwide production of crude petroleum is burned in electric power plants, the collective effective dose per year of practice is about 100 man Sv. The annual collective effective dose is tentatively estimated to be 50 man Sv, corresponding to an annual per caput effective dose of 10 nSv.

2. Peat

156. Peat is burned to produce energy in several countries, notably in Finland and Sweden [C14]. Concentrations of natural radionuclides in peat are usually similar to those in coal, but relatively high concentrations have been found to occur. In the UNSCEAR 1988 Report, the Committee tentatively estimated the normalized collective effective dose due to atmospheric releases from peat-fired power plants to be 2 man Sv $(GW\ a)^{-1}$. Since no information has been made available to the Committee on the worldwide production of electrical energy by burning peat, the collective effective dose per year of practice has not been estimated.

3. Natural gas

157. Like oil, natural gas has many applications. The main ones are domestic heating, the generation of electrical energy and as a source of heat in various industries. The annual worldwide production of natural gas is about 10^{12} m^3. Radon concentrations in natural gas at the well may vary widely around a typical value of 1 kBq m^{-3}. Owing to radioactive decay during

transfer and storage, the radon concentrations at the plant should be smaller; in the absence of data, however, no decrease has been assumed. Since about 2×10^9 m^3 of natural gas must be burned to produce 1 GW a of electrical energy, the corresponding radon emission is approximately 2 TBq and the normalized collective effective dose is 0.03 man Sv $(GW\ a)^{-1}$. Assuming that 15% of the world production of natural gas is burned in electric power plants, the collective effective dose per year of practice is about 3 man Sv. The annual collective effective dose has the same value, leading to an annual per caput effective dose of about 1 nSv.

4. Geothermal energy

158. Geothermal energy is produced in Iceland, Italy, Japan, New Zealand, the Russian Federation and the United States. Geothermal energy makes use of hot steam or water derived from high-temperature rocks deep inside the earth. Most of the activity found in geothermal fluids is due to the uranium decay chain. Isotopes of solid elements may occur in released water or land-fill, but only radon, which is released into the atmosphere when the water or steam contacts the air, is considered here. From measurements in Italy and in the United States, the Committee, in the UNSCEAR 1988 Report, estimated the average discharge of radon per unit energy generated to be 150 TBq $(GW\ a)^{-1}$ and the corresponding collective effective dose to be 2 man Sv $(GW\ a)^{-1}$. Since the annual production of electrical energy by geothermal energy is about 1.5 GW a, the annual worldwide production of geothermal energy would yield an annual collective effective dose of approximately 3 man Sv and an annual per caput effective dose of about 1 nSv.

C. USE OF PHOSPHATE ROCK

159. Phosphate rock is the starting material for the production of all phosphate products and is the main source of phosphorus for fertilizers. It can be of sedimentary, volcanic or biological origin. The world production of phosphate rock was about 130 million tonnes in 1982, the main producers being China, Morocco, the former Soviet Union and the United States. Concentrations of natural radionuclides in phosphate rock were reviewed in the UNSCEAR 1977 and 1982 Reports [U3, U4]. Concentrations of ^{232}Th and ^{40}K in phosphate rocks of all types are similar to those observed normally in soil, whereas concentrations of ^{238}U and its decay products tend to be elevated in phosphate deposits of sedimentary origin. A typical concentration of ^{238}U in sedimentary phosphate deposits is 1,500 Bq kg^{-1}. Uranium-238 and its decay products are generally found in close radioactive equilibrium in phosphate ore.

160. Exposures of members of the public result from effluent discharges of radionuclides of the ^{238}U decay series into the environment from phosphate rock mining and processing; from the use of phosphate fertilizers; and from the use of by-products and wastes.

1. Phosphate processing operations

161. Phosphate processing operations can be divided into the mining and milling of phosphate ore and the manufacture of phosphate products by either the wet process or the thermal process. Wet-process plants produce phosphoric acid, the starting material for ammonium phosphate and triple superphosphate fertilizers; in that process, phosphogypsum is produced as waste or by-product. Thermal process plants produce elemental phosphorus, which is in turn used primarily for the production of high-grade phosphoric acid, phosphate-based detergents and organic chemicals. Waste and by-products of the thermal process are slag and ferrophosphorus.

162. In the UNSCEAR 1988 Report [U1], the Committee estimated the collective effective dose from one year of discharge of radioactive materials into the atmosphere by phosphate industrial facilities around the world to be about 60 man Sv. Maximum annual individual effective doses were estimated to be about 40 μSv in the vicinity of an elemental phosphorus plant in the Netherlands, while equivalent doses in the lungs for individuals near six elemental phosphorus plants in the United States were calculated to range from 0.05 to 6 mSv.

163. Collective effective doses resulting from discharges into surface waters seem to be more important than those from atmospheric releases. In the Netherlands, all phosphogypsum produced by fertilizer plants (2 million tonnes per year) is discharged into the Rhine [K16]; these annual discharges, which contain about 0.4 TBq of ^{238}U, 2 TBq of ^{226}Ra, 0.7 TBq of ^{210}Pb and 2 TBq of ^{210}Po, were estimated to result in maximum annual individual effective doses of 150 μSv and in a collective effective dose of 170 man Sv per year to the Dutch population via the ingestion of seafood, ^{210}Po being the main contributor to the dose [K16]. In Spain, about 0.4 million tonnes per year of phosphogypsum produced in a phosphoric acid and fertilizer plant is discharged into the estuary of the Tinto and Odiel rivers [C17]; the annual effective dose to the critical group is estimated to be 60 μSv, the main pathway to man being the consumption of fish and crustacea [C17]. In France, over 3 million tonnes of phosphogypsum has been dumped into the Seine estuary [P1], but the corresponding radiation exposures have not been estimated.

2. Use of phosphate fertilizers

164. The concentrations of natural radionuclides in phosphate fertilizers were reviewed in the UNSCEAR 1982 Report. For a given radionuclide and type of fertilizer, the concentrations vary markedly from one country to another, depending on the origin of the components. Generally, the concentrations of ^{40}K and of ^{232}Th and its decay products are always low, and the concentrations of the radionuclides of the ^{238}U decay series are 5-50 times higher than in normal soil. Typical values are 4,000 and 1,000 Bq per kg P_2O_5 for ^{238}U and ^{226}Ra, respectively. The annual world consumption of phosphate fertilizers is about 30 million tonnes of P_2O_5. The worldwide use of phosphate fertilizers constitutes one of the most important sources of mobile ^{226}Ra in the environment [J6].

165. The amounts of fertilizer applied annually in the United States have been reported to range from about 30 kg P_2O_5 per hectare for barley, wheat and oats to about 150 kg P_2O_5 per hectare for potatoes and tobacco [N4]. The annual application of phosphate fertilizers represents less than 1% of the normal soil content of ^{238}U. Assuming an accumulation in the soil during the past 100 years, the mean additional absorbed dose in air above fertilized fields is about 1 nGy h^{-1}, a small fraction of the normal natural background from terrestrial sources of about 60 nGy h^{-1}. Small additional doses also occur from the ingestion of foodstuffs grown on fertilized agricultural land. In the UNSCEAR 1988 Report [U1], the collective effective dose resulting from the worldwide use of phosphate fertilizers during one year was roughly estimated to be 10,000 man Sv. Given the long duration of the practice at approximately the same rate, the numerical value of the annual collective dose is taken to be the same; the annual per caput effective dose would be about 2 μSv.

3. Use of by-products

166. The main by-products of phosphate industrial activities are phosphogypsum in wet-process fertilizer plants and calcium silicate slags in thermal process plants. Phosphogypsum currently has several commercial applications in the United States, including (a) as a fertilizer and conditioner for soils where peanuts and a variety of other crops are grown; (b) as a back-fill and road-base material in roadway and parking lot construction; (c) as an additive to concrete and concrete blocks; (d) in mine reclamation and (e) in the recovery of sulphur [C12]. The amount of phosphogypsum currently used for the above purposes in the United States represents about 5% of the total amount produced [C12]. In Europe and Japan, phosphogypsum has been used extensively in cement, wallboard and other building materials. Significant radiation exposures may occur if such by-products are used in the building industry.

167. Large quantities of phosphogypsum (about 100 million tonnes per year) are produced in wet-process phosphoric acid plants. The concentration of ^{226}Ra, which depends on the origin of the phosphate ore processed, is typically about 900 Bq kg^{-1}. Most of the phosphogypsum is considered waste and is either stored in ponds or stacks or discharged into the aquatic environment.

168. Phosphogypsum is used to some extent in the building industry as a substitute for natural gypsum in the manufacture of cement, wallboard and plaster. O'Riordan et al. [O1] estimated the additional doses that would be received by the occupants of a residential building in which 4.2 tonnes of by-product gypsum would have replaced the established materials. The additional absorbed dose rate in air from external irradiation was estimated to be 0.07 μGy h^{-1}, while the annual effective dose from inhalation of radon progeny was assessed at 0.6 mSv. Similar values of the annual effective dose from inhalation of radon progeny were estimated by O'Brien et al. [O2]. If it is assumed that 5% of the by-product gypsum is used as building material in dwellings, on average four persons live in each dwelling, and the mean life of a dwelling is 50 years, the collective effective doses resulting from one year of worldwide use of phosphogypsum in the building industry are estimated to be 10^5 man Sv from external irradiation and 2 10^5 man Sv from the inhalation of radon progeny. These estimates are highly uncertain and need to be confirmed by measurements in dwellings that have been constructed using known amounts of phosphogypsum.

169. The practice of using phosphogypsum in building materials is at least 50 years old [F9], but information is lacking on the amounts that have been used. If it is assumed that 5% of the current annual production (about 100 million tonnes) has been used in building materials in each of the last 50 years, it is found that 60 million houses of the current housing stock, sheltering about 5% of the world's population, have phosphogypsum included in their building materials. However, this figure seems to be too high. If it is instead assumed that 1% of the world's population lives in dwellings that include phosphogypsum in their building materials, the annual collective effective dose is estimated to be 5 10^4 man Sv. Dividing by the world's population of 5.3 10^9 yields a per caput annual effective dose of about 10 μSv.

170. Calcium silicate slag may be used as a component of concrete. Measured concentrations in slag samples range from 1,300 to 2,200 Bq kg^{-1} of ^{226}Ra [B11, M26]. Results from an indoor survey indicate that the gamma absorbed dose rate in air can

be as high as 0.3 μGy h^{-1} above background in dwellings constructed of concrete slabs containing 43% by weight slag [B11]. In a similar survey carried out in Canada, absorbed dose rates of up to 0.2 μGy h^{-1} were obtained [M26].

D. MINING AND MILLING OF MINERAL SANDS

171. Mineral sands, also called heavy minerals, are defined as those sands that have a specific gravity above 2.9. They originate from eroded inland rocks, traces of which were subsequently transported by surface waters towards the sea, where they were deposited by the combined action of wind, waves and sea currents. These mineral sands may occur under water, form part of sea, be part of the dunes or occur inland within a few tens of kilometres of the coast [K17]. Countries where mineral sands are mined include Australia, Bangladesh, Indonesia, Malaysia, Thailand and Viet-Nam.

172. Either dry mining or dredging techniques are employed in the mining of mineral sands deposits. The heavy minerals are extracted from the ore in two stages. In the first stage, a heavy mineral concentrate is extracted in a wet, gravity separation process. In a second stage, individual minerals are separated from the heavy mineral concentrate by means of dry electrostatic and magnetic techniques.

173. The heavy minerals of major commercial importance are ilmenite ($FeO \cdot TiO_2$), altered ilmenite, called leucoxene ($Fe_2O_3 \cdot TiO_2$), rutile (TiO_2), zircon ($ZrSiO_4$), monazite [a rare earth phosphate ($CePO_4$ YPO_4)] and, to a lesser extent, xenotime [a yttrium phosphate (YPO_4)]. Typical concentrations of ^{232}Th and ^{238}U in Australian heavy mineral sands, which are presented in Table 25, are much greater than the worldwide average concentrations in soils and rocks [K17].

174. Heavy minerals have numerous applications. The titaniferous minerals, once they have been processed into titanium oxide (TiO_2), are used as a pigment in paints, paper, plastics, cosmetics and ceramics. Rutile is made into titanium metal and then used, for example, in aircraft frames and jet engines. Zircon, and the associated minerals zirconia and zirconium, is used in the production of ceramics, refractory, foundry and abrasive materials, catalysts, paints, fuel cladding and structural materials in nuclear reactors. Monazite and xenotime rare earth minerals are used, for example, in the electronics, illumination and glass-making industries, in the production of magnets, superconductors and ceramics and as chemical catalysts and alloying agents in metallurgy [K17].

175. Information on exposures of members of the public resulting from the mining and milling of mineral sands is extremely scarce. In an assessment of an Australian plant, members of the public who worked on a property adjacent to the plant site were estimated to receive a dose slightly greater than 1 mSv a^{-1}, attributable mainly to external irradiation from heavy minerals spilled on the property [A9]. Away from the site, the main contribution to the dose received by members of the public results from the inhalation of dust from the plant; the highest doses were estimated to be about 0.25 mSv a^{-1} for five persons located 1.5-2 km from the plant [A9]. If the management of the plant is aware of the radiation impact of mineral sands and takes measures to control their emission, the doses will be much lower. In a study of potential radiation doses arising from a proposed mineral sand mine and processing plant in Australia, it was shown that doses to the critical group could be as low as a few μSv a^{-1} [H19].

E. SUMMARY

176. The extraction and processing of earth materials expose the general public to additional natural radiation when the earth materials, or their industrial products or by-products, contain above-average concentrations of naturally occurring radionuclides. Since very little information is available to assess those additional exposures, the related dose estimates are highly uncertain.

177. Some of those earth materials (coal, oil, peat etc.) are used to produce electrical energy by non-nuclear means. It is estimated that the production of 1 GW a of electrical energy results in collective effective doses of 20 man Sv from the use of coal, 2 man Sv from the use of peat and geothermal water or steam, 0.5 man Sv from the use of oil and 0.03 man Sv from the use of natural gas (Table 26). Taking into account the worldwide production of electrical energy in coal-fired power plants, the corresponding annual per caput effective dose is about 2 μSv. Annual per caput effective doses from other non-nuclear means of electrical energy production are much lower (Table 27).

178. Mineral sands, defined as those sands with a specific gravity greater than 2.9, usually exhibit concentrations of ^{232}Th and ^{238}U that are much greater than the worldwide average concentrations in soils and rocks. Information on exposures of members of the public resulting from the mining and milling of mineral sands is extremely scarce; annual effective doses received by critical groups may be about 1 mSv. Annual per caput effective doses have not been estimated.

179. The highest annual per caput effective doses to the public from the extractive industries are estimated to result from the use of phosphate by-products by the building industry (10 μSv), the domestic use of coal for cooking and heating (0.4-8 μSv), the use of coal ash in building materials (5 μSv) and the use of phosphate fertilizers (2 μSv). The annual per caput effective dose estimates are summarized in Table 27. The overall annual per caput effective dose arising from the extraction and processing of earth materials is estimated to be about 20 μSv.

CONCLUSIONS

180. Natural sources of ionizing radiation pervade the environment and cause exposures to all human beings. There are four main components of these exposures: cosmic rays, terrestrial gamma rays, ingested or inhaled long-lived radionuclides and inhaled radon isotopes. The first three may be said to form the basic natural radiation background because of the relative constancy of exposure. Exposures to radon and its decay products are much more widely variable. Radon gas diffuses from soils and building materials upon the decay of trace levels of radium that are naturally present. The levels of radon can build up, particularly in indoor closed spaces.

181. Doses from natural sources of radiation have been evaluated for general, worldwide geographic and geological conditions that result in normal doses and for unusual or atypical conditions that result in increased doses. The estimates of dose are for adults or for an age-weighted population if the doses to children and infants are significantly different.

182. The average annual effective doses worldwide for each of the four components of natural exposure are summarized in Table 28. For the three basic components, the annual value is 1.1 mSv. The inhalation of radon and thoron progeny results in an average annual effective dose of 1.3 mSv. The overall average annual effective dose is found to be 2.4 mSv. Small changes have been made in the various components of the effective dose; however, the compensatory effect of these changes is such that the total remains the same as in the UNSCEAR 1988 Report.

183. The importance of the inhalation of radon progeny is apparent from Table 28. It is the single most significant mechanism of human exposure to natural radiation in terms of both the average dose and the spread of doses. In middle and high latitudes, it is also the most amenable to control by building design, materials selection and ventilation. However, in low latitudes, little control can be exercised when outdoor and indoor atmospheres are not much different.

184. Radiation exposures resulting from the extraction and processing of earth materials have also been considered. These exposures are relatively small in comparison with the overall exposure from natural sources of ionizing radiation. The average annual effective dose worldwide arising from the extraction and processing of earth materials is estimated to be about 20 μSv. Because data related to those exposures are scarce, this dose estimate is highly uncertain.

Table 1
Properties of some cosmic-ray particles present in the earth's atmosphere
[E6, U5]

Class	*Name*		*Mass (MeV)*	*Mean life (s)*	*Principal mode of decay*
			Hadrons		
Nucleons	Proton	(p)	938.2	Stable	Stable
	Neutron	(n)	939.5	1.01 10^3	$p + e^- + \nu_e$
Mesons	Pion	($\pi^\pm$)	139.6	2.55 10^{-8}	$\mu + \nu_\mu$
		(π^0)	134.9	1.78 10^{-10}	$\gamma + \gamma$
	Kaon	($K^\pm$)	493.7	1.23 10^{-8}	
		(K_1)	497.7	0.91 10^{-10}	$\mu + \nu_\mu$
		(K_2)	497.7	5.7 10^{-8}	$\pi + \pi$
			Leptons		
	Muon	($\mu^\pm$)	105.6	2.2 10^{-6}	$e^\pm + \nu_e + \nu_\mu$
	Electron	($e^\pm$)	0.511	Stable	Stable
	Neutrino	(ν_e)	0	Stable	Stable
		(ν_μ)	0	Stable	Stable
			Photons		
	Photon	(γ)	0	Stable	Stable

Table 2
Average annual exposures to cosmic rays

Location	*Population (millions)*	*Altitude (m)*	*Annual effective dose (μSv)*		
			Ionizing	Neutron	Total
High-altitude cities					
La Paz, Bolivia	1.0	3900	1120	900	2020
Lhasa, China	0.3	3600	970	740	1710
Quito, Ecuador	11.0	2840	690	440	1130
Mexico City, Mexico	17.3	2240	530	290	820
Nairobi, Kenya	1.2	1660	410	170	580
Denver, United States	1.6	1610	400	170	570
Tehran, Iran	7.5	1180	330	110	440
Sea level			240	30	270
World average			300	80	380

Table 3
Annual intakes by ingestion of cosmogenic radionuclides and effective doses to adults

Radionuclide	*Intake (Bq a^{-1})*	*Annual effective dose (μSv)*
H-3	500	0.01
Be-7	1000	0.03
C-14	20000	12
Na-22	50	0.15

Table 4
Surveys of absorbed dose rates in air from terrestrial gamma radiation

Country/area	Population in 1990	Outdoors				Indoors				Ratio indoors to outdoors	Ref.
		Year of survey	Number of measurements	Absorbed dose rate ($nGy\ h^{-1}$)		Year of survey	Number of measurements	Absorbed dose rate ($nGy\ h^{-1}$)			
	(10^6)			Average	Range			Average	Range		
Algeria	25.0	1991	35 sites [a]	70	60-80						[B17]
Australia	16.9	1992	8 sites	93	64-123	1990	3367	103		1.11	[C11, L4]
Austria	7.6	1980	> 1000 [b]	43	20-150	1980	1900	71		1.65	[T1]
Belgium	9.9	1987	272 [c]	43	13-58	1989	300	58		1.35	[D1, S34]
Bulgaria	9.0		3670 [d]	70	48-96		1210	75	57-93	1.07	[V6]
Canada	26.5	1984	33 areas [e]	24	18-44						[G2]
Chile	13.2	1988	7 sites	60	30-90						[S3]
China	1120	1991	8805 [f]	62	2-341	1991	8805	99	11-418	1.60	[N22]
Taiwan Province	20	1989	155 sites	57	17-87						[C2]
Cuba	10.6	1990	54 sites [f]	42	26-53						[S48]
Denmark	5.1	1980	14 sites [g]	38	17-52	1987	489	63		1.66	[N6, S9, S10]
Egypt	52.4	1992	162 sites	32	8-93	1991	80		14-2100		[H22, I1]
Finland	5.0	1980	[h]	65		1983		80 [k]		1.23	[L3]
France	56.1	1985	5142 [h]	68	10-250	1985	5798	75		1.10	[M3, R2]
German Dem.Rep.	16.2	1991	2000	55	<4-430	1977	158	70		1.27	[L9]
Germany, Fed.Rep. of	61.3	1978	24739 [d]	53	4-350	1978	29996	70		1.32	[B10]
Greece	10.0	1990	724 sites	42							[S4]
Hong Kong	5.9	1990	27 sites	76	37-113						[L2]
		1992	76 sites [i]	160	100-230	1992	194	190	70-290	1.17	[T12]
Hungary	10.6	1987	123 sites [j]	55	20-130	1987	123	84	10-200	1.53	[N7]
Iceland	0.25	1982	[j]	28	11-83	1982		23	14-32	0.82	[E1]
India	853	1986	2800 [j]	55	20-1100						[N8]
Indonesia	184	1986	[j]	55	47-63						[S31]
Ireland	3.7	1980	284 [k]	42	<1-180	1985	223	62	10-140	1.48	[M4, M8]
Italy	57.1	1972	1365 [k]	57	7-500	1991	1500	86		1.51	[C3, C13]
Japan	123	1980	1127	49	5-100	1984	135	50 [l]		1.02	[A2, A3]
		1991	12 sites		66-144						[M23]
Luxembourg	0.4	1991	110	40							[K8]
Namibia	1.8	1991	274	120	80-260	1991	156	140	120-160	1.17	[S32]
Netherlands	15.0	1985	1049 [k]	32	10-60	1985	399	64	30-100	2.02	[J1, V1]
New Zealand	3.4					1988	716	20	<1-73		[R3]

Table 4 (continued)

Country/area	Population in 1990 (10^6)	Outdoors				Indoors				Ratio indoors to outdoors	Ref.
		Year of survey	Number of measurements	Absorbed dose rate (nGy h^{-1})		Year of survey	Number of measurements	Absorbed dose rate (nGy h^{-1})			
				Average	Range			Average	Range		
Norway	4.2	1977	234	73	20-1200	1965	2026	95		1.30	[S2, S10]
Mexico	88.6	1986/1991	1112 [j]	78	42-140						[C22]
Paraguay	4.3	1991	[j]	46	38-53						[F11]
Philippines	62.4	1991	1300	56	31-118						[D10]
Poland	38.4	1980	352 sites [j]	37	15-90	1984	1351		42-120		[K1, N9]
Portugal	10.3	1991	[g]	85	9-226	1991	1351	105	37-244	1.24	[A7]
Romania	24.0	1979	2372	81	32-210						[T2]
Spain	39.2	1991	1053	46	25-83	1991	100	68 [i]		1.48	[Q1, Q2]
Sudan	25.2	1991	[k]	53	26-690						[E5]
Sweden	8.4	1969-1989	[e, m, k]	56	41-69 [n]	1975-1978	1298	110	20-460	1.96	[M5, M9]
Switzerland	6.6	1964	3100 [g]	60							[H4]
United Kingdom	57.2	1988	25 areas [e]	34	8-89	1988	2300	60		1.76	[G3, W3]
United States	249	1972		46	13-100	1991	247	37 [i]		0.80	[M18, O3]
Population-weighted average				57				83		1.44	

[a] Ground survey with calcium sulphate thermoluminescent dosimeters and an ionization chamber.
[b] Ground survey in populated areas with a Geiger-Müller counter.
[c] Ground survey with thermoluminescent dosimeters, gamma spectrometers and ionization chambers.
[d] Ground survey with scintillation detectors.
[e] Aerial survey with a scintillation detector.
[f] Ground survey with scintillation detectors and ionization chambers.
[g] Ground survey with ionization chamber and gamma spectrometer.
[h] Ground survey with thermoluminescent dosimeters.
[i] Ground survey with energy-compensated Geiger-Müller counters.
[j] Ground survey with ionization chambers.
[k] Estimated.
[l] Calculated.
[m] 60% country coverage.
[n] Range of country averages.

Table 5
Activity concentrations of natural radionuclides in soil and absorbed dose rates in air

Radionuclide	*Concentration (Bq kg^{-1})*		*Dose coefficient* [a]	*Dose rate (nGy h^{-1})*	
	Mean [b]	*Range*	*(nGy h^{-1} per Bq kg^{-1})*	*Mean*	*Range*
China [N22]					
K-40	580 ± 200	12-2190	0.0414	24	0.5-90
Th-232 series	49 ± 28	1.5-440	0.623	31	0.9-270
U-238 series	40 ± 34	1.8-520	-	[c]	
Ra-226 subseries	37 ± 22	2.4-430	0.461	17	1.1-200
Total				72	2-560
United States [M1]					
K-40 [U1]	370	100-700	0.0414	15	4-29
Th-232 series	35	4-130	0.623	22	2-81
U-238 series	35	4-140	-	[c]	
Ra-226 subseries	40	8-160	0.461	18	4-74
Total				55	10-200

[a] Reference [P2, S12].
[b] Area-weighted mean for China; arithmetic mean for the United States.
[c] Dose from ^{226}Ra subseries.

Table 6
Activity concentrations of natural radionuclides in various types of soil in the Nordic countries [C14]

Type of soil	*Activity concentration (Bq kg^{-1})*		
	^{40}K	^{226}Ra	^{232}Th
Sand and silt	600-1200	5-25	4-30
Clay	600-1300	20-120	25-80
Moraine	900-1300	20-80	20-80
Soils containing alum shale	600-1000	100-1000	20-80

Table 7
Estimated absorbed dose rates in air within masonry dwellings

Material	*Concentration (Bq kg^{-1})*			*Activity utilization index* [a]	*Absorbed dose rate in air for indicated fractional mass of building material (nGy h^{-1})*				*Reference*
	C_K	C_{Ra}	C_{Th}		*1.0*	*0.75*	*0.5*	*0.25*	
Typical masonry	500	50	50	1.0	80	60	40	20	[N10]
Granite blocks	1200	90	80	1.9	140	105	70	35	[N10]
Coal ash aggregate	400	150	150	2.4	180	135	90	45	[U1]
Alum shale concrete	770	1300	67	9.0	670	500	390	170	[N10]
Phosphogypsum	60	600	20	3.9	290	220	145	70	[N10]
Natural gypsum	150	20	5	0.25	20	15	10	5	[N10]

[a] Assuming full utilization of the materials (w_m = 1).

Table 8
Conversion coefficients from air kerma to effective dose for terrestrial gamma rays
[P19, S12]

Radionuclides	*Conversion coefficient (Sv per Gy)*		
	Adults	*Children*	*Infants*
K-40	0.74	0.81	0.95
Th-232 series	0.72	0.81	0.92
U-238 series	0.69	0.78	0.91
Overall	0.72	0.80	0.93

Table 9
National estimates of the average annual effective dose from terrestrial gamma rays

Country	*Effective dose (mSv)*	*Reference*
Bulgaria	0.45	[V6]
Canada	0.23	[N2]
China	0.55	[N22]
Denmark	0.36	[C14]
Finland	0.49	[C14]
Germany	0.41	[B10, K9, L9]
Japan	0.32	[A6, F10]
Norway	0.48	[C14, S10]
Spain	0.40	[Q2]
Sweden	0.65	[M9, S10]
United Kingdom	0.35	[H3]
United States	0.28	[N2]
USSR	0.32	[B5]
Population-weighted world average	0.45	

Table 10
Reference annual intake of food and air
[I5, W4]

Intake	*Food consumption (kg a^{-1})*		
	Adults	*Children*	*Infants*
Milk products	105	110	120
Meat products	50	35	15
Grain products	140	90	45
Leafy vegetables	60	40	20
Roots and fruits	170	110	60
Fish products	15	10	5
Water and beverages	500	350	150
Intake	*Breathing rate (m^3 a^{-1})*		
	Adults	*Children*	*Infants*
Air	8000	5500	1400

Table 11
Reference activity concentrations of natural radionuclides in food and air

Intake	*Activity concentration (mBq kg^{-1})*								
	$^{238}U \rightarrow ^{234}U$	^{230}Th	^{226}Ra	^{210}Pb	^{210}Po	^{232}Th	^{228}Ra	^{228}Th	^{235}U
Milk products	1	0.5	5	40	60	0.3	5	0.3	0.05
Meat products	2	2	15	80	60	1	10	1	0.05
Grain products	20	10	80	100	100	3	60	3	1.0
Leafy vegetables	20	20	50	30	30	15	40	15	1.0
Roots and fruits	3	0.5	30	25	30	0.5	20	0.5	0.1
Fish products	30	-	100	200	2000	-	-	-	-
Water supplies	1	0.1	0.5	10	5	0.05	0.5	0.05	0.04
Intake	*Activity concentration (μBq m^{-3})*								
	$^{238}U \rightarrow ^{234}U$	^{230}Th	^{226}Ra	^{210}Pb	^{210}Po	^{232}Th	^{228}Ra	^{228}Th	^{235}U
Air	1	0.5	0.5	500	50	1	1	1	0.05

Table 12
Committed effective dose per unit activity intake of natural radionuclides for adults [I4]

Radionuclide	*Ingestion*		*Inhalation*	
	Fractional transfer to blood	*Dose coefficient (μSv Bq^{-1})*	*Class of solubility*	*Dose coefficient (μSv Bq^{-1})*
U-238	0.05	0.025	Y	30
U-234	0.05	0.03	Y	30
Th-230	0.0002	0.07	Y	50
Ra-226	0.2	0.2	W	2
Pb-210	0.2	1	D	2
Po-210	0.1	0.2	D	1
Th-232	0.0002	0.4	Y	200
Ra-228	0.2	0.3	W	1
Th-228	0.0002	0.07	Y	100
U-235	0.05	0.03	Y	30
Pa-231	0.001	2	W	200
Ac-227	0.001	2	W	300

Table 13
Average age-weighted annual intakes of natural radionuclides and associated effective doses

Radionuclide	*Ingestion*		*Inhalation*	
	Intake (Bq)	*Dose (μSv)*	*Intake (mBq)*	*Dose (μSv)*
U-238	4.9	0.12	6.9	0.21
U-234	4.9	0.15	6.9	0.21
Th-230	2.5	0.18	3.5	0.18
Ra-226	19	3.8	3.5	0.01
Pb-210	32	32	3500	7.0
Po-210	55	11	350	0.35
Th-232	1.3	0.52	6.9	1.4
Ra-228	13	3.9	6.9	0.01
Th-228	1.3	0.09	6.9	0.69
U-235	0.21	0.01	0.4	0.01
Total		52		10

Table 14
Elevated values of activity concentrations of natural radionuclides in foods

Food	*Country*	*Radionuclide*	*Activity concentration in fresh food ($mBq\ kg^{-1}$)*		*Ref.*
			Range	*Arithmetic mean*	
Cows' milk	Brazil	Ra-226	29-210	108	[A4]
		Pb-210	5-60	45	[A8]
Chicken meat	Brazil	Ra-226	37-163	86	[L10]
		Ra-228	141-355	262	
Beef	Brazil	Ra-226	30-59	44	[L10]
		Ra-228	78-111	96	
Pork	Brazil	Ra-226	7-22	13	[L10]
		Ra-228	93-137	121	
Reindeer meat	Sweden	Pb-210	400-700	550	[P7]
		Po-210	-	11000	
Cereals	India	Ra-226	up to 510	174	[L6]
		Th-228	up to 5590	536	
Corn	Brazil	Ra-226	70-229	118	[V3]
		Pb-210	100-222	144	
Rice	China	Ra-226		250	[Z1]
		Pb-210		570	
Green vegetables	India	Ra-226	325-2120	1110	[L6]
		Th-228	348-5180	1670	
Carrots	Brazil	Ra-226	329-485	411	[V3]
		Pb-210	218-318	255	
Roots and tubers	India	Ra-226	477-4780	1490	[L6]
		Th-228	70-32400	21700	
Fruits	India	Ra-226	137-688	296	[L6]
		Th-228	59-21900	2590	

Table 15
Elevated values of activity concentrations of natural radionuclides in potable waters of various sources

Source	*Country*	*Radionuclide*	*Activity concentration ($mBq\ l^{-1}$)*			*Reference*
			Range	*Arithmetic mean*	*Geometric mean*	
Bottled waters	Brazil	Ra-226	<10-130		27	[P8]
		Pb-210	<50-190		77	
	France	U-238	up to 2000	60		[P5, P9, S11] [R12, R13, R14, M19]
		Ra-226	up to 2700	60		
		Th-232	-	< 40		
	Germany	U-238	<1-140		4.4	[B12, G4, G5]
		Ra-226	<1-1800		25	
		Pb-210	3.3-53		9.0	
		Po-210	0.4-8.9		1.8	
	Indonesia	Ra-226	<1-60	22	-	[S31]
	Portugal	Ra-226	<3-2185		26.7	[B6]
		Pb-210	2-392		18.5	
Ground waters	Finland	U-238	up to 74000	4200		[S15]
		Ra-226	up to 5300	440		
		Pb-210	up to 10200	430		
		Po-210	up to 6300	220		
	Sweden	Ra-226	2-2460	45	13.7	[K4]
	Yugoslavia	Ra-226	0.5-510	60	-	[K11]

Table 16
Alpha decay properties of ^{220}Rn and ^{222}Rn with short-lived decay products
[B7, M11]

^{220}Rn					^{222}Rn			
Radionuclide	*Branch (%)*	*Half-life*	*Energy (MeV)*	*Intensity (%)*	*Radionuclide*	*Half-life*	*Energy (MeV)*	*Intensity (%)*
Rn-220		55 s	6.29	100	Rn-222	3.824 d	5.49	100
Po-216		0.15 s	6.78	100	Po-218	3.04 min	6.00	100
Pb-212		10.64 h	β, γ	-	Pb-214	26.8 min	β, γ	-
Bi-212		60.6 min	6.05	25	Bi-214	19.7 min	β, γ	-
			6.09	10	Po-214	163.7 μs	7.69	100
Po-212	64	304 ns	8.78	100				
Tl-208	36	3.10 min	β, γ	-				

Table 17
Activity concentrations of ^{226}Ra and ^{228}Ra in various types of rock
[W6]

Type of rock	*Example*	*Concentration (Bq kg^{-1})*			
		^{226}Ra		^{228}Ra	
		Arithmetic mean	*Range*	*Arithmetic mean*	*Range*
Acid intrusive	Granite	78	1-370	111	0.4-1030
Basic extrusive	Basalt	11	0.4-41	10	0.2-36
Chemical sedimentary	Limestone	45	0.4-340	60	0.1-540
Detrital sedimentary	Clay, shale, sandstone	60	1-990	50	0.8-1470
Metamorphosed igneous	Gneiss	50	1-1800	60	0.4-420
Metamorphosed sedimentary	Schist	37	1-660	49	0.4-370

Table 18
Activity concentrations of natural radionuclides in various types of rock in the Nordic countries
[C14]

Rock type	*Activity concentration (Bq kg^{-1})*		
	^{40}K	^{226}Ra	^{232}Th
Normal granite	600-1800	20-120	20-80
Thorium- and uranium-rich granite	1200-1800	100-500	40-350
Gneiss	600-1800	20-120	20-80
Diorite	300-1000	1-20	4-40
Sandstone	300-1500	5-60	4-40
Limestone	30-150	5-20	1-10
Shale	600-1800	10-120	8-60
Middle Cambrian alum shale	1000-1800	120-600	8-40
Upper Cambrian or Lower Ordovician alum shale	1000-1800	600-4500	8-40

Table 19
Parameters of emanation and diffusion of ^{222}Rn from the earth and from building materials

Material	*Representative value*	*Range*	*Ref.*
	Emanation fraction		
Rock (sieved)	0.084 [a]	0.005 - 0.40	[B8]
Soil (various)	0.23 [a]	0.02 - 0.83	[D5]
Brick (clay)	0.04 [b]	0.02 - 0.1	[S17]
Concrete (ordinary)	0.15 [c]	0.1 - 0.4	[S17]
Gypsum (natural)	0.08 [b]	0.03 -0.2	[S17]
	Porosity		
Earth	0.25	0.01-0.5	[F6, H14,
Building materials	0.15	0.01-0.7	O5, S19]
	Diffusion coefficient (m^2 s^{-1})		
Earth	5 10^{-7}	10^{-11}-10^{-6}	[F6, H14,
Building materials	1 10^{-8}	10^{-11}-10^{-6}	O5, S19]

[a] Arithmetic mean.
[b] Inferred from range.
[c] Inferred from range and mix.

Table 20
Flux density from the convection of radon and the resultant entry rates into the model building caused by an underpressure of 5 Pa with varying permeability of the subjacent earth

Circumstance	*Flux density (Bq m^{-2} s^{-1})*					*Entry rate (Bq m^{-3} h^{-1})*				
	Permeability (m^2)					*Permeability (m^2)*				
	10^{-13}	10^{-12}	10^{-11}	10^{-10}	10^{-9}	10^{-13}	10^{-12}	10^{-11}	10^{-10}	10^{-9}
Cracked floor [a]	0.0071	0.0078	0.014	0.078	0.043	10	11	20	112	62
Bare earth	0.028	0.030	0.043	0.19	0.085 [b]	40	43	62	274	122 [b]

[a] With an array of 1 cm cracks every 1 m of floor. Values averaged over whole floor.
[b] Trend adjustment of published data [W8].

Table 21
Average radon concentrations and percentage utilization of water supplies
[N18, O5]

Type of supply	*Concentration ($Bq\ m^{-3}$)*			*Utilization (%)*		
	United States	*United Kingdom*	*Reference value*	*United States*	*United Kingdom*	*Reference value*
Surface water	1100	1000	1000	50	66	60
Ground water	11500	30000	10000	32	34	30
Well water	208000	< 1000000	100000	18	< 1	10

Table 22
Illustrative radon entry rates for the model masonry building in a temperate climate

Source of radon	*Mechanism*	*Entry rate ($Bq\ m^{-3}\ h^{-1}$)*	*Percentage*
Building elements	Diffusion	10	21
Subjacent earth	Diffusion	7.5	15
	Advection	20	41
Outdoor air	Infiltration	10	20
Water supply	De-emanation	1	2
Natural gas	Consumption	0.3	1
All sources and mechanisms		49	100

Table 23
Radon concentrations in dwellings determined in indoor surveys

Country/area	*Year of survey*	*Type of survey*	*Duration of exposure*	*Number of dwellings surveyed*	*Radon concentration (Bq m^{-3})*			*Geometric standard deviation*	*Ref.*
					Arithmetic mean	*Geometric mean*	*Maximum value*		
Algeria	1987	Exploratory	60 days	50	32		137		[C9]
Argentina, 3 cities	1990	Preliminary		180	32	31	127	2.0	[G6]
Australia	1990	National	1 year	3413	12	8.7	423	2.1	[L4]
Austria, Salzburg	1980	Local	Grab samples	729	-	15	190	-	[S40, S41]
Belgium	1991	National	6 months	450	48		4000		[V8]
Canada	1977-1980	National	Grab samples	13413	34	14	1724	3.6	[L7]
Canada, Nova Scotia	1990	Regional	3 months	719	108	-	5920	3.6	[J9]
China, seven provinces	1989	Regional		3945	24	20	378	2.2	[Z2]
China, Sechuan	1990	Regional		1967	19	17	170	1.7	[C10]
China, Shenzhen	1986	Regional		69	16	14	54	2.0	[R5]
Czechoslovakia	1982	National	Grab samples	1200	140 [a]	-	20000	-	[T6, T8]
Denmark	1985	National	6 months	496	47	29	560	2.2	[S9, U15]
Egypt	1991	National		329	9.0		24		[K12]
Finland	1982	National	1 month	8150	90	64	-	3.1	[C19, C21]
France	1988	National	60 days	3006	62	41	4687	2.7	[R6, R7]
Germany (former Fed. Republic)	1984	Regional	3 months	5970	49	40	-	1.8	[S29]
Germany, Cottbus	1989	Regional	3 months	67	35	23	153	2.5	[L9]
Germany, Saxony and Thuringia	1990	Exploratory	3 days	5000	270	190	115000	2.4	[L9]
Germany (former Fed. Republic)	1991	Regional	3 days	1040	57	34	3100	2.9	[K13]
Ghana, Legon	1990	Exploratory	9 months	25			340		[O6]
Greece	1988	Exploratory	6 months	73	52		492		[G7]
Hong Kong	1991	Regional		140	41		140		[T9]
India	1991	Exploratory	3 months	1208	57	42	214	2.2	[S37]
Indonesia	1991	Exploratory		165	12		120		[S31]
Iran, 4 cities	1988	Exploratory	90 days	121	82		3070		[S26]
Ireland	1987	National	6 months	736	-	37	1700	-	[C18]
Italy	1991	National	1 year	2250	80	62		1.9	[B15, B16]
Japan	1990	National	1 year	6000	29	23		1.6	[K5]
Kuwait	1988	Exploratory	1 year	69	41		103		[M13]
Luxembourg	1991	National		2500		65			[K8]
Netherlands	1982-1984	National	1 year	1000	29	24	118	1.6	[H17,P24,P25]
New Zealand	1988	National	1 year	717	20	18	94		[R3]
Norway	1991	National	6 months	7500	60	30			[S39]
Pakistan	1991	Exploratory	2.5 months	50	30		83		[T10]
Poland	1991	Preliminary	1 year	345	38		568		[B14]
Portugal	1991	National	4 months	4200	81	37	2795		[F14]
Spain	1991	National		1700	86	43	15400	3.7	[Q2, Q3]
Sweden	1980-1982	National	2 weeks	512	108	62	3310		[M17, S42]
Sweden	1990-1991	National	3 months	1360	108	56	3900		[S43]
Switzerland	1991	National	2.5 months	1600	70		3000		[S38]
Syria, 2 areas	1990	Exploratory	6 months	77	20		72		[O7]
United Kingdom	1991		3 months	96000	20		10000		[W9]
United States	1991	National	1 year	5967	46	25		3.1	[M24, U12]
United States, New York	1988	Regional	1 year	2043	42	26	1420	2.7	[P11]
Median values					42	30		2.2	

[a] Derived from radon EEC measurements, using an equilibrium factor of 0.4.

Table 24
Average concentrations in air of radon and thoron, including their decay products, and annual effective doses

Radionuclide	*Location*	*Concentration ($Bq\ m^{-3}$)*		*Effective dose coefficient (nSv per $Bq\ h\ m^{-3}$)*		*Annual effective dose* [a] *(μSv)*	
		Gas	*EEC* [b]	*Gas*	*EEC*	*Gas*	*EEC*
Radon	Outdoors	10	8	0.17	9	3.0	130
	Indoors	40	16	0.17	9	48	1000
Total (rounded)						1200	
Thoron	Outdoors	10	0.1	0.11	10	1.9	1.8
	Indoors	3	0.3	0.11	32	2.3	67
Total (rounded)						73	

[a] Weighted for occupancy: 0.2 outdoors, 0.8 indoors.

[b] The equilibrium equivalent concentration (EEC) of radon (or thoron) is the product of the concentration of radon (or thoron) and of the equilibrium factor between radon (or thoron) and its decay products. The values of the equilibrium factor have been taken to be 0.8 outdoors and 0.4 indoors for radon. Thoron EEC values are based on measurements.

Table 25
Typical concentrations of ^{232}Th and ^{238}U in heavy mineral sands in Australia
[K17]

Mineral	*^{232}Th concentration ($Bq\ kg^{-1}$)*	*^{238}U concentration ($Bq\ kg^{-1}$)*
Ore	60-200	40
Heavy mineral concentrate	1000-1300	<100
Ilmenite	600-6000	<100-400
Leucoxene	1000-9000	250-600
Rutile	<600-4000	<100-250
Zircon	2000-3000	200-400
Monazite	600000-900000	10000-40000
Xenotime	180000	50000
Average soil and rock	40	40

Table 26
Estimates of collective effective dose per unit electrical energy generated by non-nuclear sources

Source	*Normalized collective effective dose [man Sv $(GW\ a)^{-1}$]*
Coal	20
Oil	0.5
Natural gas	0.03
Geothermal	2
Peat	2

Table 27
Estimates of annual per caput effective doses resulting from the extraction and processing of earth materials

Source	*Annual per caput effective dose (μSv)*
Coal	
Mining	0.0001-0.002
Electrical energy production	2
Domestic use	0.4-8
Use of fuel ash	5
Other non-nuclear sources of electrical energy production	
Oil	0.01
Natural gas	0.001
Geothermal	0.001
Exploitation of phosphate rock	
Industrial operations	0.04
Fertilizers	2
By-products and wastes	10

Table 28
Average annual effective dose to adults from natural sources of ionizing radiation

Component of exposure	*Annual effective dose (mSv)*	
	In areas of normal background	*In areas of elevated exposures*
Cosmic rays	0.38	2.0
Cosmogenic radionuclides	0.01	0.01
Terrestrial radiation: external exposure	0.46	4.3
Terrestrial radiation: internal exposure (excluding radon)	0.23	0.6
Terrestrial radiation: internal exposure from radon and its decay products		
Inhalation of Rn-222	1.2	10
Inhalation of Rn-220	0.07	0.1
Ingestion of Rn-222	0.005	0.1
Total	2.4	-

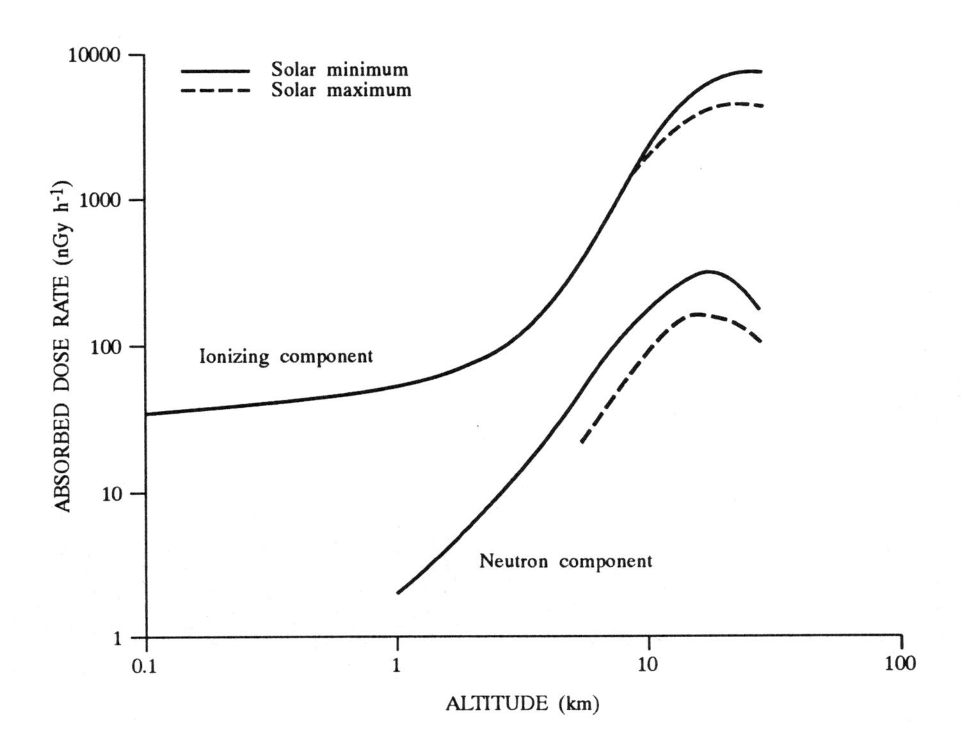

Figure I.
Absorbed dose rate in air at 50° geomagnetic latitude from the ionizing and neutron components of cosmic rays as a function of altitude.
[U3]

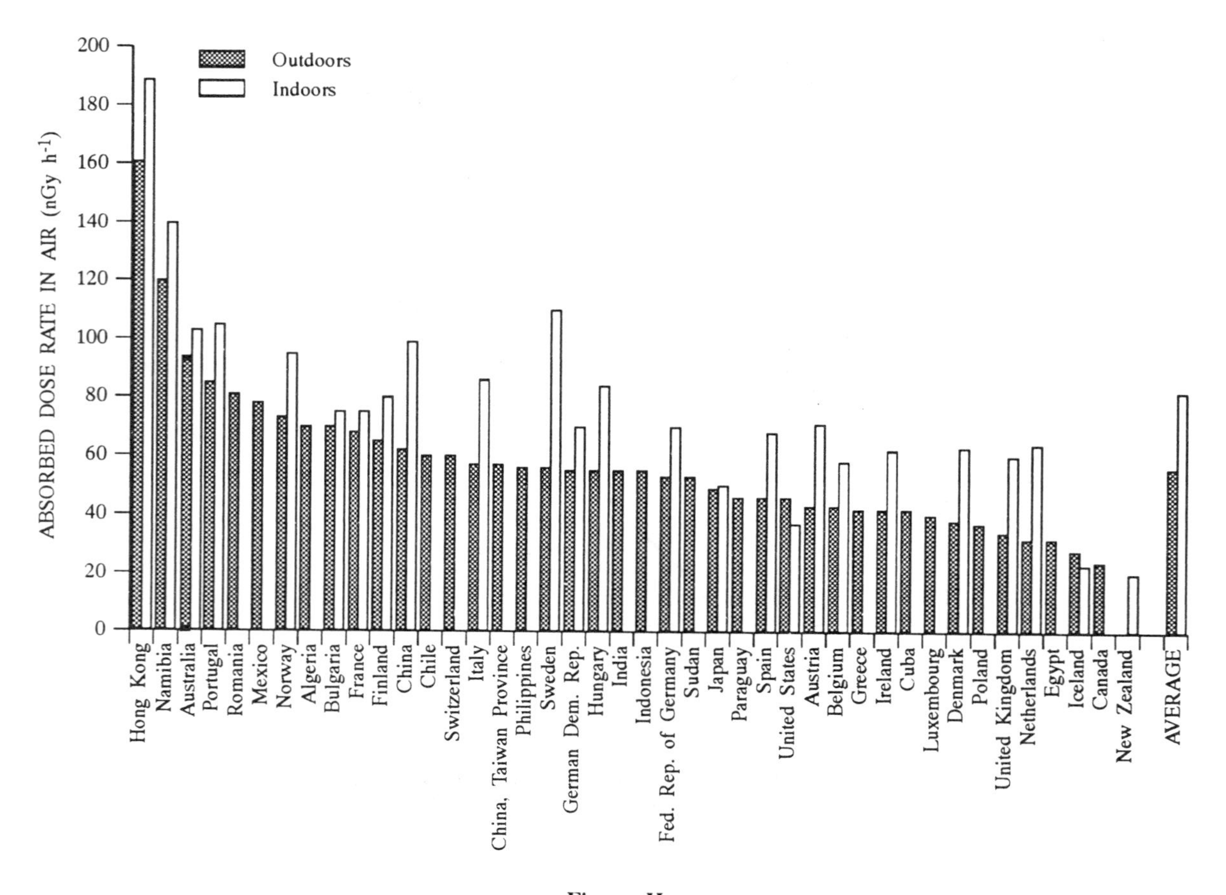

Figure II.
Absorbed dose rates in air from terrestrial gamma radiation ranked according to levels outdoors.

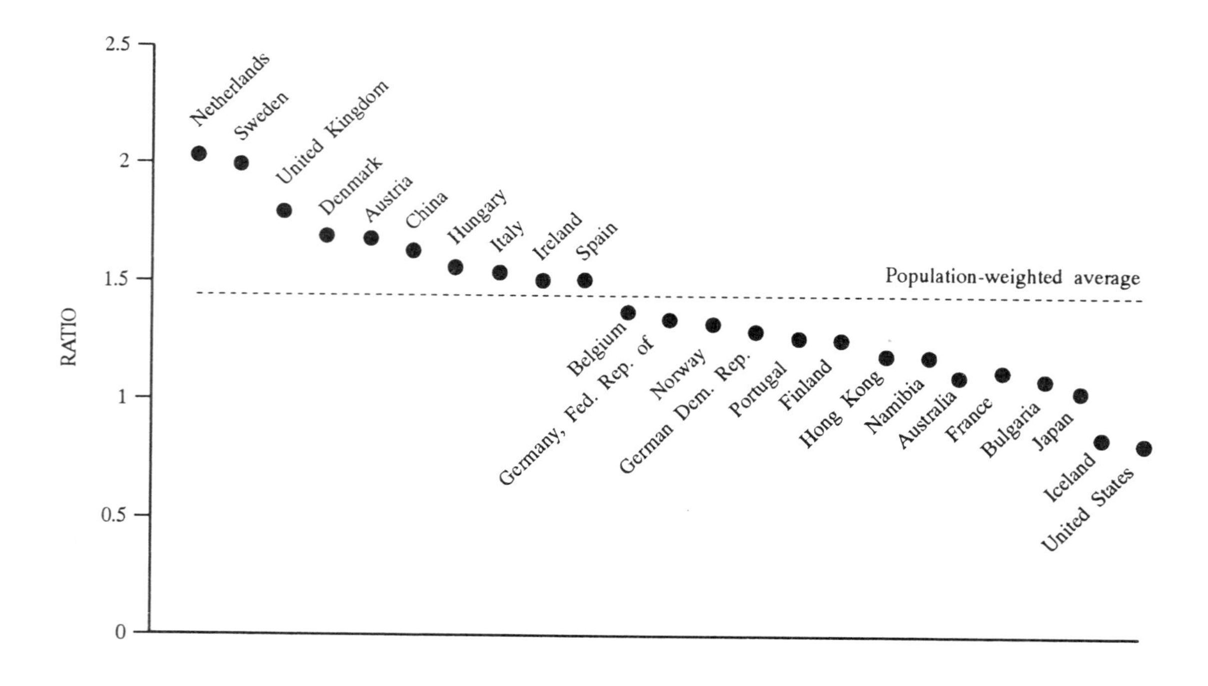

Figure III.
Ratio of indoor to outdoor absorbed dose rates in air from terrestrial radiation.

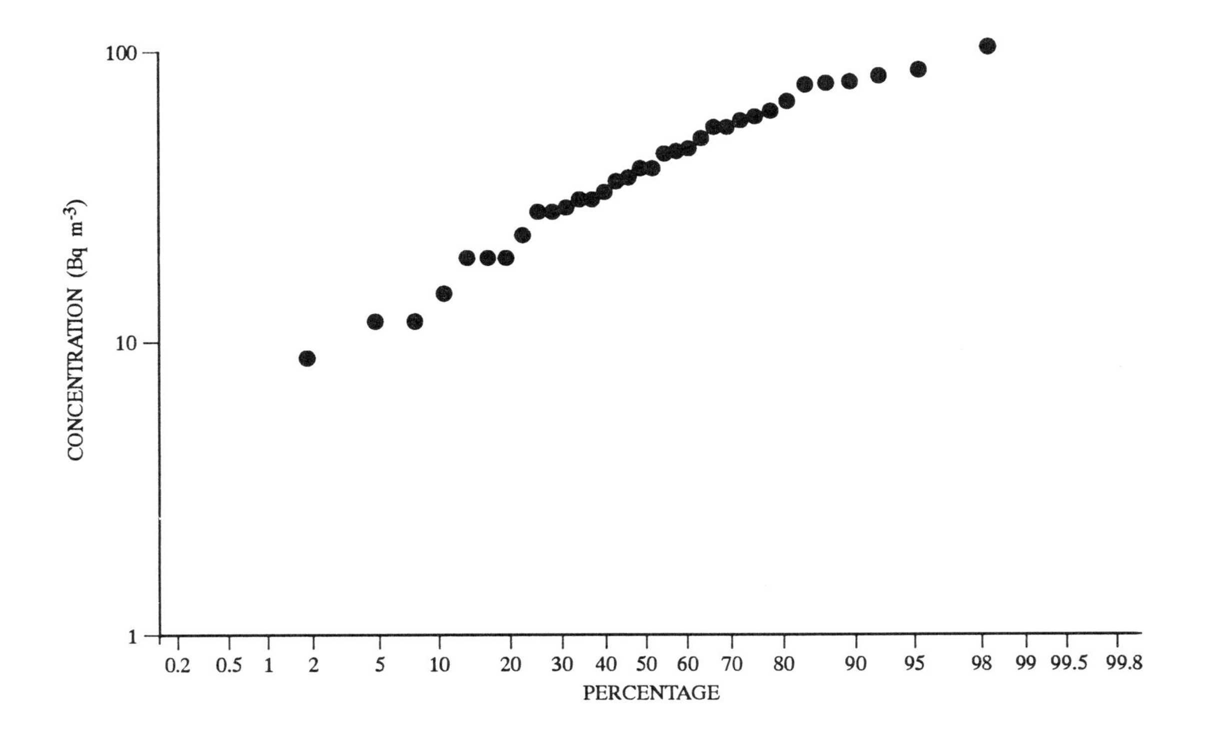

Figure IV.
Distribution of survey measurements of radon concentrations indoors.

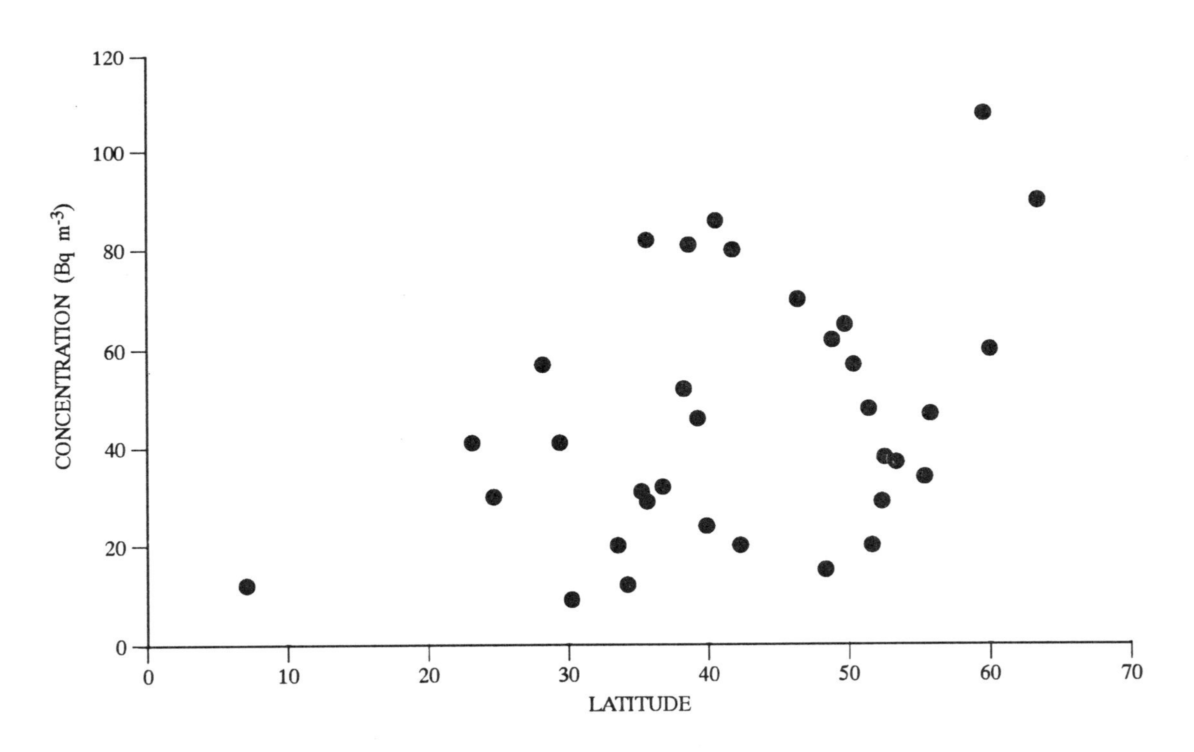

Figure V.
Radon concentrations indoors in relation to latitude.
The population-weighted average is 40 Bq m^{-3}.

References

A1 Angelo, J.A., W. Quam and R.G. Madonna. Radiation protection issues and techniques concerning extended manned space missions. p. 91-105 in: Radiation Protection in Nuclear Energy (Volume 2). IAEA, Vienna, 1988.

A2 Abe, S., K. Fujitaka and K. Fujimoto. Natural radiation in Japan. p. 1034-1048 in: Natural Radiation Environment III. CONF-780422 (1980).

A3 Abe, S., K. Fujimoto and K. Fujitaka. Relationship between indoor and outdoor gamma-ray exposure in wooden houses. Radiat. Prot. Dosim. 7: 267-269 (1984).

A4 Amaral, E.C.S., Z.L. Carvalho and J.M. Godoy. Transfer of Ra-226 and Pb-210 to forage and milk in a Brazilian high natural radioactivity region. Radiat. Prot. Dosim. 24: 119-121 (1988).

A5 Åkerblom, G., P. Andersson and B. Clavensjö. Soil gas radon - a source of indoor radon daughters. Radiat. Prot. Dosim. 7: 49-54 (1984).

A6 Abe, S., K. Fujitaka, M. Abe et al. Extensive field survey of natural radiation in Japan. J. Nucl. Sci. Technol. 18:21-45 (1981).

A7 Amaral, E.M., J.G. Alves and J.V. Carreiro. Doses to the Portuguese population due to natural gamma radiation. Radiat. Prot. Dosim. 45: 541-543 (1992).

A8 Amaral, E.C.S., E.R.R. Rochedo, H.G. Paretzke et al. The radiological impact of agricultural activities in an area of high natural radioactivity. Radiat. Prot. Dosim. 45: 289-292 (1992).

A9 Alexander, E.G., N.D. Stewart and B.J. Wallace. The radiological impact of past and present practices of the mineral sands industry in Queensland. Paper submitted to the Bulletin of the Australian Radiation Protection Society, March 1993.

B1 Bouville, A. and W.M. Lowder. Human population exposure to cosmic radiation. Radiat. Prot. Dosim. 24: 293-299 (1988).

B2 Bailey, M.R. and A. Birchall. New ICRP dosimetric model for the respiratory tract: a progress report. Radiol. Prot. Bull. 119: 13-20 (1991).

B3 Beck, H.L. The physics of environmental gamma radiation fields. p. 101-133 in: The Natural Radiation Environment II. CONF-720805-P1 (1972).

B4 Blaton-Albicka, K. and J. Pensko. Assessment of radon exhalation rates in dwellings in Poland. Health Phys. 41: 548-551 (1981).

B5 Buldakov, L.A., G.M. Avetisov, R.M. Barhudarov et al. Problems of regulating radiation exposure of the public. p. 59-63 in: Proceedings of the IVth European Congress and XIIIth Regional Congress of IRPA, Salzburg, 1986. OVS, Austria, 1988.

B6 Bettencourt, A.O., M.M.G.R. Teixeira, M.C. Fáisca et al. Natural radioactivity in Portuguese mineral waters. Radiat. Prot. Dosim. 24: 139-142 (1988).

B7 Browne, E. and R.B. Firestone (eds.). Table of Radioactive Isotopes. Wiley, New York, 1986.

B8 Barretto, P.M.C. Emanation characteristics of terrestrial and lunar materials and the radon-222 loss effect on the uranium-lead system discordance. Ph.D. Thesis. Rice University, Houston, 1973. (As quoted in [N15])

B9 Brown, K. Radiation exposure from building materials. NRPB-M69 (1982).

B10 Bundesminister des Innern. Die Strahlenexposition von aussen in der Bundesrepublik Deutschland durch natürliche Radioaktive Stoffe in Freien und in Wohnungen unter Berücksichtigung des Einflusses von Baustoffen. Bericht über ein von Bundesminister des Innern gefördertes Forschungvorhaben. 1978.

B11 Booth, G.F. The need for radiation controls in the phosphate and related industries. Health Phys. 32: 285-290 (1977).

B12 Bundesamtes für Strahlenschutz. Umweltradioaktivität Jahresbericht 1990.

B13 Baeza, A., M. del Río, C. Miró et al. Natural radioactivity in soils of the province of Cáceres (Spain). Radiat. Prot. Dosim. 45: 261-263 (1992).

B14 Biemacka, M., J. Henschke, J. Jagielak et al. Preliminary measurements of the natural ionising radiation in three types of building in Poland. in: Progress of Medical Physics, 1992. (in Polish)

B15 Bochicchio, F. Instituto Superiore di Sanità, Rome, Italy. Communication to UNSCEAR Secretariat. (1991).

B16 Bochicchio, F., G. Campos Venuti, S. Mancioppi et al. First results of the indoor natural radiation survey in Italy. Radiat. Prot. Dosim. 45: 459-463 (1992).

B17 Benkrid, M., D. Mebhah, S. Djeffal et al. Environmental gamma radiation monitoring by means of TLD and ionisation chamber. Radiat. Prot. Dosim. 45: 77-80 (1992).

C1 Curtis, S.B., W. Atwell, R. Beever et al. Radiation environments and absorbed dose estimations on manned space missions. Adv. Space Res. 6: 269-274 (1986).

C2 Chu, T-C., P-W. Weng and Y-M. Lin. Changes in per capita and collective dose equivalent due to natural radiation in Taiwan (1950-1983). Health Phys. 56: 201-217 (1989).

C3 Cardinale, A., G. Cortellessa, F. Gera et al. Distribution in the Italian population of the absorbed dose due to the natural background radiation. p. 421-440 in: The Natural Radiation Environment II. CONF-720805-P1 (1972).

C4 Commission of the European Communities. A preliminary assessment of the radiological impact of the Chernobyl reactor accident on the population of the European Community. CEC, Luxembourg, 1987.

C5 Camplin, W.C. and A. Aarkrog. Radioactivity in North European waters. p. 199-302 in: The Radiological Exposure of the Population of the European Community from Radioactivity in North European Marine Waters. Project Marina. EUR 12483EN. CEC, Luxembourg, 1990.

C6 Cliff, K.D., J.C.H. Miles and K. Brown. The incidence and origin of radon and its decay products in buildings. NRPB-R159 (1984).

C7 Collé, R., R.J. Rubin, L.I. Knab et al. Radon transport through and exhalation from building materials: a review and assessment. NBS Technical Note 1139 (1981).

C8 Cothern, C.R. and P. Milvy. Risk assessment of radon in drinking water. Trace Subst. Environ. Health 12: 68-76 (1988).

C9 Cherouati, D.E. and S. Djeffal. Measurements of radon and radon daughters in dwellings in Algiers. Radiat. Prot. Dosim. 25: 137-139 (1988).

C10 Chen, Y. Indoor radon concentrations in homes of Sichuan residents and the dose to the population exposed to radon and its daughters. p. 59-64 in: Indoor Air Quality '90. Proceedings of the 5th International Conference on Indoor Air Quality and Climate, Toronto, 1990.

C11 Clarke, P.C., M.B. Cooper, L.J. Martin et al. Environmental Radioactivity Surveillance in Australia. Results for 1992. ARL Technical Report (in preparation, 1993).

C12 Conklin, C. Potential uses of phosphogypsum and associated risks. Background Information Document. EPA 402-R92-002 (1992).

C13 Campos Venuti, G. Instituto Superiore di Sanità, Rome, Italy. Communication to the UNSCEAR Secretariat (1991).

C14 Christensen, T., H. Ehdwall and E. Stranden (eds.). Natural Radiation, Nuclear Wastes and Chemical Pollutants. Nordic Liaison Committee for Atomic Energy, Stockholm, 1990.

C15 Colangelo, C.H., M.R. Huguet, M.A. Palacios et al. Levels of polonium-210 in some beverages and tobacco. Comision Nacional de Energia Atómica, Buenos Aires. (unpublished report)

C16 Cliff, K.D., B.M.R. Green, A. Mawle et al. Thoron daughter concentrations in UK homes. Radiat. Prot. Dosim. 45: 361-366 (1992).

C17 Cancio, D., J. Gutierrez, R. Salvador et al. Evaluacion radiológica de la industria de fosfatos de Huelva. Consejo de Seguridad Nuclear. Report CIEMAT/PRIMA/UCRE/11/89 (1989).

C18 Commission of the European Communities. Radiation protection, exposure to natural radiation in dwellings of the European Community. CEC, Luxembourg, 1987.

C19 Castrén, O., K. Winqvist, I. Mäkeläinen et al. Radon measurements in Finnish houses. Radiat. Prot. Dosim. 7: 333-336 (1984).

C20 Cross, F.T., N.H. Harley and W. Hofmann. Health effects and risks from radon-222 in drinking water. Health Phys. 48: 649-670 (1985).

C21 Castrén, O. Dealing with radon in dwellings: The Finnish experience. Presented at the Second International Specialty Conference on Indoor Radon. Air Pollution Control Association, New Jersey, April 1987.

C22 Comisión Nacional de Seguridad Nuclear y Salvaguardias. Valores de la exposición a la radiación natural medidos en diferentes puntos de la República Mexicana (1991).

C23 Chittaporn, P. and N.H. Harley. Indoor and outdoor ^{222}Rn in Thailand. Health Phys. (accepted for publication, 1993).

D1 Deworm, J.P., W. Slegers, J. Gillard et al. Survey of the natural radiation of the Belgian territory as determined with different methods. Radiat. Prot. Dosim. 24: 347-351 (1988).

D2 Doi, M., S. Kobayashi and K. Fujimoto. A passive measurement technique for characterization of high-risk houses in Japan due to enhanced levels of indoor radon and thoron concentrations. Radiat. Prot. Dosim. 45: 425-430 (1992).

D3 de Planque, G. TLD measurements and model calculations of environmental radiation exposure rates. p. 987-1003 in: Natural Radiation Environment III. CONF-780422, Volume 2 (1980).

D4 Davies, D.M. Cosmic Radiation in Concorde operations and the impact of new ICRP Recommendations on commercial aviation. Radiat. Prot. Dosim. 48: 121-124 (1993).

D5 Damkjaer, A. and U. Korsbech. Measurement of the emanation of radon-222 from Danish soils. Sci. Total Environ. 45: 343-350 (1985).

D6 Dimbylow, P.J. and P. Wilkinson. The numerical solution of the diffusion equation describing the flow of radon through cracks in a concrete slab. Radiat. Prot. Dosim. 11: 229-236 (1985).

D7 Dimbylow, P.J. The solution of the pressure driven flow equation for radon ingress through cracks in concrete foundations. Radiat. Prot. Dosim. 18: 163-167 (1987).

D8 Dudney, C.S., A.R. Hawthorne, R.G. Wallace et al. Radon-222, ^{222}Rn progeny, and ^{220}Rn progeny levels in 70 homes. Health Phys. 58: 297-311 (1990).

D9 Doi, M., S. Kobayashi and K. Fujimoto. Potential risk of thoron and its progenies in the air of traditional Japanese wooden houses. p. 1339-1342 in: Worldwide Achievement in Public and Occupational Health Protection Against Radiation. Proceedings of the 8th International Conference of the International Radiation Protection Association, Montreal, Canada, May 1992.

D10 Duran, E.B., C.M. de Vera, F.M. de la Cruz et al. Outdoor exposure to natural radiation in the Philippines. Philippine Nuclear Research Institute, Quezon City, 1991.

D11 Daschil, F., W. Hofmann, P. Pfligersdorffer et al. Bestimmung der Radon- und Thoronexhalation aus Baumaterialproben. OEFZS Bericht No. A 0715 Kap. III. Seibersdorf, Austria (1985).

E1 Ennow, K.R. and S.M. Magnusson. Natural radiation in Iceland and the Faroe Islands. National Institute of Radiation Protection. SIS (1982).

E2 El-Khatib, A.M. and A.A. Abou El-Khier. Regional study of black sands radioactivity. Isotopenpraxis 24: 333-336 (1988).

E3 Eichholz, G.G., F.J. Clarke and B. Kahn. Radiation exposure from building materials. p. 1331-1346 in: Natural Radiation Environment III. CONF-780422, Volume 2 (1980).

E4 Environmental Protection Agency. Radon measurements in schools. An interim report. EPA 520/1-89-010 (1989).

E5 Elamin, O.I. National Council for Research, Khartoum Communication to the UNSCEAR Secretariat (1991).

E6 Enge, H. Introduction to Nuclear Physics. Addison-Wesley, Reading, Massachusetts, 1966.

F1 Fry, R.J.M. and D.S. Nachtwey. Radiation protection guidelines for space missions. Health Phys. 55: 159-164 (1988).

F2 Fujitaka, K. and S. Abe. Effect of partition walls and neighbouring buildings on indoor exposure rate due to cosmic-ray muons. Health Phys. 51: 647-659 (1986).

F3 Fujimoto, K. and S. Kobayashi. Shielding effect of snow cover on indoor exposure due to terrestrial gamma radiation. p. 910-913 in: Radiation Protection Practice. Proceedings of the 7th International Congress of the International Radiation Protection Association (Volume II). Pergamon Press, Sydney, 1988.

F4 Food and Agriculture Organization. FAO Food Balance Sheets, 1979-1981. FAO, Rome, 1984.

F5 Fisenne, I.M., P.M. Perry, K.M. Decker et al. The daily intake of uranium-234, 235, 238; thorium-228, 230, 232 and radium-226, 288 by New York City residents. Health Phys. 53: 357-363 (1987).

F6 Folkerts, K.H., G. Keller and H. Muth. An experimental study on diffusion and exhalation of Rn-222 and Rn-220 from building materials. Radiat. Prot. Dosim. 9: 27-34 (1984).

F7 Fisk, W.J. and R.J. Mowris. The impacts of balanced and exhaust mechanical ventilation on indoor radon. LBL-23136 (1987).

F8 Fisenne, I.M. Radon concentrations at Chester, NJ, and New York City. EML (1987).

F9 Fitzgerald, J.E. and E.L. Sensitaffar. Radiation exposure from construction materials utilizing byproduct gypsum from phosphate mining. Radioactivity in Consumer Products. NUREG/CP0001 (1978).

F10 Fujimoto, K. Significance of measurement of natural radiation in the fields of applied nuclear energy and radiation. Japanese Health Phys. 22: 411-419 (1987).

F11 Facetti, J.F. Comisión Nacional de Energia Atómica, Asunción. Communication to the UNSCEAR Secretariat (1991).

F12 Fujimoto, K. External gamma exposure to radon progeny in indoor air. J. Nucl. Sci. Technol. 22: 1001-1010 (1985).

F13 Fisenne, I.M. and P.M. Perry. Stable calcium and potassium in tissues from New York City residents. EML-455 (1986).

F14 Faísca, M.C., M.M.G. Teixeira and A.O. Bettencourt. Indoor radon concentrations in Portugal - a national survey. Radiat. Prot. Dosim. 45: 465-467 (1992).

G1 Gutiérrez, J., C. Baixeras, B. Robles et al. Indoor radon levels and dose estimation in two major Spanish cities. Radiat. Prot. Dosim. 45: 495-498 (1992).

G2 Grasty, R.L., J.M. Carson, B.W. Charbonneau et al. Natural background radiation in Canada. Geological Survey of Canada, Bulletin 360 (1984).

G3 Green, B.M.R., P.R. Lomas, E.J. Bradley et al. Gamma radiation levels outdoors in Great Britain. NRPB-R191 (1988).

G4 Gans, I. Natural radionuclides in mineral waters. Sci. Total Environ. 45: 93-99 (1985).

G5 Gans, I., H.U. Fusban, H. Wollenhaupt et al. Radium-226 und andere natürliche Radionuklide in Trinkwasser und in Getränken in der Bundesrepublik Deutschland. H4/1987. Institut für Wasser-, Boden- und Lufthygiene des Bundesgesundheitsamtes, Berlin, 1987.

G6 Gomez, J.C., A.A. Oliveira, M.I. Arnaud et al. Radon in dwellings in Argentina. p. 391-400 in: Proceedings of the International Conference on High Levels of Natural Radiation, Ramsar, 1990. IAEA, Vienna, 1993.

G7 Georgiou, E., K. Ntalles, M. Molfetas et al. Radon measurements in Greece. p. 387-390 in: Radiation Protection Practice. Proceedings of the 7th International Congress of the International Radiation Protection Association (Volume I). Pergamon Press, Sydney, 1988.

G8 Gutt, W. and P.J. Nixon. Use of waste materials in the construction industry. Analysis of the RILEM Symposium by Correspondence. Building Research Establishment Reprint R2/79 (1979).

G9 Guo, Q., M. Shimo, Y. Ikebe et al. The study of thoron and radon progeny concentrations in dwellings in Japan. Radiat. Prot. Dosim. 45: 357-359 (1992).

G10 Gadgil, A.J. Models of radon entry. Radiat. Prot. Dosim. 45: 373-380 (1992).

G11 Grasty, R.L. Summer outdoor radon variations in Canada and their relation to soil moisture. Health Phys. (accepted for publication, 1993).

H1 Hirman, J.W. Solar proton event forecasts. p. 61-70 in: Terrestrial Space Radiation and its Biological Effects. (P.D. McCormack, C.E. Swenberg and H. Bücker, eds.) Plenum Press, New York, 1988.

H2 Hajnal, F., J.E. McLaughlin, M.S. Weinstein et al. 1970 sea-level cosmic-ray neutron measurements. HASL-241 (1971).

H3 Hughes, H.J., K.B. Shaw and M.C. O'Riordan. Radiation exposure of the UK population - 1988 review. NRPB-R227 (1989).

H4 Herbst, W. Investigations of environmental radiation and its variability. p. 781-796 in: The Natural Radiation Environment. University of Chicago Press, Chicago, 1964.

H5 Hess, C.T., J. Michel, T.R. Horton et al. The occurrence of radioactivity in public water supplies in the United States. Health Phys. 48: 553-586 (1985).

H6 Horton, T.R. Nationwide occurrence of radon and other natural radioactivity in public water supplies. EPA 520/5-85-008 (1985).

H7 Holtzman, R.B. Application of radiolead to metabolic studies. in: The Biogeochemistry of Lead in the Environment. Elsevier, 1978.

H8 Hopke, P.K. A critical review of measurements of the "unattached" fraction of radon decay products. DOE/ER-0451P (1990).

H9 Harley, N.H. Lung cancer risk from exposure to environmental radon. Presented at the 3rd International Conference on Anticarcinogenesis and Radiation Protection, Dubrovnik, October 1989.

H10 Harley, N.H. and B.S. Pasternack. The beta dose to critical human tumor sites from krypton-85. Health Phys. 33: 567-575 (1977).

H11 Hopkin, S.M. and J.C. Ellis. Drinking water consumption in Great Britain. WRC-TR/137 (1980).

H12 Hewitt, J.E., L. Hughes, J.B. McCaslin et al. Exposure to cosmic-ray neutrons at commercial jet aircraft altitudes. p. 855-881 in: Natural Radiation Environment III. CONF-780422, Volume 2 (1980).

H13 Hua, J. and Y. Qingyu. The Estimation of Dose from Cosmic Radiation Received by the Population Living in Mainland Areas of China. Institute of Atomic Energy of China, Beijing, 1991.

H14 Holkko, J. and S. Liukkonen. Radon diffusion in Finnish glacial till soil. Radiat. Prot. Dosim. 45: 231-233 (1992).

H15 Hubbard, L.M., N. Hagberg and A. Enflo. Temperature effect on radon dynamics in two Swedish dwellings. Radiat. Prot. Dosim. 45: 381-386 (1992).

H16 Hopper, R.D., R.A. Levy, R.C. Rankin et al. National ambient radon study. Presented at the 1991 International Symposium on Radon and Radon Reduction Technology, Philadelphia, 1991.

H17 Hogeweg, B., B.F. Bosnjakovic and W.M. Willart. Radiation aspects of indoor environments and related radioecological problems: a study of the situation in the Netherlands. Radiat. Prot. Dosim. 7: 327-331 (1984).

H18 Hassib, G.M., M.I. Hussein, H.A. Amer et al. Assessment of radon concentration in Egyptian dwellings by using a passive technique. Atomic Energy Authority, Cairo (1992).

H19 Harrington, T. A study of potential radiation doses arising from a proposed mineral sand mine and processing plant in Victoria. Paper submitted to the Bulletin of the Australian Radiation Protection Society, March 1993.

H20 Hughes, J.S. 1992 review of UK population exposure. NRPB report (in preparation, 1993).

H21 Hopke, P.K., P. Wasiolek, N. Montassier et al. Measurement of activity-weighted size distributions of radon decay products in a normally occupied home. Radiat. Prot. Dosim. 45: 329-331 (1992).

H22 Hussein, M.I. and F.A. Kawy. Indoor gamma levels in some Egyptian cities. Atomic Energy Authority, Cairo (1992).

I1 Ibrahim, N., A. Abd El Ghani, S. Shawky et al. Measurements of radioactivity levels in soil in the Nile delta and middle Egypt. Health Phys. 64: 620-627 (1993).

I2 International Commission on Radiation Units and Measurements. Basic aspects of high energy particle interactions and radiation dosimetry. ICRU Report 28 (1978).

I3 International Civil Aviation Organization. Civil Aviation Statistics of the World. Doc 9180/15 (1990).

I4 International Commission on Radiological Protection. Annual Limits on Intakes of Radionuclides by Workers Based on the 1990 Recommendations. ICRP Publication 61. Annals of the ICRP. Pergamon Press, Oxford, 1991.

I5 International Commission on Radiological Protection. Report of the Task Group on Reference Man. ICRP Publication 23. Pergamon Press, Oxford, 1975.

I6 International Commission on Radiological Protection. 1990 Recommendations of the International Commission on Radiological Protection. ICRP Publication 60. Annals of the ICRP. Pergamon Press, Oxford, 1991.

I7 International Commission on Radiological Protection. Limits for Inhalation of Radon Daughters by Workers. ICRP Publication 32. Annals of the ICRP. Pergamon Press, Oxford, 1981.

I8 International Commission on Radiological Protection. Lung Cancer Risk from Indoor Exposures to Radon Daughters. ICRP Publication 50. Annals of the ICRP. Pergamon Press, Oxford, 1987.

J1 Julius, H.W. and R. van Dongen. Radiation doses to the population in the Netherlands, due to external natural sources. Sci. Total Environ. 45: 449-458 (1985).

J2 Jonassen, N. and J.P. McLaughlin. Exhalation of radon-222 from building materials and walls. p. 1211-1236 in: Natural Radiation Environment III. CONF-780422, Volume 2 (1980).

J3 Jacobi, W. and K. Eisfeld. Dose to tissues and effective dose equivalent by inhalation of radon-222, radon-220 and their short-lived daughters. GSF-8-626 (1980).

J4 James, A.C. A reconsideration of cells at risk and other key factors in radon daughter dosimetry. p. 400-418 in: Radon and its Decay Products: Occurrence, Properties and Health Effects. (P.K. Hopke, ed.) American Chemical Society, Washington, 1987.

J5 James, A.C., J.C. Strong, K.D. Cliff et al. The significance of equilibrium and attachment in radon daughter dosimetry. Radiat. Prot. Dosim. 24: 451-455 (1988).

J6 Jaworowski, J. Sources and the global cycle of radium. Chapter 2-2, pp. 129-142 in: The Environmental Behaviour of Radium. IAEA Technical Reports Series No. 10. Vienna, 1990.

J7 Jeffries, R.A. and J.B. Twining. Levels of radionuclides in edible tissues of organisms from Australian coastal waters. in: Proceedings of a Workshop on Environmental Radiochemistry and Radionuclide Measurement, Adelaide, 1990.

J8 Juntunen, R. Uranium and Radon in Wells Drilled Into Bedrock in Southern Finland. Report 98. Geological Survey of Finland, Espoo, 1991. (in Finnish)

J9 Jackson, J.A. Estimating radon potential from an aerial radiometric survey. Health Phys. 62:450-452 (1992).

J10 James, A.C. The dosimetry of human exposure to radon, thoron and their progeny. Part I: Quantification of lung cancer risk from indoor exposure. USDOE/EOH Radon Technological Report Series (1993).

J11 Jacobi, W. Radiation and lung cancer: problems and topics for future research. p. 15-19 in: Proceedings of the Workshop on the Future of Human Radiation Research, Schloss Elmau, 1991. BIR Report 22, London, 1991.

K1 Koperski, J. Exposure of urban populations to natural gamma background in Poland. Radiat. Prot. Dosim. 8: 163-171 (1984).

K2 Kusama, T., T. Nakagawa, M. Kai et al. Estimation of population dose from all sources in Japan. p. 14-17 in: Radiation Protection Practice. Proceedings of the 7th International Congress of the International Radiation Protection Association (Volume I). Pergamon Press, Sydney, 1988.

K3 Kauranen, P. and J.K. Miettinen. Po-210 and Pb-210 in the arctic food chain and the natural radiation exposure of Lapps. Health Phys. 16: 287-295 (1969).

K4 Kulich, J., H. Möre and G.A. Swedjemark. Radon and radium in household waters. SSI report 88-11 (1988). (in Swedish)

K5 Kobayashi, S., K. Fujimoto, T. Iwasaki et al. Nationwide survey of indoor radon concentration in Japan. p. 63-67 in: Proceedings of the Third International Symposium on Advanced Nuclear Energy Research, Mito City, Japan, 1991.

K6 Kojima, H. and S. Abe. Measurements of the total and unattached radon daughters in a house. Radiat. Prot. Dosim. 24: 241-244 (1988).

K7 Kendall, G.M., T.P. Fell and A.W. Phipps. A model to evaluate doses from radon in drinking water. Radiol. Prot. Bull. 97: 7-8 (1988).

K8 Kayser, P. Direction de la Santé, Luxembourg. Communication to the UNSCEAR Secretariat (1991).

K9 Kaul, A. Bundesamt für Strahlenschutz. Communication to the UNSCEAR Secretariat (1991).

K10 Kolb, W.A. Radiological significance of ^{227}Ac and ^{231}Pa. Health Phys. 61: 919 (1991).

K11 Kobal, I., J. Vaupotič, D. Mitić et al. Natural radioactivity of fresh waters in Slovenia, Yugoslavia. Environ. Int. 16: 141-154 (1990).

K12 Kenawy, M.A. and A.A. Morsy. Measurements of environmental radon-222 concentration in indoor and outdoors in Egypt. Nucl. Tracks Radiat. Meas. 19: 343-345 (1991).

K13 König, K. Bundesamt für Strahlenschutz. Communication to the UNSCEAR Secretariat (1991).

K14 Köksal, M., N. Celebi, N. Kiyak et al. Indoor ^{222}Rn monitoring in Turkey and ^{222}Rn levels in Istanbul houses. Health Phys. 65: 87-88 (1993).

K15 Katase, A., Y. Matsumoto, T. Sakae et al. Indoor concentrations of ^{220}Rn and its decay products. Health Phys. 54:283-286 (1988).

K16 Köster, H.W., H.P. Leenhouts, A.W. van Weers et al. Radioecological model calculations for natural radionuclides released into the environment by disposal of phosphogypsum. Sci. Total Environ. 45: 47-53 (1985).

K17 Koperski, J. Radiation protection in the mining and milling of mineral sands. Paper submitted to the Bulletin of the Australian Radiation Protection Society, March 1993.

L1 Lund, N. The abundances in the cosmic radiation. (The elements lighter than Ge.) p. 111-123 in: Cosmic Abundances of Matter. (C.J. Waddington, ed.) American Institute of Physics, New York, 1989.

L2 Leung, K.C., S.Y. Lau and C.B. Poon. Gamma radiation dose from radionuclides in Hong Kong soil. J. Environ. Radioact. 11: 279-290 (1990).

L3 Lemmelä, H. Measurements of environmental gamma radiation in Finland. Paper presented at the meeting of the Nordic Society for Radiation Protection. Geilo, Norway, 1980.

L4 Langroo, M.K., K.N. Wise, J.G. Duggleby et al. A nation-wide survey of radon and gamma radiation levels in Australian homes. Health Phys. 61: 753-761 (1991).

L5 Ladinskaya, L., Y.D. Parfenov, D.K. Popov et al. Lead-210 and polonium-210 content of air, water, foodstuffs and the human body. Arch. Environ. Health 27: 254-258 (1973).

L6 Lalit, B.Y. and V.K. Shukla. Natural radioactivity in foodstuffs from high natural radioactivity areas of southern India. p. 43-49 in: Natural Radiation Environment. (K.G. Vohra et al., eds.) Wiley Eastern Limited, New Delhi, 1982.

L7 Létourneau, E.G., R.G. McGregor and W.B. Walker. Design and interpretation of large surveys for indoor exposure to radon daughters. Radiat. Prot. Dosim. 7: 303-308 (1984).

L8 Landman, K.A. Diffusion of radon through cracks in a concrete slab. Health Phys. 43: 65-71 (1982).

L9 Lehmann, S. Bundesamt für Strahlenschutz, Berlin. Communication to the UNSCEAR Secretariat (1991).

L10 Linsalata, P., R. Morse, H. Ford et al. Th, U, Ra and rare earth element distributions in farm animal tissues from an elevated natural radiation background environment. J. Environ. Radioact. 14: 233-257 (1991).

L11 Linsalata, P., M. Eisenbud and E. Penna Franca. Ingestion estimates of Th and the light rare elements based on measurements of human feces. Health Phys. 50: 163-167 (1986).

M1 Myrick, T.E., B.A. Berven and F.F. Haywood. Determination of concentrations of selected radionuclides in surface soil in the U.S. Health Phys. 45: 631-642 (1983).

M2 Maurice, Y.T., ed. Uranium in granites. Paper 81-23 in: Proceedings of a workshop held in Ottawa, Ontario, 25-26 Nov. 1980. Canada Geological Survey; 1990.

M3 Madelmont, C., A. Rannou, H. Renouard et al. Sources externes: cosmique, tellurique et domestique. p. 61 in: Congrès sur les donneés actuelles sur la radioactivité naturelle. Monte Carlo, 1984.

M4 McAulay, I.R. and P.A. Colgan. γ-ray background radiation measurement in Ireland. Health Phys. 39: 821-826 (1980).

M5 Mellander, H. National Institute for Radiation Protection, Stockholm, Sweden. Communication to the UNSCEAR Secretariat (1990).

M6 Mason, G.C., S.B. Solomon, M.B. Cooper et al. Radiological assessment of mineral sand mining in Australia. p. 1347-1350 in: Radiation Protection Practice. Proceedings of the 7th International Congress of the International Radiation Protection Association (Volume III). Pergamon Press, Sydney, 1988.

M7 Mollah, A.S., S.C. Das, A. Begum et al. Indoor gamma radiation exposure at the Cox's Bazar coastal areas. Radiat. Prot. Dosim. 27: 43-45 (1989).

M8 McAulay, I.R. and J.P. McLaughlin. Indoor natural radiation levels in Ireland. Sci. Total Environ. 45: 319-325 (1985).

M9 Mjönes, L. Gamma radiation in Swedish dwellings. Radiat. Prot. Dosim. 15: 131-140 (1986).

M10 Miller, K.M. and A.C. George. External γ-ray dose rates from radon-222 progeny indoors. Health Phys. 54: 203-206 (1988).

M11 Martz, D.E., R.T. Harris and G.H. Langner. The half-life of Po-218. Health Phys. 57: 121-130 (1989).

M12 Mishra, U.C. and M.C. Subba Ramu. Natural radioactivity in houses and mine atmospheres in India. Radiat. Prot. Dosim. 24: 25-28 (1988).

M13 Mustafa, A.A., C.M. Vasisht and J. Sabol. Measurement and dosimetry of indoor concentrations in Kuwait. p. 246-250 in: Radiation Protection Practice. Proceedings of the 7th International Congress of the International Radiation Protection Association (Volume I). Pergamon Press, Sydney, 1988.

M14 Martz, D.E., R.J. Falco and G.H. Langer. Time-averaged exposures to ^{220}Rn and ^{222}Rn progeny in Colorado homes. Health Phys. 58: 705-713 (1990).

M15 May, H. and L.D. Marinelli. Cosmic ray contribution to the background of low-level scintillation spectrometers. p. 463-480 in: The Natural Radiation Environment. University of Chicago Press, Chicago, 1964.

M16 Montagne, C., J.P. Donne, D. Pelcot et al. Inflight radiation measurements aboard French airliners. Radiat. Prot. Dosim. 48: 79-83 (1993).

M17 Mjönes, L., A. Burén and G.A. Swedjemark. Radon concentrations in Swedish dwellings. The result of a nation-wide investigation. SSI-a 84-23 (1984).

M18 Miller, K.M. Measurements of external radiation in United States dwellings. Radiat. Prot. Dosim. 45: 535-539 (1992).

M19 Maisonneuve, J. and M-L. Remy. Les elements radioactifs naturels et les eaux thermominérales. in: Congrés sur les Données Actuelles sur la Radioactivité Naturelle, Monte Carlo. Societé Française de Radioprotection, 1984.

M20 Markkanen, M. and H. Arvela. Measurements of radon emanation from soils. Presented at the Nordic Society for Radiation Protection Annual Meeting, Ronneby, 1990.

M21 McAulay, I.R. and D. Marsh. Radium-226 concentrations in soil in the Republic of Ireland. Radiat. Prot. Dosim. 45: 265-267 (1992).

M22 Majborn, B. Seasonal variations of radon concentrations in single-family houses with different substructures. Radiat. Prot. Dosim. 45: 443-447 (1992).

M23 Megumi, K., S. Abe, M. Abe et al. Radon concentration, absorbed dose rate in air and concentration of natural radionuclides in soil in the Osaka district of Japan. Radiat. Prot. Dosim. 45: 477-482 (1992).

M24 Marcinowski, F. Nationwide survey of residential radon levels in the US. Radiat. Prot. Dosim. 45: 419-424 (1992).

M25 Mjönes, L., R. Falk, H. Mellander et al. Measurements of thoron and thoron progeny indoors in Sweden. Radiat. Prot. Dosim. 45: 349-352 (1992).

M26 McGregor, R.G. and H. Taniguchi. Radiation survey of Long Harbour, Newfoundland. Appendix F, p. 117-137 in: Task Force on Fluoride. Canadian Public Health Association, Long Harbour, (1978).

M27 Mjönes, L. Gamma radiation in dwellings. SSI-a81-18 (1981). (in Swedish)

N1 National Council on Radiation Protection and Measurements. Guidance on radiation received in space activities. NCRP Report No. 98 (1989).

N2 National Council on Radiation Protection and Measurements. Exposure of the population in the United States and Canada from natural background radiation. NCRP Report No. 94 (1987).

N3 National Council on Radiation Protection and Measurements. Neutron contamination from medical electron accelerators. NCRP Report No. 79 (1984).

N4 National Plant Food Institute. The Fertilizer Handbook. Washington, D.C., 1963.

N5 National Radiological Protection Board. Committed equivalent organ doses and committed effective doses from intakes of radionuclides. NRPB-R245 (1991).

N6 Nielsen, S.P. Terrestrial and cosmic radiation in Denmark. p. 101-110 in: Seminar on the Radiological Burden of Man from Natural Radioactivity in the Countries of the European Communities. V/2408/80. CEC, Luxembourg, 1980.

N7 Nikl, I. and L.B. Sztanyik. External indoor and outdoor gamma exposures in Hungary during the period of 1983-86. Radiat. Prot. Dosim. 24: 387-389 (1988).

N8 Nambi, K.S.V., V.N. Bapat, M. David et al. Natural background radiation and population dose distribution in India. Health Physics Division, Bhabha Atomic Research Centre, Bombay, 1986.

N9 Niewadomski, T., J. Koperski and E. Ryba. Natural radiation in Poland and its disturbance in an urban environment. Health Phys. 38: 25-32 (1980).

N10 Nuclear Energy Agency. Exposure to radiation from the natural radioactivity in building materials. Report by NEA Group of Experts. OECD, Paris, 1979.

N11 Nishikawa, T., S. Okabe and M. Aoki. Monte Carlo calculation of gamma-ray flux density due to atmospheric radon daughters. J. Nucl. Sci. Technol. 26: 525-529 (1989).

N12 Nguyen, V.D., L. Lebaron-Jacobs, P. Bouisset et al. Real time determintion of the quality factor and dose equivalent of cosmic radiation aboard French airliners. Presented at the International Congress of Aviation and Space Medicine, Tokyo, 1992.

N13 Nuclear Energy Agency. The radiological impact of the Chernobyl accident in OECD countries. OECD, Paris, 1987.

N14 Nazaroff, W.W., B.M. Moed and R.G. Sextro. Soil as a source of indoor radon: generation, migration and entry. p. 57-112 in: Radon and its Decay Products in Indoor Air. (W.W. Nazaroff and A.V. Nero, eds.) Wiley, New York, 1988.

N15 National Council on Radiation Protection and Measurements. Control of radon in houses. NCRP Report No. 103 (1989).

N16 Nazaroff, W.W. and R.G. Sextro. Technique for measuring the indoor ^{222}Rn source potential of soil. Environ. Sci. Technol. 23: 451-458 (1989).

N17 National Council on Radiation Protection and Measurements. Evaluation of occupational and environmental exposures to radon and radon daughters in the United States. NCRP Report No. 78 (1984).

N18 Nazaroff, W.W., S.M. Doyle, A.V. Nero et al. Radon entry via potable water. p. 131-157 in: Radon and its Decay Products in Indoor Air. (W.W. Nazaroff and A.V. Nero, eds.) Wiley, New York, 1988.

N19 Nero, A.V. Radon and its decay products in indoor air: an overview. p. 1-53 in: Radon and its Decay Products in Indoor Air. (W.W. Nazaroff and A.V. Nero, eds.) Wiley, New York, 1988

N20 Nero, A.V., A.J. Gadgil, W.W. Nazaroff et al. Indoor radon and decay products; concentrations, causes and control strategies. DOE/ER-0480P (1990).

N21 Nuclear Energy Agency. Dosimetry aspects of exposure to radon and thoron and decay products. NEA Expert Report. OECD, Paris, 1983.
N22 National Environmental Protection Agency. Nationwide survey of environmental radioactivity level in China (1983-1990). 90-S315-206. The People's Republic of China, 1990.
N23 Nakamura, T., Y. Uwamino, T. Ohkubo et al. Altitude variation of cosmic-ray neutrons. Health Phys. 53: 509-517 (1987).
O1 O'Riordan, M.C., M.J. Duggan, W.B. Rose et al. The radiological implications of using by-product gypsum as a building material. NRPB-R7 (1972).
O2 O'Brien, R.S., J.R. Peggie and I.S. Leith. Estimates of the radiation dose from phospho-gypsum plaster-board if used in domestic buildings. ARL/TR098 (1991).
O3 Oakley, D.T. Natural radiation exposure in the United States. USEPA ORP/SID 72-1 (1972).
O4 O'Brien, K. Human dose from radiation of terrestrial origin. p. 1163-1210 in: Natural Radiation Environment III. CONF-780422, Volume 2 (1980).
O5 O'Riordan, M.C., A.C. James and K. Brown. Some aspects of human exposure to Rn-222 decay products. Radiat. Prot. Dosim. 3: 75-82 (1982).
O6 Oppon, O.C., H.M. Aniagyei and A.W.K. Kyere. Monitoring of natural background radiation in some Ghanaian homes. p. 385-390 in: Proceedings of the International Conference on High Levels of Natural Radiation, Ramsar, 1990. IAEA, Vienna, 1993.
O7 Othman, I., M. Al-Hushari and G. Raja. Preliminary evaluation of Rn level in homes and offices in two different regions in Syria. p. 377-390 in: Proceedings of the International Conference on High Levels of Natural Radiation, Ramsar, 1990. IAEA, Vienna, 1993.
O8 O'Riordan, M.C. Human exposure to radon in homes. Documents of the NRPB, Volume 1(1) (1990).
O9 O'Brien, K., W. Friedberg, F.E. Duke et al. The exposure of aircraft crews to radiations of extraterrestrial origin. Radiat. Prot. Dosim. 45: 145-162 (1992).
O10 Oge, M. United States Environmental Protection Agency. Communication to the UNSCEAR Secretariat (1991).
P1 Pressler, J.W. By-product gypsum. p. 105-115 in: The Chemistry and Technology of Gypsum. ASTM-STP 861 (R.A. Kuntze, ed.). American Society for Testing and Material (1984).
P2 Petoussi, N., M. Zanke, K. Saito et al. Organ doses to adults and children from environmental gamma rays. p. 372-377 in: The Radioecology of Natural and Artificial Radionuclides. (W. Feldt, ed.) Verlag TüV Rheinland GmbH, Köln, 1989.
P3 Pfister, H. and H. Pauly. External radiation exposure due to natural radionuclides in phosphate fertilizers in the Federal Republic of Germany. p. 447-467 in: Seminar on the Radiological Burden of Man from Natural Radioactivity in the Countries of the European Communities. V/2408/80. CEC, Luxembourg, 1980.
P4 Pfeiffer, W.C., E. Penna-Franca, C. Costa Ribeiro et al. Measurements of environmental radiation exposure dose rates at selected sites in Brazil. An. Acad. Bras. Cienc. 53: 683-691 (1981).
P5 Pellerin, P. Resultats relatifs a la surveillance de l'environnement et a la surveillance medicale pour l'annee 1988. SCPRI, France, 1989.
P6 Paul, A.C., T. Velayudhan, P. Pillai et al. Radiation exposure at the high background area at Manavalakurichi - the changing trends. J. Environ. Radioactitity (in press, 1993).
P7 Persson, B.R. Lead-210, polonium-210 and stable lead in the food-chain lichen, reindeer and man. p. 347-367 in: The Natural Radiation Environment II. CONF-720805-P1 (1972).
P8 Pires do Rio, M.A., J.M. Godoy and E.C.S. Amaral. Ra-226, Ra-228 and Pb-210 concentrations in Brazilian mineral waters. Radiat. Prot. Dosim. 24: 159-161 (1988).
P9 Pellerin, P., M.E. Gahinet, J.P. Moroni et al. Quelques observations a propos de la radioactivite naturelle de l'alimentation en France. p. 331-348 in: Seminar on the Radiological Burden of Man from Natural Radioactivity in the Countries of the European Communities. V/2408/80. CEC, Luxembourg, 1980.
P10 Porstendörfer, J. and A. Wicke. Radon and radon daughters in dwellings. p. 189-196 in: Proceedings of the Specialist Meeting on Personnel Dosimetry and Area Monitoring Suitable for Radon and Daughter Products. OECD, Paris, 1978.
P11 Perritt, R.L., T.D. Hartwell, L.S. Sheldon et al. Radon-222 levels in New York State homes. Health Phys. 58: 147-155 (1990).
P12 Porstendörfer, J. and T.T. Mercer. Influence of nuclei concentration and humidity upon the attachment rate of atoms in the atmosphere. Atmos. Environ. 12: 2223-2228 (1978).
P13 Porstendörfer, J., A. Reineking and K.H. Becker. Free fractions, attachment rates, and plate-out rates of radon daughters in houses. p. 285-300 in: Radon and its Decay Products: Occurrence, Properties and Health Effects. (P.K. Hopke, ed.) American Chemical Society, Washington, 1987.
P14 Porstendörfer, J., A. Wicke and A. Schraub. The influence of exhalation, ventilation and deposition processes upon the concentration of radon (Rn-222), thoron (Rn-220) and their decay products in room air. Health Phys. 34: 465-473 (1978).
P15 Peterman, B.F. and C.J. Perkins. Dynamics of radioactive chemically inert gases in the human body. Radiat. Prot. Dosim. 22: 5-12 (1988).
P16 Porstendörfer, J. and A. Reineking. Indoor behaviour and characteristics of radon progeny. Radiat. Prot. Dosim. 45: 303-311 (1992).
P17 Penna-Franca, E., C. Costa-Ribeiro, P. Cullen et al. Natural radioactivity in Brazil: a comprehensive review with a model for dose-effect studies. p. 929-940 in: The Natural Radiation Environment II. CONF-720805-P2 (1972).
P18 Pinnock, W.R. Measurements of radioactivity in Jamaican building materials and gamma dose equivalents in a prototype red mud house. Health Phys. 61: 647-651 (1991).
P19 Petoussi, N., P. Jacob, M. Zankl et al. Organ doses for foetuses, babies, children and adults from environmental gamma rays. Radiat. Prot. Dosim. 37: 31-34 (1991).

P20 Pietrzak-Flis, Z. Radium-226 in Polish diet and foodstuffs. Nukleonika 27: 227-231 (1972).

P21 Pan Ziqiang, He Zhenyun, Yang Yin et al. Natural background radiation and population dose in China. China Nuclear Science and Technology report CNIC-00675 and BSPEH-0006 (1992).

P22 Pan Ziqiang. Radiological impact of coal-fired energy in China. China National Nuclear Corporation, Beijing. (1993).

P23 Pan Ziqiang. China National Nuclear Corporation, Beijing. Communation to the UNSCEAR Secretariat (1993).

P24 Put, L.W. and R.J. de Meijer. Survey of radon concentrations in Dutch dwellings. p.49-54 in: Proceedings of the 3rd International Conference on Indoor Air Quality and Climate. Stockholm, Sweden, 1984.

P25 Put, L.W., R.J. de Meijer and B. Hogeweg. Survey of radon concentrations in Dutch dwellings. Sci. Total Environ. 45: 441-448 (1985).

Q1 Quindos, L.S., P.L. Fernandez, C. Rodenas et al. Estimate of external gamma exposure outdoors in Spain. Radiat. Prot. Dosim. 45: 527-529 (1992).

Q2 Quindos, L.S., P.L. Fernandez and J. Soto. Exposure to natural sources of radiation in Spain. Presented at the International Conference on the Implications of the New ICRP Recommendations on Radiation Protection Practices and Interventions, Salamanca, 1991.

Q3 Quindos, L.S., P.L. Fernandez and J. Soto. National survey of indoor radon in Spain. Environ. Int. 17: 101-105 (1991).

R1 Reineking, A., G. Butterweck, J. Kesten et al. Thoron gas concentration and aerosol characteristics of thoron decay products. Radiat. Prot. Dosim. 45: 353-356 (1992).

R2 Rannou, A., C. Madelmont and H. Renouard. Survey of natural radiation in France. Sci. Total Environ. 45: 467-474 (1985).

R3 Robertson, M.K., M.W. Randle and L.J. Tucker. Natural radiation in New Zealand houses. NRL 1988/6 (1988).

R4 Revzan, K.L. and W.J. Fisk. Modelling radon entry into houses and basements: the influence of structural factors. LBL-28019 (1990).

R5 Ren, T., Z. Liu, L. Tang et al. Indoor radon measurements in the Shenzhen region of the People's Republic of China. Radiat. Prot. Dosim. 22: 159-164 (1988).

R6 Rannou, A. and G. Tymen. Les resultats des campagnes de mesures de radon et facteurs explicatifs. p. 42-63 in: Exposition au Radon dans les Habitations - Aspects Techniques et Sanitaires. SFRP, Paris, 1989.

R7 Rannou, A. The bare detector and results of indoor radon survey in France. in: Proceedings of the Workshop on Radon Monitoring in Radioprotection, Environmental Radioactivity and Earth Sciences, Trieste, 1989.

R8 Regulla, D. and J. David. Radiation measurements in civil aircraft. GSF-41/91 (1991).

R9 Reineking, A. and J. Porstendörfer. "Unattached" fraction of short-lived Rn decay products in indoor and outdoor environments: an improved single-screen method and results. Health Phys. 58: 715-727 (1990).

R10 Reineking, A., G. Butterweck, J. Porstendörfer et al. Intercomparison of methods for investigating the physical characteristics of radon decay products in the indoor environment. Radiat. Prot. Dosim. 45: 41-46 (1992).

R11 Ramachandran, T.V. and U.C. Mishra. Exposure to natural radiation sources of Bombay population. Indian J. Occup. Health 31: 68-72 (1988).

R12 Remy, M.-L. and N. Lemaitre. Eaux minérales et radioactivité. Hydrogéologie 4: 267-278 (1990).

R13 Remy, M.-L. and P. Pellerin. Radioactivité naturelle de 250 sources hydrominérales francaises. Bulletin Inserm T23/1 (1968).

R14 Remy, M.-L. and P. Pellerin. Quelques données générales sur la radioactivité des sources hydrominérales francaises. in: Colloque Sur Les Eaux Thermominérales, Bagnères de Luchon. Association des Géolgues du Sud-Ouest, 1981.

R15 Robé, M.C., A. Rannou and J. Le Bronec. Radon measurement in the environment in France. Radiat. Prot. Dosim. 45: 455-457 (1992).

S1 Stassinopoulos, E.G. The earth's trapped and transient space radiation environment. p. 5-35 in: Terrestrial Space Radiation and its Biological Effects. (P.D. McCormack ed.) Plenum Press, New York, 1988.

S2 Stranden, E. Population doses from environmental gamma radiation in Norway. Health Phys. 33: 319-323 (1977).

S3 Stuardo, E. Natural radiation external exposure levels in Chilean sub-antarctic and country stations. p. 926-929 in: Radiation Protection Practice. Proceedings of the 7th International Congress of the International Radiation Protection Association (Volume II). Pergamon Press, Sydney, 1988.

S4 Simopoulos, S.E. Natural Radioactivity Analysis Results of Greek Surface Soil Samples. National Technical University, MPX-3, Athens, 1990.

S5 Swedjemark, G.A. Terrestrial and cosmic radiation in Scandinavia. p. 125-147 in: Seminar on the Radiological Burden of Man from Natural Radioactivity in the Countries of the European Communities. V/2408/80. CEC, Luxembourg, 1980.

S6 Sunta, C.M., M. David, M.C. Abani et al. Analysis of dosimetry data of high natural radioactivity areas of SW coast of India. p. 35-42 in: Natural Radiation Environment. (K.G. Vohra et al., eds.). Wiley Eastern Limited, New Delhi, 1982.

S7 Sunta, C.M. A review of the studies of high background areas of the S-W coast of India. p. 71-86 in: Proceedings of the International Conference on High Levels of Natural Radiation, Ramsar, 1990. IAEA, Vienna, 1993.

S8 Snihs, J.O. National Institute of Radiation Protection, Stockholm, Sweden. Communication to the UNSCEAR Secretariat (1990).

S9 Statens Institut for Stralenhygiejne. Natural radiation in Danish homes. Riso, Denmark, 1987.

S10 Stranden, E. Natural radionuclides in the atmospheric and terrestrial environments in the Nordic countries. p. 3-8 in: The Radioecology of Natural and Terrestrial Radionuclides. (W. Feldt, ed.) Verlag TüV Rheinland, Köln, 1989.

S11 Service Central de Protection contre les Rayonnements Ionisants. Communication to the UNSCEAR Secretariat (1990).

S12 Saito, K., N. Petoussi, M. Zankl et al. Calculation of organ doses from environmental gamma rays using human phantoms and Monte Carlo methods. Part 1. Monoenergetic sources of natural radionuclides in the ground. GSF-B2/90 (1990).

S13 Smith-Briggs, J.L., E.J. Bradley and M.D. Potter. Measurement of natural radionuclides in United Kingdom diet. Sci. Total Environ. 35: 431-440 (1984).

S14 Smith-Briggs, J.L., E.J. Bradley and M.D. Poster. The ratio of lead-210 to polonium-210 in UK diet. Sci. Total Environ. 54: 127-133 (1986).

S15 Salonen, L. Natural radionuclides in ground water in Finland. Radiat. Prot. Dosim. 24: 163-166 (1988).

S16 Stein, L. Chemical properties of radon. p. 240-251 in: Radon and its Decay Products. (P.K. Hopke, ed.) ACS, Washington D.C., 1987.

S17 Stranden, E. Building materials as a source of indoor radon. p. 113-130 in: Radon and its Decay Products in Indoor Air. (W.W. Nazaroff and A.V. Nero, eds.) Wiley, New York, 1988.

S18 Stranden, E., A.K. Kolstad and B. Lind. The influence of moisture and temperature on radon exhalation. Radiat. Prot. Dosim. 7: 55-58 (1984).

S19 Schery, S.D., D.H. Gaeddert and M.H. Wilkening. Factors affecting exhalation of radon from a gravelly sandy loam. J. Geophys. Res. 89: 7299-7309 (1984).

S20 Stranden, E. and L. Berteig. Radon in dwellings and influencing factors. Health Phys. 39: 275-284 (1980).

S21 Stevens, R. Building Research Establishment, Watford, United Kingdom. Communication to the UNSCEAR Secretariat (1990).

S22 Steinhäusler, F. Radon in the environment: a global approach. p. 1549-1552 in: Worldwide Achievement in Public and Occupational Health Protection Against Radiation. Proceedings of 8th International Congress of the IRPA, Montreal, Canada, May 1992.

S23 Schery, S.D. Measurements of airborne Pb-212 and Rn-220 concentrations at varied locations within the United States. Health Phys. 49: 1061-1067 (1985).

S24 Subba Ramu, M.C., T.V. Ramachandran, T.S. Muraleedharan et al. Indoor levels of radon daughters in some high background areas of India. Radiat. Prot. Dosim. 30: 41-44 (1990).

S25 Subba Ramu, M.C., A.N. Shaikh, T.S. Muraleedharan et al. Measurements of the equilibrium factor for ^{222}Rn daughters in dwellings in India. Sci. Total Environ. 99: 49-52 (1990).

S26 Sohrabi, M. and A.R. Solaymanian. Indoor radon level measurements in Iran using AEOI passive dosimeters. p. 242-245 in: Radiation Protection Practice. Proceedings of the 7th International Congress of the International Radiation Protection Association (Volume 1). Pergamon Press, Sidney, 1988.

S27 Strong, J.C. The size of attached and unattached radon daughters in room air. J. Aerosol Sci. 19: 1327-1330 (1988).

S28 Stranden, E. and T. Strand. A dosimetric discussion based on measurements of radon daughter equilibrium and unattached fraction in different atmospheres. Radiat. Prot. Dosim. 16: 313-318 (1986).

S29 Schmier, H. and A. Wicke. Results from a survey of indoor radon exposures in the Federal Republic of Germany. Sci. Total Environ. 45: 307-310 (1985).

S30 Schuhmacher, H. and U.J. Schrewe. Dose equivalent measurements on board civil aircraft. PTB-N-13 (1993).

S31 Soekarno, S. National Atomic Energy Agency, Jakarta, Indonesia. Communication to the UNSCEAR Secretariat (1991).

S32 Steinhäusler, F. and H. Lettner. Radiometric survey in Namibia. Radiat. Prot. Dosim. 45: 553-555 (1992).

S33 Sohrabi, M. High level natural radiation areas with special regard to Ramsar. Presented at Second Workshop on Radon in Radioprotection, Environmental and Earth Sciences, ICTP, Trieste, 1991.

S34 Slegers, W. Terrestrial radiation in Belgium. Ministère Santé Publique, Brussels (1989). (unpublished report)

S35 Saito, K. External doses due to terrestrial gamma rays on the snow cover. Radiat. Prot. Dosim. 35: 31-39 (1991).

S36 Schery, S.D., S. Whittlestone, K.P. Hart et al. The flux of radon and thoron from Australian soils. J. Geophys. Res. 94: 8567-8576 (1989).

S37 Subba Ramu, M.C., A.N. Shaikh, T.S. Muraleedharan et al. Environmental radon monitoring in India and a plea for a national effort. Presented at the Conference on Particle Tracks in Solids, Jodhpur, 1991.

S38 Surbeck, H. and H. Völkle. Radon in Switzerland. Presented at the 1991 International Symposium on Radon and Radon Reduction Technology, Philadelphia, 1991.

S39 Strand, T., B.M.R. Green and P.R. Lomas. Radon in Norwegian dwellings. Radiat. Prot. Dosim. 45: 503-508 (1992).

S40 Steinhäusler, F., W. Hofmann, E. Pohl et al. Local and temporal distribution pattern of radon and daughters in an urban environment and determination of organ-dose frequency distributions with demoscopical methods. p. 1145-1162 in: Natural Radiation Environment III. CONF-780422 (1980).

S41 Steinhäusler, F. Long-term investigations in Austria of environmental natural sources of ionizing radiation and their impace on man. Ber. Nat. Med. Ver. Salzburg 6: 7-50 (1982).

S42 Swedjemark, G.A. and L. Mjönes. Radon and radon daughter concentrations in Swedish houses. Radiat. Prot. Dosim. 7: 341-345 (1984).

S43 Swedjemark, G.A., H. Mellander and L. Mjönes. Radon levels in the 1988 Swedish Housing Stock. in: Indoor Air '93. Proceedings of the 6th International Conference on Indoor Air Quality and Climate, Helsinki, 1993.

S44 Spencer, H., D. Osis, I.M. Fisenne et al. Measured intake and excretion patterns of naturally occurring ^{234}U, ^{238}U, and calcium in humans. Radiat. Res. 124: 90-95 (1990).

S45 Siotis, I. and A.D. Wrixon. Radiological consequences of the use of fly ash in building materials in Greece. Radiat. Prot. Dosim. 7: 101-105 (1984).

S46 Solomon, S.B. and T. Ren. Characterisation of indoor airborne radioactivity. Radiat. Prot. Dosim. 45: 323-327 (1992).

S47 Stranden, E. Assessment of the radiological impact of using fly ash in cement. Health Phys. 44: 145-153 (1983).

S48 Sed, L.J., O. Rodríguez, R.A. Moreno et al. Organización de la red nacional de vigilancia radiológica ambiental de la República de Cuba. Presentado en el Primer Congreso Regional sobre Seguridad Radiológica y Nuclear, Buenos Aires, 21-25 October 1991.

T1 Tschirf, E. External natural radiation exposure in Austria. p. 175-176 in: Seminar on the Radiological Burden of Man from Natural Radioactivity in the Countries of the European Communities. V/2408/80. CEC, Luxembourg, 1980.

T2 Toader, M. External irradiation from natural sources to the population of Romania. Igiena 28(3): 215-222 (1979). (in Romanian)

T3 Thomas, J., J. Hůlka and J. Salava. New houses with high radiation exposure levels. p. 177-182 in: Proceedings of the International Conference on High Levels of Natural Radiation, Ramsar, 1990. IAEA, Vienna, 1993.

T4 Tanner, A.B. Radon migration in the ground: a supplementary review. p. 5-56 in: Natural Radiation Environment III. CONF-780422, Volume 1 (1980).

T5 Toth, A., I. Fehér, S. Novotny Lakatos et al. Distribution of natural radioactive isotope concentrations and emanation factors measured on concrete and brick samples produced in Hungary. p. 1396-1406 in: Natural Radiation Environment III. CONF-780422, Volume 2 (1980).

T6 Thomas, J., E. Kunz, J. Salava et al. Current state of the indoor radon problem in the CSR. Kernenergie 32: 13-15 (1989).

T7 Tu, K.W. and A.C. George. Indoor thoron progeny measurements. EML-520 (1988).

T8 Thomas, J. A review of surveys of indoor radon measurements in Czechoslovakia. p. 1-12 in: Radon Investigations in Czechoslovakia II. Geological Survey, Prague, 1991.

T9 Tso, M.W. and J.K.C. Leung. Survey of indoor ^{222}Rn concentrations in Hong Kong. Health Phys. 60: 237-241 (1991).

T10 Tufail, M., M. Amin, W. Akhtar et al. Radon concentration in some houses of Islamabad and Rawalpindi, Pakistan. Nucl. Tracks Radiat. Meas. 19: 429-430 (1991).

T11 Tsui, K.C., M.C. Wong and B.Y. Lee. Field estimation of cosmic contribution to total external gamma radiation in Hong Kong. Environmental Radiation Monitoring, Hong Kong, Technical Report No. 4 (1991).

T12 Tso, M.W. and C.C. Li. Terrestrial gamma radiation dose in Hong Kong. Health Phys. 62: 77-81 (1992).

T13 Tymen, G., M.C. Robe and A. Rannou. Measurements of aerosol and radon daughters in five radon houses. Radiat. Prot. Dosim. 45: 319-322 (1992).

U1 United Nations. Sources, Effects and Risks of Ionizing Radiation. United Nations Scientific Committee on the Effects of Atomic Radiation, 1988 Report to the General Assembly, with annexes. United Nations sales publication E.88.IX.7. United Nations, New York, 1988.

U3 United Nations. Ionizing Radiation: Sources and Biological Effects. United Nations Scientific Committee on the Effects of Atomic Radiation, 1982 Report to the General Assembly, with annexes. United Nations sales publication E.82.IX.8. United Nations, New York, 1982.

U4 United Nations. Sources and Effects of Ionizing Radiation. United Nations Scientific Committee on the Effects of Atomic Radiation, 1977 report to the General Assembly, with annexes. United Nations sales publication E.77.IX.1. United Nations, New York, 1977.

U5 United Nations. Ionizing Radiation: Levels and Effects. Report of the United Nations Scientific Committee on the Effects of Atomic Radiation, with annexes. United Nations sales publication E.72.IX.17 and 18. United Nations, New York, 1972.

U11 United Nations. World Population Prospects 1988. United Nations, New York, 1989.

U12 United States Environmental Protection Agency. National Residential Radon Survey. EPA 402/R-92-011 (1992).

U13 United Nations. Industrial Statistics Yearbook 1985. United Nations, New York, 1987.

U14 Ulbak, K., N. Jonassen and K. Backmark. Radon exhalation from samples of concrete with different porosities and fly ash additives. Radiat. Prot. Dosim. 7: 45-48 (1984).

U15 Ulbak, K., B. Stenum, A. Sorensen et al. Results from the Danish indoor radiation survey. Radiat. Prot. Dosim. 24: 401-405 (1988).

V1 Van Dongen, R. and J.R.D. Stoute. Outdoor natural background radiation in the Netherlands. Sci. Total Environ. 45: 381-388 (1985).

V2 van de Ven-Breken, T.J., J. Brenot, S. Bonnefous et al. Consumption of food in EC countries: CEC research programme post-Chernobyl. Underlying data for derived emergency reference levels. Report 243402002. National Institute of Public Health and Environmental Protection, Bilthoven, 1990.

V3 Vasconcellos, L.M.H., E.C.S. Amaral and M.E. Vianna. Uptake of Ra-226 and Pb-210 by food crops cultivated in a region of high natural radioactivity in Brazil. J. Environ. Radioact. 5: 287-302 (1987).

V4 Vanmarcke, H., A. Janssens, F. Raes et al. The behaviour of radon daughters in the domestic environment. Effect on the effective dose equivalent. p. 301-323 in: Radon and its Decay Products: Occurrence, Properties and Health Effects. (P.K. Hopke, ed.) American Chemical Society, Washington, 1987.

V5 Vanmarcke, H., P. Berkvens and A. Poffijn. Radon versus Rn daughters. Health Phys. 56: 229-231 (1989).

V6 Vassilev, G. Irradiation of the population from the natural background. Committee on the Use of Atomic Energy for Peaceful Purposes, Sofia, 1991.

V7 Vicente, R., J.C. Dellamano and S.A. Bellintani. Radiological significance of ^{227}Ac and ^{231}Pa. Health Phys. 60: 719-720 (1991).

V8 Vanmarke, H. Studiecentrum voor Kernenergie, Mol, Belgium. Communication to the UNSCEAR Secretariat. (1991).

V9 Van der Lugt, G. and L.C. Scholten. Radon emanation from concrete and the influence of using fly ash in cement. Sci. Total Environ. 45: 143-150 (1985).

W1 Wilson, J.W. and L.W. Townsend. Radiation safety in commercial air traffic: a need for further study. Health Phys. 55: 1001-1003 (1988).

W2 Wollenberg, H.A. and A.R. Smith. A geochemical assessment of terrestrial gamma-ray absorbed dose rates. Health Phys. 58: 183-189 (1990).

W3 Wrixon, A.D., B.M.R. Green, P.R. Lomas et al. Natural radiation exposure in UK dwellings. NRPB-R190 (1988).

W4 World Health Organization. Derived Intervention Levels for Radionuclides in Food. WHO, Geneva, 1988.

W5 Weast, R.C., M.J. Astle and W.H. Beyer (eds.). Handbook of Chemistry and Physics. CRC Press, 1985.

W6 Wollenberg, H.A. Naturally occurring radioelements and terrestrial gamma-ray exposure rates: an assessment based on recent geochemical data. LBL-18714 (1984).

W7 Wilkening, M.H., W.E. Clements and D. Stanley. Radon-222 flux measurements in widely separated regions. p. 717-730 in: The Natural Radiation Environment II. CONF-720805-P2 (1972).

W8 Wrixon, A.D., S.L. Wan and K.D. Cliff. The origin of indoor radon. p. 228-231 in: Radiation Protection Practice. Proceedings of the 7th International Congress of the International Radiation Protection Association (Volume 1). Pergamon Press, Sidney, 1988.

W9 Webb, G.A.M. Exposure to radon. Radiat. Prot. Dosim. 42: 191-195 (1992).

W10 Wilson, C. Regional environmental documentation of natural radiation in Sweden. in: Proceedings of International Meeting on Radon-Radon Progeny Measurements. EPA 520/5-83/021 (1983).

Y1 Yue, Q.Y. and H. Jin. Measurement of ionization distribution in the lower atmosphere caused by cosmic ray. in: Proceedings of Workshop on Occupational and Environmental Radiation Protection, Hong Kong, 7-9 December 1987.

Z1 Zhu, H. Investigation of food radioactivity and estimation of external dose by ingestion in two Chinese high radiation areas. p. 153-162 in: Proceedings of the International Conference on High Levels of Natural Radiation, Ramsar, 1990. IAEA, Vienna, 1993.

Z2 Zuoyuan, W. Natural Radiation in China: Level and Distribution. Laboratory of Industrial Hygiene, Beijing, 1992.

ANNEX B

Exposures from man-made sources of radiation

CONTENTS

INTRODUCTION

1. Several practices and activities of man involving the production and use of radionuclides have resulted in releases of radioactive materials to the environment. Some of these activities have ceased, such as testing of nuclear weapons in the atmosphere, and some are continuing, such as electrical energy generation by nuclear reactors and radioisotope production and usage. In carrying out these activities, several accidents have occurred at nuclear installations and waste storage sites and in the transport of weapons or nuclear materials, causing in some cases significant contamination of the local environment. The purpose of this Annex is to evaluate and compare the collective doses to the local and global populations from these various man-made sources of radiation exposures.

2. Most of these subjects have been dealt with in the past by the Committee in separate assessments. Atmospheric nuclear testing and nuclear power production, in particular, have been extensively analysed. In this Annex, the evaluation procedures are summarized, and the dose calculations are extended. For nuclear power production, estimates of average releases per unit electrical energy generated are combined with data on energy generated by all reactors to evaluate the total releases of radionuclides worldwide and the collective dose from the beginning of this practice. For the first time since the Committee began its assessments of exposures from nuclear power production, there is complete reporting of radionuclides released from all reactors in operation in all countries for the latest evaluation period. The Committee acknowledges the cooperation of a great many scientists and officials who have made these data available for this evaluation.

3. A number of sources cannot be so systematically evaluated. These include releases from the use of radioisotopes in industries or hospitals, in which only trace contamination and very low doses result, and in the military fuel cycle, for which data have been restricted and the dose evaluations have therefore remained incomplete and uncertain. In this Annex the Committee considers these various sources to the extent possible to provide a comprehensive assessment of exposures from man-made sources.

4. Exposures from accidents of environmental significance are summarized here. Most of the doses resulting from these sources were evaluated in detail at the time of occurrence, in particular the doses

throughout the northern hemisphere from the Chernobyl accident, presented in the UNSCEAR 1988 Report [U1]. However, further data are becoming available on some accidents that occurred many years ago, when the full disclosure of details was not possible. This information is considered here to provide indications of the population doses that were received. Evaluations of doses to populations living near nuclear test sites have been undertaken, and some dose estimates have been provided in published reports. These results are also included in this Annex. For the various sources, the collective doses evaluated are those committed by the specific releases. If less than the complete dose commitments have been evaluated, the integration times are specified in the discussions for each type of source.

I. ATMOSPHERIC NUCLEAR TESTING

5. A very important concern of the Committee since its inception has been to evaluate the exposures caused by nuclear explosions in the atmosphere. The first atmospheric nuclear explosions took place in 1945. Subsequent testing of nuclear weapons in the atmosphere occurred until 1980, with periods of intensive testing in the years 1952-1954, 1957-1958 and 1961-1962. A limited nuclear test ban treaty (Treaty Banning Nuclear Weapon Tests in the Atmosphere, in Outer Space and Under the Water) was signed in August 1963, and much less frequent testing in the atmosphere occurred subsequently.

6. Exposures from nuclear weapons tests in the atmosphere have been reviewed by the Committee in all its previous reports until the cessation of the practice [U3-U10]. As there have been no tests in the atmosphere since October 1980, the most recent analysis prepared by the Committee, in the UNSCEAR 1982 Report [U3], remains complete and valid. These results and the generally applicable methodologies of exposure assessment are summarized here.

7. The basic quantity of radiation dose evaluations for radionuclides released to the environment is the dose commitment. Dose commitments are calculated from the input of radionuclides into the environment, using transfer coefficients relating appropriate time-integrated quantities in environmental compartments and in man. Schematic representation of the methodology used by the Committee for evaluating exposures from radionuclides released in nuclear testing is illustrated in Figure I. Transfer coefficients are used to relate input, integrated concentrations of radionuclides and dose in successive environmental compartments. For example, the transfer coefficient from diet to tissue is the ratio of the integrated concentration of the radionuclide in tissue to that in diet and is designated P_{34}. Transfers linking input to dose are determined by the sequential multiplication of transfer coefficients. Transfers by parallel pathways are assumed to be independent and are thus additive. For the transfers indicated in Figure I, the dose commitment for a specific radionuclide and a given tissue, D_c, due to an environmental input A_0 into the atmosphere is given by

$$D_c = P_{01}[P_{12}P_{23}P_{34}P_{45} + P_{14}P_{45} + P_{15} + P_{12}P_{25}]A_0 \qquad (1)$$

8. In this formula the transfer coefficient P_{01} is the integrated concentration of a radionuclide in air at a specified location or averaged for a broader region, divided by the amount released. The first term in the brackets relates the subsequent transfer to deposition, diet, tissue and dose via ingestion. The second term (P_{14} P_{45}) is the transfer from the atmosphere to tissue and dose via inhalation. The third term (P_{15}) accounts for direct (cloud gamma) irradiation from the radionuclide in air. The fourth term is the component of external irradiation from radionuclides deposited on the ground. Some minor pathways (e.g., resuspension) have not been indicated in Figure I, but these are taken into account in determining the integrated concentrations in the compartments. To this extent, the model indicates compartment interrelationships rather than mechanical transfer pathways. Although the terminology was developed for evaluations of doses from radionuclides produced in atmospheric nuclear testing, the methodology is generally applicable to any source of release of radionuclides to the air or terrestrial environment.

A. ENVIRONMENTAL INPUT

9. A nuclear device derives its explosive energy, usually expressed in kilotonnes or megatonnes of TNT equivalent, from one or both of two nuclear processes: fission of the heavy nuclides ^{235}U and ^{239}Pu in a chain reaction and fusion of the hydrogen isotopes deuterium and tritium in a thermonuclear process. Fission produces a whole spectrum of different radioactive nuclides, while fusion in principle creates

only tritium. However, because a thermonuclear device needs high pressures and temperatures to ignite it, in practice a fission device is needed as a primary stage to provide these conditions. Also in practice, the nuclear reactions do not proceed to ultimate completion, so some residual amounts of tritium will also remain. Thus, the explosion of a fusion charge always implies that at least some residual radioactive material is released. Many thermonuclear devices also produce large amounts of radioactive debris in a second fission stage, where high energy neutrons from the fusion reactions are utilized to split the atoms of a ^{238}U blanket. In some fission charges a small thermonuclear stage is used primarily to make neutrons and boost the utilization of the fissile material.

10. The exact composition of products of the fission process depends on the mixture of fissioning nuclides (^{235}U, ^{239}Pu and ^{238}U) and on the neutron energies involved. However, for the purpose of estimating dose commitments, it is sufficient to use average production values per unit fission yield. These are dominated by the ^{238}U high-energy neutron fission mode, as this type of fission was the predominant one in past atmospheric testing.

11. Neutron activation products are produced in significant amounts in fusion explosions from reactions of neutrons with surrounding materials, such as nitrogen in the air and the construction materials of the device. One very important such product is ^{14}C, which is made in the $^{14}N(n,p)^{14}C$ reaction in the atmosphere. The fusion yields are thus of interest for estimating doses from certain radionuclides. Fusion yields are also important, as they are the second part of the total yield, which governs the altitude to which the nuclear cloud rises and, as a result, the time delay before the debris reaches man.

12. A total of 520 atmospheric nuclear explosions (including 8 underwater) have occurred at a number of locations [D2, D8, Z1]. Based on a survey of published estimates of nuclear yields of different tests and measurements of deposited amounts of radioactive materials, Bennett [B5] compiled a list of individual yields of atmospheric nuclear explosions and the partitioning of debris between different parts of the atmosphere. As accurate data on individual tests have not generally been available, this information is of course somewhat uncertain. Summed yields during certain periods of time, however, do agree with reported total yields for these time intervals, and the integrated depositions of long-lived fission products are reasonably consistent with the estimates. The estimates of fission, fusion and total yields exploded in the atmosphere for each year since 1945 are illustrated in Figure II.

13. There were two main periods when most of the radioactive debris produced in nuclear explosions was injected into the atmosphere, namely 1952-1958 and 1961-1962. About 42% of all fission yield in the atmosphere was exploded in the former period and 47% in the latter, adding up to 89% for the 11-year period from 1952 through 1962. The corresponding numbers for fusion yield are 25% and 72%, respectively, giving a total of 97% for the 1952-1962 period. Less than 0.5% of the total fission yield and completely insignificant amounts of fusion yield were exploded before 1952, leaving 11% and 3%, respectively, for the period since 1962. About 90% of the fission yield was due to explosions in the northern hemisphere.

14. The total explosive yield from past atmospheric nuclear weapons tests amounts to 545 Mt, consisting of 217 Mt from fission and 328 Mt from fusion. The contributions of local, tropospheric and stratospheric fallout to total fallout are 12, 10 and 78%, respectively. Local fallout, which is loosely defined as that part of the debris that deposits on the ground in the vicinity of the test site, has not previously been considered by the Committee in its dose assessments because nuclear weapons tests were conducted in isolated areas.

15. The major radionuclides produced in atmospheric nuclear testing from the standpoint of doses delivered are listed in Table 1, along with the basic data of radioactive half-life, mode of decay, fission yield and amounts released into the atmosphere (local fallout excluded).

B. DEPOSITS ON THE EARTH'S SURFACE

16. The Committee has traditionally estimated collective effective doses committed to the populations of the 40°-50° latitude bands in the northern and southern hemispheres (zones of maximum fallout), to the population of the whole northern hemisphere and the whole southern hemisphere, and to the entire world's population. Fission products, residual radionuclides of the weapons materials and activation products have been considered in the dose assessment.

17. The committed collective effective dose to those populations from past atmospheric testing arises mainly from external irradiation from the radionuclides deposited on the earth's surface and internal exposure from radionuclides incorporated into ingested foods. Since the doses from these pathways are strongly related to the amounts of radionuclides deposited on the ground, the first step in the dose assessment

consists in estimating the deposition densities in the latitude bands considered for the radionuclides of interest. For this purpose, the Committee has relied upon extensive measurements of ^{90}Sr, ^{89}Sr and ^{95}Zr for the assessment of the activities of all radionuclides present in the environment in a solid form. This is the case for all radionuclides considered in this Section, with the exception of ^{3}H and ^{14}C.

18. The deposition of ^{90}Sr has been monitored worldwide in a network of between 50 and 200 stations operated by and in cooperation with the Environmental Measurements Laboratory (EML), formerly the Health and Safety Laboratory (HASL) [H7]. The global deposition of ^{90}Sr has also been estimated by others, such as the United Kingdom Atomic Energy Authority [C2], with a network of 8 stations in the United Kingdom, and 18 stations elsewhere. When results of these two networks are compared, the annual values are found to differ by up to 50%, but the integrated and cumulative depositions agree to within 2% [L2]. Because the United States network has been the largest and most widely distributed, the data collected by it have been adopted by the Committee. The total hemispheric annual deposition values are calculated by averaging the deposition density over all collecting stations in each 10° latitude band, multiplying by the area of the respective band and then summing all nine bands of the hemisphere [L2].

19. Data on the time-integrated deposition of ^{90}Sr in each 10° latitude band of the globe are given in Table 2. Because the last atmospheric nuclear weapons test occurred in 1980, and deposition of radioactive aerosols takes place within a few years, it can be considered that the deposition of ^{90}Sr produced by past atmospheric tests is essentially complete. Also shown in Table 2 are the areas of the latitude bands and the population distribution in these regions. The latitudinal population distribution is used to calculate the population-weighted deposition densities, which are then used as the basis for estimating the per caput doses and dose commitments from ^{90}Sr. Owing to its rather well-known geographical distribution, ^{90}Sr is used as a fallout indicator for all long-lived radionuclides (defined here as those radionuclides with a radioactive half-life greater than 100 days) from past nuclear tests; ^{90}Sr deposition values are therefore the basic information for estimating dose commitments from a number of radionuclides. For long-lived nuclides that deposit over several years, the method of using ^{90}Sr as an indicator and applying a production ratio corrected for decay can be expected to yield adequate estimates of deposition densities. The uncertainties attached to the deposition estimates increase as the physical half-life of the radionuclide considered decreases.

20. Short-lived radionuclides (in this context, nuclides with half-lives from 8 to 100 days) show different fallout patterns. These vary not only with the half-life of the radionuclide but also with its decay chain and the chemical properties of the elements involved, because they determine the type of particles that the radionuclide will tend to be incorporated into and thus its subsequent dissemination pattern. As the deposition of all short-lived nuclides that might be of interest was not measured globally during the periods of atmospheric testing, a pattern drawn mainly from data on ^{95}Zr and ^{89}Sr has been used to infer deposition of all short-lived radionuclides [U3, U4].

21. The population-weighted deposition densities of ^{95}Zr in past tests are given in the last column of Table 2. Zirconium-95 has been chosen as the indicator for short-lived nuclides because it is a comparatively well-mapped radionuclide with a suitable half-life and it is commonly used in studies of fractionation (deviations of actual radionuclide ratios in fallout compared to what can be calculated from production yields and decay). The corresponding deposition densities of other short-lived nuclides are calculated by multiplying by an empirical factor that accounts for the difference in half-life and possible fractionation phenomena. However, the error introduced can be quite large, as the empirical factors in most cases are based on rather limited data and deposition patterns have varied among tests.

22. The ratios used to derive the population-weighted deposition densities of the radionuclides formed in atmospheric nuclear tests (based on ^{90}Sr for the long-lived radionuclides, with the exception of ^{3}H and ^{14}C, and on ^{95}Zr for the short-lived radionuclides) are presented in Table 3, along with the population-weighted average deposition densities obtained by this method for the 40°-50° latitude bands of each hemisphere, for each hemisphere and for the world.

23. This method has not been used for ^{3}H or ^{14}C, because these radionuclides are readily recycled in the biosphere and become homogeneously disseminated in the hemisphere in which they are released within a time that is short in comparison to their radioactive half-lives. The interhemispheric transfer of radionuclides other than isotopes of the inert noble gases is very limited because of tropospheric wind patterns and efficient scavenging by precipitation in the tropical latitudes. The dose commitments from ^{3}H and ^{14}C are based on a comparison with the doses and production rates of these radionuclides in their natural occurrence.

24. The quotient of the deposition density (integrated deposition density rate) to the production amount (integrated release rate) of the radionuclide forms the transfer coefficient P_{02}. These values may be

determined from the data in Tables 1 and 3. The relationship of P_{02} values to the half-lives of the radionuclides is illustrated in Figure III for the temperate zone of the northern hemisphere. Owing to the pattern of atmospheric testing, the deposition densities and thus the P_{02} values are higher by a factor of about 4 in the northern hemisphere than in the southern hemisphere. The values in the temperate zones are about 1.5 times higher than the hemispheric averages. Since the residence time of particulate debris injected into the stratosphere is of the order of one to a few years, most of the longer-lived radionuclides are deposited without appreciable decay. The P_{02} values in this case are approximately 5 kBq m^{-2} per EBq released. Radioactive decay before deposition appreciably lowers the values of P_{02} for radionuclides with half-lives of less than one year. The variations seen in Figure III of P_{02} values for a few radionuclides (^{125}Sb, ^{241}Pu) illustrate the uncertainties in production and deposition estimates.

C. TRANSFER FROM DEPOSITION TO DOSE

25. The assessments of doses from different radionuclides were presented in detail in the UNSCEAR 1977 Report [U4] and the UNSCEAR 1982 Report [U3]. Measurements reported in the scientific literature on which the estimates were based and the computational techniques applied to derive doses were listed and described. The results can be summarized in terms of the transfer coefficients P_{25}, which link the time-integrated deposition density on the earth's surface to the dose commitments in the relevant organs and tissues of man. Three principal pathways are considered: external irradiation, inhalation and ingestion.

26. The ingestion pathway is of significance for radionuclides that are efficiently transferred through the chain formed by deposition to plant uptake to grazing animals (in many cases)-dietary intake and are absorbed from the gastro-intestinal tract to blood. Some delay may be introduced in these transfers. One important exception to this, however, is the short-lived radionuclide ^{131}I, which can rather quickly be transferred via the pasture-cow-milk chain to man. For most radionuclides, the intake amounts by ingestion result primarily from the initial retention by crops and pasture during deposition and only secondarily from delayed root uptake.

27. To make reliable assessments of doses through the ingestion pathway, there is a need for extensive empirical data on the concentrations of the relevant radionuclides in different types of food and the various diets in different population groups. Analyses of this kind have been made in previous reports of the Committee, especially for ^{90}Sr and ^{137}Cs, which together with ^{14}C, are the primary contributors to the ingestion dose commitments [U3, U4]. To evaluate the P_{25} transfer coefficients, regression analysis has been applied to models relating measured radionuclide concentrations in diet to the annual deposition density rates and the measured concentrations in relevant organs.

28. The transfer of ^{90}Sr and ^{137}Cs from deposition to diet has been modelled by a three-component model:

$$C_i = b_1 \dot{F}_i + b_2 \dot{F}_{i-1} + b_3 \sum_{n=1}^{\infty} e^{-\lambda n} \dot{F}_{i-n} \quad (2)$$

where C_i is the concentration of the radionuclide in a food component or in the total diet in the year i due to the deposition density rate in the year i, $\dot{F}_i$, in the previous year, $\dot{F}_{i-1}$, and in all previous years, reduced by exponential decay. The exponential decay with decay constant λ reflects both radioactive decay and environmental loss of the radionuclide. The coefficients b_i and the parameter λ are determined by regression analysis of measured deposition and diet data.

29. The transfer coefficient from deposition to diet is given by

$$P_{23} = \int_0^{\infty} C(t)\,dt \Big/ \int_0^{\infty} \dot{F}(t)\,dt \quad \text{or} \quad \sum_{i=1}^{\infty} C_i \Big/ \sum_{i=1}^{\infty} \dot{F}_i \quad (3)$$

From the above model, the transfer coefficient can be expressed as

$$P_{23} = b_1 + b_2 + b_3\, e^{-\lambda m}/(1 - e^{-\lambda m}) \quad (4)$$

where b_i are the transfer components per unit annual deposition: b_1 is the transfer in the first year, primarily from direct deposition; b_2 is the transfer in the second year from lagged use of stored foods and uptake from the surface deposit; and b_3 is the transfer via root uptake from the accumulated deposit. The units of P_{23} and b_i are Bq a kg^{-1} per Bq m^{-2}. In the exponential term, λ has units a^{-1} and m is a constant equal to one year.

30. Results of regression fitting of this fallout model to monitoring data have been presented in previous UNSCEAR Reports [U3, U4, U5]. Further analysis of the available data is presented in Table 4. The fits to the long-term monitoring results in Denmark are shown in Figure IV. Relatively minor adjustments in parameter values are needed in the fits to extended

monitoring data, indicating, in particular, that the projections of long-term transfers are confirmed.

31. Adequate representations of transfers to the total diet or to separate components of the diet are obtained for relatively uniform deposition during the year, as occurred for fallout from atmospheric weapons testing. For deposition occurring within a much shorter time period, such as following the Chernobyl accident, the transfer is dependent on the particular agricultural conditions at the time of deposition and on short-term restrictions on certain foods in the diet that may be imposed. Thus, the first-year and second-year lagged transfers of ^{137}Cs to diet in measured concentrations in 1986 and 1987 are much lower than would be expected from the fallout model. The discrepancy may have been less in other countries, depending on the agricultural conditions, than is shown for Denmark in Figure IV. In contrast to weapons fallout, the deposition of ^{90}Sr from the Chernobyl accident was much less significant than that of ^{137}Cs.

32. From the results of the transfer factor analysis given in Table 4, it is seen that transfers from widespread but relatively normal areas of transfer may vary by ±50% for total diet, with even greater variations for some specific food groups. The foods included in each major group differ in the various locations, as do the consumption amounts of these foods.

33. The transfer coefficients, P_{23}, for ^{90}Sr and ^{137}Cs are summarized in Table 5. These are the averaged results from Argentina, Denmark and the United States of the transfers to the five food categories weighted for consumption amounts. Because they come from only three locations, the average values with standard deviations are only general indications of the transfers and variations to be expected. The results are similar to the previously adopted values of P_{23}: 4 mBq a kg^{-1} per Bq m^{-2} for ^{90}Sr and 9 mBq a kg^{-1} per Bq m^{-2} for ^{137}Cs [U3].

34. Figure V shows the contributions to transfer in the various periods. For ^{90}Sr, the major component of P_{23} (50%) arises from transfer from the deposit. For ^{137}Cs, the major transfer is within the first year of deposition (45%), with diminishing transfer in the second and subsequent years following deposition. The contributions to transfers by the various food groups are indicated in Table 5. For ^{90}Sr, milk and grain products are the most significant foods. For ^{137}Cs, these categories, along with meat, account for the major part of the transfer. It is recognized that much wider variations in transfer occur in certain areas for particular soil conditions and foods. This includes the Arctic food chain (lichen-reindeer-man) and areas where the caesium-binding clay content of soils is low, thus allowing higher and more persistent uptake of ^{137}Cs to plants. In these cases, order of magnitude differences in transfer may result. More detailed evaluations of the extent of these conditions are necessary to determine the added contributions that may be made to the collective doses.

35. The transfer coefficients P_{34}, linking concentrations of radionuclides in diet to those in the body and P_{45}, linking concentrations in the body to dose, have been evaluated and the results published in the UNSCEAR 1982 Report [U3] and the UNSCEAR 1977 Report [U4]. For some radionuclides, the integrated dietary intake rates have been determined directly. Relating these values to the deposition of the radionuclide forms the transfer coefficient P_{24}. The units of this expression are Bq per Bq m^{-2}. Values of P_{23} may be transformed to this by multiplication by the consumption rate of foods, which is in effect the transfer coefficient P_{34}. As this is a convenient form for estimating dose, all radionuclides considered in the ingestion pathway evaluation are included in the listing of P_{24} values in Table 6.

36. The values of the dose per unit intake of radionuclides are, in fact, the transfer coefficients P_{45}. These have been or are being re-evaluated, based on the latest metabolic data, and compilations are available [I13, N1]. It is necessary to state the specific assumptions of absorption and retention of the radionuclides; therefore, the P_{45} values used in the evaluations given here are included in Table 7. The values of effective dose use the weighting factors defined by the ICRP in 1990 [I12].

37. The overall transfer coefficients P_{25}, linking the deposition to the dose from radionuclides produced in atmospheric nuclear testing, are compiled in Table 8. The results for the ingestion pathway have been obtained by multiplication of the transfer coefficients P_{24} in Table 6 and P_{45} in Table 7. The values of P_{25} are considered to apply as averages to large populations in the world. Adjustments are needed if applications are to be made to smaller groups for which diet or local conditions of transfer may be different.

38. For the inhalation pathway, the association is between atmospheric concentrations and dose, P_{15}, but because there is a direct relationship between atmospheric concentration and deposition, the association with dose from inhalation can also be made from the deposition amount. The expression used is

$$P_{25} = P_{14} P_{45} / P_{12} \qquad (5)$$

where P_{14} is the average breathing rate of the individual in the population, P_{45} is the dose per unit intake factor for the organ or tissue considered and P_{12} is the deposition velocity averaged over all weather conditions, including precipitation. The value of P_{14} has been taken to be 20 m^3 d^{-1}, or 7,300 m^3 a^{-1} for all populations. The values of P_{45}, in nGy Bq^{-1}, are listed in Table 7. The transfer coefficient P_{12} varies with the precipitation rate at various locations and also with the physical and chemical nature of the radionuclide considered. The average value of P_{12} for particulate material has been estimated to be 1.76 cm s^{-1}, or 5.56 10^5 m a^{-1}. Although this value is based on observations in New York City over several years [B5], measurements in the United Kingdom [C3] and Sweden [B6, D1] are in reasonable agreement, after normalization to the same annual precipitation. Furthermore, since the yearly rainfall in New York City is fairly close to the population-weighted average for the whole world, the New York value is considered adequate for global average calculations. The transfer coefficients P_{25} evaluated for the inhalation pathway are listed in Table 8.

39. In addition to experiencing internal irradiation from inhaled or ingested radionuclides, people are also irradiated externally from gamma-emitting nuclides dispersed in the air and deposited on the ground. As the debris normally spends much more time deposited on the ground than dispersed in ground-level air, the external dose due to irradiation from the earth's surface is normally much higher than the dose due to irradiation while the debris is airborne. The average ratio of the absorbed dose from ground surface contamination to that from air immersion is proportional to the half-life of the radionuclide and is, for example, of the order of 100 for short-lived ^{140}Ba and 1,000,000 for long-lived ^{137}Cs.

40. The P_{25} transfer coefficients for external irradiation have been calculated by multiplying the dose rate conversion factors for radionuclides deposited on the ground, derived from Beck [B3], by the mean lifetime of the radionuclide (half-life ÷ ln 2) and by an average factor assuming 80% indoor occupancy in buildings with a shielding factor of 0.2. The latter factor is 0.7 Sv per Gy (equivalent dose rate in the body per unit absorbed dose rate in air) times 0.36 (0.2 outdoor occupancy plus 0.8 indoor occupancy times 0.2 building shielding). The Committee has in the past [U3, U4] rounded this product to 0.3; the procedure here, however, is to postpone the rounding to the final dose estimate. For short-lived radionuclides (all except ^{137}Cs), the dose-rate conversion factor applying to a plane source is used. For ^{137}Cs, the dose-rate conversion factor applying to an exponential concentration profile in the ground of mean depth 3 cm is used. The indoor occupancy, as well as the shielding factor, varies a great deal among different populations of the world, and this is a source of uncertainty in the dose assessments for external irradiation. Also, the different dynamic behaviours of radionuclides deposited in urban and in rural environments have not been taken into account for the dose estimates from radionuclides produced in atmospheric nuclear testing. The transfer coefficients P_{25} are given in Table 8 for the effective dose commitment. The same numerical values can be expected to apply more or less to the absorbed doses in individual organs in the body; however, since the absorbed doses per unit deposition density have not been specifically evaluated, there are no values given in Table 8.

D. DOSE ESTIMATES

1. Regional and global exposure

41. The effective dose commitments from individual radionuclides in past atmospheric testing (^{3}H and ^{14}C excepted) can be calculated by multiplying the population-weighted integrated deposition density of the radionuclide in the region of interest (Table 3) by the appropriate P_{25} transfer coefficient (Table 8). As an example, the effective dose commitment due to ingestion of ^{137}Cs in the population of the 40°-50° latitude band in the temperate zone of the northern hemisphere is 5,200 Bq m^{-2} times 54.6 nSv per Bq m^{-2} = 280 μSv. The results for each radionuclide and for all pathways are given in Table 9.

42. As indicated previously, the dose commitments from ^{3}H and ^{14}C are derived from comparisons with the natural doses and production rates by cosmic rays. The dose calculations make use of the fact that the dose commitment to production ratios for those radionuclides are equal to the annual natural dose to production ratios. The annual absorbed dose in tissue from natural tritium has been estimated to be 10 nGy, resulting from an annual production per hemisphere of 37 PBq [U3]. Assuming a total release from atmospheric nuclear testing of 190 EBq to the atmosphere of the northern hemisphere and 50 EBq to that of the southern hemisphere [U3], the absorbed dose commitments in tissue from fallout tritium are as follows: northern hemisphere, $1.9\ 10^{20}$ Bq × (10^{-8} Gy a^{-1}) ÷ ($3.7\ 10^{16}$ Bq a^{-1}) = 51 μGy, and southern hemisphere, $0.5\ 10^{20}$ Bq × (10^{-8} Gy a^{-1}) ÷ ($3.7\ 10^{16}$ Bq a^{-1}) = 14 μGy. It has not been possible to account for latitudinal variations in the tritium distribution. The simplification is made in assuming fairly rapid mixing of tritium throughout the hemisphere. The effective dose commitments from ^{3}H are 51 μSv (northern hemisphere), 14 μSv (southern hemisphere) and 47 μSv (world). The global value is the population-weighted estimate, taking into account that 89% of the world population resides in the northern

hemisphere and 11% in the southern hemisphere. On the basis of the intake rates of hydrogen in water [N8], the dose commitment can be apportioned as 7% arising from inhalation and absorption through the skin and 93% from ingestion [U3].

43. Carbon-14 is produced naturally by cosmic ray neutrons impinging on nitrogen in the upper atmosphere. This means that the dose commitment from ^{14}C injected into the atmosphere by nuclear tests can be calculated in the same way as the dose commitment from tritium produced in atmospheric tests. The annual natural production of ^{14}C of about 1 PBq and the resulting equilibrium specific activity in man yields an annual dose to the gonads of 5 μGy [U3]. Based on this, it can be concluded that the 220 PBq from nuclear explosions have given a dose commitment to the gonads of all populations of (5 μGy a^{-1}) $\div$ (1 PBq a^{-1}) $\times$ 220 PBq = 1,100 μGy. In the same way, dose commitments to the lungs, bone lining cells, red bone marrow, thyroid and other tissues can be assessed as 1,300, 4,800, 5,300, 1,300 and 2,900 μGy, respectively [U3], yielding an effective dose commitment of 2,600 μSv. The corresponding collective effective dose per unit release is 120 man Sv per TBq, assuming an equilibrium world population of 10^{10} people reached in the next century and maintained over the next thousands of years. Other published estimates range between 67 and 159 man Sv per TBq [B10, I2, K2, K4, K5, M2, S1].

44. The ^{14}C doses are due to ingested and inhaled carbon. On the basis of the relative intake and retention of carbon in these pathways, the dose commitments from ingestion are estimated to be 10^4 times larger than those arising from inhalation [K4]. The dose commitments from ^{14}C are delivered over a very long time period. From calculations based on an environmental compartment model for ^{14}C that comprises 25 discrete carbon reservoirs (Figure VI) and takes into account the dilution of ^{14}C by stable carbon released during fossil fuel combustion, it is estimated that only 5% of the dose commitment is delivered in the first 100 years after the release of ^{14}C; about 71% of the dose commitment will have been delivered during 10^4 years after the release of ^{14}C [M2]. The deep ocean, divided into 18 compartments, accounts for the slow recycling of ^{14}C into the biosphere.

45. The effective dose commitments from atmospheric nuclear testing for all of the 22 radionuclides considered for the populations of the world and of the 40°-50° latitude bands of each hemisphere are presented in Table 9. The total effective dose commitments are 4.4 and 3.1 mSv in the 40°-50° latitude bands of the northern and southern hemispheres, respectively, and the global average is 3.7 mSv.

46. The summary listing in Table 10 for the world population shows that ^{14}C is the dominant contributor to the total effective dose commitment, accounting for 70% of the effective dose commitment to the world's population. However, if only 10% of the ^{14}C dose commitment is included in the comparison, that is, if the dose commitments are truncated approximately to the year 2200, at which time all other radionuclides will have delivered almost all of their dose, ^{14}C contributes only 19% to the truncated effective dose commitment to the world's population. Besides ^{14}C, the most important contributors to the effective dose commitment to the world population are ^{137}Cs, ^{95}Zr-^{95}Nb, ^{90}Sr, ^{106}Ru, ^{54}Mn, ^{144}Ce, ^{131}I and ^{3}H.

47. Including all of the ^{14}C dose, 16% of the total effective dose commitment to the world population is delivered through external irradiation, 4% through inhalation and 80% through ingestion. Including only 10% of the ^{14}C dose, the corresponding numbers are 44%, 10% and 46%, respectively. Thus, ingestion is the most important pathway, if ^{14}C is fully included, while ingestion and external irradiation are about equally important, if only 10% of effective dose commitment from ^{14}C is included. In both cases inhalation contributes substantially less.

48. As the explosive power in past atmospheric tests has been estimated to be 545 Mt, it may be concluded that the past tests have given an average complete effective dose commitment of about 7 μSv Mt^{-1} to the world population. Of this, about 5 μSv Mt^{-1} is due to ^{14}C and about 2 μSv Mt^{-1} to fission products. The transuranium elements have contributed about 0.1 μSv Mt^{-1}. Normalizing the fission product dose commitment to the total fission yield exploded of 217 Mt gives an estimate of about 5 μSv Mt^{-1} fission.

49. A summary of the global collective effective doses committed from past atmospheric nuclear tests is given in Table 11. For these calculations, some assumptions about the global population have been made. For inhalation exposure and other exposures from radionuclides with half-lives of less than a few years, the population of the world has been taken to be 3.2 10^9 persons, as it was in the early 1960s during maximum fallout. For ^{3}H, ^{90}Sr, ^{137}Cs and ^{241}Pu, a global population of 4 10^9 persons has been applied, and for the very long-lived ^{14}C, ^{239}Pu, ^{240}Pu and ^{241}Am, the projected global population has been assumed to be 1 10^{10} persons.

50. In Table 11 the radionuclides are listed in order of their decreasing contributions to the collective effective dose. The order is essentially the same as in Table 10, with ^{14}C being the dominant contributor and ^{137}Cs, ^{90}Sr, ^{95}Zr and ^{106}Ru following. The total global

impact of all atmospheric nuclear explosions carried out for test purposes in the past is 3 10^7 man Sv.

2. Local exposure

51. Populations living near the sites where nuclear weapons tests took place received relatively higher doses than the average values assessed above. In the United States, about 100 surface or near-surface tests were conducted at the Nevada test site between 1951 and 1962, with a total explosive fission yield of approximately 1 Mt. Dose reconstructions have been undertaken for the populations living in the vicinity of the Nevada test site during the period of atmospheric testing [C7, W1]. The local population size was 180,000 persons. Preliminary results indicate that thyroid doses of up to 1 Gy may have been received by children. The collective dose from external exposure has been estimated to be approximately 500 man Sv [A5]. Ninety per cent of the collective dose was received during the years 1953-1957.

52. Following the nuclear test Bravo at Bikini in the Pacific test site of the United States, residents of Rongelap and Utirik Atolls were exposed to unexpected fallout. The islands are 210 and 570 km, respectively, east of Bikini. Eighty-two individuals were evacuated from Rongelap 51 hours after the explosion and 159 persons were removed from Utirik within 78 hours. External exposures, mainly from short-lived radionuclides, ranged from 1.9 Sv on Rongelap (67 persons, including 3 in utero), 1.1 Sv on nearby Allingnae Atoll (19 persons, including 1 in utero) and 0.1 Sv on Utirik (167 persons, including 8 in utero) [L3]. The collective dose was thus of the order of 160 man Sv. Doses to the thyroid, caused by several isotopes of iodine, tellurium and by external gamma radiation, were estimated to be 12, 22 and 52 Gy on average and 42, 82 and 200 Gy maximum to adults and children of 9 years and 1 year, respectively, on Rongelap [L3].

53. At the Semipalatinsk test site in the Kazakh region of the former USSR, atmospheric tests were conducted from 1949 through 1962, and about 300 underground tests were conducted from 1964 until 1989 [T5]. In total, 10,000 people in settlements bordering the testing site were exposed to some extent. The collective dose due to external irradiation was estimated to be 2,600 man Sv, 80% of which resulting from testing in the period 1949-1953, due to external irradiation and 2,000 man Sv due to internal exposure from the ingestion intake of radionuclides [T5]. The collective absorbed dose to the thyroid was of the order of 10,000 man Gy.

54. The United Kingdom conducted a programme of nuclear warhead development tests between 1953 and 1963 in Australia, at the Monte Bello Islands and at Emu and Maralinga on the mainland. In all, twelve major nuclear tests involving atomic explosions with total yields of about 100 kt, 16 kt and 60 kt were performed at the three sites, respectively [D3]. The collective effective dose to the Australian population from these test series has been estimated to be 700 man Sv [W3]. In addition, several hundred smaller scale experiments were performed at Maralinga [D3] which resulted in the dispersal of about 24 kg of ^{239}Pu over some hundreds of square kilometres. This area remains contaminated and potential doses to future inhabitants of the Maralinga and Emu areas have been assessed with a view to rehabilitation of the two sites [D3, H3, W2]. Annual effective doses of several millisievert would be expected to result from continuous occupancy within the two areas, with maximums of several hundred millisievert in the immediate vicinity of the two sites.

II. UNDERGROUND NUCLEAR TESTS

55. About 1,400 nuclear test explosions have been carried out beneath the earth's surface. Particularly since 1963, when the limited nuclear test ban treaty banning atmospheric tests was agreed, the practice became more frequent. Prohibiting atmospheric tests was a crucial step in lessening the doses to the world's population from tests of weapons. In fact, a well-contained under-ground nuclear explosion delivers extremely low doses or dose commitments to any group of people. However, there have been occasions when, owing to venting or the diffusion of gases, radioactive materials leaked from underground tests, resulting in the dissemination of radioactive debris over at least regional distances.

A. WEAPONS TESTS

56. Estimates of annual yields and numbers of underground tests have been compiled from data collected by the National Defence Research Establishment in Sweden [N10]. The total annual yields are

presented in Table 12. The basis for these estimates are either announcements made by the testing nation or simple calculations employing a formula of the following form:

$$\text{yield (kt)} = 10^{(M-a)/b} \qquad (6)$$

where M stands for the seismic surface or body wave magnitude and a and b are constants that vary with wave type, explosion location and observing laboratory. The total yield of underground tests is estimated to be 90 Mt, or about one sixth of the total yield exploded in the atmosphere.

57. More than 500 tests were conducted underground at the Nevada test site in the United States, but only 32 are reported to have led to off-site contamination as a result of venting [H4]. Table 13 shows, as an example, the atmospheric releases of ^{131}I from these 32 underground tests. The total amount of ^{131}I released into the atmosphere was about 5 PBq, which is five orders of magnitude smaller than the amount produced by atmospheric testing (6.5 10^5 PBq, from Table 1). The amount of ^{131}I or of any other radionuclide released into the atmosphere by underground tests carried out at sites other than the Nevada test site is not available.

58. The collective effective dose per unit release of ^{131}I would be expected to be much greater for the venting of underground tests than for atmospheric tests, because the release from underground tests occurs at ground level instead of higher in the atmosphere. Estimates of collective effective dose per unit release to the lower layers of the atmosphere were made in the UNSCEAR 1988 Report [U1]; these estimates are 1 10^{-13} man Sv per Bq for ^{131}I released in the Chernobyl accident and 4 10^{-13} man Sv per Bq for ^{131}I released from nuclear power stations. In order to account for the low population densities in the vicinity of weapons tests sites, it is assumed that a lower figure, 1 10^{-14} man Sv per Bq, is appropriate for releases of ^{131}I from underground tests. This figure, combined with a release of 5 PBq, leads to a collective effective dose from ^{131}I releases from venting underground tests carried out at the Nevada test site of 50 man Sv. Extrapolating to the total number of underground tests (1,400) at all locations would indicate that 15 PBq, in total, of ^{131}I has been released, and the collective dose is of the order of 150 man Sv. In comparison, the corresponding collective effective dose from ^{131}I from past atmospheric tests is estimated to be 164,000 man Sv (Table 11).

59. Other than these rather unusual events, where amounts of radioactive materials have been collected on filters, it is reasonable to assume that a few high-yield underground tests have leaked radioactive gases such as tritium or noble gases such as ^{133}Xe. There have been suggestions that observed peak concentrations in atmospheric tritium (HT or HTO) and ^{37}Ar (produced in $^{40}Ca(n,\alpha)^{37}Ar$ reactions underground) could have been due to leakages from underground explosions [B7, L5, M1]. Traces of short-lived radionuclides resulting from tests in the USSR were observed in Finland and Sweden in 1966 [K1, P2] and in 1971 [E1, K6]. The collective dose to the population of Sweden was estimated to be 3 man Sv from the venting of an underground test at Semipalatinsk in 1966 and 0.1 man Sv or less on seven other occasions when radionuclides from underground tests were detected in that country [D10].

60. The total ^{131}I produced in the underground explosions could be estimated to be 90 Mt total yield times the normalized fission production of 4,200 PBq Mt^{-1} (Table 1), which is 380 EBq. The fractional release is thus 4 10^{-5} of the amount produced. This same estimate of the release fraction may be applied to the noble gases, of which ^{133}Xe is the predominant radionuclide. The normalized fission production of ^{133}Xe is 14.5 EBq Mt^{-1} (6.54% fission yield [R1], adjusted for the half-life and yield of ^{90}Sr production given in Table 1). Total production of ^{133}Xe in underground tests is then estimated to be 1,300 EBq, of which 50 PBq may have been released (90 Mt × 14.5 EBq Mt^{-1} × 4 10^{-5}). The normalized collective dose from noble gases estimated for surface releases (applied to releases from nuclear power reactors) is 0.1 man Sv PBq^{-1} [U1]. The collective dose due to noble gases released from underground tests is then 50 PBq × 0.1 man Sv PBq^{-1} = 5 man Sv. This estimate is very uncertain. The collective dose per unit release may be overestimated because of the remote locations of the test sites; however, there is even greater uncertainty in the release fraction.

61. The same estimation procedures applied to ^3H produced in underground testing would indicate a total release of 10^{-4} PBq and a collective dose of 0.001 man Sv. This is a negligible component of the collective dose under the assumptions made. The analysis indicates that releases of ^{131}I are of the most significance and that the total collective dose from released radioactive materials from the 1,400 underground tests conducted thus far is of the order of 200 man Sv. Evaluations have not yet been made of potential exposures resulting from residual debris underground at the sites of the explosions.

B. PEACEFUL NUCLEAR EXPLOSIONS

62. It is to be expected that shallow underground explosions conducted for excavation purposes or deeper underground explosions in mining operations

also involve releases of radioactive materials to the environment. Programmes to develop applications of peaceful nuclear explosions were carried out during the 1960s in the United States and USSR. About 100 test explosions were performed. The presumed advantages of nuclear explosions have, however, been outweighed by the residual contamination and other disadvantages.

63. Doses to local or global populations from peaceful nuclear explosions have resulted primarily from cratering experiments. There were 6 such tests at the Nevada Test Site between 1962 and 1968 and a reported 9 experiments worldwide [U5]. The collective dose to the local population (180,000 persons) living near the Nevada site has been estimated to be 3 man Sv from the Sedan 104 kt cratering experiment in 1962 [A5]. The total from all tests, peaceful and military, conducted at the Nevada site from 1961 to 1975 was 5.7 man Sv [A5]. Therefore the total local collective dose from peaceful nuclear explosions can be estimated to be no more than 5 man Sv at Nevada and perhaps 10 man Sv worldwide.

64. The long-range dose commitment from the Schooner cratering experiment in the United States in 1968 was estimated in the UNSCEAR 1972 Report [U5]. Tungsten-181, formed in the neutron shield used to minimize the formation of activation products, was detected in several locations in Europe after this event. The effective dose commitment was estimated to be 12 nSv from radionuclides other than ^{3}H in the population of the 40°-50° latitude band of the northern hemisphere (630 million persons at the time) [U5]. The estimated release of ^{3}H of 15 PBq [U5] would have resulted in a dose commitment of 4 nSv (0.27 nGy PBq^{-1} from comparison with natural ^{3}H dose and release in the northern hemisphere) in the population of the northern hemisphere (3,160 million persons at the time). The collective dose from this test is thus estimated to be 20 man Sv. If it may be considered that this result is representative of the other cratering experiments, the collective dose worldwide from cratering experiments is 180 man Sv. The collective dose from peaceful nuclear explosions is thus estimated to be the same order of magnitude as that from venting underground military tests.

III. NUCLEAR WEAPONS FABRICATION

65. The production of radioactive materials for military use and the fabrication of weapons has involved routine and accidental releases of radionuclides and exposures of local or regional populations. These dose commitments and collective doses have not been estimated before by the Committee because no data were available. Some of the secrecy of this industry is being reduced, however, and information on discharges and doses from recent (and, in some cases earlier) operations is being provided. With this information and some rough estimates of the total amounts of radioactive materials produced, the doses from the weapons industry can be estimated.

66. The radioactive components of nuclear weapons are the fissile nuclides ^{239}Pu and ^{235}U; the fertile nuclide ^{238}U, which fissions only if irradiated by high-energy neutrons; tritium; and in some presumably older constructions small amounts of materials such as ^{210}Po, which are used to initiate the chain reaction in the fission bomb. Tritium is used in boosted fission bombs, where the efficiency is increased by neutrons from a comparatively small thermonuclear reaction fuelled by tritium. Tritium is probably also used in the main thermonuclear stage of some types of hydrogen bombs.

67. Doses arise in several stages of the nuclear weapons production line. As in the nuclear energy fuel cycle, production starts with the mining and milling of uranium. After that there is the need to convert the uranium to uranium hexafluoride gas, which is the form of uranium used at the gas diffusion or centrifugation plant where the ^{235}U content is enriched. If this process is carried to enrichments of the order of 90%, weapons-grade uranium is produced, which can be used directly to fabricate nuclear weapons components. Alternatively, the enrichment can be omitted or carried to only a few per cent. The uranium is then used to fuel reactors, which coupled to reprocessing and purification yields plutonium and tritium for the weapons. Some doses also derive from the weapons fabrication and assembly, as well as from the maintenance, transportation and recycling of weapons. Doses resulting from routine releases are considered in this Chapter.

A. PRODUCTION AMOUNTS

68. The total amounts of radioactive materials produced for weapons use are not known from directly reported information. An assessment has been made of plutonium in present weapons stockpiles by consider-

ing the amounts of long-lived fission products in high-level waste in the United States and by analysing the global atmospheric inventory of ^{85}Kr [H5]. Krypton-85 is a noble gas and a long-lived fission product that is released to the atmosphere when reactor fuel is reprocessed, for example, to extract plutonium. Correcting the global inventory mainly for the hitherto modest civilian reprocessing yields a number that may be seen to be a measure of the global plutonium stockpile. The estimated stockpiles in the United States and the former USSR were estimated to be around 100 tonnes in each country.

69. According to United Nations studies in 1981 and 1990 on nuclear weapons, the nuclear arsenals comprise more than 40,000 weapons with a total explosive yield of 13,000 Mt [U11, U12]. If it is assumed that the first fission stage in all these weapons is based on plutonium, a total inventory of weapons plutonium of 200 tonnes implies that, on average, 5 kg is used in each device. This is a reasonable figure [E5], which thus lends some credibility to the estimated total production.

70. Tritium is also produced for weapons use. It decays with a half-life of 12.32 years, which means that tritium must be produced continually to preserve the weapons stockpile. It has been estimated for the United States that an annual production of 3 kg of tritium is just enough to balance the decay [C11], and from this the total amount of tritium in the United States stockpile can be easily calculated to be about 55 kg. The world tritium stockpile can then be assumed to be twice as much, or around 110 kg. If it is assumed that this tritium was first produced in the early 1960s and has been maintained since then, a total tritium production of $110 + 30 \times 6 = 290$ kg results. If a further reasonable assumption is made, that is, that tritium is produced at the same (atom)rate as plutonium in the reactor, these 0.29 tonnes of tritium are equivalent to a production of (239/3) 0.29 = 23 tonnes of plutonium.

B. RELEASES AND DOSE ESTIMATES

71. In the United States, weapons production activities have been centred at locations reporting mainly through four regional offices of the Department of Energy: Albuquerque, Oak Ridge, Richland and Savannah River. Doses reported from these centres between 1976 and 1982 are considered to contribute about 90% of the population dose from activities related to weapons research and production. Little information is available on doses or releases before 1976. Efforts are being made, however, to reconstruct doses to the public living near nuclear installations, and some data from earlier periods are becoming available.

72. The Hanford nuclear weapons facility in the United States released substantial quantities of radioactive materials into the atmosphere and the Columbia River from its plutonium production reactors and fuel reprocessing facilities. Two plutonium production reactors started operating at Hanford in December 1944. Two fuel reprocessing plants began extracting plutonium in the same month, and a third production reactor was added in 1945 [C5]. The atmospheric releases of ^{131}I from reprocessing facilities were estimated from the quantity of reactor fuel reprocessed and the time interval between removal from the reactors and reprocessing. Table 14 presents the estimated annual releases of ^{131}I into the atmosphere from 1944 to 1956 [C5]. The largest releases of ^{131}I occurred between 1944 and 1946 during the effort to develop and produce the first arsenal of nuclear weapons. At that time, fuel rods were reprocessed soon after their removal from the reactors in order to maximize plutonium production, and there was no filtering or chemical processing of ^{131}I before atmospheric release. About 18 PBq of ^{131}I was released into the atmosphere between 1944 and 1946, while the release from 1947 to 1956 amounted to about 2 PBq (Table 14). The total atmospheric release of ^{131}I was 20 PBq between 1944 and 1956. Preliminary calculations indicate that the maximum thyroid doses were of the order of 10 Gy in 1945 [C5]. The collective effective doses, based on a value of 4 10^{-13} man Sv per Bq of ^{131}I released from nuclear installations and a population density of 25 persons per km^2 [U1, W4], are roughly estimated to be 7,000 man Sv for 1944-1946 and 1,000 man Sv for 1947-1956. These figures do not include the contributions from other radionuclides in the airborne discharges, which have not yet been reported, or from the liquid releases to the Columbia River. The dose reconstruction effort, which is scheduled to be finished in 1994, will produce more complete and accurate dose estimates.

73. The Chelyabinsk-40 centre, located near the town of Kyshtym, was the first Soviet nuclear installation dedicated to the production of plutonium for military purposes. A uranium-graphite reactor with an open cooling water system was commissioned in June 1948, and a fuel reprocessing plant started operating in December 1948 [N5]. Liquid releases to the Techa River from 1949 to 1956 amounted to 100 PBq, with 95% of this release being discharged from March 1950 to November 1951 [K7]. The main contributors to the activity associated with the radioactive materials released were ^{89}Sr (8.8%), ^{90}Sr (11.6%), ^{137}Cs (12.2%), rare-earth isotopes (26.8%), ^{95}Zr-^{95}Nb (13.6%) and ruthenium isotopes (25.9%) [K7]. These

large releases appear to have resulted in large part from a lack of waste treatment capability and from the storage of radioactive wastes in open, unlined earthen reservoirs [T4]. A hydrological isolation system, including a small reservoir called Lake Karachay, was built after 1952 to contain the low- and intermediate-level wastes.

74. The population along the Techa River was exposed to both external and internal irradiation. External irradiation was caused by gamma radiation from ^{137}Cs, ^{106}Ru and ^{95}Zr in the flood-plain areas, in vegetable gardens near the houses, and inside the houses. Internal irradiation was mainly due to the consumption of water and of local foodstuffs contaminated with ^{89}Sr, ^{90}Sr, ^{137}Cs and some other radionuclides. Tissue and effective doses, presented in Table 15, have been estimated for the populations living along the 240-km-long Techa River [A4]. Average cumulative effective doses are estimated to have ranged up to 1,400 mSv in the village of Metlino, located 7 km downstream from the point of discharge. The evacuation of the population of that village started in 1953; from 1955 to 1960, inhabitants of another 19 settlements were moved away from the river. Altogether, 7,500 persons were evacuated [K7]. It appears from Table 15 that all villages along the Techa River within about 50 km of the plutonium production centre were evacuated. The collective effective dose can be assessed from the distribution of estimated cumulative effective doses to individuals, which are as follows [A4]: 0-50 mSv, 10% of population; 50-100 mSv, 44%; 100-200 mSv, 18%; 200-250 mSv, 15%; 250-500 mSv, 2%; 500-1,000 mSv, 3%; and >1,000 mSv, 8%. Assuming that the 11% of the exposed population who received cumulative effective doses greater than 500 mSv is identical with the 7,500 persons who were evacuated, the collective effective dose received by the population living along the Techa River is about 15,000 man Sv. This value does not include the contributions from the airborne discharges, which have not been reported, or from the contamination of the Iset River, into which the Techa River discharges its waters.

75. These data from Hanford and Chelyabinsk give some indications of doses from the earlier practice of nuclear weapons fabrication, but it is difficult to extrapolate this information to the total weapons industry. Another method of estimating dose is to relate the radioactive material production amounts to the doses involved in producing and utilizing nuclear fuels in the civilian fuel cycle. Plutonium production reactors, which are optimized for the purpose, produce about 1 g of ^{239}Pu per MW d (thermal power), which, if a thermal conversion of 0.33 is assumed, can be expressed, for comparison, as 1.1 tonne per GW a of electrical power. This means that the plutonium and tritium in present arsenals correspond to (200 + 23)/1.1 = about 200 GW a (electrical power) of reactor operation. According to the UNSCEAR 1988 Report [U1], 1 GW a of electrical power in the civilian fuel cycle yields a collective dose of 4 man Sv locally and regionally and 200 man Sv globally. The total collective effective dose committed from weapons plutonium and tritium production may thus be estimated to be 800 man Sv locally and regionally and 40,000 man Sv globally.

76. The estimated annual collective doses from weapons production activities in the United States, as reflected in reports of the Department of Energy for the four main locations between 1976 and 1982, were 5.8, 8.2, 5.2, 2.2, 2.4, 2.3 and 1.7 man Sv, respectively [D7]. The United States nuclear weapons stockpile grew by the mid-1960s to somewhat above 30,000 weapons [C12]. Since then, as older weapons have been retired, the stockpile has decreased, to some 25,000 weapons. However, some of the retired weapons have been replaced, and tritium has been produced continually to balance the radioactive decay. From the reported variation with time of the annual doses since 1976, it can be assumed that the collective dose per year of practice increases as one goes back in time. Assuming that the mean annual population dose commitment from 1965 to 1990 was 10 man Sv and that during this period, on average, 1,000 weapons were produced annually, an average population dose commitment of 0.01 man Sv for each weapon produced is estimated. With a total United States production of 30,000 + (20 × 1,000) = 50,000 weapons, the total estimate would be 500 man Sv. With similar doses from weapons production in the Soviet Union, the collective dose committed to the local and regional population from nuclear weapons production in the world would become 1,000 man Sv, in agreement with the estimate based on plutonium and tritium production in the previous paragraph.

77. This estimate of about 1,000 man Sv for the local and regional collective dose from the global nuclear weapons industry in more recent practice is admittedly uncertain, as it is based on many assumptions and few data. The global component of the collective effective dose is also rather uncertain, as it mainly arises from radon releases from mill tailings in the next 10^4 years. The amounts of enriched uranium produced for weapons purposes are not known, and this part of the military fuel cycle has not yet been assessed. However, even if the committed collective dose from nuclear weapons research, development and production is taken to be roughly 100,000 man Sv, this represents less than 1% of the committed collective dose from atmospheric testing, which according to Table 11 was about 3 10^7 man Sv.

IV. NUCLEAR POWER PRODUCTION

78. The generation of electrical energy by nuclear reactors has continually increased since the beginning of this practice in the 1950s. In 1989, the electrical energy generated by nuclear reactors amounted to 212 GW a, representing 17% of the world's electrical energy generated in that year and 5% of the world's energy consumption [I7].

79. The nuclear fuel cycle includes the mining and milling of uranium ore, its conversion to nuclear fuel material, which usually includes the enrichment of the isotopic content of ^{235}U, the fabrication of fuel elements, the production of energy in the nuclear reactor, the storage of irradiated fuel or its reprocessing with the recycling of the fissile and fertile materials recovered, and the storage and disposal of radioactive wastes. Radioactive materials are transported between installations in the entire fuel cycle.

80. Radiation exposures of members of the public resulting from effluent discharges of radioactive materials from installations of the nuclear fuel cycle were assessed in previous UNSCEAR Reports [U1, U3, U4, U5], in which discharge data for 1970-1974, 1975-1979 and 1980-1984 were included. In this Annex, similar data are presented for the years 1985-1989, as well as the trend with time of the normalized annual releases since 1970. The doses are estimated using the same environmental and dosimetric models as in the UNSCEAR 1988 Report [U1]. In this Chapter doses to the public from routine effluent discharges are considered.

81. The doses to the exposed individuals vary widely from installation to installation and from one location to another, and the individual dose generally decreases rapidly with distance from a given source. In this Annex, an indication is given of the range of individual doses associated with each type of installation. To evaluate the total impact of radionuclides released at each stage of the nuclear fuel cycle, results are normalized in terms of the collective effective dose per unit quantity of electrical energy produced, expressed as man Sv per GW a. The estimated amounts of natural uranium, uranium oxide (U_3O_8), fuel, and units of enrichment required to generate 1 GW a of electrical energy are presented in Table 16 for several reactor types [O2, O3].

A. MINING AND MILLING

82. Uranium mining operations involve the removal from the ground of large quantities of ore containing uranium and its decay products at concentrations of between a tenth of a per cent and a few per cent. In comparison, the average concentrations of uranium in soils of normal natural background areas are of the order of 1 ppm. Uranium is mined using underground or open-pit techniques. The annual quantities of uranium produced in 1975-1989 are presented in Table 17 [O2]. The total amount of uranium produced worldwide remained fairly stable between 1985 and 1990, at about 50,000 tonnes, extracted from about 20 million tonnes of ore. Milling operations involve the processing of these large quantities of ore to extract the uranium in a partially refined form, known as yellow cake.

1. Effluents

83. Radon is the most important radionuclide released from uranium mines. Data on radon emissions from mines in Australia, Canada and the German Democratic Republic for the period 1985-1989 are collected in Table 18. Releases normalized to the production of uranium oxide (U_3O_8) ranged from 1 to 2,000 GBq t^{-1} and were, for most mines, much greater in Canada and in the German Democratic Republic than in Australia. The production-weighted average of the normalized radon release is 300 GBq t^{-1} of uranium oxide. Since about 250 t uranium oxide are required to produce 1 GW a of electrical energy (Table 16), the average radon release, normalized to the generation of electri-cal energy, is approximately 75 TBq $(GW\ a)^{-1}$. This is greater, by a factor of almost 4, than the value adopted in the UNSCEAR 1982 Report and the UNSCEAR 1988 Report. Previous data have been both limited and variable. The present database is somewhat more extensive, and a production-weighted average has been calculated.

84. Releases of natural radionuclides in uranium milling have been reported for mills in Australia and Canada. Results for airborne releases are shown in Table 19. The releases normalized to electrical energy generated are comparable to values adopted in the UNSCEAR 1982 Report and the UNSCEAR 1988 Report. Some variability is inherent, given the limited data available. Mill sites in dry areas give rise to effectively no liquid effluents. The run-off water of mills in wet climates, however, will contain radionuclides and may need treatment before release into watercourses. Liquid releases have been reported for two Canadian uranium mills and are presented in Table 20. There is no obvious explanation for the relatively large amounts of uranium in releases, compared to the other radionuclides of that decay series.

85. The extraction of uranium during milling is made as complete as possible but cannot reach 100%. Typically, the residual tailings from the mill will contain from 0.001% to 0.01% uranium, depending on the grade of ore and the extraction process. More importantly, mill tailings contain the totality of the decay products of ^{234}U that were present in the ore extracted from the mine. Because the two precursors of ^{222}Rn are present in the mill tailings, namely ^{226}Ra, with a half-life of 1,600 years, and ^{230}Th, with a half-life of 80,000 years, mill tailings constitute a long-term source of atmospheric ^{222}Rn. Tailings are discharged from mills into open, uncontained piles or behind engineered dams or dikes with solid or water cover. All tailings piles act as sources of airborne releases of ^{222}Rn, although the release rates can be low if the tailings are covered with water.

86. Measurements over bare tailings piles [A8, B8, C8, S8] show that the exhalation rate of ^{222}Rn is about 1 Bq m^{-2} s^{-1} per Bq g^{-1} of ^{226}Ra. Since the concentration of ^{226}Ra in uranium ore with 1% U_3O_8 is approximately equal to 100 Bq g^{-1}, the release rates of ^{222}Rn over bare tailings resulting from the treatment of uranium ore with 0.1%-3% U_3O_8 are expected to range between 10 and 300 Bq m^{-2} s^{-1}; taking the current average ore grade to be 0.2% U_3O_8, the average exhalation rate of ^{222}Rn is expected to be 20 Bq m^{-2} s^{-1}. Reported emission rates of ^{222}Rn for 1985-1989 from mill tailings in Argentina, Australia, Canada and the German Democratic Republic are presented in Table 21. The emission rates per unit area range from 0.1 to 43 Bq m^{-2} s^{-1}, with most of the values centred on 10 Bq m^{-2} s^{-1}, which is an improvement over the emission rates expected from bare tailings. Assuming, as in the UNSCEAR 1988 Report, that the production of a uranium mine generates tailings of about 1 ha (GW a)$^{-1}$ and that the release rates of ^{222}Rn remain unchanged during five years, a typical emission rate per unit area of 10 Bq m^{-2} s^{-1} corresponds to a normalized release of ^{222}Rn of about 20 TBq (GW a)$^{-1}$. This applies to mill tailings of an operating mill.

87. It is likely that further treatment will be carried out to minimize the releases of ^{222}Rn from abandoned tailings piles. As reported in the UNSCEAR 1988 Report, several techniques were analysed in a study by the Nuclear Energy Agency of the Organization for Economic Cooperation and Development (OECD) [O1] for a number of sites. The radon exhalation rate varied by factors of more than 10^6, according to the treatment assumed, showing that this is clearly a crucial parameter in the assessment of the impact of tailings piles. In the UNSCEAR 1988 Report, it was assumed that some reasonably impermeable cover would be used and that the radon exhalation rate from abandoned tailings piles would be 3 Bq m^{-2} s^{-1}. Because of the assumed protection against erosion and of the long radioactive half-life of ^{230}Th, the radon exhalation rate would remain essentially unchanged over at least 10,000 years and would only decrease by a factor of 2 over the next 80,000 years. Further treatment of the abandoned tailings piles by future generations in the next millennium would probably cause a variation in the exhalation rate, which could be either a decrease or an increase. Two extreme options can be envisaged:

(a) to uncover the tailings piles so that the radon exhalation rate would be increased to its initial value of about 20 Bq m^{-2} s^{-1};
(b) to treat the tailings in such a way that the resulting exhalation rate is decreased to 0.02 Bq m^{-2} s^{-1}, which is the average value corresponding to soils in normal background areas.

88. In this Annex, it is assumed that the average ^{222}Rn exhalation rate from abandoned tailings piles is 3 Bq m^{-2} s^{-1} [corresponding to a normalized emission rate of 1 TBq a^{-1} (GW a)$^{-1}$] and that this value will remain unchanged over the next 10,000 years. These assumptions of the long-term release of radon are the same as in the UNSCEAR 1988 Report [U1]. It is, however, recognized that the ^{222}Rn exhalation rate could range between 0.02 and 20 Bq m^{-2} s^{-1} any time in the next 10,000 years and beyond. Normalized releases of radionuclides assumed for the mining and milling operations are summarized in Table 22.

2. Dose estimates

89. In the dose estimation procedure used in the UNSCEAR 1988 Report, a reference mine and mill site was considered with population densities of 3 km^{-2} at 0-100 km and 25 km^{-2} at 100-2,000 km. The collective doses resulting from airborne discharges were then calculated using an atmospheric dispersion model with the characteristics of a semi-arid area and an effective release height of 10 m. The resultant collective effective doses per unit release are shown in Table 22, along with the collective effective doses per unit electrical energy generated for the radionuclides released during the operation of the model mine and mill and from the abandoned tailings piles. The total collective effective dose per unit electrical energy generated is estimated to be 1.5 man Sv (GW a)$^{-1}$ during the operation of the mine and mill and to be essentially due to the radon releases. This is greater by a factor of 3 than the estimate given in the UNSCEAR 1988 Report, since additional data have indicated higher average normalized releases. The uncertainties exist not only from normalized releases but also from conditions of the model site and the population

distributions. There may be wide deviations from the above assumptions for actual sites. The doses from liquid effluents are negligible in comparison to the doses from airborne effluents.

90. The collective effective dose per unit electrical energy generated that is due to the releases of radon from abandoned tailings piles is estimated to be delivered at a rate of 0.015 man Sv $(GW a)^{-1}$ per year of release. The rate of release as a function of time is assumed to be constant, and given the very long radioactive half-lives of the radon precursors, the normalized collective effective dose committed is proportional to the assumed duration of the release. Taking this period to be 10,000 years for the sake of illustration, the result is an estimated 150 man Sv $(GW a)^{-1}$. This figure is highly dependent on future management practices; its estimated range is from 1 to 1,000 man Sv $(GW a)^{-1}$.

B. URANIUM FUEL FABRICATION

91. The uranium ore concentrate produced at the mills is further processed and purified and converted to uranium tetrafluoride (UF_4), and then to uranium hexafluoride (UF_6) if it is to be enriched in the isotope ^{235}U, before being converted into uranium oxide or metal and fabricated into fuel elements. Uranium enrichment is not needed for gas-cooled, graphite-moderated reactors (GCRs) or heavy-water-cooled, heavy-water-moderated reactors (HWRs). Enrichments of 2%-5% are required for light-water-moderated and cooled reactors (PWRs and BWRs) and for advanced gas-cooled, graphite-moderated reactors (AGRs).

1. Effluents

92. Available data on airborne and liquid discharges from installations of this stage of the fuel cycle are given in Table 23. Emissions of radionuclides from the conversion, enrichment, and fuel fabrication processes are generally small and consist essentially of the long-lived uranium isotopes, ^{234}U, ^{235}U, and ^{238}U, along with ^{234}Th and ^{234m}Pa, which are the short-lived decay products of ^{238}U. The long half-life of ^{230}Th prevents the activity build-up of any other radionuclide of the ^{238}U series. The solid wastes arising during uranium fuel fabrication are trivial in quantity by comparison with those from the uranium mines and mills.

93. The normalized effluent discharges from model fuel conversion, enrichment and fabrication facilities, which are taken to be the same as in the 1988 UNSCEAR Report, are presented in Table 24.

2. Dose estimates

94. Collective doses resulting from the airborne releases were estimated for the model facility specified in the UNSCEAR 1988 Report, with a constant population density of 25 km^{-2} out to 2,000 km. The normalized collective effective dose is estimated to be 2.8 10^{-3} man Sv $(GW a)^{-1}$, with inhalation the most important pathway of exposure. The collective doses due to liquid discharges are much less than those from airborne discharges, as was assessed in the UNSCEAR 1982 Report for the same relative releases.

C. REACTOR OPERATION

95. Nearly all the electrical energy generated by nuclear means is produced in thermal reactors. The fast neutrons produced by the fission process are slowed down to thermal energies by use of a moderator. The most common materials used as moderators are light water (in PWRs and in BWRs), heavy water (in HWRs) and graphite (in GCRs and light-water-cooled, graphite-moderated reactors [LWGRs]). The electrical energy generated by these various types of reactors from 1970 to the end of 1989 is illustrated in Figure VII. During this period the number of nuclear reactors increased from 77 to 426; the installed capacity, from 20 to 318 GW; and the energy generated, from 9 to 212 GW a [I10]. Basic data on nuclear reactors in operation in 1985-1989 are presented in Table 25.

96. The uranium fuel for the nuclear reactors is contained in discrete pins, which prevent leakage of the radioactive fission products into the coolant circuit. The heat generated in the fuel pins by the slowing down of the fission fragments is removed by forced convection, the most usual coolants being light water (in PWRs, BWRs and LWGRs), heavy water (in HWRs), and carbon dioxide (in GCRs). The thermal energy carried by the coolant is then transformed into electrical energy by means of turbine generators.

97. In addition to the reactor types mentioned above, there are five fast breeder reactors (FBRs) in operation in the world. In that type of reactor, fission is induced by fast neutrons, there is no moderator and the coolant is a liquid metal. The main advantage of the FBR lies in its ability to produce more nuclear fuel than it consumes.

1. Effluents

98. During the production of power by a nuclear reactor, radioactive fission products are formed within the fuel and neutron activation products in structural

and cladding materials. Radioactive contamination of the coolant occurs because fission products diffuse into the coolant from the small fraction of fuel with defective cladding, and particles arising from the corrosion of structural and cladding materials are activated as they are carried through the core. All reactors have treatment systems for the removal of radionuclides from gaseous and liquid wastes.

99. The amounts of different radioactive materials released from the reactors depend on the reactor type, its design and the specific waste treatment plant installed. As in the previous UNSCEAR Reports, annual release data have been compiled for each type of reactor. Annual releases are reported in this Annex for the period 1985-1989. These include:

(a) noble gases (argon, krypton and xenon) released to atmosphere (Table 26); the radionuclide compositions of the noble gases discharged from PWRs and BWRs in the United States in 1988 are given in Tables 27 and 28, respectively;
(b) tritium in airborne effluents (Table 29);
(c) carbon-14 released to the atmosphere, available for a few reactors (Table 30);
(d) iodine-131 in airborne effluents (Table 31); releases of other radioactive isotopes of iodine from PWRs and BWRs in the United States in 1988 are presented in Table 32;
(e) particulates in airborne effluents (Table 33);
(f) tritium in liquid effluents (Table 34);
(g) radionuclides other than tritium in liquid effluents (Table 35); the radionuclide compositions of the activities released in liquid effluents from PWRs and BWRs in the United States in 1988 are given in Tables 36 and 37, respectively.

100. For each effluent category, the reported discharges from individual reactors in a given year vary over several orders of magnitude according to design, type of waste treatment, and level of irregular operations and maintenance. Even for reactors of the same type, the variations are enormous. As an example, the statistical distribution of the ^{131}I released from PWRs in the United States during 1988 is illustrated in Figure VIII. For the distribution assumed to be lognormal, a very large geometric standard deviation of 13 is obtained. Neither the amount of electrical energy generated nor the age of the reactor appears to have a clear effect on the quantities of radioactive materials released in a given year. The normalized releases of radionuclides in airborne effluents from PWRs in the United States in 1988 are illustrated in Figure IX. Both the total and normalized releases seem to be independent of the amount of electrical energy generated in that year or of the age of the reactor. This may indicate that effluent treatments in all reactors are maintained to current standards.

101. The trends in normalized releases from all reactors worldwide of the major components of radionuclides in airborne and liquid effluents are illustrated in Figures X to XVI. Deviations from the general patterns may reflect abnormal operation, special maintenance or the like in specific reactors. Some variability may also reflect data that are too incomplete to provide representative averages. The data become increasingly incomplete for years before 1985. For the period 1985-1989, although some components of discharges are not measured, the reporting of available data is nearly complete for all reactors in operation in the world.

102. Because of the variability in annual releases, normalized releases have been averaged over five-year periods in order to assess the collective doses. The normalized releases for the data available since 1970 are presented in Table 38. Data are available for all types of reactors and effluent categories for 1985 1989, except ^{131}I discharged from FBRs. A release equal to that from PWRs is assumed. Estimated values only are available for ^{3}H releases from LWGRs [I14]. For some earlier periods the data are less complete for some reactor types. In order to include estimates for those periods as well, the more recent data or the data for PWRs are used.

103. The trends in the principal components of releases from reactors, averaged over all reactor types and over five-year time periods from 1970 to 1989, are shown in Figure XVII. Atmospheric discharges of noble gases and iodines, as well as liquid discharges of radionuclides other than tritium, have been decreasing, and there have been less obvious changes for the other components. The downward trends no doubt reflect improvements in the quality of nuclear fuel as well as in the performance and standards of reactors in operation.

104. The estimates of normalized release of radionuclides from reactors may be combined with the electrical energy generated to obtain estimates of the total releases from all reactor operations in the world. A record of energy generation by reactors worldwide is compiled by the International Atomic Energy Agency (IAEA) [I10]. Since this record is not complete, especially for earlier years of operating experience in some countries, data provided separately to the Committee and a few estimated values have been added to provide the summary listing given in Table 39. The average normalized release values in Table 38 are assumed to be the most representative and are applied throughout each five-year period. The total releases from all reactors for the entire period of their usage, during which time 1,844 GW a of electrical energy was generated, and the average normalized releases are given in Table 40.

2. Local and regional dose estimates

105. National authorities usually require that environmental monitoring programmes be carried out in the vicinity of a nuclear reactor. In general, the activity concentrations of radionuclides in effluent discharges are too low to be measurable except close to the point of discharge. Dose estimates for the population therefore rely on modelling the environmental transfer and transport of radioactive materials.

106. In the UNSCEAR 1982 Report and the UNSCEAR 1988 Report, the Committee used a model site that is most representative of northern Europe and the north-eastern United States, since those areas contain a large proportion of all power-producing reactors. The cumulative population within 2,000 km of the model site is about 250 million, giving an average population density of 20 km^{-2}. Within 50 km of the site, the population density is taken to be 400 km^{-2} in order to reflect siting practices. This model site has also been used in this Annex, along with the environmental and dosimetric models of the UNSCEAR 1988 Report. With the exception of ^{3}H and ^{14}C, most of the collective doses are delivered to populations in local and regional areas surrounding the model site. The collective effective dose per unit release for the radionuclides or for the radionuclide compositions representative for each reactor type are presented in Table 41.

107. Estimates of collective effective dose per unit electrical energy generated resulting from effluent discharges from reactors in 1985-1989 are given in Table 42. These are obtained by multiplying the normalized releases (Table 38) by the collective effective dose per unit release (Table 41). The total for all reactor operation is 1.4 man Sv $(GW\ a)^{-1}$.

108. A similar procedure may be used to evaluate the collective dose from the entire period of reactor operation. The average normalized releases in five-year periods (Table 38) are multiplied by the annual energy generation of the different reactor types (Table 39) and by the factors of collective dose per unit release (Table 41). The results for each reactor type are combined in Table 43. The total collective effective dose from all reactor operations through 1989 is estimated to have been 3,700 man Sv. The contributions by each reactor type (not indicated, but determined from the calculation) are 45% from HWRs, 29% from BWRs, 14% from PWRs, 9% from LWGRs, 4% from GCRs and 0.3% from FBRs.

109. The estimated collective effective doses from effluent discharges from reactors have changed over the course of time, as the amounts of electrical energy generated and the released amounts per unit energy generated have changed. Figure XVIII shows the trends for the various effluent categories. The collective doses from atmospheric discharges of noble gases and of iodine and from liquid discharges of radionuclides other than tritium decreased or remained stable from before 1970 through 1985-1989. The other components of the local and regional collective dose increased with time as the quantity of electrical energy generated increased, also shown in Figure XVIII.

110. Individual doses resulting from routine releases of radioactive effluents from reactors are usually low. For the model site, the annual effective doses to most exposed individuals are estimated to be 1 μSv for PWRs, 7 μSv for BWRs, 10 μSv for HWRs, 10 μSv for GCRs, 20 μSv for LWGRs and 0.1 μSv for FBRs.

D. FUEL REPROCESSING

111. At the fuel reprocessing stage of the nuclear fuel cycle, the elements uranium and plutonium in the irradiated nuclear fuel are recovered to be used again in fission reactors. Spent fuel elements are preferably stored under water for a minimum of four to five months, in order to ensure that the short-lived ^{131}I decays to a very low level. Since one reprocessing plant can serve a large number of nuclear reactors, the quantities of radionuclides passing through the plant are high in absolute terms.

112. Reprocessing is, at present, carried out in only a few countries and is limited to a small portion of the irradiated fuel. Known reprocessing capacities, as summarized in Table 44, amount to about 3,300 t of uranium per annum. The annual throughputs of irradiated fuel from civilian power programmes to fuel reprocessing plants in France, Japan and the United Kingdom are illustrated in Figure XIX. In the 1980s the total throughput at these plants ranged from an equivalent of 5 to 8.5 GW a of electrical energy, representing 5% of the annual worldwide nuclear electrical energy production in that period. The fraction of irradiated fuel that is reprocessed has been decreasing slightly with time, as energy production has expanded somewhat more than the throughput of fuel at the reprocessing plants. The fractional amounts reprocessed in terms of energy production equivalent were 0.078, 0.066 and 0.04 during 1975-1979, 1980-1984 and 1985-1989, respectively. The data for years before 1975 are incomplete.

113. Several countries have taken decisions not to reprocess fuel. In these countries, the fuel will either be disposed of or stored retrievably; in the latter case the possibility of reprocessing at some later date

would not be precluded. The current strategy for the management of spent fuel in different countries is summarized in Table 45; in each case the amount of irradiated fuel produced in 1990 is indicated, based on the amount of nuclear energy generated in that year. For the countries included in Table 45, the generation of spent oxide fuel in 1990 was about 11,000 t of uranium.

1. Effluents

114. The radionuclides of principal concern in effluents from reprocessing plants are the long-lived nuclides: ^{3}H, ^{14}C, ^{85}Kr, ^{129}I, ^{134}Cs, ^{137}Cs and isotopes of transuranium elements. The reported releases of radionuclides to the atmosphere and to the sea from the Sellafield, Cap de La Hague and Tokai-Mura reprocessing plants for 1985-1989 are listed in Table 46. In this Table, the values for the electrical energy generated that correspond to the annual throughput of fuel were estimated from the ^{85}Kr discharges, using production rates of 14 PBq (GW a)$^{-1}$ for GCRs and 11.5 PBq (GW a)$^{-1}$ for PWRs. The variations with time of the normalized releases of ^{3}H and ^{137}Cs in liquid effluents from the Cap de La Hague and Sellafield reprocessing plants are illustrated in Figure XX. The annual total releases follow a similar pattern. Discharges of tritium have been increasing slightly, but ^{137}Cs releases have been decreasing. Stricter controls on releases from the Sellafield plant have, since the early 1980s, reduced the ^{137}Cs releases to levels comparable to those from the Cap de La Hague plant. The normalized releases from the Tokai-Mura plant have been comparable to those from the European plants for ^{3}H but several orders of magnitude less for ^{137}Cs.

115. The data in Table 46, along with those quoted in previous UNSCEAR Reports [U1, U3, U4] and additional data from Japan [N13], have been used to determine the average normalized releases of radionuclides during the five-year periods. The limited data prior to 1975 have been combined with later data to provide estimates for 1970-1979. The values are given in Table 47. The normalization is relevant to the equivalent energy production of the fuel reprocessed. Tritium releases in liquid effluents increased in the most recent five-year period, but there have been decreases for most other radionuclides, particularly for ^{137}Cs (by a factor of 80), for ^{90}Sr (by a factor of 13) and for ^{106}Ru (by a factor of 9).

116. The total amounts of radionuclides released from fuel reprocessing can be estimated by completing the record of amounts of fuel reprocessed prior to 1975. For this purpose the ratio of 0.078 times the annual electrical energy generated by reactors has been used. The energy generated by reactors was given in Table 39. The fuel reprocessed (energy equivalent) times the average normalized releases of Table 47 give estimates of the total annual releases, which are shown in Table 48. Whenever the measured results from all three reprocessing plants in France, Japan and the United Kingdom were available, those results, instead of estimated values, were used in Table 48. Measured results were available for ^{3}H and ^{85}Kr in airborne effluents and ^{3}H, ^{90}Sr, ^{106}Ru, ^{137}Cs in liquid effluents since 1975, for ^{129}I in airborne effluents in 1980-1984 and in liquid effluents in 1983-1986. The average normalized releases for the entire period of fuel reprocessing operations given in Table 48 correspond to 1,844 GW a of electrical energy generated and an amount of fuel reprocessed equivalent to 101 GW a.

2. Local and regional dose estimates

117. The collective doses from the reprocessing of nuclear fuel arise from local and regional exposures and from exposures to the globally dispersed radionuclides. Estimates of the local and regional dose commitments are given in this Section and the global contribution in Section E. The local and regional collective doses per unit release of radionuclides were evaluated in the UNSCEAR 1988 Report [U1]. These values are included in Table 49 along with the normalized release amounts derived in Table 46. The product of these two quantities gives the collective effective dose per unit energy equivalent of fuel reprocessed. Since the total fuel reprocessed in 1985-1990 was 4% of the total, the collective dose normalized to the total energy generated in the period is less by the factor 0.04. The total normalized collective effective dose (relative to total energy generated) is 0.05 man Sv (GW a)$^{-1}$ from airborne effluents and 0.2 man Sv (GW a)$^{-1}$ from liquid effluents.

118. The evaluation of the collective dose for the entire period of fuel reprocessing is straightforward from the estimates of annual releases of radionuclides presented in Table 48. The quantities in this table are multiplied by the factors of collective dose per unit release in Table 49. The results are presented in Table 50. The collective dose from the start of the reprocessing practice is estimated to be 4,600 man Sv. The main components (over 90%) of the dose are ^{137}Cs and ^{106}Ru in liquid effluents.

119. Annual individual doses to critical groups have been evaluated for the three reprocessing plants for which release data are available. Individual doses for Sellafield have been derived from environmental monitoring data, combined with information on the habits of local critical groups [C4]. The main path-

ways considered are the consumption of locally caught fish and shellfish, whole body external irradiation from intertidal areas and external irradiation of the skin of fishermen while handling nets and pots. Annual individual doses to critical groups by the ingestion pathway peaked at about 3.5 mSv in the early 1980s and later declined, to about 0.2 mSv in 1986. The estimated annual individual doses to the critical group for whole body exposure to external irradiation also peaked in the early 1980s at about 1 mSv and decreased to about 0.3 mSv in 1986. Finally, the measured beta dose rates from nets and pots have suggested that skin exposure to fishermen would be no more than 0.1 mSv a^{-1} [C4]. The exposure pathways for critical groups are similar for the fuel reprocessing plant at Cap de La Hague. The estimated annual individual doses for 1986 are 0.2 mSv for the consumption of fish and shellfish and 0.05 mSv for whole body external irradiation. The annual doses to critical groups near the Tokai-Mura reprocessing plant are of the order of 1 μSv [S3].

E. GLOBALLY DISPERSED RADIONUCLIDES

120. The radionuclides giving rise to global collective doses are those that are sufficiently long-lived and that migrate readily through the environment, achieving widespread distribution. The radionuclides of interest are ^{3}H, ^{14}C, ^{85}Kr and ^{129}I. The very long-lived ^{129}I poses a special problem because of the uncertainties involved in the prediction of population size, dietary habits and environmental pathways over periods of tens of millions of years. In this Annex, the global dose commitments are truncated at 10,000 years. By that time, ^{3}H and ^{85}Kr have decayed to insignificant levels and ^{14}C has decayed to about 30% of its initial value. Results for alternative integration periods were presented in the UNSCEAR 1988 Report [U1]. The limit of 10,000 years was chosen to correspond to the maximum period of integrity of tailings piles from which ^{230}Th continues to support ^{222}Rn emanation. Beyond 10,000 years either complete erosion or massive covering of the tailings would occur due to the expected intervention of an ice age. The uncertainties of dose calculations become exceedingly great as integration periods are extended over thousands of years.

121. The collective effective dose per unit electrical energy generated is evaluated in Table 51. The normalized release from reactors and reprocessing plants, the latter less by a factor of 0.04 when normalized for the total energy generated, representing the fraction of fuel reprocessed, is multiplied by the factors of collective dose per unit release. For tritium, the collective dose per unit release to air is taken to correspond to the quotient of the annual dose rate to the hemispheric production rate of natural tritium (10 nSv a^{-1} ÷ 37 PBq) times the world population of the northern hemisphere ($5\ 10^{9} \times 0.89$). The result is 0.0012 man Sv TBq^{-1}. For release to sea, calculations with a global circulation model have shown that the normalized collective dose is a factor of 10 less [N8]. For ^{14}C, the collective dose per unit release is taken to be 85 man Sv TBq^{-1}, which over the 10,000-year period is 71% of the normalized collective dose committed for all time (see paragraph 44). For ^{85}Kr and ^{129}I, the collective dose factors are taken to be as evaluated in the UNSCEAR 1988 Report [U1]. The normalized collective dose, truncated at 10,000 years, from globally dispersed radionuclides is 53 man Sv $(GW\ a)^{-1}$ and is due almost entirely to ^{14}C.

122. The total collective effective dose from globally dispersed radionuclides for the entire period of nuclear power production can be evaluated by multiplying the total release of these radionuclides by the collective dose per unit release. The results of this calculation are given in Table 52. The total is 123,000 man Sv, over 99% of which is due to ^{14}C.

F. SOLID WASTE DISPOSAL AND TRANSPORT

123. The solid wastes that arise from reactor operations as well as from the handling, processing and disposal of spent fuel are generally characterized as low-level wastes, intermediate-level wastes, and high-level wastes. Low-level wastes and intermediate-level wastes are generally disposed of by shallow burial. Burial facilities range from simple trenches or pits containing untreated wastes and capped with soil (typically used for low-level wastes) to concrete structures containing conditioned wastes and capped with soil (typically used for intermediate-level wastes). Some low-level wastes were disposed of at sea at more than 50 sites from 1946 to 1982 [I11]. Various solutions are envisaged for the disposal of high-level wastes, but none have yet been implemented. Decommissioned reactors will become part of solid waste management programmes in the future. Several reactors have been shut down, but none have yet been dismantled or transformed into a waste disposal site as yet.

124. Doses from solid waste disposal are usually assumed to result from the migration of radionuclides through the burial site into groundwater. The normalized collective effective dose attributable to wastes from reactor operation is almost entirely due to ^{14}C and roughly amounts to 0.5 man Sv $(GW\ a)^{-1}$; the corresponding value for wastes from the handling and processing of spent fuel is 0.05 man Sv $(GW\ a)^{-1}$.

These estimates are highly uncertain as they depend critically on the assumptions used for the containment of the solid wastes and for the site characteristics.

125. Materials of various types are transported between the installations involved in the nuclear fuel cycle. Members of the public in the vicinity of the trucks, boats or trains carrying the radioactive materials are exposed to small doses of external irradiation. On the basis of fragmentary data, the normalized collective effective dose was estimated to be 0.1 man Sv $(GW\ a)^{-1}$ in the UNSCEAR 1988 Report. The same value is used in this Annex.

G. SUMMARY OF DOSE ESTIMATES

126. A summary of the main contributions to the total collective effective dose, normalized per unit electrical energy generated, is shown in Table 53. The local and regional normalized collective effective doses, which are effectively received within one or two years of discharge, amount to 3 man Sv $(GW\ a)^{-1}$ and are principally due to routine atmospheric releases during reactor and mining operations. Even though the contributions from the various components of the nuclear fuel cycle are different from those reported in the UNSCEAR 1988 Report, the total remains the same, as the decreases in the dose estimates from reactor operation and fuel reprocessing have been compensated by increases in the dose estimates from mining and milling. Globally dispersed radionuclides in effluents from the nuclear fuel cycle and long-term releases from solid waste disposal result in small exposures to members of the public over a very long time (10,000 years or more). The normalized collective effective dose received within 10,000 years amounts to about 200 man Sv $(GW\ a)^{-1}$ and is mainly due to the release of radon from mill tailings and to the release of ^{14}C from fuel reprocessing plants and from reactors.

127. The assessment of the local and regional collective dose for the entire period of nuclear power production has been determined for reactor operation, 3,700 man Sv (Table 43), and for fuel reprocessing, 4,600 man Sv (Table 50). It can be assumed that the normalized collective effective dose from mining and milling, given as 1.5 man Sv $(GW\ a)^{-1}$ in Table 53, is also representative of earlier periods. The total collective dose from this portion of the fuel cycle is thus 1.5 man Sv $(GW\ a)^{-1} \times 1,844$ GW a = 2,700 man Sv. The total for the entire fuel cycle is 2,700 + 3,700 + 4,600 = 11,300 man Sv. The average normalized collective dose for the entire period of the practice is estimated to be 11,000 man Sv ÷ 1,844 GW a = 6 man Sv $(GW\ a)^{-1}$. This long-term average is higher than the value for present practice owing to the declining releases from reactors and fuel reprocessing operations.

128. The estimation of collective effective doses from globally dispersed radionuclides and from long-term releases from solid waste disposal is rather speculative, as it depends heavily on future waste management practices and on the evolution of the world's population over the next 10,000 years. Multiplying the figure of 200 man Sv $(GW\ a)^{-1}$ obtained in this Annex as well as in the UNSCEAR 1988 Report by 1,844 GW a yields a collective effective dose from these sources of about 400,000 man Sv. About 25% of the total is due to ^{14}C released from reactors and reprocessing plants (Table 52) and the remainder to radon released from mill tailings.

V. RADIOISOTOPE PRODUCTION AND USE

129. Radionuclides are used for a variety of purposes in industry, medicine and research [I6], and both the number of uses and the quantities used have been continually increasing. For example, in Japan, the number of establishments using radionuclides and/or radiation generators has grown over the years, from about 100 in 1960 to about 5,000 in 1990 [J2]. Exposures of the public may result from activities associated with the production, use and waste disposal of the radioactive materials. The doses from the use of radioisotopes in consumer products were considered in the UNSCEAR 1982 Report [U3]. The doses evaluated in this Chapter are those resulting from releases to the environment, which may occur during production, use or disposal. Radionuclides produced for sealed sources are not considered, since they are not normally released. Radiopharmaceuticals, ^{14}C and ^{3}H are usually eventually released, and with some approximation the total production can give an estimate of the total release.

A. PRODUCTION AMOUNTS AND RELEASES

130. The amounts of radioisotopes produced for commercial or medical purposes are not well documented. Likewise, the releases during production

or use are not widely reported. The evaluation of doses must therefore remain rather approximate, with only preliminary, very uncertain results having been used. Statistics on radioisotope production and use are available only for Japan [J2]. Table 54 gives the annual uses of radioisotopes in 1989 in hospitals, schools, research institutions and industries. From the population of Japan (118.9 million) the usage per 10^6 population may be determined: for example, 5.2, 6.1, 14 and 34 GBq per 10^6 population for ^{14}C, ^{125}I, ^{3}H and ^{131}I, respectively.

131. The production of compounds labelled with ^{14}C has been estimated for the United States in 1978 to be about 7 TBq [N9], corresponding to 30 GBq per 10^6 population. This is six times the normalized usage in Japan. The production amount of ^{14}C in the United Kingdom is not available, but the reported releases in airborne and liquid effluents from the commercial production plant were reported to be 3.2 TBq in 1987 [H6]. This corresponds to 55 GBq per 10^6 population. The net production must be substantially greater. It is, however, supporting users in many other countries as well as in the United Kingdom. By assuming that 10% of the ^{14}C is lost at production and normalizing to the population of Europe (roughly 10 times that of the United Kingdom), the estimate of normalized production becomes 50 GBq per 10^6 population.

132. To obtain approximate figures of production, usage and ultimate release amounts, the ^{14}C estimate of the United States is assumed and applied at the rates of 100% to the population of developed countries (1.2 10^9 population) and 10% to the population of developing countries (3.7 10^9 population). The annual production and release of radioisotopes relative to ^{14}C are determined from the values given in Table 54 for Japan. Thus, for example, the production of ^{3}H and ^{131}I is three and six times greater, respectively, than the production of ^{14}C.

133. The annual global production and ultimate release of these radionuclides may be estimated to be 30 GBq per 10^6 population (^{14}C) times an equivalent world population of 1.6 10^9 persons times the relative production fractions. The results for several radionuclides are given in Table 55. Other radionuclides not included in this Table, especially those in solid form, are unlikely to be released or widely dispersed from the end-uses.

134. Additional data on the production and release of radioisotopes are available for ^{131}I administered to patients in medical facilities. The total amount of ^{131}I produced for medical purposes in Sweden during 1986 was 0.9 TBq [N15]. Radioactive discharges of ^{131}I from hospitals in Australia in 1988-1989 have been reported as 2.9 TBq [A9]. These amounts, corresponding to 110 and 190 GBq per 10^6 population, give some corroboration to the value used in Table 55 (200 GBq per 10^6 population). About two thirds of orally administered ^{131}I is excreted via the urine of treated patients in the first day [E2]; however, only very low concentrations of ^{131}I have been measured in surface waters in Germany [A7] and in the sewage systems of cities in Sweden [E2] and in the United States [S5]. Waste treatment systems in hospitals with hold-up tanks may reduce the amounts of ^{131}I discharged in liquid effluents to 5 10^{-4} of amounts administered to patients [J3].

B. DOSE ESTIMATES

135. Since the environmental levels of radioisotopes used for medical, educational or industrial purposes are in general undetectable, only approximate, calculated estimates can be made of the collective doses. The results are given in Table 55. The estimates assume no partial retention of the radionuclides in end-products and no hold-up prior to wide dispersion and the exposure of local, regional or global populations. This could result in overestimated doses, significantly so for radioiodines that have short half-lives. The dose coefficients listed in Table 55 are those derived and used for radionuclides produced and released in nuclear power production. Tritium and the noble gases are assumed to be released to the atmosphere, ^{14}C to be released in both airborne and liquid effluents and ^{131}I and ^{125}I to be released to rivers. There could be occasional release of iodine in airborne effluents, for example from incineration of waste materials. This would be easily detected, but since it is so seldom reported, it can be assumed that this is not an important source of release. The dose coefficient for ^{125}I is based on age-weighted dose-per-unit-intake values [N1] and the ^{125}I half-life of 13 hours, with other model parameters the same as for ^{131}I.

136. The total local and regional collective effective dose from releases of radioisotopes used in one year in medical and industrial applications is of the order of 100 man Sv. If it can be assumed that the practice of these radioisotope uses has been building up over the past 40 years, the collective dose committed from all past releases would be 20 times the present annual value, or 2,000 man Sv in total. The global component of the collective effective dose, arising almost entirely from ^{14}C, is 4,000 man Sv from one year of radioisotope usage and 80,000 man Sv committed from the entire practice to date. The contribution of this source to man-made exposures in general is thus relatively unimportant on an annual basis. The doses from ^{14}C are at low dose rate but extend over a long period of time.

VI. ACCIDENTS

137. A number of accidents have occurred at both civilian and military nuclear installations and in the transport of nuclear materials. In some cases, there was substantial contamination of the environment. These accidents are discussed in this Chapter, and the magnitude of population doses incurred are estimated.

A. CIVILIAN NUCLEAR REACTORS

138. The two principal accidents involving installations of the civilian nuclear fuel cycle took place at the Three Mile Island reactor in the United States in March 1979 and at Chernobyl in the USSR in April 1986.

1. Three Mile Island

139. The accident at Three Mile Island has been the subject of many reports, particularly from the United States Nuclear Regulatory Commission and the President's Commission [K3]. The cause of the accident was the failure to close a pressure relief valve, which led to severe damage of uncooled fuel. The accident re eased large amounts of radioactive materials from failed fuel to the containment, but the environmental releases were relatively small (about 370 PBq of noble gases, mainly ^{133}Xe, and 550 GBq of ^{131}I into the atmosphere).

140. Individual doses averaged 15 μSv within 80 km of the plant, and the maximum effected dose that any member of the public could have received is estimated to have been 850 μSv from external gamma irradiation [K3]. The collective effective dose due to the release has been estimated to be 20 man Sv within 80 km of the plant [K3]. The contribution to the effective dose commitment due to ^{133}Xe dispersion beyond 80 km may have been equal to that within 80 km [U3], which gives a total of 40 man Sv.

2. Chernobyl

141. The worldwide exposures from the Chernobyl accident were evaluated in detail in the UNSCEAR 1988 Report [U1]. In the course of a low-power engineering test, uncontrollable instabilities developed and caused explosions and fire, which damaged the reactor and allowed radioactive gases and particles to be released into the environment. The fire was extinguished and the releases stopped by the tenth day after the accident. The death toll within three months of the accident was 30, all of them members of the operating staff of the reactor or of the fire-fighting crew.

142. The total release of radioactive materials is estimated to have been 1-2 EBq [I3], the principal radionuclides being ^{131}I (630 PBq), ^{134}Cs (35 PBq) and ^{137}Cs (70 PBq) [I15]. The proportional amounts dispersed beyond the USSR were determined to be 34% for ^{131}I and 56% for ^{137}Cs [I15].

143. About 115,000 residents were relocated from a 30 km exclusion zone surrounding the reactor. The external radiation doses to most of those evacuated was less than 0.25 Sv, although a few in the most contaminated areas might have received doses up to 0.3-0.4 Sv. The collective dose from external radiation to the evacuees is estimated to have been 16,000 man Sv. Individual thyroid doses to children may have been 2.5 Gy and higher in some cases, with an average thyroid dose of 0.3 Gy and a collective thyroid dose of 400,000 man Gy [C10].

144. The radiation situation beyond the 30 km zone surrounding the reactor was determined primarily by the wind directions. When rainfall occurred at the time that the radioactive cloud was passing, the deposition density of ^{137}Cs and other fission radionuclides was enhanced. In the USSR, an area of about 10,000 km^2 was contaminated with ^{137}Cs to levels in excess of 560 kBq m^{-2}, and an area of 21,000 km^2 received upwards of 190 kBq m^{-2} [I15]. A government commission determined that 786 settlements, located in Belarus, the Russian Federation, and Ukraine, with a population of 270,000, were to be considered as "strict control zones". Protective measures preventing the consumption of contaminated foodstuffs were applied in the strict control zones. The average effective dose received by the populations in the strict control zones is estimated to have been 37 mSv in the year following the accident and 23 mSv in 1987-1989 [I15]. An international review project was conducted in 1990 to investigate environmental levels, doses and the health of residents of unevacuated settlements [I1]. The project corroborated results of measurements and dose evaluations. Diet and body measurements showed that agricultural practices and protective measures were effective in limiting exposures. The doses determined by whole body counting were less than expected from calculation by environmental models. Estimation of thyroid doses requires interpretation of early direct measurements and calculation of presumed ^{131}I intakes; these doses are thus subject to considerable uncertainties.

145. Detailed information on environmental contamination levels and radiation doses received by populations in the northern hemisphere was made available to the Committee by many countries, either

directly to the UNSCEAR secretariat or in published reports. This information enabled the Committee, in the UNSCEAR 1988 Report [U1], to calculate first-year radiation doses in the USSR, all other European countries and a few other countries in the northern hemisphere. The projected doses beyond the first year were based on the environmental behaviour of ^{137}Cs determined in many years of measurements following atmospheric nuclear testing.

146. The collective effective dose from the Chernobyl accident was estimated to be approximately 600,000 man Sv [U1]. Of this amount, 40% is expected to be received in the territory of the former USSR, 57% in the rest of Europe and 3% in other countries of the northern hemisphere.

B. MILITARY INSTALLATIONS

147. There have been two accidents at military plants that are known to have caused measurable exposures of the public: an accident at Kyshtym in the southern Ural Mountains of the USSR in September 1957 and the Windscale reactor accident in the United Kingdom in October of the same year.

1. Kyshtym

148. In the early 1950s high-level radioactive wastes from the Chelyabinsk-40 plutonium production centre near Kyshtym were stored in water-cooled tanks encased in concrete. The corrosion and failure of process monitoring equipment led to a breakdown in the cooling system of a 300 m^3 tank, allowing the 70-80 tonnes of waste, stored mainly in the form of nitrate and acetate compounds and containing about 1 EBq of radioactive materials, to heat up. The water in the tank evaporated, and as the sediments dried out, they reached temperatures of 330-350°C. On 29 September 1957 the contents of the tank exploded with a power estimated to have been equivalent to 70-100 tonnes of TNT [R3]. About 90% of the radioactive materials contained in the tank deposited locally, while the remainder (about 100 PBq) was dispersed away from the site of the explosion [A4, B11, B12, N2, N3, R3, T1, T4]. The main contributors to the total activity associated with the radioactive materials released were ^{144}Ce + ^{144}Pr (66%), ^{95}Zr + ^{95}Nb (24.9%), ^{90}Sr + ^{90}Y (5.4%) and ^{106}Ru + ^{106}Rh (3.7%). In addition, ^{137}Cs (0.036%), ^{89}Sr (traces), ^{147}Pm (traces), ^{155}Eu (traces) and $^{239,240}Pu$ (traces) were also released [B11]. With the exception of caesium, the radionuclide composition is similar to that of fission products that had been cooled for about one year. Waste treatment at the reprocessing plant involved concentrating the radionuclides by means of precipitation with sodium hydroxide. Caesium was practically the only element with radionuclides that remained in the solution; it was later concentrated separately [R3].

149. The radioactive cloud reached a height of about 1 km. Wind conditions were relatively stable during the dispersion of the cloud over a relatively flat surface, and there was no precipitation. This resulted in an oblong fallout area, extending to about 300 km from the plant, with a clearly defined axis and monotonic decrease in the deposition density along the axis and perpendicular to it. Virtually all of the deposition occurred within 11 h. The boundaries of the contaminated area were taken to correspond to a ^{90}Sr deposition density of 4 kBq m^{-2}, twice the level of global fallout.

150. Redistribution of the deposited radionuclides occurred to some extent, most noticeably in the first few days after the accident. The main sources of the redistribution were the crowns of trees and the soil surfaces. On the whole, the delineation of the fallout area was practically complete by 1958, when wind migration was redistributing less than 1% of the original fallout. Over the next 30 years, wind transfer did not affect appreciably the distribution of the contamination [T1]. The contaminated area was estimated to comprise between 15,000 and 23,000 km^2, with a population of about 270,000, in the provinces Chelyabinsk, Sverdlovsk and Tyumen [B11, N3]. There were 1,154 people in areas with a ^{90}Sr deposition density greater than 40 MBq m^{-2}, 1,500 in areas with a deposition greater than 4 MBq m^{-2} and 10,000 in areas with a deposition greater than 70 kBq m^{-2} [B11, N3].

151. External irradiation was the main route of exposure during the first few months after the accident; subsequently, the ingestion of ^{90}Sr in foodstuffs became predominant. During the initial period, the dose rate in air was about 1.3 μGy h^{-1} from gamma emitting radionuclides in areas with a ^{90}Sr deposition density of 40 kBq m^{-2}, with maximum values of about 5 mGy h^{-1} near the plant, where the deposition density of ^{90}Sr reached 150 MBq m^{-2} [B11]. Within 10 days of the accident 1,154 persons [B11, B12, N3, R3] were evacuated from the settlements in the most severely affected area, which had a ^{90}Sr deposition density greater than 40 MBq m^{-2}. Subsequently, monitoring of the radioactive contamination levels in foodstuffs and agricultural produce was carried out to assure that an annual ^{90}Sr intake of 50 kBq a^{-1} would not be exceeded. A ban on foods was imposed with concentration limits of ^{90}Sr relative to the mass of calcium in foods of 7.4 Bq g^{-1} initially and 2.4 Bq g^{-1} at a subsequent period. This led to the destruction of more than 10,000 tonnes of agricultural produce in the first two years following the accident and to the

decision to carry out a further systematic evacuation of the population from areas with a ^{90}Sr deposition density greater than 150 kBq m^{-2} [R3]. The resettlement, which began 8 months after the accident, was completed 18 months after the accident. Altogether, 10,730 persons were evacuated [B11]. The collective dose is evaluated in Table 56. The average dose received by the population group evacuated within 10 days of the accident was 170 mSv from external irradiation and 1,500 mSv to the gastro-intestinal tract; the average effective dose was 520 mSv. The collective dose received by the evacuated individuals amounted to about 1,300 man Sv.

152. The doses received by the populations that were not evacuated are also presented in Table 56. About half of the effective dose had been delivered within one year, more than 90% within 10 years and nearly all within 30 years of the accident. The effective dose per unit deposition density was estimated to be 320 μSv per kBq m^{-2} over 30 years, with just over 20% due to external irradiation. The collective effective doses received by the non-evacuated population (about 260,000 persons) have been reported to be 1,100 man Sv [N3] and about 5,000 man Sv [B1]. It is difficult to judge the validity of these figures, as the information on the correspondence of ^{90}Sr deposition densities with populations is very coarse. However, it is indicated that average effective doses received over 30 years are estimated to have been 20 mSv for a group of about 10,000 people living in areas with a ^{90}Sr deposition density between 40 and 70 kBq m^{-2} and 4 mSv for a group of 2,000 people living in areas with a deposition density between 4 and 40 kBq m^{-2} [B11]. On the basis of the relationship between population and the deposition density of ^{90}Sr described above, it can be assumed that the number of people living in areas with deposition densities between 40 and 70 kBq m^{-2} was 10,000 and that the number of people living in areas with deposition densities between 4 and 40 kBq m^{-2} was 250,000, resulting in a collective effective dose over 30 years of 1,200 man Sv.

153. A less serious accident occurred in 1967, as a consequence of the disposal of radioactive wastes containing 4 EBq of ^{90}Sr and ^{137}Cs radioactive wastes in Lake Karachay [A3, N4, T4]. On that occasion, dust from the lake bed or the shore-line, containing about 20 TBq of ^{90}Sr and ^{137}Cs, was dispersed by the wind over an area of 1,800 km^2 and to a distance of up to 75 km. The contaminated territory included portions under the radioactive plume of the 1957 accident. The maximum deposition density of ^{90}Sr was 0.4 MBq m^{-2}, and the $^{137}Cs/^{90}Sr$ activity ratio was 3. Specific information on the doses resulting from that accident is not available; it is expected that they are included in the doses from the much more serious accident that occurred in 1957 at the same site. However, because the $^{137}Cs/^{90}Sr$ activity ratios were very different in the 1957 and 1967 accidents, it would be possible, as evidenced by recent measurements [A3], to separate the contributions from the two accidents by analysing soil samples.

2. Windscale

154. The accident at Windscale in October 1957 began during a routine release of the Wigner energy stored in the graphite of the gas-cooled reactor. Owing to errors in operation, the fuel became overheated and caught fire. The fire lasted for about three days. Major releases of radionuclides occurred mainly in two periods: when the air flow was re-started through the core soon after the accident started, in an attempt to cool it, and when water was pumped into the reactor to extinguish the fire on the second day of the accident [C13]. The release of ^{131}I is estimated to have been 740 TBq, accompanied by 22 TBq of ^{137}Cs, 3 TBq of ^{106}Ru and 1.2 PBq of ^{133}Xe [C10]. In addition to the fission products, other radionuclides were released, the most notable being ^{210}Po, which was being produced by neutron irradiation of bismuth ingots in the core. The release of ^{210}Po amounted to 8.8 TBq [C10, C14]. The Windscale reactor has not been used again since.

155. The contamination of pasture land was widespread, the majority of the released radioactive materials having passed south-south-east of Windscale, in the direction of London, and eventually over Belgium before having turned northwards, to Norway. At the time of accident, the radionuclide identified as being of principal concern was ^{131}I, and the main pathway to man was identified as the ingestion of cow's milk. The prompt imposition of a ban on milk supplies had the effect of reducing ^{131}I intakes via the pasture-cow-milk-pathway [C10]. Extensive environmental measurements were made in the United Kingdom at the time of the accident. Maximum doses to persons close to the site were estimated to have been of the order of 10 mGy to the thyroid of adults and perhaps 100 mGy to the thyroid of children [B2, C9]. Thyroid doses to adults in Leeds and London were estimated from measurements of ^{131}I in the thyroids to have been 1 mGy and 0.4 mGy, respectively [B2], with young children having received doses twice as great.

156. The collective effective dose received in the United Kingdom and in Europe from all radionuclides and pathways was estimated to have been 2,000 man Sv, of which about 900 man Sv was due to inhalation and 800 man Sv was due to the ingestion of milk and other foodstuffs. External irradiation from

ground deposits of radionuclides was estimated to have contributed 300 man Sv. The main contributors to the collective effective dose were ^{131}I (37%) and ^{210}Po (37%), followed by ^{137}Cs (15%) [C10].

C. TRANSPORT OF NUCLEAR WEAPONS

157. Fourteen accidents involving aircraft carrying nuclear weapons or components of nuclear weapons are known to have occurred, the two most publicized being the aircraft crash near Palomares, Spain, in January 1966 and the crash at Thule, Greenland, in January 1968. Appreciable amounts of ^{239}Pu were released locally to the environment. A number of nuclear weapons have also been lost at sea.

158. The accident at Palomares, on the Mediterranean coast, occurred on 17 January 1966, when two United States military planes collided in the process of a mid-air refuelling operation. The parachutes of two of the four thermonuclear weapons carried by one of the planes failed to deploy, resulting in the detonation of their conventional explosives and the release of their fissile material upon hitting the ground. Partial ignition of the fissile material formed a cloud that contaminated 2.26 km^2 of uncultivated farm land and urban land with ^{239}Pu and ^{240}Pu [I16-I20]. The other two bombs were recovered intact, one in a dry river bed near the mouth of the Almanzora River and the other in the sea.

159. Where the deposition density of alpha emitters was greater than 1.2 MBq m^{-2} (an area of 22,000 m^2), the contaminated vegetation and a surface layer of soil, approximately 10 cm deep, were collected, separated and disposed of as radioactive waste. Arable land with levels below 1.2 MBq m^{-2} was irrigated, ploughed to a depth of 30 cm, harrowed and mixed. On rocky hillsides, where ploughing was not possible, soil with a plutonium level greater than 0.12 MBq m^{-2} was removed to some extent with hand tools [I17].

160. Estimates of the doses from inhalation and from ingestion have been derived from measured concentrations of ^{239}Pu and ^{240}Pu in ground-level air, in agricultural foodstuffs and in people. The urine and lungs of Palomares inhabitants have been sampled and measured for plutonium since 1966. Of the 714 people examined up to 1988, only 124 showed concentrations of plutonium in urine greater than the minimum detectable activity. Iranzo et al. [I18] estimated that the 70-year committed effective doses for 55 of these people ranged from 20 to 200 mSv owing to the acute inhalation of radioactive particles at the time of the accident or immediately afterwards. The highest estimated 70-year committed effective dose was 240 mSv to a one-year-old child [I18]. From data in this reference, the collective effective dose due to acute inhalation of radioactive particles immediately after the accident can be estimated to have been about 1 man Sv.

161. The resuspension of soil particles has been monitored since 1966 at four locations [I17]. The average annual concentrations of ^{239}Pu and ^{240}Pu during the period 1966-1980 were 5.5 μBq m^{-3} at the location representative of the urban centre and 52 μBq m^{-3} at the location representative of the most exposed farming area [I17]. The corresponding 50-year effective dose per year of intake by inhalation of radioactive particles resuspended from soil are 4 and 35 μSv per year of intake for people in the urban area and in the most exposed farming area, respectively. Assuming that (a) the total number of persons exposed is 714; (b) 90% of that exposed population resides in the urban area and the remainder in the most exposed farming area; and (c) the amount of ^{239}Pu and ^{240}Pu available for resuspension decreases exponentially with a half-time of 100 years, the collective effective dose due to the resuspension of radioactive particles is roughly estimated to be 1 man Sv.

162. The main crops in the cultivated area of the Palomares region are tomatoes, barley and alfalfa [I20]. From the plutonium concentrations in those products, it can be inferred that resuspension of the plutonium particles in soil plays a more important role than absorption through root uptake in the contamination of agricultural products cultivated in the area [I20]. Iranzo et al. [I20] estimated that the individual committed effective dose due to a yearly consumption of unwashed contaminated tomatoes would be 1.5 μSv and that the collective effective dose from a yearly consumption of tomatoes grown on one hectare of contaminated soils would be 10^{-4} man Sv. Assuming that (a) the cultivated area used for the production of tomatoes is 100 hectares (1 km^2) and (b) the amount of plutonium available for the contamination of agricultural crops decreases exponentially with a half-time of 100 years (reflecting the predominant role of resuspension), the collective effective dose due to the ingestion of tomatoes contaminated as a result of the accident is crudely estimated to be about 1 man Sv. The contamination of barley and alfalfa also results in the contamination of products used for human consumption (milk and meat), but the doses due to ingestion of those products are much lower than those due to the ingestion of tomatoes because of the filtering effect of the animals.

163. Some of the plutonium deposited on land was transferred to the Mediterranean Sea when the Almanzora River, which flows through the village of Palomares, flooded [G1]. This transfer, however, is not significant from a radiological point of view.

164. Near Thule, the high-explosive components of four weapons detonated in an airplane crash, contaminating about 0.2 km^2. About 10 TBq of plutonium was recovered in the surface layer of the snow pack, and about 1 TBq was estimated to be trapped in the ice [L1]. A radioecological investigation conducted during the summer of 1968, when the ice had broken up, showed that the accident had measurably raised the plutonium level in the marine environment as far as 20 km from the point of impact. The highest concentrations were found in bottom sediments, in bivalves and in crustacea. Larger animals such as birds, seals and walruses showed plutonium levels hardly different from the fallout background [A1, A2].

165. Accidents have also happened during the transport of nuclear weapons by sea. At least 48 nuclear weapons and 11 reactors have been reported to be lying on the ocean floor [E3]. The most serious losses were two nuclear-powered submarines, each carrying several nuclear weapons; one sank off the coast of Bermuda in October 1986 and the other in the Norwegian Sea in April 1989. Another loss occurred near the coast of Japan in 1965, when an airplane with a 1 Mt hydrogen bomb rolled off an aircraft carrier. No information has been reported on the number of deaths or on the extent of environmental contamination associated with those accidents that resulted in the loss of nuclear weapons. However, some information is available about an accident that took place aboard a missile-carrying nuclear submarine in July 1961 in the Atlantic Ocean [K8]. In that accident, a depressurization in the primary coolant of one of the two nuclear reactors led to substantial radioactive contamination in the submarine and to a reactor shutdown. To prevent reactor meltdown, a temporary emergency cooling system was fabricated; this required welding work to be carried out in the reactor compartment itself, which led to eight deaths within a few weeks of the accident [K8].

D. SATELLITE RE-ENTRY

166. In 1964, when a SNAP-9A satellite containing ^{238}Pu as a power source re-entered the atmosphere and then burned up, about 600 TBq of that radionuclide were injected into the stratosphere [H1]. A similar device re-entered the atmosphere intact, produced no releases and fell into the Pacific Ocean in April 1970. Another generator fell into waters off the coast of California in May 1968, when a weather satellite exploded during launch. It was recovered in October 1968. In January 1978, the Cosmos 954 satellite re-entered the atmosphere, partially burned and scattered debris in the Northwest Territories of Canada. Detailed information on the characteristics of the radioisotopes and reactor-powered devices used in satellites, as well as on the malfunctions that have occurred, has been gathered by OECD [O4].

167. The collective dose from the SNAP-9A re-entry may be evaluated by applying transfer coefficients to the released amount. The transfer coefficient P_{25} from deposition of ^{238}Pu to dose via the ingestion pathway has been estimated to be 0.6 nSv per Bq m^{-2} (Table 8). The transfer coefficient P_{02} for ^{238}Pu, which has a half-life 87.7 years, would be expected to be 5 kBq m^{-2} per EBq released (Figure III) for temperate latitudes. The dose commitment for these latitudes would then be estimated to be 0.6 PBq $\times P_{02} \times P_{25}$ = 1.8 nSv. The hemisphere average is less by a factor of 1.5 and the opposite hemisphere average is less by a factor of 4. Since re-entry was in the southern hemi phere, the averages for the hemispheres are 1.2 nSv (south) and 0.3 nSv (north). The population-weighted world average is 0.4 nSv (89% of the population lives in the northern hemisphere). For the relatively long half-life of ^{238}Pu, a world population of 6 10^9 may be taken to apply to this exposure [U3]. The collective effective dose from the ingestion pathway due to the re-entry of the SNAP-9A is thus estimated to be 2.4 man Sv.

168. The transfer coefficient P_{25} for the inhalation pathway has an estimated value of 800 nSv per Bq m^{-2} (Table 8). The dose commitment for the southern hemisphere temperate region is thus 0.6 PBq $\times P_{02} \times P_{25}$ = 2,400 nSv. The average values for the hemispheres are then 1,600 nSv (southern hemisphere), 400 nSv (northern hemisphere) and 530 nSv (world). The collective dose from the inhalation pathway, with a population of 4 10^9 applicable at the time of re-entry, is 2,100 man Sv. The inhalation pathway is the dominant contributor to the collective dose. This is comparable to the collective effective dose derived for ^{238}Pu produced in atmospheric nuclear testing, which released 0.33 PBq, about half the total of the satellite re-entry, but with injection mostly into the atmosphere of the northern hemisphere.

169. Similar procedures may be used to estimate the collective dose from the Cosmos 954 re-entry. The fuel core was estimated to contain 20 kg of enriched uranium [G3]. With a steady power output of 100 kW over the 128 day lifetime of the satellite, the burn-up of the fuel was estimated to be 2 10^{18} fissions per gram of uranium [G3]. The estimated radionuclide inventory in the core at re-entry is presented in Table 57 [T6]. From analysis of recovered debris, it has been assumed that 75% of the radionuclide amounts were dispersed in the high atmosphere on re-entry of the space craft and 25% was deposited on the ground in the uninhabited impact area. The absence of the volatile elements iodine and caesium in surface samples indicates that 100% of the radionuclides of

these elements were dispersed on burn-up of the fuel core in the atmosphere. The collective dose is estimated in Table 57 from the widely dispersed material using the transfer factors of Figure III and Table 8. The result is 16 man Sv, mainly to the population of the northern hemisphere from ^{137}Cs and ^{90}Sr and over a longer term from ^{239}Pu.

E. INDUSTRIAL AND MEDICAL SOURCES

170. Three notable accidents involving small sealed sources used for industrial or medical purposes have occurred since 1982 [U1]. In December 1983, at Ciudad Juarez, Mexico, a non-licensed teletherapy source containing 16.7 TBq of ^{60}Co was sold to a scrapyard [M4]. It is believed that the source was broken and that its 6,000 pellets began to be dispersed during transport [M4]. The consequences of this accident were the contamination of thousands of tonnes of metallic products that were sold in Mexico and the United States, as well as the contamination of several foundries and streets and hundreds of houses. About one thousand people were exposed to substantial levels of radiation. It is estimated that seven persons received between 3 and 7 Sv; 73 persons received between 0.25 and 3 Sv, and 700 persons received between 0.005 and 0.25 Sv [M4]. There were no deaths.

171. In 1984, at Mohammedia, Morocco, a source of ^{192}Ir used to make radiographs of welds at a construction site became detached from the take-up line to its shielded container. The source dropped to the ground and was noticed by a passer-by, who took it home. Eight persons, an entire family, died from the radiation over-exposure, having suffered doses of 8-25 Sv [I4, S10]. Estimates of doses to the individuals are unavailable, so only a rough approximation can be made of the collective dose. Assuming 10 Sv on average to each person, the collective dose to those who died would have been 80 man Sv.

172. In September 1987, at Goiania, Brazil, a 50.9 TBq ^{137}Cs source was inadvertently removed from a therapy unit and dismantled by junk dealers [C6, I5, R4, V1]. The therapy unit was located in the abandoned and partly demolished Goiania Radiotherapy Institute. The dismantling of the source resulted in localized contamination of an inhabited area of the city. As the result of the direct handling of the source or parts of it, either during its dismantling or subsequently, 129 people were exposed, either externally or internally. Some suffered very high external contamination owing to the way they had handled the caesium powder, such as having daubed their skin. Internal exposures resulted from eating with contaminated hands. The dose estimates varied from zero up to 5.3 Sv. Fifty-four persons were hospitalized and four died [I5]. The estimated collective doses were 56.3 man Sv from external exposures and 3.7 man Sv from internal exposures, including 14.9 man Sv (external) and 2.3 man Sv (internal) to the four persons who died [D9]. In the course of the decontamination programme, seven houses were demolished and large amounts of soil had to be removed. The total volume of waste removed was 3,100 m^3 [V1].

CONCLUSIONS

173. A number of events, activities or practices involving radiation sources have resulted in the release of radioactive materials to the environment. The consequent exposures of the population have been evaluated in this Annex. Estimates have been made of the total amounts of radioactive materials released in the event or since the beginning of the practice and of the collective doses that have been received or committed.

174. The most significant cause of exposure has been the testing of nuclear weapons in the atmosphere. A large number of tests were performed in the 1950s and to the end of 1962, with less frequent testing occurring until 1980, when the practice stopped altogether. The Committee has repeatedly evaluated the exposures from this source. The extensive measurements allow a rather systematic and complete assessment to be made. In this Annex the transfer coefficients that describe the movement of radionuclides in the environment to man and to the dose are summarized, extended and updated. The collective effective dose committed to the world population by atmospheric nuclear testing is estimated to be 3 10^7 man Sv. Of this total, 86% is due to long-term, low-level exposure from ^{14}C. Over the next 10,000 years a collective dose of 2.2 10^7 man Sv will have been received. This value is recorded in Table 58, which summarizes the estimated collective doses from all sources.

175. The underground testing of nuclear weapons does not generally cause the population to be exposed to radiation. It is only when there is some leakage or venting of gases or aerosols, as has occurred on some occasions, that relatively low exposures may result. The Committee estimates the collective effective dose

from underground testing to be of the order of 200 man Sv.

176. The Committee has not previously estimated the exposures of populations that result from the production of materials and the fabrication of nuclear weapons. Data are still not readily available, but initial estimates of collective doses have been made, namely of the order of 24,000 man Sv to local and regional populations and 40,000 man Sv from global, long-term exposure. Efforts are under way to reconstruct exposures that occurred in the early years of this activity, so some refinement and extension of the estimates can be anticipated.

177. A major activity utilizing radioactive materials is the generation of electrical energy with nuclear reactors. The release of radionuclides during routine operation of the nuclear fuel cycle is relatively low, however, and the doses can only be calculated using representative models for the sites and the dispersion processes through the environment. The releases and collective doses since the beginning of the practice in the 1950s have been at least two orders of magnitude less than those for atmospheric nuclear testing. The global, long-term collective effective dose to be received within 10,000 years is estimated to be 400,000 man Sv. Twenty-five per cent of this is due to ^{14}C released from reactors and reprocessing plants and 75% is due to ^{222}Rn released from uranium mill tailings piles.

178. A number of radioisotopes are used for industrial, educational and medical purposes. Those used in solid forms may not be released from end-uses; however, the gases, tritium, ^{14}C and radioiodines can be expected to be eventually released and dispersed. Data are generally unavailable on production amounts and release fractions of the radionuclides. Based on assumed values, the Committee estimates the global, long-term collective effective dose from this source to be 80,000 man Sv, with negligible contributions from all radionuclides except ^{14}C.

179. The accidents that have resulted in environmental contamination and exposures of population groups include those at civilian nuclear reactors (Three Mile Island and Chernobyl), at military installations (Windscale and Kyshtym), those that occurred in the transport of nuclear weapons (Thule and Palomares) and in satellite re-entry (SNAP-9A and Cosmos 954) and those that involved the loss or misuse of industrial and medical sources (Ciudad Juarez, Mohammedia and Goiania). With the exception of the Chernobyl accident and the re-entry of satellites, the environmental contamination has been localized, and for all except the Chernobyl accident the collective radiation doses have been relatively low. Nevertheless, injuries and deaths have resulted from some of these accidents.

180. The total collective dose from all sources of man-made environmental exposures is dominated by atmospheric nuclear testing. This source contributes 95% of the total collective dose indicated in Table 58. The annual collective effective dose to the world's population from natural sources of radiation exposure of 12,000,000 man Sv may help to put these estimates into perspective. Atmospheric nuclear testing was equivalent to three years of natural exposure of the world population at the time of the exposures. Other sources, of the order of a few tens or hundreds of thousands of man sievert, are comparable to hours or days of natural background exposure. The Committee has made the estimates in Table 58 with the objective of documenting each source of exposure and providing a perspective on the magnitudes of radionuclide releases and collective doses involved.

Table 1
Radionuclides produced and globally dispersed in atmospheric nuclear testing

Radio-nuclide	*Half-life* [E7]	*Decay mode*	*Fission yield* (%) [H2]	*Estimates of amounts released into the atmosphere (excluding local fallout)* [a]		
				Total (EBq)	*Normalized release* ($PBq\ Mt^{-1}$)	
					Fission	*Fusion*
H-3	12.32 a	ß	-	240	0.026	740
C-14	5730 a	ß	-	0.22	[b]	0.67
Mn-54	312.5 d	EC,γ	-	5.2	-	15.9
Fe-55	2.74 a	EC	-	2	-	6.1
Sr-89	50.55 d	ß	2.56	91.4	590	-
Sr-90	28.6 a	ß	3.50	0.604	3.90	-
Y-91	58.51 d	ß	3.76	116	748	-
Zr-95	64.03 d	ß,γ	5.07	143	922	-
Ru-103	39.25 d	ß,γ	5.20	238	1540	-
Ru-106	371.6 d	ß,γ	2.44	11.8	76.4	-
Sb-125	2.73 a	ß,γ	0.29	0.524	3.38	-
I-131	8.02 d	ß,γ	2.90	651	4200	-
Cs-137	30.14 a	ß,γ	5.57	0.912	5.89	-
Ba-140	12.75 d	ß,γ	5.18	732	4730	-
Ce-141	32.50 d	ß,γ	4.58	254	1640	-
Ce-144	284.9 d	ß,γ	4.69	29.6	191	-
Pu-239	24100 a	α,γ	-	0.00652	-	-
Pu-240	6560 a	α,γ	-	0.00435	-	-
Pu-241	14.4 a	ß	-	0.142	-	-

a For the non-gaseous fission products a total non-local fission explosion yield of 155 Mt, obtained from measured ^{90}Sr deposition, was assumed in deriving the total amounts released.

b For simplicity it is assumed that all ^{14}C is due to fusion, as fusion produces up to 6 times more neutrons than fission for the same energy release. The production reaction is $^{14}N(n,p)^{14}C$.

Table 2
Latitudinal distribution of ^{90}Sr and ^{95}Zr deposition from atmospheric nuclear testing

Latitude band (*degrees*)	*Area of band* (*10^{12} m^2*)	*Population distribution* (*%*)	*Integrated deposition (PBq)* ^{90}Sr	*Integrated deposition density (Bq m^{-2})* ^{90}Sr	*Integrated deposition density (Bq m^{-2})* ^{95}Zr
Northern hemisphere					
80-90	3.9	0	1.0	260	
70-80	11.6	0	7.9	680	
60-70	18.9	0.4	32.9	1740	
50-60	25.6	13.7	73.9	2890	
40-50	31.5	15.5	101.6	3230	38000
30-40	36.4	20.4	85.3	2340	
20-30	40.2	32.7	71.2	1770	
10-20	42.8	11.0	50.9	1190	
0-10	44.1	6.3	35.7	810	
Total	255	100	460	2140 [a]	25000 [a]
Southern hemisphere					
0-10	44.1	54.0	21.0	480	
10-20	42.8	26.7	17.8	420	
20-30	40.8	14.9	28.1	700	
30-40	36.4	13.0	27.6	760	
40-50	31.5	0.9	28.1	890	8300
50-60	25.6	0.5	12.1	470	
60-70	18.9	0	6.7	350	
70-80	11.6	0	2.5	220	
80-90	3.9	0	0.3	80	
Total	255	100	144	540 [a]	5000 [a]
Global	510	89 (northern) 11 (southern)	604	1960 [a]	23000 [a]

[a] Population-weighted values.

Table 3
Estimates of population-weighted deposition densities of the major radionuclides produced in atmospheric testing (^{3}H and ^{14}C not included)

Radio-nuclide	*Ratio to ^{90}Sr*	*Ratio to ^{95}Zr*	*Population-weighted deposition density (Bq m^{-2})*				
			Northern hemisphere		*Southern hemisphere*		*World*
			40°-50°	*Entire*	*40°-50°*	*Entire*	
Mn-54	2.9		9400	6200	2600	1600	5700
Fe-55	2.1		6800	4500	1900	1100	4100
Sr-89		0.52	20000	13000	4300	2600	12000
Sr-90	1.0		3230	2140	890	540	1960
Y-91		0.66	25000	17000	5000	3300	15000
Zr-95		1.0	38000	25000	8300	5000	23000
Nb-95		1.7	64000	43000	14000	8500	39000
Ru-103		0.75	28000	19000	6200	3800	17000
Ru-106	7.5		24000	16000	6700	4100	15000
Sb-125	0.89		2900	1900	790	480	1700
I-131		0.50	19000	13000	4200	2500	11000
Cs-137	1.6		5200	3400	1400	860	3100
Ba-140		0.62	23000	16000	5100	3100	14000
Ce-141		0.55	21000	14000	4600	2800	13000
Ce-144	15		48000	32000	13000	8100	29000
Pu-238	0.00046		1.5	0.98	0.41	0.25	0.90
Pu-239	0.011		35	23	10	6	22
Pu-240	0.0072		23	15	6	4	14
Pu-241	0.23		730	480	200	120	440
Am-241	0.0077 [a]		25	17	7	4	15

[a] Upon decay of ^{241}Pu.

Table 4
Components of the transfer coefficient P_{23} from deposition density to diet for ^{90}Sr and ^{137}Cs

Country	*^{90}Sr*					*^{137}Cs*				
	Transfer factor parameters [a]y					*Transfer factor parameters [a]*				
	b_1	b_2	b_3	λ	P_{23}	b_1	b_2	b_3	λ	P_{23}
Milk products										
Argentina	1.2	1.1	0.1	0.1	3.7	7.7	0	0.2	0.1	8.8
Denmark	1.5	0.9	0.3	0.1	4.9	3.0	2.1	0.06	0.08	5.9
United States	0.7	0.3	0.2	0.1	2.6	3.4	1.8	0.2	0.3	5.7
Average					3.7					6.8
Grain products										
Argentina	1.6	1.5	0.06	0.02	6	2.0	6.9	0		8.9
Denmark	3.1	9.8	0.1	0.02	17.2	3.4	23.2	0.0003	4.3	26.6
United States	0.7	1.5	0.2	0.08	4.1	2.1	8.0	0.3	0.2	11.7
Average					9.1					15.7
Vegetables										
Argentina	0.02	0	0.1	0.26	0.4	2.1	2.3	0		4.4
Denmark	0.4	0	0.1	0.05	3.1	2.4	0	0.02	0.02	3.3
United States	0.3	0.06	0.3	0.08	4.0	1.2	0	0.1	0.19	1.8
Average					2.5					3.2
Fruit										
Argentina	0.3	0.2	0.04	0.09	1.0	0.5	2.6	0		3.1
Denmark	0.9	0.005	0.05	0.05	2.0	1.8	1.2	0.1	0.3	3.5
United States	0.1	0	0.1	0.06	2.5	1.6	0.0	1.1	0.5	3.3
Average					1.8					3.3
Meat										
Argentina	0.7	0.8	0.03	0.02	3	22.1	0	3.7	0.7	26.2
Denmark	0.5	0.04	0.04	0.09	0.9	13.4	0	80.3	2.0	26.2
United States	0.002	0.1	0.04	0.1	0.4	1.5	0	17.7	1.3	7.9
Average					1.4					
Total diet										
Sum of weighted components [b]										
Argentina	0.8	0.7	0.07		2.7	4.9	2.5	0.3		8.0
Denmark	1.3	1.9	0.2		5.6	4.4	4.5	12.1		11.4
United States	0.4	0.3	0.2		2.6	2.2	1.7	3.3		5.8
Average					3.6					8.4
Fit on total diet										
Argentina	1.1	0.6	0.04	0.03	3.0	6.3	1.8	0		8.1
Denmark	1.3	2.0	0.1	0.06	5.5	4.1	6.5	0.02	0.02	11.4
United States	0.5	0.4	0.2	0.08	3.0	1.6	2.0	0.8	0.4	5.1
Average					3.8					8.2

[a] The transfer coefficients for the first year, b_1, second year, b_2, and subsequent years, b_3, and the total transfer factor, P_{23}, have the units mBq a kg^{-1} per Bq m^{-2}. The units of the exponential decay constant, λ, are a^{-1}. The regression fits are for the periods: Argentina 1964-1979, Denmark 1962-1985 and United States 1960-1983 (^{90}Sr, New York) and 1961-1977 (^{137}Cs, Chicago).

[b] Fractional amounts by weight of the five food groups, milk products, grain products, vegetables, fruit and meat, in the total diet are, respectively, [U3]:
Argentina: 0.26, 0.2, 0.24, 0.2, 0.08 (^{90}Sr); 0.26, 0.2,0.31, 0.16, 0.08 (^{137}Cs);
Denmark: 0.35, 0.16, 0.24, 0.1, 0.15 (^{90}Sr and ^{137}Cs)
United States: 0.31, 0.15, 0.19, 0.15, 0.19 (^{90}Sr) in New York; 0.33, 0.14, 0.19. 0.17, 0.17 (^{137}Cs) in Chicago.

Table 5
Transfer of fallout ^{90}Sr and ^{137}Cs from deposition to diet [a]

Component	*Transfer factor [b]*	*Contribution to total transfer*	*Contribution to component transfer from food categories (%)*				
			Milk	*Grain*	*Vegetables*	*Fruit*	*Meat*
^{90}Sr							
Direct deposition	0.8 ± 0.4	22%	43%	38%	6%	8%	5%
Lagged transfer	1.0 ± 0.8	27%	23%	72%	0.4%	2%	3%
Transfer from deposit	1.8 ± 0.6	51%	32%	28%	26%	10%	4%
Total transfer	3.6 ± 1.7	100%	32%	42%	15%	7%	4%
^{137}Cs							
Direct deposition	3.8 ± 1.4	45%	36%	11%	13%	5%	35%
Lagged transfer	2.9 ± 1.5	35%	15%	71%	8%	6%	0%
Transfer from deposit	1.7 ± 1.0	20%	15%	4%	7%	7%	67%
Total transfer	8.4 ± 2.8	100%	25%	30%	10%	6%	29%

a Average consumption-weighted results for Argentina, Denmark and the United States.
b The units are mBq a kg^{-1} per Bq m^{-2}.

Table 6
Transfer coefficients P_{24} from deposition to intake into the body by ingestion for fallout radionuclides derived from measurements in the temperate zone of the northern hemisphere

Radio-nuclide	*Deposition density [a] (Bq m^{-2})*	*Integrated intake rate (Bq)*	*Transfer coefficient (Bq per Bq m^{-2})*
Fe-55	4500	55000 [b]	10
Sr-89	20000	700 [c]	0.03
Sr-90	3230	6140 [d]	1.9
I-131	19000	1370 [e]	0.07 [f]
Cs-137	5200	21800 [d]	4.2
Ba-140	23000	120 [c]	0.005
Pu-238	1.5	0.075 [e]	0.05 [g]
Pu-239	35	24 [e]	0.7 [g]
Pu-240	23	16 [e]	0.7 [g]
Pu-241	730	29 [e]	0.04 [g]
Am-241	25	5 [e]	0.2 [g]

a Values from Table 3 (40°-50°) except for Fe-55 (entire) northern hemisphere.
b Inferred from estimated dose to red bone marrow in the northern hemisphere of 6 μGy [U3, U4] and dose to red bone marrow per unit intake by ingestion of 0.11 nGy Bq^{-1} [N1].
c Value from [U3]; measurements only for milk.
d Inferred from transfer coefficient value (Bq a kg^{-1} per Bq m^{-2}) in Table 4 times an average food consumption rate of 500 kg a^{-1}.
e Inferred from transfer coefficient value and deposition density.
f Derived from P_{23} value of 0.63 mBq a l^{-1} per Bq m^{-2} [U3] for transfer to milk times an average milk consumption rate of 0.3 l d^{-1}.
g Derived in [U3].

Table 7
Transfer coefficients P_{45} from intake to dose for radionuclides produced in atmospheric nuclear testing [a] [N1]

Radio-nuclide	*Absorption fraction*	*Committed equivalent dose per unit intake (nSv Bq^{-1})*								*Effective dose per unit intake (nSv Bq^{-1})*
		Bone surfaces	*Breast*	*Colon*	*Gonads*	*Liver*	*Lungs*	*Red bone marrow*	*Thyroid*	
Ingestion										
Fe-55	0.1	0.11	0.10	0.31	0.11	0.35	0.10	0.11	0.11	0.15
Sr-89	0.3	4.8	0.26	21	0.26	0.26	0.26	3.3	0.26	3.4
Sr-90	0.3	390	1.3	19	1.3	1.3	1.3	180	1.3	28
I-131 [b]	1.0	0.15	0.20	0.09	0.09	0.10	0.18	0.16	1218	61
Cs-137	1.0	12	12	14	13.5	14	13	13	13	13
Ba-140	0.1	0.53	0.16	26	0.565	0.12	0.069	0.42	0.056	3.7
Pu-238	0.00001	160	0.00018	57	2.3	29	0.00009	13	0.00008	12
Pu-239	0.00001	180	0.00012	53	2.6	31	0.00008	14	0.00008	12
Pu-240	0.00001	180	0.00018	53	2.6	31	0.00008	14	0.00007	13
Pu-241	0.00001	3.5	0.000003	0.27	0.056	0.53	0.000005	0.28	.000001	0.14
Am-241	0.0005	9000	0.016	59	130	1600	0.017	720	0.0066	290
Inhalation [c]										
Mn-54	0.1	1.3	0.85	1.3	0.49	2.4	6.4	1.1	0.74	1.7
Fe-55	0.1	0.18	0.17	0.28	0.18	0.58	1.0	0.18	0.19	0.33
Sr-89	0.01	0.16	0.0086	14	0.0086	0.0086	83	0.11	0.0086	12
Sr-90	0.01	65	0.24	20	0.24	0.24	2900	30	0.24	350
Y-91	0.0001	0.32	0.0089	15	0.0073	0.32	99	0.32	0.0084	14
Zr-95	0.002	2.3	1.2	3.9	0.33	2.1	40	1.3	1.2	6.3
Nb-95	0.01	0.51	0.4	1.9	0.24	0.66	8.3	0.44	0.36	1.6
Ru-103	0.05	0.24	0.31	3.1	0.19	0.50	16	0.32	0.26	2.5
Ru-106	0.05	1.6	1.8	37	1.2	2.3	1000	1.8	1.7	130
Sb-125	0.01	1.1	0.41	3.3	0.23	0.85	22	0.53	0.33	3.4
I-131	1.0	0.052	0.073	0.025	0.024	0.037	0.65	0.057	270	13
Cs-137	1.0	7.9	7.8	9	8.3	8.6	8.7	8.2	8.0	8.5
Ba-140	0.1	2.3	0.3	4.4	0.37	0.3	1.7	1.2	0.27	1.1
Ce-141	0.0003	0.26	0.044	4.1	0.031	0.26	17	0.085	0.025	2.6
Ce-144	0.0003	4.9	0.35	34	0.22	26	790	2.9	0.29	100
Pu-238	0.00001	720000	0.44	33	10000	130000	310000	58000	0.38	61000
Pu-239	0.00001	820000	0.39	31	12000	150000	320000	66000	0.37	64000
Pu-240	0.00001	820000	0.43	31	12000	150000	320000	66000	0.37	64000
Pu-241	0.00001	18000	0.023	0.18	270	3000	3100	1400	0.093	930
Am-241	0.0005	2200000	2.7	32	32000	380000	18000	170000	1.6	70000

[a] Values are for adults except for ingestion of ^{131}I; the absorption fractions correspond to values used in previous UNSCEAR assessments [U1, U3]; the committed equivalent doses (from [N1]) are for a period of 50 years after intake for adults and to age 70 years for children (for ingestion of ^{131}I).

[b] ^{131}I: age and milk consumption weighted values; 0-1 year, 1-9 years, 9-19 years, and adult age groups are 2, 16, 20, 62% of population with milk consumption 330, 180, 150, 90 l a^{-1}, respectively; the dose factors for the four age groups are the average for 3-month-old and 1-year-old children; for 5-year-old children; for 15-year-old children; and for adults.

[c] Absorption assumptions are Class D (days): ^{131}I, ^{137}Cs and ^{140}Ba; Class W (weeks): ^{54}Mn, ^{55}Fe, ^{125}Sb and ^{241}Am; and Class Y: (years) all other radionuclides.

Table 8
Transfer coefficients P_{25} from deposition to dose for radionuclides produced in atmospheric nuclear testing

Radio-nuclide	*Transfer coefficient to equivalent dose (nSv per Bq m^-2^)*								*Transfer coefficient for effective dose (nSv per Bq m^-2^)*
	Bone surfaces	*Breast*	*Colon*	*Gonads*	*Liver*	*Lungs*	*Red bone marrow*	*Thyroid*	
					Ingestion				
Fe-55	1.5	1.3	4.1	1.5	4.7	1.3	1.5	1.5	2.0
Sr-89	0.17	0.0091	0.74	0.0091	0.0091	0.0091	0.12	0.0091	0.12
Sr-90	722	2.4	35	2.4	2.4	2.4	330	2.4	52
I-131	0.011	0.014	0.0063	0.0059	0.0069	0.012	0.011	84	4.2
Cs-137	50	50	59	57	59	55	55	55	55
Ba-140	0.0026	0.00077	0.13	0.0027	0.00058	0.00033	0.0020	0.00027	0.018
Pu-238	8.0	a	2.9	0.12	1.5	a	0.65	a	0.60
Pu-239	130	0.00008	37	1.8	22	0.00005	9.8	37	8.4
Pu-240	130	0.00013	37	1.8	22	0.00006	9.8	0.00005	9.1
Pu-241	0.14	a	0.011	0.0022	a	a	0.011	a	0.0056
Am-241	1800	0.0032	12	26	320	0.0034	140	0.00132	58
					Inhalation				
Mn-54	0.017	0.011	0.017	0.0064	0.032	0.084	0.014	0.010	0.022
Fe-55	0.0024	0.0022	0.0037	0.0024	0.0076	0.013	0.0024	0.0025	0.0043
Sr-89	0.0021	0.0001	0.18	0.0001	0.0001	1.1	0.0014	0.0001	0.16
Sr-90	0.85	0.0032	0.26	0.0032	0.0032	38	0.39	0.0032	4.6
Y-91	0.0042	0.0001	0.20	0.0001	0.0042	1.3	0.0042	0.0001	0.18
Zr-95	0.030	0.016	0.051	0.0043	0.028	0.53	0.017	0.016	0.083
Nb-95	0.0067	0.0053	0.025	0.0032	0.0087	0.11	0.0058	0.0047	0.021
Ru-103	0.0032	0.0041	0.041	0.0025	0.0066	0.21	0.0042	0.0034	0.033
Ru-106	0.021	0.024	0.49	0.016	0.030	13	0.024	0.022	1.7
Sb-125	0.014	0.0054	0.043	0.0030	0.011	0.29	0.0070	0.0043	0.045
I-131	0.0007	0.0010	0.0003	0.0003	0.0005	0.0085	0.0008	3.5	0.17
Cs-137	0.10	0.10	0.12	0.11	0.11	0.11	0.11	0.11	0.11
Ba-140	0.030	0.0039	0.058	0.0049	0.0039	0.022	0.016	0.0035	0.014
Ce-141	0.003	0.0006	0.054	0.0004	0.0034	0.22	0.0011	0.0003	0.034
Ce-144	0.06	0.0046	0.45	0.0028	0.34	10	0.038	0.0038	1.3
Pu-238	9450	0.0058	0.43	130	1710	4100	760	0.0050	800
Pu-239	10800	0.0051	0.41	160	1970	4200	870	0.0049	840
Pu-240	10800	0.0056	0.41	160	1970	4200	870	0.0049	840
Pu-241	236	0.0003	0.0024	3.5	39	41	18	0.0012	12
Am-241	28900	0.035	0.42	420	4990	240	2230	0.021	920
					External exposure				
Mn-54									9.9
Zr-95									3.7
Nb-95									1.0
Ru-103									0.72
Ru-106									2.9
Sb-125									16
I-131									0.12
Cs-137									97
Ba-140									1.1
Ce-141									0.081
Ce-144									0.47

[a] Less than 0.00001.

Table 9
Effective dose commitments from radionuclides produced in atmospheric nuclear testing

Radio-nuclide	Effective dose commitment (μSv)											
	North temperate zone (40°-50°)				South temperate zone (40°-50°)				World population			
	External	Ingestion	Inhalation	Total	External	Ingestion	Inhalation	Total	External	Ingestion	Inhalation	Total
H-3		48	3.6	51		13	0.95	14		44	3.3	47
C-14		2600	0.26	2600		2600	0.26	2600		2600	0.26	2600
Mn-54	93		0.21	94	26		0.06	26	57		0.13	57
Fe-55		14	0.03	14		3.8	0.01	3.8		8.2	0.02	8.2
Sr-89		2.3	3.1	5.5		0.51	0.68	1.2		1.4	1.9	3.3
Sr-90		170	15	180		46	4.1	50		102	9.0	111
Y-91			4.6	4.6			1.0	1.0			2.8	2.8
Zr-95	140		3.1	144	31		0.69	32	85		1.9	87
Nb-95	67		1.4	68	15		0.30	15	40		0.82	41
Ru-103	20		0.93	21	4.5		0.20	4.7	12		0.56	13
Ru-106	70		41	110	20		11	31	44		26	69
Sb-125	47		0.13	47	13		0.04	13	27		0.08	28
I-131	2.3	79	3.2	85	0.50	17	0.71	19	1.4	48	2.0	51
Cs-137	510	280	0.58	790	140	76	0.16	210	300	170	0.35	470
Ba-140	25	0.42	0.34	26	5.6	0.09	0.07	5.8	15	0.25	0.21	16
Ce-141	1.7		0.71	2.4	0.37		0.16	0.53	1.0		0.43	1.5
Ce-144	23		63	86	6.1		17	23	14		38	52
Pu-238		0.0009	1.2	1.2		0.0002	0.30	0.30		0.0005	0.72	0.72
Pu-239		0.29	29	30		0.08	8.4	8.5		0.18	18	18
Pu-240		0.21	19	20		0.05	5.0	5.1		0.13	12	12
Pu-241		0.004	8.9	8.9		0.001	2.4	2.4		0.003	5.4	5.4
Am-241		1.5	23	24		0.41	6.4	6.8		0.87	14	15
Total (rounded)	1000	3190	220	4400	260	2760	60	3100	600	2980	140	3700

Table 10
Contributions to the total effective dose commitment to the world population from atmospheric nuclear testing

Radio-nuclide	*Effective dose commitment (μSv)*	*Contribution to total (%)*		*Radio-nuclide*	*Effective dose commitment (μSv)*	*Contribution to total (%)*	
		Including 100% ^{14}C	*Including 10% ^{14}C*			*Including 100% ^{14}C*	*Including 10% ^{14}C*
C-14	2580	70	19	Pu-239	18	0.5	1.3
Cs-137	470	13	35	Ba-140	16	0.4	1.2
Sr-90	110	3.0	8.1	Am-241	15	0.4	1.1
Zr-95	87	2.4	6.4	Ru-103	13	0.3	0.9
Ru-106	69	1.9	5.1	Pu-240	12	0.3	0.9
Mn-54	57	1.5	4.2	Fe-55	8	0.2	0.6
Ce-144	52	1.4	3.8	Pu-241	5	0.1	0.4
I-131	51	1.4	3.8	Sr-89	3	0.09	0.2
H-3	47	1.3	3.5	Y-91	3	0.08	0.2
Nb-95	41	1.1	3.0	Ce-141	1	0.04	0.1
Sb-125	28	0.7	2.0	Pu-238	1	0.02	0.05
Total effective dose commitment				3700 μSv			

Table 11
Collective effective dose to the world population committed by atmospheric nuclear testing

Radio-nuclide	*Collective effective dose (1000 man Sv)*				*Contribution to total (%)*	
	External	*Ingestion*	*Inhalation*	*Total*	*Including 100% ^{14}C*	*Including 10% ^{14}C [a]*
C-14		25800	2.6	25800	86	39
Cs-137	1210	677	1.1	1890	6.3	28
Sr-90		406	29	435	1.5	6.6
Zr-95	272		6.1	278	0.93	4.2
Ru-106	140		82	222	0.74	3.3
H-3		176	13	189	0.63	2.8
Mn-54	181		0.4	181	0.61	2.7
Ce-144	44		122	165	0.55	2.5
I-131	4.4	154	6.3	164	0.55	2.5
Nb-95	129		2.6	131	0.44	2.0
Sb-125	88		0.2	88	0.30	1.3
Pu-239		1.8	56	58	0.20	0.88
Am-241		8.7	44	53	0.18	0.80
Ba-140	49	0.81	0.66	51	0.17	0.77
Ru-103	39		1.8	41	0.14	0.62
Pu-240		1.3	38	39	0.13	0.59
Fe-55		26	0.06	26	0.09	0.40
Pu-241		0.01	17	17	0.06	0.26
Sr-89		4.5	6.0	11	0.04	0.16
Y-91			8.9	8.9	0.03	0.13
Ce-141	3.3		1.4	4.7	0.02	0.07
Pu-238		0.003	2.3	2.3	0.01	0.03
Total (rounded)	2160	27200	440	30000	100	100

[a] Corresponds to dose delivered by ^{14}C before the year 2200.

Table 12
Estimated number and yields of underground nuclear explosions
[N10, S2]

Year	*Number of explosions*	*Yield (Mt)*	*Year*	*Number of explosions*	*Yield (Mt)*	*Year*	*Number of explosions*	*Yield (Mt)*
1957	5	0.002	1969	55	4.1	1981	51	1.8
1958	15	0.03	1970	52	6.6	1982	58	1.8
1959			1971	36	6.9	1983	56	1.2
1960			1972	40	2.5	1984	58	2.3
1961	12	0.1	1973	30	7.7	1985	35	1.2
1962	61	1.0	1974	34	4.2	1986	23	0.8
1963	43	1.0	1975	38	7.5	1987	47	2.2
1964	48	1.0	1976	42	5.4	1988	40	1.6
1965	51	1.8	1977	45	3.5	1989	27	0.7
1966	59	3.7	1978	55	2.7	1990	18	1.1
1967	51	2.2	1979	54	3.9	1991	14	0.3
1968	60	4.8	1980	51	2.9	1992	8	1.1
Total			1352 test explosions			Total yield 90 Mt		

Table 13
Atmospheric releases of iodine-131 to the atmosphere from underground tests carried out at the Nevada test site in the United States
[H4]

Name of test	*Year of test*	*Atmospheric release (TBq)*
Antler	1961	0.2
Feather	1961	0.04
Pampas	1962	0.0004
Platte	1962	0.4
Eel	1962	0.4
Des Moines	1962	1200
Bandicoot	1962	330
Yuba	1963	0.0008
Eagle	1963	0.08
Pike	1964	13
Alva	1964	0.001
Drill	1964	0.5
Parrot	1964	0.2
Alpaca	1965	0.0009
Tee	1965	0.06
Diluted Waters	1965	0.7
Red Hot	1966	7
Pin Stripe	1966	7
Double Play	1966	4
Derringer	1966	0.009
Nash	1967	0.5
Midi Mist	1967	0.01
Hupmobile	1968	4
Pod	1969	0.03
Scuttle	1969	0.0001
Snubber	1970	0.2
Mint Leaf	1970	3
Baneberry	1970	3000
Diagonal Line	1971	0.05
Riola	1980	0.02
Total (rounded)		5000

Table 14
Estimated annual releases of ^{131}I to the atmosphere from the Hanford plutonium production plant in the United States [C5]

Year	Annual release (TBq)	Year	Annual release (TBq)	Year	Annual release (TBq)
1944	1800	1947	900	1952	40
1945	13000	1948	40	1953	25
1946	2800	1949	230	1954	20
		1950	100	1955	30
		1951	630	1956	15
Total 1944-1946	17600	Total 1947-1956		2030	

Table 15
Estimated cumulative doses from radionuclides released into the Techa River from the Chelyabinsk plutonium production plant in the former USSR
[A4]

Village	Distance downstream from the point of discharge (km)	Absorbed dose (mGy)				Effective dose (mSv)
		Red bone marrow	Bone lining cells	G.I. tract	Other	
Metlino [a]	7	1640	2260	1400	1270	1400
Techa-Vrod [a]	18	1270	1480	1190	1150	1190
Asanovo [a]	27	1270	1900	1040	900	1000
Nadirovo [a]	49	950	1800	620	440	560
Muslyumovo	78	610	1430	290	120	240
Brodokalmak	109	140	310	70	33	58
Russkaya Techa	138	220	530	100	37	82
Novopetropavloskoe	152	280	680	130	43	100
Schutikha	202	80	180	26	22	36
Zatechenskoe	237	170	400	84	32	66

[a] Village was evacuated.

Table 16
Estimated uranium and fuel requirements to generate 1 GW a of electrical energy
[O2, O3]

Reactor type	Amount required for 1 GW year			
	Natural uranium (t)	Uranium oxide [a] (t)	Enrichment (SWU) [b]	Fuel (t)
LWR [c]	220	260	130000	37
HWR [d]	180	210	-	180
Magnox [e]	330	390	-	330
AGR [f]	220	260	130000	38

[a] Derived from the amounts of natural uranium using a U_3O_8: heavy metal ratio of 1:18.
[b] Separative work units.
[c] Assuming average fuel irradiation of 30 GWd/tU (thermal energy), thermal efficiency of 33% and an average fuel enrichment of 3% with 0.25% tails.
[d] Assuming a fuel irradiation of 7.3 GWd/tU (thermal energy) and a thermal efficiency of 30%.
[e] Assuming a fuel irradiation of 4.5 GWd/tU (thermal energy) and a thermal efficiency of 26%.
[f] Assuming an average fuel irradiation of 24 GWd/tU (thermal energy), a thermal efficiency of 40% and average enrichment of 2.7% and tails of 0.25%.

Table 17
Production of uranium
[O2]

Country	Annual production of uranium (t) [a]														
	1975	*1976*	*1977*	*1978*	*1979*	*1980*	*1981*	*1982*	*1983*	*1984*	*1985*	*1986*	*1987*	*1988*	*1989* [b]
Argentina	22	40	100	126	134	187	123	155	172	129	126	173	95	142	150
Australia		359	356	516	705	1561	2922	4422	3211	4324	3206	4154	3780	3532	3800
Belgium						20	40	45	45	40	40	40	40	40	40
Brazil				35			4	242	189	117	115	115	0	0	0
Canada	3560	4850	5790	6800	6820	7150	7720	8080	7140	11170	10880	11720	12440	12400	11000
France	1731	1871	2097	2183	2362	2634	2552	2859	3271	3168	3189	3248	3376	3394	3190
Gabon	800	850	907	1022	1100	1033	1022	970	1006	918	940	900	800	930	950
Germany, Fed. Rep.of	57	38	15	35	25	35	36	34	47	32	30	26	53	38	30
India	200	200	200	200	200	200	200	200	200	200	200	200	200	200	200
Japan	3	2	1	2	2	5	3	5	4	4	7	6	8	0	0
Namibia		654	2340	2697	3840	4042	3971	3776	3719	3700	3400	3300	3500	3600	3600
Niger	1306	1460	1609	2060	3620	4128	4363	4259	3426	3276	3181	3110	2970	2970	3000
Pakistan	30	30	30	30	30	30	30	30	30	30	30	30	30	30	30
Portugal	115	88	95	98	114	82	102	113	104	115	119	110	141	144	150
South Africa	2488	2758	3360	3961	4797	6146	6131	5816	6060	5732	4880	4602	3963	3850	2900
Spain	136	170	177	191	190	190	178	150	170	196	201	215	223	228	216
United States	8900	9800	11500	14200	14400	16800	14800	10300	8200	5700	4300	5200	5000	5050	4600
Yugoslavia											30	59	72	80	85
Total	19348	23170	28577	34121	38339	44243	44197	41456	36994	38851	34874	37208	36691	36628	33941

[a] Data only include uranium produced in WOCA (World Outside Centrally planned economies Area). Estimate of uranium production in non-WOCA countries in 1990 is about 18,000 t uranium per year with a decreasing trend; the main producers are believed to be China, Czechoslovakia, the German Democratic Republic and the USSR [I4].

[b] Data for 1989 are estimates.

Table 18
Radon emissions from uranium mines
[A6, A9, D4, N12, O5, R2, W5]

Mine	*Year*	*Ore grade (% of U_3O_8)*	*Production of U_3O_8* [a] *(t)*	*Emission of ^{222}Rn (TBq)*	*Normalized emission of ^{222}Rn (GBq t^{-1})*
		Australia			
Ranger	1985	0.32	4500	45 [b]	10 [c]
	1986	0.35	4700	73 [b]	16 [c]
	1987	0.38	5000	89 [b]	18 [c]
	1988	0.42	6400	120 [b]	19 [c]
	1989	0.41	6000	130	22
Olympic [d]	1988	0.11	600	16	27
	1989	0.11	1200	32	27
Nabariek [e]	1985	1.42	1600	21	13
	1986	1.42	1600	21	13
	1987	1.42	1600	21	13
	1988	1.42	900	12	13
		Canada [f]			
Amok	1985	0.37	860	1	1.2
	1986	0.40	850	1	1.2
	1987	0.42	870	1	1.2
	1988	0.49	900	1	1.1
	1989	0.57	740	1	1.4
Rabbit Lake	1985	0.22	890	1600	1800
	1986	0.46	1500	1600	1100
	1987	0.51	2300	1600	680
	1988	0.72	2800	1600	560
	1989	0.84	2011	1600	760
Denison Mine	1985	0.08	2600	1100	500
	1986	0.08	2040	1100	530
	1987	0.08	1900	1100	570
	1988	0.08	2060	1100	520
	1989	0.08	2000	1100	540
Panel Mine	1985	0.10	990	96	97
	1986	0.10	980	96	98
	1987	0.09	820	96	120
	1988	0.08	780	96	120
	1989	0.09	850	96	110
Stanleigh Mine	1985	0.07	810	120	150
	1986	0.07	750	120	160
	1987	0.07	500	120	240
	1988	0.07	460	120	270
	1989	0.09	570	120	210
		German Democratic Republic			
Thuringian Mines	1985	0.092	3600	540	150
	1986	0.092	3500	610	170
	1987	0.091	3500	660	190
	1988	0.091	3400	730	210
	1989	0.090	3300	690	210
Aue	1985	0.483	840	1600	1900
	1986	0.466	750	1700	2300
	1987	0.475	710	1400	2000
	1988	0.463	710	1400	1950
	1989	0.481	690	650	2000
Königstein	1985	-	670	160	240
	1986	-	605	300	500
	1987	-	540	300	560
	1988	-	520	260	500
	1989	-	500	250	500

Table 18 (continued)

Mine	Year	Ore grade (% of U_3O_8)	Production of U_3O_8 [a] (t)	Emission of ^{222}Rn (TBq)	Normalized emission of ^{222}Rn ($GBq\ t^{-1}$)
Freital	1985	0.097	160	10	61
	1986	0.100	180	8	45
	1987	0.116	190	7	36
	1988	0.112	170	6	36
	1989	0.111	130	5	40

[a] The mill throughput was used when the mine throughput was not available.
[b] Estimated from 1989 value.
[c] Estimated from 1989 value, normalized to U_3O_8 production.
[d] Metallurgical plant; production commenced in June 1988.
[e] Mining ceased in 1990. Mill feed was taken from stockpile, and tailings were returned to mine pit.
[f] Emission of radon estimated from annual average concentration in exhaust air.

Table 19
Radionuclides released in airborne effluents from uranium mills
[A6, N12, O5, R2]

Mine	Year	Ore grade (%)	Ore throughput (Mt)	U_3O_8 production (t)	Annual emission (GBq)					
					^{210}Pb	^{210}Po	^{222}Rn	^{226}Ra	^{230}Th	^{238}U
Australia										
Ranger	1985	0.32	1	3200			43000			1.2
	1986	0.35	0.97	3400			46000			1
	1987	0.38	0.87	3300			44000			0.8
	1988	0.42	0.78	3300			44000			0.8
	1989	0.41	0.98	4000			54000			2
Olympic [a]	1988	0.11	0.5	550	10	85	8000	0.05	0.05	0.1
	1989	0.11	1.1	1200	21	190	16000	0.1	0.1	0.2
Nabariek [b]	1985	1.42	0.12	1700			21000			0.7
	1986	1.42	0.12	1700			21000			0.7
	1987	1.42	0.12	1700			21000			0.7
	1988	1.42	0.07	990			12000			0.4
Canada										
Key Lake	1985	0.28	0.19	530	0.0004				0.0004	0.02
	1986	0.23	0.25	580						
	1987	0.19	0.28	530	0.11			0.002	0.011	31.5
	1988	0.2	0.24	480						
	1989	0.24	0.24	580	0.009			0.024	0.041	0.85
Rabbit Lake	1985-1989	0.53	0.36	1900			9200			
Total release (GBq)					0.12 [c]	[c]	339200	0.18	0.20	41.0
U_3O_8 production (t)					1640		27000	2870	3400	26700
Normalized release ($GBq\ t^{-1}$)					0.00007		13	0.00006	0.00006	0.0015
Normalized release [$GBq\ (GW\ a)^{-1}$]					0.02		3000	0.02	0.02	0.4

[a] Metallurgical plant; production commenced in June 1988; emissions of ^{210}Pb and ^{210}Po are for the particular process and are not representative of normal milling.
[b] Mill operations ceased in July 1988.
[c] Data for Olympic mill are not generally representative and are, therefore, not included in total.

Table 20
Radionuclides released in liquid effluents from uranium mills
[A6]

Mine	*Year*	*Ore grade (%)*	*Ore throughput (Mt)*	*U_3O_8 production (t)*	*Annual emission (GBq)*			
					^{210}Pb	*^{226}Ra*	*^{230}Th*	*^{238}U*
Canada								
Amok	1987	0.42	0.206	865	0.3	0.13	0.25	16
	1988	0.49	0.183	897	0.1	0.02	0.035	6.5
	1988	0.57	0.13	741	0.05	0.01	0.029	7.6
Key Lake	1985	2.72	0.195	5304	0.34	0.23	0.61	1.7
	1986	2.31	0.249	5752	0.16	0.19	0.16	1.1
	1987	1.87	0.282	5273	0.15	0.19	0.06	1.3
	1988	1.94	0.242	4695	0.06	1.2	0.11	0.5
	1989	2.40	0.243	5832	0.07	0.17	0.07	0.7
Total release (GBq)					1.23	2.14	1.32	35.40
U_3O_8 production (t)					29400	29400	29400	29400
Normalized release (GBq t^{-1})					0.00004	0.00007	0.00005	0.0012
Normalized release [GBq (GW a)$^{-1}$]					0.01	0.02	0.01	0.3

Table 21
Radon emissions from uranium mill tailing piles

Mill	*Year*	*Tailings area (ha)*	*Emission rate* ($Bq\ m^{-2}\ s^{-1}$)	*^{222}Rn emission (TBq)*
Argentina [C18]				
San Rafael	1986	5.0	8.2	13
	1987	5.0	11.5	18
Los Adobes	1986	7.0	8.1	18
Don Otto	1986	7.5	43.1	100
Los Gigantes	1985	5.0	0.7	1
	1986	5.0	0.8	1
La Estela	1986	1.0	11.0	3
Malargue	1985	3.0	10.7	10
	1986	3.0	12.3	11
	1987	3.0	10.2	9.5
Australia [A9, C8, D4, L4, 05, R2]				
Ranger [a]	1985	0 / 360 [d]	0 / 0.1 [b]	11
	1986	0 / 360 [b]	0 / 0.1 [b]	11
	1987	0 / 360 [b]	0 / 0.1 [b]	11
	1988	110 / 250 [b]	0.9 / 0.1 [b]	40
	1989	120 / 240 [b]	0.9 / 0.1 [b]	45
Olympic [b]	1988	75	1.6	6
	1989	75	1.6	13
Nabariek [c]	1985	6.2	0.1	0.2
	1986	6.2	0.1	0.2
	1987	6.2	2.1	4.2
	1988	6.2	2.1	4.2
	1989	6.2	2.1	4.2
Canada [A6]				
Key Lake	1985-1989	36	6	68
Rabbit Lake				
Tailings pond	1985-1989	53	3.7	62
Open pit	1985-1989	11.5	20	73
Panel mine	1985	55	10	173
	1986	60	10	189
	1987	67	10	211
	1988	74	10	233
	1989	80	10	252
Stanleigh mine	1985	35	10	110
	1986	38	10	120
	1987	43	10	136
	1988	47	10	148
	1989	50	10	158
Quirke mine	1985	107	10	337
	1986	111	10	350
	1987	115	10	363
	1988	121	10	382
	1989	127	10	400
German Democratic Republic [W5]				
Crossen	1989	230 [e]	12 [f]	450
Seelingsstädt	1989	250 [e]	12 [f]	500

[a] Subaqueous tailings deposition until 1988, then combination of subaqueous and subaerial tailings deposition.
[b] Subaerial tailings deposition, using a rotational cycle to produce layering of tailings.
[c] Subaqueous tailings deposition prior to 1987; subaerial tailings deposition thereafter.
[d] Subaerial/subaqueous values.
[e] About 50% of the tailing piles are covered with water.
[f] Subaerial value.

Table 22
Normalized releases of radionuclides in airborne effluents and collective doses from a model uranium mine and mill [a]

Radio-nuclide	*Normalized release [GBq (GW a)$^{-1}$]*				*Collective dose per unit release (man Sv TBq^{-1})*	*Normalized collective effective dose [man Sv (GW a)$^{-1}$]*			
	Mine	*Mill*	*Mill tailings*			*Mine*	*Mill*	*Mill tailings*	
			In operation	*Abandoned*				*In operation*	*Abandoned*
Pb-210		0.02			1		0.00002		
Po-210		0.02			1		0.00002		
Rn-222	75000	3000	20000	1000 [b]	0.015	1.1	0.045	0.3 [c]	150 [d]
Ra-226		0.02			0.6		0.00001		
Th-230		0.02			30		0.0006		
U-234		0.4			8		0.003		
U-238		0.4			7		0.003		

[a] Normalized emissions in liquid effluents (0.01 for ^{210}Po, ^{210}Pb and ^{230}Th; 0.02 for ^{226}Ra; 0.3 for ^{234}U and ^{238}U) contribute negligibly to the collective dose.
[b] Annual activity released; the rate of activity is assumed to remain constant over more than 10,000 years.
[c] Dose commitment corresponding to a five-year release.
[d] Dose commitment corresponding to a 10,000-year release.

Table 23
Uranium-238 released in effluents from fuel conversion, enrichment and fabrication plants
[A6, B13, M3]

Installation	*Year*	*Airborne discharges (GBq)* ^{238}U	*Liquid discharges (GBq)* ^{238}U
Canada			
Blind River refinery Capacity: 18,000 t of uranium as UO_3	1985 1986 1987 1988 1989	0.9 1.0 1.1 1.0 0.9	0.2 0.08 0.1 0.2 0.1
Port Hope UO_2 plant Capacity: 2,800 t of uranium as UO_2	1986 1987 1988 1989	0.4 0.6 0.4 0.2	0 0 0 0
Port Hope UF_6 plant Capacity: 10,000 t of uranium as UF_6	1986 1987 1988 1989	3.1 2.6 2.5 0.7	5.3 2.6 3.7 2.6
Toronto fuel fabriaction plant Capacity: 1,050 t of uranium as UO_2	1987 1988 1989	< 0.001 < 0.001 < 0.001	0.02 0.02 0.02
Port Hope fuel fabrication plant Capacity: 900 t of uranium as UO_2	1987 1988 1989	0.001 0.001 0.001	0.01 0.01 0.01

		Airborne discharges (GBq)			*Liquid discharges (GBq)*	
		Uranium	*Uranic α*	*Uranic β*	*Uranic α*	*Uranic β*
Republic of Korea						
Korea Nuclear Fuel Company (fabrication)	1988 1989		0.07 0.3	0.3 0.1	0.009 0.03	0.013 0.013

Table 23 (continued)

Installation		*Airborne discharges (GBq)*			*Liquid discharges (GBq)*	
		Uranium	*Uranic α*	*Uranic β*	*Uranic α*	*Uranic β*
United Kingdom						
Capenhurst (enrichment)	1985	0.006			0.9	0.9
	1986	0.01			2	2
	1987	0.02			3	3
	1988	0.02			1.7	1.7
	1989				< 0.9	< 0.9
Springfields (conversion, fabrication)	1985		1	1	700	160000
	1986		1	1	600	115000
	1987		1	1	500	77000
	1988		1	1	400	110000
	1989		1	2	400	114000

Table 24
Normalized releases of radionuclides from model fuel conversion, enrichment and fabrication facility

Radio-nuclide	*Atmospheric discharges [MBq (GW a)$^{-1}$] from*			*Aquatic discharges [MBq (GW a)$^{-1}$] from*		
	Conversion	*Enrichment*	*Fabrication*	*Conversion*	*Enrichment*	*Fabrication*
Ra-226				0.11		
Th-228	0.022					
Th-230	0.4					
Th-232	0.022					
Th-234	130	1.3	0.34			170
U-234	130	1.3	0.34	94	10	170
U-235	6.1	0.06	0.0014	4.3	0.5	1.4
U-238	130	1.3	0.34	94	10	170

Table 25
Worldwide installed capacity and electrical energy generated
[19]

Country	*Reactor*	*Start-up year*	*Capacity (GW)*	*Electrical energy generated (GW a)*				
				1985	*1986*	*1987*	*1988*	*1989*
PWRs								
Belgium	Doel 1-4	1974/85	2.71	1.893	2.232	2.062	2.275	2.079
	Tihange 1-4	1975/85	2.791	1.440	2.026	2.483	2.386	2.388
Brazil	Angra 1	1982	0.626	0.362	0.015	0.104	0.065	0.194
Bulgaria	Kozloduy-1-2	1974/75	0.816	0.677	0.606	0.639	0.548	0.555
	Kozloduy-3-4	1980/82	0.816	0.712	0.669	0.659	0.687	0.601
	Kozloduy-5	1987	0.953	- [a]	-	0.016	0.449	0.383
China, Taiwan Province	Maanshan 1	1984	0.89	0.355	0.190	0.541	0.587	0.619
	Maanshan 2	1985	0.89	0.484	0.308	0.735	0.619	0.603
Czechoslovakia	Bohunice 1-4	1978/85	1.632	0.993	1.242	1.220	1.217	1.290
	Dukovany 1-4	1985/87	1.632	0.228	0.654	1.139	1.261	1.327
Finland	Loviisa 1-2	1977/80	0.89	0.816	0.765	0.819	0.794	0.814
France	Belleville 1-2	1987/88	2.62	-	-	0.071	0.955	1.559
	Blayais 1-4	1981/83	3.64	2.921	2.887	2.509	2.228	2.704
	Bugey 2-5	1978/79	3.64	2.605	2.658	2.140	1.952	2.273
	Cattenom 1-2	1986/87	2.6	-	0.025	0.998	1.532	0.978
	Chinon B1-B4	1982/87	3.55	1.257	1.499	1.674	2.125	2.340
	Chooz-A (Ardennes)	1967	0.305	0.193	0.156	0.094	0.198	0.186
	Cruas 1-4	1983/84	3.555	2.547	2.541	2.392	2.025	2.555
	Dampierre 1-4	1980/81	3.56	2.742	2.762	2.295	2.118	2.655
	Fessenheim 1-2	1977	1.76	1.366	1.277	1.276	1.168	1.016
	Flamanville 1-2	1985/86	2.66	0	0.792	1.631	1.630	1.552
	Gravelines 1-6	1980/85	5.46	3.952	4.098	3.617	3.694	3.882
	Nogent 1-2	1987/88	2.62	-	-	0.055	0.886	1.215
	Paluel 1-4	1984/86	5.32	1.586	4.577	5.537	4.836	5.667
	St. Alban 1-2	1985/86	2.67	0.147	0.891	1.490	1.113	1.473
	St. Laurent B1-2	1981	1.795	1.247	1.272	1.168	1.236	1.329
	Tricastin 1-4	1980/81	3.66	2.946	2.771	2.587	2.309	2.575
Germany, Fed. Rep. of	Biblis A-B	1974/76	2.386	1.752	1.563	1.494	1.322	1.324
	Brokdorf	1986	1.326	-	0.034	1.082	0.980	1.026
	Emsland	1988	1.242	-	-	-	0.650	1.125
	Grafenrheinfeld	1981	1.235	1.112	0.995	0.954	1.005	1.073
	Greifswald	1973/79	1.632	1.117	1.117	1.117	1.117	1.129
	Grohnde	1984	1.3	1.241	1.165	1.101	1.165	1.173
	Isar 2	1988	1.31	-	-	-	0.688	0.882
	Mülheim-Kärlich	1986	1.219	-	0.155	0.332	0.688	0
	Neckarwestheim 1-2	1976/89	2.02	0.703	0.474	0.616	0.602	1.449
	Obrigheim	1968	0.34	0.296	0.304	0.283	0.299	0.292
	Philippsburg 2	1984	1.268	1.068	1.168	1.098	1.109	1.105
	Stade	1972	0.64	0.555	0.573	0.506	0.507	0.478
	Unterweser	1978	1.23	1.134	0.831	0.990	1.040	1.055
Hungary	Paks 1-4	1982/87	1.66	0.696	0.797	1.179	1.441	1.490
Italy	Enrico Fermi	1964	0.26	0.148	0.230	0.018	0	0
Japan	Genkai 1-2	1975/80	1.058	0.793	0.856	0.872	0.665	0.619
	Ikata 1-2	1977/81	1.076	0.841	0.961	0.965	0.808	0.835
	Mihama 1-3	1970/76	1.57	1.154	1.468	1.124	1.091	1.178
	Ohi 1-2	1977/78	2.24	1.443	1.712	1.788	1.072	1.435
	Sendai 1-2	1983/85	1.692	0.994	1.379	1.392	1.495	1.413
	Takahama 1-4	1974/84	3.22	2.471	2.485	2.391	2.215	2.472
	Tomari-1	1988	0.55	-	-	-	0.006	0.412
	Tsuruga-2	1986	1.115	-	0.177	0.999	0.906	0.857
Netherlands	Borssele	1973	0.481	0.372	0.408	0.337	0.346	0.391
Republic of Korea	Kori 1	1977	0.556	0.361	0.374	0.520	0.254	0.312
	Kori 2	1983	0.605	0.426	0.450	0.487	0.514	0.578
	Kori 3-4	1985	1.79	0.201	1.218	1.332	1.373	1.458

Table 25 (continued)

Country	*Reactor*	*Start-up year*	*Capacity (GW)*	*Electrical energy generated (GW a)*				
				1985	*1986*	*1987*	*1988*	*1989*
Republic of Korea (continued)	Ulchin 1-2	1988/89	1.84	-	-	-	0.114	0.831
	Yonggwang 1-2	1986	1.8	-	0.282	1.172	1.425	1.388
South Africa	Koeberg 1-2	1984/85	1.844	0.616	1.008	0.710	1.201	1.269
Spain	Almaraz 1-2	1981/83	1.86	1.263	1.284	1.552	1.449	1.496
	Asco 1	1983	0.93	0.506	0.586	0.730	0.761	0.771
	Asco 2	1985	0.93	0.030	0.613	0.680	0.784	0.768
	José Cabrera 1	1968	0.153	0.032	0.120	0.125	0.130	0.129
	Trillo 1	1988	1.04	-	-	-	0.179	0.816
	Vandellos 2	1987	0.996	-	-	0.005	0.582	0.670
Sweden	Ringhals 2	1974	0.8	0.490	0.453	0.481	0.481	0.413
	Ringhals 3	1980	0.915	0.695	0.712	0.704	0.702	0.665
	Ringhals 4	1982	0.915	0.676	0.641	0.647	0.758	0.632
Switzerland	Beznau 1-2	1969/71	0.7	0.601	0.601	0.572	0.593	0.579
	Gösgen	1979	0.94	0.770	0.771	0.789	0.783	0.785
USSR	Armenia 1-2	1976/79	0.752	0.601	0.343	0.540	0.550	0.150
	Balakovo 1-3	1985/88	2.85	0.006	0.594	1.090	2.240	2.150
	Kalinin 1-2	1984/86	1.9	0.543	0.657	1.522	1.400	1.500
	Khmelnitski 1	1987	0.95	-	-	0.005	0.450	0.710
	Kola 1-4	1973/84	1.644	1.349	1.355	1.460	1.440	1.430
	Novovoronezh 3-5	1971/80	1.72	1.907	1.380	1.710	1.310	1.280
	Rovno 1-3	1980/86	1.695	1.210	0.696	1.302	1.380	1.440
	South Ukraine 1-3	1982/89	2.85	1.503	1.408	0.916	1.240	1.000
	Zaporozhe 1-5	1984/89	4.75	0.559	1.279	2.236	2.850	2.430
United States	Arkansas One-1	1974	0.836	0.593	0.410	0.544	0.452	0.386
	Arkansas One-2	1978	0.858	0.537	0.607	0.754	0.565	0.625
	Beaver Valley 1-2	1976/87	1.643	0.674	0.546	0.726	1.309	0.953
	Braidwood 1	1987	1.12	-	-	0.166	0.391	0.531
	Braidwood 2	1988	1.12	-	-	-	0.154	0.815
	Byron 1-2	1985/87	2.21	0.194	0.844	1.054	1.445	1.714
	Callaway 1	1984	1.118	0.918	0.822	0.722	0.930	0.953
	Calvert Cliffs 1-2	1975/76	1.65	1.138	1.465	1.153	1.343	0.319
	Catawba 1	1985	1.129	0.393	0.594	0.731	0.872	0.888
	Catawba 2	1986	1.129	-	0.151	0.818	0.620	0.745
	Crystal River 3	1977	0.821	0.327	0.303	0.413	0.658	0.334
	Davis-Besse 1	1977	0.86	0.222	0	0.578	0.133	0.836
	Diablo Canyon 1-2	1984/85	2.16	0.659	1.378	1.600	1.315	1.805
	Donald Cook 1-2	1975/78	2.08	0.890	1.254	1.148	1.118	1.381
	Farley 1	1977	0.824	0.670	0.655	0.736	0.674	0.688
	Farley 2	1981	0.83	0.625	0.680	0.561	0.748	0.642
	Fort Calhoun 1	1973	0.478	0.350	0.412	0.349	0.300	0.376
	H. B. Robinson 2	1970	0.665	0.598	0.548	0.484	0.363	0.319
	Haddam Neck	1967	0.565	0.529	0.244	0.290	0.378	0.338
	Indian Point 1-2	1962/73	0.864	0.761	0.437	0.588	0.692	0.511
	Indian Point 3	1976	0.965	0.540	0.631	0.554	0.766	0.567
	Kewaunee	1974	0.503	0.422	0.440	0.458	0.447	0.427
	Maine Yankee	1972	0.81	0.611	0.713	0.462	0.526	0.792
	McGuire 1	1981	1.129	0.774	0.591	0.839	0.845	0.891
	McGuire 2	1983	1.129	0.640	0.710	0.865	0.920	0.847
	Millstone 2	1975	0.863	0.401	0.590	0.787	0.655	0.544
	Millstone 3	1986	1.142	-	0.669	0.770	0.877	0.809
	North Anna 1-2	1978/80	1.83	1.440	1.408	1.053	1.687	1.164
	Oconee 1-2-3	1973/74	2.538	1.939	1.902	1.867	2.134	2.088
	Palisades	1971	0.73	0.605	0.096	0.301	0.392	0.415
	Palo Verde 1	1985	1.221	0.129	0.715	0.601	0.761	0.205
	Palo Verde 2	1986	1.221	-	0.303	0.935	0.770	0.536
	Palo Verde 3	1987	1.221	-	-	-	1.146	0.152
	Point Beach 1-2	1970/72	0.97	0.794	0.821	0.819	0.862	0.810
	Prairie Island 1-2	1973/74	1.003	0.832	0.876	0.919	0.880	0.945
	R. E. Ginna	1969	0.47	0.413	0.412	0.434	0.403	0.351
	Rancho Seco 1	1974	0.873	0.221	0	0	0.326	0.165
	Salem 1	1976	1.106	1.028	0.809	0.710	0.847	0.709
	Salem 2	1981	1.106	0.575	0.607	0.705	0.683	0.893
	San Onofre 1	1967	0.436	0.281	0.101	0.309	0.158	0.135
	San Onofre 2-3	1982/83	2.15	1.017	1.499	1.572	1.729	1.607
	Sequoyah 1-2	1980/81	2.296	1.107	0	0	0.464	1.783

Table 25 (continued)

Country	*Reactor*	*Start-up year*	*Capacity (GW)*	*Electrical energy generated (GW a)*				
				1985	*1986*	*1987*	*1988*	*1989*
United States (continued)	Shearon Harris 1	1987	0.86	-	-	0.386	0.610	0.644
	South Texas 1	1988	1.25	-	-	-	0.319	0.720
	South Texas 2	1989	1.25	-	-	-	-	0.346
	St. Lucie 1	1976	0.839	0.670	0.805	0.653	0.714	0.793
	St. Lucie 2	1983	0.839	0.697	0.702	0.679	0.846	0.621
	Surry 1-2	1972/73	1.562	1.106	1.026	1.076	0.714	0.464
	Three Mile Island 1	1974	0.808	0.093	0.550	0.575	0.624	0.824
	Three Mile Island 2	1978	0	0	0	0	0	0
	Trojan	1975	1.095	0.789	0.810	0.498	0.724	0.633
	Turkey Point 3	1972	0.666	0.391	0.515	0.101	0.396	0.412
	Turkey Point 4	1973	0.666	0.591	0.199	0.303	0.373	0.241
	Virgil C. Summer 1	1982	0.885	0.598	0.817	0.590	0.579	0.618
	Vogtle 1, 2	1987/89	2.166	-	-	0.447	0.776	0.994
	Waterford 3	1985	1.075	0.317	0.834	0.849	0.748	0.869
	Wolf Creek	1985	1.135	0.435	0.795	0.742	0.762	1.108
	Yankee NPS	1960	0.167	0.135	0.159	0.130	0.128	0.149
	Zion 1-2	1973	2.08	1.138	1.400	1.278	1.484	1.449
Yugoslavia	Krsko	1981	0.62	0.439	0.436	0.488	0.449	0.508
Total annual electrical energy generated (GW a)			199.54	95.01	106.94	119.15	130.10	137.79
BWRs								
China, Taiwan Province	Chin Shan 1	1977	0.604	0.431	0.469	0.456	0.401	0.318
	Chin Shan 2	1978	0.604	0.490	0.433	0.427	0.426	0.349
	Kuosheng 1	1981	0.951	0.677	0.833	0.729	0.638	0.608
	Kuosheng 2	1982	0.951	0.708	0.717	0.741	0.685	0.597
Finland	TVO 1-2	1978/80	0.71	1.236	1.290	1.297	1.312	1.242
Germany, Fed. Rep. of	Brunsbüttel	1976	0.771	0.642	0.643	0.597	0.581	0.468
	Gundremmingen B,C	1984	2.488	2.089	1.863	1.798	1.659	2.002
	Isar 1	1977	0.87	0.723	0.818	0.644	0.594	0.594
	Krümmel	1983	1.26	1.062	1.083	1.048	1.052	0.941
	Philippsburg 1	1979	0.864	0.699	0.596	0.741	0.708	0.703
	Würgassen	1971	0.64	0.530	0.551	0.540	0.531	0.432
India	Tarapur-1,2	1969	0.30	0.212	0.212	0.155	0.217	0.140
Italy	Caorso	1981	0.86	0.454	0.605	0	0	0
Japan	Fukushima Daiichi 1-6	1970/79	4.546	2.930	3.260	3.271	3.296	3.173
	Fukushima Daini 1-4	1981/86	4.286	2.426	2.474	3.067	3.309	2.718
	Hamaoka 1-3	1974/86	2.377	1.008	0.886	1.813	1.475	1.724
	Kashiwazaki Kariwa 1,5	1984/89	2.134	0.566	0.765	1.050	0.794	0.854
	Onagawa-1	1983	0.497	0.372	0.384	0.361	0.389	0.344
	Shimane 1-2	1973/88	1.23	0.433	0.243	0.344	0.419	0.967
	Tokai 2	1978	1.08	0.794	0.662	0.804	0.695	0.963
	Tsuruga 1	1969	0.341	0.194	0.261	0.268	0.254	0.281
Mexico	Laguna Verde (Mark)	1989	0.65	-	-	-	-	0.036
Netherlands	Dodewaard	1968	0.05	0.049	0.046	0.047	0.049	0.041
Spain	Confrentes	1984	0.939	0.701	0.761	0.786	0.815	0.805
	S. Maria de Garona	1971	0.46	0.198	0.390	0.293	0.307	0.401
Sweden	Barsebeck 1	1975	0.6	0.468	0.499	0.520	0.501	0.494
	Barsebeck 2	1976	0.6	0.492	0.471	0.508	0.501	0.480
	Forsmark 1	1980	0.97	0.638	0.835	0.741	0.782	0.701
	Forsmark 2	1981	0.97	0.655	0.798	0.748	0.796	0.678
	Forsmark 3	1985	1.068	0.474	0.921	0.804	0.852	0.841
	Oskarshamn 1	1971	0.442	0.314	0.358	0.369	0.327	0.363
	Oskarshamn 2	1974	0.605	0.455	0.488	0.483	0.504	0.452
	Oskarshamn 3	1985	1.16	0.439	0.957	0.806	0.835	0.889
	Ringhals 1	1974	0.75	0.590	0.510	0.556	0.536	0.554
Switzerland	Leibstadt	1984	0.99	0.773	0.773	0.823	0.842	0.799
	Mühleberg	1972	0.322	0.285	0.241	0.281	0.285	0.262

Table 25 (continued)

Country	*Reactor*	*Start-up year*	*Capacity (GW)*	*Electrical energy generated (GW a)*				
				1985	*1986*	*1987*	*1988*	*1989*
United States	Big Rock Point	1962	0.067	0.041	0.058	0.043	0.044	0.048
	Browns Ferry 1-3	1973/76	3.195	0.357	0	0	0	0
	Brunswick 1-2	1975/76	1.58	0.795	1.017	1.113	0.957	0.958
	Clinton 1	1987	0.946	-	-	0.186	0.669	0.327
	Cooper	1974	0.764	0.122	0.463	0.630	0.480	0.547
	Dresden 2-3	1970/71	1.545	0.857	0.703	0.886	0.970	1.127
	Duane Arnold-1	1974	0.538	0.222	0.364	0.291	0.402	0.359
	Enrico Fermi 2	1986	1.093	-	0	0.159	0.463	0.597
	Fitzpatrick	1975	0.757	0.476	0.687	0.479	0.497	0.703
	Grand Gulf 1	1984	1.142	0.493	0.468	0.882	1.095	0.896
	Hatch 1-2	1974/78	1.525	1.157	0.829	1.237	0.956	1.213
	Hope Creek 1	1986	1.031	-	0.118	0.834	0.739	0.755
	Humboldt Bay 3	1963						
	Lacrosse	1968	0.048	0.037	0.018	0.015		
	Lasalle 1-2	1982/84	2.072	0.948	0.894	0.991	1.269	1.448
	Limerick 1	1985	1.055	0.133	0.823	0.610	0.762	0.599
	Millstone 1	1970	0.654	0.524	0.599	0.500	0.632	0.530
	Monticello	1971	0.536	0.489	0.386	0.404	0.522	0.303
	Nine Mile Point 1	1969	0.61	0.563	0.359	0.527		
	Nine Mile Point 2	1987	1.072	-	-	0.030	0.290	0.490
	Oyster Creek	1969	0.62	0.428	0.150	0.355	0.405	0.275
	Peach Bottom 2-3	1974	2.086	0.651	1.342	0.355	0	0.471
	Perry 1	1986	1.141	-	-	0.095	0.826	0.612
	Pilgrim 1	1972	0.67	0.565	0.117	0	0	0.195
	Quad Cities 1-2	1972	1.538	1.214	1.045	1.074	1.123	1.144
	River Bend 1	1985	0.936	0.003	0.342	0.567	0.828	0.546
	Susquehanna 1-2	1982/84	2.07	1.439	1.290	1.682	1.635	1.514
	Vermont Yankee	1972	0.504	0.342	0.235	0.404	0.470	0.412
	WPPSS-2	1984	1.095	0.591	0.592	0.685	0.685	0.700
Total annual electrical energy generated (GW a)			73.58	37.65	40.00	42.95	44.09	43.98
			HWRs					
Argentina	Atucha-1	1974	0.335	0.168	0.252	0.160	0.092	0
	Embalse	1983	0.6	0.431	0.350	0.522	0.521	0.532
Canada	Bruce 1-4	1977/78	3.394	2.558	2.447	2.167	2.008	1.830
	Bruce 5-8	1984/87	3.371	1.297	2.061	2.592	2.698	3.005
	Gentilly-2	1982	0.64	0.364	0.433	0.532	0.603	0.556
	Pickering 1-4	1971/73	2.06	0.710	0.783	0.919	0.872	1.205
	Pickering 5-8	1982/86	2.064	1.227	1.670	1.786	1.934	1.719
	Point Lepreau	1982	0.635	0.619	0.596	0.583	0.609	0.601
India	Kalpakkam 1-2	1983	0.44	0.094	0.176	0.247	0.217	0.096
	Rajasthan 1-2	1972/80	0.414	0.135	0.123	0.137	0.184	0.159
Pakistan	Karachi	1971	0.125	0.030	0.060	0.035	0.022	0.0080
Republic of Korea	Wolsong 1	1982	0.629	0.599	0.505	0.589	0.504	0.577
Total annual electrical energy generated (GW a)			14.58	8.20	9.40	10.24	10.24	10.28
			GCRs					
France	Bugey 1	1972	0.54	0.317	0.179	0.211	0.289	0.203
	Chinon A2-3	1965/66	0.54	0.081	0	0.012	0.109	0.150
	St. Laurent A1-2	1969/71	0.84	0.461	0.514	0.492	0.628	0.316
Japan	Tokai-1	1965	0.159	0.098	0.099	0.092	0.116	0.053
Spain	Vandellos 1	1972	0.48	0.334	0.338	0.346	0.349	0.280
United Kingdom	Berkeley	1962	0.138	0.118	0.091	0.109	0.142	0.050
	Bradwell	1962	0.245	0.213	0.181	0.213	0.194	0.092
	Calder Hall	1956	0.198	0.164	0.161	0.153	0.149	0.159
	Chapelcross	1959	0.192	0.163	0.166	0.168	0.164	0.156
	Dungeness A	1965	0.424	0.381	0.300	0.349	0.238	0.251
	Dungeness B1-2	1983/85	0.72	0.278	0.277	0.111	0.260	0.100
	Hartlepool A1-A2	1983/84	0.84	0.156	0.319	0.241	0.221	0.464
	Heysham 1A-B, 2A-B	1983/88	2.07	0.254	0.272	0.467	0.665	1.322

Table 25 (continued)

Country	Reactor	Start-up year	Capacity (GW)	Electrical energy generated (GW a)				
				1985	1986	1987	1988	1989
United Kingdom (continued)	Hinkley Point A	1965	0.47	0.401	0.406	0.423	0.416	0.315
	Hinkley Point B, A-B	1976	1.12	0.855	0.764	0.549	0.819	0.763
	Hunterston A1	1964	0.3	0.256	0.261	0.259	0.227	0.231
	Hunterston B1-2	1976/77	1.15	0.931	0.935	0.901	0.868	0.878
	Oldbury-A	1967	0.434	0.379	0.378	0.368	0.385	0.333
	Sizewell-A	1966	0.42	0.307	0.227	0.315	0.305	0.296
	Torness A-B	1988/89	1.25	-	-	-	0.261	0.662
	Trawsfynydd	1965	0.39	0.368	0.334	0.353	0.230	0.297
	Wylfa	1971	0.84	0.763	0.468	0.514	0.705	0.755
Total annual electrical energy generated (GW a)			13.76	7.28	6.67	6.64	7.74	8.13
LWGRs								
USSR	Beloyarsky 2	1967	0.146	0.174		0.117	0.100	0.081
	Bilibino 1-4	1974/76	0.044	0.040	0.039	0.040	0.035	0.033
	Chernobyl 1-4	1977/81	2.775	3.335	0.240	1.549	2.240	2.310
	Ignalina 1-2	1983/87	2.76	1.082	1.128	1.540	1.460	1.900
	Kursk 1-4	1976/85	3.7	2.370	2.776	2.950	3.270	2.940
	Leningrad 1-4	1973/81	3.7	3.200	3.356	3.273	3.170	3.110
	Smolensk 1-3	1982/89	1.85	1.207	1.198	1.577	1.650	1.620
Total annual electrical energy generated (GW a)			14.98	11.41	8.74	11.05	11.93	11.994
FBRs								
France	Creys-Malville	1985	1.2	0	0.106	0.093	0	0.201
	Phenix	1973	0.233	0.132	0.173	0.178	0.168	0.069
USSR	Beloyarsky 3	1980	0.56	0.435	0.392	0.445	0.429	0.422
United Kingdom	Dounreay	1975	0.25	0.102	0.102	0.096	0.070	0.119
Total annual electrical energy generated (GW a)			2.243	0.669	0.773	0.811	0.668	0.810

[a] A dash indicates that the reactor is not yet in operation.

Table 26
Noble gases released from reactors in airborne effluents

Country	*Reactor*	*Release (GBq)*				
		1985	*1986*	*1987*	*1988*	*1989*
PWRs						
Belgium [M6]	Doel 1-4	77900	17800	8000	24300	3400
	Tihange 1-4	15200	49700	30400	49500	13100
Brazil [C1]	Angra 1	300	80	800	200	9900
Bulgaria [C16]	Kozloduy-1-2	99000	47000	198000	84000	125000
	Kozloduy-3-4	80000	42000	61000	88000	114000
	Kozloduy-5	- [a]	-		433000	528000
China, Taiwan Province [T2]	Maanshan 1-2	73.4	537	3600	2150	1760
Czechoslovakia [N11]	Bohunice 1-4	66900	45700	37100	37200	38900
	Dukovany 1-4	1200	4100	5900	6400	3000
Finland [F2]	Loviisa 1-2	1100	1000.0	1100	1100	1100
France [E4]	Belleville 1-2	-	-	28000	85000	44000
	Blayais 1-4	430000	370000	110000	130000	140000
	Bugey 2-5	110000	93000	53000	45000	39000
	Cattenom 1-2	-	2600	40000	54000	59000
	Chinon B1-B4	170000	210000	49000	42000	48000
	Chooz-A (Ardennes)	160000	240000	15000	31000	69000
	Cruas 1-4	270000	150000	18000	16000	21000
	Dampierre 1-4	280000	270000	160000	140000	170000
	Fessenheim 1-2	94000	100000	44000	11000	10000
	Flamanville 1-2	36000	240000	24000	8600	7000
	Gravelines 1-6	330000	310000	110000	110000	81000
	Nogent 1-2	-	-	3200	18000	26000
	Paluel 1-4	340000	590000	220000	160000	150000
	St. Alban 1-2	7800	33000	15000	16000	9900
	St. Laurent B1-2	130000	100000	11000	8500	22000
	Tricastin 1-4	130000	130000	28000	27000	41000
Germany, Federal Republic of [B4, B9, S7]	Biblis A-B	14000	28100	40300	20700	3490
	Brokdorf	-	7.4	0	0.1	280
	Emsland	-	-	-	77	94
	Grafenrheinfeld	12	10	0.53	190	14000
	Greifswald	190000	160000	230000	280000	540000
	Grohnde	51	50	3800	10000	3800
	Isar 2	-	-	-	11	38
	Mülheim-Kärlich	-	0	0	0	0
	Neckarwestheim 1-2	11000	12000	11000	21000	18600
	Obrigheim	970	620	460	650	650
	Philippsburg 2	5300	500	830	2600	3100
	Stade	34000	190000	82000	38000	9900
	Unterweser	5600	8400	4700	3400	3700
Hungary [F3]	Paks 1-4	108000	194000	328000	133000	176000
Italy [C22]	Enrico Fermi (Trino)	28	18000	1590	0.03	0.07
Japan [J1]	Genkai 1-2	1300	1400	1000	1100	690
	Ikata 1-2	48	19	7.4	6.3	5.9
	Mihama 1-3	1400	1400	930	270	250
	Ohi 1-2	1300	3700	1500	930	1000
	Sendai 1-2	67	41	41	36	40
	Takahama 1-4	2000	630	480	1100	350
	Tomari-1	-	-	-	0	0.17
	Tsuruga-2	-	85	0.85	5.9	8.6
Netherlands [M5]	Borssele	600	4000	200	1200	2300
Republic of Korea [M3]	Kori 1	6660	8670	2440	0000	2380
	Kori 2	1430	1520	527	121	0
	Kori 3-4	24800	34800	28900	18500	22600
	Ulchin 1-2	-	-	-	6	405
	Yonggwang 1-2	-	1781	11730	12356	5030

Table 26 (continued)

Country	*Reactor*	*Release (GBq)*				
		1985	*1986*	*1987*	*1988*	*1989*
South Africa [C20]	Koeberg 1-2		207000	33700	55000	50800
Spain [C21]	Almaraz 1-2	169000	270000	6590	29800	3950
	Asco 1	4760	10800	9650	57100	84900
	Asco 2	1590	18500	14400	62100	60600
	José Cabrera 1	41500	141000	142000	99400	96900
	Trillo 1	-	-	-	300	2990
	Vandellos 2	-	-	0	17600	26300
Sweden [N14]	Ringhals 2	3600	10100	14000	15000	5400
	Ringhals 3	9100	63200	31000	620	6800
	Ringhals 4	490	26400	76000	57300	6000
Switzerland [D5, D6]	Beznau 1-2	14500	32000	18000	18000	44000
	Gösgen	15000	7000	4200	6800	12000
USSR [G2, I14]	Armenia 1-2	66000	55400	577000	57700	62200
	Balakovo 1-3	0	66200	173000	173000	60500
	Kalinin 1-2	270000	270000	248000	56700	51300
	Khmelnitski 1	-	-	-	119000	96200
	Kola 1-4	1040000	544000	564000	415000	423000
	Novovoronezh 3-5	43000	41000	27200	29700	32400
	Rovno 1-3	88100	99900	55500	241000	136000
	South Ukraine 1-3	200000	123000		41400	47100
	Zaporozhe 1-5	110000	407000	275000	110000	78700
United States [T3]	Arkansas One-1	300000	63300	12100	45900	86200
	Arkansas One-2	330000	128000	7620	79900	102000
	Beaver Valley 1-2	1450	2800	8330	3480	5800
	Braidwood 1	-	-	10.4	1550	43300
	Braidwood 2	-	-	-	1410	18800
	Byron 1-2	10320	23500	48100	65900	30200
	Callaway 1	61800	192000	107000	25500	26700
	Calvert Cliffs 1-2	147000	283000	168000	211000	121000
	Catawba 1	10200	50300	89200	57700	11700
	Catawba 2	-	50300	89200	57700	11700
	Crystal River 3	38900	102000	40700	126000	167000
	Davis-Besse 1	4370	0.02	14100	4030	14000
	Diablo Canyon 1-2	21200	85900	26400	12100	12400
	Donald Cook 1-2	183000	12200	32400	9550	4300
	Farley 1	62900	47400	48100	35500	3700
	Farley 2	24500	68100	26700	21900	5900
	Fort Calhoun 1	54800	21000	15700	29000	6100
	H. B. Robinson 2	79200	24400	28500	38500	1000
	Haddam Neck	102000	86200	132000	94400	633000
	Indian Point 1-2	69600	75900	173000	8400	3200
	Indian Point 3	57000	71400	67300	11500	11600
	Kewaunee	1840	2420	1180	1080	2400
	Maine Yankee	16300	39600	28900	2660	750
	McGuire 1	71400	38900	75500	72200	26600
	McGuire 2	71400	38900	75500	72200	26600
	Millstone 2	14800	3700	14700	23500	9100
	Millstone 3	-	884	3890	3120	11000
	North Anna 1-2	298000	211000	38900	17900	53300
	Oconee 1-2-3	870000	899000	389000	958000	332000
	Palisades	136000	64000	64800	89900	5600
	Palo Verde 1	9360	98800	47000	68100	23700
	Palo Verde 2	-	72900	202000	110000	15900
	Palo Verde 3	-	-	0.93	5030	30900
	Point Beach 1-2	4290	1030	1780	2990	560
	Prairie Island 1-2	1700	1120	32.4	5.25	6400
	R. E. Ginna	15000	7730	6550	1910	18900
	Rancho Seco 1	173000	3440	0.80	56200	74000
	Salem 1	62200	51400	135000	19600	51400
	Salem 2	42600	31700	39200	43700	2700
	San Onofre 1	142000	15200	36300	111000	33500
	San Onofre 2-3	936000	305000	807000	189000	91000
	Sequoyah 1-2	169000	44.8	0	8330	142000
	Shearon Harris 1	-	-		83300	42600
	South Texas 1	-	-	-	31700	16500
	South Texas 2	-	-	-	-	4300

Table 26 (continued)

Country	*Reactor*	*Release (GBq)*				
		1985	*1986*	*1987*	*1988*	*1989*
United States (continued)	St. Lucie 1	1880000	1230000	230000	52500	168000
	St. Lucie 2	353000	369000	318000	339000	82100
	Surry 1-2	76600	73600	11400	13500	5100
	Three Mile Island 1	4000	141000	29200	69200	77700
	Three Mile Island 2	0	10.4	0	16.3	0
	Trojan	40700	34900	9440	15700	22000
	Turkey Point 3	48800	135000	34700	46300	62900
	Turkey Point 4	66600	37400	29100	48500	63300
	Virgil C. Summer 1	5180	514	23500	12300	67300
	Vogtle 1-2	-	-	3960	4260	20200
	Waterford 3	304000	414000	208000	196000	20700
	Wolf Creek	6360	1170	6400	29300	23700
	Yankee NPS	54400	18900	14200	7620	4500
	Zion 1-2	144000	118000	4370	48500	41400
Yugoslavia [F1]	Krsko	0	0	0	0	0
Total release (GBq)		12900000	12000000	8320000	7640000	6970000
Normalized release [GBq (GW a)$^{-1}$]		137000	112000	70600	58700	50600
Average normalized release 1985-1989 [GBq (GW a)$^{-1}$]		81000				
BWRs						
China, Taiwan Province [T2]	Chin Shan 1-2	499000	254000	84000	62200	46900
	Kuosheng 1-2	407	136	4510	7840	5330
Finland [F2]	TVO 1-2	0	5800	6000	180	19000
Germany, Federal Republic of [B4, B9]	Brunsbüttel	19000	820	6600	23000	7900
	Gundremmingen B,C	21	4800	19000	3900	15000
	Isar 1	27000	1900	860	860	360
	Krümmel	950	210	14000	9700	1000
	Philippsburg 1	35	29	760	480	10
	Würgassen	11000	9300	2900	3100	1400
India	Tarapur-1,2					
Italy [C22]	Caorso	420	1360	3470	5550	1060
Japan [J1]	Fukushima Daiichi 1-6	740	290	190	4.1	0
	Fukushima Daini 1-4	0	0	0.0034	0	0
	Hamaoka 1-3	0	0	0	0	0
	Kashiwazaki Kariwa 1,5	0	0	0	0	0
	Onagawa-1	0	0	0	0	0
	Shimane 1-2	0	0	0	0	0
	Tokai 2	0	0	150	0	0
	Tsuruga 1	1.6	3.1	1.7	0	0.26
Mexico [C19]	Laguna Verde (Mark II)	-	-	-	-	0
Netherlands [M5]	Dodewaard	9800	11000	4300	3200	5400
Spain [C21]	Confrentes	49500	59200	113000	97500	49500
	S. Maria de Garona	70500	76400	58600	68200	74700
Sweden [N14]	Barsebeck 1	160	640	630	530	5800
	Barsebeck 2	290	80700	980	528000	1560000
	Forsmark 1	70800	81	330	740	304000
	Forsmark 2	232000	265000	199000	278000	721000
	Forsmark 3	660	24600	4850	11500	10300
	Oskarshamn 1	533000	508000	301000	305000	201000
	Oskarshamn 2	30400	25000	14500	15900000	2410000
	Oskarshamn 3	17200	265000	49000	106000	131000
	Ringhals 1	1280000	1240000	482000	490000	132000
Switzerland [D5, D6]	Leibstadt	12	1800	160	13000	63000
	Mühleberg	83000	620000	1400	200000	120000
United States [T3]	Big Rock Point	2320000	2320000	309000	287000	262000
	Browns Ferry 1-3	977000	83600	11.9	0	0

Table 26 (continued)

Country	*Reactor*	*Release (GBq)*				
		1985	*1986*	*1987*	*1988*	*1989*
United States (continued)	Brunswick 1-2	648000	1670000	977000	58500	50300
	Clinton 1	-	-	253	161	480
	Cooper	51400	63600	44400	67000	12700
	Dresden 2-3	109000	16200	10200	6220	1360
	Duane Arnold-1	9290	11500	8100	26100	1620
	Enrico Fermi 2	-	0	0	41.1	6070
	Fitzpatrick	540000	98100	175000	144000	20700
	Grand Gulf 1	5590	4960	7700	3490	5330
	Hatch 1-2	466000	733000	781000	128000	18600
	Hope Creek 1	-	1410	44000	6510	12400
	Humboldt Bay 3	0	0	0	2400	240
	Lacrosse	317000	131000	86200	0	0
	Lasalle 1-2	7220	110000	241000	140000	40000
	Limerick 1	0	13.7	892	6250	9550
	Millstone 1	41100	122000	216000	32400	6700
	Monticello	138000	131000	146000	218000	147000
	Nine Mile Point 1	36400	18200	7300	666	0.006
	Nine Mile Point 2	-	-	222	1490	3120
	Oyster Creek	1540000	2840000	125000	187000	12000
	Peach Bottom 2-3	4770000	1030000	426000	44000	97700
	Perry 1	-	45.5	392	46300	7100
	Pilgrim 1	121000	4660	0	0	25100
	Quad Cities 1-2	109000	54800	13800	139	10600
	River Bend 1		62900	51.4	75.9	3070
	Susquehanna 1-2	19100	8700	4550	2680	4400
	Vermont Yankee	127000	57720	0	0	38100
	WPPSS-2	7840	6140	19800	33400	202000
Total release (GBq)		15300000	13000000	5020000	19600000	6880000
Normalized release [GBq (GW a)$^{-1}$]		409000	328000	117000	446000	157000
Average normalized release 1985-1989 [GBq (GW a)$^{-1}$]		290000				
HWRs						
Argentina [C15, C18]	Atucha-1	5500	6200	1400	3500	600
	Embalse	150000	420000	310000	96000	130000
Canada [A6]	Bruce 1-4	789000	558000	519000	1500000	491000
	Bruce 5-8	106000	127000	139000	154000	106000
	Gentilly-2	120000	50000	49000	83000	0
	Pickering 1-4	192000	183000	289000	233000	340000
	Pickering 5-8	176000	269000	231000	215000	218000
	Point Lepreau	800	5000	100	300	0
India	Kalpakkam 1-2 Rajasthan 1-2	*Not reported*				
Pakistan	Karachi	*Not reported*				
Republic of Korea [M3]	Wolsong 1	137900	125400	151300	171800	91000
Total release (GBq)		1680000	1740000	1690000	2460000	1380000
Normalized release [GBq (GW a)$^{-1}$]		210000	192000	172000	250000	137000
Average normalized release 1985-1989 [GBq (GW a)$^{-1}$]		191000				
GCRs						
France [E4]	Bugey 1	130000	122000	37000	53000	96000
	Chinon A2-3	25000	0	5000	36000	63000
	St. Laurent A1-2	244000	256000	118000	179000	140000
Japan [J1]	Tokai-1	280000	280000	230000	260000	210000
Spain [C21]	Vandellos 1	45200	18600	29500	27600	12000
United Kingdom [N6, P1, S4]	Berkeley	340000	240000	290000	380000	70000
	Bradwell	740000	630000	730000	680000	320000

Table 26 (continued)

Country	*Reactor*	*Release (GBq)*				
		1985	*1986*	*1987*	*1988*	*1989*
United Kingdom (continued)	Calder Hall					2530000
	Chapelcross	3000000	3000000	3100000	3000000	3000000
	Dungeness A	1200000	1000000	1100000	760000	830000
	Dungeness B1-2	20000	50000	10000	20000	7200
	Hartlepool A1-A2	10000	20000	10000	10000	20000
	Heysham 1A-B, 2A-B	10000	10000	10000	10000	7600
	Hinkley Point A	3100000	3100000	3700000	3200000	2400000
	Hinkley Point B, A,B	70000	140000	120000	110000	69000
	Hunterston A1	725000	735000	730000	640000	650000
	Hunterston B1-2	56000	32000	46000	59000	37000
	Oldbury-A	130000	70000	160000	180000	150000
	Sizewell-A	1700000	1400000	1900000	1800000	1800000
	Torness A-B	-	-	-	4300	4600
	Trawsfynydd	5000000	5000000	5000000	900000	1600000
	Wylfa	70000	70000	5000	70000	70000
Total release (GBq)		16900000	16200000	17300000	12400000	14100000
Normalized release [GBq (GW a)$^{-1}$]		2370000	2480000	2670000	1630000	1730000
Average normalized release 1985-1989 [GBq (GW a)$^{-1}$]		2150000				
LWGRs						
USSR [G2, I14]	Beloyarsky 2					12700000
	Bilibino 1-4					307000
	Chernobyl 1-4	2550000				3120000
	Ignalina 1-2	4900000	3170000	1170000	2460000	2260000
	Kursk 1-4	2330000	8510000	6970000	6200000	7030000
	Leningrad 1-4	7830000	4700000	4440000	3510000	2930000
	Smolensk 1-3	2910000	3490000	3940000	2130000	3250000
Total release (GBq)		20500000	19900000	16500000	14300000	31600000
Normalized release [GBq (GW a)$^{-1}$]		1800000	2300000	1800000	1500000	2600000
Average normalized release 1985-1989 [GBq (GW a)$^{-1}$]		2000000				
FBRs						
France [S6]	Creys-Malville	5000	38000	29000	31000	36000
	Phenix	5200	6300	6100	5100	4600
USSR	Beloyarsky 3					
United Kingdom	Dounreay					
Total release (GBq)		10200	44300	35100	36100	40600
Normalized release [GBq (GW a)$^{-1}$]		77000	160000	130000	210000	150000
Average normalized release 1985-1989 [GBq (GW a)$^{-1}$]		150000				

[a] A dash indicates that the reactor was not yet in operation.

Table 27
Isotopic composition of noble gases released from PWRs in the United States, 1988 [T3]

Reactor	Release (TBq)										
	^{41}Ar [a]	^{85}Kr	^{85m}Kr	^{87}Kr	^{88}Kr	^{131m}Xe	^{133}Xe	^{133m}Xe	^{135}Xe	^{135m}Xe	^{138}Xe [b]
Arkansas One 1	- [c]	0.119	0.137	-	-	0.0618	42.9	0.0374	2.96	-	-
Arkansas One 2	0.00073	0.00066	0.00907	0.00043	0.00321	1.42	66.2	0.0833	12.2	-	-
Beaver Valley 1-2	0.0112	2.35	0	-	-	0.139	0.858	0.00107	0.125	0.00087	-
Braidwood 1	0.0123	0.0066	0.00069	0.00002	0.0006	0.0197	1.49	0.00999	0.0141	-	-
Braidwood 2	0.0290	0.00054	0.00044	0	0.00002	0.0327	1.35	0.00403	0.00138	-	-
Byron 1-2	0.0243	0.392	0.0147	0.00021	0.00936	0.249	64.0	0.463	0.633	-	-
Callaway 1	0.0226	3.03	0.0925	-	0.0269	0.0888	20.7	0.0947	1.38	-	-
Calvert Cliffs 1-2	0.00225	11.6	1.65	0.336	0.165	0.944	181	1.44	13.8	0.00012	-
Catawba 1	0.222	0.0770	0.0342	0.00485	0.0381	0.451	55.9	0.574	0.666	0.00021	0.00013
Catawba 2	0.222	0.0770	0.0342	0.00485	0.0381	0.451	55.9	0.574	0.666	0.00021	0.00013
Crystal River 3	-	0.907	0.255	-	-	1.59	121	0.150	2.67	-	-
Davis-Besse 1	-	0.183	-	-	0.0369	0.00071	3.77	0.00588	0.0414	-	-
Diablo Canyon 1-2	0.0766	0.333	0.00381	0.00006	0.00429	0.577	10.7	0.0339	0.433	0.00016	0.00004
Donald C. Cook 1-2	0.0144	0.0562	0.00537	0.0047	0.0261	0.0299	9.07	0.0463	0.300	0.005	0.00385
Fort Calhoun	0.0640	0.225	0.00027	-	-	0.633	27.9	0.126	0.0599	-	-
H.B. Robinson 2	0.176	4.26	0.172	0.00577	0.0102	0.166	31.0	0.244	2.23	0.00287	-
Haddam Neck	0.0264	7.18	0.125	0.114	0.168	0.150	84.0	0.285	2.01	0.0202	0.0503
Harris 1	0.0131	-	1.80	0.599	3.00	-	71.8	1.20	4.18	-	0.599
Indian Point 1-2	0.0274	-	0.00799	0.00169	0.0106	-	7.59	0.0161	0.418	0.0185	0.00013
Indian Point 3	0.0133	0.121	0.0054	0.00219	0.0077	0.308	10.6	0.0747	0.305	0.00049	0.00012
Joseph M. Farley 1	0.973	25.4	0.0226	0.00232	0.00747	0.0426	6.77	0.0807	2.23	0	0.00304
Joseph M. Farley 2	1.32	16.9	-	-	-	-	2.74	0.00703	0.881	-	0.00197
Kewaunee	0.0028	0.00696	0.00007	-	-	0.00005	0.238	0.00053	0.00184	-	-
Maine Yankee	-	0.0577	0.00013	-	0	0.00334	2.48	0.0183	0.101	-	-
McGuire 1	0.324	1.37	0.182	0.0261	0.172	0.396	66.2	0.903	2.62	0.00051	0.00004
McGuire 2	0.324	1.37	0.182	0.0261	0.172	0.396	66.2	0.903	2.62	0.00051	0.00004
Millstone 2	-	0.157	0	-	-	0.0907	27.1	0.0633	4.77	-	-
Millstone 3	-	-	0.00008	-	-	0.00751	2.87	0.0186	0.221	-	-
North Anna 1-2	0.00003	0.135	0.0011	0.00001	0.00002	0.0722	17.5	0.0216	0.0962	-	-
Oconee 1-3	0.189	62.5	0.357	0.0566	0.325	13.8	866	6.92	6.92	0.0466	-
Palisades	0.0337	0.0981	0.0298	0.0662	0.0766	0.0257	88.8	0.0264	0.179	0.242	0.164

Table 27 (continued)

Reactor	*Release (TBq)*										
	^{41}Ar [a]	^{85}Kr	^{85m}Kr	^{87}Kr	^{88}Kr	^{131m}Xe	^{133}Xe	^{133m}Xe	^{135}Xe	^{135m}Xe	^{138}Xe [b]
Palo Verde 1	0.0208	0.955	0.0158	0.00003	0.00129	0.259	58.1	0.230	2.54	-	5.88
Palo Verde 2	0.0640	1.62	0.037	0.00067	0.0925	2.04	104	0.411	1.54	-	0.00149
Palo Verde 3	0.291	0.00244	0.00403	-	0.00114	0.00899	4.55	0.00411	0.154	-	0.00001
Point Beach 1-2	0.0725	0.0364	0.0271	0.0548	0.0625	-	2.23	0.0124	0.131	0.0940	0.266
Prairie Island 1-2	-	0.00455	-	-	-	-	0.0007	0	0.00002	-	-
R.E. Ginna	0.0440	-	0.00364	0.00592	0.00795	0.00729	1.28	0.00104	0.466	0.0655	0.0240
Rancho Seco 1	0.00088	0.0744	0.109	0.00018	0.0881	0.566	54.0	0.357	0.936	0.00001	-
Salem 1	0.00028	0.0407	0.0133	-	-	0.290	18.5	0.0366	0.703	0.00001	-
Salem 2	0.00057	0.0673	0.114	0.0209	0.154	0.0981	41.4	0.225	1.27	0.185	-
San Onofre 1	0.00021	0.426	0.137	0.0094	0.0426	0.145	105	0.988	3.27	0.00004	-
San Onofre 2-3	0.640	0.592	1.21	0.223	0.316	0.570	174	0.235	11.8	0.120	0.0346
Sequoyah 1-2	0.00921	0.0744	0.00648	-	0.00055	0.0403	7.99	0.0788	0.136	-	-
South Texas 1	28.1	-	0.00633	0.00814	0.0119	-	3.54	0.00218	0.0474	0.00173	-
St. Lucie 1	0.112	-	0.195	0.00618	0.248	0.00043	44.4	0.202	7.51	-	-
St. Lucie 2	0.0696	0.0355	2.76	0.0137	1.18	0.128	296	3.22	35.2	-	-
Summer 1	0.0138	0.151	0.0751	0.00019	0.108	0.0562	11.0	0.0392	0.840	-	-
Surry 1-2	0.0451	0.153	0	0.00034	0.00055	0.0729	13.1	0.0223	0.169	0.00024	-
Three Mile Island 1	0.120	0.320	0.0496	0.00002	0.00407	0.437	66.2	0.533	1.33	0.00001	-
Three Mile Island 2	-	0.0163	-	-	-	-	-	-	-	-	-
Trojan	0.0313	0.101	0.0131	0.0036	0.00433	0.0929	14.2	0.0503	0.239	0.0264	0.0094
Turkey Point 3	0.0312	0.0511	0.0221	0.00031	0.00148	0.577	44.4	0.257	0.692	-	-
Turkey Point 4	1.08	0.0559	0.0235	0.00027	0.00284	0.511	45.5	0.278	0.718	-	-
Vogtle 1	1.17	0	0	-	0.00001	-	2.87	0.00201	0.232	-	-
Waterford 3	0.0195	0.477	0.0133	-	0.00581	0.648	188	0.189	6.96	-	-
Wolf Creek 1	0.0360	0.0433	0.0283	0.00001	0.0407	0.151	28.0	0.283	0.696	-	-
Yankee Rowe 1	0.0320	0.152	0.0718	0.0625	0.131	0.0407	3.77	0.0766	1.44	1.76	0.0303
Zion 1-2	0.00385	0.126	0.00042	-	0.00048	0.0238	51.4	0.0132	2.05	-	-
Total release (TBq)	36.1	145	10.1	1.66	6.80	28.9	3400	22.2	147	2.59	7.07
Normalized activity [TBq (GW a)$^{-1}$]	0.87	3.5	0.24	0.040	0.16	0.69	82	0.53	3.5	0.062	0.17

[a] Discharge of ^{37}Ar from one reactor (Yankee Rowe 1): 0.0263 TBq, resulting in a normalized activity of 0.00063 TBq (GW a)$^{-1}$.
[b] Discharges of ^{137}Xe from two reactors (Haddam Neck: 0.0135 TBq; Trojan: 0.00762 TBq), resulting in a normalized activity of 0.00051 TBq (GW a)$^{-1}$.
[c] A dash indicates no value reported.

Table 28
Isotopic composition of noble gases released from BWRs in the United States, 1988 [T3]

Reactor	Release (TBq)												
	^{41}Ar	^{83m}Kr	^{85}Kr	^{85m}Kr	^{87}Kr	^{88}Kr	^{89}Kr [a]	^{131m}Xe	^{133}Xe	^{133m}Xe	^{135}Xe	^{135m}Xe	^{137}Xe	^{138}Xe [b]
Big Rock Point	- [c]	-	-	4.18	20.8	13.1	-	-	1.58	-	19.7	33.9	-	140
Browns Ferry 1-3	-	-	-	-	-	-	-	-	-	-	-	-	-	-
Brunswick 1-2	0.803	-	-	2.62	0.396	2.26	-	-	16.1	0.0418	22.6	3.13	8.51	1.87
Clinton 1	-	-	-	-	-	-	-	-	-	-	0.161	-	-	-
Cooper	-	0.511	2.83	0.999	3.17	3.27	14.1	-	4.85	0.0426	4.85	1.75	17.0	13.8
Dresden 1-3	-	-	0.00048	0.0320	0	0.0607	-	-	0.833	-	4.14	0.272	-	0.866
Duane Arnold	-	-	0.00028	0.581	0.781	1.19	-	-	8.47	0.0270	13.4	0.847	-	0.762
Edwin I. Hatch 1-2	0.496	-	3.26	6.77	3.09	6.66	-	2.52	87.3	0.0925	9.99	4.44	0.0121	3.37
Fermi 2	-	-	-	0.0158	-	-	-	-	-	-	0.0253	-	-	-
Grand Gulf 1	0.0747	-	-	0.023	0.0422	0.0251	3.16	-	0.00105	-	0.0400	0.0341	-	0.0947
Hope Creek 1	-	0.0651	-	0.0651	0.261	0.261	1.76	-	0.130	-	0.329	0.392	2.02	1.24
Humboldt Bay 3	-	-	2.40	-	-	-	-	-	-	-	-	-	-	-
James A. Fitzpatrick	0.496	-	-	15.4	6.14	20.7	-	0.466	52.2	2.19	38.9	1.91	-	5.55
Lacrosse	-	-	-	-	-	-	-	-	-	-	-	-	-	-
Lasalle 1-2	0.307	-	0.0017	19.4	0.0103	24.3	-	-	89.5	-	6.73	-	-	-
Limerick 1	-	-	0	-	-	-	-	-	3.96	0.00365	1.57	0.751	-	-
Millstone 1	-	-	7.36	0.178	1.17	0.0929	-	-	15.0	-	1.97	1.33	-	5.40
Monticello	-	0.470	6.25	0.470	2.37	1.54	41.1	0.304	59.9	0.295	2.29	3.19	53.7	40.0
Nine Mile Point 1	-	-	0.00001	-	-	-	-	-	0.544	-	0.122	-	-	-
Nine Mile Point 2	0.221	-	0.00001	0.0122	0.0280	0.0176	-	-	0	-	0.0314	0.110	0.310	0.759
Oyster Creek 1	-	-	-	12.6	28.6	32.8	-	-	33.3	-	66.2	5.96	-	7.55
Peach Bottom 2-3	-	-	-	-	-	-	-	-	-	-	-	-	-	-
Perry 1	0.0381	-	-	1.95	0.105	0.655	-	0.0984	29.2	0.540	9.21	4.07	0.0295	0.247
Pilgrim 1	-	-	-	-	-	-	-	-	-	-	-	-	-	-
Quad-Cities 1-2	-	-	-	-	-	0.0625	-	-	0.0636	-	0.0132	-	-	-
River Bend 1	-	-	-	-	-	-	-	-	-	-	0.0759	-	-	-
Susquehanna 1-2	-	-	-	-	-	-	-	-	2.68	-	-	-	-	-
Vermont Yankee	-	-	-	-	-	-	-	-	-	-	-	-	-	-
WNP-2	0.0229	-	0.00126	1.62	0.614	1.92	-	0.231	20.9	1.48	4.26	1.67	-	0.611
Total release (TBq)	2.46	1.05	22.1	66.9	67.5	109	60.1	3.61	427	4.71	207	63.7	81.5	221
Normalized activity [TBq (GW a)$^{-1}$]	0.15	0.063	1.3	4.0	4.0	6.5	3.6	0.22	26	0.28	12	3.8	4.9	13

[a] Discharge of ^{90}Kr from one reactor (Monticello): 1.3875 TBq, resulting in a normalized activity of 0.08299 TBq (GW a)$^{-1}$.
[b] Discharge of ^{139}Xe from one reactor (Monticello): 4.107 TBq, resulting in a normalized activity of 0.24566 TBq (GW a)$^{-1}$.
[c] A dash indicates no value reported.

Table 29
Tritium released from reactors in airborne effluents

Country	*Reactor*	*Release (GBq)*				
		1985	*1986*	*1987*	*1988*	*1989*
PWRs						
Belgium [M6]	Doel 1-4	540	580	630	1580	1410
	Tihange 1-4	0	0	0	0	0
Brazil [C1]	Angra 1	8.4	47.9	29.9	82	160
Bulgaria [C16]	Kozloduy-1-5	*Not reported*				
China, Taiwan Province [T2]	Maanshan 1-2	22.4	184	422	740	947
Czechoslovakia [N11]	Bohunice 1-4	370	3400	2400	1600	1480
	Dukovany 1-4	37	190	404	404	409
Finland [F2]	Loviisa 1-2	2900	1800	1800	1700	1100
France [E4]	Belleville 1-2 Blayais 1-4 Bugey 2-5 Cattenom 1-2 Chinon B1-B4 Chooz-A (Ardennes) Cruas 1-4 Dampierre 1-4 Fessenheim 1-2 Flamanville 1-2 Gravelines 1-6 Nogent 1-2 Paluel 1-4 St. Alban 1-2 St. Laurent B1-2 Tricastin 1-4	*Included with noble gases*				
Germany, Federal Republic of [B4, B9, S7]	Biblis A-B	3640	1800	720	670	1000
	Brokdorf	- [a]	4	89	180	100
	Emsland	-	-	-	230	500
	Grafenrheinfeld	640	700	710	500	500
	Greifswald					
	Grohnde	45	200	440	580	500
	Isar 2	-	-	-	220	400
	Mülheim-Kärlich	-	3	48	520	300
	Neckarwestheim 1-2	420	1200	980	610	1000
	Obrigheim	340	200	170	160	200
	Philippsburg 2	140	400	1000	1100	1100
	Stade	830	1100	1600	760	800
	Unterweser	1700	1800	1300	1300	800
Hungary [F3]	Paks 1-4	760	570	1000	610	680
Italy [C22]	Enrico Fermi (Trino)	370	300	180	43	31
Japan [J1]	Genkai 1-2 Ikata 1-2 Mihama 1-3 Ohi 1-2 Sendai 1-2 Takahama 1-4 Tomari-1 Tsuruga-2	*Not measured*				
Netherlands [M5]	Borssele	330	500	390	480	340
Republic of Korea [M3]	Kori 1				5	2
	Kori 2	65		167	10	357
	Kori 3-4					3260
	Ulchin 1-2	-	-	-	2	98
	Yonggwang 1-2	-	48	593	1260	650
South Africa [C20]	Koeberg 1-2				1190	2330

Table 29 (continued)

Country	Reactor	Release (GBq)				
		1985	1986	1987	1988	1989
Spain [C21]	Almaraz 1-2	100	160	1050	1360	2070
	Asco 1	280	350	480	1370	1680
	Asco 2	4	230	250	200	270
	José Cabrera 1	510	270	580	260	1530
	Trillo 1	-	-	-	20	0
	Vandellos 2	-	-	0	20	70
Sweden [N14]	Ringhals 2 Ringhals 3 Ringhals 4	*Not measured*				
Switzerland [D5, D6]	Beznau 1-2 Gösgen	*Not measured*				
USSR [G2, I14]	Armenia 1-2 Balakovo 1-3 Kalinin 1-2 Khmelnitski 1 Kola 1-4 Novovoronezh 3-5 Rovno 1-3 South Ukraine 1-3 Zaporozhe 1-5	*Reported to be ≈ 0*				
United States [T3]	Arkansas One-1	355	223	250	128	600
	Arkansas One-2	127	81.4	177	185	460
	Beaver Valley 1-2	570	733	2630	1600	2980
	Braidwood 1	-	-	1.64	101	320
	Braidwood 2	-	-	-	98.4	140
	Byron 1-2	34.5	19.8	36.3	59.9	6810
	Callaway 1	190	759	825	566	1440
	Calvert Cliffs 1-2	121	137	35.5	1160	750
	Catawba 1	5.74	105	551	1120	880
	Catawba 2	-	105	551	1120	880
	Crystal River 3	762	614	544	367	1270
	Davis-Besse 1	607	381	344	1850	700
	Diablo Canyon 1-2	366	574	788	2420	1410
	Donald Cook 1-2	803	247	426	223	650
	Farley 1	4292	3411	1469	4290	4260
	Farley 2	12210	4551	4107	2210	3450
	Fort Calhoun 1	35.3	51.1	113	142	140
	H. B. Robinson 2	3275	127	514	283	620
	Haddam Neck	3286	357	2327	3400	5070
	Indian Point 1-2	64.8	114	31.4	62.5	11
	Indian Point 3	67.0	137	121	169	82
	Kewaunee	315	1939	1340	265	370
	Maine Yankee	101	224	113	238	470
	McGuire 1	932	1130	925	888	980
	McGuire 2	932	1130	925	888	980
	Millstone 2	4630	4290	4920	3850	2420
	Millstone 3	-	30600	2340	2650	680
	North Anna 1-2	330	2710	640	3490	4510
	Oconee 1-2-3	1580	1600	3960	1700	4370
	Palisades	158	116	118	154	410
	Palo Verde 1	151	16900	9880	15700	5770
	Palo Verde 2	-	3620	13800	10400	13300
	Palo Verde 3	-	-	115	14100	6770
	Point Beach 1-2	2480	4440	4370	4660	5250
	Prairie Island 1-2	2700	4180	2280	5590	4370
	R. E. Ginna	3200	2850	6730	6220	3200
	Rancho Seco 1	1230	910	485	648	1390
	Salem 1	947	2360	7360	14800	7360
	Salem 2	1110	5770	18200	13700	8070
	San Onofre 1	1070	63	559	759	1250
	San Onofre 2-3	295	559	3120	699	1500
	Sequoyah 1-2	3620	1040	544	507	2080
	Shearon Harris 1	-	-	0	0	0
	South Texas 1	-	-	-	636	230
	South Texas 2	-	-	-	-	440
	St. Lucie 1	14800	1510	2830	5400	11500
	St. Lucie 2	5990	1490	2530	3160	2880

Table 29 (continued)

Country	*Reactor*	*Release (GBq)*				
		1985	*1986*	*1987*	*1988*	*1989*
United States (continued)	Surry 1-2	1210	1070	1130	1030	1020
	Three Mile Island 1	0.87	910	36.1	223	180
	Three Mile Island 2	733	1480	1310	422	530
	Trojan	884	1090	1040	2380	2700
	Turkey Point 3	8440	11000	15100	7440	160
	Turkey Point 4	5810	11000	15100	7440	160
	Virgil C. Summer 1	10.2	0.06	20.1	55.9	3.9
	Vogtle 1-2	-	-	2090	3080	33700
	Waterford 3	0	4480	22800	9100	4660
	Wolf Creek	1530	1950	2770	5400	4550
	Yankee NPS	195	381	3130	169	250
	Zion 1-2	688	2600	3070	13700	2560
Yugoslavia [F1]	Krsko	2200	1530	2470	345	590
Total release (GBq)		110000	156000	191000	203000	201000
Normalized release [GBq (GW a)$^{-1}$]		2230	2920	3140	2850	2620
Average normalized release 1985-1989[GBq (GW a)$^{-1}$]		2800				
BWRs						
China, Taiwan Province [T2]	Chin Shan 1-2	1280	1650	1260	237	334
	Kuosheng 1-2	35.7	259	323	5110	1100
Finland [F2]	TVO 1-2	140	200	150	150	110
Germany, Federal Republic of [B4, B9]	Brunsbüttel	470	240	230	150	140
	Gundremmingen B,C	76	120	140	140	220
	Isar 1	520	520	230	320	410
	Krümmel	510	730	260	230	100
	Philippsburg 1	120	16	31	51	69
	Würgassen	1000	410	450	660	920
India	Tarapur-1,2					
Italy [C22]	Caorso	545	40	20	8	2
Japan [J1]	Fukushima Daiichi 1-6	*Not measured*				
	Fukushima Daini 1-4					
	Hamaoka 1-3					
	Kashiwazaki Kariwa 1,5					
	Onagawa-1					
	Shimane 1-2					
	Tokai 2					
	Tsuruga 1					
Mexico [C19]	Laguna Verde (Mark II)	-	-	-	-	1120
Netherlands [M5]	Dodewaard	130	180	100	140	140
Spain [C21]	Confrentes	41	70	190	170	80
	S. Maria de Garona	250	190	210	320	620
Sweden [N14]	Barsebeck 1	*Not measured*				
	Barsebeck 2					
	Forsmark 1					
	Forsmark 2					
	Forsmark 3					
	Oskarshamn 1					
	Oskarshamn 2					
	Oskarshamn 3					
	Ringhals 1					
Switzerland [D5, D6]	Leibstadt	*Not measured*				
	Mühleberg					
United States [T3]	Big Rock Point	932	352	256	196	190
	Browns Ferry 1-3	277	108	43.7	21.9	7.4
	Brunswick 1-2	141	262	224	205	340
	Clinton 1	-	-	9.69	326	32

Table 29 (continued)

Country	*Reactor*	*Release (GBq)*				
		1985	*1986*	*1987*	*1988*	*1989*
United States (continued)	Cooper	18.6	14.4	0	0	0
	Dresden 2-3	1800	344	696	962	540
	Duane Arnold-1	729	533	562	881	610
	Enrico Fermi 2	-	0	0	0	0
	Fitzpatrick	87.0	350	396	411	470
	Grand Gulf 1	78.1	103	121	138	120
	Hatch 1-2	984	1230	2620	1810	2000
	Hope Creek 1	-	170	170000	6030	1020
	Humboldt Bay 3	1.47	1.47	1.46	1.47	1.50
	Lacrosse	1290	448	529	47.4	39
	Lasalle 1-2	85.1	396	1240	0.12	22
	Limerick 1	0	0	5660	2370	660
	Millstone 1	3070	2420	6920	2670	4260
	Monticello	2710	2170	4480	3020	3420
	Nine Mile Point 1	1220	2950	1720	147	290
	Nine Mile Point 2	-	-	0.91	320	370
	Oyster Creek	451	714	291	463	380
	Peach Bottom 2-3	1420	973	1100	260	210
	Perry 1	-	55.1	710	174	0
	Pilgrim 1	240	175	21.3	5.92	180
	Quad Cities 1-2	1930	2510	2510	1670	2890
	River Bend 1		22.6	157	107	220
	Susquehanna 1-2	2880	1580	1730	759	2130
	Vermont Yankee	327	105	418	1624	2050
	WPPSS-2	286	192	810	318	620
Total release (GBq)		26100	22800	207000	32600	28400
Normalized release [GBq (GW a)$^{-1}$]		1130	950	8200	1230	1080
Average normalized release 1985-1989 [GBq (GW a)$^{-1}$]		2500				
HWRs						
Argentina [C15, C18]	Atucha-1	250000	320000	460000	810000	700000
	Embalse	30000	27000	33000	49000	86000
Canada [A6]	Bruce 1-4	1481000	1809000	2116000	2120000	2324000
	Bruce 5-8	98000	164000	462000	480000	760000
	Gentilly-2	49000	137000	123000	117000	137000
	Pickering 1-4	385000	346000	654000	962000	1184000
	Pickering 5-8	144000	187000	231000	196000	278000
	Point Lepreau	110000	200000	220000	220000	210000
India [B14]	Kalpakkam 1-2	167000	653000	727000	1338000	1148000
	Rajasthan 1-2	637000	667000	1123000	1032000	1476000
Pakistan [P3]	Karachi	235000	183000	199000	117000	1430000
Republic of Korea [M3]	Wolsong 1	89720	241600	313300	299000	225600
Total release (GBq)		3680000	4930000	6660000	7740000	9960000
Normalized release [GBq (GW a)$^{-1}$]		446000	522000	649000	754000	968000
Average normalized release 1985-1989 [GBq (GW a)$^{-1}$]		480000				
GCRs						
France [E4]	Bugey 1	*Included with noble gases*				
	Chinon A2-3					
	St. Laurent A1-2					
Japan [J1]	Tokai-1	*Not measured*				
Spain [C21]	Vandellos 1	25000	7310	9	16	18
United Kingdom [N6, P1, S4]	Berkeley					2500
	Bradwell					
	Calder Hall					
	Chapelcross					

Table 29 (continued)

Country	*Reactor*	*Release (GBq)*				
		1985	*1986*	*1987*	*1988*	*1989*
United Kingdom (continued)	Dungeness A					
	Dungeness B1-2					
	Hartlepool A1-A2					
	Heysham 1A-B, 2A-B					
	Hinkley Point A					
	Hinkley Point B, A,B					
	Hunterston A1	1200	1500	2000	4100	1000
	Hunterston B1-2	5500	8200	6000	5500	5400
	Oldbury-A	400				
	Sizewell-A					
	Torness A-B	-	-	-	1000	3200
	Trawsfynydd					
	Wylfa					
Total release (GBq)		32100	17000	8010	10600	12100
Normalized release [GBq (GW a)$^{-1}$]		16900	11100	5320	6230	5480
Average normalized release 1985-1989 [GBq (GW a)$^{-1}$]		9020				
LWGRs						
USSR [G2, I14]	Beloyarsky 2 Bilibino 1-4 Chernobyl 1-4 Ignalina 1-2 Kursk 1-4 Leningrad 1-4 Smolensk 1-3	*Only average normalized release reported*				
Total release (GBq)						
Normalized release [GBq (GW a)$^{-1}$]						
Average normalized release 1985-1989 [GBq (GW a)$^{-1}$]		26000				
FBRs						
France	Creys-Malville Phenix					
USSR	Beloyarsky 3					
United Kingdom [N6]	Dounreay		13600	190	23000	350
Total release (GBq)			13600	190	23000	350
Normalized release [GBq (GW a)$^{-1}$]			130000	2000	330000	2900
Average normalized release 1985-1989 [GBq (GW a)$^{-1}$]		96000				

[a] A dash indicates that the reactor was not yet in operation.

Table 30
Carbon-14 discharged as CO_2 from reactors into the atmosphere

Country	*Reactor*	*Release (GBq)*				
		1985	*1986*	*1987*	*1988*	*1989*
PWRs						
Finland [F2]	Loviisa 1,2	320	300	320	83	300
Germany, Federal Republic of [B4, B9]	Biblis A-B	28	53	44	45	46
	Brokdorf	-	-	12	86	180
	Emsland	-	-	-	29	100
	Grafenrheinfeld	91	95	92	75	230
	Grohnde	17	-	58	61	88
	Isar 2	-	-	-	370	380
	Mülheim-Kärlich	-	10	20	26	7.4
	Neckarwestheim 1-2	30	32	49	63	93
	Obrigheim	13	20	13	9.9	9.1
	Philippsburg 2	5.6	69	54	48	71
	Stade	49	55	12	46	19
	Unterweser	75	26	28	46	33
Hungary [F3]	Paks 1, 2, 3, 4				65	59
Yugoslavia [F1]	Krsko	529	270	454	208	356
Total release (GBq)		1160	930	1160	1260	1960
Normalized release [GBq (GW a)$^{-1}$]		130	130	120	99	140
Average normalized release [GBq (GW a)$^{-1}$]		120				
BWRs						
Germany, Federal Republic of [B4, B9]	Brunsbüttel	260	720	420	590	280
	Gundremmingen	770	750	810	740	940
	Isar	320	350	330	390	400
	Kahl			0	0	0
	Krümmel	190	410	440	320	77
	Lingen			0	0	0
	Philippsburg 1	250	270	320	350	69
	Würgassen	360	340	180	190	170
Total release (GBq)		2150	2840	2500	2580	1940
Normalized release [GBq (GW a)$^{-1}$]		370	510	470	500	380
Average normalized release [GBq (GW a)$^{-1}$]		450				
HWRs						
Argentina [C15, C18]	Atucha	370	381	268	146	0
	Embalse	385	318	472	458	467
Canada [A6]	Pickering A		13300	13000	11800	4400
	Pt. Lepreau	234	443	333	36	43
Total release (GBq)		990	14400	14100	12400	4910
Normalized release [GBq (GW a)$^{-1}$]		810	7300	6400	5900	2100
Average normalized release [GBq (GW a)$^{-1}$]		4800				
GCRs						
United Kingdom [N6, S4]	Heysham 1A-B, 2A-B				76	528
	Hunterston A1					77
	Hunterston B1-2					1000
Total release (GBq)					76	1610
Normalized release [GBq (GW a)$^{-1}$]					110	660
Average normalized release [GBq (GW a)$^{-1}$]		540				

Table 31
Iodine-131 released from reactors in airborne effluents

Country	*Reactor*	*Release (GBq)*				
		1985	*1986*	*1987*	*1988*	*1989*
PWRs						
Belgium [M6]	Doel 1-4	0.56	0.22	0.042	0.15	0.18
	Tihange 1-4	0.16	0.6	0.14	1.36	0.31
Brazil [C1]	Angra 1	0	0	0	0	0
Bulgaria [C16]	Kozloduy-1-2	5.08	3.08	13.7	4.58	1.07
	Kozloduy-3-4	3.73	2.73	4.92	2.32	1.67
	Kozloduy-5	- [a]	-		0.60	1.38
China, Taiwan Province [T2]	Maanshan 1-2	0.0057	0.00004	0	0.024	0
Czechoslovakia [N11]	Bohunice 1-4	2.2	2.4	1.8	1.4	1.48
	Dukovany 1-4	0.09	1.7	1.7	0.93	2.11
Finland [F2]	Loviisa 1-2	0.0067	0	0.038	0.08	0.24
France [E4]	Belleville 1-2	*Included with particulates*				
	Blayais 1-4					
	Bugey 2-5					
	Cattenom 1-2					
	Chinon B1-B4					
	Chooz-A (Ardennes)					
	Cruas 1-4					
	Dampierre 1-4					
	Fessenheim 1-2					
	Flamanville 1-2					
	Gravelines 1-6					
	Nogent 1-2					
	Paluel 1-4					
	St. Alban 1-2					
	St. Laurent B1-2					
	Tricastin 1-4					
Germany, Federal Republic of [B4, B9, S7]	Biblis A-B	0.1	0.037	0.055	0.078	0.021
	Brokdorf	-		0	0	0
	Emsland	-	-	-	0	0
	Grafenrheinfeld	0.00007	0.13	0.00002	0	0.011
	Greifswald	3.9	5.7	8.6	10.3	6.7
	Grohnde		0.0042	0.0029	0.00091	0.0082
	Isar 2	-	-	-	0	0
	Mülheim-Kärlich	-	0.084	0.00012	0.00091	0
	Neckarwestheim 1-2	0.018	0.16	0.00014	0.00013	0.012
	Obrigheim	0.005	0.00044	0.00004	0.00019	0
	Philippsburg 2	0.003	0.00035	0.00092	0.00047	0.00065
	Stade	0.039	0.095	0.072	0.01	0.033
	Unterweser	0.0005	0.011	0.0041	0.0056	0.003
Hungary [F3]	Paks 1-4	0.1	0.12	0.22	0.22	0.22
Italy [C22]	Enrico Fermi (Trino)	0.00019	0.0015	0.00099		
Japan [J1]	Genkai 1-2	0	0.0085	0	0	0
	Ikata 1-2	0.00005	0.034	0	0	0
	Mihama 1-3	0.027	0.067	0.0037	0.0013	0.0025
	Ohi 1-2	0.0059	0.23	0.0016	0.056	0.0012
	Sendai 1-2	0	0.011	0	0	0
	Takahama 1-4	0.021	0.11	0.0027	0.02	0.00022
	Tomari-1	-	-	-	0	0
	Tsuruga-2	-	0.033	0.001	0	0
Netherlands [M5]	Borssele	0.0025	0.011	0.002	0	0.0085
Republic of Korea [M3]	Kori 1	1.51	0.54		0	0.013
	Kori 2		0.004	0.002	0.013	
	Kori 3-4	0.028	0.052	0.2	0.174	0.096
	Ulchin 1-2	-	-	-		0.0007
	Yonggwang 1-2	-		0.00004	0.013	0.0004

Table 31 (continued)

Country	*Reactor*	*Release (GBq)*				
		1985	*1986*	*1987*	*1988*	*1989*
South Africa [C20]	Koeberg 1-2		0.18	0.38	1.5	1.183
Spain [C21]	Almaraz 1-2	0.295	0.315	0	0.004	0.002
	Asco 1	0.114	0.04	0.015	0.1	0.183
	Asco 2	0.006	0.003	0.003	0.013	0.019
	José Cabrera 1	1.18	0.199	0.393	0.234	0.848
	Trillo 1	-	-	-	0.015	0.027
	Vandellos 2	-	-	0	0.2	0.09
Sweden [N14]	Ringhals 2	0.053	0.097	0.29	0.48	0.09
	Ringhals 3	0.0024	0.53	0.57	0.063	0.01
	Ringhals 4	0.0036	0.1	1.1	1.6	0.03
Switzerland [D5, D6]	Beznau 1-2	0.0093	0.021	0.024	0.07	0.6
	Gösgen	0.078	0.0093	0.0034	0.007	0.029
USSR [G2, I14]	Armenia 1-2	7.5	4.05	1.11	5.81	5.55
	Balakovo 1-3	0	0.44	1.89	2.03	0.22
	Kalinin 1-2	0.13	0.95	3.38	0.27	1.35
	Khmelnitski 1	-	-	0	0.078	0.30
	Kola 1-4	0.54	0.77	1.60	1.13	6.35
	Novovoronezh 3-5	0.67	12.2	0.068	0.14	0.027
	Rovno 1-3	0.085	0.20	3.11	4.18	1.23
	South Ukraine 1-3	0.047	0.17		0.021	
	Zaporozhe 1-5	0.141	0.052	4.07		0.23
United States [T3]	Arkansas One-1	0.12	0.14	0.0088	0.030	0.02
	Arkansas One-2	0.11	0.0060	0.0009	0.0098	0.017
	Beaver Valley 1-2	0.016	0.18	0.45	0.046	0.0014
	Braidwood 1	-	-	0.0003	0.012	0.0085
	Braidwood 2	-	-	-	0.0028	0.0081
	Byron 1-2	0.078	2.01	0.34	0.47	0.028
	Callaway 1	0.011	0.043	0.015	0.0007	0.0057
	Calvert Cliffs 1-2	1.92	3.22	3.39	4.63	1.776
	Catawba 1	0.021	0.095	0.047	0.028	0.025
	Catawba 2	-	0.095	0.047	0.028	0.025
	Crystal River 3	0.015	0.025	0.081	0.037	0.075
	Davis-Besse 1	0.019		0.040	0.018	0.11
	Diablo Canyon 1-2	0.0089	0.051	0.068	0.026	0.034
	Donald Cook 1-2	3.81	0.60	1.97	0.25	0.024
	Farley 1	0.21	0.027	0.0098	0.044	0.0013
	Farley 2	0.011	0.050	0.0054	0.00009	0.00002
	Fort Calhoun 1	0.26	0.052	0.19	0.011	0.0047
	H. B. Robinson 2	0.50	0.36	0.77	0.040	0.00011
	Haddam Neck	0.028	0.29	0.021	1.35	0.53
	Indian Point 1-2	0.047	0.069	0.065	0.0015	0.046
	Indian Point 3	0.067	0.15	0.076	0.13	0.05
	Kewaunee	0.0014	0.0013	0.0023	0.013	0.46
	Maine Yankee	0.011	0.080	0.048	0.016	0.007
	McGuire 1	0.30	0.17	0.30	0.21	0.13
	McGuire 2	0.30	0.17	0.30	0.21	0.13
	Millstone 2	0.22	0.20	0.24	1.88	1.4
	Millstone 3	-	0.0093	0.071	0.35	0.45
	North Anna 1-2	0.90	0.79	0.47	0.058	0.14
	Oconee 1-2-3	0.14	0.86	0.51	3.07	0.83
	Palisades	0.76	0.032	0.77	0.75	0.47
	Palo Verde 1	0.053	0.29	2.09	0.058	0.022
	Palo Verde 2	-	0.11	0.50	1.68	0.11
	Palo Verde 3	-	-		0.0046	0.22
	Point Beach 1-2	0.13	0.041	0.11	0.020	0.012
	Prairie Island 1-2	0.27	0.081	0	0.00004	0.00017
	R. E. Ginna	0.036	0.010	0.084	0.0016	0.017
	Rancho Seco 1	0.24	0.055	0	0.0073	0.0098
	Salem 1	0.20	0.043	0.061	0.025	0.13
	Salem 2	0.017	0.12	0.058	0.033	0.003
	San Onofre 1	0.042	0.0074	0.015	0.38	0.077
	San Onofre 2-3	16.4	5.88	15.1	2.77	17.5
	Sequoyah 1-2	0.095	0	0	0.0013	0.011
	Shearon Harris 1	-	-	0		0.00003
	South Texas 1	-	-	-	0.030	0.13
	South Texas 2	-	-	-	-	

Table 31 (continued)

Country	*Reactor*	*Release (GBq)*				
		1985	*1986*	*1987*	*1988*	*1989*
United States (continued)	St. Lucie 1	6.70	9.95	1.46	0.24	0.21
	St. Lucie 2	3.96	1.55	2.04	1.05	0.31
	Surry 1-2	0.94	0.65	0.67	0.35	0.014
	Three Mile Island 1	0	0.0012	0.0047	0.047	0.3
	Three Mile Island 2	0	0.0002	0		
	Trojan	0.19	0.24	0.068	0.11	0.1576
	Turkey Point 3	0.26	0.64	0.42	0.14	0.011
	Turkey Point 4	0.26	0.072	0.47	0.14	0.01055
	Virgil C. Summer 1	0.0007	0.0011	0.017	0.084	0.06
	Vogtle 1-2	-	-	0.0005	0.0004	0.003
	Waterford 3	0.13	0.19	0.031	0.032	0.024
	Wolf Creek	0.00006	0.0078	0.0008	0.0021	0.00065
	Yankee NPS	0.026	0.0070	0.0010	0.0019	0.0033
	Zion 1-2	0.070	0.11	0.0082	0.043	0.075
Yugoslavia [F1]	Krsko	10.9	13	10.5	16.3	12
Total release (GBq)		79.2	81.3	93.5	77.5	72.2
Normalized release [GBq (GW a)$^{-1}$]		1.1	1.0	1.1	0.80	0.71
Average normalized release 1985-1989 [GBq (GW a)$^{-1}$]		0.93				
BWRs						
China, Taiwan Province [T2]	Chin Shan 1-2	30.1	20.9	5.74	7.14	3.96
	Kuosheng 1-2	0.0044	0.00033	0.0047	0.33	0.26
Finland [F2]	TVO 1-2	0.0030	0.078	0.036	0.0025	0.12
Germany, Federal Republic of [B4, B9]	Brunsbüttel	0.2	0.044	0.04	0.088	0.076
	Gundremmingen B,C	0.093	0.46	0.11	0.018	0.012
	Isar 1	0.011	0.54	0.12	0.15	0.0083
	Krümmel	0.011	0.0057	0.092	0.13	0.08
	Philippsburg 1	0.019	0.011	0.00092	0.12	0.0063
	Würgassen	0.8	0.4	0.25	0.16	0.3
India	Tarapur 1-2	*Not reported*				
Italy [C22]	Caorso	0.20	0.50	0.02	0.03	0.007
Japan [J1]	Fukushima Daiichi 1-6	0.13	0.37	0.035	0.041	0.0096
	Fukushima Daini 1-4	0	0.089	0.00001	0	0.00001
	Hamaoka 1-3	0.0029	0.093	0.00067	0.00048	0
	Kashiwazaki Kariwa 1,5	0	0.063	0	0	0
	Onagawa-1	0	0.015	0	0.00037	0
	Shimane 1-2	0	0.035	0	0	0
	Tokai 2	0	0.018	0.07	0	0
	Tsuruga 1	0.0002	0.011	0.00026	0	0
Mexico [C19]	Laguna Verde (Mark II)	-	-	-	-	0.0001
Netherlands [M5]	Dodewaard	0.05	0.04	0.03	0.04	0.04
Spain [C21]	Confrentes	0.118	0.17	1.61	1.83	0.14
	S. Maria de Garona	0.013	0.14	0.12	0.16	0.03
Sweden [N14]	Barsebeck 1	0.03	0.030	0.012	0.034	0.05
	Barsebeck 2	0.01	0.067	0.008	0.037	0.2
	Forsmark 1	0.01	0.18	0.023	0.017	0.03
	Forsmark 2	0.66	0.21	0.053	0.081	0.16
	Forsmark 3	0.03	2.40	0.64	0.86	1.1
	Oskarshamn 1	0.20	0.24	0.082	0.14	0.1
	Oskarshamn 2	0.05	0.45	0.055	5.60	1.6
	Oskarshamn 3	0.002	2.80	0.13	32.00	0.88
	Ringhals 1	5.70	0.86	0.31	0.41	0.47
Switzerland [D5, D6]	Leibstadt	0.00	0.70	0.00	0.52	2
	Mühleberg	0.06	5.40	0.04	0.57	0.46
United States [T3]	Big Rock Point	2.56	1.00	0.16	0.08	0.096
	Browns Ferry 1-3	0.44	0.06	0		

Table 31 (continued)

Country	*Reactor*	*Release (GBq)*				
		1985	*1986*	*1987*	*1988*	*1989*
United States (continued)	Brunswick 1-2	1.48	0.56	1.85	0.84	0.56
	Clinton 1	-	-	0.00	0.01	0.0062
	Cooper	0.09	0.28	0.19	0.36	0.19
	Dresden 2-3	2.29	0.47	0.67	4.03	0.17
	Duane Arnold-1	0.03	0.26	1.67	0.25	0.0068
	Enrico Fermi 2	-	0.00	0.00	0.01	
	Fitzpatrick	1.73	0.44	1.09	0.62	0.023
	Grand Gulf 1	0.01	0.00	0.11	0.00	0.023
	Hatch 1-2	0.22	0.87	13.10	0.35	0.12
	Hope Creek 1	-				
	Humboldt Bay 3	0.00	0.00	0.00		
	Lacrosse	0.18	0.20	0.07		
	Lasalle 1-2	0.31	2.42	0.58	0.29	0.21
	Limerick 1		0.00	0.00	0.21	0.13
	Millstone 1	0.43	0.40	0.69	0.11	0.087
	Monticello	2.49	2.13	5.85	1.59	3.36
	Nine Mile Point 1	0.83	0.28	0.25		
	Nine Mile Point 2	-	-	0.00	0.00	0.017
	Oyster Creek	109	24.3	3.24	1.95	1.49
	Peach Bottom 2-3	2.20	3.20	0.56		0.032
	Perry 1	-	-	0.00	1.67	0.31
	Pilgrim 1	1.78	0.30	0.01		0.19
	Quad Cities 1-2	1.78	0.76	0.76	0.22	0.096
	River Bend 1		0.00	0.00	0.02	0.001
	Susquehanna 1-2	0.04	0.00	0.00	0.03	0.019
	Vermont Yankee	0.01	0.00	0.37	0.13	0.2
	WPPSS-2	0.07	0.15	0.24	3.33	1.43
Total release (GBq)		167	75.4	41.1	66.6	20.9
Normalized release [GBq (GW a)$^{-1}$]		4.5	1.9	0.98	1.5	0.49
Average normalized release 1985-1989 [GBq (GW a)$^{-1}$]		1.8				
HWRs						
Argentina [C15, C18]	Atucha-1	0.59	0.59	0.065	0.23	0.0013
	Embalse	0.23	2.5	0.0019	0.37	0
Canada [A6]	Bruce 1-4	0	0.1	0.1	0.1	0
	Bruce 5-8	0.1	0.1	0.1	0.1	0.1
	Gentilly-2	0	0.2	0	0	0
	Pickering 1-4	0.1	0.1	0.1	0.9	1.1
	Pickering 5-8	0	0.1	0.1	0.1	0.1
	Point Lepreau	0	0	0	0.1	0
India	Kalpakkam 1-2 Rajasthan 1-2	*Not reported*				
Pakistan [P3]	Karachi	0.015	0.041			
Republic of Korea [M3]	Wolsong 1					0.00004
Total release (GBq)		1.04	3.73	0.47	1.90	1.30
Normalized release [GBq (GW a)$^{-1}$]		0.14	0.43	0.050	0.20	0.13
Average normalized release 1985-1989 [GBq (GW a)$^{-1}$]		0.19				
GCRs						
France [E4]	Bugey 1 Chinon A2-3 St. Laurent A1-2	*Included with particulates*				
Japan [J1]	Tokai-1	0.0017	0.016	0.0031	0.00081	0
Spain [C21]	Vandellos 1	0.002	0.017	0.011	0.047	0.099
United Kingdom [N6, P1, S4]	Berkeley Bradwell					

Table 31 (continued)

Country	*Reactor*	*Release (GBq)*				
		1985	*1986*	*1987*	*1988*	*1989*
United Kingdom (continued)	Calder Hall					0.63
	Chapelcross					
	Dungeness A					
	Dungeness B1-2	1.9	1.9	1.9	1.9	1.9
	Hartlepool A1-A2	0.2	0.3	0.3	0.3	0.3
	Heysham 1A-B, 2A-B	0.9	1.2	1.2	1.2	1.2
	Hinkley Point A					
	Hinkley Point B, A,B	0.4	0.4	0.4	0.4	0.4
	Hunterston A1					
	Hunterston B1-2	2.3	0.1	0.1	0.1	
	Oldbury-A					
	Sizewell-A					
	Torness A-B	-	-	-		
	Trawsfynydd					
	Wylfa					
Total release (GBq)		5.70	3.93	3.91	3.95	4.53
Normalized release [GBq (GW a)$^{-1}$]		2.0	1.3	1.4	1.2	1.1
Average normalized release 1985-1989 [GBq (GW a)$^{-1}$]		1.4				
LWGRs						
USSR [G2, I14]	Beloyarsky 2					17.2
	Bilibino 1-4					0
	Chernobyl 1-4	8.10				13.4
	Ignalina 1-2	80.0	149	11.9	77.3	2.63
	Kursk 1-4	64.8	35.1	39.2	16.2	5.4
	Leningrad 1-4	45.9	29.7	27.0	13.5	2.7
	Smolensk 1-3	4.3	13.5	18.9	8.17	4.2
Total release (GBq)		203	227	97.0	115	45.5
Normalized release [GBq (GW a)$^{-1}$]		18	27	10	12	3.8
Average normalized release 1985-1989 [GBq (GW a)$^{-1}$]		14				
FBRs						
France [S6]	Creys-Malville Phenix	*Not reported*				
USSR [I14]	Beloyarsky 3	*Not reported*				
United Kingdom [N6]	Dounreay	*Not reported*				
Total release (GBq)						
Normalized release [GBq (GW a)$^{-1}$]						
Average normalized release 1985-1989 [GBq (GW a)$^{-1}$]						

[a] A dash indicates that the reactor was not yet in operation.

Table 32
Isotopic composition of iodine released from reactors in the United States, 1988
[T3]

Reactor	*Release (GBq)*				
	^{131}I	^{132}I	^{133}I	^{134}I	^{135}I
PWRs					
Arkansas One 1	0.030	0.00016	0.00111	-	-
Arkansas One 2	0.00981	0.00008	0.00142	-	-
Beaver Valley 1-2	0.0459	- [a]	0.00659	-	0.00079
Braidwood 1	0.0119	-	0.0047	0.888	-
Braidwood 2	0.00282	-	0.00058	-	0.00012
Byron 1-2	0.474	0.0165	0.138	0.00093	0.0414
Callaway 1	0.00069	-	-	-	-
Calvert Cliffs 1-2	4.63	-	4.33	-	0.00332
Catawba 1	0.0282	0.00009	0.0167	0.00005	0.00007
Catawba 2	0.0282	0.00009	0.0167	0.00005	0.00007
Crystal River 3	0.0365	-	0.00269	-	-
Davis-Besse 1	0.0176	-	0.00607	-	-
Diablo Canyon 1-2	0.0259	-	0.0134	-	-
Donald C. Cook 1-2	0.251	-	0.0301	-	0.00246
Fort Calhoun	0.0114	-	0.0847	-	-
H.B. Robinson 2	0.0396	-	0.0252	-	-
Haddam Neck	1.35	-	0.0944	-	1.44
Harris 1	-	0.00013	-	-	-
Indian Point 1-2	0.00149	-	0.110	-	-
Indian Point 3	0.126	-	0.0202	-	-
Joseph M. Farley 1	0.0437	-	0.00005	-	-
Joseph M. Farley 2	0.00009	-	0	-	-
Kewaunee	0.0128	0.196	0.00093	-	-
Maine Yankee	0.0164	-	0.004	-	-
McGuire 1	0.206	0.0444	0.0677	0	0.00003
McGuire 2	0.206	0.0444	0.0677	0	0.00003
Millstone 2	1.88	-	0.966	-	-
Millstone 3	0.350	-	0.1647	-	-
North Anna 1-2	0.0577	0.00025	0.448	-	0.00044
Oconee 1-3	3.07	0.0540	0.707	0.00692	0.174
Palisades	0.747	0.0263	0.172	-	0.0187
Palo Verde 1	0.0577	-	0.0188	-	0.0258
Palo Verde 2	1.68	0.0001	0.0247	-	0.00042
Palo Verde 3	0.00455	0.00025	0.00474	-	0.00041
Point Beach 1-2	0.0201	0.0177	0.0566	-	0.0034
Prairie Island 1-2	0.00004	-	0.00074	-	-
R.E. Ginna	0.0016	-	0.104	-	-
Rancho Seco 1	0.00733	-	0.00155	-	-
Salem 1	0.0249	-	-	-	-
Salem 2	0.0326	-	-	-	-
San Onofre 1	0.381	0.144	0.0396	-	0.0198
San Onofre 2-3	2.77	0.0167	0.599	-	0.0692
Sequoyah 1-2	0.00134	-	-	-	-
South Texas 1	0.0303	-	0.00947	-	-
St. Lucie 1	0.237	1.584	1.58	-	-
St. Lucie 2	1.055	-	1.44	-	-
Summer 1	0.0844	0.00851	0.0418	0.00008	0.00389
Surry 1-2	0.354	0.0403	0.174	0.00034	0.0154
Three Mile Island 1	0.0466	0.00012	0.0285	-	0.0414
Three Mile Island 2	-	-	-	-	-
Trojan	0.107	0.00001	0.0377	-	0.00026
Turkey Point 3	0.144	-	0.157	-	0.0729
Turkey Point 4	0.142	-	0.156	-	0.0729
Vogtle 1	0.00035	-	0.00179	-	-
Waterford 3	0.0322	-	0.0002	-	-
Wolf Creek 1	0.00209	-	-	-	-
Yankee Rowe 1	0.00186	-	0.0006	-	0.00006
Zion 1-2	0.0426	0.0611	0.0151	0.00973	0.00673
Total release (GBq)	20.1	2.25	11.1	0.91	2.01
Normalized activity [GBq (GW a)$^{-1}$]	0.50	0.054	0.29	0.022	0.048

Table 32 (continued)

Reactor	*Release (GBq)*				
	^{131}I	^{132}I	^{133}I	^{134}I	^{135}I
BWRs					
Big Rock Point	0.0796	-	0.759	-	0.929
Browns Ferry 1-3	-	-	-	-	-
Brunswick 1-2	0.840	1.41	1.61	0.840	1.69
Clinton 1	0.00907	-	0.0177	0.00285	-
Cooper	0.365	0.00342	0.0747	-	0.0414
Dresden 1-3	4.03	-	1.447	-	2.49
Duane Arnold	0.246	-	0.0725	-	0.0117
Edwin I. Hatch 1 -2	0.347	-	0.995	-	0.910
Fermi 2	0.015	0.00037	0.236	-	0.00312
Grand Gulf 1	0.00225	-	0.0109	-	-
Hope Creek 1	-	-	-	-	-
Humboldt Bay 3	-	-	-	-	-
James A. Fitzpatrick	0.622	-	1.77	-	-
Lacrosse	-	-	-	-	-
Lasalle 1-2	0.289	0.888	14.9	0.115	1.43
Limerick 1	0.208	-	0.136	-	-
Millstone 1	0.110	-	0.537	-	-
Monticello	1.59	-	7.84	-	7.14
Nine Mile Point 1	-	-	-	-	-
Nine Mile Point 2	0.00094	-	0.00858	-	-
Oyster Creek 1	1.95	-	8.66	-	7.4
Peach Bottom 2-3	-	-	-	-	-
Perry 1	1.67	0.00246	1.24	-	0.0182
Pilgrim 1	-	-	-	-	-
Quad-Cities 1-2	0.225	-	1.32	-	3.38
River Bend 1	0.0177	-	0.176	-	-
Susquehanna 1-2	0.0262	-	-	-	-
Vermont Yankee	0.128	-	0.184	-	-
WNP-2	3.33	0.249	1.49	-	0.0503
Total release (GBq)	16.1	2.54	43.5	0.95	25.5
Normalized activity [GBq (GW a)$^{-1}$]	0.96	0.15	2.6	0.057	1.5

[a] A dash indicates no value reported.

Table 33
Particulates released from reactors in airborne effluents

Country	*Reactor*	*Release (GBq)*				
		1985	*1986*	*1987*	*1988*	*1989*
PWRs						
Belgium [M6]	Doel 1-4	0.33	0.53	0.18	0.12	0.03
	Tihange 1-4	0.025	0.073	0.062	0.095	0.071
Brazil [C1]	Angra 1	0.0007	0	0	0	0
Bulgaria [C16]	Kozloduy-1-2	1.56	1.21	5.28	1.96	1.32
	Kozloduy-2					
	Kozloduy-3-4	1.74	3.16	0.90	0.74	0.74
	Kozloduy-4					
	Kozloduy-5	- [a]	-		0.41	1.19
China, Taiwan Province [T2]	Maanshan 1-2	0.038	0.0030	0	0.018	0.033
Czechoslovakia [N11]	Bohunice 1-4	1.73	0.44	0.16	0.2	0.38
	Dukovany 1-4	0.031	0.06	0.08	0.04	0.172
Finland [F2]	Loviisa 1-2	0.043	0.091	0.068	0.058	1.8
France [E4]	Belleville 1-2	-	-	0.013	0.082	0.13
	Blayais 1-4	2.5	2.6	0.33	0.41	0.72
	Bugey 2-5	0.7	1.5	0.84	0.85	0.69
	Cattenom 1-2	-	0.0041	0.3	0.19	0.18
	Chinon B1-B4	0.3	1.1	1.5	0.36	0.56
	Chooz-A (Ardennes)	0.07	0.26	0.096	0.1	0.19
	Cruas 1-4	0.07	0.28	0.093	0.069	0.09
	Dampierre 1-4	1.5	7.1	0.59	0.41	0.75
	Fessenheim 1-2	0.12	0.17	0.11	0.026	0.025
	Flamanville 1-2		0.089	0.097	0.29	0.1
	Gravelines 1-6	1.9	2.1	1.7	0.69	1.1
	Nogent 1-2	-	-	0.0047	0.084	0.096
	Paluel 1-4	0.26	0.48	0.59	0.43	0.51
	St. Alban 1-2	0.033	0.18	0.11	0.083	0.11
	St. Laurent B1-2	0.7	1.5	0.6	0.52	0.44
	Tricastin 1-4	0.6	0.7	0.22	0.18	0.23
Germany, Federal Republic of [B4, B9, S7]	Biblis A-B	0.31	0.1	0.17	0.32	0.077
	Brokdorf	-	0	0.00003	0.00023	0
	Emsland	-	-	-	0	0.00032
	Grafenrheinfeld	0.002	0	0.0017	0.0014	0.00096
	Greifswald	0.5	0.5	0.5	0.6	0.6
	Grohnde		0.00054	0.00069	0.00065	0.00088
	Isar 2	-	-	-	0.00014	0.00005
	Mülheim-Kärlich	-	0	0	0	0
	Neckarwestheim 1-2	0.014	0.022	0.012	0.0063	0.0044
	Obrigheim	0.024	0.032	0.012	0.014	0.013
	Philippsburg 2		0.00005	90.0001	0.00013	0.0011
	Stade	0.028	0.026	0.013	0.031	0.052
	Unterweser	0.008	0.0056	0.0076	0.0028	0.0014
Hungary [F3]	Paks 1-4	0.12	1.02	2.21	1.57	4.12
Italy [C22]	Enrico Fermi (Trino)	0.00067	0.0045	0.0017	0.0009	0.0006
Japan [J1]	Genkai 1-2	*Not measured*				
	Ikata 1-2					
	Mihama 1-3					
	Ohi 1-2					
	Sendai 1-2					
	Takahama 1-4					
	Tomari-1					
	Tsuruga-2					
Netherlands [M5]	Borssele	0	0.004	0	0	0
Republic of Korea [M3]	Kori 1	0.13	0.14	0.015	0.009	0.034
	Kori 2	0.002	0.003	0.003	0.001	0.0002
	Kori 3-4		0.002	0.016	0.0001	0.001

Table 33 (continued)

Country	*Reactor*	*Release (GBq)*				
		1985	*1986*	*1987*	*1988*	*1989*
Republic of Korea (continued)	Ulchin 1-2	-	-	-	0	0.139
	Yonggwang 1-2	-	0.00007	0.001	0.007	0.002
South Africa [C20]	Koeberg 1-2		0.005	0.0007	0	0.0002
Spain [C21]	Almaraz 1-2	2.47	0.67	0.003	0.04	0.05
	Asco 1	0.06	2.24	4.45	0.04	0.04
	Asco 2	0.007	0.01	0.02	0.03	0.03
	José Cabrera 1	0.23	0.1	0.08	0.12	0.18
	Trillo 1	-	-	-	0.005	0.005
	Vandellos 2	-	-	0	0.0002	0.01
Sweden [N14]	Ringhals 2	0.008	0.006	0.005	0.012	0.0045
	Ringhals 3	0.004	0.002	0.011	0.006	0.0034
	Ringhals 4	0.001	0.002	0.012	0.008	0.0058
Switzerland [D5, D6]	Beznau 1-2	0.0009	0.0007	0.00085	0.011	0.00065
	Gösgen	0.01	0.0057	0.00078	0.0023	0.0014
USSR [G2, I14]	Armenia 1-2	7.50	7.48	24.3	32.4	31.9
	Balakovo 1-3	0	104	0.43	0.49	0.15
	Kalinin 1-2	0.009	0.088	0.059	0.19	0.05
	Khmelnitski 1	-	-			0.063
	Kola 1-4	0.22	0.43	0.91	0.89	11.3
	Novovoronezh 3-5	27.8	28.1	3.10	5.31	1.32
	Rovno 1-3		0.74	0.84	0.14	0.20
	South Ukraine 1-3	0.19	2.43		0.16	
	Zaporozhe 1-5	0.00072	0.041	0.044	0.067	0.19
United States [T3]	Arkansas One-1	0.012	0.0067	0.0024	0.0080	0.01
	Arkansas One-2	0.010	0.0027	0.0010	0.0058	0.005
	Beaver Valley 1-2	0.043	0.11	0.052	0.085	0.4086
	Braidwood 1	-	-	0.0002	0.89089	0.0009
	Braidwood 2	-	-	-	0.0007	0.0029
	Byron 1-2	0.0026	0.011	0.0048	0	0.001
	Callaway 1	0.0006	0.0011	0.0014	0.012	0.0004
	Calvert Cliffs 1-2	0.059	0.0074	0.0037	0.41	0.004
	Catawba 1	0	0.15	0.23	0.12	0.003
	Catawba 2	-	0.15	0.23	0.12	0.003
	Crystal River 3	0.012	0.013	0.048	0.0097	0
	Davis-Besse 1	0		0.0059	0	0.003
	Diablo Canyon 1-2	0	0.0026	0.019	0.022	0.002
	Donald Cook 1-2	2.78	0.25	0.41	0.079	1.246
	Farley 1	0.0004	0.0029	0.0043	0.016	0
	Farley 2	0.0003	0	0.0002	0.00001	0.00001
	Fort Calhoun 1	0.0081	0.0026	0	0.0001	0
	H. B. Robinson 2	0.0074	0.0078	0	0.0011	0.00509
	Haddam Neck	0.014	0.056	0.029	0.019	0.03
	Indian Point 1-2	210	309	0.52	0.34	0.094
	Indian Point 3	0.0033	0.0033	0.0007	0.0004	0.0003
	Kewaunee	0.0089	0.21	0.45	0.38	0.19
	Maine Yankee	0.0042	0.020	0.044	0.0010	0.0018
	McGuire 1	0.18	0.96	1.95	0.021	0.01
	McGuire 2	0.18	0.96	1.95	0.021	0.01
	Millstone 2	0.020	0.0026	0.0004	0.019	0
	Millstone 3	-	0.0044	0.12	0.016	0.02
	North Anna 1-2	2.27	0.052	0.17	0.027	0.02
	Oconee 1-2-3	0.044	0.75	4.89	2.96	0.49
	Palisades	1.06	0.080	0.25	0.23	0.17
	Palo Verde 1	0.0004	0.0022	0.056	0.0096	0.006
	Palo Verde 2	-	0.015	0	0.048	0.002
	Palo Verde 3	-	-		0.00004	0.02
	Point Beach 1-2	0.21	0.021	0	0.062	0.108
	Prairie Island 1-2	0.0011	0.0007	0.0086	0.0028	0.00061
	R. E. Ginna	0.0003	0.0046	0.24	0.0005	0.014
	Rancho Seco 1	0.053	0.0004	0.00006	0.010	0.0002
	Salem 1	1.44	0	0	0.054	0.004
	Salem 2	3.29	0	0.0019	0.0041	0.029
	San Onofre 1	0.0011	0.0004	0.0003	0.019	0.005
	San Onofre 2-3	0.19	0.11	0.41	0.096	0.001
	Sequoyah 1-2	0.022	0.058	0.019	0.0057	0.005

Table 33 (continued)

Country	*Reactor*	*Release (GBq)*				
		1985	*1986*	*1987*	*1988*	*1989*
United States (continued)	Shearon Harris 1	-	-	0.0002	1.00	0.00003
	South Texas 1	-	-	-	0	0.02
	South Texas 2	-	-	-	-	0.053
	St. Lucie 1	22.6	0	0	0	0.003
	St. Lucie 2	3.15	0.0074	0.0037	0.0037	0
	Surry 1-2	0.044	0.13	0.10	0.39	0.046
	Three Mile Island 1	0.0011	0.013	0	0	0
	Three Mile Island 2	0.0017	0.0060	0.0027	1.00	0.00013
	Trojan	0.016	0.017	0.028	0.040	0.0014
	Turkey Point 3	0.030	0.074	0.041	0.034	0.099
	Turkey Point 4	0.030	0.019	0.041	0.034	0.00051
	Virgil C. Summer 1	0.0002	0	0.0095	0.0019	0
	Vogtle 1-2	-	-	0.0003	0.0003	0.043
	Waterford 3	0	0.0059	0.0068	0.014	0.004
	Wolf Creek	0	0	0.0072	0.001	0.0002
	Yankee NPS	0.0020	0.0005	0.0005	0.0003	0.0034
	Zion 1-2	0.87	1.54	0.14	0.48	0.013
Yugoslavia [F1]	Krsko	0.535	0.102	0.396	0.1	0.073
Total release (GBq)		303	487	154	60	65
Normalized release [GBq (GW a)$^{-1}$]		3.6	5.0	1.4	0.50	0.51
Average normalized release 1985-1989 [GBq (GW a)$^{-1}$]		2.0				
BWRs						
China, Taiwan Province [T2]	Chin Shan 1-2	7.51	8.21	0.63	0.60	0.37
	Kuosheng 1-2	0.036	0.0056	0.0027	0.027	0.021
Finland [F2]	TVO 1-2	1.1	0.95	0.2	0.2	0.18
Germany, Federal Republic of [B4, B9]	Brunsbüttel	0.021	0.008	0.03	0.023	0.052
	Gundremmingen B,C	0	0.031	0.0034	0.0031	0
	Isar 1	0.15	0.23	0.019	0.028	0.0085
	Krümmel	0.052	0.035	0.022	0.0025	0.0054
	Philippsburg 1	0.11	0.029	0.02	0.017	0.013
	Würgassen	0.22	0.22	0.21	0.24	0.28
India	Tarapur-1					
	Tarapur-2					
Italy [C22]	Caorso	0.68	0.33	0.069	0.03	0.036
Japan [J1]	Fukushima Daiichi 1-6	*Not measured*				
	Fukushima Daini 1-4					
	Hamaoka 1-3					
	Kashiwazaki Kariwa 1,5					
	Onagawa-1					
	Shimane 1-2					
	Tokai 2					
	Tsuruga 1					
Mexico [C19]	Laguna Verde (Mark II)	-	-	-	-	0.0122
Netherlands [M5]	Dodewaard	0.062	0.028	0.019	0.038	0.041
Spain [C21]	Confrentes	0.16	0.13	0.07	0.15	0.1
	S. Maria de Garona	0.27	0.15	0.23	0.14	0.05
Sweden [N14]	Barsebeck 1	3.96	0.45	0.3	0.066	0.2
	Barsebeck 2	0.2	0.22	0.087	0.124	48
	Forsmark 1	15.4	1.4	0.54	0.25	0.2
	Forsmark 2	5.21	7.7	2.3	0.94	0.6
	Forsmark 3	0.45	103	156	112	61
	Oskarshamn 1	6.15	7.9	2.5	4.5	7.3
	Oskarshamn 2	1.5	0.32	1	179	64
	Oskarshamn 3	0.013	1.7	0.026	79	14
	Ringhals 1	0.93	4.19	0.35	1.95	87

Table 33 (continued)

Country	*Reactor*	*Release (GBq)*				
		1985	*1986*	*1987*	*1988*	*1989*
Switzerland [D5, D6]	Leibstadt	0.0012	0.00038	0.037	0.012	0.056
	Mühleberg	0.07	12	0.19	0.13	0.078
United States [T3]	Big Rock Point	0.49	1.80	0.93	1.80	0.084
	Browns Ferry 1-3	0.48	0.039	0.066	1.07	0.0069
	Brunswick 1-2	0.85	1.17	4.88	5.71	1.23
	Clinton 1	-	-	0.0080	2.19	0.34
	Cooper	0.76	0.15	0.80	0.39	0.0046
	Dresden 2-3	3.48	2.16	4.70	4.66	42.4
	Duane Arnold-1	0.30	2.45	3.40	0.33	0.11
	Enrico Fermi 2	-	0.00001	0.32	0.088	0.62
	Fitzpatrick	4.45	2.76	3.94	1.97	2.61
	Grand Gulf 1	0.020	0.013	0.048	0.016	0.017
	Hatch 1-2	2.50	0.35	0.59	1.24	0.09
	Hope Creek 1	-				0
	Humboldt Bay 3	0.0028	0.0061	0.0025	1.01	0.0014
	Lacrosse	0.096	0.020	0.016	1.00	0.00048
	Lasalle 1-2	0.55	0.20	1.26	0.21	0.09
	Limerick 1		0.28	0.043	0.038	0.15
	Millstone 1	1.49	1.35	0.23	0.17	0.26
	Monticello	1.19	0.40	0.56	1.33	0.86
	Nine Mile Point 1	0.45	0.37	0.35	1.07	0.11
	Nine Mile Point 2	-	-	191	0.025	0.17
	Oyster Creek	3.33	1.55	0.60	0.40	0.39
	Peach Bottom 2-3	0.34	0.21	0.185	1.06	0.098
	Perry 1	-	0.00004	0.0003	0.041	0.01
	Pilgrim 1	0.32	0.16	0.0175	1.01	0.02
	Quad Cities 1-2	20.6	3.35	2.72	0.69	1.4
	River Bend 1		0.0009	0.011	0.018	0.014
	Susquehanna 1-2	0.94	0.12	0.22	0.041	0.022
	Vermont Yankee	0.20	0.47	0.10	0.12	0.13
	WPPSS-2	8.92	2.44	2.61	15.02	2.9
Total release (GBq)		96.1	171	385	422	338
Normalized release [GBq (GW a)$^{-1}$]		3.3	5.6	12.4	13.0	10.3
Average normalized release 1985-1989 [GBq (GW a)$^{-1}$]		9.1				
HWRs						
Argentina [C15, C18]	Atucha-1	0.022	0.0044	0.014	0.0023	0.00075
	Embalse	0.22	0.039	0.95	0.089	0
Canada [A6]	Bruce 1-4	0.3	0.4	0.8	1	0.1
	Bruce 5-8	0.2	0.3	0.3	0.2	0.2
	Gentilly-2	0	0	0	0	0
	Pickering 1-4	0	1.1	1.1	0.8	1
	Pickering 5-8	0	0	0	0	0
	Point Lepreau	0	0	0	0	0
India [B14]	Kalpakkam 1-2					
	Rajasthan 1-2	0.22	0.20	0.35	0.35	0.15
Pakistan	Karachi	*Not reported*				
Republic of Korea [M3]	Wolsong 1	0.006				0.006
Total release (GBq)		0.97	2.04	3.51	2.44	1.46
Normalized release [GBq (GW a)$^{-1}$]		0.12	0.23	0.37	0.26	0.14
Average normalized release 1985-1989 [GBq (GW a)$^{-1}$]		0.23				
GCRs						
France [E4]	Bugey 1	0.2	0.15	0.13	0.12	0.33
	Chinon A2-3	0.1	0.5	1.3	0.25	0.21
	St. Laurent A1-2	1.2	1.3	0.5	0.4	0.26
Japan [J1]	Tokai-1					

Table 33 (continued)

Country	*Reactor*	*Release (GBq)*				
		1985	*1986*	*1987*	*1988*	*1989*
Spain [C21]	Vandellos 1	0.05	0.07	0.08	0.19	0.27
United Kingdom [N6, P1, S4]	Berkeley	0	0	0	0.03	0.006
	Bradwell	0.1	0.1	0.1	0.08	0.06
	Calder Hall					0.6
	Chapelcross					
	Dungeness A	0.2	0.2	0.2	0.2	0.2
	Dungeness B1-2	0.1	0.3	0.1	0.1	0.1
	Hartlepool A1-A2	0	0	0	0.04	0.04
	Heysham 1A-B, 2A-B	0	0	0.1	0.05	0.05
	Hinkley Point A	0.3	0.3	0.3	0.3	0.3
	Hinkley Point B, A,B	0.5	0.6	0.6	0.5	0.5
	Hunterston A1	0	0.065	0.084	0.098	0.11
	Hunterston B1-2	0.2	0.22	0.27	0.14	0.083
	Oldbury-A	0.2	0.2	0.3	0.1	0.1
	Sizewell-A	0.5	1.4	0.4	0.6	0.5
	Torness A-B	-	-	-	0.17	0.023
	Trawsfynydd	0.5	0.5	0.6	0.3	0.2
	Wylfa	0.1	0.1	0.1	0.2	0.1
Total release (GBq)		4.25	6.01	5.16	3.87	4.04
Normalized release [GBq (GW a)$^{-1}$]		0.62	0.96	0.83	0.53	0.51
Average normalized release 1985-1989 [GBq (GW a)$^{-1}$]		0.68				
LWGRs						
USSR [G2, I14]	Beloyarsky 2					28.5
	Bilibino 1-4					0
	Chernobyl 1-4	14.8				49.7
	Ignalina 1-2	38.0	8.78	3.33	3.55	1.74
	Kursk 1-4	153	48.6	91.8	43.2	20.3
	Leningrad 1-4	9.45	7.29	5.40	4.05	9.45
	Smolensk 1-3	4.40	12.2	8.64	11.2	4.86
Total release (GBq)		220	76.9	109	62.0	115
Normalized release [GBq (GW a)$^{-1}$]		20	9.1	12	6.5	9.6
Average normalized release 1985-1989 [GBq (GW a)$^{-1}$]		12				
FBRs						
France [S6]	Creys-Malville	0.002	0.04	0.007	0.007	0.008
	Phenix	0.03	0.02	0.02	0.02	0.02
USSR	Beloyarsky 3					
United Kingdom [N6]	Dounreay		0.013	0.010	0.032	0.056
Total release (GBq)		0.032	0.073	0.037	0.059	0.084
Normalized release [GBq (GW a)$^{-1}$]		0.24	0.19	0.10	0.25	0.22
Average normalized release 1985-1989 [GBq (GW a)$^{-1}$]		0.19				

[a] A dash indicates that the reactor was not yet in operation.

Table 34
Tritium released from reactors in liquid effluents

Country	Reactor	Release (GBq)				
		1985	1986	1987	1988	1989
PWRs						
Belgium [M6]	Doel 1-4	46700	44300	49400	72800	56800
	Tihange 1-4	46200	54500	58000	69200	49600
Brazil [C1]	Angra 1	*Not reported*				
Bulgaria [C16]	Kozloduy 1-5	*Not reported*				
China, Taiwan Province [T2]	Maanshan 1-2	6600	4120	15400	14600	17400
Czechoslovakia [N11]	Bohunice 1-4	12560	14590	13650	8280	10440
	Dukovany 1-4	6900	2800	13700	14600	18000
Finland [F2]	Loviisa 1-2	9300	13000	13000	16000	15000
France [E4]	Belleville 1-2	- [a]	-	200	19000	29000
	Blayais 1-4	80000	87000	78000	63000	60000
	Bugey 2-5	79000	87000	64000	62000	51000
	Cattenom 1-2	-	100	12000	23000	24000
	Chinon B1-B4	22000	40000	48000	50000	47000
	Chooz-A (Ardennes)	98000	111000	107000	71000	110000
	Cruas 1-4	57000	48000	50000	49000	36000
	Dampierre 1-4	67000	77000	57000	54000	64000
	Fessenheim 1-2	30000	38000	36000	33000	24000
	Flamanville 1-2	100	7000	42000	36000	33000
	Gravelines 1-6	95000	114000	97000	82000	91000
	Nogent 1-2	-	-	1000	15000	22000
	Paluel 1-4	31000	68000	86000	100000	100000
	St. Alban 1-2	3000	16000	29000	21000	37000
	St. Laurent B1-2	30000	40000	43000	31000	43000
	Tricastin 1-4	72000	61000	54000	55000	54000
Germany, Federal Republic of [B4, B9, S7]	Biblis A-B	33000	29000	24000	24000	25000
	Brokdorf	-	100	25000	940	13000
	Emsland	-	-	-	1700	13000
	Grafenrheinfeld	22000	14000	16000	14000	14000
	Greifswald					
	Grohnde	7200	8000	16000	13000	13000
	Isar 2	-	-	-	1800	7100
	Mülheim-Kärlich	-	1900	4900	10000	1700
	Neckarwestheim 1-2	13000	11000	12000	7400	17800
	Obrigheim	5300	4100	5700	3800	4400
	Philippsburg 2	13000	22000	13000	13000	21000
	Stade	6200	7100	6100	6000	4600
	Unterweser	27000	14000	14000	12000	15000
Hungary [F3]	Paks 1-4	8600	7200	11800	16400	14900
Italy [C22]	Enrico Fermi (Trino)	23800	69	5350	63	67
Japan [J1]	Genkai 1-2	21000	32000	29000	17000	26000
	Ikata 1-2	31000	33000	33000	21000	34000
	Mihama 1-3	16000	22000	24000	21000	13000
	Ohi 1-2	29000	41000	33000	30000	26000
	Sendai 1-2	20000	27000	34000	41000	38000
	Takahama 1-4	37000	44000	48000	70000	40000
	Tomari-1	-	-	-	440	2100
	Tsuruga-2	-	5600	23300	4070	12000
Netherlands [M5]	Borssele	5700	8400	4600	6900	5700
Republic of Korea [M3]	Kori 1	18900	10900		7810	16000
	Kori 2	10800	14000	18300	12100	25700
	Kori 3-4	12200	24800	26600	30300	32600
	Ulchin 1-2	-	-	-	2430	6900
	Yonggwang 1-2	-	3970	17700	7740	35100
South Africa [C20]	Koeberg 1-2		15100	10800	32400	37300

Table 34 (continued)

Country	*Reactor*	*Release (GBq)*				
		1985	*1986*	*1987*	*1988*	*1989*
Spain [C21]	Almaraz 1-2	36100	15000	31100	47000	49000
	Asco 1	9130	11000	13000	18400	16100
	Asco 2	3180	20000	16200	18300	23500
	José Cabrera 1	2540	1180	20	10	2150
	Trillo 1	-	-	-	677	10200
	Vandellos 2	-	-	0.4	4680	10600
Sweden [N14]	Ringhals 2	19500	13400	30500	13100	12600
	Ringhals 3	10800	19600	19200	20000	23000
	Ringhals 4	14600	13500	14600	19100	21700
Switzerland [D5, D6]	Beznau 1-2	34000	41000	37000	22000	10000
	Gösgen	23000	15000	12000	14000	12000
USSR [G2, I14]	Armenia 1-2	*Average normalized release estimated to be 30000 GBq (GW a)$^{-1}$*				
	Balakovo 1-3					
	Kalinin 1-2					
	Khmelnitski 1					
	Kola 1-4					
	Novovoronezh 3-5					
	Rovno 1-3					
	South Ukraine 1-3					
	Zaporozhe 1-5					
United States [T3]	Arkansas One-1	12100	7840	5550	9250	14097
	Arkansas One-2	8920	8510	13000	9030	16280
	Beaver Valley 1-2	5550	7620	21200	15100	22977
	Braidwood 1	-	-	1520	10100	20646
	Braidwood 2	-	-	-	9030	20646
	Byron 1-2	9660	2480	15200	37400	47730
	Callaway 1	21800	16100	16600	33000	22533
	Calvert Cliffs 1-2	17900	27200	27300	23100	8732
	Catawba 1	6480	4370	13500	13100	16465
	Catawba 2	-	4370	13500	13100	16465
	Crystal River 3	6510	6400	13200	18900	12728
	Davis-Besse 1	2490	773	9100	1300	8843
	Diablo Canyon 1-2	15800	25800	25600	15900	34595
	Donald Cook 1-2	42200	25700	72900	40700	32338
	Farley 1	22300	26400	23600	19100	25863
	Farley 2	18600	23000	18700	27900	22496
	Fort Calhoun 1	6180	6810	8440	8580	8436
	H. B. Robinson 2	11400	12700	10100	19800	6068
	Haddam Neck	213000	95500	117000	43700	178000
	Indian Point 1-2	13000	12400	20800	16200	20720
	Indian Point 3	12600	21000	12600	21200	12897
	Kewaunee	14000	10900	13000	12300	12617
	Maine Yankee	6810	13000	4370	10800	15614
	McGuire 1	14900	16900	18200	19600	15651
	McGuire 2	14900	16900	18200	19600	15651
	Millstone 2	6140	10400	10600	9580	13542
	Millstone 3	-	20000	21800	20200	25789
	North Anna 1-2	54800	57700	30900	71800	51800
	Oconee 1-2-3	45900	49600	35100	26300	37740
	Palisades	15900	2340	4400	10500	2982
	Palo Verde 1	0	0	0	0	0
	Palo Verde 2	-	0	0	0	0
	Palo Verde 3	-	-	0	0	0
	Point Beach 1-2	29800	30000	26200	13200	20683
	Prairie Island 1-2	25800	24800	16500	15000	17168
	R. E. Ginna	18500	13200	20900	12900	21904
	Rancho Seco 1	3330	2410	677	3740	2697
	Salem 1	34200	15200	14000	23500	22533
	Salem 2	21300	16200	24500	13600	18907
	San Onofre 1	88100	16800	84000	56600	35594
	San Onofre 2-3	17600	27400	30300	23800	48100
	Sequoyah 1-2	23400	9100	4400	7440	42550
	Shearon Harris 1	-	-	9180	14800	16946
	South Texas 1	-	-	-	7360	11729
	South Texas 2	-	-	-	-	10064
	St. Lucie 1	10600	10300	12500	10200	14985
	St. Lucie 2	13500	10300	12500	10200	14985

Table 34 (continued)

Country	*Reactor*	*Release (GBq)*				
		1985	*1986*	*1987*	*1988*	*1989*
United States (continued)	Surry 1-2	28800	32300	30200	18300	15873
	Three Mile Island 1	335	6250	7290	11200	13801
	Three Mile Island 2	0.08	0.06	0.05	0.2	0.036
	Trojan	9810	5290	6480	13900	11800
	Turkey Point 3	16000	13500	9950	11100	8473
	Turkey Point 4	16000	13500	9950	11100	8473
	Virgil C. Summer 1	11500	13900	27200	27900	25345
	Vogtle 1-2	-	-	11900	14400	33966
	Waterford 3	940	15900	19400	18600	13256
	Wolf Creek	6770	13900	11700	15000	21756
	Yankee NPS	8440	6510	8100	7250	6216
	Zion 1-2	24300	26400	24300	35900	38739
Yugoslavia [F1]	Krsko	10900	13000	10500	16300	12000
Total release (GBq)		2350000	2350000	2650000	2580000	2970000
Normalized release [GBq (GW a)$^{-1}$]		28000	24200	25100	22600	24200
Average normalized release 1985-1989 [GBq (GW a)$^{-1}$]		25000				
BWRs						
China, Taiwan Province [T2]	Chin Shan 1-2	174	233	673	205	1720
	Kuosheng 1-2	95.1	112	944	529	1150
Finland [F2]	TVO 1-2	1200	1600	1900	1300	1300
Germany, Federal Republic of [B4, B9]	Brunsbüttel	870	500	500	510	270
	Gundremmingen B,C	1200	1200	1600	1200	1500
	Isar 1	470	650	750	810	510
	Krümmel	760	1000	950	880	690
	Philippsburg 1	900	770	620	550	480
	Würgassen	710	490	390	410	960
India	Tarapur-1					
	Tarapur-2					
Italy [C22]	Caorso	1120	1200	97	29	6.3
Japan [J1]	Fukushima Daiichi 1-6	4100	3400	2300	2600	2600
	Fukushima Daini 1-4	410	440	700	960	1500
	Hamaoka 1-3	2400	1700	1700	1500	1300
	Kashiwazaki Kariwa 1,5	44	16	36	0	170
	Onagawa-1	24	41	63	110	75
	Shimane 1-2	310	120	280	130	280
	Tokai 2	590	740	520	480	1100
	Tsuruga 1	350	410	350	440	240
Mexico [C19]	Laguna Verde (Mark II)	-	-	-	-	1120
Netherlands [M5]	Dodewaard	170	270	170	150	200
Spain [C21]	Confrentes	540	120	70	30	70
	S. Maria de Garona	250	100	160	490	60
Sweden [N14]	Barsebeck 1	290	950	490	280	400
	Barsebeck 2	290	950	490	280	400
	Forsmark 1	580	441	630	705	760
	Forsmark 2	580	441	630	705	760
	Forsmark 3	150	1060	330	390	550
	Oskarshamn 1	260	386	610	735	490
	Oskarshamn 2	260	386	610	735	490
	Oskarshamn 3	110	330	335	430	220
	Ringhals 1	525	527	533	639	665
Switzerland [D5, D6]	Leibstadt	270	400	320	300	440
	Mühleberg	260	520	440	410	540
United States [T3]	Big Rock Point	47.0	13.0	21.7	12.8	23.6
	Browns Ferry 1-3	1230	293	75.1	54.0	0.7
	Brunswick 1-2	366	214	714	1150	25.9

Table 34 (continued)

Country	*Reactor*	*Release (GBq)*				
		1985	*1986*	*1987*	*1988*	*1989*
United States (continued)	Clinton 1	-	-	69.2	107	55.1
	Cooper	187	206	186	154	202
	Dresden 2-3	276	470	825	636	677
	Duane Arnold-1	1.32	0	0	0	0
	Enrico Fermi 2	-	11.1	38.9	34.5	48.1
	Fitzpatrick	155	185	91.8	328	27.1
	Grand Gulf 1	191	544	677	496	488
	Hatch 1-2	2120	1060	1040	1630	1690
	Hope Creek 1	-	0.26	353	346	870
	Humboldt Bay 3	40.0	2.47	0.03	0.03	0.042
	Lacrosse	4740	2130	1720	170	103
	Lasalle 1-2	14.4	5.07	40.7	64.8	39.6
	Limerick 1	42.6	76.2	223	0	999
	Millstone 1	662	197	659	1400	1690
	Monticello	0	0	0	0	0
	Nine Mile Point 1	0	81.0	0	0	0
	Nine Mile Point 2	-	-	17.1	293	300
	Oyster Creek	0	39.6	72.5	599	147
	Peach Bottom 2-3	1870	1650	1720	359	740
	Perry 1	-	0.1	108	272	258
	Pilgrim 1	289	370	119	21.2	87.7
	Quad Cities 1-2	126	238	256	269	1077
	River Bend 1		169	256	357	592
	Susquehanna 1-2	338	570	692	537	1014
	Vermont Yankee	0	0	0	0	0
	WPPSS-2	555	4700	2080	51.1	75.1
Total release (GBq)		33500	34700	32200	28300	34200
Normalized release [GBq (GW a)$^{-1}$]		900	870	750	640	780
Average normalized release 1985-1989 [GBq (GW a)$^{-1}$]		790				
HWRs						
Argentina [C15, C18]	Atucha-1	320000	280000	360000	590000	300000
	Embalse	16000	79000	160000	170000	220000
Canada [A6]	Bruce 1-4	1066000	1376000	1110000	1550000	1639000
	Bruce 5-8	31000	42000	520000	58000	48000
	Gentilly-2	31000	42000	520000	58000	48000
	Pickering 1-4	333000	84000	444000	592000	592000
	Pickering 5-8	377000	844000	1687000	1073000	85000
	Point Lepreau	24000	110000	96000	120000	320000
India [B14]	Kalpakkam 1-2	16870	30450	30410	63200	90690
	Rajasthan 1-2	6470	15380	4950	28670	23550
Pakistan [P3]	Karachi	36800	49000	39600	25400	10000
Republic of Korea [M3]	Wolsong 1	12000	36810	50780	74520	60440
Total release (GBq)		2270000	2990000	5020000	4400000	3440000
Normalized release [GBq (GW a)$^{-1}$]		276000	316000	489000	429000	334000
Average normalized release 1985-1989 [GBq (GW a)$^{-1}$]		374000				
GCRs						
France [E4]	Bugey 1	17000	2000	100	9000	0
	Chinon A2-3	500	300	0	3000	1000
	St. Laurent A1-2	5000				
Japan [J1]	Tokai-1	31	0.2	22	0.05	5.2
Spain [C21]	Vandellos 1	6210	283	3530	7480	83.4
United Kingdom [N6, P1, S4]	Berkeley	500	100	1200	270	3530
	Bradwell	1300	6200	1600	790	960
	Calder Hall					

Table 34 (continued)

Country	*Reactor*	*Release (GBq)*				
		1985	*1986*	*1987*	*1988*	*1989*
United Kingdom (continued)	Chapelcross	900	200	700	550	630
	Dungeness A	800	2400	200	340	200
	Dungeness B1-2	46400	29700	6800	22900	16200
	Hartlepool A1-A2	22400	45800	31900	33800	112000
	Heysham 1A-B, 2A-B	24700	58200	82900	112000	195000
	Hinkley Point A	22600	2100	5400	2760	1140
	Hinkley Point B, A,B	336000	257000	169000	272000	266000
	Hunterston A1	1900	1100	1300	2200	760
	Hunterston B1-2	342000	366000	269000	292000	333000
	Oldbury-A	800	900	900	890	720
	Sizewell-A	9900	3100	2300	760	2100
	Torness A-B	-	-	-		
	Trawsfynydd	2400	600	3800	550	490
	Wylfa	7000	8700	6200	7300	3000
Total release (GBq)		848000	785000	587000	769000	937000
Normalized release [GBq (GW a)$^{-1}$]		119000	131000	97800	115000	134000
Average normalized release 1985-1989 [GBq (GW a)$^{-1}$]		120000				
LWGRs						
USSR [G2, I14]	Beloyarsky 2 Bilibino 1-4 Chernobyl 1-4 Ignalina 1-2 Kursk 1-4 Leningrad 1-4 Smolensk 1-3	*Only average normalized release reported*				
Total release (GBq)						
Normalized release [GBq (GW a)$^{-1}$]						
Average normalized release 1985-1989 [GBq (GW a)$^{-1}$]		11000				
FBRs						
France [S6]	Creys-Malville	0	300	100	0	2900
	Phenix	0	0	0	0	0
USSR	Beloyarsky 3					
United Kingdom	Dounreay					
Total release (GBq)		0	300	100	0	2900
Normalized release [GBq (GW a)$^{-1}$]		0	1100	370	0	11000
Average normalized release 1985-1989 [GBq (GW a)$^{-1}$]		3000				

[a] A dash indicates that the reactor was not yet in operation.

Table 35
Radionuclides excluding tritium released from reactors in liquid effluents

Country	*Reactor*	*Release (GBq)*				
		1985	*1986*	*1987*	*1988*	*1989*
PWRs						
Belgium [M6]	Doel 1-4	14.0	21.3	3.7	11.0	22.5
	Tihange 1-4	52.4	57.3	62.2	57.4	77.3
Brazil [C1]	Angra 1	*Not reported*				
Bulgaria [C16]	Kozloduy-1-2	0.81	0.83	0.71	0.88	0.83
	Kozloduy-3-4	0.78	0.65	0.76	0.80	0.60
	Kozloduy-5	- [a]	-		1.24	1.09
China, Taiwan Province [T2]	Maanshan 1-2	3.3	2.95	1.01	0.23	1.61
Czechoslovakia [N11]	Bohunice 1-4	0.64	0.33	0.81	0.22	0.08
	Dukovany 1-4	0.012	0.036	0.021	0.30	0.30
Finland [F2]	Loviisa 1-2	18	17	13	15	21
France [E4]	Belleville 1-2	-	-	1	3	24
	Blayais 1-4	87	104	75	75	56
	Bugey 2-5	177	176	168	117	160
	Cattenom 1-2	-	0.4	8	3	10
	Chinon B1-B4	61	89	56	63	56
	Chooz-A (Ardennes)	8	9	10	7	17
	Cruas 1-4	26	19	12	11	11
	Dampierre 1-4	222	138	212	75	35
	Fessenheim 1-2	37	42	27	28	23
	Flamanville 1-2	0.5	39	62	111	23
	Gravelines 1-6	120	153	109	96	130
	Nogent 1-2	-	-	1	6	22
	Paluel 1-4	98	175	160	54	57
	St. Alban 1-2	6	73	88	30	23
	St. Laurent B1-2	369	58	17	10	18
	Tricastin 1-4	140	62	53	35	36
Germany, Federal Republic of [B4, B9, S7]	Biblis A-B	2.4	2.3	3.8	0.12	1.26
	Brokdorf	-	0	0	0	0
	Emsland	-	-	-	0.023	0.013
	Grafenrheinfeld	0.035	0.15	0.071	0.054	0.068
	Greifswald					
	Grohnde	0.11	0.011	0.084	0.082	0.25
	Isar 2	-	-	-	0.0039	0.02
	Mülheim-Kärlich	-	0.25	0.13	0.019	0.38
	Neckarwestheim 1-2	0.3	0.16	0.1	0.033	0.07
	Obrigheim	0.77	0.58	0.41	0.38	0.41
	Philippsburg 2	0.047	0.25	0.32	0.69	0.29
	Stade	1.2	1.5	1.3	1	0.56
	Unterweser	0.72	0.23	0.23	0.1	0.23
Hungary [F3]	Paks 1-4	1.31	1.09	3.19	2.04	2.91
Italy [C22]	Enrico Fermi (Trino)	61	42	54	3.6	2.2
Japan [J1]	Genkai 1-2	0	0	0	0	0
	Ikata 1-2	0	0	0	0	0
	Mihama 1-3	0.022	0.015	0.017	0.021	0.0065
	Ohi 1-2	0.021	0.016	0.0044	0.00021	0
	Sendai 1-2	0	0	0	0	0
	Takahama 1-4	0.0081	0.013	0.0027	0	0
	Tomari-1	-	-	-	0	0
	Tsuruga-2	-	0.00013	0.0017	0.00014	0.00059
Netherlands [M5]	Borssele	5.7	2.7	1.9	3.0	3.7
Republic of Korea [M3]	Kori 1	0.33	0.85	0.71	3.09	2.09
	Kori 2	0.80	0.63	0.33	0.23	0.14
	Kori 3-4	0.60	3.35	4.31	0.40	0.26
	Ulchin 1-2	-	-	-	2.15	1.73
	Yonggwang 1-2	-	0.214	1.69	2.09	1.34

Table 35 (continued)

Country	*Reactor*	*Release (GBq)*				
		1985	*1986*	*1987*	*1988*	*1989*
South Africa [C20]	Koeberg 1-2		3.36	7.8	1.47	1.69
Spain [C21]	Almaraz 1-2	75.4	30.1	7.7	18.9	18.7
	Asco 1	70.6	97.7	89.1	264	103
	Asco 2	1.88	84.1	217	316	75.6
	José Cabrera 1	9.76	173	11	20	44.9
	Trillo 1	-	-	-	3.59	1.1
	Vandellos 2	-	-	0.03	8.34	24.6
Sweden [N14]	Ringhals 2	47.5	102	102	48.8	52.5
	Ringhals 3	20.9	57.8	26.7	82.0	37.7
	Ringhals 4	58.7	26.9	46.1	46.8	41.4
Switzerland [D5, D6]	Beznau 1-2	8.9	0.00001	8	5.9	21
	Gösgen	0.16	0.089	0.0026	0.0081	0.0096
USSR [G2, I14]	Armenia 1-2					
	Balakovo 1-3					
	Kalinin 1-2					
	Khmelnitski 1	-	-			
	Kola 1-4					
	Novovoronezh 3-5					
	Rovno 1-3					
	South Ukraine 1-3					
	Zaporozhe 1-5					
United States [T3]	Arkansas One-1	131	188	90.7	138	75.5
	Arkansas One-2	161	127	68.5	165	98.1
	Beaver Valley 1-2	4.18	4.40	24.8	3.77	20.2
	Braidwood 1	-	-	1.85	317	92.5
	Braidwood 2	-	-	-	112	93.2
	Byron 1-2	603	150	91.8	51.8	23.5
	Callaway 1	0.18	1.42	18.2	2.86	0.37
	Calvert Cliffs 1-2	88.1	66.2	192	97.7	76.6
	Catawba 1	46.6	14.1	24.2	20.1	12.7
	Catawba 2	-	14.1	24.2	20.1	12.7
	Crystal River 3	55.9	30.0	35.3	8.55	8.73
	Davis-Besse 1	6.85	2.28	2.41	6.22	6.81
	Diablo Canyon 1-2	118	411	106	74	59.6
	Donald Cook 1-2	83.6	12.4	74	16.4	29.8
	Farley 1	2.49	3.77	1.88	2.95	2.7
	Farley 2	1.39	3.06	1.71	3.16	2.72
	Fort Calhoun 1	10.6	3.10	7.51	11.4	20.8
	H. B. Robinson 2	34.8	9.657	27.2	35.7	10.4
	Haddam Neck	3.12	11.47	15.8	25.4	14.4
	Indian Point 1-2	68.5	134	223	105	23.6
	Indian Point 3	15.5	7.22	12.8	11.9	21.9
	Kewaunee	50.0	19.7	47.7	18.5	45.1
	Maine Yankee	1.15	11.1	32.6	12.9	6.77
	McGuire 1	23.0	28.6	58.1	95.1	57
	McGuire 2	23.0	28.6	58.1	95.1	57
	Millstone 2	170	166	151	329	392
	Millstone 3	-	111	200	117	220
	North Anna 1-2	188	34.8	49.2	16.0	42.9
	Oconee 1-2-3	154	112	107	115	141
	Palisades	2.16	5.18	3.42	1.27	0.14
	Palo Verde 1	0	0	0	0	0
	Palo Verde 2	-	0	0	0	0
	Palo Verde 3	-	-	0	0	0
	Point Beach 1-2	70.3	592	27.9	3.54	2.06
	Prairie Island 1-2	1.02	22.2	2.23	9.44	6.4
	R. E. Ginna	19.3	2.39	2.18	1.27	3
	Rancho Seco 1	0.27	0.054	0.021	0.21	0.08
	Salem 1	107	161	123	119	115
	Salem 2	104	226	151	120	132
	San Onofre 1	288	31.5	31.2	26.3	25.4
	San Onofre 2-3	414	30.3	19.9	42.9	34
	Sequoyah 1-2	53.7	6.11	17.2	16.6	13.1
	Shearon Harris 1	-	-	33.6	2.97	8.95
	South Texas 1	-	-	-	8.29	112
	South Texas 2	-	-	-	-	0.43

Table 35 (continued)

Country	*Reactor*	*Release (GBq)*				
		1985	*1986*	*1987*	*1988*	*1989*
United States (continued)	St. Lucie 1	101	93.6	22.0	9.77	9.47
	St. Lucie 2	102	89.9	20.1	9.58	9.36
	Surry 1-2	316	324	191	89.2	143
	Three Mile Island 1	0.23	0.52	1.63	1.72	0.6
	Three Mile Island 2	0.0066	0.0069	0.0043	0.041	0.012
	Trojan	17.2	9.77	7.73	7.44	5.96
	Turkey Point 3	16.6	9.36	13.8	12.1	5.85
	Turkey Point 4	16.6	9.36	13.8	12.1	5.85
	Virgil C. Summer 1	26.2	12.1	18.1	27.9	50.7
	Vogtle 1-2	-	-	21.3	61.4	14.9
	Waterford 3	10.7	149	47.4	52.2	47.4
	Wolf Creek	23.5	83.6	10.7	14.0	26.8
	Yankee NPS	0.63	0.50	0.58	2.63	0.18
	Zion 1-2	87.7	59.2	58.1	132	127
Yugoslavia [F1]	Krsko	13.4	4.54	1.88	1.71	0.63
Total release (GBq)		5650	5500	4320	4460	3840
Normalized release [GBq (GW a)$^{-1}$]		66	56	40	38	31
Average normalized release 1985-1989 [GBq (GW a)$^{-1}$]		45				
BWRs						
China, Taiwan Province [T2]	Chin Shan 1-2	10.1	10.1	12.0	8.77	14.6
	Kuosheng 1-2	8.84	3.81	115	41.4	91.8
Finland [F2]	TVO 1-2	14	35	36	17	33
Germany, Federal Republic of [B4, B9]	Brunsbüttel	0.81	0.49	0.4	1.1	0.35
	Gundremmingen B,C	2.7	4.8	0.84	0.54	0.22
	Isar 1	0.54	0.87	0.56	1.6	0.27
	Krümmel	0.36	0.042	0.013	0.062	0.022
	Philippsburg 1	0.78	0.97	0.56	0.5	0.44
	Würgassen	1.9	1.2	0.55	1.1	0.96
India	Tarapur-1					
	Tarapur-2					
Italy [C22]	Caorso	20	58	16	15	12
Japan [J1]	Fukushima Daiichi 1-6	0.037	0.01	0.0067	0	0
	Fukushima Daini 1-4	0	0	0	0	0
	Hamaoka 1-3	0.056	0.03	0.014	0.012	0.011
	Kashiwazaki Kariwa 1,5	0	0	0	0	0.00073
	Onagawa-1	0	0	0	0	0
	Shimane 1-2	0.007	0.0089	0.0081	0.0059	0.0034
	Tokai 2	0.13	0.12	0	0	0
	Tsuruga 1	0.019	0.012	0.0093	0.011	0.0036
Mexico [C19]	Laguna Verde (Mark II)	-	-	-	-	15.03
Netherlands [M5]	Dodewaard	15	9.6	14	11	11
Spain [C21]	Confrentes	0.96	0.63	0.38	1.26	0.24
	S. Maria de Garona	8	1.13	1.19	2.09	0.32
Sweden [N14]	Barsebeck 1	32.4	80	33.4	12.8	14.4
	Barsebeck 2	32.4	80	33.4	12.8	14.4
	Forsmark 1	180	233	122	163	185
	Forsmark 2	180	233	122	163	185
	Forsmark 3	20	174	14	4	4
	Oskarshamn 1	30	41	29	49	149
	Oskarshamn 2	30	41	29	49	149
	Oskarshamn 3	2	3	2	7	13
	Ringhals 1	54.8	63.4	42.9	30.4	56.5
Switzerland [D5, D6]	Leibstadt	0.6	0.0004	0.026	0.41	0.48
	Mühleberg	2.4	13	6.6	14	4.6

Table 35 (continued)

Country	*Reactor*	*Release (GBq)*				
		1985	*1986*	*1987*	*1988*	*1989*
United States [T3]	Big Rock Point	5.66	2.62	10.1	8.07	8.58
	Browns Ferry 1-3	49.6	19.9	12.0	8.95	6.33
	Brunswick 1-2	4.26	4.66	26.5	30.8	57.7
	Clinton 1	-	-	0.57	4.07	0.64
	Cooper	481	273.8	83.3	86.2	81
	Dresden 2-3	75.1	7.92	14.0	4.29	24.2
	Duane Arnold-1	0.030	0	0	0	0
	Enrico Fermi 2	-	0.14	0.78	2.74	6.22
	Fitzpatrick	6.66	0.71	2.90	1.80	2.02
	Grand Gulf 1	7.88	11.1	13.5	14.7	11.8
	Hatch 1-2	27.5	29.2	30.2	36.4	9.18
	Hope Creek 1	-	28.0	59.9	26.8	38.9
	Humboldt Bay 3	4.63	1.74	0.44	0.28	0.31
	Lacrosse	67.7	185	42.9	16.5	6.25
	Lasalle 1-2	142	0.66	32.9	407	14.8
	Limerick 1	0.81	0.21	2.76	0	4.14
	Millstone 1	17.2	28.6	42.2	40.0	33.5
	Monticello	0	0	0	0	0
	Nine Mile Point 1	0	0.025	0	0	0
	Nine Mile Point 2	-	-	48.1	114	8.14
	Oyster Creek	0	0	0.25	0.99	1.85
	Peach Bottom 2-3	79.9	17.0	12.2	7.47	4.18
	Perry 1	-	0.14	0.54	9.25	42.9
	Pilgrim 1	39.2	7.81	54.4	1.32	0.92
	Quad Cities 1-2	54.0	8.73	2.63	2.07	17.9
	River Bend 1		3.92	2.95	20.6	41.1
	Susquehanna 1-2	23.5	29.3	11.5	3.51	3.77
	Vermont Yankee	0	0	0	0	0
	WPPSS-2	0.40	0.86	0.45	0.23	1.86
Total release (GBq)		1740	1750	1140	1460	1380
Normalized release [GBq (GW a)$^{-1}$]		46	44	27	33	32
Average normalized release 1985-1989 [GBq (GW a)$^{-1}$]		36				
HWRs						
Argentina [C15, C18]	Atucha-1	51	42	100	96	59
	Embalse	1.9	7.1	4.5	2.7	5.8
Canada [A6]	Bruce 1-4	90	120	50	130	20
	Bruce 5-8	7	13	3	8	9
	Gentilly-2	9.7	3.5	12	2.8	1.1
	Pickering 1-4	32	20	23	23	44
	Pickering 5-8	10	20	20	60	10
	Point Lepreau	1.6	1.1	0.4	1.9	1.1
India [B14]	Kalpakkam 1-2	13.4	23.2	46.0	48.1	27.6
	Rajasthan 1-2	2.81	3.50	0.39	3.05	4.53
Pakistan [P3]	Karachi	38.1	20.0	40.0	44.0	13.0
Republic of Korea [M3]	Wolsong 1	0.72	2.56	1.54	1.23	0.16
Total release (GBq)		258	276	301	421	195
Normalized release [GBq (GW a)$^{-1}$]		31	29	29	41	19
Average normalized release 1985-1989 [GBq (GW a)$^{-1}$]		30				
GCRs						
France [E4]	Bugey 1	43	76	35	15	4
	Chinon A2-3	5	11	5	2	3
	St. Laurent A1-2	57				
Japan [J1]	Tokai-1	0.1	0.059	0.067	0.031	0.015
Spain [C21]	Vandellos 1	154	133	129	97.6	12.6

Table 35 (continued)

Country	*Reactor*	*Release (GBq)*				
		1985	*1986*	*1987*	*1988*	*1989*
United Kingdom [N6, P1, S4]	Berkeley	290	320	240	330	230
	Bradwell	1510	720	710	440	395
	Calder Hall					
	Chapelcross	2000	86	500	170	220
	Dungeness A	2190	3100	570	410	230
	Dungeness B1-2	38	76	18	51	2.5
	Hartlepool A1-A2	18	65	34	24	22
	Heysham 1A-B, 2A-B	9	15	24	33	57
	Hinkley Point A	3720	450	960	500	900
	Hinkley Point B, A,B	50	39	19	26	32
	Hunterston A1	3.6	1.6	1.1	1	0.62
	Hunterston B1-2	90	40	30	30	40
	Oldbury-A	1120	690	560	830	410
	Sizewell-A	1010	760	710	460	360
	Torness A-B	-	-	-		
	Trawsfynydd	430	200	180	380	280
	Wylfa	48	61	58	75	64
Total release (GBq)		12800	6840	4780	3870	3260
Normalized release [GBq (GW a)$^{-1}$]		1800	1140	800	580	470
Average normalized release 1985-1989 [GBq (GW a)$^{-1}$]		960				
LWGRs						
USSR [G2, I14]	Beloyarsky 2 Bilibino 1-4 Chernobyl 1-4 Ignalina 1-2 Kursk 1-4 Leningrad 1-4 Smolensk 1-3	*Not reported*				
Total release (GBq)						
Normalized release [GBq (GW a)$^{-1}$]						
Average normalized release 1985-1989 [GBq (GW a)$^{-1}$]						
FBRs						
France [S6]	Creys-Malville	0	31	0.1	0.1	0.1
	Phenix	0	0	0	0	0
USSR	Beloyarsky 3					
United Kingdom	Dounreay					
Total release (GBq)		0	31	0.1	0.1	0.1
Normalized release [GBq (GW a)$^{-1}$]		0	110	0.4	0.6	0.4
Average normalized release 1985-1989 [GBq (GW a)$^{-1}$]		30				

[a] A dash indicates that the reactor was not yet in operation.

Table 36
Composition of radionuclides, excluding tritium, released in liquid effluents from PWRs in the United States, 1988 [T3]

PART A

Reactor	Release (GBq)														
	^{24}Na	^{51}Cr	^{54}Mn	^{55}Fe	^{56}Mn	^{57}Co	^{58}Co	^{59}Fe	^{60}Co	^{65}Zn	^{89}Sr	^{90}Sr	^{92}Sr	^{95}Nb	^{95}Zr
Arkansas One 1	0.0366	1.17	10.8	16.0	- [a]	0.0659	30.3	0.151	3.34	0.118	0.699	0.0155	0.123	0.291	0.164
Arkansas One 2	0.588	6.18	5.96	1.72	-	0.00337	25.7	0.280	2.49	-	0.0511	0.00163	0.340	2.36	1.68
Beaver Valley 1-2	0.00053	0.00102	0.0216	0.562	-	0.0077	1.65	-	0.784	0.00086	-	-	-	0.00039	-
Braidwood 1	0.102	0.206	7.92	-	-	0.250	297	0.213	5.18	-	0.0247	-	-	0.0648	0.0355
Braidwood 2	0.0944	0.206	5.99	-	-	0.130	96.9	0.0951	3.22	-	-	-	-	0.0629	0.0338
Byron 1-2	0.00048	6.99	1.08	-	-	0.0385	22.1	1.02	11.1	0.0301	-	-	-	1.44	0.899
Callaway 1	-	-	0.0696	0.555	-	0.00152	0.139	0.00053	0.389	-	0.174	0.0688	-	0.0211	0.00633
Calvert Cliffs 1-2	0.0455	3.16	0.326	-	-	0.00981	17.7	0.00799	1.22	-	0.136	0.0182	-	1.17	0.614
Catawba 1	0.0124	1.94	0.792	6.73	-	0.0176	4.33	0.377	2.00	0.0149	0.00225	0.0005	0.00205	0.241	0.152
Catawba 2	0.0124	1.94	0.792	6.73	-	0.0176	4.33	0.377	2.00	0.0149	0.00225	0.0005	0.00205	0.241	0.152
Crystal River 3	-	0.0214	0.118	0.525	-	-	1.62	-	1.47	-	0.156	0.00773	0.321	0.0311	0.00633
Davis-Besse 1	-	0.00507	0.0336	1.428	-	0.0115	1.21	0.00028	2.09	0.00017	0.00426	0.00131	-	-	0.0107
Diablo Canyon 1-2	0.0277	0.692	1.33	13.0	0	0.108	31.6	0.210	7.4	0.00334	0.0725	0.00514	0	-	0.360
Donald C.Cook 1-2	0.0150	0.263	0.884	1.37	-	0.0183	2.70	-	2.49	0.0659	0.0136	0.00607	-	0.0054	0.0054
Fort Calhoun	-	0.0121	0.644	-	-	0.00128	1.59	-	0.302	-	0.1125	0.0157	-	0.0108	0.00161
H.B. Robinson 2	0.00351	0.707	0.37	18.3	-	0.0228	5.96	0.0367	5.25	0.00158	-	0.0011	0.00004	0.0344	0.00585
Haddam Neck	-	-	0.107	2.00	-	0.00507	0.696	-	3.81	-	0.00333	0.0411	-	0.00107	0.00107
Harris 1	-	1.61	0.186	0.0781	-	0.00288	2.27	0.0276	0.241	-	-	0.00009	-	0.0142	0.0142
Indian Point 1-2	-	7.81	0.353	24.8	-	0.0137	17.9	0.257	16.9	0.00239	0.00714	0.00083	-	0.592	0.0936
Indian Point 3	0.00268	0.662	0.0566	4.33	-	0.00045	1.47	0.167	0.562	-	0.00018	-	-	0.0345	0.00795
Joseph M. Farley 1	0.00037	0.264	0.0187	0.364	-	0.00071	0.264	0.00551	0.511	0.00025	-	0.00064	-	0.107	0.0288
Joseph M. Farley 2	0.00286	0.199	0.0253	0.755	-	0.00024	0.240	0.0100	0.522	0.00038	-	-	-	0.104	0.0214
Kewaunee	0.0114	0.309	0.186	2.93	-	0.0134	9.92	0.0718	2.32	-	0.0474	0.00052	-	0.0503	0.0353
Maine Yankee	-	0.548	0.0216	1.61	-	0.00309	2.32	0.00903	1.84	-	0.257	0.00455	-	0.0186	0.0186
McGuire 1	0.074	11.1	3.05	15.4	0.00011	0.135	38.1	0.662	13.7	0.110	0.00287	0.00035	0.0426	2.24	1.35
McGuire 2	0.074	11.1	3.05	15.4	0.00011	0.135	38.1	0.662	13.7	0.110	0.00287	0.00035	0.0426	2.24	1.35
Millstone 2	0.0488	12.6	2.92	9.92	-	0.381	154	0.37	71.0	-	0.255	0.0829	0.492	1.02	0.474
Millstone 3	0.688	1.32	14.5	8.95	-	0.221	29.6	0.773	22.8	0.0747	0.0229	0.00466	0.525	2.11	0.784
North Anna 1-2	0.2446	-	0.0829	-	-	-	0.618	-	4.96	-	-	-	0.00681	0.129	0.0158
Oconee 1-3	0.0788	8.84	0.310	3.12	-	0.0429	23.2	0.112	4.48	-	0.0225	0.00588	0.340	1.81	1.12
Palisades	-	0.0212	0.0181	-	-	-	0.253	-	0.302	-	0.0951	0.0258	-	0.0014	-

Table 36 (continued)

Reactor	*Release (GBq)*														
	^{24}Na	^{51}Cr	^{54}Mn	^{55}Fe	^{56}Mn	^{57}Co	^{58}Co	^{59}Fe	^{60}Co	^{65}Zn	^{89}Sr	^{90}Sr	^{92}Sr	^{95}Nb	^{95}Zr
Palo Verde 1	-	-	-	-	-	-	-	-	-	-	-	-	-	-	-
Palo Verde 2	-	-	-	-	-	-	-	-	-	-	-	-	-	-	-
Palo Verde 3	-	-	-	-	-	-	-	-	-	-	-	-	-	-	-
Point Beach 1-2	1.41	0.00196	0.0057	-	-	0.00188	0.252	-	0.755	-	0.0992	0.0130	-	0.00596	-
Prairie Island 1-2	0.00068	0.0607	0.0148	8.33	-	0.00008	0.313	0.114	0.148	0.00127	0.0844	0.00237	0.00041	0.0112	0.00168
R.E. Ginna	-	0.00999	0.00496	0.00091	-	-	0.0318	-	0.0596	-	0.00418	0.00167	-	0.00171	0.00171
Rancho Seco 1	-	-	0.00095	-	-	-	0.0003	-	0.0451	-	-	0.00069	-	-	-
Salem 1	0.511	0.881	3.74	11.0	-	0.148	47.0	0.00984	10.2	0.0203	0.463	0.0873	0.00073	0.566	0.455
Salem 2	0.385	0.117	6.44	13.0	0.11914	0.168	48.8	0.00108	11.0	-	0.625	0.152	0.0130	0.242	0.117
San Onofre 1	-	0.157	0.0194	0.153	-	0.00145	1.91	0.0067	0.829	0.00152	0.0013	0.00374	-	0.00696	0.0115
San Onofre 2-3	0.0144	0.518	0.796	1.02	-	0.0248	8.73	0.0309	0.810	0.00051	0.400	0.00303	-	0.403	0.211
Sequoyah 1-2	-	0.00106	0.0607	2.71	-	0.0022	0.00296	-	9.07	-	0.0170	0.0122	-	0.00013	-
South Texas 1	0.00157	0.718	0.122	-	-	-	5.37	0.0414	0.123	-	-	-	-	0.134	0.137
St. Lucie 1	0.00455	0.655	0.0481	1.22	-	0.00018	2.27	0.00121	1.82	-	-	0.0303	-	0.275	0.144
St. Lucie 2	0.00455	0.655	0.0481	1.22	-	0.00018	2.27	0.00121	1.82	-	-	0.00099	-	0.275	0.144
Summer 1	0.00984	1.02	0.636	2.26	-	0.0332	8.66	0.0677	2.65	0.0240	-	-	-	0.315	0.315
Surry 1-2	0.0246	5.96	0.411	10.5	-	0.0259	12.5	0.245	16.4	0.00329	-	-	0.00022	0.448	0.229
Three Mile Island 1	-	0.0714	0.00287	0.282	-	-	0.847	0.00065	0.0231	-	0.00083	0.00013	-	0.0111	0.00422
Three Mile Island 2	-	-	-	-	-	-	-	-	-	-	-	0.0224	-	-	-
Trojan	-	0.755	0.0470	2.78	-	0.00186	0.936	0.0250	1.30	-	0.0814	0.0140	-	0.223	0.121
Turkey Point 3	0.00092	0.289	0.555	1.72	-	0.00012	0.966	0.0186	6.81	0.00063	0.00722	0.00194	-	0.00825	0.0023
Turkey Point 4	0.00092	0.289	0.555	1.72	-	0.00012	0.966	0.0186	6.81	0.00063	0.00722	0.00194	-	0.00825	0.0023
Vogtle 1	0.144	9.69	1.75	7.29	-	0.0836	35.1	1.18	1.92	0.0522	-	-	-	1.15	0.736
Waterford 3	0.0522	2.38	0.278	4.70	-	0.0266	18.9	0.303	1.47	0.00622	0.0163	0.00042	0.0121	1.03	0.599
Wolf Creek 1	0.00016	0.729	0.448	2.83	-	0.0261	5.44	0.322	2.34	0.0128	0.103	0.00117	0.00647	0.196	0.0681
Yankee Rowe 1	-	0.0374	0.00307	0.151	-	-	0.00433	0.00869	0.00544	0.00932	0.0295	0.0131	-	0.00374	0.00374
Zion 1-2	0.0966	9.81	0.659	2.72	-	0.0659	47.0	1.06	29.7	-	-	-	-	1.74	1.10
Total release (GBq)	4.83	115	78.7	232	0.12	2.27	1110	9.36	315	0.68	4.10	0.67	2.27	23.5	13.9
Normalized activity [GBq (GW a)$^{-1}$]	0.12	2.8	1.9	5.6	0.0029	0.054	26.7	0.22	7.6	0.016	0.099	0.016	0.055	0.56	0.33

Table 36 (continued)

PART B

Reactor	Release (GBq)														
	^{97}Nb	^{97}Zr	^{99}Mo	^{99m}Tc	^{103}Ru	^{106}Ru	^{110m}Ag	^{113}Sn	^{122}Sb	^{124}Sb	^{125}Sb	^{131}I	^{132}I	^{132}Te	^{133}I
Arkansas One 1	0.0129	0.0134	0.230	0.159	0.00729	0.0275	29.3	0.0283	0.0123	1.01	12.2	7.4	0.0150	-	0.103
Arkansas One 2	0.0137	0.0168	1.51	1.57	0.0799	0.0143	34.2	0.249	0.366	2.87	24.5	4.96	0.0855	0.0710	1.08
Beaver Valley 1-2	0.0105	-	0.00072	0.00071	0.0002	-	0.0662	-	-	0.0366	0.466	0.0134	-	-	0.00331
Braidwood 1	-	0.555	0.00377	-	-	-	0.00166	0.00095	-	1.67	0.0455	0.692	2.43	-	0.0477
Braidwood 2	-	0.555	0.00377	-	-	-	-	0.00095	-	0.209	0.0455	0.644	2.42	-	0.0474
Byron 1-2	-	-	0.00747	0.00085	0.0310	-	0.00118	0.0198	-	0.0356	0.529	0.999	0.0374	-	0.0357
Callaway 1	-	-	-	-	-	0.0356	0.00015	0.00028	-	0.00052	-	0.0122	-	-	0.00012
Calvert Cliffs 1-2	0.648	-	0.00355	0.134	0.111	-	2.67	0.0803	-	0.759	6.29	10.3	0.0633	0.0250	0.940
Catawba 1	0.0300	-	0.00198	0.0125	0.0114	0.0189	0.0117	0.0361	0.0540	0.271	0.847	0.362	0.0057	-	0.0810
Catawba 2	0.0300	-	0.00198	0.0125	0.0114	0.0189	0.0117	0.0361	0.0540	0.271	0.847	0.362	0.0057	-	0.0810
Crystal River 3	-	0.0400	0.00257	0.0338	-	0.144	0.914	-	-	-	-	0.117	-	-	0.0161
Davis-Besse 1	-	-	-	0.00023	-	-	1.28	0.0081	-	-	0.109	0.00925	-	-	-
Diablo Canyon 1-2	-	-	0.0588	-	0.00488	-	0.0115	0.0120	0.0109	0.234	2.82	2.35	0.00082	0.0130	0.629
Donald C. Cook 1-2	-	0.0253	-	0.00327	-	-	0.995	0.00995	-	0.0733	1.72	1.46	-	-	0.0422
Fort Calhoun	-	-	0.00488	0.0248	0.00385	-	0.0414	-	-	0.0309	2.58	0.855	-	-	0.0392
H.B. Robinson 2	0.0574	-	-	0.00559	-	0.0044	0.463	0.00168	-	1.45	2.42	0.0156	-	-	0.00205
Haddam Neck	-	-	-	-	-	-	0.00067	-	-	0.0147	0.0323	1.39	2.82	-	3.69
Harris 1	-	-	-	0.00059	0.00021	-	-	0.00329	0.00043	0.0109	0.0244	0.0109	-	-	0.00097
Indian Point 1-2	-	-	-	-	0.00692	0.0150	0.323	-	-	1.65	10.9	1.14	1.02	-	5.77
Indian Point 3	-	-	-	0.00574	-	-	0.511	0.00352	-	0.138	1.22	1.10	0.00046	-	0.0150
Joseph M. Farley 1	-	0.00032	0.00032	0.00152	0.0341	0.0511	0.177	-	-	0.0206	0.818	0.0107	0.0796	0.00356	0.00016
Joseph M. Farley 2	-	0.00043	-	0.00083	0.0267	0.0477	0.210	-	-	0.0278	0.855	0.00226	0.0231	0.00451	0.00075
Kewaunee	-	-	-	-	-	-	0.858	0.0292	0.0233	0.562	0.426	0.0500	0.00215	-	0.0120
Maine Yankee	-	-	0.00067	0.00096	0.0217	-	0.283	0.00932	-	3.40	1.18	0.0821	-	-	0.00053
McGuire 1	0.180	0.00131	0.0302	0.120	0.122	0.146	0.511	0.267	0.00958	0.277	2.48	2.35	0.0147	-	0.283
McGuire 2	0.180	0.00131	0.0302	0.120	0.122	0.146	0.511	0.267	0.00958	0.277	2.48	2.35	0.0147	-	0.283
Millstone 2	2.13	-	-	0.00122	0.100	0.381	1.30	-	-	3.16	3.92	3.92	0.0363	-	0.814
Millstone 3	2.68	-	0.327	0.190	-	0.101	1.23	-	-	0.146	0.744	9.84	0.500	-	1.82
North Anna 1-2	-	0.107	-	0.0733	-	0.525	4.11	-	0.00329	0.0114	2.31	0.448	0.00677	-	0.870

Table 36 (continued)

Reactor	Release (GBq)														
	^{97}Nb	^{97}Zr	^{99}Mo	^{99m}Tc	^{103}Ru	^{106}Ru	^{110m}Ag	^{113}Sn	^{122}Sb	^{124}Sb	^{125}Sb	^{131}I	^{132}I	^{132}Te	^{133}I
Oconee 1-3	1.99	-	0.0807	0.227	0.999	0.422	12.0	-	0.111	4.18	36.8	4.70	0.0651	-	1.09
Palisades	-	-	-	-	-	-	-	-	-	-	-	0.0169	-	-	-
Palo Verde 1	-	-	-	-	-	-	-	-	-	-	-	-	-	-	-
Palo Verde 2	-	-	-	-	-	-	-	-	-	-	-	-	-	-	-
Palo Verde 3	-	-	-	-	-	-	-	-	-	-	-	-	-	-	-
Point Beach 1-2	0.00039	0.00064	0.00137	0.00122	0.00217	0.00385	0.0365	0.0119	-	0.00866	0.037	0.0518	0.0377	0.00027	0.448
Prairie Island 1-2	0.00257	0.00153	-	-	-	-	0.0747	0.0459	0.00327	0.0718	0.129	-	-	-	-
R.E. Ginna	-	-	0.00411	-	-	-	0.00551	-	-	-	-	0.369	0.00221	-	0.243
Rancho Seco 1	-	-	0.0111	-	-	0.00079	-	-	-	-	-	0.0335	-	-	0.00258
Salem 1	0.903	0.507	0.0581	0.176	0.0596	0.0140	0.184	0.00163	0.202	2.33	3.46	2.05	0.360	0.0006	1.04
Salem 2	0.256	-	0.0044	0.121	0.0507	-	0.385	0.00381	0.137	2.03	3.42	5.00	1.73	0.00548	3.27
San Onofre 1	-	-	0.0385	0.0186	0.0184	0.0228	0.00892	0.00058	-	0.0305	0.0143	6.36	0.00164	0.00202	2.74
San Onofre 2-3	0.00296	-	0.433	0.440	0.0155	0.0290	0.0884	0.0236	-	0.130	0.777	15.0	0.00048	0.00574	4.26
Sequoyah 1-2	0.00007	0.00253	-	0.00396	-	-	0.00696	-	-	-	0.810	0.0599	-	0.00008	0.00228
South Texas 1	-	0.00023	0.00296	0.00367	-	-	-	-	-	-	-	0.186	-	-	0.00289
St. Lucie 1	0.0884	-	-	0.00098	0.0234	-	0.0548	0.0129	0.0323	0.525	1.10	0.288	0.00222	0.00418	0.0320
St. Lucie 2	0.0884	-	-	0.00098	0.0234	-	0.0548	0.0129	0.0323	0.525	1.10	0.269	0.00222	0.00418	0.0320
Summer 1	-	0.00006	0.0181	0.0407	0.0429	0.0362	0.00651	0.0135	-	0.211	0.662	1.72	0.437	-	0.914
Surry 1-2	-	-	0.00548	0.00707	0.137	-	0.270	-	-	1.48	13.6	3.09	0.0285	0.0295	0.0581
Three Mile Island 1	-	-	-	-	0.00024	-	0.0570	-	-	-	0.00807	0.0714	-	-	-
Three Mile Island 2	-	-	-	-	-	-	-	-	-	-	-	-	-	-	-
Trojan	-	-	0.00054	0.00057	0.0973	0.670	0.0707	0.0113	-	-	0.119	0.00977	-	-	-
Turkey Point 3	0.00012	-	0.0179	0.0179	0.00258	-	0.0792	-	-	0.0955	0.673	0.0851	-	-	0.00943
Turkey Point 4	0.00012	-	0.0179	0.0179	0.00258	-	0.0792	-	-	0.0955	0.673	0.0537	-	-	0.00232
Vogtle 1	0.0004	0.00056	0.0381	0.0459	0.00124	-	-	-	0.0440	0.844	0.592	0.102	-	0.0017	0.176
Waterford 3	0.0651	0.0122	0.0385	0.0392	0.0810	0.0714	0.381	0.403	0.629	1.93	4.44	3.7	0.0145	0.0319	0.161
Wolf Creek 1	0.0599	-	0.0744	0.00134	-	-	0.128	0.0607	-	0.0755	0.662	0.0522	-	-	0.00016
Yankee Rowe 1	-	-	0.0316	0.00175	0.0047	-	0.0044	-	-	0.00463	0.013 3	0.0194	-	-	0.00396
Zion 1-2	-	-	0.00403	0.0107	0.126	-	7.73	0.366	-	2.42	11.1	0.862	0.729	0.0666	0.178
Total (GBq)	9.43	1.84	3.10	3.64	2.38	2.94	102	2.03	1.73	35.6	163	97.4	13.0	0.27	31.4
Normalized activity [GBq (GW a)$^{-1}$]	0.23	0.044	0.074	0.087	0.057	0.071	2.4	0.049	0.042	0.85	3.9	2.3	0.31	0.0065	0.75

Table 36 (continued)

PART C

Reactor	Release (GBq)													
	^{134}Cs	^{134}I	^{135}I	^{136}Cs	^{137}Cs	^{138}Cs	^{139}Ba	^{140}Ba	^{140}La	^{141}Ce	^{143}Ce	^{144}Ce	^{187}W	^{239}Np
Arkansas One 1	2.53	-	0.00189	0.00115	5.92	0.0559	-	0.00433	0.232	-	-	-	-	-
Arkansas One 2	4.37	-	0.0895	-	16.2	0.0692	-	-	0.107	-	-	0.0448	0.0500	-
Beaver Valley 1-2	0.0407	-	-	-	0.0899	-	-	0.00013	0.00013	-	-	0.00083	-	-
Braidwood 1	0.0710	0.0533	0.00121	0.00474	0.326	-	-	0.0350	0.0350	-	-	-	0.00135	-
Braidwood 2	0.0710	0.0455	0.00051	0.00474	0.326	-	-	0.0252	0.0252	-	-	-	0.00135	-
Byron 1-2	1.65	-	0.0134	0.0301	2.02	-	-	0.161	0.161	-	-	-	-	-
Callaway 1	0.477	-	-	-	0.747	-	-	0.00054	-	-	-	0.164	-	-
Calvert Cliffs 1-2	16.6	-	0.0247	0.171	34.4	-	-	0.00064	0.0121	0.0212	-	0.0818	-	-
Catawba 1	0.219	-	0.0035	0.00158	0.342	0.247	0.00046	0.00233	0.0533	0.00033	0.0001	-	0.00138	0.00084
Catawba 2	0.219	-	0.0035	0.00158	0.342	0.247	0.00046	0.00233	0.0533	0.00033	0.0001	-	0.00138	0.00084
Crystal River 3	0.217	-	-	-	0.485	-	0.0102	-	0.0362	-	-	-	-	-
Davis-Besse 1	0.0229	-	-	-	0.0622	-	-	-	0.00178	-	-	0.0252	-	-
Diablo Canyon 1-2	6.03	0	0.0414	0.0718	7.03	0	0	-	0.0762	0.00009	-	0.00199	0.00006	-
Donald C. Cook 1-2	1.08	-	-	0.122	1.40	-	-	0.0105	0.0105	-	-	-	-	-
Fort Calhoun	1.34	-	-	0.0022	3.66	-	-	0.00966	0.124	-	-	-	-	-
H.B. Robinson 2	0.0766	-	-	-	0.187	0.0101	0.0135	-	-	-	-	0	-	-
Haddam Neck	0.279	4.92	4.66	-	0.899	-	-	0.00015	0.00015	-	-	-	-	-
Harris 1	-	-	-	-	0.0077	-	-	0.00086	0.00086	-	-	-	-	-
Indian Point 1-2	0.451	0.318	3.59	-	2.11	-	-	0.0529	0.269	-	-	0.00488	-	-
Indian Point 3	0.722	-	-	0.00533	0.692	-	-	-	0.0197	-	-	-	-	-
Joseph M. Farley 1	0.0331	-	0.00007	0.00211	0.121	-	-	-	0.0081	0.00518	-	0.00914	-	0.00029
Joseph M. Farley 2	0.00369	-	0.00008	0.00315	0.0369	-	-	0.00054	0.00529	0.00358	-	0.00821	-	0.00086
Kewaunee	0.228	-	0.00096	0.0071	0.293	-	-	-	0.00273	-	-	-	-	-
Maine Yankee	0.172	-	-	-	1.07	-	-	0.0237	0.0237	0.00249	-	0.00172	-	-
McGuire 1	0.259	0.00866	0.747	0.00655	0.459	0.258	0.00258	0.0115	0.109	0.0522	0.0130	0.129	0.00003	0.0929
McGuire 2	0.259	0.00866	0.747	0.00655	0.459	0.258	0.00258	0.0115	0.109	0.0522	0.0130	0.129	0.00003	0.0929
Millstone 2	13.3	-	0.0611	0.184	42.2	-	0.0507	0.429	0.400	-	-	0.00548	-	-
Millstone 3	5.85	0.0659	0.0396	0.296	8.47	-	-	-	-	-	-	-	-	-
North Anna 1-2	0.303	-	0.463	-	0.714	-	0.00707	-	-	-	0.00243	-	-	-

Table 36 (continued)

Reactor	Release (GBq)													
	^{134}Cs	^{134}I	^{135}I	^{136}Cs	^{137}Cs	^{138}Cs	^{139}Ba	^{140}Ba	^{140}La	^{141}Ce	^{143}Ce	^{144}Ce	^{187}W	^{239}Np
Oconee 1-3	1.49	-	-	0.0559	3.26	0.0670	1.79	0.0209	0.611	0.239	-	0.759	0.00736	0.149
Palisades	0.0225	-	-	-	0.773	-	-	-	-	-	-	-	-	-
Palo Verde 1	-	-	-	-	-	-	-	-	-	-	-	-	-	-
Palo Verde 2	-	-	-	-	-	-	-	-	-	-	-	-	-	-
Palo Verde 3	-	-	-	-	-	-	-	-	-	-	-	-	-	-
Point Beach 1-2	0.0184	0.00844	0.0166	-	0.319	-	0.00914	0.00227	-	-	-	0.0176	0.00126	-
Prairie Island 1-2	-	-	-	-	0.00008	0.00053	-	-	-	-	-	-	-	-
R.E. Ginna	0.132	0.0018	0.0918	-	0.300	-	-	-	-	-	-	-	-	-
Rancho Seco 1	0.0163	-	-	0.0144	0.103	-	-	-	-	-	-	-	-	-
Salem 1	4.85	0.407	0.622	0.00344	4.96	2.84	-	0.0104	0.0144	0.0492	-	0.699	0.463	-
Salem 2	3.53	1.29	0.703	0.0814	4.00	0.703	-	0.0581	0.0381	0.0644	-	0.0829	0.0236	0.144
San Onofre 1	5.88	-	1.34	0.151	6.62	0.0077	-	0.0209	0.00529	0.00288	-	0.0177	-	0.0255
San Onofre 2-3	2.06	-	-	0.192	4.40	-	0.00396	0.170	0.144	0.00238	0.00071	0.0529	-	-
Sequoyah 1-2	1.01	-	-	-	2.78	-	0.00006	-	-	-	0.00015	0.00071	-	-
South Texas 1	-	-	-	-	-	-	-	-	-	-	-	-	0.00081	-
St. Lucie 1	0.407	0.00161	-	-	0.644	-	-	-	0.0422	0.00205	-	-	0.00202	-
St. Lucie 2	0.374	0.00161	-	-	0.592	-	-	-	0.0422	0.00205	-	-	0.00202	-
Summer 1	3.74	0.168	0.607	0.119	2.66	0.0261	-	0.0411	-	0.0116	-	0.0588	-	0.00023
Surry 1-2	5.03	0.00154	0.00215	0.020	18.4	0.00067	-	0.328	0.115	0.00171	-	0.00448	-	0.00141
Three Mile Island 1	0.112	-	-	0.00244	0.231	-	-	-	0.00101	-	-	-	-	-
Three Mile Island 2	0.00014	-	-	-	0.0192	-	-	-	-	-	-	-	-	-
Trojan	0.0115	-	-	-	0.0293	-	-	-	0.00881	0.00744	-	0.108	-	-
Turkey Point 3	0.169	-	-	0.270	0.385	-	0.0105	-	0.0796	-	-	-	-	-
Turkey Point 4	0.169	-	-	0.270	0.385	-	0.0105	-	0.0796	-	-	-	-	-
Vogtle 1	-	-	0.0514	-	0.00574	-	0.00133	-	0.0217	-	-	-	0.0958	-
Waterford 3	2.47	-	-	0.0139	3.89	0.115	0.172	0.00088	0.239	0.0130	-	0.0522	0.0292	0.180
Wolf Creek 1	0.0440	0.00014	-	-	0.0725	0.0120	0.00108	-	0.0025	0.00377	-	0.0540	-	-
Yankee Rowe 1	0.0666	-	-	0.00403	0.0788	-	-	0.00814	0.00814	0.00662	-	0.0300	-	-
Zion 1-2	5.40	0.0836	0.0110	0.323	7.51	-	-	0.00044	0.110	-	-	-	-	-
Total release (GBq)	93.9	7.39	13.9	2.44	194	4.92	2.08	1.44	3.43	0.54	0.03	2.54	0.68	0.68
Normalized activity [GBq (GW a)$^{-1}$]	2.3	0.18	0.33	0.059	4.6	0.12	0.050	0.035	0.082	0.013	0.00071	0.061	0.016	0.017

[a] A dash indicates no value reported.

Table 37
Composition of radionuclides, excluding tritium, released in liquid effluents from BWRs in the United States, 1988 [T3]

PART A

Reactor	Release (GBq)													
	^{24}Na	^{51}Cr	^{54}Mn	^{55}Fe	^{56}Mn	^{57}Co	^{58}Co	^{59}Fe	^{60}Co	^{65}Zn	^{89}Sr	^{90}Sr	^{92}Sr	^{95}Nb	^{95}Zr
Big Rock Point	- [a]	0.0392	1.68	-	-	-	0.0366	0.223	2.11	0.0921	0.0260	0.139	0.00027	-	-
Browns Ferry 1-3	-	0.00095	0.00781	-	-	0.00026	-	-	1.69	0.256	-	-	-	-	-
Brunswick 1-2	533	5.29	5.96	1.21	0.00181	0.0003	1.44	0.400	8.55	-	0.0907	0.00235	0.00903	0.00087	-
Clinton 1	0.0305	2.92	0.455	0.0666	-	-	0.270	0.0185	0.225	0.00075	0.0455	0.00141	-	0.00012	0.00012
Cooper	0.588	5.33	10.4	2.76	-	-	3.27	0.037	40.3	-	3.06	0.259	-	-	-
Dresden 1-3	-	0.0252	0.260	0.444	-	-	0.0133	0.0287	2.93	-	0.00008	0.00633	-	0	0
Duane Arnold	-	-	-	-	-	-	-	-	-	-	-	-	-	-	-
Edwin I. Hatch 1-2	0.496	0.284	0.488	-	0.0141	-	0.124	0.0287	1.60	5.07	0.0277	-	0.0293	0.0196	0.00525
Fermi 2	0.120	1.07	0.155	-	-	-	0.241	0.0777	0.0818	0.0892	0.00918	0.0004	-	0.00821	0.00659
Grand Gulf 1	0.0463	11.5	1.06	0.180	0.0008	-	0.239	0.107	0.999	-	0.0414	-	0.0064	0.00533	0.00533
Hope Creek 1	4.63	3.42	1.19	8.66	-	-	0.280	0.411	0.562	7.10	-	-	0.00097	0.00128	-
Humboldt Bay 3	-	-	-	-	-	-	-	-	0.0347	-	-	0.00562	-	-	-
James A. Fitzpatrick	0.0188	0.0105	0.396	-	-	-	0.0407	0.00403	0.659	0.0130	-	-	-	-	-
Lacrosse	-	-	0.877	3.89	-	0.00181	0.0022	-	9.07	0.0361	0.0159	0.0581	-	0.00135	0.00135
Lasalle 1-2	0.918	261	42.9	9.84	-	-	12.3	19.5	55.5	2.20	0.0176	0.00118	-	0.234	0.0389
Limerick 1	-	-	-	-	-	-	-	-	-	-	-	-	-	-	-
Millstone 1	0.0781	0.0599	1.35	2.32	-	-	0.0318	0.00136	32.8	0.316	0.0224	0.0670	-	-	-
Monticello	-	-	-	-	-	-	-	-	-	-	-	-	-	-	-
Nine Mile Point 1	-	-	-	-	-	-	-	-	-	-	-	-	-	-	-
Nine Mile Point 2	2.30	40.0	13.6	0	-	-	28.3	6.73	15.7	7.03	-	-	-	-	-
Oyster Creek 1	-	0.181	0.0245	-	-	-	0.0437	-	0.507	-	0.0311	0.00077	-	-	-
Peach Bottom 2-3	-	-	0.00063	-	-	-	-	-	-	-	0.00999	0.0211	-	-	-
Perry 1	0.00662	6.07	0.936	0.173	0.0175	-	0.392	0.265	1.04	-	0.0511	0.00225	-	-	-
Pilgrim 1	-	-	0.00507	0.0836	-	-	-	-	0.326	-	-	0.00054	-	-	-
Quad-Cities 1-2	0.0132	0.659	0.0670	0.119	-	-	0.0562	-	0.655	0.00895	0.0269	0.00784	-	-	-
River Bend 1	-	17.7	0.736	0.625	-	-	0.252	0.0836	1.22	0.0881	-	-	-	0.00013	0.00013
Susquehanna 1-2	0.186	1.64	0.714	0.507	-	-	0.0064	0.0137	0.342	0.0255	-	-	-	-	-
Vermont Yankee	-	-	-	-	-	-	-	-	-	-	-	-	-	-	-
WNP-2	-	0.0381	0.00237	0.00178	-	-	0.00555	-	0.0369	0.074	0.00155	0.00007	-	0.00122	0.00122
Total release (GBq)	5340	357	83.2	30.9	0.03	0.002	47.4	27.9	177	22.4	3.4	0.57	0.046	0.272	0.059
Normalized activity [GBq (GW a)$^{-1}$]	320	21	5.0	1.9	0.0021	0.00014	2.8	1.7	11	1.3	0.21	0.034	0.0028	0.016	0.0035

Table 37 (continued)

PART B

Reactor	*Release (GBq)*													
	97Nb	*^{97}Zr*	*^{99}Mo*	*^{99m}Tc*	*^{103}Ru*	*^{106}Ru*	*^{110m}Ag*	*^{122}Sb*	*^{124}Sb*	*^{125}Sb*	*^{131}I*	*^{132}I*	*^{132}Te*	*^{133}I*
Big Rock Point	-	-	0.0003	-	-	-	0.0327	-	0.0184	-	0.00799	-	-	0.0197
Browns Ferry 1-3	-	-	0.0125	0.0125	-	-	-	-	-	0.0426	-	-	-	-
Brunswick 1-2	-	-	0.0577	0.179	-	-	0.0162	-	0.00133	0.00459	0.485	0.00999	0.0389	0.221
Clinton 1	-	-	0.0057	0.0174	-	-	-	0.00089	0.00133	-	-	-	-	-
Cooper	-	-	0.0176	0.437	-	-	0.365	-	-	0.0636	2.55	-	-	0.125
Dresden 1-3	-	-	-	-	-	-	-	-	0.00001	-	0.00092	-	-	-
Duane Arnold	-	-	-	-	-	-	-	-	-	-	-	-	-	-
Edwin I. Hatch 1-2	0.131	-	0.0171	0.106	-	-	-	-	-	0.194	0.836	0.0158	-	0.341
Fermi 2	-	-	0.0570	0.0910	0.127	-	0.00044	-	-	-	-	-	-	0.00455
Grand Gulf 1	-	0.00047	0.00574	0.0167	-	0.00873	0.0403	-	-	-	0.00067	-	-	0.00082
Hope Creek 1	0.0107	0.0105	0.0141	0.0437	0.00057	-	-	0.00032	-	-	0.00081	-	0.00059	0.0129
Humboldt Bay 3	-	-	-	-	-	-	-	-	-	-	-	-	-	-
James A. Fitzpatrick	-	-	-	-	-	-	-	-	0.00144	-	0.0218	-	-	0.0107
Lacrosse	-	-	-	-	-	-	0.0208	-	-	-	-	-	-	-
Lasalle 1-2	-	-	-	0.0007	-	-	0.265	-	-	-	1.23	-	-	-
Limerick 1	-	-	-	-	-	-	-	-	-	-	-	-	-	-
Millstone 1	-	-	-	0.0177	0.00017	-	-	-	-	-	0.0474	-	-	0.0411
Monticello	-	-	-	-	-	-	-	-	-	-	-	-	-	-
Nine Mile Point 1	-	-	-	-	-	-	-	-	-	-	-	-	-	-
Nine Mile Point 2	-	-	0.0206	0.0194	-	-	-	-	-	-	-	-	-	-
Oyster Creek 1	-	-	-	0.0153	-	-	-	-	-	-	0.00199	-	-	-
Peach Bottom 2-3	-	-	-	-	-	-	0.00629	-	-	-	-	-	-	-
Perry 1	-	-	-	0.00566	-	-	0.116	-	0.00105	-	0.101	-	-	0.00503
Pilgrim 1	-	-	-	-	-	-	-	-	-	-	-	-	-	-
Quad-Cities 1-2	-	-	0.00115	-	-	-	0.0596	-	-	-	0.00078	-	-	0.00066
River Bend 1	0.0751	-	0.0329	0.0340	-	-	0.0170	0.00138	0.273	-	-	-	-	-
Susquehanna 1-2	-	-	-	-	-	-	0.0403	-	-	-	-	-	-	-
Vermont Yankee	-	-	-	-	-	-	-	-	-	-	-	-	-	-
WNP-2	-	-	-	-	-	-	0.0289	-	-	-	0.00777	-	-	-
Total release (GBq)	0.216	0.0110	0.242	0.995	0.127	0.0087	1.01	0.00259	0.297	0.304	5.29	0.025	0.039	0.782
Normalized activity [GBq (GW a)$^{-1}$]	0.013	0.00066	0.015	0.060	0.0076	0.00052	0.060	0.00015	0.018	0.018	0.32	0.0015	0.0024	0.047

Table 37 (continued)

PART C

Reactor	Release (GBq)													
	^{134}Cs	^{134}I	^{135}I	^{136}Cs	^{137}Cs	^{138}Cs	^{139}Ba	^{140}Ba	^{140}La	^{141}Ce	^{143}Ce	^{144}Ce	^{187}W	^{239}Np
Big Rock Point	0.145	-	0.0102	-	1.37	-	-	-	-	-	-	-	-	-
Browns Ferry 1-3	1.36	-	-	-	5.59	-	-	-	-	-	-	-	-	-
Brunswick 1-2	1.27	0.00126	0.107	0.0105	4.48	-	-	0.0025	0.0025	-	-	0.0318	0.00825	0.294
Clinton 1	-	-	-	-	-	-	-	-	-	-	-	-	-	-
Cooper	5.96	-	-	0.0074	10.2	-	-	0.0777	0.0825	-	-	-	-	-
Dresden 1-3	-	-	-	-	0.592	0.0125	-	-	0.00004	-	-	-	-	-
Duane Arnold	-	-	-	-	-	-	-	-	-	-	-	-	-	-
Edwin I. Hatch 1-2	9.88	0.253	0.134	0.116	14.9	0.0107	0.0134	0.0131	0.00603	0.00364	-	0.0094	-	0.252
Fermi 2	-	-	-	-	-	-	-	-	-	-	-	0.0662	-	-
Grand Gulf 1	0.0147	-	0.0007	-	0.0138	0.00056	-	-	-	0.00079	-	-	0.00396	-
Hope Creek 1	-	-	-	-	0.00005	-	0.00304	-	-	0.00045	0.00013	-	-	0.00163
Humboldt Bay 3	0.00081	-	-	-	0.240	-	-	-	-	-	-	-	-	-
James A. Fitzpatrick	0.171	-	0.0022	-	0.418	-	-	-	-	-	-	-	-	0.0124
Lacrosse	0.0566	-	-	-	2.52	-	-	-	-	-	-	0.00463	-	-
Lasalle 1-2	0.681	-	-	0.0722	1.82	0.0777	-	0.00017	0.00017	0.0281	-	-	-	-
Limerick 1	-	-	-	-	-	-	-	-	-	-	-	-	-	-
Millstone 1	0.0426	-	-	-	2.85	-	-	-	-	-	-	0.00025	-	-
Monticello	-	-	-	-	-	-	-	-	-	-	-	-	-	-
Nine Mile Point 1	-	-	-	-	-	-	-	-	-	-	-	-	-	-
Nine Mile Point 2	-	-	-	-	-	-	-	-	-	-	-	-	0.0074	-
Oyster Creek 1	0.0140	-	-	-	0.147	-	-	-	0.0244	-	-	-	-	-
Peach Bottom 2-3	1.62	-	-	-	2.81	-	-	-	-	-	-	-	-	-
Perry 1	-	-	-	-	0.00411	-	-	-	0.0204	-	-	-	-	-
Pilgrim 1	0.0140	-	-	-	0.588	-	-	-	-	-	-	-	-	-
Quad-Cities 1-2	0.00677	-	-	-	0.348	-	-	-	0.0018	-	-	-	-	-
River Bend 1	-	-	-	-	-	-	-	-	-	-	-	0.00625	0.0114	-
Susquehanna 1-2	0.0155	-	-	-	0.0148	-	-	-	-	-	-	-	-	-
Vermont Yankee	-	-	-	-	-	-	-	-	-	-	-	-	-	-
WNP-2	0.0107	-	-	-	0.0138	-	-	-	-	-	-	-	-	-
Total release (GBq)	21.3	0.254	0.254	0.206	49.0	0.101	0.0164	0.093	0.138	0.033	0.00013	0.119	0.0310	0.560
Normalized activity [GBq (GW a)$^{-1}$]	1.3	0.015	0.015	0.012	2.9	0.0061	0.00098	0.0056	0.0082	0.0020	0.00001	0.0071	0.0019	0.034

[a] A dash indicates no value reported.

Table 38
Average releases of radionuclides from reactors per unit electrical energy generated

Years	Normalized release [TBq (GW a)$^{-1}$]						
	PWRs	BWRs	GCRs	HWRs	LWGRs	FBRs	Total [a]
Noble gases							
1970-1974	530	44000	580	4800	5000 [b]	150 [b]	13000
1975-1979	430	8800	3200	460	5000 [b]	150 [b]	3300
1980-1984	220	2200	2300	210	5500	150 [b]	1200
1985-1989	81	290	2100	190	2000	150	330
Tritium							
1970-1974	5.4	1.8	9.9	680	26 [b]	96 [b]	48
1975-1979	7.8	3.4	7.6 [b]	540	26 [b]	96 [b]	38
1980-1984	5.9	3.4	5.4	670	26 [b]	96 [b]	44
1985-1989	2.8	2.5	9.0	480	26 [b]	96	30
Carbon-14							
1970-1974	0.22 [b]	0.52 [b]	0.22 [b]	6.3 [b]	1.3 [b]	0.12 [b]	0.71
1975-1979	0.22	0.52 [c]	0.22 [b]	6.3 [b]	1.3 [b]	0.12 [b]	0.70
1980-1984	0.35	0.33	0.35 [b]	6.3	1.3 [b]	0.12 [b]	0.75
1985-1989	0.12	0.45	0.54	4.8	1.3	0.12 [b]	0.52
Iodine-131							
1970-1974	0.0033	0.15	0.0014 [b]	0.0014	0.080 [b]	0.0033 [b]	0.047
1975-1979	0.0050	0.41	0.0014 [b]	0.0031	0.080 [b]	0.0050 [b]	0.12
1980-1984	0.0018	0.0093	0.0014	0.0002	0.080	0.0018 [b]	0.0089
1985-1989	0.0009	0.0018	0.0014	0.0002	0.014	0.0009 [b]	0.0018
Particulates							
1970-1974	0.018 [c]	0.040 [c]	0.0010 [b]	0.00004 [b]	0.015 [b]	0.0002 [b]	0.019
1975-1979	0.0022	0.053	0.0010	0.00004	0.015 [b]	0.0002 [b]	0.017
1980-1984	0.0045	0.043	0.0014	0.00004	0.016	0.0002 [b]	0.014
1985-1989	0.0020	0.0091	0.0007	0.0002	0.012	0.0002	0.0040
Tritium (liquid)							
1970-1974	11	3.9	9.9	180	11 [b]	2.9 [b]	19
1975-1979	38	1.4	25	350	11 [b]	2.9 [b]	42
1980-1984	27	2.1	96	290	11 [b]	2.9 [b]	38
1985-1989	25	0.79	120	370	11 [b]	2.9	41
Other (liquid)							
1970-1974	0.20 [b]	2.0 [c]	5.5 [c]	0.60	0.20 [b]	0.20 [b]	2.1
1975-1979	0.18	0.29	4.8	0.47	0.18 [b]	0.18 [b]	0.70
1980-1984	0.13	0.12	4.5	0.026	0.13 [b]	0.13 [b]	0.38
1985-1989	0.045	0.036	0.96	0.030	0.045 [b]	0.028	0.079

[a] Weighted by the fraction of energy generated by the reactor types.
[b] Estimated value.
[c] Data available for one year only.

Table 39
Electrical energy generated by nuclear reactors worldwide

Year	Electrical energy generated (GW a)						
	PWRs	*BWRs*	*GCRs*	*HWRs*	*LWGRs*	*FBRs*	*Total*
Before 1970	5.53	3.18	18.92	0.41	0.74	0	28.8
1970	2.54	1.53	3.67	0.18	0.17	0	8.1
1971	4.07	3.47	4.16	0.57	0.17	0.008	12.5
1972	5.52	5.30	5.15	0.85	0.17	0.006	17.0
1973	7.90	6.63	4.44	1.82	0.82	0.005	21.6
1974	12.12	8.20	5.28	2.02	0.84	0.11	28.6
1975	20.34	10.16	5.19	1.93	1.49	0.15	39.3
1976	22.70	13.38	5.55	2.45	2.15	0.11	46.3
1977	29.84	14.14	5.88	2.74	2.79	0.036	55.4
1978	34.00	18.86	5.68	3.81	3.44	0.17	66.0
1979	33.37	20.89	5.79	4.60	4.74	0.22	69.6
1980	40.08	21.18	5.56	4.81	4.74	0.55	76.9
1981	50.94	22.93	5.38	5.19	6.03	0.58	91.0
1982	56.06	25.20	6.00	5.03	6.68	0.52	99.5
1983	63.92	26.04	6.48	6.52	8.94	0.54	112.4
1984	78.80	31.27	7.00	7.29	8.87	0.61	133.8
1985	94.82	37.76	7.46	8.29	11.41	0.67	160.4
1986	105.3	40.07	6.89	9.53	8.74	0.77	171.3
1987	117.3	43.15	6.86	10.33	11.05	0.81	189.5
1988	128.6	44.21	7.93	10.77	11.93	0.67	204.1
1989	135.9	44.23	8.13	10.33	11.99	0.81	211.4
Total	1050	442	137	99.5	108	7.4	1844

Table 40
Estimated releases of radionuclides from reactors worldwide

Year	Release (TBq)						
	Noble gases	^{3}H	^{14}C	^{131}I	*Particulates*	*Tritium (liquid)*	*Other (liquid)*
Before 1970	160000	519	10.6	0.59	0.26	341	112
1970	72500	179	3.5	0.26	0.11	104	23.9
1971	161000	462	7.5	0.56	0.22	203	31.0
1972	244000	670	10.7	0.85	0.32	285	40.6
1973	312000	1360	18.8	1.11	0.42	490	40.5
1974	385000	1540	22.0	1.36	0.56	587	49.3
1975	123000	1330	25.1	4.40	0.61	1610	32.6
1976	157000	1650	31.5	5.79	0.79	1900	36.1
1977	172000	1880	36.2	6.19	0.86	2290	39.5
1978	218000	2540	47.2	8.20	1.12	2830	41.3
1979	243000	3000	54.8	9.13	1.25	3110	42.9
1980	94200	3740	59.7	0.66	1.18	3110	33.7
1981	107000	4100	68.1	0.79	1.32	3510	34.7
1982	118000	4040	70.7	0.88	1.46	3680	38.5
1983	135000	5160	86.3	1.08	1.56	4390	42.1
1984	151000	5780	98.1	1.15	1.86	5080	47.1
1985	59600	4700	86.8	0.32	0.68	6520	13.6
1986	54700	5330	91.3	0.30	0.69	7150	13.5
1987	61300	5820	101	0.35	0.77	7780	14.2
1988	66700	6080	107	0.38	0.81	8360	15.9
1989	67800	5910	106	0.38	0.83	8410	16.4
Total release (TBq)	3160000	65800	1140	44.7	17.7	71700	759
Average normalized release [TBq $(GW\ a)^{-1}$]	1720	36	0.62	0.024	0.010	39	0.41

Table 41
Collective dose per unit release of radionuclides from reactors

Type of release	*Radionuclide*	*Composition for reactor type*	*Collective dose per unit release (man Sv PBq^{-1})*
Airborne	Noble gases	PWR BWR GCR	0.12 [a b] 0.26 0.011
	Tritium		11
	Carbon-14		1800 [c]
	Iodines [d]	PWR BWR GCR	340 520 [a] 510 [b]
	Particulates		5400
Liquid	Tritium		0.81
	Other than tritium	PWR BWR GCR	20 [a b] 170 40

[a] Also assumed for LWGRs and FBRs.
[b] Also assumed for HWRs.
[c] Local and regional.
[d] Expressed in terms of ^{131}I released.

Table 42
Normalized collective effective doses from radionuclides released from reactors, 1985-1989

Reactor type	*Electrical energy generated (%)*	*Collective effective dose per unit electrical energy generated [man Sv (GW a)$^{-1}$]*						
		Airborne effluents					*Liquid effluents*	
		Noble gases	*^{3}H*	*^{14}C [a]*	*^{131}I*	*Particulates*	*^{3}H*	*Other*
PWR	62.13	0.010	0.030	0.22	0.0003	0.011	0.020	0.0009
BWR	22.35	0.075	0.028	0.81	0.0009	0.049	0.0006	0.0061
GCR	3.98	0.024	0.099	0.97	0.0007	0.0038	0.097	0.038
HWR	5.26	0.023	5.3	8.6	0.0001	0.0011	0.30	0.0006
LWGR	5.88	0.24	0.29	2.3	0.0069	0.065	0.0089	0.0009
FBR	0.40	0.018	1.1	0.22	0.0005	0.0010	0.0023	0.0006
Weighted average		0.039	0.33	0.94	0.0008	0.022	0.033	0.004
Total		1.4						

[a] Local and regional components only.

Table 43
Collective effective dose from radionuclides released from reactors worldwide

Year	*Collective effective dose (man Sv)*							
	Noble gases	*Tritium*	^{14}C	^{131}I	*Particulates*	*Tritium (liquid)*	*Other (liquid)*	*Total*
Before 1970	38	5.7	19	0.30	1.4	0.28	5.3	70
1970	18	2.0	6.3	0.13	0.61	0.08	1.3	28
1971	41	5.1	13	0.29	1.2	0.16	2.1	63
1972	62	7.4	19	0.44	1.7	0.23	3.0	94
1973	78	15	34	0.57	2.3	0.40	3.3	133
1974	96	17	40	0.70	3.0	0.48	4.0	161
1975	25	15	45	2.3	3.3	1.3	1.6	94
1976	33	18	57	3.0	4.3	1.5	1.8	119
1977	36	21	65	3.2	4.6	1.9	2.0	133
1978	47	28	85	4.2	6.1	2.3	2.2	175
1979	53	33	99	4.7	6.7	2.5	2.3	201
1980	16	41	107	0.32	6.4	2.5	1.5	176
1981	18	45	123	0.39	7.2	2.8	1.6	198
1982	20	44	127	0.43	7.9	3.0	1.7	205
1983	22	57	155	0.53	8.5	3.6	1.9	249
1984	26	64	177	0.57	10	4.1	2.1	283
1985	6.9	52	156	0.15	3.7	5.3	0.62	225
1986	6.6	59	164	0.14	3.7	5.8	0.62	240
1987	7.5	64	182	0.16	4.1	6.3	0.65	264
1988	7.9	67	192	0.17	4.4	6.8	0.71	279
1989	8.0	65	190	0.17	4.5	6.8	0.72	275
Total	668	724	2055	23	95	58	41	3665

Table 44
Fuel reprocessing capacities in 1989
[18]

Fuel reprocessing plant	*Reprocessing capacity ($t\ a^{-1}$)*		
	Metal	*Oxide*	*FBR*
France			
Marcoule UP1 (GCR fuel)	600		
Cap de La Hague UP2 (LWR fuel)		400	
Marcoule APM			5
Germany, Federal Republic of			
Karlsruhe		35	
Japan			
Tokai-Mura		210	
India			
Tarapur (HWR and LWR fuel)		100	
Trombay (Reseach reactor fuel)	50		
USSR			
Kyshtym		400	
United Kingdom			
Sellafield (Magnox reactor fuel)	1500		
Dounreay			1
Total	2150	1145	6

Table 45
Management strategies for spent fuel [a]
[I8]

Country	Interim storage	Final storage	Reprocessing	*Indicative amounts of spent fuel generated in 1990 (t a^{-1})*			
				All countries		*Countries with an intent to reprocess*	
				Metal	*Oxide [b]*	*Metal*	*Oxide [b]*
Argentina [c]	×		×		170		170
Belgium			×		170		170
Brazil	×				9		
Bulgaria			×		57		57
Canada [c]		×			2500		
China			×				
Czechoslovakia			×		10		10
Finland	×		×		8		8
France			×	150	1200	150	1200
Germany	×		×		670		670
Hungary			×		54		54
India [d]			×		200		200
Japan			×	33	1000	33	1000
Mexico	×				24		
Netherlands			×		14		14
Pakistan [c]	×				23		
Republic of Korea [d]	×				300		
South Africa	×				36		
Spain	×				230		
Sweden	×	×			340		
Switzerland			×		100		100
USSR			×		420		420
United Kingdom			×	1300	140	1300	140
United States		×			2900		
Yugoslavia	×				19		
Total (rounded)				1500	11000	1500	4900

[a] Based on energy generated in 1990 and the data in Table 16.
[b] LWR oxide fuel unless otherwise indicated.
[c] HWR fuel.
[d] In the case of India, about 190 t, in the case of the Republic of Korea, about 100 t is HWR fuel.

Table 46
Radionuclides released in effluents from fuel reprocessing plants, 1985-1989
[B13, C17, N7, N13, S3, S9]

Reprocessing plant	*Year*	*Electrical energy generated (GW)*	*Release (TBq)*											
			Airborne effluents						*Liquid effluents*					
			^{3}H	^{14}C	^{85}Kr	^{129}I	^{131}I	^{137}Cs	^{3}H	^{14}C	^{90}Sr	^{106}Ru	^{129}I	^{137}Cs
France Cap de La Hague	1985	6.11	32		70300				2600	0.7	76	440	0.13	29
	1986	2.52	6		29000				2300	0.7	78	470	0.13	29
	1987	3.04	15		35000				3000		65			7.6
	1988	2.35	21		27000				2500		48			8.5
	1989	3.65	25		42000				3700		41			13
United Kingdom Sellafield	1985	1.70	268	7.0	23800	0.007	0.002	0.002	1062	1.3	52	81	< 0.1	325
	1986	3.81	171	5.4	53300	0.03	0.003	0.007	2150	2.6	18.3	28	0.12	17.9
	1987	2.43	78.3	9.5	34000	0.019	0.004	0.004	1375	2.1	15.0	22.1	0.1	11.8
	1988	2.84	185.6	3.6	39800	0.024	0.002	0.005	1724	3.0	10.1	23.6	0.13	13.3
	1989	3.69	677	3.9	51700	0.024	0.002	0.004	2144	2.0	9.2	25.0	0.17	28.6
Japan Tokai-Mura	1985	1.2	2.8		10000	0.0010	[a]		260		0.000002	[a]	[a]	0.00008
	1986	1.2	2.7		13000	0.0023	[a]		240		0.000025	[a]	[a]	0.00017
	1987	0.93	3.7		12000	0.00014	[a]		260		0.000009	[a]	[a]	0.00015
	1988	0.17	2.5		2700	0.00009	[a]		74		[a]	[a]	[a]	0.00009
	1989	1.1	3.7		9800	0.00024	[a]		240		[a]	[a]	[a]	0.00004
Total release (TBq)			1494	29.4	453400	0.108	0.013	0.022	23630	12.4	412.6	1090	0.880	483.7
Electrical energy generated (GW a)			36.74	14.47	36.74	19.07	19.07	14.47	36.74	23.1	36.74	27.70	27.70	36.74
Normalized release [TBq $(GW\ a)^{-1}$]			41	2.0	12300	0.0057	0.0007	0.0015	643	0.54	11	39	0.032	13

[a] Less than detection limit.

Table 47
Normalized releases of radionuclides from fuel reprocessing plants

Years	*Normalized release [TBq (GW a)$^{-1}$] [a]*					
	Airborne effluents					
	^{3}H	^{14}C	^{85}Kr	^{129}I	^{131}I	^{137}Cs
1970-1979	88	1.8	14200	0.002	0.098	0.11
1980-1984	52	3.4	12700	0.004	0.019	0.038
1985-1989	41	2.0	12300	0.006	0.0007	0.002
	Liquid effluents					
	^{3}H	^{14}C	^{90}Sr	^{106}Ru	^{129}I	^{137}Cs
1970-1979	400	0.54 [b]	140	340	0.046	1000
1980-1984	405	0.54 [b]	48	120	0.040	270
1985-1989	643	0.54	11	39	0.032	13

[a] Normalization is for energy equivalent of fuel reprocessed.
[b] Estimated value.

Table 48
Estimated releases of radionuclides from fuel reprocessing plants worldwide

Year	Fuel reprocessed (GW a)	Release in airborne effluents (TBq)						Release in liquid effluents (TBq)					
		^{3}H	^{14}C	^{85}Kr	^{129}I	^{131}I	^{137}Cs	^{3}H	^{14}C	^{90}Sr	^{106}Ru	^{129}I	^{137}Cs
Before 1970	2.2	198	4.0	32000	0.004	0.22	0.25	898	1.2	306	753	0.10	2250
1970	0.6	56	1.1	8990	0.001	0.06	0.07	252	0.34	86	212	0.03	633
1971	1.0	86	1.7	13800	0.002	0.10	0.11	389	0.52	133	326	0.04	975
1972	1.3	117	2.3	18900	0.002	0.13	0.15	530	0.71	181	444	0.06	1330
1973	1.7	149	3.0	24000	0.003	0.17	0.19	674	0.90	230	565	0.08	1690
1974	2.2	197	3.9	31800	0.004	0.22	0.25	891	1.2	304	747	0.10	2240
1975	4.8	447	8.5	68000	0.008	0.47	0.53	1810	2.6	541	1590	0.22	5260
1976	4.0	446	7.1	57000	0.007	0.40	0.45	1460	2.2	421	1320	0.18	4320
1977	3.9	307	7.0	58800	0.007	0.39	0.44	1250	2.1	500	1360	0.18	4530
1978	4.0	227	7.1	56800	0.007	0.39	0.44	1810	2.2	737	1610	0.18	4130
1979	4.8	422	8.4	68100	0.008	0.47	0.53	1840	2.6	367	1140	0.22	2620
1980	5.5	265	19	68900	0.03	0.10	0.21	1980	2.9	381	727	0.22	3000
1981	7.4	473	25	95600	0.02	0.14	0.28	2810	4.0	304	861	0.29	2400
1982	8.2	370	28	103600	0.03	0.16	0.31	2760	4.4	405	890	0.33	2050
1983	7.5	278	25	93800	0.03	0.14	0.28	3000	4.0	346	890	0.30	1220
1984	5.1	358	17	65400	0.04	0.10	0.19	3080	2.7	182	699	0.20	464
1985	9.0	303	18	104100	0.05	0.006	0.014	3920	4.8	128	521	0.23	354
1986	7.5	180	15	95300	0.04	0.005	0.011	4690	4.0	96	498	0.25	47
1987	6.4	97	13	81000	0.04	0.004	0.010	4640	3.4	80	252	0.20	19
1988	5.4	209	11	68700	0.03	0.004	0.008	4300	2.9	58	211	0.17	22
1989	8.4	706	17	103500	0.05	0.004	0.013	6080	4.5	50	332	0.27	42
Total	101	5890	243	1318000	0.41	3.7	4.7	49100	54	5840	15900	3.9	39600
Average normalized release for fuel reprocessed [TBq (GW a)$^{-1}$]		58	2.4	13000	0.0040	0.036	0.047	490	0.54	58	160	0.038	390
Average normalized release for energy generated [TBq (GW a)$^{-1}$]		3.2	0.13	720	0.0002	0.002	0.003	27	0.029	3.2	8.6	0.002	21

Table 49
Normalized local and regional collective effective dose from fuel reprocessing, 1985-1989

Radio-nuclide	*Normalized release* [a] *[TBq (GW a)$^{-1}$]*	*Collective dose per unit release (man Sv TBq^{-1})*	*Normalized collective dose [man Sv (GW a)$^{-1}$]*	
			For fuel reprocessed	*For energy generated* [b]
Airborne effluents				
H-3	41	0.0027	0.11	0.004
C-14	2.0	0.4	0.81	0.033
Kr-85	12300	0.0000074	0.091	0.004
I-129	0.0057	44	0.25	0.010
I-131	0.0007	0.4	0.0003	0.00001
Cs-137	0.0015	11	0.017	0.0007
Total				0.05
Liquid effluents				
H-3	643	0.0000018	0.0012	0.00005
C-14	0.54	0.4	0.21	0.009
Sr-90	11	0.012	0.13	0.005
Ru-106	39	0.07	2.8	0.11
I-129	0.032	-	-	-
Cs-137	13	0.08	1.1	0.042
Total				0.17

[a] Normalized for the energy equivalent of fuel reprocessed.
[b] The fraction of fuel reprocessed during 1985-1989 was 0.04.

Table 50
Estimated local and regional collective dose from radionuclides released from fuel reprocessing plants worldwide

Year	Collective effective dose (man Sv)											
	Airborne						Liquid					
	^{3}H	^{14}C	^{85}Kr	^{129}I	^{131}I	^{137}Cs	^{3}H	^{14}C	^{90}Sr	^{106}Ru	^{129}I	^{137}Cs
Before 1970	0.5	1.6	0.24	0.17	0.088	2.7	0.002	0.5	3.7	53	0	180
1970	0.2	0.4	0.07	0.05	0.025	0.8	0.0005	0.1	1.0	15	0	51
1971	0.2	0.7	0.10	0.07	0.038	1.2	0.0007	0.2	1.6	23	0	78
1972	0.3	0.9	0.14	0.10	0.052	1.6	0.001	0.3	2.2	31	0	106
1973	0.4	1.2	0.18	0.13	0.066	2.1	0.001	0.4	2.8	40	0	135
1974	0.5	1.6	0.23	0.17	0.088	2.7	0.002	0.5	3.6	52	0	179
1975	1.2	3.4	0.50	0.36	0.19	5.9	0.003	1.0	6.5	111	0	421
1976	1.2	2.9	0.42	0.30	0.16	4.9	0.003	0.9	5.1	92	0	346
1977	0.8	2.8	0.44	0.30	0.15	4.8	0.002	0.8	6.0	95	0	362
1978	0.6	2.8	0.42	0.30	0.16	4.9	0.003	0.9	8.8	113	0	330
1979	1.1	3.4	0.50	0.36	0.19	5.8	0.003	1.0	4.4	80	0	210
1980	0.7	7.4	0.51	1.47	0.042	2.3	0.004	1.2	4.6	51	0	240
1981	1.3	10.1	0.71	0.93	0.056	3.1	0.005	1.6	3.6	60	0	192
1982	1.0	11.1	0.77	1.16	0.062	3.4	0.005	1.8	4.9	62	0	164
1983	0.7	10.1	0.69	1.31	0.057	3.1	0.005	1.6	4.1	62	0	98
1984	1.0	7.0	0.48	1.63	0.039	2.1	0.006	1.1	2.2	49	0	37
1985	0.8	7.3	0.77	2.24	0.002	0.2	0.007	1.9	1.5	36	0	28
1986	0.5	6.1	0.71	1.87	0.002	0.1	0.008	1.6	1.2	35	0	3.8
1987	0.3	5.2	0.60	1.59	0.002	0.1	0.008	1.4	1.0	18	0	1.6
1988	0.6	4.4	0.51	1.33	0.001	0.1	0.008	1.2	0.7	15	0	1.7
1989	1.9	6.9	0.77	2.10	0.002	0.1	0.011	1.8	0.6	23	0	3.3
Total	16	97	9.8	18	1.5	52	0.09	22	70	1110	0	3200
Total	4600											

Table 51
Normalized collective effective dose from globally dispersed radionuclides for a time period of 10,000 years

Radio-nuclide	*Normalized activity released [TBq (GW a)$^{-1}$]*			*Collective dose per unit release (man Sv TBq^{-1})*	*Normalized collective dose [man Sv (GW a)$^{-1}$]*
	Reactors [a]	*Reprocessing plants* [b]	*Total* [c]		
H-3	71	684 [d]	98	0.0012 [e f]	0.09
C-14	0.52	2.54	0.62	85 [g]	53
Kr-85		12300	490	0.0002 [f]	0.1
I-129		0.038	0.0015	4 [g]	0.006
Total					53

[a] Normalization for total energy generated.
[b] Normalization for fuel reprocessed.
[c] Normalization for total energy generated; the contribution from reprocessing plants is weighted according to the fraction of fuel reprocessed (0.04).
[d] Release to sea: 643 TBq (GW a)$^{-1}$; remainder released to air.
[e] For release to air or fresh water; less by a factor of 10 for release to sea.
[f] For world population of 5 10^9 at time of release.
[g] For world population of 10^{10}.

Table 52
Estimated releases of globally dispersed radionuclides and collective effective dose for a time period of 10,000 years

Year	*Release (TBq)*			
	^{3}H	*^{14}C*	*^{85}Kr*	*^{129}I*
Before 1970	1960	15.8	32000	0.11
1970	592	5.0	8990	0.030
1971	1140	9.7	13800	0.046
1972	1600	13.8	18900	0.063
1973	2670	22.6	24000	0.080
1974	3210	27.1	31800	0.11
1975	5200	36.2	68000	0.23
1976	5460	40.8	57000	0.19
1977	5720	45.3	58800	0.19
1978	7400	56.4	56800	0.19
1979	8370	65.8	68100	0.23
1980	9090	81.2	68900	0.25
1981	10900	97.3	95600	0.32
1982	10900	103	103600	0.35
1983	12800	116	93800	0.33
1984	14300	118	65400	0.24
1985	15500	110	104100	0.28
1986	17400	111	95300	0.29
1987	18300	117	81000	0.24
1988	19000	120	68700	0.20
1989	21100	127	103500	0.32
Total release (TBq)	193000	1440	1318000	4.3
Dose commitment per unit release (nGy TBq^{-1})	0.00027 [a]	8.5	0.000043	0.4
Population	[b]	10^{10}	[b]	10^{10}
Collective effective dose (man Sv)	180	122000	260	17
Total collective effective dose (man Sv)	123000			

[a] Release to atmosphere or fresh water; factor of 10 less for release to sea surface.
[b] Global population in year of release (1970 3.7 10^9, 1975 4.1 10^9, 1980 4.5 10^9, 1985 4.9 10^9, 1989 5.2 10^9); assuming 3.6 10^9 persons for releases before 1970.

Table 53
Normalized collective effective dose to members of the public from radionuclides released in effluents from the nuclear fuel cycle

Source	*Normalized collective effective dose [man Sv (GW a)$^{-1}$]*
Local and regional component	
Mining	1.1
Milling	0.05
Mine and mill tailings (releases over 5 years)	0.3
Fuel fabrication	0.003
Reactor operation	
Atmospheric	1.3
Aquatic	0.04
Reprocessing	
Atmospheric	0.05
Aquatic	0.2
Transportation	0.1
Total (rounded)	3
Solid waste disposal and global component	
Mine and mill tailings (releases of radon over 10,000 years)	150
Reactor operation	
Low-level waste disposal	0.00005
Intermediate-level waste disposal	0.5
Reprocessing solid waste disposal	0.05
Globally dispersed radionuclides (truncated to 10,000 years)	50
Total (rounded)	200

Table 54
Unsealed radioisotopes used in Japan in 1989
[J2]

Radio-nuclide	Quantities of radioisotopes used (GBq)				
	Hospitals and clinics	*Educational organizations*	*Research institutions*	*Industry and other*	*Total*
H-3	25	334	1168	123	1650
C-14	13	16	469	118	616
P-32	24	407	543	21	995
S-35	10	111	134	8	263
Ca-45	2	11	6	1	20
Cr-51	25	114	79	8	236
Fe-59	6	0.7	1	0.3	8
Ga-67	16660	0.6	0.2	1.2	16660
Se-75	10	(0.05)	(0.1)	-	10
Kr-81m [a]	813	-	-	-	813
Kr-85	-	-	14	202	216
Tc-99m [a]	163200	22	12	265	163500
Tc-99m [b]	63770	1	(0.4)	75	63840
In-111	344	0.2)	(0.07)	(0.07)	344
I-123	8353	4	(0.5)	2	8359
I-125	273	133	174	149	729
I-131	3964	12	32	3	4011
Xe-133	32060	33	3	3	32100
Pm-147	-	-	-	75850	75850
Tl-201	15200	(0.4)	1	2	15200

[a] Generator.
[b] Solution.

Table 55
Production and dose estimates for radioisotopes used in medical, educational and industrial applications

Radio-nuclide	Annual normalized production [a] (GBq per 10^6 population)	Annual global production [b] and release (PBq)	Collective dose coefficient (man Sv PBq^{-1})	Annual collective effective dose (man Sv)
H-3	80	0.13	11	1.4
C-14	30	0.05	1800 [c]	86 [c]
Kr-85	10	0.02	0.18	0.004
I-123	400	0.7	0.022	0.01
I-125	40	0.06	120	7
I-131	200	0.3	30	9
Xe-133	1600	2.6	0.14	0.4
Total				100

[a] Developed countries only.
[b] Equivalent to 1.6 10^9 population (1.2 10^9 times 100% usage in developed countries plus 3.7 10^9 times 10% usage in developing countries).
[c] Local and regional (short-term) dose. Long-term collective dose coefficient is 85,000 man Sv PBq^{-1} and annual collective effective dose is 4,000 man Sv.

Table 56
Collective effective dose from the Kyshtym accident

Number of individuals	*Deposition density of ^{90}Sr in regions (kBq m^{-2})*	*Average effective dose (mSv)*		*Collective dose (man Sv)*
		External	*Total*	
Evacuated population				
1150 [a]	20000	170	520	600
280 [b]	2400	140	440	120
2000 [b]	670	39	120	240
4200 [c]	330	19	56	235
3100 [d]	120	6.8	23	70
Total				1300
Non-evacuated population				
10000	40-70		20	200
250000	4-40		4	1000
Total				1200

[a] Evacuated 7-10 days after the accident.
[b] Evacuated 250 days after the accident.
[c] Evacuated 350 days after the accident.
[d] Evacuated 670 days after the accident.

Table 57
Estimates of collective effective dose from re-entry to the atmosphere and burn-up of the Cosmos 954 satellite

Radionuclide	*Core inventory at re-entry [T6] (TBq)*	*Transfer coefficient P_{02} [a] (Bq m^{-2} per EBq)*	*Deposition [a b] (Bq m^{-2})*	*Transfer coefficient P_{25} [c] (nSv per Bq m^{-2})*	*Dose commitment [d] (nSv)*	*Collective effective dose [e] (man Sv)*
Sr-90	3.1	5300	0.012	56.6	0.70	2.0
Zr-95	310	270	0.063	3.78	0.24	0.62
Nb-95	220	270	0.045	1.02	0.045	0.12
Ru-103	120	120	0.011	0.75	0.008	0.02
Ru-106	5.4	2000	0.008	4.6	0.04	0.10
I-131	180	29	0.005	4.5	0.02	0.06
Cs-137	3.2	5400	0.017	143	2.5	7.1
Ba-140	400	31	0.009	1.13	0.01	0.03
Ce-141	340	83	0.021	0.12	0.002	0.01
Ce-144	93	1600	0.11	1.8	0.20	0.52
Pu-239	0.27	5400	0.001	848	0.93	5.7
Total						16

[a] For temperate latitudes of the northern hemisphere.
[b] Assuming 100% of ^{131}I and ^{137}Cs and 75% of other radionuclides in core inventory at the time of re-entry were released to the atmosphere.
[c] From Table 8, all pathways combined.
[d] Average value for temperate latitudes of northern hemisphere; divide by 1.5 to obtain average for northern hemisphere; divide northern hemisphere average value by 4 to obtain average value for southern hemisphere.
[e] Assuming global population of 4.3 10^9 distributed 89% in northern hemisphere and 11% in southern hemisphere; for ^{239}Pu, the global population is assumed to be 10^{10}.

Table 58
Estimates of radionuclide released and collective effective dose from man-made environmental sources of radiation

Source	*Release (PBq)*						*Collective effective dose* [a] *(man Sv)*	
	^{3}H	^{14}C	*Noble gases*	^{90}Sr	^{131}I	^{137}Cs	*Local and regional*	*Global*
Atmospheric nuclear testing								
Global	240000	220		604	650000	910		22300000
Local								
Semipalatinsk							4600	
Nevada							500 [b]	
Australia							700	
Pacific test site							160 [b]	
Underground nuclear testing			50		15		200	
Nuclear weapons fabrication								
Early practice								
Hanford							8000 [c]	
Chelyabinsk							15000 [d]	
Later practice							1000 30000 [e]	10000
Nuclear power production								
Milling and mining							2700	
Reactor operation	140	1.1	3200		0.04		3700	
Fuel reprocessing	57	0.3	1200	6.9	0.004	40	4600	
Fuel cycle							300000 [e]	100000
Radioisotope production and use	2.6	1.0	52		6.0		2000	80000
Accidents								
Three Mile Island			370		0.0006		40	
Chernobyl					630	70		600000
Kyshtym				5.4		0.04	2500	
Windscale			1.2		0.7	0.02	2000	
Palomares							3	
Thule							0	
SNAP 9A								2100
Cosmos 954				0.003	0.2	0.003		20
Ciudad Juarez							150	
Mohammedia							80	
Goiania						0.05	60	
Total							380000	23100000
Total collective effective dose (man Sv)							23500000	

[a] Truncated at 10,000 years.
[b] External dose only.
[c] From release of ^{131}I to the atmosphere.
[d] From releases of radionuclides into the Techa River.
[e] Long-term collective dose from release of ^{222}Rn from tailings.

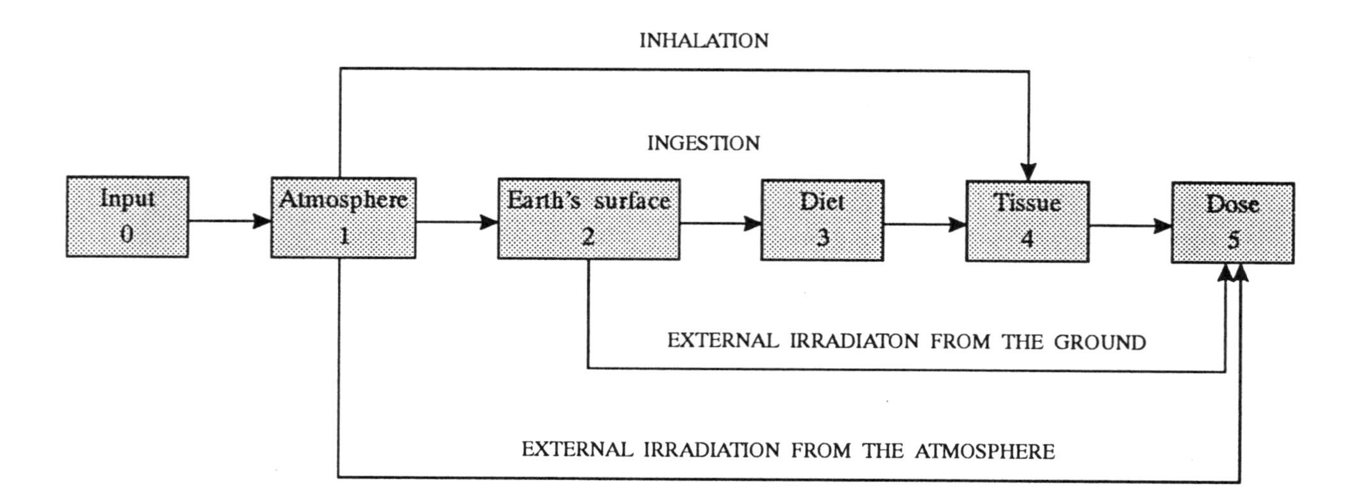

Figure I.
Compartment model used to assess doses from releases of radioactive materials to the atmosphere from nuclear testing.

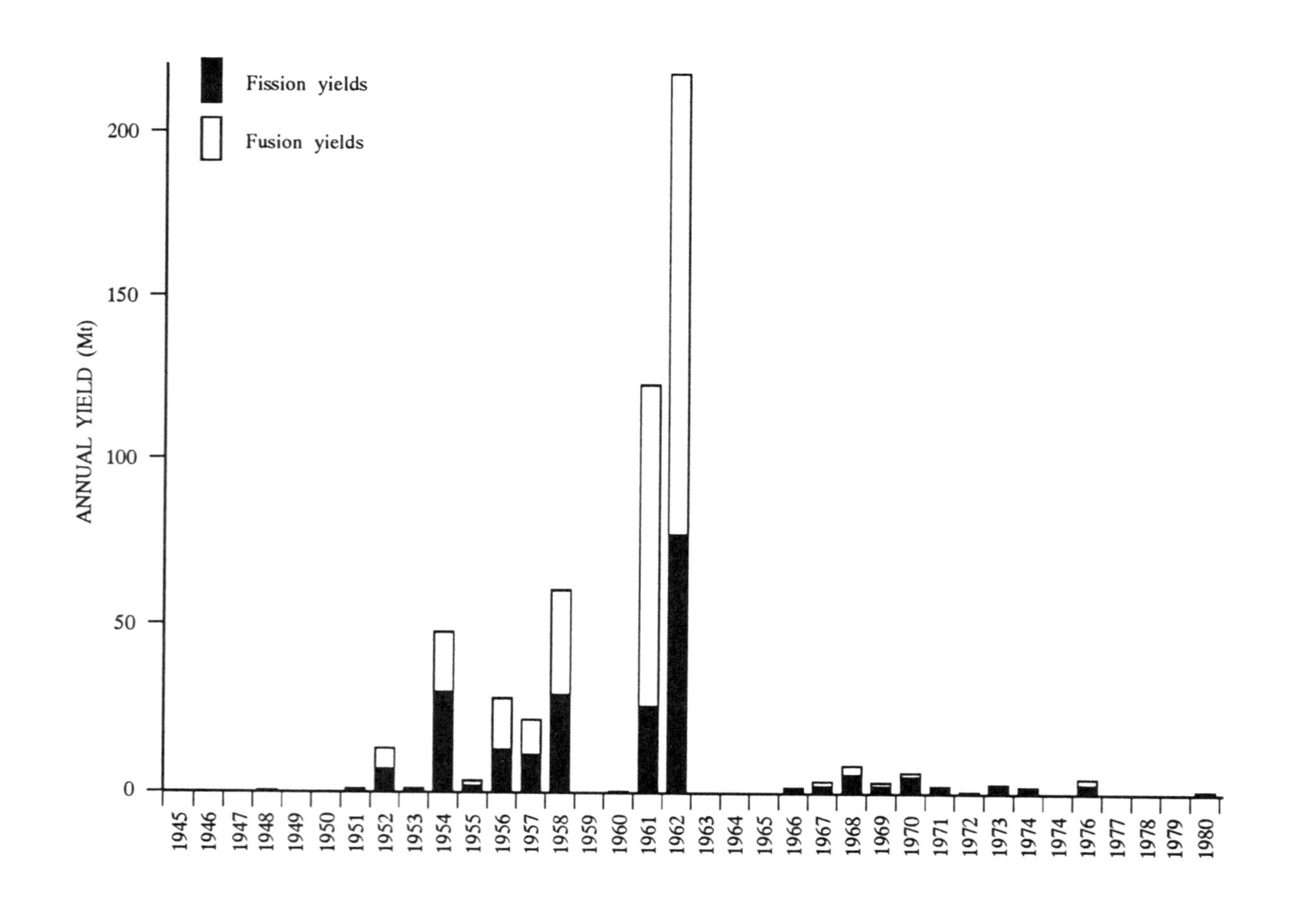

Figure II.
Fission and fusion yields of atmospheric nuclear explosions.
[B5]

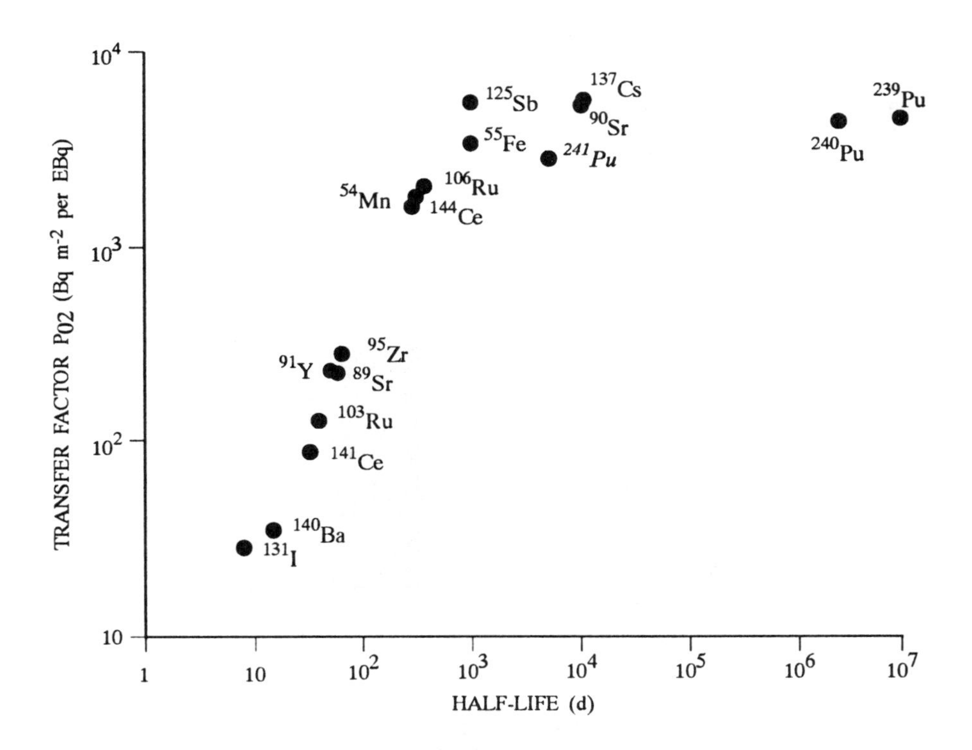

Figure III.
Transfer factor P_{02} from production of radionuclides in atmospheric nuclear testing to deposition on the earth's surface in the temperate zone of the northern hemisphere.

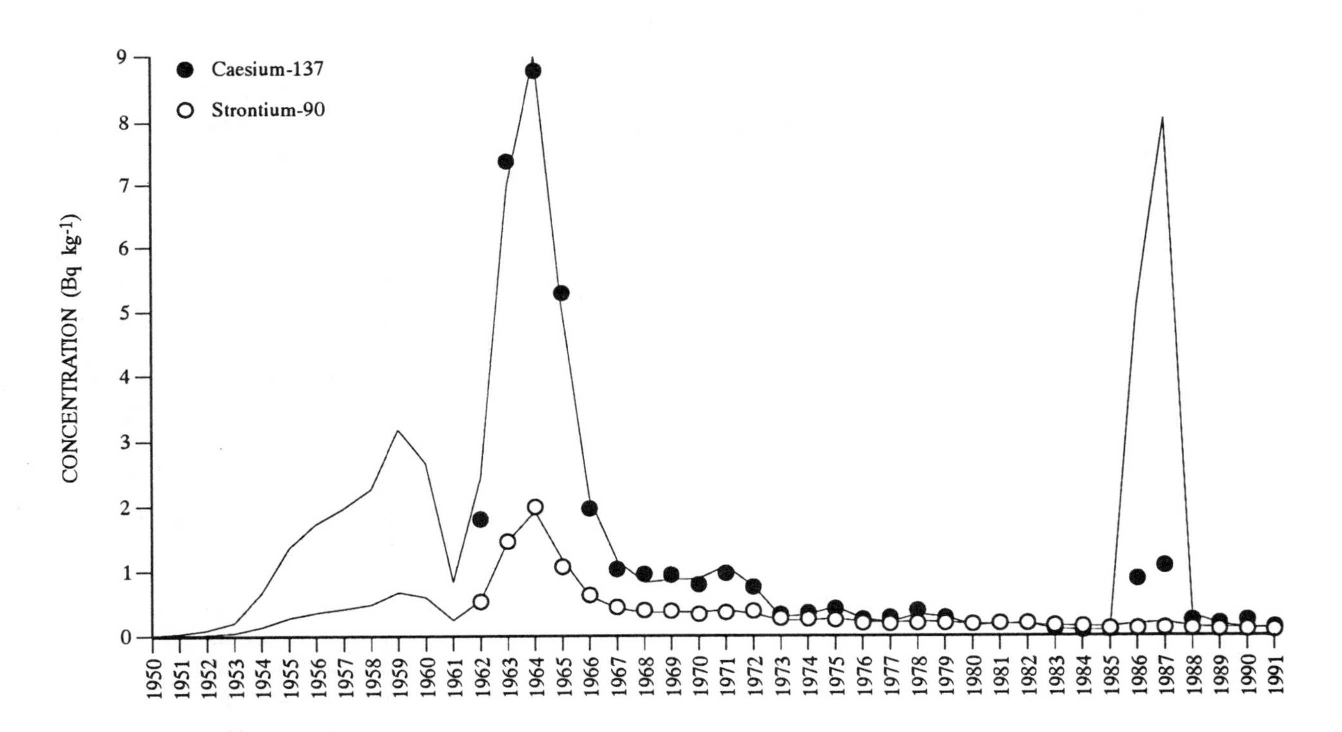

Figure IV.
Strontium-90 and caesium-137 in the total diet of Denmark.
Points: measured values; lines: results of application of regression models to the annual deposition densities.

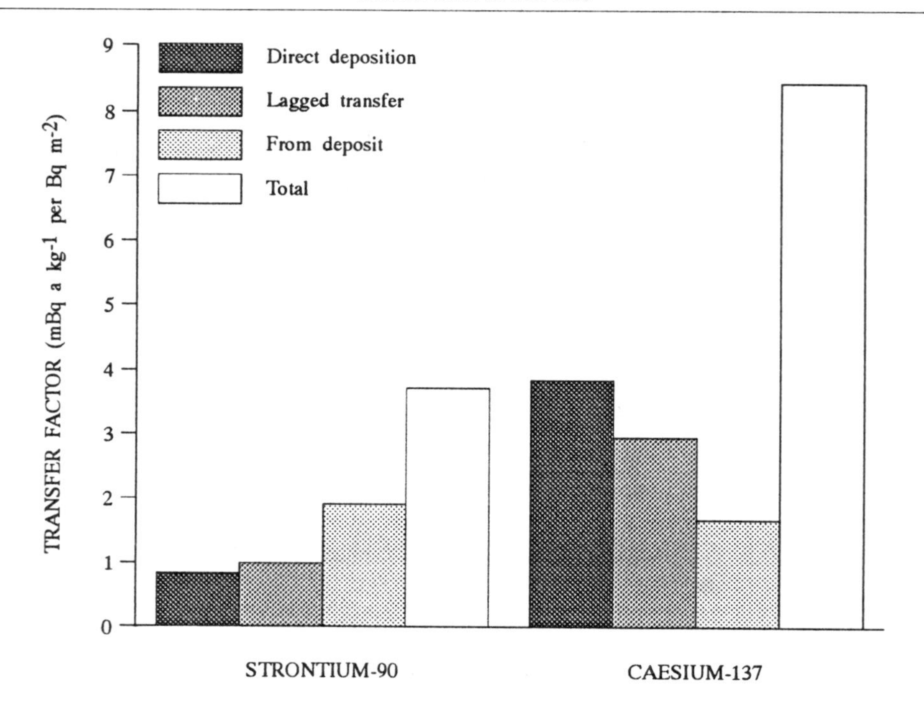

Figure V.
Contributions to strontium-90 and caesium-137 in total diet per unit deposition density derived from regression model results of measurements in Argentina, Denmark and the United States.

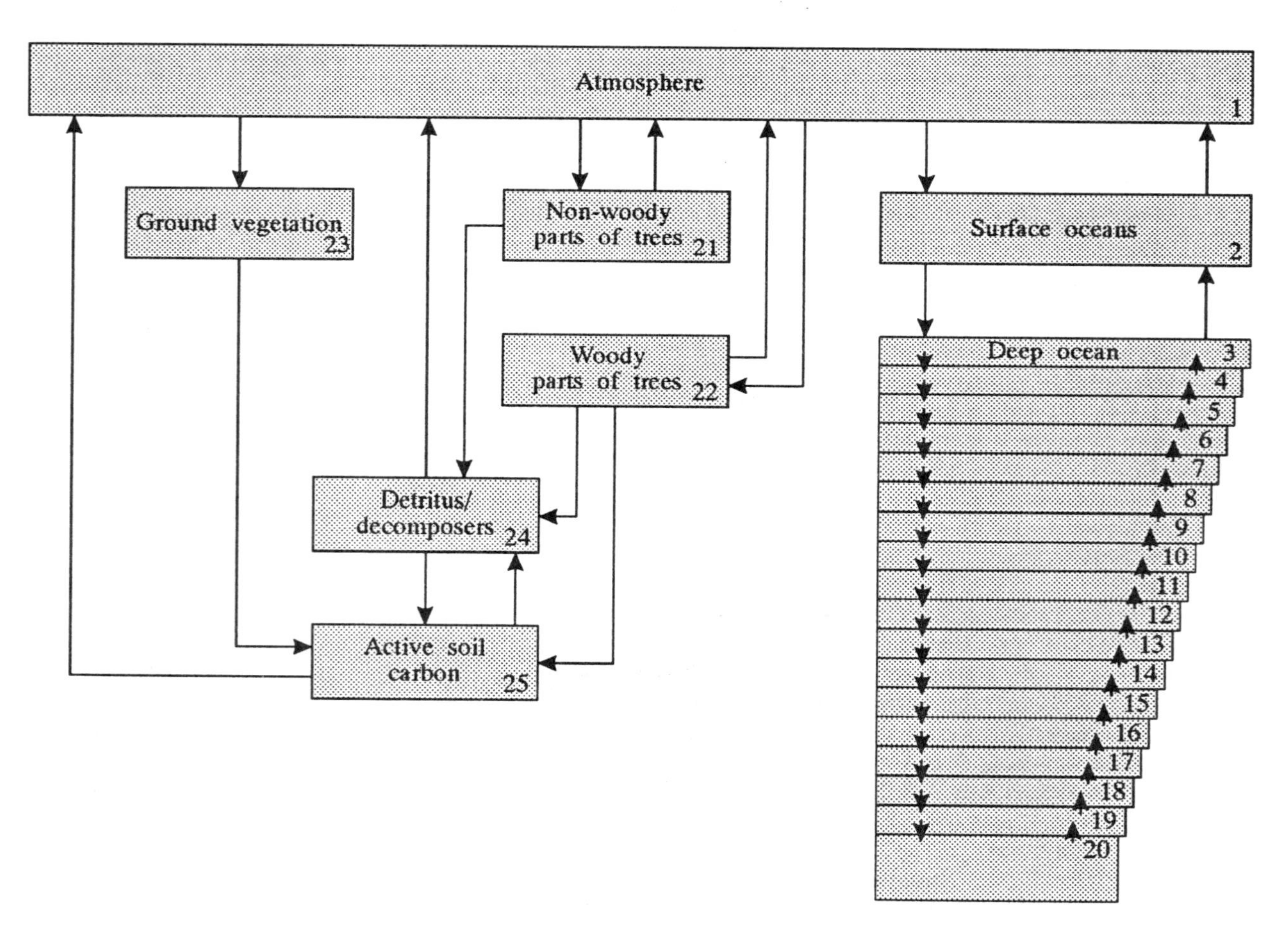

Figure VI.
Environmental compartment model of the carbon cycle.
[E6]

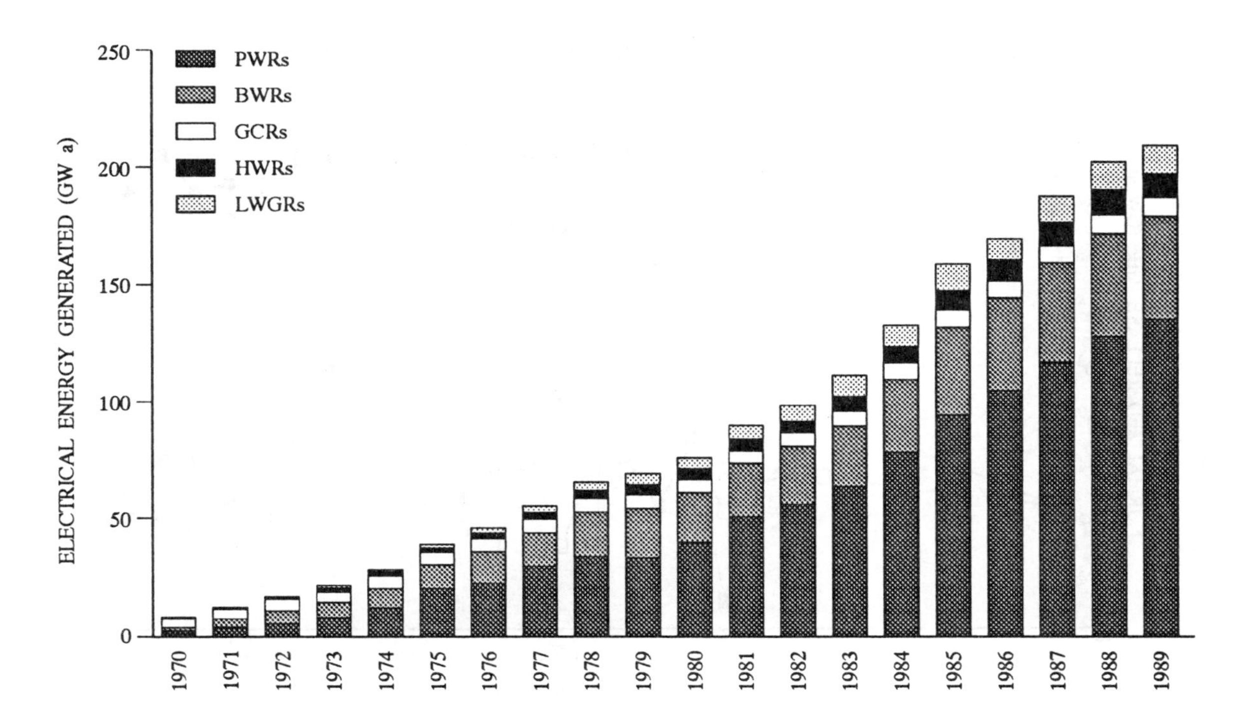

Figure VII.
Contributions by reactor types to total electrical energy generated worldwide by nuclear means.

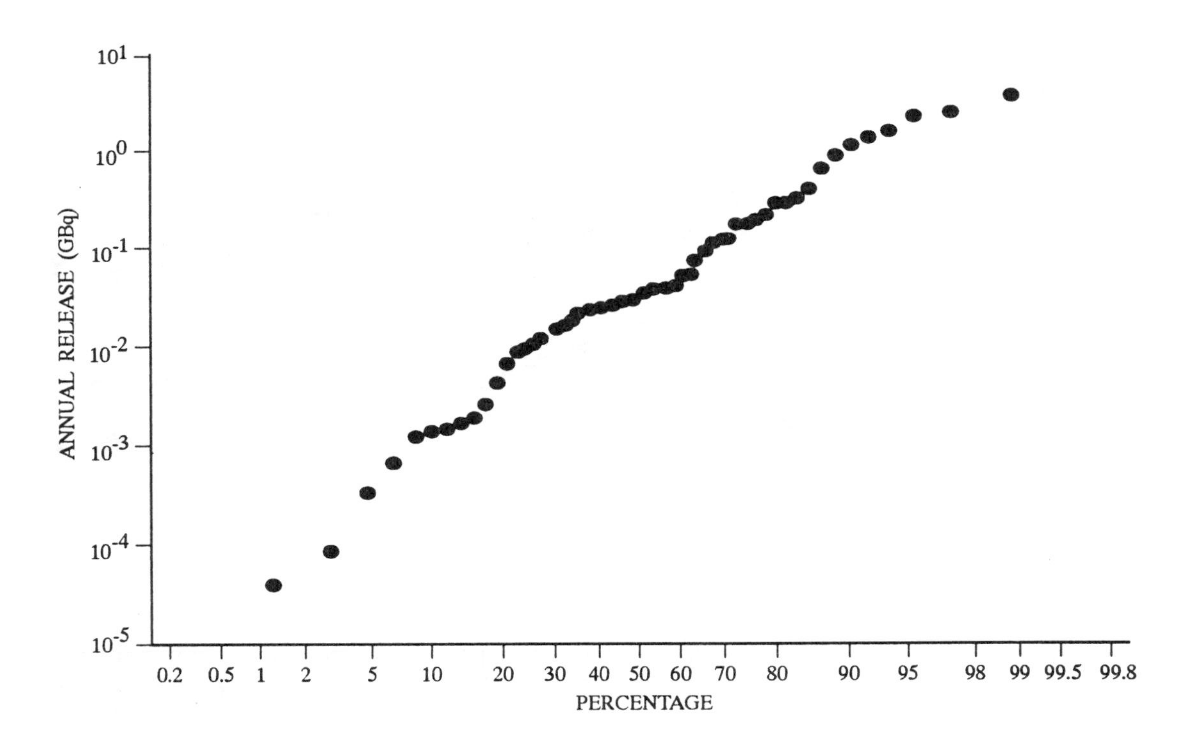

Figure VIII.
Distribution of annual releases of iodine-131 in airborne effluents from PWRs in the United States, 1988.
(Number of values: 56; geometric mean: 0.038 GBq; geometric SD: 13.)
[T3]

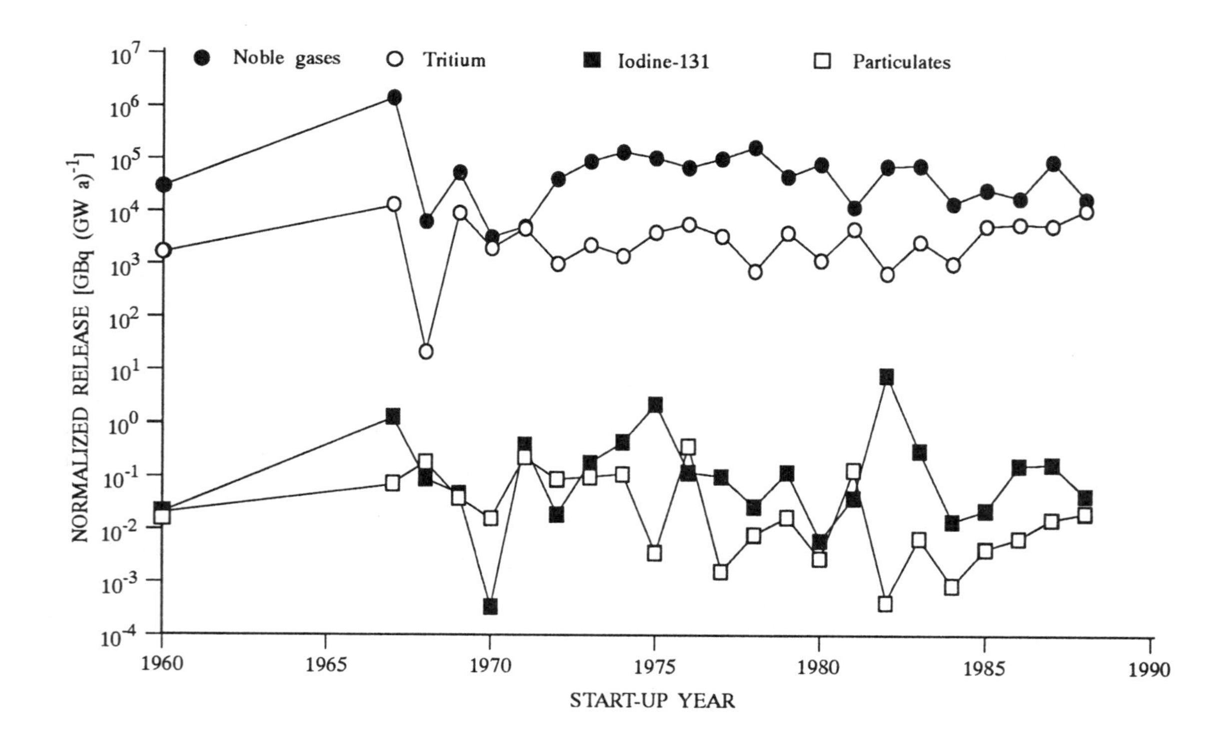

Figure IX.
Normalized release of radionuclides from PWRs in the United States during 1988, averaged for reactors of the same age (start-up year).

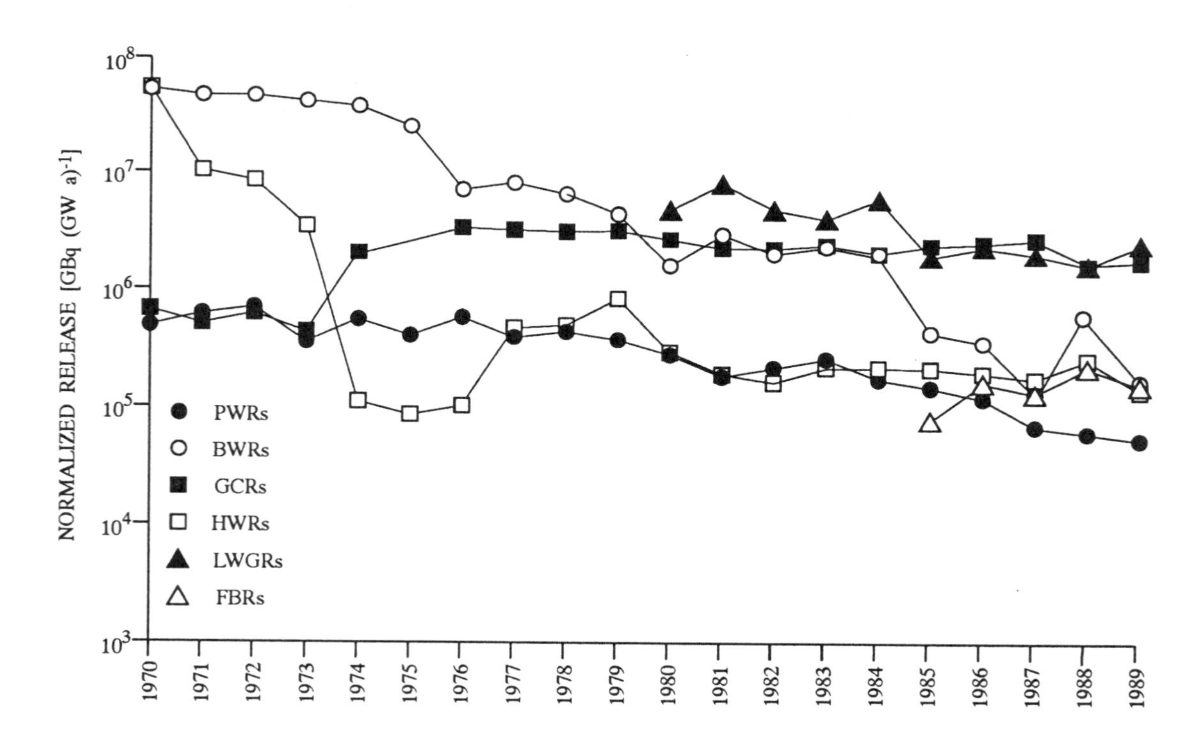

Figure X.
Trends in release of noble gases in airborne effluents from reactors.

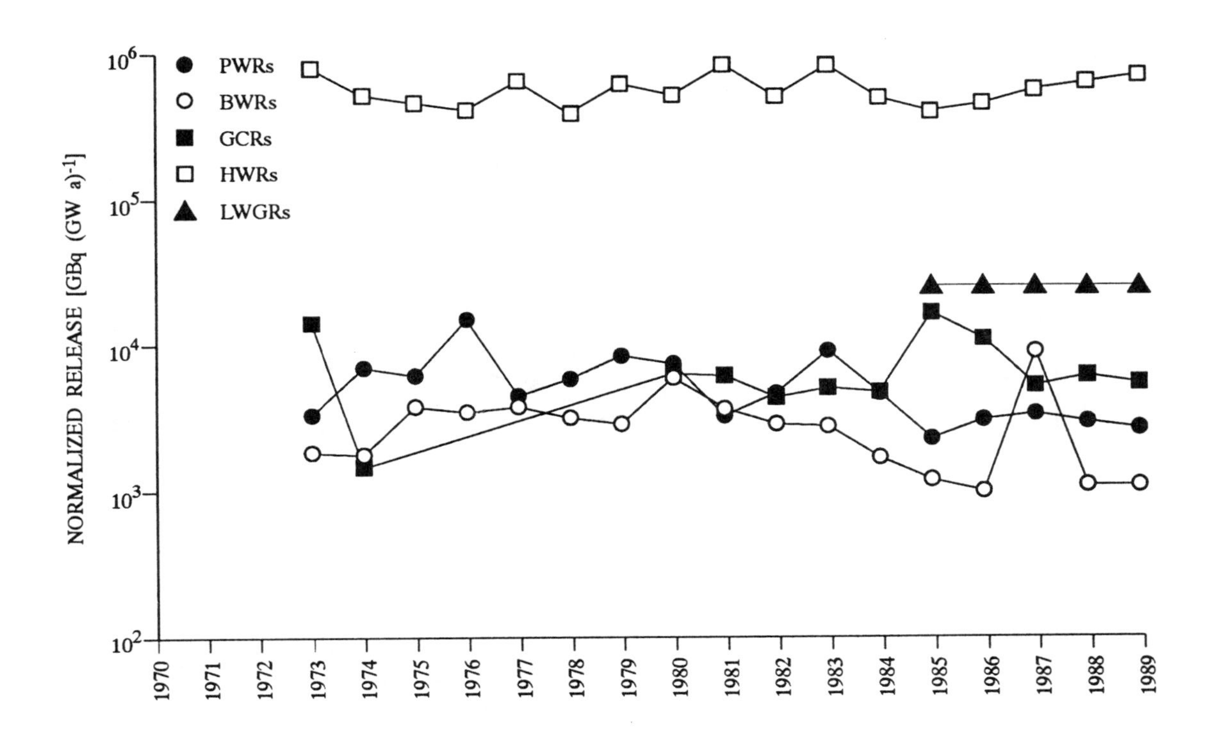

Figure XI.
Trends in release of tritium in airborne effluents from reactors.
For LWGRs, only estimated average value is available.

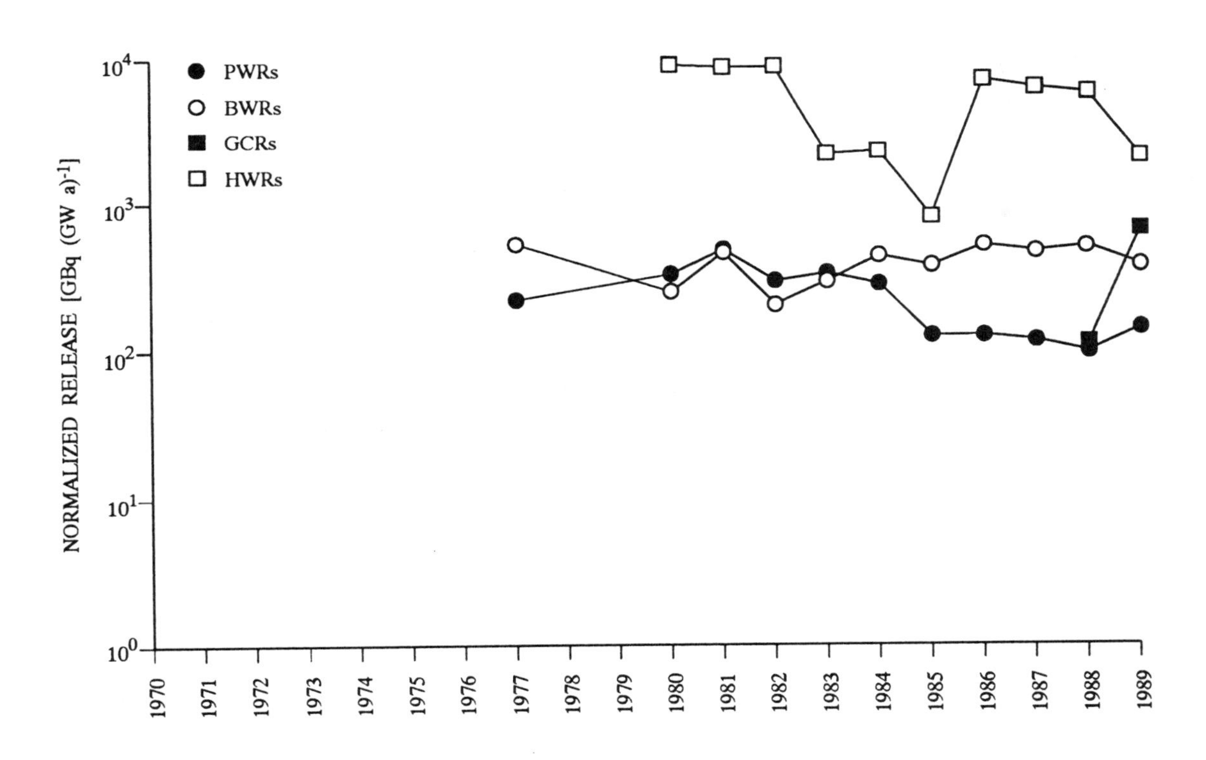

Figure XII.
Trends in release of carbon-14 in airborne effluents from reactors.

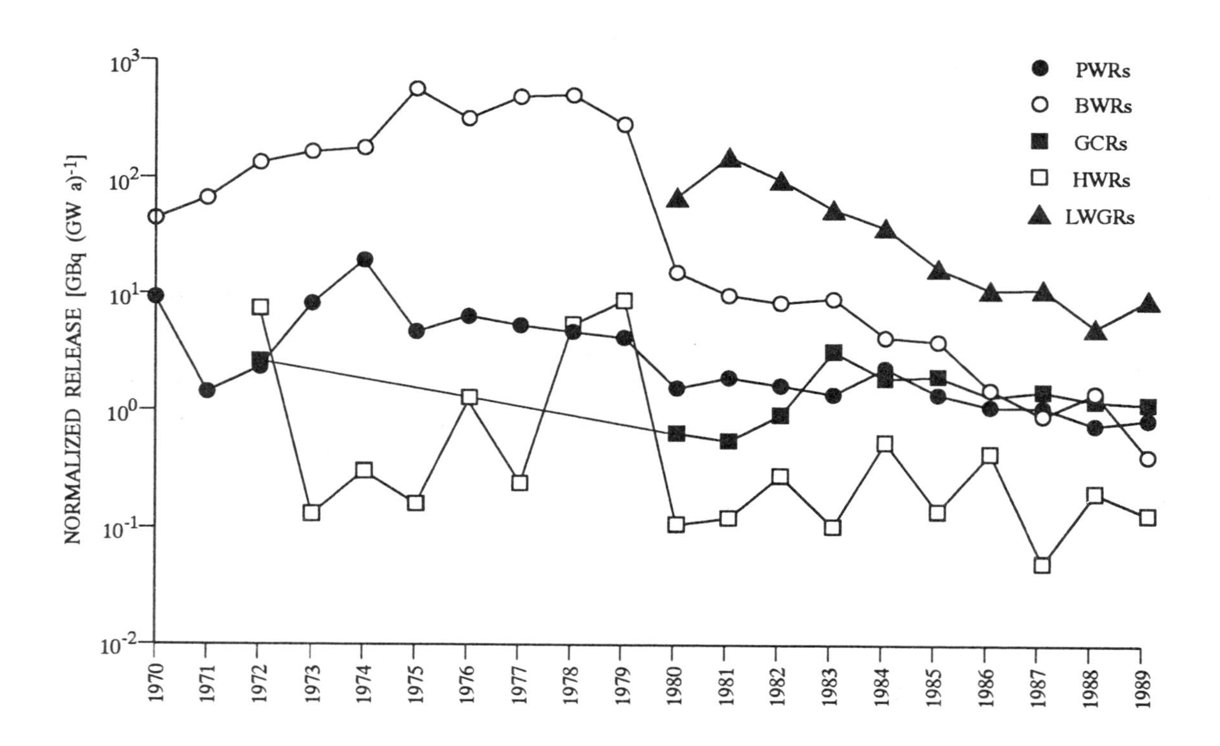

Figure XIII.
Trends in release of iodine-131 in airborne effluents from reactors.

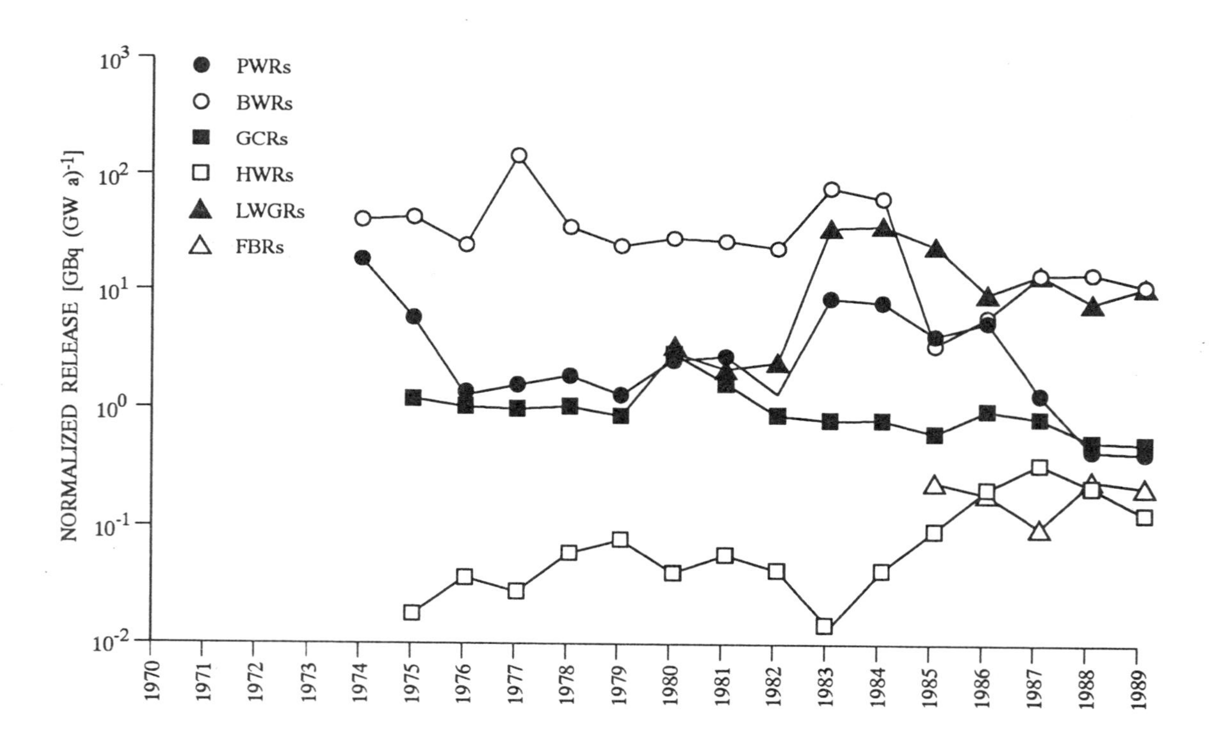

Figure XIV.
Trends in release of particulates in airborne effluents from reactors.

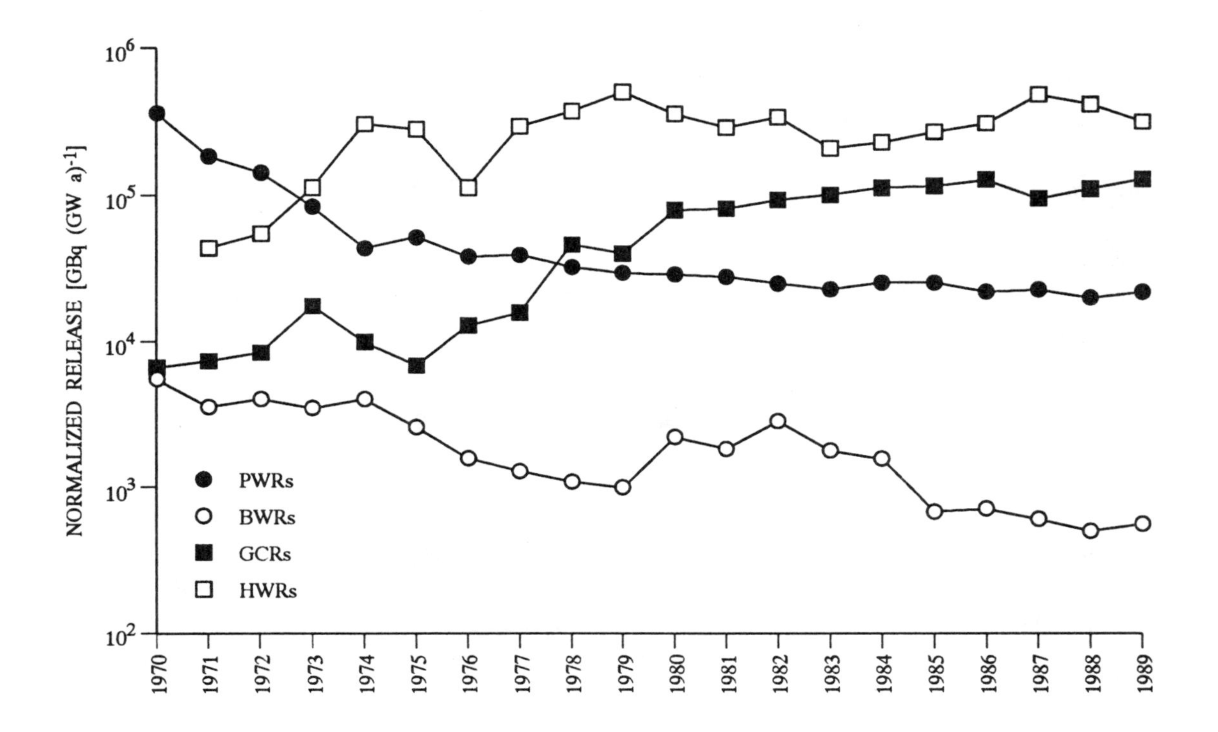

Figure XV.
Trends in release of tritium in liquid effluents from reactors.

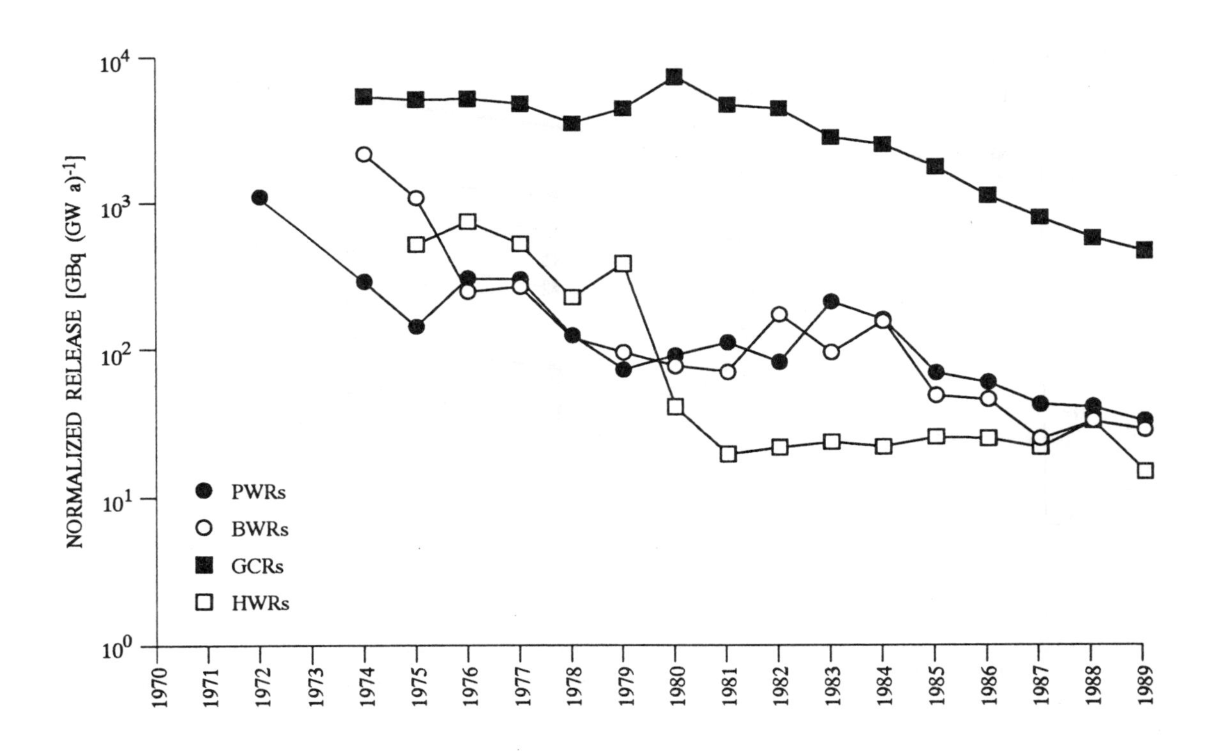

Figure XVI.
Trends in release of radionuclides excluding tritium in liquid effluents from reactors.

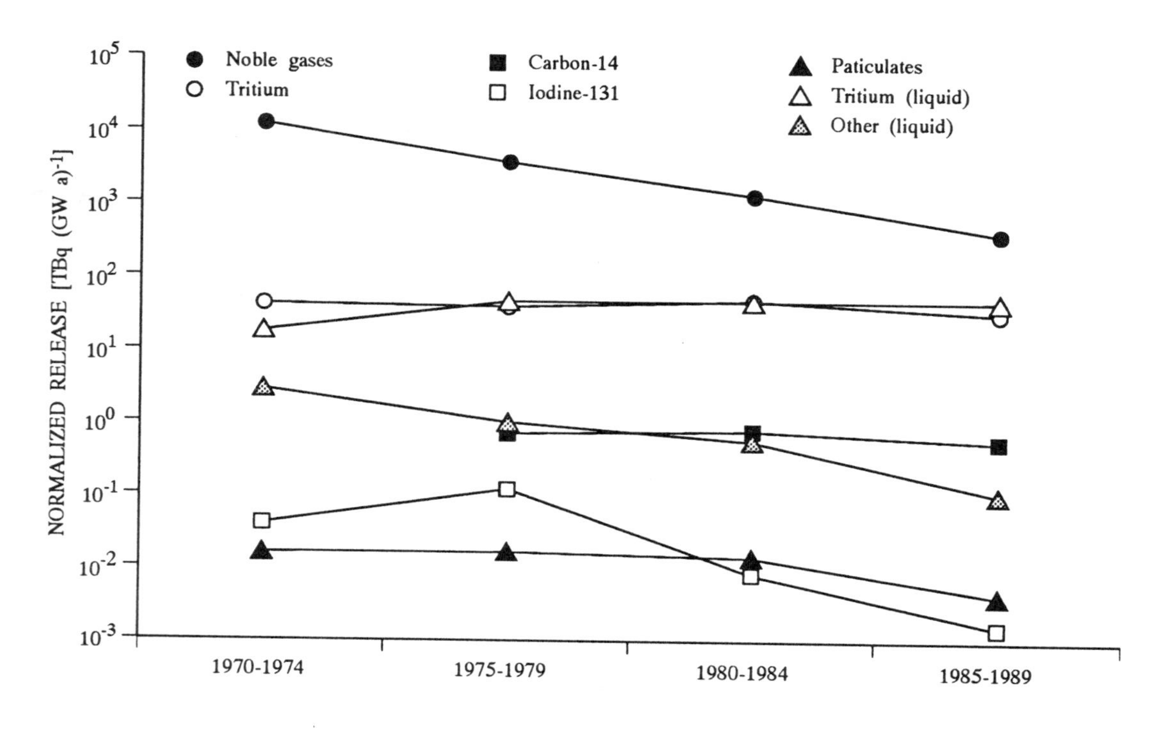

Figure XVII.
Normalized release of radionuclides averaged over five-year periods for all reactors.

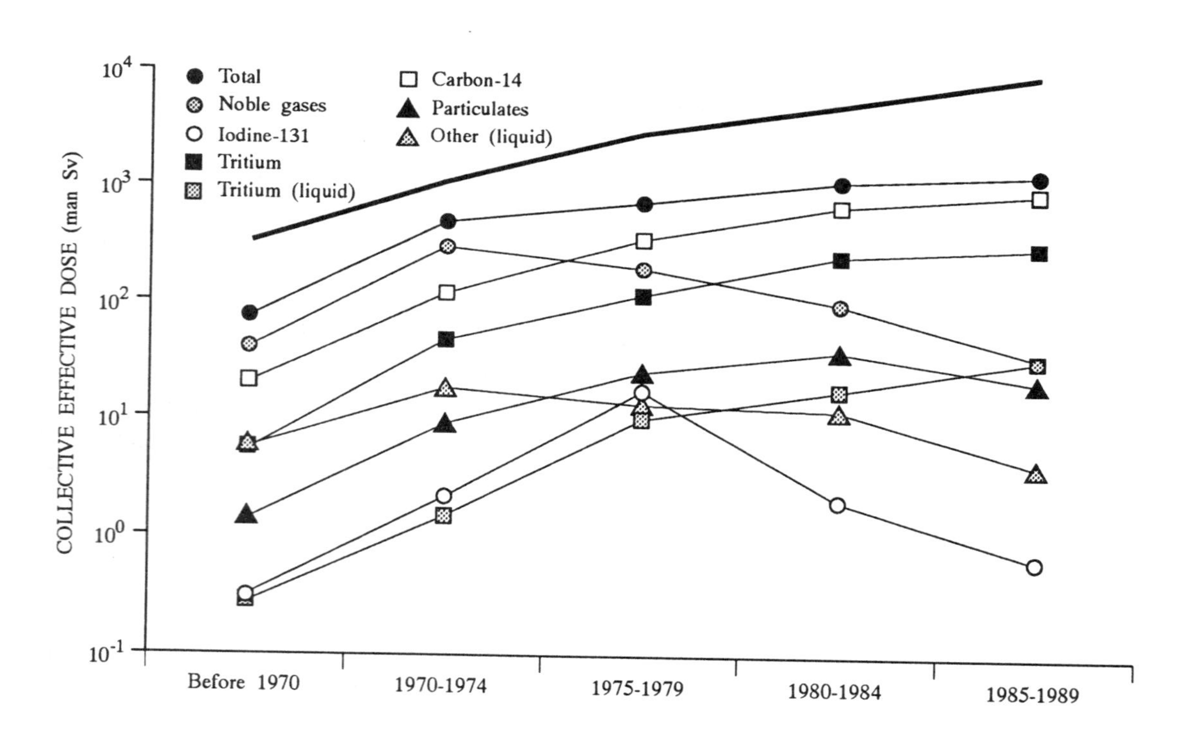

Figure XVIII.
Local and regional collective effective dose from release of radionuclides from reactors. The trend in the total electrical energy generated by nuclear means is indicated by the heavy line (numerical values on left axis apply with units 0.1 GW a).

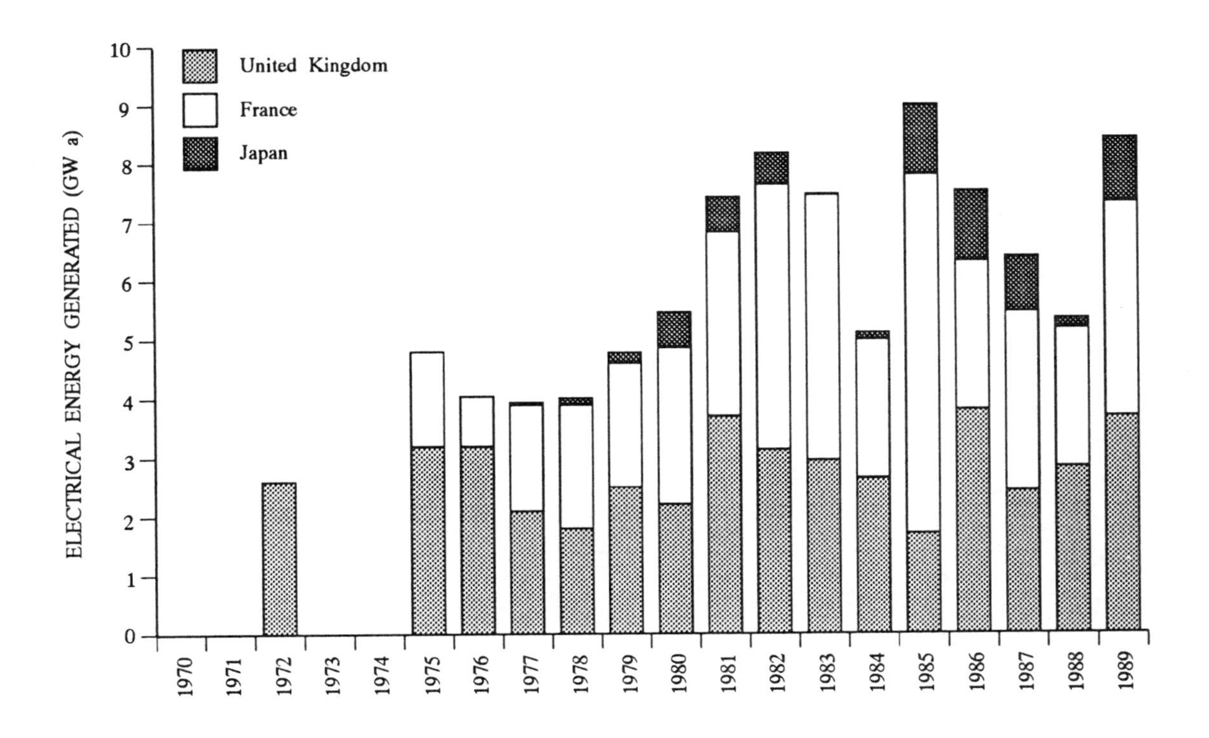

Figure XIX.
Nuclear fuel reprocessed wordwide.
Data before 1975 are incomplete.

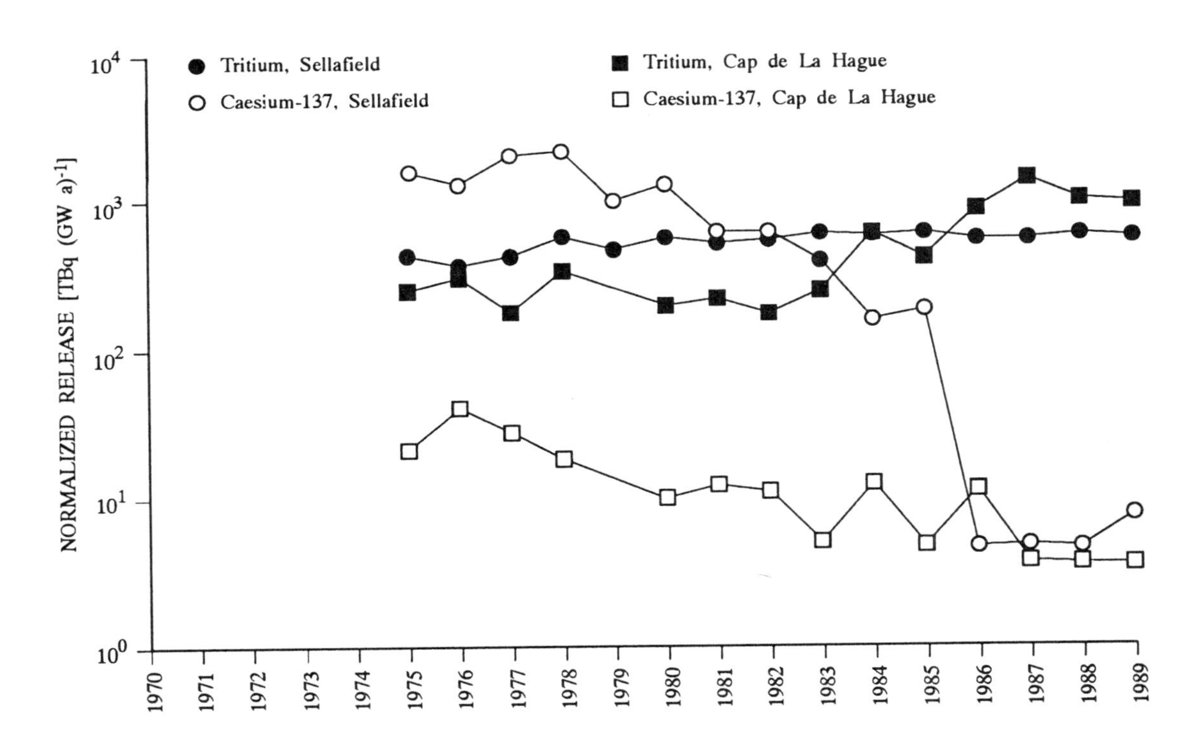

Figure XX.
Trends in normalized releases of tritium and caesium-137 in liquid effluents from fuel reprocessing plants at Cap de La Hague in France and Sellafield in the United Kingdom.

References

A1 Aarkrog, A. Radioecological investigations. p. 74-79 in: Project Crested Ice. A Joint Danish-American Report on the Crash Near Thule Airbase on 21 January 1968 of a B-52 Bomber Carrying Nuclear Weapons. Riso-R-213 (1970).

A2 Aarkrog, A. Radioecological investigations of plutonium in an arctic marine environment. Health Phys. 20: 31-47 (1971).

A3 Aarkrog, A., H. Dahlgaard, M. Frissel et al. Sources of anthropogenic radionuclides in the Southern Urals. J. Environ. Radioact. 15: 69-80 (1992).

A4 Akleev, A.V., P.V. Goloschapov, M.O. Degteva et al. Central Institute for Atomic Science and Technology, Moscow. Radioactive contamination in the southern Urals and human health effects. Communication to the UNSCEAR Secretariat (1991).

A5 Anspaugh, L.R., Y.E. Ricker, S.C. Black et al. Historical estimates of external γ exposure and collective external γ exposure from testing at the Nevada Test Site. II. Test series after Hardtack II, 1958, and summary. Health Phys. 59: 525-532 (1990).

A6 Atomic Energy Control Board, Canada. Communication from J.W. Beare (1991).

A7 Arndt, J., I. Gans and H. Rühle. Erfassung der Belastung der Gewässer durch Jod-131 - Abgaben aus der Nuklearmedizin. p. 225-237 in: Tagungsbericht Radioaktivität und Umwelt. Band I. Norderney, 1978.

A8 As, D. Van, A. Grundling, S. Redding et al. An assessment of the population dose due to radon-222 from mine tailings on the Witwatersrand. Radiation-Risk-Protection. p. 254-257 in: Proceedings of the 6th International Congress of the International Radiation Protection Association, Berlin, 1984.

A9 Australian Radiation Laboratory. Communication from S.B. Solomon (1991).

B1 Balonov, M.I. Radiological consequences of the Chernobyl NPP accident in comparison with those of the Kyshtym and Windscale radiation accidents. p. 749-767 in: Proceedings of Seminar on Comparative Assessment of the Environmental Impact of Radionuclides Released during Three Major Nuclear Accidents: Kyshtym, Windscale, Chernobyl. EUR-13574 (1990).

B2 Baverstock, K.F. and J. Vennart. Emergency reference levels for reactor accidents: a re-examination of the Windscale reactor accident. Health Phys. 30: 339-344 (1976).

B3 Beck, H.L. Exposure rate conversion factors for radionuclides deposited on the ground. EML-378 (1980).

B4 Bundesamt für Strahlenschutz, Germany. Communication from A. Kaul (1990).

B5 Bennett, B.G. Environmental aspects of americium. EML-348 (1978).

B6 Bernström, B. Radioactivity from nuclear explosions in ground-level air and precipitation in Sweden. NaI (Tl) measurements from 1972 to the end of 1975. FOA/C40080-T2(A1) (1978) and EML-349 (1979).

B7 Bernström, B. Tritium in atmospheric hydrogen gas at a Swedish sampling station at Hagfors. FOA/C40062-T2 (1977).

B8 Bigu, J., M. Grenier, N.K. Dave et al. Study of radon flux and other radiation variables from uranium mine tailings areas. Uranium 1: 257-277 (1984).

B9 Bundesminister fur Umwelt, Naturschutz und Reaktorsicherheit. Umweltpolitik. Berichte der Bundesregierung an den Deutschen Bundestag über Umweltradioaktivität und Strahlenbelastung in den Jahren 1986, 1987, 1988 und 1989.

B10 Bush, R.P., I.F. White and G.M. Smith. Carbon-14 waste management. AERE-R10543 (1983).

B11 Buldakov, L.A., S.N. Demin, V.A. Kostyuchenko et al. Medical consequences of the radiation accident in the Southern Urals in 1957. p. 419-431 in: Proceedings of a Symposium on Recovery Operations in the Event of a Nuclear Accident or Radiological Emergency. STI/PUB/826. IAEA, Vienna, 1990.

B12 Burnazyan, A.I. (ed.). Results of Studies and Experience in Elimination of the Consequences of Accidental Contamination of a Territory with the Products of Uranium Fission. Energoatomizdat, Moscow, 1990.

B13 British Nuclear Fuels plc. Annual report on radioactive discharges and monitoring of the environment for 1987, 1988 and 1989. Health and Safety Directorate, United Kingdom (1988, 1989 and 1990).

B14 Bhabbha Atomic Research Centre, India. Communication to the UNSCEAR Secretariat from D. Gopinath (1993).

C1 Comisao Nacional de Energia Nuclear, Brazil. Communication from A.S. Paschoa (1991).

C2 Cambray, R.S., G.N.J. Lewis, K. Playford et al. Radioactive fallout in air and rain: results to the end of 1982. AERE-R10859 (1983).

C3 Cambray, R.S., E.M.R. Fisher, W.L. Brooks et al. Radioactive fallout in air and rain: results to the middle of 1970. AERE-R6556 (1970).

C4 Camplin, W.C. Critical group doses from anthropogenic sources. p. 253-268 in: Seminar on the Radiological Exposure of the Population of the European Community from Radioactivity in North European Marine Waters, Bruges, June 1989. Project MARINA. CEC Report XI/4669/89 (1989).

C5 Cate, S., A.J. Ruttenber and A.W. Conklin. Feasibility of an epidemiologic study of thyroid neoplasia in persons exposed to radionuclides from the Hanford nuclear facility between 1944 and 1956. Health Phys. 59: 169-178 (1990).

C6 Carvalho, A.B. The psychological impact of the radiological accident in Goiania. p. 463-477 in: Proceedings of a Symposium on Recovery Operations in the Event of a Nuclear Accident or Radiological Emergency. STI/PUB/826. IAEA, Vienna, 1990.

C7 Church, B.W., D.L. Wheeler, C.M. Campbell et al. Overview of the Department of Energy's off-site radiation exposure review project (ORERP). Health Phys. 59: 503-510 (1990).

C8 Ciallella, H.E., O.D. Jordan, A.A. Oliveira et al. Radon emanation measurements from uranium ore tailings in Argentina. Radiation protection practice. p. 373-376 in: Proceedings of the 7th International

Congress of the International Radiation Protection Association, Sydney, 1988.

C9 Clarke, R.H. An analysis of the 1957 Windscale accident using the reactor safety code WEERIE. Ann. Nucl. Sci. Eng. 1: 73-82 (1974).

C10 Clarke, R.H. Current radiation risk estimates and implications for the health consequences of Windscale, TMI and Chernobyl accidents. p. 102-118 in: Medical Response to Effects of Ionizing Radiation. (W.A. Crosbie and J.H. Gittus, eds.) Elsevier Applied Science, 1989.

C11 Cochran, T.B., M.M. Hoenig and W.M. Arkin. Nuclear weapons materials. Science 215: 1344 (1982).

C12 Cochran, T.B., M.M. Hoenig and W.M. Arkin. Nuclear weapons databook. U.S. Nuclear Forces and Capabilities (Volume I). Ballinger Publishing Co., New York, 1984.

C13 Crick, M.J. and G.S. Linsley. An assessment of the radiological impact of the 1957 Windscale reactor fire. NRPB-R135 (1982).

C14 Crick, M.J. and G.S. Linsley. An assessment of the radiological impact of the Windscale reactor fire, October 1957. Int. J. Radiat. Biol. 46: 479-506 (1984).

C15 Curti, A.R. and A.A. Oliveira. Impacto radiológico ambiental debido a la operación de las centrales nucleares argentinas. Rev. Soc. Argent. Radioprotección 2: (1991).

C16 Committee on the Use of Atomic Energy for Peaceful Purposes, Bulgaria. Communication to the UNSCEAR Secretariat from Y. Yanev (1992).

C17 Camplin, W.C. and A. Aarkrog. Radioactivity in North European Waters: Report of Working Group II of CEC Project MARINA. Fisheries Research Data Report No. 20, Lowestoft, 1989.

C18 Comisión Nacional de Energía Atómica, Argentina. Communication to the UNSCEAR Secretariat from E. Palacios (1990/1992).

C19 Comisión Nacional de Seguridad Nuclear y Salvaguardias, Mexico. Communication to the UNSCEAR Secretariat from E. Araico (1990).

C20 Council for Nuclear Safety, South Africa. Communication to the UNSCEAR Secretariat from N.H. Keenan (1990).

C21 Consejo de Seguridad Nuclear, Spain. Communication to the UNSCEAR Secretariat from J. Butragueno (1992).

C22 Comitato Nazionale per la Ricerca e per lo Sviluppo dell'Energia Nucleare e delle Energie Alternative (ENEA), Italy. Communication to the UNSCEAR Secretariat from C. Rollo (1992).

D1 DeGeer, L.E., R. Arntsing, I. Vintersved et al. Particulate radioactivity, mainly from nuclear explosions, in air and precipitation in Sweden mid-year 1975 to mid-year 1977. FOA/C40089-T2(A1) (1978) and p. I-49-I-124 in: EML-349 (1979).

D2 Dubasov, U.V., A.M. Matushenko, N.P. Pilonov et al. Semipalatinsk Test Site: Estimated Radiological Consequences. Information Bulletin. Centre for Public Information on Atomic Energy, Moscow, 1993.

D3 Department of Primary Industries and Energy, Australia. Rehabilitation of Former Nuclear Test Sites in Australia. Australian Government Publishing Service, Canberra, 1990.

D4 Department of Mines and Energy, Australia. Radon daughters in tropical northern Australia and the environmental impact of uranium mining. Communication from J. Kvasnika (1990).

D5 Division Principale de la Securité des Installations Nucléaires. Les installations nucleaires en Suisse en 1989. HSK-AN-2210 et KSA-AN-1550 (1990).

D6 Division Principale de la Securité des Installations Nucléaires, Suisse. Emissionen aus Kernanlagen und daraus resultierende Dosen für die Umgebungsbevölkerung im Jahre 1985. HSK-AN-1736 or KSA-AN-1207 (1986); im Jahre 1986. HSK-AN-1882 or KSA-AN-1293 (1987); im Jahre 1987: HSK-AN-2003 or KSA-AN-1388 (1988); im Jahre 1988: HSK-AN 2203 or KSA-AN-1540 (1989); im Jahre 1989: HSK-AN-2224 or KSA-AN-1560 (1990).

D7 Department of Energy, United States. Summary of Environmental Reports. Department of Energy Sites, January - December 1982. DOE/EP-0049 and earlier reports in the same series.

D8 Department of Energy, United States. Announced United States nuclear tests. NVO-209 (1985).

D9 Dunstana, R., J. Lipsztein, C. de Oliveria et al. ^{137}Cs internal contamination of members of the public involved in an accident in Brazil and the efficacy of Russian blue treatment. Health Phys. (1993, in press).

D10 De Geer, L.E. Observations in Sweden of venting underground nuclear explosions. Symposium on Underground Nuclear Weapons Testing: Potential Environmental Impacts and their Containment, Ottawa, 1991.

E1 Eriksen, B. Investigation of airborne radioactive materials originating from underground nuclear explosion in USSR, 23 March 1971. FOA/C4502-A1, Stockholm (1972).

E2 Erlandsson, B. and S. Mattsson. Medically used radionuclides in sewage sludge. Water, Air Soil Pollut. 9: 199-206 (1978).

E3 Eriksen, V.O. Sunken Nuclear Submarines. A Threat to the Environment? Norwegian University Press, 1991.

E4 Electricité de France. Environnement, année 1991. Rapport d'Activité, Annexe IX. Département Sécurité Radioprotection Environnement (1992).

E5 Environment and Natural Resources Policy Division. Nuclear Proliferation Factbook. Congressional Research Service, United States Library of Congress, Washington, 1977.

E6 Emanuel, W.R., G.G. Killough, G. Post et al. Computer implementation of a globally averaged model of the world carbon cycle. DOE/NBB-0062 (1984).

E7 Evaluated Nuclear Structure Data File (ENSDF). Edited and maintained by the National Nuclear Data Center, Brookhaven National Laboratory. ENSDF 8/2/83 (1983).

F1 Federal Secretariat for Energy and Industry, Yugoslavia (former). Communication to the UNSCEAR Secretariat from S. Spasic (1991).

F2 Finland, Finnish Centre for Radiation and Nuclear Safety. Communication to the UNSCEAR Secretariat from O. Vilkamo (1992).

F3 Frederic Joliot-Curie National Research Institute for Radiobiology and Radiohygiene, Hungary. Communication by L.B. Sztanyik (1991).

G1 Gasco, C., E. Iranzo and L. Romero. Transuranics transfer in a Spanish marine ecosystem. Paper presented at the Third International Conference on Low-level Measurements of Actinides and Long-lived Radionuclides in Biological and Environmental Samples. Bombay, India, 1991.

G2 Guser, N., M. Golavko, O. Shamov et al. The effluents of radioactive gases and aerosols by nuclear power stations. At. Energ. 74: 361-365 (1993).

G3 Gummer, W.K., F.R. Capbell, G.B. Knight et al. Cosmos 954. The occurrence and nature of recovered debris. Info-0006. Atomic Energy Control Board, Ottawa (1980).

H1 Harley, J.H. Possible plutonium-238 distribution from a satellite failure. p. I-38-I-42 in: HASL-149 (1964).

H2 Harley, N., I. Fisenne, L.D.Y. Ong et al. Fission yield and fission product decay. p. 251-260 in: HASL-164 (1965).

H3 Haywood, S.M. and J. Smith. Assessment of the potential radiological impact of residual contamination in the Maralinga and Emu areas. NRPB-R237 (1990).

H4 Hicks, H.G. Radiochemical data collected on events from which radioactivity escaped beyond the borders of the Nevada Test Site range complex. UCRL-52934 (1981).

H5 von Hippel, F. and B. Levi. Controlling the source. Verification of a cut-off in the production of plutonium and high-enriched uranium for nuclear weapons. PU/CEES 167. Princeton University, 1984.

H6 Hughes, J.S., K.B. Shaw and M.C. O'Riordan. Radiation exposure of the UK population - 1988 review. NRPB-R227 (1988).

H7 Health and Safety Laboratory. Final tabulation of monthly ^{90}Sr fallout data: 1954-1976. HASL-329 (1977).

I1 International Advisory Committee. The International Chernobyl Project, Technical Report. IAEA, Vienna (1991).

I2 International Atomic Energy Agency. The radiological impact of radionuclides dispersed on a regional and global scale: methods for assessment and their application. IAEA-TRS-250. Vienna, 1985.

I3 International Atomic Energy Agency. Summary Report on the Post-Accident Review Meeting on the Chernobyl Accident. Safety Series No. 75-INSAG-1. IAEA, Vienna, 1986.

I4 International Atomic Energy Agency. Nuclear Safety Review for 1984 and 1985. IAEA, Vienna, 1986.

I5 International Atomic Energy Agency. The radiological accident in Goiania. IAEA, Vienna, 1988.

I6 International Atomic Energy Agency. Isotopes in day to day life. IAEA/PI/A.6E 84-00924. IAEA, Vienna, 1984.

I7 International Atomic Energy Agency. Energy, electricity and nuclear power estimates for the period up to 2005. Reference Data Series No. 1. IAEA, Vienna, 1990.

I8 International Atomic Energy Agency. Nuclear Power, Nuclear Fuel Cycle and Waste Management: Status and Trends 1990. Part C of the IAEA Yearbook 1990. IAEA, Vienna, 1990.

I9 International Atomic Energy Agency. Operating Experience in Nuclear Power Stations in Member States in 1990. IAEA, Vienna, 1991.

I10 International Atomic Energy Agency. Power Reactor Information System. IAEA, Vienna, 1992.

I11 International Atomic Energy Agency. Inventory of radioactive material entering the marine environment: Sea disposal of radioactive waste. IAEA-TECDOC-588. IAEA, Vienna, 1991.

I12 International Commission on Radiological Protection. 1990 Recommendations of the International Commission on Radiological Protection. ICRP Publication 60. Annals of the ICRP 21(1-3). Pergamon Press, Oxford, 1991.

I13 International Commission on Radiological Protection. Age-dependent doses to members of the public from intake of radionuclides. ICRP Publication 56. Annals of the ICRP 20(2). Pergamon Press, Oxford, 1989.

I14 Institute of Biophysics, Moscow. Communication to the UNSCEAR Secretariat from O. Pavlovsky (1991) and L. Ilyin (1992).

I15 Ilyin, L.A., M.I. Balonov, L.A. Buldakov et al. Radiocontamination patterns and possible health consequences of the accident at the Chernobyl nuclear power station. J. Radiol. Prot. 10: 3-29 (1990).

I16 Iranzo, E. First results from the programme of action following the Palomares accident. p. 446-455 in: Radiological Protection of the Public in a Nuclear Mass Disaster. Interlaken, Switzerland, 1968.

I17 Iranzo, E., S. Salvador and C.E. Iranzo. Air concentrations of ^{239}Pu and ^{240}Pu and potential doses to persons living near Pu-contaminated areas in Palomares, Spain. Health Phys. 52: 453-461 (1987).

I18 Iranzo, E., A. Espinosa and C.E. Iranzo. Dose estimation by bioassay for population involved in an accident with Plutonium release. Paper presented at the Second Conference on Radiation Protection and Dosimetry. Orlando, Florida, 1988.

I19 Iranzo, E., P. Rivas, E. Mingarro et al. Distribution and migration of Plutonium in soils of an accidentally contaminated environment. Radiochim. Acta 52/53: 249-256 (1991).

I20 Iranzo, E., A. Espinosa and C.E. Iranzo. Evaluation of remedial actions taken in agricultural area contaminated by transuranides. 4th International Symposium of Radioecology: Impact of Nuclear Origin Accidents on Environment. Cadarache, France, March 1988.

J1 Japan Nuclear Safety Policy Division, Nuclear Safety Bureau, Science and Technology Agency. Radioactive effluents from nuclear facilities in Japan, 1985-1989. Communication to the UNSCEAR Secretariat (1992).

J2 Japan Radioisotope Association, Nuclear Safety Bureau, Science and Technology Agency. Statistics on the use of radiation in Japan 1989 (1989).

J3 Junker, D. Nuclear medicine: Personnel exposure to radiation and release of activity to the environment. Nucl. Med. 30: 141-148 (1991).

K1 Kauranen, P., A. Kulmala and R. Mattsson. Fission products of unusual composition in Finland. Nature 216: 238-241 (1967).

K2 Kelly, G.N., J.A. Jones, P.M. Bryant et al. The predicted radiation exposure of the population of the European Community resulting from discharges of krypton-85, tritium, carbon-14 and iodine-129 from the nuclear power industry to the year 2050. CEC V/2676/75 (1975).

K3 Kemeny, J.G. The President's Commission on the accident at Three Mile Island. Pergamon Press, 1979.

K4 Killough, G.G. and P. Rohwer. A new look at the dosimetry of C-14 released to the atmosphere as carbon dioxide. Health Phys. 34: 141-159 (1978).

K5 Killough, G.G. A dynamic model for estimating radiation dose to the world population from releases of C-14 to the atmosphere. Health Phys. 38: 269-300 (1980).

K6 Kolb, W. Tungsten-181 and short-lived fission products in ground-level air in North Germany and North Norway. Nature 232: 552-553 (1971).

K7 Kosenko, M.M. Medical Effects of population exposure to radiation as a result of radiation accidents in the Southern Urals. Abstract. Dissertation for the Degree of Doctor of Medical Sciences. Institute of Biophysics, USSR Ministry of Health, Moscow, 1991.

K8 Kuznetzov, G. Twenty-five years before Chernobyl. p. 129-131 in: Proceedings of Seminar on Comparative Assessment of the Environmental Impact of Radionuclides Released during Three Major Nuclear Accidents: Kyshtym, Windscale, Chernobyl. EUR-13574 (1990).

L1 Langham, W.H. Technical and laboratory support. p. 36-41 in: Project Crested Ice. A Joint Danish-American Report on the Crash Near Thule Airbase on 21 January 1968 of a B-52 Bomber Carrying Nuclear Weapons. Riso-R-213 (1970).

L2 Larsen, R.J. Worldwide deposition of Sr-90 through 1981, and through 1983. EML-415 and EML-444 (1983 and 1985).

L3 Lessard, E., R. Miltenberger, R. Conard et al. Thyroid absorbed dose for people at Rongelap, Utirik and Sifo on March 1, 1954. BNL 51882 (1985).

L4 Leach, V.A., K.H. Lokan and L.J. Martin. A study of radiation parameters at the Nabarlek mine, NT. ARL/TR 028 (1980).

L5 Loosli, H., H. Oeschger, R. Studer et al. Atmospheric concentrations and mixing of argon-37. p. 24-39 in: Noble Gases. CONF-730915 (1973).

M1 Mason, A.S. and H.G. Ostlund. Atmospheric HT and HTO 1975-1976. University of Miami, Rosenstiel School of Marine and Atmospheric Sciences, 1977.

M2 McCartney, M., M.S. Baxter and E.M. Scott. Carbon-14 discharges from the nuclear fuel cycle: I. Global effects. J. Environ. Radioact. 8: 143-155 (1988).

M3 Ministry of Science and Technology, Republic of Korea. Response to UNSCEAR Questionnaire on occupational exposure in industry. Korea Electric Power Corporation (1990).

M4 Molina, G. Lessons learned during the recovery operations in the Ciudad Juarez accident. p. 517-524 in: Proceedings of a Symposium on Recovery Operations in the Event of a Nuclear Accident or Radiological Emergency. STI/PUB/826. IAEA, Vienna, 1990.

M5 Ministry of Housing, Physical Planning and Environment, Netherlands. Results from routine release of radionuclides from nuclear power installations in the Netherlands. Report 1990/45 (1990). (in Dutch)

M6 Ministère de la Santé Publique et de l'Environnement, Belgium. Communication to the UNSCEAR Secretariat from J.M. Lambotte (1991/1992).

N1 National Radiological Protection Board. Committed equivalent organ doses and committed effective doses from intakes of radionuclides. NRPB-M288 (1991).

N2 Nikipelov, B.V., G.N. Romanov, L.A. Buldakov et al. Accident in the Southern Urals on 29 September 1957. Document provided to the IAEA by the Chairman of the USSR State Committee on the Utilization of Atomic Energy and circulated by the IAEA as INFCIRC/368 (28 July 1989).

N3 Nikipelov, B.V., E.I. Mikerin, G.N. Romanov et al. The radiation accident in the Southern Urals in 1957 and the cleanup measures implemented. p. 373-403 in: Proceedings of a Symposium on Recovery Operations in the Event of a Nuclear Accident or Radiological Emergency. STI/PUB/826. IAEA, Vienna, 1990.

N4 Nikipelov, B.V., A.S. Nikiforov, O.L. Kedrovsky et al. Practical rehabilitation of territories contaminated as a result of implementation of nuclear material production defense programs. VNIPI prom-technologii, Moscow, 1992.

N5 Nikipelov, B., A. Lyzlov and N. Koshurnikova. An experience of the first enterprise of the nuclear industry (levels of exposure and health of workers). Priroda 2: 30-38 (1990).

N6 National Radiological Protection Board. UK power reactor discharges 1989. Communication to the UNSCEAR Secretariat from R.H. Clarke (1992).

N7 National Radiological Protection Board. Communication to the UNSCEAR Secretariat from A. Mayall (1990).

N8 National Council on Radiation Protection and Measurements. Tritium in the environment. NCRP Report No. 62 (1979).

N9 National Council on Radiation Protection and Measurements. Carbon-14 in the environment. NCRP Report No. 81 (1985).

N10 National Defence Research Establishment (FOA), Division of Hydroacoustics and Seismology, Sweden. Communication to the UNSCEAR Secretariat from L.E. DeGeer (1992).

N11 National Institute of Public Health, Centre of Radiation Hygiene, Prague, Czechoslovakia. Communication to the UNSCEAR Secretariat (1992).

N12 Nabarlek Uranium Mine, Australia. Communication to the UNSCEAR Secretariat from I. Marshman (1990).

N13 National Institute of Radiological Sciences, Japan. Communication to the UNSCEAR Secretariat from H. Matsudaira (1992).

N14 National Institute of Radiation Protection, Sweden. Activity releases and ocupational exposure in the nuclear power industry. SSI-rapport 86-09 (1986), 87-19 (1987), 88-20 (1988) and 89-12 (1989).

N15 National Institute of Radiation Protection, Sweden. Communication to the UNSCEAR Secretariat from G. Bengtsson (1990).

O1 Organization for Economic Co-operation and Development, Nuclear Energy Agency. Long-term radiological aspects of management of wastes from uranium mining and milling. OECD/NEA (1984).

O2 Organization for Economic Co-operation and Development, Nuclear Energy Agency, and the International Atomic Energy Agency. Uranium - Resources, Production and Demand, 1989. OECD, Paris, 1990.

O3 Organization for Economic Co-operation and Development, Nuclear Energy Agency, and the International Atomic Energy Agency. Nuclear Energy and its Fuel Cycle. Report by an Expert Group. OECD, Paris, 1987.

O4 Organization for Economic Co-operation and Development. Emergency Preparedness for Nuclear-Powered Satellites. Stockholm, Sweden, 1989.

O5 Olympic Dam Operations, Australia. Communication to the UNSCEAR Secretariat from F. Harris (1990).

P1 Pepper, R.B. et al. Report on radioactive discharges, associated environmental monitoring and personal radiation doses resulting from operation of CEGB nuclear sites during 1986. EGB/HSD Report, HS/R222/87 (1987) and HS/R230/88 (1988).

P2 Persson, G. Fractionation phenomena in activity from an underground nuclear explosion. Health Phys. 16: 515-523 (1968).

P3 Pakistan Atomic Energy Commission. Communication to the UNSCEAR Secretariat from K. Munir-Samad (1993).

R1 Rider, B.F. Compilation of fission product yields. General Electric Co., Vallecitos Nuclear Center Report. NEDO-12154-3B ENDF-292 (1980).

R2 Ranger Uranium Mine, Australia. Communication to the UNSCEAR Secretariat from R. Auty (1990).

R3 Romanov, G.N., B.V. Nikipelov and E.G. Drozhko. The Kyshtym accident: causes, scale and radiation characteristics. p. 25-40 in: Proceedings of Seminar on Comparative Assessment of the Environmental Impact of Radionuclides Released during Three Major Nuclear Accidents: Kyshtym, Windscale, Chernobyl. EUR-13574 (1990).

R4 Rozental, J.J., C.E. de Almedia and A.H. Mendonca. Aspects of the initial and recovery phases of the radiological accident in Goiania, Brazil. p. 3-22 in: Proceedings of a Symposium on Recovery Operations in the Event of a Nuclear Accident or Radiological Emergency. STI/PUB/826. IAEA, Vienna, 1990.

S1 Schwibach, J., H. Riedel and J. Bretschneider. Investigations into the emission of Carbon-14 compounds from nuclear facilities, its measurement and the radiation exposure resulting from the emission. CEC V/3062/78 (1978).

S2 Stockholm International Peace Research Institute, SIPRI. Yearbook 1991.

S3 Shinohara, K. and T. Asano. Environmental dose assessment for low-level radioactive effluents discharged from Tokai reprocessing plant. Health Phys. 62 (1): 58-64 (1992).

S4 Short, A. and A.R. Davies. Report on radioactive discharge, and environmental monitoring at nuclear sites during 1988 and during 1989. Nuclear Electric Health and Safety Department, United Kingdom. HS/R242/89 (1989) and HS/R251/90 (1990).

S5 Sodd, V.J., R.J. Velten and E.L. Saenger. Concentrations of the medically useful radionuclides, technetium-99m and iodine-131 at a large metro-politan waste water treatment plant. Health Phys. 28: 355-359 (1975).

S6 Service Central de Protection contre les Rayonnements Ionisants, France. Communication to the UNSCEAR Secretariat from P. Pellerin (1992).

S7 Staatliches Amt für Atomsicherheit und Strahlenschutz. Interim Annual Reports of the National Board for Atomic Safety and Radiation Protection. SAAS, Germany (East) (1991).

S8 Strong, K.P., D.M. Levins and A.G. Fane. Radon diffusion through uranium tailings and earth cover. p. 713-719 in: Radiation Hazards in Mining. Society of Mining, New York, 1982.

S9 Service Central de Protection contre les Rayonnements Ionisants, France. Communication to the UNSCEAR Secretariat from J. Moroni (1992).

S10 Service Central de Protection contre les Rayonnements Ionisants, France. Annual Report, 1984.

T1 Ternovskij, I.A., G.N. Romanov, E.A. Fedorov et al. Radioactive cloud trace formation dynamics after the radiation accident in the Southern Urals in 1957: Migration processes. p. 433-437 in: Proceedings of a Symposium on Recovery Operations in the Event of a Nuclear Accident or Radiological Emergency. STI/PUB/826. IAEA, Vienna, 1990.

T2 Taiwan Power Company. Communication to the UNSCEAR Secretariat (1992).

T3 Tichler, J., K. Norden and J. Congemi. Radioactive materials released from nuclear power plants. Annual Reports 1985 to 1989. NUREG/CR-2907 and BNL-NUREG-51581, Volumes 6 to 10 (1988-1992).

T4 Trabalka, J.R. and S.I. Auerbach. One western perspective of the 1957 Soviet nuclear accident. p. 41-6999 in: Proceedings of Seminar on Comparative Assessment of the Environmental Impact of Radionuclides Released during Three Major Nuclear Accidents: Kyshtym, Windscale, Chernobyl. EUR-13574 (1990).

T5 Tsyb, A.F., V.F. Stepanenko, V.A. Pitkevich et al. Around the Semipalatinsk testing ground: radioecological situation and exposure of population in the Semipalatinsk region (based on the materials of the Interagency Commission report). J. Radiat. Med. 12: (1990).

T6 Tracy, B.L., F.A. Prantl and J.M. Quinn. Health impact of radioactive debris from the satellite cosmos 954. Health Phys. 47: 225-233 (1984).

U1 United Nations. Sources, Effects and Risks of Ionizing Radiation. United Nations Scientific Committee on the Effects of Atomic Radiation, 1988 Report to the General Assembly, with annexes. United Nations sales publication E.88.IX.7. United Nations, New York, 1988.

U3 United Nations. Ionizing Radiation: Sources and Biological Effects. United Nations Scientific Committee on the Effects of Atomic Radiation, 1982 Report to the General Assembly, with annexes. United Nations sales publication E.82.IX.8. United Nations, New York, 1982.

U4 United Nations. Sources and Effects of Ionizing Radiation. United Nations Scientific Committee on the Effects of Atomic Radiation, 1977 report to the General Assembly, with annexes. United Nations sales publication E.77.IX.1. United Nations, New York, 1977.

U5 United Nations. Ionizing Radiation: Levels and Effects. Report of the United Nations Scientific Committee on the Effects of Atomic Radiation, with annexes. United Nations sales publication E.72.IX.17 and 18. United Nations, New York, 1972.

U6 United Nations. Report of the United Nations Scientific Committee on the Effects of Atomic Radiation. Official Records of the General Assembly, Twenty-fourth Session, Supplement No. 13 (A/7613). New York, 1969.

U7 United Nations. Report of the United Nations Scientific Committee on the Effects of Atomic Radiation. Official Records of the General Assembly, Twenty-first Session, Supplement No. 14 (A/6314). New York, 1966.

U8 United Nations. Report of the United Nations Scientific Committee on the Effects of Atomic Radiation. Official Records of the General Assembly, Nineteenth Session, Supplement No. 14 (A/5814). New York, 1964.

U9 United Nations. Report of the United Nations Scientific Committee on the Effects of Atomic Radiation. Official Records of the General Assembly, Seventeenth Session, Supplement No. 16 (A/5216). New York, 1962.

U10 United Nations. Report of the United Nations Scientific Committee on the Effects of Atomic Radiation. Official Records of the General Assembly, Thirteenth Session, Supplement No. 17 (A/3838). New York, 1958.

U11 United Nations. Comprehensive study on nuclear weapons. The Secretary General's report to the General Assembly. United Nations sales publication E.81.I.11. United Nations, New York, 1981.

U12 United Nations. Comprehensive study on nuclear weapons. The Secretary-General's report to the General Assembly. Document A/45/373 (18 September 1990). United Nations, New York, 1990.

V1 Vinhas, L.A. Decontamination of the highly contaminated sites in the Goiania radiological accident. p. 39-47 in: Proceedings of a Symposium on Recovery Operations in the Event of a Nuclear Accident or Radiological Emergency. STI/PUB/826. IAEA, Vienna, 1990.

W1 Wachholz, B.W. Overview of the National Cancer Institute's activities related to exposure of the public to fallout from the Nevada test site. Health Phys. 59: 511-514 (1990).

W2 Williams, G.A. Inhalation hazard assessment at Maralinga and Emu. ARL/TR-087 (1990).

W3 Wise, K.N. and J.R. Moroney. Public health impact of fallout from British nuclear weapons tests in Australia, 1952-1957. Australian Radiation Laboratory, ARL/TR-105 (1992).

W4 World Health Organization. Selected radionuclides: tritium, carbon-14, krypton-85, strontium-90, iodine, caesium-137, radon, plutonium. Environmental Health Criteria 25. WHO, Geneva, 1983.

W5 Wismut AG, Germany (East). Communication to the UNSCEAR Secretariat from S. Richter (1991).

Z1 Zander, I. and R. Araskog. Nuclear explosions 1945-1972, basic data. FOA/A4505-A1 (1973).

ANNEX C

Medical radiation exposures

CONTENTS

INTRODUCTION

1. Ionizing radiation is widely used for both the diagnosis and treatment of injuries and disease. As a result of this practice, individuals and populations receive significant exposure to radiation, although they normally receive in return the direct benefits in health care. Nevertheless, there is a continuing need to analyse the frequencies, doses and trends of diagnostic and therapeutic medical radiation procedures worldwide. Such information permits the evaluation of regional differences in medical radiation usage, comparisons with other sources of radiation, the identification of areas of concern, and the estimation of presumed detriment. It can also be used by ministries of health and other bodies involved in optimization and other aspects of radiation protection.

2. The Committee has repeatedly assessed exposures from the medical uses of radiation. The available data have been evaluated and extrapolated to worldwide usage. In the UNSCEAR 1988 Report [U1], the Committee estimated that medical radiation exposures ranged from 0.4 to 1 mSv annually per caput. Exposures from medical radiation, which amount to less than half the exposure to natural background radiation, exceed those from all other man-made sources.

3. The purpose of this Annex is to provide an updated review and assessment of medical radiation exposures worldwide. Within this framework, there are specific objectives, such as to determine temporal and

regional trends in doses and practices; to assess how the introduction of new techniques, radiation protection measures or quality assurance programmes affect these trends; to evaluate the variations in dose for given procedures and for total practices as well as the reasons for such variations; and to examine the age distributions of patients subjected to various procedures. While some of these objectives are descriptive, they could also serve as quantitative inputs for analysis, e.g. risk-benefit analyses.

4. Medical radiation exposures arise from the diagnostic use of x rays and other external radiation sources and internally administered radioisotopes as well as from the therapeutic use of external and sealed internal sources of radiation and radiopharmaceuticals. The basic information needed for assessing medical radiation exposures is the frequency of each type of diagnostic or therapeutic procedure and the doses to all parts of the body. Since there are considerable variations in values from country to country, comprehensive data are required to make the assessment complete and accurate. From data assembled in a consistent manner over time, important trends should be apparent in exposures from medical radiation usage.

5. One impediment to the accurate assessment of medical radiation exposures has been the incompleteness or unavailability of data for many regions of the world. To improve this situation, the Committee sent a questionnaire on medical radiation usage to all States Members of the United Nations. Information was requested on examination and treatment facilities; the number, age- and sex-distribution of patients; and doses from procedures. Not all countries were able to provide the information requested, but the responses received constitute a valuable database for the Committee's evaluation, supplementing published scientific papers and reports and permitting a more complete and accurate analysis of medical radiation exposures. The Committee gratefully acknowledges the response of so many countries to the UNSCEAR Survey of Medical Radiation Usage and Exposures. The countries are listed in Part A of the References.

I. ANALYSIS OF MEDICAL EXPOSURES

6. Ionizing radiation is used for two main purposes in medicine: diagnosis and therapy. Of these, diagnosis is much more common and is experienced by many more people. The doses to persons being examined are usually quite low. Radiation therapy, by contrast, is used mainly to treat cancer patients. While a high dose delivered to a limited, predetermined location is required to kill malignant tissue, it is necessary to restrict the irradiation of surrounding normal tissues.

7. Radiation exposures from medical examinations and treatments are determined by the type and frequency of the procedure and by the doses to tissues in the radiation fields. Because of the great regional differences in the availability of medical radiation services, it is necessary to have an extensive database to evaluate the radiation exposures worldwide. Although more countries are now collecting statistics on medical radiation usage, the Committee is still forced to make rather large extrapolations to determine the total dose to all people. The availability of medical radiation data and the procedures for extrapolation and dose evaluations are discussed in this Chapter.

A. MEDICAL RADIATION USAGE

8. Not all countries are able to provide statistics on medical radiation exposures. To supplement the data that were available, the Committee undertook a survey in 1990-1991 of medical radiation usage and exposures worldwide. Questionnaires were sent to 140 countries, and over 50 responded. The data contained in these responses, combined with data in published papers, cover more medical radiation services and exposures than the data available for previous Reports of the Committee and thus permit improved worldwide dose estimates.

9. An analogous survey, but limited to six common types of x-ray examination in 24 x-ray departments in 10 European countries, was carried out by the Commission of the European Communities [M23]. Hitherto, that survey has served mainly for optimizing x-ray examination procedures rather than for describing the impact on the population of the doses from the examinations [M23, M26]. A survey of x-ray examinations in the USSR is described in a preliminary report [N4]. Two related surveys, one in China [Z6] and one in India [S40], based on sound statistical sampling have been made available to the Committee.

10. The improved database does not obviate the need for extrapolation of the available data, especially for the least developed regions of the world. In the UNSCEAR 1988 Report [U1], a good correlation was shown to exist between the number of x-ray examinations per unit of population and the number of

physicians per unit of population. Accordingly, data on diagnostic x-ray frequencies in a small number of countries could be extrapolated to estimate diagnostic x-ray frequencies in all regions of the world, based on a more widely available statistic, the number of physicians per unit population. Countries were categorized as to level of health care, based on the population per physician [U1]. In countries of health-care level I, there is at least one physician for every 1,000 population; health-care level II, one physician for 1,000-3,000 population; health-care level III, one for 3,000-10,000 population and health-care level IV, one for more than 10,000 population.

11. Although there will in future be greater reliance on the direct reporting of examination or treatment frequencies, the grouping of countries according to level of health care is retained here for the analysis of medical radiation exposures. The use of health-care levels has several advantages: it gives a basis for extrapolating data on medical radiation usage to the entire world; it allows comparing trends for different levels of health care; and it is consistent with the analysis in the UNSCEAR 1988 Report [U1].

12. The World Health Organization (WHO) has carried out two major surveys of physician densities (number of physicians per 1,000 population) [U18, W1]. The first set of data centred on the year 1977 and the second on 1984. The 1977 data were used by the Committee to evaluate medical radiation exposures for the UNSCEAR 1988 Report [U1]. It should be noted that there are uncertainties in the WHO data because physicians are defined differently in different countries.

13. There may well also be questions of the validity of assigning an average health-care level to an entire country, for such a value may obscure wide variations. As an example, Brazil, at level II (it has one physician per 1,035 population), is geographically and demographically heterogeneous, and its level of development varies greatly [C14, D4]. Urban areas such as Brasilia (one physician per 500 population) are typical of level I, while the states of Acre and Maranhao (one physician per 3,000 population) approach level III. Large countries at level I may also contain less-developed areas, and in most countries, there are differences in the availability of medical radiation in urban and rural areas. Since the correlation between medical radiation facilities and number of physicians is not absolute, the availability of medical radiology in a particular country may be better or worse than indicated by its health-care level, particularly during periods of rapid development. Ecuador moved from level II to level I between the two WHO surveys, but the density of equipment and frequencies of examination and treatment are still typical of level II countries.

14. As health care improves, it can be expected that the distribution of the world population in the four health-care categories will shift. In the 1977 survey, the distribution was as follows: 29%, 35%, 23% and 13% in levels I-IV, respectively. In the 1984 survey, it was 27%, 50%, 15% and 8%. The most significant change was the increase in the proportion of people living in countries at level II, as improvements in health care caused countries formerly at levels III and IV to move up. Using the 1984 WHO survey to determine a country's health-care level and taking into account population growth, the number of people in each health-care level in 1990 was as follows: level I, 1,350 million; level II, 2,630 million; level III, 850 million; and level IV, 460 million.

15. Table 1 indicates the level of health care and the population of the 93 countries appearing in subsequent tables or otherwise discussed in this Annex. The table also lists the information obtained by the UNSCEAR Survey of Medical Radiation Usage and Exposures on the number of radiologists and the number of x-ray units, therapy units and nuclear medicine clinics. The availability of medical radiation services in the four health-care levels of the world is summarized in Table 2, which gives the number of radiologists and the number of facilities per 1,000 population. Table 3 lists the numbers of diagnostic examinations and therapeutic treatments. While some of the respondents gave the number of patients, others may have given the number of examinations and procedures. Although the one may be a first approximation of the other, the two quantities can differ by a factor of 3 or more, depending on the procedure.

16. There are some general limitations in data obtained in surveys of medical radiation uses and exposures. Thus, estimates of countrywide values are often based on extensive extrapolations from small samples. Some data are very coarsely rounded, while others may be spuriously precise. Varying definitions (of, for example, "radiologist", "examination" or "x-ray unit") and different ways of categorizing individual procedures contribute to the variations and inexactness of all data. In some cases, national x-ray statistics may be confounded by statistics on ultrasound examinations, entered as "radiological" procedures. These uncertainties underlie the data obtained in the UNSCEAR Survey of Medical Radiation Usage and Exposures. Although the data in the Tables are given to two or sometimes even three significant figures, the statistical precision is obviously almost always less.

17. These uncertainties notwithstanding, a reasonable degree of compilation and analysis seemed feasible. The number of responses from level I countries and the completeness of these responses, should give

adequate statistical reliability. With data available for China and India, the representativeness of data on level II countries is also quite high. For countries with less-developed medical services the precision is lower, but on a worldwide basis, this has little impact on the estimation of the per caput effective dose or the collective dose from medical radiation usage.

18. Medical radiation facilities are very unevenly distributed throughout the world. Table 2 shows that the numbers of facilities per 1,000 population are from 20 to 1,000 times smaller in countries of health-care level IV than of level I, the numbers differing by a factor of up to 50 between different health-care levels. Within health-care levels there is generally a closer relationship between the number of facilities and the size of the population, but even here the variations are notable.

19. The trends observed in medical radiation facilities are uneven. At levels II-IV the availability of facilities has generally been increasing with time. At level I the number of medical and dental x-ray units and therapeutic x-ray units per unit population have decreased somewhat. Since the countries constituting the health-care level may be different for the different periods, some caution must be exercised in attributing real differences.

20. The data in Tables 2 and 3 can be used to estimate the total numbers of medical radiation facilities and usage in the world. These results are given in Table 4. The average normalized quantities have been applied to the total population of each region. The main point to note is that level I, with 25% of the world population, accounts for some 70% of the diagnostic x-ray examinations and for 90% of the patients for therapy and nuclear medicine treatments. There is still a far from equitable distribution of medical radiation services in the world.

B. DOSE EVALUATION

21. Doses to tissues and organs from medical radiation exposures are evaluated in terms of absorbed dose. For x-ray examinations, the dose without backscatter at the entrance side of the patient is specified by the air kerma. The effect of backscatter is included in the specification of the entrance surface dose. To facilitate the summary of results and the comparison with exposures from other sources of radiation, it has been the practice of the Committee to evaluate effective doses from the procedures. Along with its simplifying advantages, this quantity has limitations when applied to medical radiation exposures.

22. Earlier assessments by the Committee of medical radiation exposures in the UNSCEAR 1958, 1962 and 1972 Reports [U5, U9, U10] stressed the genetically significant dose. This gave some common measure for the uneven dose distributions from various procedures and also recognized that the age distribution of patients or individuals examined differed from that of the general population. The doses to bone marrow were also evaluated. Doses to additional organs were estimated in the UNSCEAR 1977 Report [U4]. Beginning with the UNSCEAR 1982 Report [U3] and continuing in the UNSCEAR 1988 Report [U1], the effective dose equivalent was evaluated. The Committee's decision to express patient doses in terms of effective dose is based mainly on the potential for comparisons this provides. Effective doses permit, in principle at least, comparisons between time periods, countries, health-care levels, medical methods and sources of radiation.

23. It is not possible to obtain a correct estimate of detriment from multiplication of effective doses to patients by the nominal fatality probability coefficients given by ICRP [I8]. This has several reasons [D13]. In the first place, patients are by their very nature a group which can expect to benefit from medical radiation exposure. Thus, for patients, radiation-induced detriment cannot be computed or regarded as, for example, an occupational hazard. Any analysis would not be fair without consideration of the increase in health obtained from the medical radiation usage. This is usually easily done in individual cases, but there are no general methods to compare overall hazards and benefits.

24. Another difficulty is that patients, because of their health status, may respond differently to the radiation exposures than the base population. Methods of deriving separate risk estimates for patients, which would take account of their health status, have not yet been fully developed [H17, H34]. Furthermore, the age and sex distribution of patients will rarely match that of the population for whom the nominal fatality probability coefficients of ICRP [I8] were derived. Several ways to adjust for different age and sex distributions have been suggested [S47, V9], but these have not been applied to the data in this Annex, since the purpose of using effective dose here is not to provide input for calculations of estimated detriment, but to facilitate comparisons between exposed groups.

25. Most, but not all, of the values given in this Annex were calculated as effective dose equivalents. Therefore, throughout this Annex, a distinction is made between effective dose equivalents, H_E [I1] and effective doses, E [I8]. Typical values are indicated for specific examinations. Average effective doses or effective dose equivalents refer to the arithmetical average among examined patients. Per caput doses refer to the arithmetical average in the entire popula-

tion (including non-examined individuals). Both of these may refer to specific examinations or to total doses for an entire medical radiation practice. When average or per caput doses from different countries are combined, this is normally done on a population-weighted basis.

26. The relationship between E and H_E is discussed in a number of publications [H36, L22, R27, S44, W28, Z7]. The results of dose calculations are included in Table 5. Generally lower values of effective dose compared to effective dose equivalent are obtained for examinations of the chest and skull, for mammography and for computed tomography. Higher values are obtained for examinations of the abdomen and gastro-intestinal tract. The specific values are not always consistent in the various calculations. In particular, Huda et al. [H36] obtained lower E/H_E estimates for the chest and skull and higher estimates for the abdomen than other authors. This difference is mainly attributable to the way the "remainder" dose was computed for H_E [L22, H29]. However, while the range of E/H_E values of Huda et al. [H36] is widest, with individual values ranging from 0.24 to 2.1, their average value for all examinations of 0.9 seems similar to average E/H_E values from other sources. Thus, although E/H_E values for specific types of examination may deviate from unity, the total effective doses for diagnostic x-ray examinations should be fairly similar whether computed with the 1977 or the 1990 weighting factors. This has been verified for a range of typical examinations in several countries. The E/H_E values ranged from 0.93 to 1.13, a variation that is certainly no greater than the variation in effective dose resulting from differences between countries in average patient size [G21, M43]. The average of all E/H_E values is 1.01, supporting the notion that effective doses for entire practices, such as diagnostic x-ray examinations, should be insensitive to the choice of weighting factors, even if individual examinations deviate somewhat more. It should be noted, however, that the correlation between energy imparted and effective dose becomes weaker with the ICRP 1990 [I8] weighting factors [H36].

27. The situation is similar for nuclear medicine examinations [H36, G21, G22, J8]. The average of all E/H_E values is, as for x-ray examinations, around 0.9 (Table 5). E/H_E values exceeding 1 occur mainly when the thyroid is exposed. Values of the effective dose equivalent (H_E) for most radiopharmaceuticals are listed in ICRP Publication 53 [I5]; values of the effective dose (E) for these substances are also available [I14, J9].

28. Since organ doses are in most cases not measured but calculated, the underlying assumptions and models used affect the numerical results for both organ doses and effective doses. The influence of the models for the radiation source, the human body, the radiation transport calculation and the definition of dose equivalent have been investigated in several papers [B2, D2, V7, Z15].

29. When cited papers state exposure only (expressed in C kg^{-1} or in non-SI units), this has been converted to surface air kerma using the relationship that 2.58 10^{-4} C kg^{-1} is equivalent to 8.7 10^{-3} Gy. For therapy, effective doses are not easily used for purposes of comparison. Although effective doses to radiotherapy patients are briefly discussed in this Annex, the impact of therapy is primarily described by the number of patients treated and the age- and sex-distribution of these patients.

C. BENEFITS AND RISKS

30. Exposures to patients in medical diagnostic examinations and treatments are made in anticipation of the direct benefits to be received by the patient. Usually the risk to the individual is small in comparison with the benefit, and it is easy to justify the exposure. Risk can be assessed for the exposed populations, although the procedures are not so straightforward. The dose quantities to be used in detriment evaluations were considered in the previous Section. Some general considerations on benefits and risks in medical uses of radiation are presented below.

31. In diagnostic radiography, the dose must be sufficient to obtain the desired information. If too low a dose is chosen, the image may be of unacceptably low quality [G19]. Within a relatively narrow dose band, the amount of information is generally correlated with the dose used. This is, of course, not the case when high doses are simply the result of unsatisfactory technique, for example, too large a field, the incorrect positioning of the patient or incorrect film processing (underdevelopment) in x-ray examinations. Even quite small deviations from satisfactory techniques can remove the correlation [L19]. But to some extent, there is a positive correlation between dose and information for a given technique: doses that are too low permit random noise to blur the images so that they are not clinically useful [G2]. Particularly in fluoroscopy, images may appear to improve in quality with increasing dose to the patient [B4].

32. In therapy, it is necessary that deterministic effects be induced in the target organ. In consequence, the dose to the target organ must usually exceed some threshold. Below this threshold, no benefit at all is likely to result. Above the threshold, the dose imparted to the target volume must be delivered within a

narrow range, since higher doses do not produce an extra benefit but may cause serious injury or death. This description is simplified, since the height of the threshold can be manipulated in various ways, such as with concurrent chemotherapy, but it indicates that the amount of benefit is not linearly correlated with the dose in radiotherapy.

33. The risks associated with the diagnostic uses of ionizing radiation are normally limited to late stochastic effects, which are estimated to occur at a frequency of perhaps 0.01% for an average examination (deterministic skin damage may occur after fluoroscopy in extreme cases). At the individual level, these risks are almost always small compared to the benefit of diagnosis and treatment. They may also help to avert a competing risk; for instance, cardiac fluoroscopy could entail entrance surface doses of several gray, possibly even inducing deterministic skin damage, but might obviate the need for open heart surgery. In contrast, the risks associated with radiotherapy treatment involve deterministic effects, which must be induced to a sufficient extent, and also late stochastic effects, which can occur in about 10% of therapy courses [W10]. In fact, second cancers in radiotherapy patients are important sources of data for the assessment of radiation risks.

34. From a radiation protection point of view, doses should be maintained as low as reasonably achievable. This means that exposures above clinically acceptable minimum doses, must be avoided. There is much potential for reducing the risks associated with medical radiation exposures for diagnostic or therapeutic purposes. While radiation protection is outside the scope of this Annex, the considerations involved influence the doses encountered and therefore merit mention here. The Annex discusses some ways of reducing doses from specific procedures. In particular, quality control programmes are setting targets for facilities whose doses are excessive, thereby reducing average doses.

35. Mass screening programmes continue to come under scrutiny, and in most countries mass lung screening programmes have been reduced or eliminated. Mammography screening programmes, however, are expanding. Nationwide breast screening programmes and policies are in effect in Finland, the Netherlands, Sweden and the United Kingdom. Several other European countries, Australia, New Zealand and several provinces in Canada have decided to start such programmes [V17]. The benefits of such programmes are diminished if the screening procedures subsequently induce breast cancers. Since the frequency of breast cancer increases with age and the radiosensitivity of the breast decreases with age, the relative benefit of screening is much greater in older women. The question of suitable age to start screening and how often to repeat it (in other words, the question of when the benefit outweighs the detriment) has been studied by several authors [A6, A8, D3, D6, I10, M25, V1, W11]. These considerations apply only to mass screening programmes. In clinical examinations of women in whom breast cancer is already suspected, correctly performed mammography will virtually always be beneficial.

36. There is certainly merit in seeking to restrict doses when the radiological procedures are readily available. For most of the developing countries, however, the more important need may be to expand the availability of medical radiation services. Health will improve with such an expansion, and therefore an increased collective dose to the population due to higher examination frequency would be justified. Even here, however, it is important to maintain equipment in proper order and to introduce modern techniques to optimize the radiation exposures that are made for medical purposes.

D. SUMMARY

37. Medical radiation facilities are very unevenly distributed in the world. Four levels of health care have been defined, based on physician densities. Level I comprises countries with fewer than 1,000 persons per physician, level II countries have 1,000-3,000, level III, 3,000-10,000 and level IV, more than 10,000 persons per physician. Some 26% of the world population resides in level I countries, 50% in level II, 16% in level III and 9% in level IV countries. The data provided in response to the UNSCEAR Survey of Medical Radiation Usage and Exposures indicate that in 1990, there were 210,000 radiologists worldwide, 720,000 diagnostic x-ray units, 1.6 billion x-ray examinations performed and 6 million patients undergoing some form of radiotherapy. Some 70% of these medical radiation services were available in countries of health-care level I and the remaining 30% to the three quarters of the world population that live in countries of health-care levels II-IV.

38. Medical irradiation entails benefits to the patient as well as detriment from the radiation exposure. Radiation protection is not in itself a subject of this Annex, but its effect on medical exposure is discussed where relevant. Doses to patients are described in terms of effective dose or effective dose equivalent, depending on which of these quantities were available. The quantity effective dose (or effective dose equivalent) was chosen to facilitate comparisons, but it is not used in any calculations aimed at assessments of detriment to patients. Instead, effective doses have

been supplemented, where possible, with basic data on entrance surface doses or administered activity to facilitate comparisons. For therapy patients, no single type of dose quantity permits a valid determination of radiological impact, so the assessment of this practice is based primarily on the numbers of patients receiving various treatments, with effective dose used as supplementary information.

II. DIAGNOSTIC X RAY EXAMINATIONS

39. Of the medical uses of radiation, the examination of patients with x rays for diagnostic purposes is by far the most frequent practice. Such examinations are performed in all kinds of health care establishments, including hospitals and medical clinics but also, e.g. chiropractic and podiatric clinics in many countries.

40. Although the doses from diagnostic x-ray examinations are generally relatively low, the magnitude of the practice makes for a significant radiological impact. National data on diagnostic medical x-ray examinations, provided in response to the UNSCEAR Survey of Medical Radiation Usage and Exposures and supplemented with published data, are evaluated in this Chapter.

41. Although the frequencies of examinations and dose data are becoming available for many more countries than in earlier UNSCEAR Reports, it is important to remember the limitations of these data. Often, estimates in the Tables are based on quite small and not necessarily unbiased samples. Minor differences between countries or examinations should therefore not be overinterpreted. In general, values for examinations and procedures are given to two significant figures, while summary data are shown with one significant figure.

A. FREQUENCIES OF EXAMINATIONS

42. Annual numbers of diagnostic medical x-ray examinations reported by different countries span several orders of magnitude. They are shown in relation to the population of the country and its level of health care in Figure I; data for 1985-1990 are used for level I and data for 1980-1990 are used for levels II-IV to encompass a greater number of countries. Countries of health-care level I fall on the upper edge of the distribution; countries of lower health-care levels show fewer examinations at the same relative populations. When the same data (numbers of examinations) are plotted against the number of physicians, a much tighter correlation is evident. Only four countries fall somewhat below the general distribution: Ecuador, Honduras, Myanmar and Peru. It could be that the pattern of examinations is different in these countries, but it is more likely that the number of examinations has been underestimated. For instance, information from private practice is often unavailable. It could also be that the number of physicians has been overestimated; the definition of a physician is not standard, so this possibility should also be considered. On the whole, however, using the number of physicians as the basis for extrapolating from averaged reported data to the number of examinations worldwide seems well founded.

43. The total annual frequencies (number of examinations per 1,000 population) of all diagnostic medical x-ray examinations performed in a country are listed in Table 6 and illustrated in Figure II. The distribution of frequencies at each level is approximately log-normal. The range in level I countries is a factor of 6 (200-1,280 examinations per 1,000 population) and an order of magnitude or more in levels II and III (15-520 and 10-180 examinations per 1,000 population, respectively). Only one value is available for level IV from the present survey (Rwanda: 9 examinations per 1,000 population); this has been supplemented in this Figure by values available for Cote d'Ivoire and Nigeria for 1977 (40 and 25 examinations per 1,000 population). Examination frequencies for individual patients or years may of course deviate considerably from these annual average values. Repeated examinations of small subsets of the population are discussed in Section II.F.3.

44. Most data on examination frequencies were obtained by surveys or registrations that were complete enough to give representative results. In some cases, however, only small samplings were available that may not adequately reflect the availability of medical radiation services in the country. The frequency for Turkey, for example, is based on data from a single urban centre serving only 1% of the population of the country. This very likely explains why it is so different from the frequencies in other countries of health-care level II, and this should be recognized in

deriving the average values. In other cases, samples may be adequate in size but not completely representative. For example, the frequency for Brazil seems to be based on public hospitals only.

45. There are questions about the results for other countries as well. According to the 1984 WHO survey of the number of physicians in various countries [U18], Ecuador has moved from level II to the borderline of level I. The frequency of examinations remains, however, clearly typical of level II, so the classification has not yet been changed in this analysis.

46. There is no question about the health-care level for the United States, but the value for examination frequency in 1985-1990 of 800 per 1,000 population rests on considerable extrapolation. Some information indicates that the estimate could be an underestimate by up to 60% [B10, G8, M2]. Comprehensive statistics on medical radiation are often inadequate for collective dose evaluation. Many countries emphasize the delivery of medical services and pay less attention to the collection of data that might be needed to evaluate the collective radiological impact, which is anyway a secondary consideration. That said, however, estimates of examination frequencies are more broadly based than ever and are contributing to more reliable estimates of worldwide values.

47. The population-weighted frequencies of examinations in 57 countries are summarized in Table 6. Since the values for some larger countries are usually above the median values, slightly higher values are derived for the population-weighted averages. These values are 890 and 120 examinations per 1,000 population in countries of health-care levels I and II, respectively, for 1985-1990 and 64 examinations per 1,000 population in countries of health-care levels III and IV combined. Average frequencies of examination have generally been increasing. Data are not available to show trends in individual countries to any great extent, except at level I. Examinations in Thailand (level III) increased by 50% between the first period and the successive periods, and examinations in China increased by 30% between the second and third periods. At health-care level I, a few countries showed downward trends: Czechoslovakia, Finland, the Netherlands, Norway, Romania and Sweden. Increases were apparent for Canada, Cuba, the Federal Republic of Germany, France, Japan and Malta.

48. Data on specific types of examinations are summarized in Table 7. The average frequencies are the population-weighted values (i.e. the total number of examinations divided by the total population of reporting countries). They are best suited for the evaluation of collective doses. These and other statistical parameters are summarized in Table 8. The standard deviations on the unweighted average values may be used to identify unusually high or low frequencies of examinations. For example, examinations of the chest in the RSFSR of the former Soviet Union, examinations of the abdomen and gastro-intestinal tract and computed tomography in Japan and urography, angiography and mammography in the Federal Republic of Germany exceeded the average values in 1985-1990 by more than two times the standard deviations. There may be medical or other explanations for the greater frequency of specific examinations.

49. The trends in examination frequencies are illustrated in Figure III. These are the population-weighted averages of available data. The composition of the groups may vary from one period to another, thus affecting the comparisons. Countries of health-care level I are well represented. At level II, China and India are represented in the more recent periods, which helps the reliability of results. Too few data are available for countries of health-care levels III and IV to give reliable averages.

50. The main type of examination at all levels is that of the chest. This examination made up 60% of the total in level I countries during 1985-1990 and 70% in all other countries. Examinations of extremities, the remainder of the skeleton and the digestive system (abdomen and gastro-intestinal tract) accounted for just over 10% each of the total in level I countries and just under 10% in other countries. This leaves about 10% for other more specialized examinations in countries of health-care level I and only a few per cent for these examinations in all other countries.

51. Almost all examinations are being performed with increasing frequency, especially in countries of health-care levels II-IV. There are differences between countries with respect to the most prominent trends, however. In countries of health-care level II-IV the largest increase is in examinations of the chest (from 10 to 100 and from 20 to 50 examinations per 1,000 population in levels II and III-IV, respectively). In countries of health-care level I, the most notable increases are in computed tomography and examinations of the skull and abdomen. Mammography examinations increased threefold in level I countries in 1985-1990, compared with earlier periods.

52. A decreasing trend is noted for examinations of the chest in level I countries. This could be the result of the decreasing emphasis on mass screening programmes. Examinations of the extremities, the spine and the gastro-intestinal tract and urography-cholecystography reached stable levels during the last two five-year periods.

53. There are wide variations in examination frequencies between countries, even if they are geographically close and culturally and economically similar. The total frequencies of examinations in European countries differ by a factor of 3. A comparative investigation in France, Italy and the United Kingdom found differences which indicate that medical exposures are not justified in the same way in these countries [C2]. The frequencies of x-ray examinations in the Nordic countries varied by over 50% in 1982 from 500 to 800 per 1,000 population [S14], with the highest frequency in Finland, primarily because more radiological examinations took place outside of hospitals at health centres and private clinics. The frequency of colon examinations is fairly similar in the five Nordic countries, while stomach examinations are more frequent in Norway, primarily because endoscopy is less used. Cholecystography is performed about twice as frequently in Sweden as in other Nordic countries, presumably because there are fewer radiologists who could perform ultrasonographic examinations. Sweden has the highest frequency of mammography, because the Government recommends screening, while Denmark and Norway have no screening apart from minor research projects.

54. Statistics may be less accessible in health care systems where medical care is largely private and thus decentralized. They may also be less reliable; for instance, the increase in the number of x-ray examinations at hospitals in the United States could be due to a shift from private clinics to hospitals, making the change more apparent than real [N1]. While comparisons may be indicative, they must always be treated very cautiously. The definitions, methods of examination, methods of measurement and other conditions may vary greatly between studies. Thus, similarities and differences may be spurious and conclusions may be false, even in the rare cases where a formal analysis of statistical significance seems technically feasible. There may also be regional differences within countries. The frequencies of diagnostic x-ray examinations in the different republics of the former USSR are estimated to have ranged from 500 to over 1,100 per 1,000 population in 1987 [S18]. Thus, even with centrally organized health care systems, differences may occur.

55. Computed tomography is rapidly becoming a very important diagnostic technique. The number of computed tomography scanners in the United States in 1980 was 6.7 per million population, while the figure for Japan was 25 per million in 1984. In the United States, the number of computed tomography scanners in hospitals increased from 3 million in 1980 to 12.3 million in 1990 [M2]. In New Zealand, there were about 5 per million in early 1988, expected to be 20 per million within a few years [P11]. A study in Manitoba, Canada, showed the number of computed tomography scans steadily increasing, from 200 per month in 1977 to 1,500 per month in 1987 [H4]. The number of computed tomography scanners in the United Kingdom has increased from 1 scanner in 1972 to over 200 in 1990 [S42]. The relative frequency of such examinations in the United Kingdom is now estimated to be over 20 per 1,000 population [S42], contributing 20% of the collective effective dose from x-ray examinations [S43].

56. The data in Table 8 show an unweighted average value of 22 computed tomography examinations per 1,000 population in countries of health-care level I, with more than 30 per 1,000 population in Australia and the Federal Republic of Germany, 50 per 1,000 population in Belgium and 97 per 1,000 population in Japan. In the UNSCEAR 1988 Report [U1], the average frequency of computed tomography examinations in countries of health-care level I was estimated to be 9 per 1,000 population. An upward revision would, therefore, seem justified. The procedure is used at negligible frequency in all countries of health-care levels II-IV: some 2 examinations per 1,000 population, at most, with many countries reporting none of these examinations.

B. AGE- AND SEX-DISTRIBUTIONS

57. The age- and sex-distribution of patients in diagnostic x-ray examinations, and the population-weighted averages of these for each of the health-care levels, are given in Table 9. Broadly speaking, patients subjected to x-ray examinations are older than randomly chosen members of the public. This does not necessarily mean that x-ray examinations of children are rare. Many examinations are in fact rather frequent in children (in particular, those of the chest, the extremities, the skull, the pelvis/hips and the abdomen, and urography).

58. For level II-IV countries, the fraction of the patients that are children is larger than for level I countries. This difference is statistically significant. However, the frequency of child examinations may still be lower than in level I countries, since the total examination frequency is much lower. Although the detail is not given in Table 9, reports indicate that the examination of infants and young children is not infrequent. The per caput effective dose equivalent to children in the Federal Republic of Germany in 1983 was estimated to be 30% of the effective dose equivalent to an adult [M15].

59. These general conclusions from Table 9 are in agreement with observations in the UNSCEAR 1988

Report [U1], where it was also pointed out that the greater proportion of children in the populations of countries of health-care levels II-IV is reflected in a higher share (compared to level I countries) of children among examined patients. The differences in population age structure appear to be sufficient to explain the differences in patient age. The average ages for countries contributing data for Table 9 could be roughly calculated to be 34 years at level I, 27 years at level II and 24 years at level III. Similarly, the roughly calculated average ages for patients are 44, 36 and 38 years. Thus, the average person in a level II or III country is 7-10 years younger than the average person in a level I country, and the average patient in level II or III countries is 6-8 years younger than the average patient in a level I country.

60. The sex distributions do not deviate widely from the distribution of males and females in the population. The excess of women undergoing cholecystography in countries of health-care level I is well known and may possibly be related to diet. Likewise, the excess of women in level I countries having lower gastro-intestinal tract examinations was recognized in the UNSCEAR 1988 Report [U1]. The excess of women in countries of health-care level I having pelvis/hip examinations is probably associated with femoral fractures and hip joint replacements in older women. The data indicate consistently fewer female patients in level II and level III countries than in level I countries, which, if correct, may reflect an uneven distribution of medical care in different countries.

C. DOSES IN EXAMINATIONS

61. Estimates of doses to patients in diagnostic x-ray examinations, derived largely from the UNSCEAR Survey of Medical Radiation Usage and Exposures, are listed in Table 10. The primary quantity shown is average entrance surface dose, ESD, per examination. The dose-area product, DAP, was reported in one or two cases, but these values are not included in the Table. Both quantities are readily measurable. When reported in response to the UNSCEAR Survey of Medical Radiation Usage and Exposures, effective doses (or effective dose equivalents) are also listed in Table 10. Effective dose can be calculated from ESD or DAP if the projection, tube kilovoltage and beam filtration are known [B23, G23, H27, J3, R23, R24, R28, S45] and, if necessary, corrected for patient size and anatomy [L24, L25, S46]. A reasonable approximation of effective dose without such detailed information is possible from DAP [L23] but difficult from ESD. In the absence of such data, effective doses were not calculated.

62. Population-weighted average values of effective dose equivalent for specific examinations are summarized in Table 11 and illustrated in Figure IV. In line with earlier studies, average doses are comparatively high for gastro-intestinal tract examinations, about 4-7 mSv at health-care level I. Angiography and computed tomography also confer relatively high doses, about 4-7 mSv. Urography doses are about 3 mSv. Cholecystography and lumbosacral spinal examinations give doses of 1.5-2 mSv. Effective dose equivalents from examinations of the abdomen or of the pelvis/hip are of about 1 mSv. Fluoroscopic chest examinations are also associated with doses around 1 mSv, while chest radiography gives average doses of 0.14 mSv, and fluorographic mass miniature examinations, 0.5 mSv. Examinations of the skull or extremities cause average effective dose equivalents of 0.05-0.15 mSv. The average for mammography, 1 mSv, may be spuriously high due to a very high value (9.5 mSv) reported from Czechoslovakia (values of about 0.5 mSv are reported from several countries).

63. The average effective dose equivalents in countries of health-care level I, illustrated in Figure IV, indicate that, for the same examination, the doses were consistently higher in 1970-1979 than in 1980-1990. This does not necessarily mean, however, that per caput effective dose equivalents are decreasing, since the spectrum of examination changes as well. Computed tomography was already mentioned above as one example of the developments that affect collective doses appreciably.

64. Comparison of the average doses from examination in countries of health-care levels I and II in 1980-1990 is also illustrated in Figure IV (earlier data are not available for level II, and data are altogether insufficient for levels III and IV). No consistent difference is apparent: reported doses for level II are about twice those for level I for examinations of the lumbosacral spine, pelvis and hip, 20% higher than level I doses for upper gastro-intestinal tract examinations, similar to level I doses for cholecystography and for skull examinations; half the level I doses for urography and for examinations of the extremities; and less than half the level I doses for examinations of the chest, abdomen and the lower gastro-intestinal tract. While based on only two countries (China and India), the averages for level II refer to a large population. Nevertheless, apparent differences between health-care levels should be interpreted very cautiously. Some reported differences between China and India are bigger than the apparent differences between the averages of different health-care levels. It seems highly likely that dose differences of similar magnitude occur within these large countries. Conditions in China or India may also be quite different from conditions in other countries of

level II or in countries of level III or IV, where the more frequent use of fluoroscopy may cause higher doses.

65. Numerous factors of technique contribute to the dose variation observed. Several such factors are listed in Table 12, which compiles both general information [N5] and information originally aimed at mammography [R18, S56] but relevant also in a general context. Patient size is not listed in Table 12, since it is not a controllable factor of technique, but it contributes appreciably to variation [L24, L25, V3], also between countries. For instance, the weight of the reference Japanese adult male is 61.5 kg and the female 51.5 kg [T5], compared with 70 kg (male) and 60 kg (female) of the ICRP reference man [I2].

66. Variations in dose for specific procedures are discussed in more detail below. These include (a) fluoroscopy, because of its significant impact on procedures and per caput doses; (b) computed tomography, because of its rapid growth; (c) chest examinations, since they are so frequent; (d) mammography, with a view to its use in screening programmes; (e) chiropractic examinations, since they are not well known; and (f) neonatal and child examinations, because these patients may be more radiosensitive than adults.

1. Fluoroscopy

67. Traditional fluoroscopy (in which a fluorescent screen receives an image) and photofluorography (in which the image on the screen is recorded photographically or electronically) often cause high absorbed doses in the patient. There are two reasons for this: dose rates may be high and exposure times may be long. There are wide variations in patient exposures, even for the same type of examination, between patients, between equipment and between radiologists (see, e.g. [R1]). Modern equipment with image intensifiers may mean that fluoroscopy and photofluorography do not cause relatively higher doses. The imaging properties of image intensifiers have improved, and the input screen size can now be large. Based on these technical developments, a dose reduction of about one half was possible with large-screen image intensifier photofluorography instead of screen/film radiography (with full-size images) in posterior/anterior (PA) projection in scoliosis examinations [M5]. A Swiss study of older and newer fluoroscopy units for chest screening purposes revealed a 30-fold range in dose rates. Entrance surface doses ranging from 0.1 mGy for the most modern unit to 2.2 mGy for an old mobile unit were observed, the lower value being one third of the entrance surface dose observed in the same study for screen/film radiography [M37]. Nonetheless, modern equipment may also have a potential for high doses, but for somewhat different reasons. For instance, high-level fluoroscopic boost options for image enhancement can contribute to high doses and may be easily activated, e.g. by a simple foot pedal [C12].

68. Thus, fluoroscopy can cause a high dose to an examined patient. Furthermore, its widespread use in countries of health-care levels II-IV contributes to high collective patient doses [U1]. But where the Basic Radiology System developed by the World Health Organization [W3] is installed, there seems to be a potential for substantial dose reductions, which are not yet reflected in reported data (see Table 10). Trials at a Swedish hospital [H7] indicate that doses for common examinations could be reduced by 80% [C2] or even more in comparison with older fluorographic systems. Trials in Colombia [W3], which show doses less than half of those observed in the United States, seem to corroborate these results. Furthermore, the effective dose equivalents for specific examinations (see Table 10) do not appear to be consistently higher in level II countries than in level I countries. For levels III and IV, information is insufficient to draw any conclusion, but higher doses may be suspected, owing to, for one thing, the absence of stable voltage in many countries [B18].

69. Interventional radiology describes procedures in which the physician utilizes radiology for guidance before, during or after surgery or in relation to other examinations or treatments. Some examples are the placement of catheters for drainage, stone extraction, recanalization, the dilatation or occlusion of vessels and the infusion of pharmaceuticals, as well as the needle biopsy of various lesions. The dilatation of vessels by percutaneous transluminal angioplasty may be peripheral (PTA) or cardiac (PTCA). Most of these procedures require lengthy periods of fluoroscopy and may impart high doses to patients and staff. On the other hand, the frequency of these often life-saving procedures is low. The total frequency of interventional radiology in Nordic countries varies from 0.3 to 0.8 per 1,000 population [S14]. Of these, the higher values are obtained in countries with a high frequency of percutaneous nephrostomy. PTCA, with potentially very high doses, is practised at a rate of 0.03 to 0.05 procedures per 1,000 population [S14]. The number of PTCA procedures in the United States increased to an estimated 400,000 in 1990 [K29].

70. Average effective dose equivalents in interventional radiology were determined by Diaz-Romero et al. [D18] for 1,389 patients at Tenerife, Canary Islands. The results included an adjustment factor of 0.85 to take account of the age distribution of patients (see Section I.B and [H4]). After recalcula-

tion to remove the adjustment factor, the effective dose equivalents (H_E) ranged from 1.9 mSv (for nephro-urinary procedures) to 15 mSv (for abdominal arteriography). Some specific dose data and other information are given below for cardiac, cerebral and nephro-urogenital interventional radiology, as well as for other types of fluoroscopy. Gonad doses for some interventional radiology procedures are available [V14]. Fluoroscopically guided fallopian tube recanalization as a treatment for infertility has been attracting interest recently. Average absorbed ovarian doses of 8.5 ± 5.6 mGy (corresponding to an effective dose equivalent of about 2 mSv) were recorded by Hedgpeth et al. [H45].

71. The greatest radiation dose to individual patients in fluoroscopy is associated with the imaging of the heart (interventional or otherwise). Skin doses in cardiac angiography often approach 1 Gy, and during coronary angioplasty skin doses between 1 and 5 Gy were recorded for 31 patients in an Australian study [H1]. A maximum skin dose of 43 Gy (for 1 hour of fluoroscopy and 2 minutes of digital subtraction angiography) is quoted in Finland [P12], corresponding to an effective dose equivalent of about 1,400 mSv. This was a unique case, and typical skin doses were around 1 Gy (corresponding to an effective dose equivalent of about 10 mSv). In a French study, Moroni et al. [M30] highlighted some special situations with very long exposure times in angiography or catheterization, such as the sampling of pancreatic hormone to detect mute cancer or hepatic embolizations. Entrance surface doses of 2 Gy and gonad doses (outside the primary beam) of 3.2 mGy were observed in single examinations. A study in the United Kingdom [T9] reported that entrance surface doses of up to 1 Gy were in the normal range for digital subtraction angiography (including the associated fluoroscopy).

72. Some variations are difficult to assess. Patient doses differed significantly between cardiologists in one hospital in the Netherlands, but not in another one [K1]. Digital subtraction angiography (DSA) with pulsed high dose-rate fluoroscopy should permit patient doses to be reduced to about one third of the dose in conventional angiography. To some extent, however, this may be offset by more liberal use of the procedure [J6, P2]. The range of entrance surface doses and organ absorbed doses in angiography enumerated in two reviews [S37, V14] are summarized in Table 13. For cerebral angiography during the embolization of arteriovenous malformations, effective dose equivalents to patients of 6-43 mSv were recorded [B29] for entrance surface doses of 170-1,400 mGy, a range exceeding that given in Table 13. In another study [F3], effective dose equivalents in cerebral angiography ranged from 2.7 to 23 mSv (average: 10.6 mSv). Of this dose, fluoroscopy contributed 67%, cut films 26% and DSA 7%. Absorbed doses to organs in the head in conventional and DSA in the Federal Republic of Germany were given in [G17]. DSA caused lower orbital doses; conventional angiography produced lower doses in the cervical marrow, the cerebellum and the parotid glands.

73. While imaging of the heart causes high individual doses, the collective dose is mainly influenced by the much more frequent fluoroscopic examinations of the gastro-intestinal tract. In the United States, these cause average effective dose equivalents per examination of 2.4 mSv (upper gastro-intestinal tract examination) and 4.1 mSv (barium enema). Due to the frequent use of these examinations, they produce annual collective effective dose equivalents of 18,500 and 19,900 man Sv, respectively. Together, this is over 40% of the annual collective dose due to diagnostic x rays in the United States [N1]. Fluoroscopy time in gastro-intestinal tract examinations is an important source of dose variation [H33]. Screening time can be reduced significantly with no loss of examination quality [H14]. This, coupled with radiation protection attention [B4, S54], means that decreasing doses per examination are to be expected. Of course, examinations causing very low doses have little impact even if they are frequent. Fluoroscopy of the extremities produces absorbed doses of a few milligray [C11] and effective dose equivalents of 0.1 mSv or less.

74. In Japan, effective dose equivalents per examination of the upper gastro-intestinal tract were found to be 2.1 mSv for radiography and 2.8 mSv for fluoroscopy, with a total of 5 mSv when both procedures were utilized. Owing to the frequent use of these examinations, they cause annual collective effective dose equivalents of about 35,200 man Sv (radiography) and about 43,400 man Sv (fluoroscopy). This is about 43% of the total annual collective effective dose equivalent from all x-ray diagnostic examinations in Japan [M4]. Suleiman et al. [S34] reported the following absorbed doses for upper gastro-intestinal tract examinations in the United States, apparently indicating somewhat lower effective dose equivalents than in Japan: thyroid, 0.2-3.5 mGy, lung, 0.9-4.2 mGy, red bone marrow, 0.8-5.4 mGy and uterus, 0.2-1.0 mGy (all numbers refer to the sum of radiography and fluoroscopy). In another survey in the United States, enteroclysis caused entrance surface doses three times higher than dedicated peroral small bowel study (123 ± 60 mGy as opposed to 46 ± 21 mGy) [T14].

75. In extracorporeal shock-wave lithotripsy, fluoroscopic x-ray imaging is used to localize renal stones. One estimate from the United States of a likely surface air kerma was about 225 mGy [L1]. Other estimates, also from the United States, gave surface

doses of 10-300 mGy, with average female gonadal doses of about 1 mGy [B1, G13]. The dose increased with increasing stone burden and patient weight, and stones in the ureter resulted in higher average doses than renal stones [C8]. The introduction of a radiation control programme in the United States permitted exposure reductions of between 20% and 60% [G5]. An investigation in Canada produced similar values, with an average entrance surface dose of 140 mGy, corresponding to an effective dose equivalent of about 0.8 mSv [H5]. Average surface doses of 30-34 mGy were observed in Taiwan [C20]. The authors attributed their relatively low doses to, among other things, small average patient size, which permitted low current for spot films.

76. An alternative to extracorporeal lithotripsy is percutaneous lithotomy. In this procedure, fluoroscopy is used to localize the renal stones for extraction. A Swedish study reported an average effective dose equivalent to the patient of 4.2 mSv (range: 0.60-8.3 mSv) [G4]. In Finland, percutaneous nephrostomy (which is a part of percutaneous lithotripsy) generated entrance surface doses to patients of 160 mGy [V13]. Thus, the newer technique of extracorporeal lithotripsy does not seem to cause higher radiation exposure; if anything it does the reverse [V13]. An investigation in the United Kingdom [R3] gave similar results. Extracorporeal renal stone lithotripsy has been much more successful than the corresponding technique for gallstones [M33]. Although gallstones are more frequent, only a limited number of patients are suited to such treatments [Z5], so the frequency of this procedure is not expected to increase markedly.

77. Numerous suggestions for reducing doses in fluoroscopy have been made. During placement of feeding tubes, a procedure that is not diagnostic and does not require an image of high quality, order-of-magnitude dose reductions (from entrance surface doses of about 300 mGy) were achieved by removing the anti-scatter grid and increasing the iris of the video camera [R20]. Similar reductions were possible for nasoenteral tube placements [R13]. This is of significance, since many of the patients in question are exposed to these procedures repeatedly. A broader overview of measures to reduce doses in fluoroscopy has been published [I13].

2. Computed tomography

78. In computed tomography (CT), the conditions of exposure are quite different from those in conventional x-ray imaging. This has required the development of specific techniques for assessing patient dose from computed tomography. Usually, the dose in a single CT slice is estimated using either the computed tomography dose index (CTDI) or the multiple-scan average dose (MSAD) [C23, C24]. CTDI is defined as the integral along the axial, z, direction of a single-slice dose profile, D(z), divided by the nominal slice width. MSAD is the average dose across the central slice from several contiguous slices. These two parameters are related, and, under certain conditions, are identical for 7 mm thick slices. For thicker slices, MSAD underestimates CTDI, by 10%-15% for a 10 mm slice [C23]. Entries under ESD in Table 10 are actually such slice doses, as indicated in a footnote. From slice doses, organ doses and, ultimately, effective doses can be estimated [J7, S43, Z16]. Studies in the Nationwide Evaluation of X-ray Trends (NEXT) programme in the United States in 1990 [C23] indicated MSADs in examinations of the head of, usually, 34-55 mGy, although doses as high as 140 mGy were encountered.

79. The dose per examination by computed tomography varies with the type of examination. On average, the effective dose equivalent to patients undergoing such examinations was 3.2 mSv in a study in Manitoba, Canada, in 1987 [H4]. Since there were 18.2 examinations per 1,000 inhabitants in Manitoba, computed tomography contributed 0.06 mSv to the annual per caput dose from medical exposure. Effective doses, as well as effective dose equivalents, in 1989 for specific examinations and for all computed tomography in the United Kingdom were compiled by Shrimpton et al. [S43]. On average, the effective dose is lower than the effective dose equivalent by a factor of 0.7, with ratios for specific examinations ranging from 0.5 to 1.5. Only for the cervical spine is the ratio greater than unity. Their results, and associated data on examination frequency [S42], are summarized in Table 14. Absorbed organ doses recorded in the same project are given by Jones and Shrimpton [J7]. Detailed information on eye lens and gonadal doses during computed tomography were given by Rosenkranz et al. [R2].

80. In computed tomography, the absorbed dose for a given examination varied by a factor of 3 in New Zealand [P11], and a factor of 5 in Sweden [M1] and the United Kingdom [C9]. In Japan, the effective dose equivalent for the same examination varied by a factor of up to 3.5, depending on the scanner unit [N8]. Table 15 summarizes some of the dose data obtained in that study. Panzer et al. [P3] noted even greater variation, by a factor of up to 10, with 122 scanners in the Federal Republic of Germany. Researchers in the USSR found that some dose variability was unavoidable due to the clinical situation [A1], but apparently some of the variation could be removed. This would be important, since the general use of computed tomography is increasing at the same time as doses per examination are also increasing [H4]. Siddle et al.

discussed variation between scanner units [S29] and between procedures [S30] in Australia in connection with the risk of causing cataracts in the eye lens. They concluded that while neither scanner variation nor procedure variation led to doses approaching the threshold for cataracts in their studies, a potential for such doses does exist. A low-dose technique for computed tomography orbital volume measurements reduces lens doses from over 100 to 11 mGy [M24].

81. In some cases, the dose from a computed tomography examination is lower than the dose from similar examinations with conventional techniques. For instance, conventional myelography of the lumbar spine gives effective doses equivalents that are five to nine times higher than those for computed tomography of the same region (H_E = 9-18 mSv compared to 1-2 mSv), while effective dose equivalents are similar for the two techniques for cervical spine myelography (about 2 mSv) [H28]. However, patient doses from computed tomography examinations are typically an order of magnitude higher than those from conventional x-ray diagnostic examination, as reported in the Federal Republic of Germany [P10] and in the United Kingdom [S43].

82. Fetal doses in computed tomography examinations of pregnant patients were evaluated by Felmlee et al. [F6] and Panzer et al. [P9]. Both articles provide the necessary formulae for dose calculation. Felmlee et al. concluded that clinically required head scans can be performed with little or no dose to the fetus, and that the prudent use of body scans can be considered.

83. Several European countries are at present collaborating on quality assurance measures to reduce the variability in doses from comparable computed tomography scans [C9]. Such efforts at reduction are expected to reduce average doses (or rather, since both the number of examinations and the dose per examination are increasing for other reasons, as detailed above, to limit the rate of increase). Equipment failure can, of course, increase doses; as an example, the accidental loss of filtration increased entrance surface doses in head and body scans by some 25% [Y2].

3. Chest examinations

84. Individual doses are usually low in radiographic chest examinations. Digital computed radiography could permit even smaller doses than screen/film radiography (although some effort might be required to achieve acceptable image quality) [J10, K24, L19, M34]. As an example of doses in conventional chest radiography, the effective dose equivalent averaged over all chest x-ray units in Manitoba, Canada, and over all projections in 1987 was 0.07 mSv [H24]. The authors stressed that lateral projections (taken in addition to posterior/anterior or anterior/posterior in 70% of the Manitoba examinations) contributed most to the effective dose equivalent for a chest examination. For posterior/anterior only, the average entrance surface dose was 0.12 mGy, corresponding to an effective dose equivalent of about 0.02 mSv. For lateral projections, an average entrance surface dose of 0.59 mGy (corresponding to an effective dose equivalent of about 0.06 mSv) was calculated based on phantom measurements [H6].

85. A collaborative study in Sweden and the United States [L6] found that the entrance surface air kerma for posterior/anterior chest projections was 0.16 mGy in Sweden and 0.14 mGy in the United States (all Swedish facilities and 75% of United States facilities use scatter suppression, mostly grids and in a few cases air gap). These similar average doses are the result of quite different underlying conditions. Since grids typically increase the dose by a factor of 2 or 3, an even higher dose could have been expected in Sweden. Slower screen/film systems in Sweden would act in the same direction. On the other hand, in Sweden, higher tube voltage, more appropriate total filtration, the absence of single-phase units, overprocessing and a mandatory quality assurance programme all act in the direction of lower doses. As a rough approximation, the air kerma values divided by 0.75 correspond to entrance surface doses with backscatter. Using this approximation, the entrance surface doses are $0.16 \div 0.75 = 0.21$ mGy in Sweden and $0.14 \div 0.75 = 0.19$ mGy in the United States. Thus, they are of the same order of magnitude as the doses in Manitoba. As usual, there was considerable variation around the averages. In Sweden, the air kerma values ranged from 0.022 to 0.58 mGy, a 26-fold difference [L6], while in the United States they ranged from 0.004 to 0.70 mGy, a 175-fold difference [R14].

86. Studies within the Nationwide Evaluation of X-ray Trends (NEXT) programme of chest examinations in United States hospitals in 1984 and private practices in 1986 [R14] showed no overall difference in doses (an entrance surface air kerma of 0.14 mGy in both cases). Fewer private practices use scatter suppression grids. For each technique (with or without grid), doses were slightly higher in private practices. One of the causes of higher doses may be that 41% of the private practices, as opposed to 17% of the hospitals, underprocessed their films.

87. In spite of low doses, chest examinations contribute 5,100 man Sv annually in the United States, over 5% of the collective effective dose equivalent from medical x-ray usage, reflecting the fact that this is the most frequent type of x-ray examination apart

from dental x-ray examinations [N1]. Some countries conduct extensive chest screening programmes, often with photofluoroscopy rather than radiography. For conventional equipment, photofluorography causes doses at least some five times higher than radiography in chest examinations [U1], and depending on the type of fluoroscopy, the duration etc., it can cause doses 10 times higher [U1].

88. Entrance surface doses in chest radiography have been studied in Hunan Province, China (health-care level II) [Y1]. For photofluorography, the average dose was 6.1 mGy, while for full-size image radiography, the dose was 0.6 mGy. The average entrance surface dose during fluoroscopy was 9.6 mGy.

4. Mammography

89. Mammography is used in two contexts: for clinical examinations in order to investigate suspected breast cancers and for the mass screening of healthy women in order to detect such cancers. The preferred dose quantity in mammography is the mean absorbed dose in glandular tissue [I11, N14]. A summary of recent results of dose studies in mammography in countries of health-care level I is given in Table 16. The average of mean glandular doses ranged from 0.6 to 4.8 mGy per film. Reported effective dose equivalents spanned an even wider range: results of the UNSCEAR Survey of Medical Radiation Usage and Exposures gave an average effective dose equivalent of about 1 mSv and a range of 0.03-9.5 mSv. Since mammography is probably subject to more quality control and standardization than many other examinations, at least in countries where there are mammography screening programmes in effect [K16, L10, N12, P15, T11, Z8], the degree of variation is remarkable.

90. For a state-of-the-art screening programme, 1 mGy may be a representative breast dose (2-3 mGy if an anti-scatter grid is used). The dose varies with breast thickness [T20, W32] and composition [A15]. There are, as noted in the UNSCEAR 1988 Report [U1], considerable performance variations between systems, e.g. in Italy [C1] and the United States [K2, P1]. One source of variation is lack of a quality assurance programme. In the report from Italy cited in Table 16 [R19], it is observed that with the criteria used by the authors, 24% of the centres surveyed used too high a dose, 24% had a poor image quality and 14% had both high doses and poor images, illustrating the potential for quality assurance. To meet this need, the Commission of the European Communities has introduced European guidelines for quality assurance in mammography screening [C19]. In Washington State, United States, 30%-70% of 131 mammography centres were not in compliance with various quality assurance recommendations [F7]. This subject is further discussed in Section II.F.4. An important difference exists between xeromammographic systems (typical mean absorbed breast dose: 4 mGy) and screen/film systems (typical value 1 mGy) [H42, L17, R18]. The screen/film value is, in fact, an average of results without anti-scatter grids (0.6 mGy) and with grids (1.3 mGy); the latter, in turn, is an average of moving grid (1.1 mGy) and stationary grid (1.5 mGy) [D17].

91. In a study in Italy, low-dose plates permitted the surface air kerma to be reduced by 15%, to 4.4 mGy; a further 15% reduction was possible with an increased film-focus distance [C1]. In the United States, 15 new mammographic units of 8 different models were tested, using identical screen/film combinations with and without grids [K2]. The mean glandular dose varied between 0.4 and 2.2 mGy with a grid, 0.4 and 2.1 mGy without a grid, at 28 kVp. In another study in the United States, four different screen/film systems were tested [P1]. The mean glandular dose varied from 0.6 to 3.2 mGy at 25 kVp and from 0.5 to 1.8 mGy at 30 kVp. Five different types of film were tested in a study in the United States of the effects of prolonged exposure, delayed processing and increased film darkening [K21]. Each of these increased dose, by 20%-30%, and optimal viewing density was different for each film type. The Nationwide Evaluation of X-ray Trends (NEXT) programme, also in the United States, observed average mean glandular doses of 0.93 mGy in 1985 and 1.6 mGy in 1988 for screen/film mammography [R12]. For xeromammography, the values were 3.9 mGy in 1984 and 4.3 mGy in 1988. In 1985, 36% of facilities had an unacceptable image quality, but by 1988 this proportion had dropped to 13%.

5. Chiropractic examinations

92. X-ray examinations are also performed in connection with chiropractic, either at the chiropractic office or by a collaborating medical radiologist. The main types of examination are cervical spine, thoracic spine and lumbar spine. In the province of Manitoba, Canada, the entrance surface doses for these three types of examinations were 0.6, 1.8 and 3.5 mGy, respectively, corresponding to effective dose equivalents of 0.03, 0.24 and 0.41 mSv per examination and collective effective dose equivalents of 0.4, 0.8 and 6.2 man Sv for a population of 1 million [H8]. This averaged 0.22 mSv per patient and gave a per caput effective dose equivalent of 0.007 mSv. These values agree closely with corresponding values for the United States [N1] and indicate that chiropractic examinations do not make a significant contribution to either individual or the collective radiation dose.

93. Nevertheless, these averages do not reflect the extent of the dose variation encountered among chiropractic offices. In the Manitoba study, the ratio of maximum to minimum dose was as great as 23 [H8]. This is similar in magnitude to the variations found in medical diagnostic radiology [S23]. In its response to the UNSCEAR Survey of Medical Radiation Usage and Exposures, the National Radiation Laboratory of New Zealand pointed out that entrance surface doses may be difficult to interpret, because chiropractors use a complex system of plane and wedge filters and diaphragms to obtain even irradiation of contrasting tissue regions. According to the Laboratory, the filter and diaphragm systems lead to doses lower than those obtained in approximately equivalent medical procedures.

6. Neonatal and child examinations

94. The pattern of diagnostic examinations is such that children may get higher doses than adults. For instance, a study in the Netherlands reported the highest doses per examined patient for persons under age 5 years or between ages 25 and 50 years. The reason was that the most frequent examinations were abdomen, lumbar spine, intravenous pyelogram and computed tomography of the head, all of which cause doses in the middle to upper range [V16]. Furthermore, the exposure conditions and field sizes must be adapted, otherwise the effective dose from examinations of infants would be higher than that to an adult. This also applies to high-dose procedures, such as interventional cardiac catheterization, which is used on infants with a variety of congenital heart diseases [W16]. Phantoms [V11] and tables are available for the determination of absorbed organ doses to children in various x-ray examinations [T12]. With theoretical methods, Zankl et al. [Z2, Z15] obtained organ doses for an infant and a child for the most common radiographic examinations and demonstrated the strong dependence of organ doses on body size [V3]. Lindskoug [L11] provided tables of suitable exposure parameter settings.

95. Fetal doses in computed tomography were discussed above in Section II.C.2. Fetal absorbed doses in Japan during screening of the upper gastrointestinal tract ranged from 0.3 to 5.5 mGy [O2]. To the extent that pelvimetry is performed by x rays instead of ultrasound, doses (including possible fetal doses) are decreasing where computed tomography scanners are available, but not using their computed tomography feature. Pelvimetry with Scan Projection Tomography (a non-tomographic survey view with the scanner) causes doses about one tenth of those with conventional x rays [G9, W33].

96. For premature infants, chest examinations can be medically very important. Weingärtner et al. [W2] stressed the importance of suitable equipment and careful patient referral for x-ray imaging for this sensitive group of patients. Faulkner et al. [F4] listed various ways to reduce doses per film but also pointed out that neonates may be subjected to large numbers of examinations during their stay in hospital. They also mentioned that the average dose to the infant patient is determined mainly by the number of examinations, which depends on clinical symptoms. In the UNSCEAR 1988 Report [U1], other examinations of neonates (barium, computed tomography, angiocardiography) were discussed.

97. Ruiz et al. [R22] studied entrance surface doses to children of different age groups from frequent simple examinations of the abdomen, hip and pelvis, skull, spine and chest. The ranges of doses they observed in the Madrid area to children less than 1 year of age (AP projection) were 0.8-1.7 mGy (abdomen), 0.8-1.3 mGy (pelvis), 1.1-3.2 mGy (skull) and 0.1-0.5 mGy (chest). The variations observed, as well as the fact that skull doses for some examinations exceeded suggested reference values for adults [M38], were said to demonstrate the need for quality assurance programmes. Similar data collected from the United Kingdom [C22] showed that some skull doses exceeded the CEC reference dose values.

98. A study covering 11 member States of the European Community [S19], which considered typical x-ray examinations performed on infants (abdomen, skull, chest, spine, pelvis), showed large variations in entrance surface doses, far greater than the known and expected variations for corresponding examinations of adults. The maximum entrance surface doses for the abdomen, skull, chest and spine were almost 50 times higher than the minimum doses, and for the pelvis, a 76-fold difference was found. The study had been standardized on the size of the infant so that no additional variation was introduced. It should be possible to remove some of the dose variation, which would presumably lead to lower average doses to infants in future x-ray examinations.

99. Most of the patients subjected to scoliosis radiography are females between 10 and 16 years of age, and many of them are examined repeatedly, perhaps 20 times in all, for prolonged periods, so that considerable doses result from the total course of examinations. It is likely, however, that technical improvements will reduce doses per examination. As an example, the filtration systems common in chiropractic practice can reduce doses to scoliosis patients significantly [A2]. Computed radiography seems to reduce doses by about an order of magnitude, both with large-screen image intensifiers [M5] and with photostimulable phosphor imaging plates [K12, K22]. A disadvantage is that neither

technique permits the entire cervical, thoracic and lumbar spine of a tall teenager to be shown on a single image [M5, K22]. One study in Sweden found that the effective dose equivalent with state-of-the-art technique was 0.07 mSv for one examination. Other techniques gave up to 10 times higher doses. Published figures indicated that certain techniques could give doses a further order of magnitude higher [H39].

100. Several authors have examined the utility of filtration in paediatric radiology. For abdominal examinations of 10-year-old children, niobium filtration neither impaired the image quality substantially nor reduced doses significantly [J4]. Rare earth (erbium, hafnium) filters have been received with mixed reviews for paediatric radiology (and for general radiology; they are discussed below with respect to dental examinations). Although they do permit dose reductions of 20%-25% with unimpaired image quality, the cost is high [D12, S39, W15]. Adams [A9] advocated rare earth filters but also pointed out that a number of other items in a quality assurance programme are at least as important. A more advanced technical development, computed radiography using photostimulable phosphor imaging plates, permits dose reductions of 30%-50%, compared to screen/film systems, in various examinations of children, infants and premature babies [B24]. An added benefit is that the findings can be highlighted using image post-processing.

101. In computed tomography, paediatric body scans using ceramic detectors allow 50% dose reductions compared to xenon detectors, with a negligible reduction of image quality [P17]. Naidich et al. [N9] addressed the potential for low-dose computed tomography of children, comparing a 10 mA setting to the more routine 140 mA (at 120 kVp) for lung examinations. In spite of increased image noise and loss of low-contrast detail, the low-dose examination produced images of acceptable quality.

D. DENTAL X-RAY EXAMINATIONS

102. Although the effective dose to a patient from an oral radiographic examination is low, the frequency of examinations is high enough to warrant study of dose distributions. Country-by-country frequencies of dental examinations are listed in Table 17, and the entrance surface doses and effective doses or effective dose equivalents per examination, mainly for intraoral films, are listed in Table 18. Representative frequencies of dental examination were estimated in the UNSCEAR 1988 Report [U1] to be 250 and 4 per 1,000 population in countries of health-care levels I and II, respectively. Since then many additional studies have been performed, providing a wider basis for estimates. The population-weighted average examination frequency for countries of health-care levels I, II and III for 1985-1990 were, according to Table 17, 350, 2.5 and 1.7 per 1,000 population, respectively. Some data were collected on age- and sex-distributions, but these appear too scattered to warrant formal analysis. It is noted, however, that dental examinations of children are rather frequent.

103. In the UNSCEAR 1988 Report [U1], the average effective dose equivalent for a procedure involving about two dental film exposures was estimated to be 0.03 mSv. The population-weighted average effective dose equivalent per examination for countries of health-care level I in 1985-1990, calculated from the data of Table 18, was about 0.03 mSv (the weighted per caput effective dose equivalent is about 0.01 mSv). For countries of health-care levels II-IV, the effective dose equivalent per examination is probably much higher; according to Table 18, the average dose per examination was 0.2 mSv at level II (based mainly on Brazil) and 0.32 mSv at level III (based on Myanmar). These averages correspond, however, to per caput effective dose equivalents of only 0.001 mSv at level II and 0.0003 mSv at level III, due to the low examination frequencies.

104. For dental x-ray examinations, the collective effective dose equivalent in Sweden was estimated to be 79 man Sv in 1984 [S1], while a similar estimate for Finland in 1981-1985 was 15 man Sv [H2]. The population of Sweden, 8.3 million in 1984, is twice that of Finland. However, individual doses were slightly higher in Finland. The results mainly reflect differences in examination frequency; the examination frequency in Sweden is rather high, 1.9 films per inhabitant in 1986, due to a national dental service programme that provides relatively frequent examinations.

105. In contrast, the dental x-ray collective effective dose equivalent of 2,000 man Sv in France in 1984 [B5] cannot be explained just by the larger population of France (54.9 million in 1984) or by the examination frequency (0.5 films per inhabitant in 1984 [B5]). Instead, the difference arises from the average doses per examination, which are at least 2-3 times higher than in the Nordic countries [B5]. Benedittini et al. [B5] noted that the bitewing entrance surface air kerma was halved in the United States between 1973 and 1981, and that the value of 6.9 mGy in France in 1984 was comparable to the value of 5.7 mGy in the United States in 1973. According to the authors, an important explanatory factor is that there is no nationwide quality assurance programme for dental radiography in France, while quality assurance programmes have been implemented in the United States [B5].

106. Doses due to intraoral examinations span an order of magnitude, with effective dose equivalents for a complete mouth examination ranging from 0.02 to 0.28 mSv, according to a survey in the Netherlands [V2]. For rotational panoramic radiography of an adult female, Gibbs et al. estimate the effective dose equivalent to be 0.01-0.03 mSv [G12]. A later study in the Netherlands [V10] found a fourfold difference in average entrance surface doses for various bitewing radiography techniques (2.5-9 mGy), and a 35-fold range for individual measurements (0.9-31 mGy). A review of recent studies in countries of health-care level I found effective dose equivalents for single intraoral exposures from 0.001 to 0.05 mSv and for panoramic exposures from 0.007 to 0.08 mSv [S33]. A similar review [W30] that calculated effective doses using ICRP 1990 weighting factors found a range of values for full-mouth examinations of 0.03-0.14 mSv, average 0.08 mSv, and a range for panoramic examination of 0.003-0.016 mSv, average 0.007 mSv.

107. With such small effective doses, treatment courses involving several examinations over a longer period will also cause relatively small doses. Sewerin [S11] estimated the total effective dose equivalent to a patient during a seven-year treatment with osseo-integrated implants, with concomitant x-ray examinations, to be about 1.7 mSv. The study assumed, however, that two-dimensional imaging is sufficient in pre-operative examinations. Often, cross-sectional information is requested, using computed tomography of the skull, which gives doses that are higher by several orders of magnitude [C10]. The extent to which computed radiography is needed in this situation is somewhat controversial [M36, S32], but given its increasing availability, computed tomography will presumably be used more often in the future. The doses in computed tomography of the mouth region can be higher than in conventional dental x-ray examinations [K13, S55] and similar to those in other computed tomography examinations of the head and neck.

108. The average organ doses encountered in various dental x-ray examinations in France are summarized in Table 19 [B5]. The doses were determined by means of a phantom and are presented here because of the detailed anatomical subdivision. A few doses are in the range one to several milligray, but most are less than 0.2 mGy. Absorbed doses to the thyroid and the eye lens in a study in the United States [T13] were quite similar to those in Table 19. According to another study in France [P14], entrance surface doses were about 15 mGy for intraoral films and about 10 mGy for panoramic examination. Since image quality is slightly inferior with panoramic examinations and since rectangular collimation, lead-backed film and lead aprons are likely to reduce the thyroid doses from intraoral films [B26], panoramic examination is not expected to supplant intraoral films. Nonetheless, the frequency of panoramic examinations merits study. In a number of countries, they are used to screen orthodontal anomalies in children [W19].

109. Computation and interpretation of the effective dose or effective dose equivalent are not entirely straightforward for oral radiology [H38, S3]. This was particularly problematic before the ICRP recommendations of 1990 [I8] were published, since most of the organs exposed belonged to the "remainder" group, for which the ICRP 1977 recommendations [I1] provided only average weighting factors. As an illustration, when the effective dose equivalent [I1] was calculated for a single bitewing film with 60-70 kVp machines in New Zealand, the result was 0.067 mSv. When effective dose was calculated from the same data according to the ICRP recommendations of 1990 [I8], which provide specific weighting factors for some additional organs, the result was only 0.005 mSv, about 7% of the former value [W12].

110. Maruyama [M31] obtained a similar result in Japan: effective doses calculated with 1990 weighting factors [I8] were 53%-86% of the effective dose equivalents calculated with 1977 [I1] weighting factors. However, this calculation was quite sensitive to whether the skin was considered a target organ. If it was, the trend was reversed, and the effective doses were about twice the effective dose equivalents [M31]. Velders et al. [V12] in the Netherlands obtained bitewing effective dose equivalents of 2-11 μSv for various parameter combinations and effective doses of 1-4 μSv.

111. Several reviews in the United Kingdom, the United States and elsewhere summarize recent developments in dental x-ray exposure reduction [B27, H44, K3, K4, K25, T2, T3, T7]. For instance, in panoramic radiography, exposures were reduced 34%-79% with rare earth intensifying screens and heavy metal filtration, and image quality was the same or better [K3, S10]. However, the advantages of rare earth and other thin K-edge filters are not uncontested. Byrne et al. [B25] in Canada found a surface air kerma reduction for intraoral films of about 15% (as opposed to the filter manufacturer's claim of 40%), but thyroid dose was actually increased. MacDonald-Jankowski et al. in the United Kingdom confirmed the surface air kerma reduction but noted the possible disadvantages (unsharp images due to movement and x-ray tube wear) of the associated prolongation of exposure time [M35]. In a subsequent study [M42], the authors concluded that while thin K-edge filters reduced entrance surface dose and, to a certain extent, total dose to the head, orbital dose might be increased.

112. White et al. [W31] regarded niobium filtration, with a 20%-30% dose reduction, compatible with acceptable images on D-speed film. With faster (E-speed) film, niobium filtration significantly degraded the quality of the image. Other theoretical and practical studies suggest the limitations of niobium filtration [J12, M21].

113. Exposure varies widely with technique, also in less frequently performed examinations. Correctly performed [B28], video fluorographic examination of velopharyngeal function causes one tenth of the dose obtained with cinefluorography, which causes entrance surface doses in the 6-30 mGy range [I3].

E. WORLDWIDE EXPOSURES

114. The collective effective dose equivalent from diagnostic medical x-ray examinations performed worldwide is presented in Table 20. Estimates of the frequencies of each examination and the average doses have been combined to determine the collective dose for each health-care level and for the entire world. The average frequencies of examinations given in Table 7 have been used to indicate the relative frequencies, with the total corresponding to the population-weighted average for all examinations (Table 8). The data for level IV are insufficient for separate analysis and are instead included with those of level III.

115. The average doses per examination were derived from data in Table 10 and listed in Table 11. Where estimates of dose were not available for level II countries, they were assumed to be the same as for level I countries. Moreover, for lack of data, the doses in level III-IV are assumed to be the same as doses in level II. The data for level II are the population-weighted data reported for China and India, which may be expected to be representative. However, some doses are less than the more widely based averages for level I; recognizing that the values in level II are unlikely to be lower than those in level I and in order not to underestimate the collective dose, the higher values (i.e. level I values) have been assumed also for level II. This applies to examinations of the chest (radiographic and fluoroscopic), extremities, skull, abdomen and lower gastro-intestinal tract and to urography.

116. The estimate of the collective dose from all diagnostic x-ray examinations performed in one year on the world population of 1990 is 1,600,000 man Sv. The corresponding estimate in the UNSCEAR 1988 Report [U1] was 1,760,000 man Sv. The difference may well be no more than a sampling effect. The results for level I are little changed. The per caput effective dose (and effective dose equivalent) is 0.9 mSv, compared to 1.0 mSv in the earlier analysis. However, the value of 0.9 mSv includes data of 1980 for the United States, which probably underestimate the present examination frequency [M2]. For level II, the estimated per caput effective dose has been reduced, from 0.2 mSv to 0.1 mSv. Few data had been available for the earlier analysis, but the situation is much improved now that data from both China and India are available. For levels III and IV the previous range of 0.03-0.07 mSv, again based on very few data, has now been set at 0.04 mSv. There is still uncertainty in the collective doses from levels II-IV, but their significance is less than that of level I, which alone contributes 78% of the estimated worldwide collective dose.

117. Previous uncertainties regarding the use of fluoroscopy in developing countries are lessened now that data are available for China. While chest photofluoroscopy is still a common examination, accounting for 43% of all examinations in the country (Table 7), the effective dose per examination is now reported to be 0.3 mSv (although 1.0 mSv has been used in Table 20), compared with 3.4 mSv reported previously [U1]. Assuming that the higher dose still prevails would increase the estimated collective dose worldwide to 1,940,000 man Sv.

118. Specific examinations contribute to the total collective dose from diagnostic medical x-ray examinations as shown in Table 21. The examinations are listed in decreasing order of their contribution to the worldwide collective dose. The most prominent contributors in level I are upper gastro-intestinal tract, computed tomography, chest mass miniature, spine and lower gastro-intestinal tract. The doses are relatively high for the examinations of the gastro-intestinal tract, and together upper and lower gastro-intestinal tract examinations contribute more than 30% of the collective dose in level I and 19%-22% in levels II-IV. The importance of chest fluoroscopy in level II countries is apparent (it contributed 42% of the total collective dose). The relative frequency of this examination in levels III and IV was less than in levels I and II, but it was also the highest contributor to the total collective dose at this level. Other examinations of the chest were important in level II (mass miniature) and levels III and IV (radiography). Examinations of the abdomen and pelvis/hip were more important in levels II-IV than in level I, but computed tomography contributed much less to the total collective dose at the lower health-care levels.

119. Doses from all diagnostic x-ray examinations have been evaluated in a number of countries. The resulting effective dose equivalents, provided in responses to the UNSCEAR Survey of Medical Radiation Usage and Exposures or available in published

are summarized in Table 22. In a few cases, effective doses or effective dose equivalents for all examinations were calculated from data provided for specific examinations in Tables 7 and 10. Table 22 indicates that the latest annual effective dose equivalent per caput attributable to x-ray examinations in countries of health-care level I ranged from 0.3 to 2.2 mSv.

120. The population-weighted per caput effective dose equivalent in health-care level I countries, based on Table 22, for 1980-1990 is 1 mSv. This is the same value as that given in the UNSCEAR 1988 Report [U1] for available data reported for 1976-1984. The data for Canada, Czechoslovakia and the United States in Table 22 are for 1980. Updated values might have increased the 1980-1990 average somewhat, especially in view of the increasing trends in computed tomography [M2]. Thus, the weighted average for 1982-1990 is 1.2 mSv. The unweighted average and median values of data for level I reported in Table 22 are both about 0.8 mSv. This agrees with the fact that relatively high doses are reported from Japan and the former USSR (RSFSR only), both of which have large populations.

121. The reported estimates of effective dose or effective dose equivalent from diagnostic medical x-ray examinations are less extensive for levels II-IV than for level I. An overall range of 0.02-0.2 mSv is evident from the data in Table 22. The values at the lower end of the range were underestimated when fluoroscopy was not included. The estimates at the upper end of the range were made before 1980. It can only be said that the estimates of collective dose based on the frequencies of examinations and average doses in Table 20 appear reasonable. The per caput doses in that analysis were 0.1 mSv in level II and 0.04 mSv in levels III-IV.

122. The estimated annual per caput and collective effective dose (equivalent) from diagnostic x-ray examinations, taking results of the different sampling methods used into account, are summarized in Table 23. The collective dose totals are the values rounded subsequent to calculation. The values for the medical examinations for levels II-IV are those determined in Table 20. The per caput effective doses and the collective dose from dental examinations were determined from average frequencies and doses cited in Section II.D. These doses are less by a factor of 100 than those from medical examinations. The total collective dose from diagnostic x-ray examinations worldwide is just over 1.6 million man Sv.

F. TRENDS

123. It is anticipated that both the total number of diagnostic x-ray examinations and the frequency of examinations per unit population will increase worldwide for simple demographic reasons, at least up to the year 2000 and probably to 2025 [U1]. There are three main reasons for this expectation:

(a) population growth. Even if the relative frequency of examinations per unit population remained constant, the absolute number of examinations would grow by 60% from 1988 to 2025 as a result of population increase;

(b) growing urbanization. In general, urban populations have more access to health care and a much higher frequency of radiological examinations than rural ones, and the percentage of the urban population is expected to rise from 41% to 65% between 1988 and 2025;

(c) ageing of the population, particularly in Europe. Since the older population accounts for a disproportionately high utilization of medical radiation procedures, the ageing of populations leads to increasing examination frequencies. However, in Africa and Latin America, the proportion of young persons will increase. Although the frequency of examinations increases as the population ages, an older population would be less at risk for stochastic effects because of the time periods required for their induction.

124. In general terms, these factors governing long-term trends in examination frequencies and doses are likely to remain valid. For specific countries and groups of countries, over a shorter period and for specific examinations, trends may be more complex and difficult to discern, analyse or forecast.

125. It was mentioned above that according to the UNSCEAR Survey of Medical Radiation Usage and Exposures, the total frequency of all x-ray examinations at health-care level I increased from 810 per 1,000 population in the mid-1970s to 890 per 1,000 population in 1985-1990, representing a 4% increase in the population-weighted average per 5-year period. The unweighted average increased by 2% per 5-year period (not statistically significant). This observation is supported by independent estimates that there should be at least a slowing in the rate of increase of frequencies in the future compared to the 1970s [S7, S14]. The composition of the examination types changes, however: there are, for example, fewer chest examinations and more computed tomography in recent years.

126. Trends in individual countries deviate from the average. Increasing total frequencies of x-ray examinations are evident in France (+18% per five-year period), the Federal Republic of Germany (+10%), Japan (+13%), Malta (+69%), United King-

dom (+10%) and particularly in Cuba (+342%). Some differences may reflect changes in survey methods that give more complete results rather than real changes in examination frequencies. Decreasing total frequencies of examinations are reported in Finland (-10% per 5-year period), Norway (-16%) and Romania (-16%). The Netherlands [B21, B22] and also the Russian Federation show first increasing, then decreasing trends, with peak examination frequencies in the early 1980s. In Japan, the increase is due chiefly to radiographic examinations; the increased use of fluoroscopy has been relatively moderate since 1970, with a slight decline since 1987 [M32].

127. In countries of health-care levels II-IV, the frequency of examinations appears to be increasing, with a 1985-1990 population-weighted frequency of about 100 per 1,000 population. Unweighted averages increased by some 25% per 5-year period, and the trend appears to be statistically significant. In the few countries that could supply data for more than one time period, trends are less scattered than at health-care level I. Very clear increases occur in Ecuador and in India. Decreasing examination frequencies were reported for Brazil and Nicaragua.

128. One reason for slower rates of increase or slight decreases in examination frequencies in countries of health-care level I is that newer modalities, such as magnetic resonance tomography, endoscopy and ultrasonography, are replacing some x-ray examinations. X-ray examinations continue, however, to be the most important imaging method, accounting for 79% of diagnostic images in Europe in 1988 and a projected 77% in 1993 [H40]. Hill [H40] expects the relative use of computed tomography and of nuclear medicine examinations to remain constant, at 2% each. This prediction appears low for computed tomography considering its rapid increase, which more than offsets the decrease of other examinations in the United Kingdom [S42], even if a constant percentage may mean an increased number in some countries. Finally, Hill expects the share of ultrasound examinations to increase from 17% to 19% and that of magnetic resonance imaging to remain constant, at 1% [H40], although the interpretation of these percentages is hampered by the omission of endoscopy.

129. Broadly, the UNSCEAR Survey of Medical Radiation Usage and Exposures shows that doses per examination are decreasing for most procedures in countries of health-care level I (not enough information is available from other countries to draw conclusions about trends). This generalization is supported by independent reports from, for example, Australia [H37], the Federal Republic of Germany [G7], Japan [M4], Sweden [V4], the United States [S6] and the USSR [S18]. The decrease from the 1930s to the 1980s may be by a factor of 5-15, and that 1970 to 1980, by a factor of 1.5-3 [G7, H15, V19].

130. The trends for specific procedures or countries are more complicated. Table 10 indicates decreasing doses per procedure in Australia, Finland and Sweden; decreasing doses for gastro-intestinal tract imaging (important, since they are at the upper end of the dose range) but not for other examinations in Czechoslovakia; and no strong change in Romania. Trends in computed tomography doses cannot be discerned directly from Table 10, but as was shown in Section II.C.2, these doses are increasing. Hence, the total dose for all x-ray examinations per examined patient may be unchanged or only slightly decreased. This agrees with the impression of doses per examined patient in Table 11. The population-weighted annual per caput effective dose equivalent is 0.93 mSv for 1985-1990 from analyses of frequencies and doses (Table 20) and 1.2 mSv for 1982-1990 from available estimates from countries (Table 22), indicating that there has been no significant change for countries of health-care level I from the estimate of 1 mSv given in the UNSCEAR 1988 Report [U1].

131. The rapid development of more powerful yet cheaper computers is revolutionizing all imaging methods, with and without ionizing radiation. As an example, data obtained in computed tomography (or magnetic resonance tomography or nuclear medicine) can now be assembled into three-dimensional pictures that can easily be rotated by the analyst [F12, F13, T17, W17]. This may permit lower doses per examination; with pelvic trauma, for example, a three-dimensional examination obviates the need for plain radiographs to supplement a computed tomographic examination [S9], eliminating an average entrance surface dose of 23 mGy per examination. Thus, new information is obtained, and more uses of these techniques become possible.

132. The transition to digital systems in industrialized countries is likely to continue. At present 15%-30% of examinations are digital [B9, O3]. Digital radiography uses large image intensifiers or photostimulable phosphor imaging plates. Chest examinations using digital techniques can produce substantial savings of time and money for film, chemicals and archiving [K23]. While the quality of the image with a large image intensifier is not as good as with full-size images on film, the difference can be small enough to be clinically negligible. If fluoroscopy is not used, an image intensifier can reduce patient exposure to one third that of full-size images on film [K23, M16] or, in situations such as peripheral angiography, to one tenth [P21].

133. The alternative technology of imaging plates with photostimulable phosphor [T10] seems to have been more widely adopted in Japan than large image intensifier computed radiography. Worldwide, about 1,000 such systems had been installed by the end of 1991, 700 of them in Japan [B9]. This system also permits substantial dose reductions, partly because it separates the two functions of detection and display, which are combined in conventional radiographical film [W5]. For chest radiography, exposure was 20%-44% of the standard exposure with a screen/film combination [R17, S24, S25] or even 15% in paediatric chest imaging [K19]. In examinations of the upper gastro-intestinal tract, exposure was 32% of that with a screen/film combination [S26]. For urethrocystography the dose-area product was reduced from 13 mGy cm^2 to 1.3 mGy cm^2 [Z9]. As the technology improves, digital imaging is also becoming a method of choice in difficult situations like cardiac imaging [D15].

134. Digital computed radiography with imaging plates not only gives a potential for lower doses per image but also permits more sophisticated experiments in dose reduction. Using stacked imaging plates, such experiments can also be made in the course of actual diagnosis on patients without undue exposure [R17]. However, persistent anecdotal evidence (see, e.g. [J5, F8]) indicates that some of the dose reduction per image in computed radiography may be offset by a tendency of radiologists to obtain more images per patient than they would have done with conventional screen/film systems. Also, while over- or under-exposure shows up in conventional radiology as incorrect blackening of the film, considerable over-exposure can go undetected in a digital system unless exposure is specifically monitored [B9, W5].

135. The use of rare earth intensifying screens is one of the more important technical developments leading to lower doses per examination. While such screens are by no means new, having been available since the early 1970s, they are not yet utilized in all relevant situations. For instance, sample studies indicate that fewer than 50% of the radiographic examinations in the United Kingdom were carried out with rare earth screens in 1986 [N5]. Other factors remaining constant, a complete transition to rare earth screens would reduce the collective effective dose from x-ray examinations in the United Kingdom by 3,000 man Sv [N5]. It seems highly likely that rare earth screens will continue to be more widely used, reducing the doses per examination.

136. The ICRP recommendations of 1990 [I8] suggest that dose constraints or investigation levels should be considered for some common diagnostic procedures. While this is not to be construed as advocating the introduction of limits for medical exposures, it is likely that implementation [C16, N5] of the recommendations would truncate the upper end of the dose range for many examinations. Since doses per examination vary by a factor of 10 or more, even in a single hospital [H37, O7], such a truncation could be expected to reduce average doses.

137. National recommendations are also likely to lead to reduced doses. Screen/film speed is the overriding cause of patient dose variation in the United Kingdom, and fluoroscopy time in gastro-intestinal tract examinations is the second biggest cause [H33]. A United Kingdom report [N5] gives detailed recommendations for reducing patient doses (a second report [N11] deals specifically with computed tomography). It estimates that about half of the current collective effective dose to patients from x rays could be avoided. This conclusion is drawn in spite of the relatively low frequency of examinations (about twice as many examinations per caput are performed in France and the United States).

138. Recommendations to restrict doses raise a number of questions: more stringent referral criteria are a subject of some dispute [F1, K7, K8], the value of access to old radiographs may be limited [O1] and the benefits of rare earth filtration are challenged. However, since it has been suggested that in the United Kingdom the collective effective dose from diagnostic x rays could be halved [N5], there is probably a potential for similar dose reductions in many countries. If this potential is realized, as it probably will be in a number of countries, doses will go down.

1. Specific x-ray examinations and techniques

139. Fluoroscopy and photofluorography usually cause higher doses than screen/film radiography, particularly with older equipment, and are thus largely being replaced in industrialized countries. It is less clear if, or how quickly, this change will occur in developing countries. There, the higher cost of screen/film radiography is a more important consideration than in industrialized countries [T8]. In Tunisia, where over 50% of the equipment is fluoroscopic, the technique is thought to be excessively utilized [G16]. The authors judge that 60%-70% of the general practitioners equipped with fluoroscopy use the examination only to please patients, not for diagnostic advantage. Information campaigns are under way to reduce the demand for fluoroscopy.

140. In general, chest screening is becoming less frequent. For conventional posterior/anterior chest examinations with full-size images on film, doses are decreasing. In Manitoba, Canada, the average entrance surface dose decreased from 0.3 mGy in 1979 to

0.07-0.12 mGy in 1987 [H6, H24]. Some techniques may give a higher dose to patients, however. The difference in transmission between mediastinum and lungs is a complication that can be alleviated with shaped filters or with image processing in computed radiology. Alternatively, the problem can be circumvented by beam modulation, a technique that produces high image quality but with an increase in dose of up to 25% compared to air-gap screen/film systems [A10]. Beam modulation may, however, obviate the need for additional examinations, which could reduce patient dose for the entire diagnostic procedure. However, such specialized equipment is not expected to be in wide usage in the near future.

141. The growing use of computed tomography has been noted, with greater numbers of scanners and higher frequencies of examination in countries of health-care level I [C9, N5, S14]. In the United States, computed tomography is the most frequently performed x-ray examination in hospitals, accounting for 56% of the total examinations [G8]; including all other medical centres and practices, computed tomography constitutes some 9% of all examinations [B10]. Furthermore, the number of slices imaged on each patient has risen as the time required to perform scans and reconstruct images has decreased: However, since little change has occurred in the dose required per slice, the dose per examination is likely to have increased substantially [N5]. Indeed, the average effective dose equivalent due to a body scan at the Mayo Clinic in the United States was 15.6 mSv (range: 9-60 mSv) in 1988 [V8]; in 1980, the comparable figure for the United States was 1.1 mSv [N1].

142. About half of the computed tomographies in the Nordic countries in 1987 were head examinations [S14]. Computed tomography has largely replaced encephalography and cerebral angiography that was performed in cases of trauma, tumours or apoplectic strokes. In these applications, magnetic resonance tomographs may tend to replace computed tomography, although the latter is expected to remain an important tool, along with ultrasound, for abdominal examinations. Likewise, computed tomography will probably remain important in oncology, for therapy planning and for follow-up examinations after treatments [S14]. Judging from United Kingdom statistics, computed tomography now contributes more than any other single type of diagnostic procedure to the collective dose from x-ray examinations (about 20%), and the trend is still rising [S42, S43].

143. As indicated in the UNSCEAR 1988 Report [U1], the number of skull x-ray examinations increased significantly between 1964 and 1980. The more recent data in Tables 7 and 8 reflects mixed trends, but a report from the United States [M18] shows that several investigators suspected overutilization of skull radiography because of concerns of possible malpractice suits. The attention drawn to this may have altered this trend. Also, plain film skull examinations are increasingly being replaced by computed tomography examinations.

144. The number of countries with mammography screening programmes has been increasing [C6, M9, R6, T1, V6]. While doses per examination are reasonably low, with surface doses now in the range of 1 mGy [V1], the impact of mammography screening on the collective dose is not negligible. For instance, it is estimated that, when fully implemented, a nationwide screening programme in Sweden will increase the collective effective dose equivalent due to diagnostic x rays by about 5% [V4]. However, because doses per examination are decreasing, the collective dose does not increase as fast as the number of examinations. For instance, in Manitoba, Canada, the number of examinations in a population of about 1 million increased from 4,800 in 1978 to 24,000 in 1988, i.e. about fivefold. The collective breast dose has also increased, but at a much slower rate, from 40 man Gy in 1978 to 97 man Gy in 1988 [H31] (the average breast dose decreased by 50% during that period).

145. In dental radiology, the trend is very clearly towards reduced doses per examination [G3, K4, S1]. Thus, the absorbed dose to the parotid glands for common radiographic techniques decreased by one order of magnitude for every 20-year period between 1920 and 1980 [B15]. This trend is expected to continue. Goren et al. [G3] reported a dose reduction by half in the United States but noted that only 13% of surveyed dental practices used high-speed class E films. According to them, if such films were used at all dental practices, the dose would again be halved. However, it must be noted that the slower class D film is sometimes used owing to its higher average film contrast [W12]. Nevertheless, some dose reduction attributable to the use of class E film is expected. Other factors, such as reduced beam size, are also expected to lead to dose reductions. Digital computed dental radiology exists, but apparently the resolution and latitude are still inferior to that of standard dental film [W18]. The relatively bulky sensors may impede projections and the small image area hampers the evaluation of bone lesions and neutralizes dose reductions because more views are required [G20]. Thus, the technique is not expected to spread rapidly in the near future.

2. Alternatives to x-ray examination

146. Conventional radiology still dominates clinical radiology (over 80% of all examinations in the Nordic countries are done using conventional methods), and

no radical decrease in the need for conventional radiology is expected [S14]. Nevertheless, in many cases, the information needed clinically can be obtained in more than one way. Besides diagnostic x-ray examination, there may be methods in nuclear medicine, or endoscopy, ultrasonography, magnetic resonance tomography or other alternatives. Of these, ultrasonography is the most rapidly growing imaging modality, with sales of equipment growing 20% annually, an estimated 60,000-90,000 units in operation worldwide and some 60-90 million examinations annually [M8]. This corresponds to 4%-6% of the 1,600 million x-ray examinations performed annually worldwide. To some extent, x-ray examinations causing high individual doses are being replaced. For instance, magnetic resonance tomography, or sometimes transcranial-Doppler sonography, may be substituted for cranial angiography [R8].

147. An example of a diagnostic situation where nuclear medicine is an alternative to x rays is provided by non-cutaneous melanomas. A study in Italy indicated that radioimmunoscintigraphy, using monoclonal antibodies labelled with ^{111}In or ^{99m}Tc, had a significantly higher diagnostic sensitivity than conventional x-ray examinations [C9]. The investigators plan to compare radiation doses and to perform cost-benefit analyses.

148. The increasing use of alternative methods is not always accompanied by a corresponding decrease in conventional x-ray usage. The use of diagnostic ultrasound during pregnancy more than doubled in the United States between 1980 and 1987 [C5]. Prenatal x-ray examinations are rare, but considering that radiation exposure of the fetus can now be avoided, it might have been expected that they would be even rarer instead of having remained about the same during the period. A possible explanation is that the use of x rays is related to the number of Caesarean sections, since pelvic x-ray examinations are still used to assess the need for such delivery [C5]. Trends in obstetric radiography are discussed further in the following Section.

149. In contrast, urography does seem to indicate decreasing use of x rays as there is increasing access to ultrasound. The frequency of x-ray urography examinations was 16.8 per 1,000 inhabitants in Italy in 1978 and 10.5 per 1,000 in 1988 [C9]. Doses per examination in Italy were 7.1 mSv in 1983 and 4.8 mSv in 1988, corresponding to per caput doses of 0.09 and 0.05 mSv, respectively [C9]. It should be noted that not only ultrasound but also more sensitive screen/film combinations and fewer films per examination contribute to the decreasing doses per caput [C9]. Furthermore, computed tomography is also replacing urography, and an important reason for the decrease in the number of urographies is that indications, e.g. for calculus checking, have changed [S14]. Some contrast urography has been replaced by scintigraphy and other methods in nuclear medicine, which usually impart effective doses that are an order of magnitude or so lower [N10, W21].

150. According to the same report [S14], urethrocystography and hysterosalpingography have also decreased, at least in the Nordic countries in the 1980s. In Sweden, the number of cholecystographies decreased by about 70% after 1975, to some 2.4 per 1,000 inhabitants in 1987 (a 72% decrease from 1970-1974 to 5 per 1,000 in 1985-1989). This decrease was due to the replacement of cholecystography with ultrasonography. The other Nordic countries have even lower current frequencies of cholecystography: a frequency of 0.4 per 1,000 inhabitants was reported for Norway in 1988.

151. Some trends in x-ray diagnostics, ultrasonography and endoscopy have been investigated in the Federal Republic of Germany [K9]. For abdominal or total body (paediatric) examinations, there were marked decreases (30%-60%) during 1978-1984 in x-ray diagnostic examinations in hospitals and corresponding increases in sonographic examinations. Abdominal x-ray examinations also decreased by about 60%, while endoscopy increased (mainly gastroscopy, but also some coloscopy). During a similar period, 1981-1984, the frequency of abdominal x-ray examinations made by radiologists in private practice (who rarely use sonography) increased, but by the relatively small amount of about 20% [K9]. It was also found that orthopaedic practitioners in the Federal Republic of Germany were increasingly favouring sonography for screening and follow-up examinations of hip joint diseases in infants [K9]. Before the introduction of hip joint sonography, 1.45 x-ray exposures were taken per examined infant; in 1984; after the introduction of sonography, 0.95 x-ray exposures per infant were taken. In the United States, the number of ultra-sonographic examinations in radiology departments of hospitals increased from 3.5 million in 1980 to 12.1 million in 1990 [M2]. During the same period, the number of x-ray examinations also increased from 114 million in 1980 to 181 million in 1990.

152. Endoscopy not only complements but to a large extent replaces x-ray examination of the gastrointestinal tract, as was observed in the Netherlands [G15]. In Sweden the number of x-ray examinations of the stomach also decreased, from 187,000 in 1975 to 33,000 in 1987, and will presumably decrease further, as endoscopy is now available at almost all Swedish hospitals [S14]. In contrast, colon examinations remained relatively constant over the period,

partly because coloscopy is more painful for the patient and more difficult to manage. These trends may not be universal, even in countries of health-care level I (see Table 7).

153. The number of magnetic resonance tomographs has almost doubled each year in the United States [S5]. According to one estimate, which is almost certainly too low, the total number of units in operation worldwide was about 1,200 in 1989, with 800 of these in the United States, 150 in Japan, 60 in the Federal Republic of Germany, 30 in France, 30 in Italy, 24 in the United Kingdom and 40 in other countries [B11]. Another estimate, based on interviews with all suppliers of such tomographs, indicated that about 3,500 units were in operation worldwide in January 1990. Of these, about 1,800 were in the United States and 550 in Japan. About 375 units were mobile [S12]. With regard to the examination profile, 48% of the magnetic resonance tomographies in Sweden in 1989 involved the brain and 36% the back [S12]. Other applications included studies of the abdomen, joints and limbs. Recently, magnetic resonance mammography has also become available [K5].

154. In spite of this development, computed tomographs using x rays also continue to increase. Smathers [S6] believes that magnetic resonance tomography will largely supplant computed tomography. Equally, it can be postulated that, instead of decreasing, as Smathers believes, computed tomography will continue to increase and eventually reach a plateau. In fact, the use of computed tomography of the skull has been increasing at such a pace in several countries that the use of magnetic resonance tomography of the skull has been decreasing. This particular trend is not expected to continue for long, since if it did, measures would be presumably taken to limit the possible overuse of computed tomography.

3. Particular patient groups

155. Trends in obstetric radiography are a source of particular concern because of the risks to the irradiated fetus. It has been suggested that the abdominal irradiation of pregnant women has been virtually replaced by other diagnostic techniques [M6]. This notion is supported to some degree by a Swedish study, which shows that the number of x-ray examinations during pregnancy in 1987 was 38% of the number in 1975 [S14]. In the United Kingdom the number of x-ray examinations during pregnancy did not seem to be lower in 1970-1981 than in 1950-1959 or 1960-1969 [G6], but the number of films per examination did decrease, and the timing of x-ray examinations shifted towards late pregnancy with practically no first trimester exposures after 1972. Gilman et al. [G6] estimated that 12% of all pregnant women in the United Kingdom had been examined with x rays in 1976-1981. An independent study by the National Radiological Protection Board (NRPB) [K14] gave an estimate of 4.2% in 1977. The difference may be due in part to the NRPB estimate being low and in part to a statistical uncertainty of the Gilman estimate [K14]. According to Gilman et al. [G6], the withdrawal of the so-called "10-day rule" of ICRP [I9] may lead to an increase in the frequency of x-ray examinations of pregnant women.

156. From time to time concern is expressed about the undue medical exposure of children [D9]. It may be expected that various radiation protection recommendations will be introduced in response to such concern; as a result, the rate of increase of examinations of children may be restrained in the future. The pattern may be more complex in developing countries: as shown in Table 9, the fraction of examinations performed on children is larger in developing countries than in industrialized countries (an exception are hip/femur examinations, which are performed on a higher fraction of children in level I countries than in countries of levels II-IV).

157. In most cases, while a smaller fraction of the patients at health-care level I are children, the frequency of examination of children is still greater than at other health-care levels because the total x-ray examination frequency is high. However, because chest fluoroscopy is frequent at all health-care levels and because there is a higher fraction of children among patients at lower health-care levels, the frequency of examination for children under 16 is about 2, 12 and 4 per 1,000 population at levels I, II and III, respectively. It was mentioned in Section II.B that the higher fraction of children among patients in levels II and III countries is probably due partly to the demographic structure in developing countries, where a greater part of the population consists of children. Since the frequencies of examinations are generally increasing in developing countries, the frequency of examinations of children can also be expected to increase.

158. A somewhat different kind of exposure occurs if x-ray examinations are performed intentionally on persons who are not really patients. For instance, healthy persons may be subjected to examination in connection with employment or for insurance purposes. Thus, an estimated 1 million pre-employment lumbar spinal x-ray examinations were performed in the United States in 1978 [M17], corresponding to 4.4 examinations per 1,000 population. Due to their dubious predictive value [M17], these examinations are being eliminated in several countries, albeit at differing rates. There were 140,000 employment-

related x-ray examinations in the United Kingdom in 1983 [W9], representing as many as 2.5 per 1,000 population. These examinations (mostly of the chest) caused a collective effective dose equivalent of about 5 man Sv, corresponding to a per caput dose of about 0.1 μSv.

159. In connection with the increased incidence of osteoporotic fractures among elderly persons, bone densitometry has become an important tool for measuring bone mineral content, especially in industrialized countries. There are two types of bone absorptiometers besides computed tomography: single photon absorptiometry (SPA) and dual photon absorptiometry (DPA). SPA is mainly used for cortical bone, DPA mainly for cancellous bone. Formerly, ^{153}Gd was used as a photon source, but more recent equipment is based on x rays [W13] or ^{125}I. The entrance surface dose sustained by the patient in an examination of this type is about 0.02-0.05 mGy for x-ray equipment [K15, H41], corresponding to an effective dose equivalent of about 0.8 μSv, and 0.01-0.18 mGy for ^{153}Gd equipment, with the lower doses in more recent tests [S27]. Computed tomography can also be used, but the effective dose equivalents may be up to three orders of magnitude greater [K15].

160. The Committee is aware that small subsets of the population of patients are subjected to repeated examinations to an extent that allows substantially higher doses than average. It has, however, proved difficult to obtain data illustrating the full extent of this variation. A well-known study of breast cancer incidence in tuberculosis patients in Massachusetts involved 2,573 women who had been examined by x-ray fluoroscopy on average 88 times, with an average of the mean absorbed dose to the breast of 790 mGy [B30]. However, it is believed that this study is not representative of current conditions. It might be expected that many of the patients concerned were old, meaning that the potential for expression of late effects of radiation should be limited. However, scoliosis patients are routinely subjected to periodic examinations in childhood [D10]. Some premature babies may be subjected to repeated chest x-ray examinations. Preston-Martin et al. [P18] assert that patients with parotid gland tumours had experienced a greater amount of prior radiography (mostly dental) than controls.

161. In theory, it should be possible to compile further statistics on multiple examinations in countries such as Germany, where a document is available to patients on request for the recording of radiological procedures (*Röntgenpaß*). In reality, few patients seem to avail themselves of this opportunity [B31], so the information to be had may be limited. A study at major hospitals in Nürnberg and Munich indicated that of those patients undergoing x-ray examinations, which was two thirds of all admitted patients, about 52% had 4 or more films taken, including 12% with more than 20 films and 1% with more than 100 films [S16]. The county council of Stockholm, Sweden, keeps a computerized record of all patients, based on social security number [B37]. The record shows that no more than nine patients, i.e. 0.001% of the population concerned, had 14 or more examinations in 20 years. In the United Kingdom, about 1% of the population accumulated a lifetime effective dose equivalent due to diagnostic x rays of more than 100 mSv [H15]. The maximum dose encountered in the study was about 200 mSv. Most of the patients with the highest doses had no more than 10-15 examinations, albeit almost always they included several examinations of the lower gastro-intestinal tract and urographic examinations. In a Canadian case study [R5], a 60-year-old male had 29 different examinations between 1957 and 1983, apparently resulting in an effective dose equivalent of 283 mSv, 41% of which came from fluoroscopy.

4. Effects of quality assurance programmes

162. The technical and physical parameters involved in quality assurance are discussed at length in a British Institute of Radiology Report [M7]. Standardized methods, guides, training and involvement of manufacturers must be implemented in quality assurance. The standards adopted in several countries for diagnostic x-ray examinations describe indications and contraindications for procedures, patient preparation, contrast agent, positioning, technical parameters (e.g. voltage, grid, screens), number of views, other possible examinations and special regulations for radiation protection. A complementary report on the optimization of image quality and patient exposure [M19] puts quality assurance in diagnostic radiology in a wider perspective (see also [G19]). A report from the United States [N3] discusses quality assurance for all types of diagnostic imaging equipment. Numerous authors stress the importance of patient dose surveys in auditing the optimization process, so that not only theoretical output from technical parameters but also actual results are assessed [B9, F2, N5, N11, V9].

163. Quality assurance programmes for x-ray diagnostics were begun in the United States in the early 1970s and became firmly established in 1980, when federal recommendations were made [B33]. Their success is easily explained: they have led to both economic savings and dose reductions [B34, P5]. Nonetheless, such programmes are likely to gain still wider acceptance in the future, as evidenced by a survey of over 2,000 automatic film processors in the United States, which revealed underprocessing in 9%

of mammography facilities, 33% of hospitals and 42% of private practices [S53]. In dental radiology in the United States, quality assurance programmes became generally accepted more recently: about 80% of the dental hygiene programmes surveyed had some sort of programme in 1990, as opposed to about 50% in 1985 [F10]. Quality assurance programmes are likely to become established all over the world (see, e.g. [P4]). In fact, the cost reductions attainable should make quality assurance even more attractive in developing countries [B9].

164. The introduction of quality assurance is expected to decrease doses per examination worldwide, as it results in lower doses per projection, fewer retakes and fewer unnecessary examinations [G18, N5]. Mikušová et al. [M39] attributed 15-18-fold variation in entrance surface doses in gastro-intestinal tract examinations to the lack of a quality assurance programme and calculated that effective doses in such examinations can be reduced 70% or more. They stated that their results showed the need of a quality assurance programme in Czechoslovakia.

165. It is difficult to predict the pace at which quality assurance will be introduced in different countries. Data from the UNSCEAR Survey of Medical Radiation Usage and Exposures are summarized in Table 24. It appears that quality assurance is relatively well established for x-ray diagnostics, even in developing countries (although a few responses from countries of health-care level I mention a reluctance to accept quality assurance). Note that in Canada and in the United States, while there are only recommendations at the national level, there are provincial or state regulations that are legally binding.

166. Some observations on the effect of quality assurance can be quoted. In the United States, per caput doses in dental radiography are decreasing. In Spain, quality assurance programmes are being started in collaboration with the Commission of European Communities, which has adopted [M22, M38] the reference dose levels originally suggested by Shrimpton et al. [S38] and chosen as guidelines in the United Kingdom [N5]. Before quality assurance was implemented, entrance doses were up to five times higher than these maximum values, but with quality assurance at least some of the causes of higher doses could immediately be successfully corrected [C9, V18]. For lower gastro-intestinal tract examinations in the Madrid area, effective dose equivalents at one centre were 0.8 ± 0.1 mSv, while they ranged from 5.5 ± 1.0 to 14.1 ± 2.2 mSv at four others [C13]. The authors concluded that quality assurance programmes should yield significant dose reductions. In Sweden, mandatory quality assurance requirements were introduced in 1981 and are an important explanatory factor behind dose reductions [G19].

167. Several quality assurance programmes of varying scope are in effect in European countries and elsewhere [B35, D5, E4, G19, H21, L4, V15, W4]. For a discussion of patient exposure criteria in the European Community, see [H46, M38, W20]. The Commission of the European Communities has prepared two documents to provide guidance for optimization of image quality and patient dose in adult and paediatric radiology [C3, C17]. Organ doses under optimal exposure conditions are available for examinations of adults [P7]. As shown in Denmark [H12] with respect to fluoroscopic systems, such programmes need not depend on the availability of health physicists; provided a suitable test protocol is devised, radiographers on site can perform very useful quality assurance. A study by the European Federation of Medical Physicists [C4] tabulated the occurrence in 20 European countries of assessment protocols (17 countries had from 5 to 13 protocols for equipment, 16 countries had from 2 to 10 protocols for image quality), of routine quality assurance procedures (6 countries required quality assurance procedures at regular intervals, 12 others required such procedures occasionally or at least on installation); and of auxiliary equipment checks; and it recorded the implementation of various recommendations.

168. Reject and repeat rates, which reflect the quality of radiographs, have been reported by many groups but rarely from developing countries. Bassey et al. [B32] provide an analysis from Nigeria (health-care level III since 1980). At first, the repeat rate was 12.4%. As a result of increasing awareness and corrective actions in response to the project, the repeat rate dropped rapidly, to an average of 2.5% (average for the entire year analysed: 3.7%). The authors noted that a formal quality assurance programme would reduce repeat rates and exposures further. As such, these repeat rates were not particularly high, in fact, 3.7% is low compared to the United Kingdom [N5]. But, as the authors say, criteria for repeating may differ, and films of marginal quality may have been accepted in Nigeria for economic or practical reasons [B32].

169. Quality assurance can certainly be applied not only in hospitals but also in general medical practice, although general practitioners may be less aware of quality assurance methods. In New Zealand, a study using an anthropomorphic ankle phantom examined by 22 general practitioners resulted in 2 fully acceptable sets of radiographs, 8 deficient sets and 12 rejected sets, 4 of which were completely undiagnostic [L5]. Nevertheless, the authors were not overly concerned, since the range and number of radiographic procedures performed in general practice is small and presents very little radiation hazard to patients and staff.

G. SUMMARY

170. For countries of health-care level I, the population-weighted average annual frequency of diagnostic x-ray examinations in 1985-1990 was 890 per 1,000 population, rather similar to the estimate in the UNSCEAR 1988 Report [U1] of 800 per 1,000 population. Examination frequencies in individual countries of health-care level I ranged from 320 to 1,290 per 1,000 population, and both increasing and decreasing national trends are evident. For health-care levels II-IV, data are less comprehensive, but at a first approximation the average frequency is 120 examinations per 1,000 population at level II and 64 per 1,000 population for levels III and IV combined. While the total x-ray examination frequency seems to be relatively constant at health-care level I, indications are that the frequencies of examinations are increasing at levels II-IV. During the 1980s, some 60% of all examinations were of the chest, 15% of the extremities, 10% of other skeleton and 10% of the digestive system. The pattern of examinations varies with time and with health-care level.

171. Broadly speaking, the total examination frequencies are expected to continue to increase at all health care levels. There are two main reasons for this: the increasing proportion of older people in populations and increasing urbanization. The increasing availability of alternative modalities, in particular ultrasound, may, however, limit somewhat the rate of increase. Patients subjected to x-ray examination are, on average, older than randomly chosen members of the public. Nonetheless, many examinations are rather frequently performed on children under 16 years of age. With the exception of hip/femur examinations, a greater fraction of examined patients are children in countries of health-care level II and III, perhaps because those countries have younger populations. However, examination frequencies exceed those of health-care level I only in the case of chest fluoroscopy.

172. The doses to patients from diagnostic x-ray examinations vary widely. In certain cardiac procedures, entrance surface doses of several gray occur. High doses are delivered in fluoroscopy with conventional equipment. This does not mean that fluoroscopy is an unfavourable procedure, even from the restricted view of dose limitation, since with modern image intensifiers low doses can be achieved. Fluoroscopy during extracorporeal lithotripsy causes smaller doses than those encountered in conventional renal stone extraction. Computed tomography is being used more frequently, and effective doses (at present averaging about 5 mSv per examination) are increasing. Chest x-ray doses are decreasing, with effective doses per examination now often under 0.1 mSv, but the vast number performed still causes chest examination to contribute several tens of per cent of the collective effective dose. Mammography examinations now give low absorbed doses to breasts, often under 1 mGy, but extended screening programmes, commonly aimed at all women over age 40 years, could add several per cent to collective doses. Dental x rays often entail effective doses less than 0.1 mSv per examination but affect large groups, and thus add a per cent or so to the collective dose. Chiropractic x-ray examinations cause low doses per examination and affect few people. Children are a particularly sensitive group. Chest examination of neonates and scoliosis testing of teenage girls were mentioned as problem areas.

173. Per caput annual effective dose equivalents from the diagnostic use of x rays reported from a number of countries of health-care level I ranged from 0.3 to 2.2 mSv. For countries of health-care level I, the population-weighted average of values from 1982 to 1990 is 1.2 mSv. The estimate of per caput dose from analysis of population-weighted frequencies and doses of examinations is 0.9 mSv, which is little different from the estimate of 1.0 mSv given in the UNSCEAR 1988 Report. For countries of health-care level II, which have a population of 2.6 billion, information is still limited, yet more complete than for the UNSCEAR 1988 Report [U1]. The estimated per caput effective dose equivalent is 0.1 mSv (1988 estimate: 0.2-1.0 mSv). Doses at health-care levels III and IV (0.04 mSv) are more uncertain, but they do not much affect the worldwide average due to the low examination frequencies.

174. These overall trends are derived from non-homogeneous data. Both examination frequencies and patient doses vary rather widely, between neighbouring countries and even within countries. Also, similar total examination frequencies or total effective doses may be composed in different ways in different countries. Particular importance is attached to the trends for computed tomography, which is characterized by increasing examination frequency as well as increasing doses. Quality assurance programmes have amply demonstrated that dose variation can be decreased and unnecessary exposure reduced.

175. The estimates of average individual and collective doses to the world population from diagnostic medical x-ray examinations (0.3 mSv and 1.6 million man Sv) are at the lower end of the ranges suggested in the UNSCEAR 1988 Report [U1] (0.35-1.0 mSv and 1.8-5 million man Sv). There is, at present, somewhat less uncertainty about the frequencies and doses from fluoroscopy examination in countries of health-care levels II-IV. The doses from dental x-ray examinations are less than those from medical x-ray examinations by two orders of magnitude.

III. DIAGNOSTIC USE OF RADIOPHARMACEUTICALS

176. The rapid pace of change in nuclear medicine makes assessment difficult, but a few trends can be identified. Of the many different radionuclides used in nuclear medicine examinations, ^{99m}Tc and ^{131}I are the most important. As a rule, the dose per procedure is less for ^{99m}Tc, which has a shorter half-life, so it is preferred and used in the majority of cases. Even so, the usage of ^{131}I is great enough to make an important nominal contribution to the collective dose. In 1986, for example, only 13% of all nuclear medicine examinations in Sweden employed ^{131}I, but it contributed 51% of the collective dose of 420 man Sv [V4]. By comparison, 56% of the examinations in 1971 were made with ^{131}I, which contributed 92% of the collective dose of 520 man Sv. In the USSR, 77% of all examinations in 1981 utilized ^{131}I [N4]. The most commonly used radionuclide in developing countries is ^{131}I, and this is the main reason the average effective dose per examination is higher in these countries than in industrialized countries.

A. FREQUENCIES OF EXAMINATIONS

177. The frequencies of diagnostic nuclear medicine examinations performed in countries are listed in Table 25 (total frequency) and Table 26 (frequency of the main types of examinations). The results are mainly from the UNSCEAR Survey of Medical Radiation Usage and Exposures, supplemented with published data. As a first approximation, the total frequency of all nuclear medicine examinations is about 16 per 1,000 population in countries of health-care level I, 0.5 per 1,000 population in countries at level II, 0.3 per 1,000 population at level III, and 0.1 per 1,000 population at level IV. The number of countries at levels III and IV reporting information is much too small to be considered representative. The distributions of available data for 1985-1990 are illustrated in Figure V.

178. Generally higher examination frequencies (20-40 per 1,000 population) are reported for Belgium, Czechoslovakia, the Federal Republic of Germany, Luxembourg and the United States. The reasons for the higher frequency seem to differ: there are many liver/spleen and renal examinations in Czechoslovakia; many bone examinations, lung perfusions and thyroid scans in the Federal Republic of Germany; many cardiovascular examinations and lung perfusions in the United States; and all examinations are more frequent in Belgium and Luxembourg. Although the total nuclear medicine examination frequency in Canada (13 examinations per 1,000 population) is typical of health-care level I countries, there are about 10 times as many brain examinations (4 per 1,000 population) as the average for health-care level I (0.4 per 1,000 population). In some countries, all practitioners are permitted to use radiopharmaceuticals, while in many other countries, they are available only in hospitals or clinics.

179. In nuclear medicine, not only the total examination frequencies but also the patterns of examinations appear to differ more than the frequencies and patterns of x-ray examinations. Averages for the main kinds of examination at different health-care levels are given in Table 27 and illustrated in Figure VI, which shows that bone and cardiovascular examinations are the most frequent. However, these averages may conceal widely differing practices. Some such differences are discussed below. Three types of average measure are given in Table 27: the population-weighted average, the unweighted average with its standard deviation, and median values. Of these, the population-weighted averages are the most relevant for purposes of collective dose estimation, while unweighted averages and medians may be of interest when individual countries are compared to others.

180. Huda et al. [H17] point out differences between North American and European countries: ^{99m}Tc is used more frequently in Manitoba, in Canada, and in the United States. Examinations of the brain are less frequent in Europe than in North America, and cardiovascular examinations are somewhat less frequent. Within Europe there are no differences in examination frequencies between Sweden and the Federal Republic of Germany [H18, K10]. However, the use of ^{99m}Tc is as common in the Federal Republic of Germany as in North America but not as common in Sweden. There could, of course, be local deviations from this pattern within North America. The data for the United States are averaged over a large number of states; the data for Manitoba and Nova Scotia quoted in the text and Tables refer to only small parts of Canada, so that the extrapolations made from these must be regarded as tentative approximations.

181. Intra-regional differences in examination patterns may occur even where nuclear medicine has a similar total radiological impact. For instance, the Netherlands and Sweden are similar in many respects, and the impact of diagnostic nuclear medicine is similar in the two countries. Nevertheless, there are several important differences between the two countries [B3, V4]. Thus, while the use of ^{99m}Tc is similar (used in 65%

of examinations in the Netherlands and 63% in Sweden), much more ^{123}I and much less ^{131}I are used in the Netherlands than in Sweden (in 10.1% and 3.0% of examinations in the Netherlands compared with 0.6% and 14.1% of examinations in Sweden). The use of ^{201}Tl is more common in the Netherlands than in Sweden (6.8% and 2.5% of examinations, respectively).

182. The use of ^{51}Cr also differs in countries with similar nuclear medicine practice. Renal clearance with ^{51}Cr are important in Sweden (9.1% of examinations), but the radionuclide is hardly used at all in the Netherlands (0.2% of examinations). Canada [H17] and Germany [K10], with somewhat higher per caput doses from nuclear medicine, report little or no use of ^{51}Cr-EDTA, although other ^{51}Cr radiopharmaceuticals are used in Canada (sodium chromate and chromic chloride); ^{99m}Tc rather than ^{51}Cr is used for inulin and creatinine clearance measurements of the glomerular filtration rate.

183. Figure VI shows that nuclear medicine examinations in countries of health-care level I are more frequent by an order of magnitude or more than in countries of lower health-care levels. Only for thyroid uptake studies are the relative differences not quite so great. At health-care level I some 30% of examinations were of bone, some 20% were of the lung and some 15% were cardiovascular. These examinations are all being performed more frequently. The percentages of brain (5%), liver/spleen (5%-10%), renal (5%-10%) and thyroid (15%) examinations are decreasing. Trends in individual countries may deviate from this general pattern. Generally, the data indicate increased frequencies with time in the total number of nuclear medicine examinations. Myanmar reports a steadily decreasing examination frequency, from 0.54 per 1,000 population in 1976-1980 to 0.11 per 1,000 population in 1985-1990.

184. Nuclear medicine is continuing to develop in China, and more than 800 hospitals now practice nuclear medicine [W7]. The most frequent imaging procedures are liver scintigraphy, thyroid imaging, and lung, kidney, bone, brain and heart imaging, in that order [W7]. The most common function tests are thyroid uptake, renogram and cardiac function [W7]. In function tests, ^{99m}Tc is the most frequently used isotope [L14, W7]. Thus, the data cited in the UNSCEAR 1988 Report [U1], according to which ^{99m}Tc was not used in China, were not representative. Wang and Liu [W7] regard ^{113m}In as the primary alternative when ^{99m}Tc is unavailable and stress that the long half-life of the ^{113}Sn parent makes ^{113m}In generators suitable in developing countries, where low cost and long transport times are important considerations. Nonetheless, ^{131}I is still a big contributor to effective dose in China [Z6] and in India.

185. Information from other developing countries is very limited. In Tunisia, diagnostic nuclear medicine *in vivo* is practised at one clinic in Tunis, which is equipped with scintiscanners. Radionuclides are brought from France on a regular basis, which ensures supply but excludes short-lived isotopes [M13]. In Nigeria, with a population of about 100 million, one scanner is available in Lagos. About 79% of the 1,000 patients referred in 1982-1984 had thyroid-related pathology, and most of the other examinations concerned the liver, the brain or bone [F5]. In Zaire, with a population of 30 million, one nuclear medicine facility exists in Kinshasa, but apparently work there is hampered by many very difficult problems [I6].

186. Most of the examinations in nuclear medicine are performed on adult patients. For instance, 98% of all examinations in the United States are performed on patients who are at least 15 years old (and 90% were 30 years or older) [U1]. Examinations of children appear to be somewhat more frequent in eastern Europe [D1, U1]. There is no particular type of examination specifically aimed at children, apart perhaps from neonatal hypothyroidism screening, which is performed by radioimmunoassay *in vitro* and thus causes no patient dose [I6].

187. The age- and sex-distributions of patients subjected to diagnostic nuclear medicine examinations are given in Table 28. On average, the population examined is older than the general population and also older than those receiving x-ray examinations. Relatively high proportions of renal examinations are performed on children in countries of health-care level I. At health-care level II, bone and brain examinations of children are relatively frequent. The proportion of children examined is higher in countries at health-care levels II-IV, as was also the case for diagnostic x-ray examinations, but the difference between health-care levels is smaller than for x-ray examinations. As with x-ray examinations, the excess of children among examined patients may well depend on demographic factors (there are more children in these countries). Since total nuclear medicine examination frequencies are much lower at health-care levels II-IV, the frequency of examined children is consistently smaller at these health-care levels than at level I, in spite of the higher percentage of children among examined persons.

188. As expected, more women have thyroid examinations and more men have cardiovascular examinations (with the exception of China). Otherwise, the sex distributions appear to be fairly standard.

B. DOSES IN EXAMINATIONS

189. The average amounts of radioisotope compounds administered for some important procedures in diagnostic nuclear medicine are listed in Table 29. Only the major radiopharmaceuticals reported in use are included. The listing must necessarily compress the information received, which was of uneven detail to begin with, making it difficult to calculate effective doses. Some comments are, however, relevant.

190. The activity administered per examination seems to be more standardized than the factors that influence dose in diagnostic x-ray examinations. This is also true for different levels of health care. Thus, the vast differences in dose per examination between countries of different levels are due to the choice of radiopharmaceuticals not to different amounts of activity for any given procedure.

191. Thyroid examinations contribute as much as half of the collective dose from all diagnostic nuclear medicine procedures. Typical effective dose equivalents in the province of Manitoba, Canada, in 1981-1985 were 3.9 mSv for ^{131}I, 1.2 mSv for ^{123}I and 1.5 mSv for ^{99m}Tc. The substitution of other nuclides for ^{131}I in most cases reduced the estimated collective dose by a factor of 3.6 [H35]. Cardiovascular examinations caused comparatively high doses, from about 10 mSv (^{99m}Tc erythrocytes) to about 20 mSv (^{201}Tl chloride). Brain examinations with ^{99m}Tc gluconate caused 8-10 mSv, bone examinations with ^{99m}Tc phosphate up to about 7 mSv.

192. Tomographic investigations with single photon emission computed tomography (SPECT) require, on average, higher activities per examination than similar planar examinations. Consequently, SPECT tests could lead to higher patient doses [E1], at least for examinations such as myocardial scintigraphy, regional cerebral blood flow, bone scintigraphy, liver scintigraphy, radionuclide ventriculography and tests with tagged monoclonal antibodies. In principle, positron emission tomography (PET) should also require high activities per examination, but the doses do not seem to be extremely high, at least not with ^{18}F substances, which result in effective dose equivalents of up to 6 mSv per procedure [M43].

193. Examinations of children form an important part of the evaluation of patient doses, since the dose per unit activity can be much higher for children than for adults [I5, T6]. Two important differences between children and adults should be taken into account when considering the use of radiopharmaceuticals and evaluating doses. Physiological differences such as differing body weights can lead to a different (higher or lower) effective dose for children after administration of a given amount of activity [S15, T6]. Age-related dose coefficients [I5, I14] take these physiological differences into account. Another difference is the greater sensitivity of children, reflected in the higher risks per unit dose. As mentioned in Section I.B., this could in principle also be taken into account.

194. Absorbed doses, effective dose equivalents and effective doses per unit activity of various radiopharmaceuticals administered to patients have been derived and are listed in ICRP Publication 53 (for H_E) [I5] and in its Addendum (for E) [I14]. Supplementary information can be found in the MIRD (medical internal radiation dose) reports, most recently on ^{99m}Tc-labelled bone imaging agents [W6], red blood cells [A5], ^{111}In-labelled platelets [R21] and ^{99m}Tc-DTPA aerosol [A13]. Some MIRD estimates may be inexact, [K26, T15], particularly with respect to Auger emitters [H25, K27, S48].

195. There is not yet a wide basis for calculating effective doses from nuclear medicine examinations. For instance, individual differences in metabolism could contribute to variability. Furthermore, individual organ doses may vary with disease conditions, although effective dose may be a more robust quantity. Table 30 lists typical effective dose equivalents from examinations. The effective dose equivalents were calculated using the dose factors in ICRP Publication 53 [I5], but patient ages or sizes were not considered. There are three further sources of variation in estimated effective doses (effective dose equivalents):

(a) each examination category represents several types of procedure. Perhaps the most extreme example is kidney examinations: renograms are occasionally made with ^{125}I-hippurate with a typical effective dose of 0.01 mSv while renal scintigraphy with ^{99m}Tc gives at least 1 mSv per examination;
(b) a given procedure can be done with different radionuclides. A good example is thyroid scintigraphy: performed with ^{99m}Tc, the effective doses are under 1 mSv; performed with ^{131}I, they approach 100 mSv. The difference is important since ^{99m}Tc is typically less accessible in developing countries;
(c) the amount of activity administered for a procedure differs; this, however, is not a major source of variation in doses.

196. In principle, it is desirable for analytical purposes to specify the age distributions of patients; however, these are likely to be different for each type of examination. To illustrate the dependence of dose on age,

Table 31 provides the average and per caput effective dose equivalents from the average activities administered and the frequencies of examinations determined for Manitoba, Canada [H17]. The age-dependent doses per unit activity administered were taken from ICRP Publication 53 [I5].

197. The effective dose equivalents to children in Table 31 were computed with age-related dose conversion factors where possible, but when no data were available it was assumed that the activity administered to a child was the same as that to an adult. The effective dose to children per unit activity can be much higher than that to adults, and examinations of children are not all that rare. This is particularly true in the case of renal examinations, which constitute some 10% of all procedures.

198. Doses to unborn children after the administration of radiopharmaceuticals to pregnant patients may, according to Cox et al. [C18], be seriously underestimated by current methodology. Although their primary concern is with therapeutic administrations, they also discuss lung perfusion scintigrams using ^{99m}Tc albumin aggregates, which they believe is the most frequent examination in pregnant women. In their opinion, it results in a uterine dose of 10 mSv rather than the 0.3 mSv calculated by conventional methods.

C. WORLDWIDE EXPOSURES

199. Representative frequencies of nuclear medicine examinations for each health-care level and doses per examination cannot be well established from the available data. Nevertheless, the approximate values do give an indication of the collective dose from this practice. This analysis is shown in Table 32. The population-weighted frequencies of examinations were derived in Table 26 and listed in Table 27. The effective dose equivalents from typical examinations were given in Table 31, with the values for adults being used in Table 32. Higher doses were indicated in Table 30 for China for thyroid scans and liver/spleen examinations whenever the preferred isotope, ^{99m}Tc, was not available. It is not known how often this occurs, but in order not to underestimate the collective dose, the higher doses have been assumed for these examinations in health-care levels II-IV. The product of frequency and dose per examination gives the estimated collective effective dose from each examination.

200. The collective effective dose equivalent from nuclear medicine examinations worldwide is estimated to be 156,000 man Sv, with 127,000, 20,000 and 10,000 man Sv from health-care levels I, II and III-IV, respectively. Most of the collective dose (81%) is received at level I. The dose per examination averages 5.7 mSv at level I, but it is about four times higher at levels II-IV. The per caput dose is 0.09 mSv at level I but is, because of much lower frequencies, an order of magnitude less at levels II-IV.

201. The contributions of the various examinations to the collective doses are given in Table 33. At health-care level I, cardiovascular and bone scans account for 70% of the collective dose. Because of the high dose assumed for thyroid scans at level II-IV, this examination is by far the largest contributor to total collective dose from nuclear medicine in these countries.

202. This analysis of collective dose is very approximate since only a single typical examination has been assumed in each case, and the representativeness of the frequencies and doses applied cannot be established. It does, however, indicate that the collective dose from nuclear medicine examinations worldwide is about 10% of that from diagnostic medical x-ray examinations.

203. Estimates of collective dose from nuclear medicine examinations in a number of countries have been published or supplied in direct response to the UNSCEAR Survey of Radiation Usage and Exposures. These estimates are summarized in Table 34. Because the conditions, assumptions and methods underlying these results vary widely, direct comparison may not always be valid.

204. The collective doses shown in Table 34 can be compared with total medical radiation doses to determine the relative contribution of doses from nuclear medicine examinations. The collective effective dose equivalent from nuclear medicine examinations in the United States in 1982, 32,100 man Sv, amounted to about 35% of the 92,000 man Sv from diagnostic x-ray usage [N1]. In contrast, the 1,000 man Sv from nuclear medicine in the United Kingdom in 1982 constituted only about 5% of the 20,000 man Sv from diagnostic x-ray usage.

205. Alternative estimates could be derived for the effective dose equivalent from nuclear medicine examinations in Canada by extrapolating the estimates for Manitoba and Quebec to the entire country. These results would be 3,200 and 9,900 man Sv, respectively, to be compared with the estimate given in Table 34, 4,200 man Sv. The difference in the three estimates stems mainly from different assumptions about the number of examinations [L7]. Of the 260 nuclear medicine clinics in Canada, over half are located in Ontario and only 10 in Manitoba [L12], so extrapolation from Manitoba may be uncertain. The

arithmetic average of the three estimates of dose per examination is 5.1 mSv, which is similar to the value derived in Table 32 for level I countries.

206. Maruyama et al. studied the usage of radiopharmaceuticals in Japan in 1982 [M10, M11, M12]. They provided detailed age- and sex-distributions of patients for each radiopharmaceutical used in several general procedures (e.g. renogram, scintigram, blood flow) [M10]. They also derived age- and sex-specific organ-dose conversion factors and a set of sex-specific effective dose equivalents for each radiopharmaceutical used [M11]. Most of the numeric values were fairly similar to the values in ICRP Publication 53 [I5]. This comprehensive material underlies the entry for Japan in Table 34. The distribution of the collective dose over age groups and for different radiopharmaceuticals is given by Maruyama et al. [M12].

207. The per caput effective dose equivalents in Table 34 vary by two orders of magnitude, partly owing to variation in examination frequencies. In contrast, most of the effective dose equivalents per examined patient fall within a fairly narrow range, 2-5 mSv, in countries of health-care level I. The exceptions, with effective dose equivalents in the 10-30 mSv range, are countries in which the use of long-lived radionuclides, such as ^{131}I and ^{198}Au, is proportionally higher. Doses in Poland are in the upper range, with an effective dose equivalent per examination which is three times that observed in India. The main reason is that half of all examinations are performed with ^{131}I, resulting in some 20 mSv per examination. The range of the average effective dose equivalent per examination in China (15-34 mSv) [Z6] encompasses the value derived in Table 32 (20 mSv).

208. For countries of health-care level I, a population-weighted annual per caput effective dose equivalent of 0.073 mSv can be derived from Table 34. This gives some corroboration to the value derived in Table 32. In the UNSCEAR 1988 Report [U1] the estimated value was 0.05 mSv, although weighting for population would, in fact, have given 0.07 mSv. The present estimate (0.09 mSv) is hardly different, but as it is based on data from more countries, it is more reliable.

209. For health-care level II, the previous estimate of the per caput dose from nuclear medicine examinations was 0.004 mSv [U1]. The present estimate, 0.008 mSv, is again more soundly based, especially because there are data from China and India. There are still inadequate data for levels III and IV. With the frequency of all examinations only slightly less than for level II and the important thyroid scans comparable in frequency, the similar per caput dose derived for level III should mean that the collective dose will not be underestimated.

210. Annual per caput and collective effective dose equivalents from nuclear medicine examinations worldwide are summarized in Table 35. The total collective dose from the practice (160,000 man Sv) is about twice as great as the estimate in the UNSCEAR 1988 Report [U1]. Even the present estimate is highly approximate, but the underlying database has been strengthened.

D. TRENDS

211. The number of diagnostic nuclear medicine examinations increased in industrialized countries in the 1970s, but remained relatively constant in the 1980s [H17, H18]. However, the frequency of nuclear medicine examinations in hospitals in the United States increased from 5.6 million in 1980 to 7.5 million in 1990 [M2]. The frequency of examinations is expected to increase in developing countries. The data from the UNSCEAR Survey of Medical Radiation Usage and Exposures are too incomplete to allow quantifying trends.

212. One of the important developments is that new ^{99m}Tc-labelled compounds are replacing established compounds containing other radionuclides in level I and to some extent level II countries [P13]. Usually, this leads to lower doses per examination. Other important trends are the introduction of complex biological agents (such as radiolabelled monoclonal antibodies) for novel imaging applications and the proliferation of new compounds for studies with positron emission tomography (PET). These developments can be expected to lead to more examinations per caput. The proliferation of single photon emission computed tomography (SPECT) and positron emission tomography are also expected to lead to the wider use of three-dimensional rendering [H23, P22, W17], as was already discussed for x rays in Section II.F. Computed x-ray tomography and magnetic resonance tomography both provide higher resolution, however, which means that purely anatomical imaging is not an important procedure in current nuclear medicine practice [E2]. Instead, measurements of flow and biochemical reactions are important.

1. Specific methods in nuclear medicine

213. While the total number of nuclear medicine examinations may have remained relatively constant in industrialized countries from 1980 to 1990, the choice or pattern certainly has changed. As an example, data from Sweden [H18, V4] reveal a very complex pattern. The two most important changes concern the relative use of ^{99m}Tc (19% of all tests in 1971, 65% in 1987) and ^{131}I (52% in 1971 and 12% in 1987).

Gold-198 was phased out in 1977. The use of ^{125}I is decreasing, while that of ^{51}Cr, ^{123}I and ^{201}Tl is increasing. All of these trends refer specifically to the one country studied. While the trend in relative use of ^{99m}Tc and ^{131}I is presumably widespread, there may be national differences for other radionuclides. For instance, the use of ^{201}Tl (and of ^{111}In) is probably decreasing in the Federal Republic of Germany. In particular, myocardial scintigraphy with ^{201}Tl is being replaced with antimyosine immune scintigraphy, radionuclide ventriculography and other methods that give lower patient doses [B7]. One reason for national differences is the varying availability of radionuclides with short half-life (this factor is particularly relevant in developing countries).

214. The field of paediatric nuclear medicine will possibly grow [P13]. Table 28 shows that renal imaging is the most frequent examination in children, at least in countries at health-care level I. For adults, distributions vary, but on average, bone scans appear to be the most common examination. MAG-3, a recently introduced ^{99m}Tc-labelled mimic of hippuran (which is labelled with iodine) is particularly suitable for paediatric renal imaging [H22, P13]. Since ^{99m}Tc gives smaller doses than iodine, doses are not expected to increase at the same rate as the number of examinations.

215. Radioactively labelled monoclonal antibodies are a valuable diagnostic tool for finding tumours and metastases through radioimmunoscintigraphy. Their use for therapeutic purposes is mentioned in Chapter V. In a diagnostic context, they are associated with relatively high effective dose equivalents: 34 mSv (for ^{111}In), 30 mSv (^{131}I) and 7 mSv (^{99m}Tc) [R15].

216. Single photon emission computed tomography has evolved rapidly since the early 1980s, when it was still rare [P22]. Not only it is now a standard method for tumour localization but it is also used in a variety of applications, such as functional brain studies [H23], cardiac studies, bone imaging and abdominal imaging [P22]. It can also be used in conjunction with labelled monoclonal antibodies. In contrast to the very expensive positron emission tomography technique, single photon emission computed tomography may be affordable in at least some developing countries [P23], in particular if personal computer algorithms for tomography gain wider acceptance, permitting significant reductions in equipment costs [S49].

217. Positron emission tomography provides quantitative, locational, functional and biochemical information that would be difficult to obtain by other means [B13]. While positron emission tomography began as a technique for brain studies [J2], it is now used also for myocardial examination and oncological work [R11, T16]. Whole-body imaging in oncology is an expected development [D14]. The use of labelled anticancer drugs will allow *in vivo* dosimetry, an application likely to become important in the treatment of diffuse disease [O4]. However, there are two problems: equipment is costly, and the short-lived isotopes used require cyclotron facilities nearby.

218. Ott [O4] has stressed that it is hardly necessary to have a cyclotron at each hospital; regional cyclotron facilities within one or two hours distance could serve many users in densely populated areas. While positron cameras are expected to become less expensive, Ott did not foresee a price reduction by more than half in the near future [O4]. Some university institutions have been able to fabricate cameras at low costs [O4, S8], but the cyclotron requirement is likely to continue to keep positron emission tomography generally inaccessible to developing countries. In industrialized countries, the number of positron emission tomography centres is likely to grow rapidly. There were 99 of them in 1991 and 122 in 1992 [G14]; 80% of these were in the United States (75) and Japan (21) in 1992, with 2 each in Australia, the Federal Republic of Germany and Sweden and 5 each in Belgium, Canada, Italy and the United Kingdom. Generator-produced positron emitters may contribute to further growth. They would allow limited positron emission tomography studies without having to invest in a cyclotron [T16]. Generators producing ^{82}Rb from ^{82}Sr are already available, and a ^{62}Cu (from ^{62}Zn) generator is being developed.

219. Hill [H40] expects a rapid increase in the use of positron emission tomography for general imaging purposes. He points out that gamma camera images are greatly inferior to other radiological images in terms of spatial resolution, contrast discrimination and acquisition speed, because the collimator of the gamma camera reduces photon efficiency by at least three orders of magnitude and introduces scatter. Hill stresses that while positron emission tomography lends itself to high-level studies of human metabolism, it should also be an appropriate tool for nuclear medicine in general [H40]. Since the extra information gained with the most advanced positron emission tomography techniques is not necessarily of clinical significance [W29], radiation protection considerations will presumably restrain some of the future growth of positron emission tomography.

220. Limited access to positron emission tomography is likely to restrict this nuclear medicine usage in developing countries in the near future. However, this does not mean that nuclear medicine will be non-existent. Some advanced methods, such as three-dimensional rendering, may be available with reasonable investment costs. However, the high cost of

radiopharmaceuticals, as well as infrastructure problems that limit the availability of short-lived radionuclides, will presumably lead to other examination patterns than in industrialized countries. Thus, radionuclide imaging will presumably not grow very fast, since there are alternatives [I6]. However, there are no obvious alternatives to functional studies which may spread somewhat faster [I6, I7]. Diagnostic *in vitro* analysis with ready-made radioimmunoassay kits is likely to increase, since the technique will work under various conditions and is useful in diagnosis of parasitic infections, which are important in developing countries [I6, I15].

221. It should not be assumed that the evolution of nuclear medicine practice will be similar in all developing countries. On the contrary, there are great differences between individual countries [I6, I7]. At this stage, however, the quantity of nuclear medicine performed seems to be small in most developing countries, even if the methods that do find use differ greatly from country to country. Of course, there are local interruptions in the practice of nuclear medicine, caused not so much by equipment failure as by the erratic supply of radionuclides [I6, I7]. The potential of diagnostic nuclear medicine to detect diseases at an earlier stage and, accordingly, to reduce the direct and indirect costs of illness will presumably encourage developing countries to increase the availability of nuclear medicine, in spite of the difficulties.

2. Alternatives to nuclear medicine

222. The main alternative to nuclear medicine examinations is ultrasonography. Liver scintigraphy with ^{99m}Tc and renal localization with ^{125}I are tending to be replaced by ultrasonography [V4]. The frequency of thyroid scintigraphies in the Federal Republic of Germany decreased by 40% from 1978 to 1984, and at the same time the frequency of thyroid ultrasonic examinations increased by 272% [K9]. Scintigraphy is still the basic procedure for thyroid examination, while ultrasound is used for screening. Ultrasonography is used not only for thyroid and abdominal studies but also increasingly for cardiovascular, renal, locomotive (including hip-joint in children), infant skull, gynaecological and ear, nose and throat examinations.

223. The trend is, however, not universal, In private radiology practices ultrasound equipment is less common. In this case the frequencies of nuclear medicine procedures (e.g. thyroid and bone scintigraphies) have been steadily increasing [K9].

224. Echocardiography is generally regarded as useful for the screening of patients with suspected early cardiomyopathy, while angiography with radiopharmaceuticals is expected to remain the normal procedure when the disease has progressed [C9]. Magnetic resonance tomography is expected to complement (and to some extent supplant) computed tomography with x rays, as was discussed in this context in Section II.F.2. But it can also be regarded as an alternative to some types of radionuclide imaging, including single photon emission computed tomography [S6].

3. Effects of quality assurance programmes

225. Quality assurance programmes, first introduced by the World Health Organization around 1980, are well established for nuclear medicine use in countries of health-care level I. Early efforts in the United States, in particular, helped to establish these programmes [S28]. Table 24 summarizes the regulations and recommendations in countries responding to the UNSCEAR Survey of Medical Radiation Usage and Exposures. It should be noted that responses to the survey are not always consistent, perhaps reflecting differences at the state and federal levels in countries. Bäuml [B40] has compiled references to quality assurance methods and their implementation and results. Further discussion of quality control procedures in nuclear medicine is given in an NCRP report from the United States [N3] and, for radiopharmaceuticals, in an Australian Radiation Laboratory Report [B38].

226. Results of quality assurance testing demonstrate the need for such programmes. This is illustrated by tests of 125 batches of 32 different types of radiopharmaceutical in Australia 1989 [B39]. No less than 23 batches (18%) failed to meet full specifications. A test in Sweden of 81 of the 91 gamma cameras in the country revealed inferior properties for general planar imaging in a third of the cameras, considerable variations in bone imaging and insufficient uniformity in a third of the single photon emission computed tomography systems [L13].

E. SUMMARY

227. In diagnostic nuclear medicine practice, the two most important isotopes are ^{99m}Tc, the use of which is increasing, and ^{131}I, the use of which is decreasing rapidly but which still contributes much to the collective dose. In industrialized countries, the per caput doses due to exposures of patients in nuclear medicine examinations range from 0.02 to 0.2 mSv (population-weighted per caput effective dose equivalent: 0.09 mSv). The dose per examination is a few millisievert in most industrialized countries and 10-40 mSv in developing countries. The difference is due to the more frequent use of long-lived radionuclides in developing countries.

228. Examination frequencies and, hence, per caput doses are higher in North America than in Europe and much higher in industrialized countries than in developing countries. In countries with similar per caput doses, there can still be important differences in choice of procedure. In industrialized countries, examination frequencies are probably no longer increasing as quickly as they did 10 years ago. One of the reasons for this is the competing use of computed tomography and ultrasonography. New techniques, such as positron emission tomography, are expected to become established in industrialized countries. In developing countries, *in vitro* kits as well as some functional study procedures are likely to find increasing use.

229. The estimated effective dose equivalents from diagnostic nuclear medicine examinations for different levels of health care and worldwide are summarized in Table 35. For health-care level I, the annual per caput dose has been adjusted from the previous estimate [U1] of 0.05 mSv, to 0.09 mSv. Access to important new data from China and India permit an improved estimate of the annual per caput effective dose equivalent for countries of health-care level II, now estimated to be 0.008 mSv (previous estimate: 0.004 mSv). For health-care levels III and IV, per caput doses are assumed to be comparable to those in level II. However, because of the low examination frequencies, this estimate has little influence on the collective dose. The estimated per caput effective dose equivalent worldwide is now 0.03 mSv annually, and the estimated collective dose from the practice is 160,000 man Sv. This is twice the 1988 estimate, but it is still only 10% of the estimated collective dose from diagnostic x-ray examinations.

IV. THERAPEUTIC USE OF RADIATION

230. In teletherapy, an external source of radiation allows a beam of photons to be directed towards the patient. For deep-seated tumours, high energy photons are obtained primarily from ^{60}Co sources or linear accelerators [P8]. Older ^{137}Cs sources are being replaced for various reasons. Other, less common types of teletherapy apparatus are mentioned in Section IV.D. For the teletherapy of superficial tumours, x rays are utilized. Very soft Bucky x rays are used for skin disorders. In brachytherapy [T18], sealed radioactive sources are inserted into a body cavity (intracavitary or intraluminal application), placed on the surface of a tumour or on the skin (superficial application), or implanted through a tumour (interstitial therapy). Commonly used sources are ^{198}Au or ^{125}I for permanent implants, ^{137}Cs or ^{192}Ir for low-dose-rate temporary applications, and ^{60}Co or ^{192}Ir for high-dose-rate temporary applications (in the case of ^{60}Co or ^{192}Ir, always using remote afterloading). Older ^{226}Ra sources for low-dose-rate temporary applications are now much less used.

231. In therapy, the objective is to deliver a radiation dose to the patient. Neither individual nor collective effective doses are directly relevant for comparisons with doses from other sources, not even with diagnostic procedures. Furthermore, although they are mentioned below, per caput doses of any kind are difficult to interpret, since they result from averaging very high doses to very few people over an entire population. In the present context, the radiological impact of therapy can perhaps best be described simply by the number of patients and the target doses. Such information was collected in the UNSCEAR Survey of Medical Radiation Usage and Exposures. Effective doses are also discussed below, but the limitations are stressed. Although the numbers of treatments are discussed in this Annex, the data are assumed to refer to the overall courses of treatment and, therefore, to the numbers of treated patients.

A. FREQUENCIES OF TREATMENTS

232. The frequencies of radiotherapeutic treatments reported in response to the UNSCEAR Survey of Medical Radiation Usage and Exposures are given in Table 36 (total frequency) and Table 37 (frequencies of major treatments). In a few cases, it is not clear whether the number of treatments (which may be several dozen per treated patient) or the number of patients was reported. Some totals may be underestimates because certain treatments were excluded. The population-weighted average frequencies of treatments are somewhat less than those given in the UNSCEAR 1988 Report [U1]. The data were dominated at level I by the United Kingdom and the United States, both of which reported 2.4 treatments per 1,000 population but which are missing from the 1985-1990 period. China and India, with lower frequencies, have been added to the listing for level II for 1985-1990. The distributions of the total frequencies of radiotherapy treatments in countries are illustrated in Figure VII. The average annual frequencies of the main types of treatments are shown in Figure VIII.

233. Results from individual countries seem at times to be inconsistent. In many cases, the sums of reported frequencies of specific treatments in Table 37 deviate considerably from the totals listed in Table 36, which may be smaller or larger. The varying number of countries in the periods reported and the different types of treatment included under the broad categories introduce uncertainty and make it difficult to compare results. For the Nordic countries, the total frequencies are believed to be based on better statistics, while the frequencies for specific therapies are extrapolations from small samples. Turkey reports very high frequencies of treatment for leukaemia, lymphoma, Wilms' tumour and neuroblastoma compared to breast, respiratory system or female genital organ therapies. These frequencies, from one hospital, may reflect a non-random selection of patients. In some countries, there are large differences between regions. As one example, which is probably typical of many countries, adequate facilities and advanced services are available at Lima, Peru, but access to radiotherapy is much less satisfactory in rural areas [Z11, Z12, Z13, Z14].

234. Although there are uncertainties in specific data, the general trend agrees with earlier data, which suggested increased teletherapy treatment frequencies in most countries. The number of teletherapy machines in developing countries is considered to be only one tenth the number that would be justified by cancer incidences [R7].

235. Marked variation has been noted between the Nordic countries, in spite of their homogeneity [L16]. This variation is not fully evident from Table 36. Thus, in 1987 according to Lote et al. [L16], 25%-26% of cancer patients in Denmark and Norway received megavoltage radiotherapy, as compared with 36%-38% in Finland, Iceland and Sweden. The number of radiation fields given per patient was 45 in Finland and 34-37 in the other Nordic countries.

236. The age- and sex-distributions of radiotherapy patients are given in Table 38. In general, the age distributions conform with expectations. Thus, Wilms' tumour patients and neuroblastoma patients are usually under age 15 years, leukaemia and lymphoma patients are of all ages, and patients with other cancers are usually over age 15 years, with a sizable fraction over 40. The sex distributions are also as expected. Overall, neither age- nor sex-distributions differ significantly between health-care levels. Some specific deviations may be mentioned, however: for leukaemia, the 0-15 years age group is very small in Myanmar, for no obvious reason. This may be a random fluctuation. The age distribution for lymphoma patients includes a significantly higher proportion of children in countries of health-care level II than in countries of health-care levels I and III, where the proportions are not significantly different. This may reflect the distributions of Burkitt's lymphoma and of Hodgkin's disease.

B. DOSES IN TREATMENTS

237. Information on target organ doses and entrance surface doses in teletherapy and brachytherapy treatments is given in Table 39. The doses used differ, but no particular difference distinguishes the levels of health care from one another.

238. Absorbed doses in tissues or organs other than the target of the treatment could be used in assessment of patient doses, although general comparisons would be difficult. Some such absorbed doses were listed in the UNSCEAR 1982 Report [U3], but effective dose equivalents were not evaluated for four reasons:

(a) the proportionality between dose and response assumed for effective dose or effective dose equivalent calculations does not hold if organ doses exceed a few gray;
(b) the short life expectancy of the patients invalidates assumptions underlying the choice of organ weighting factors for effective dose or effective dose equivalent calculations;
(c) little is known about the dose distribution outside the target volume;
(d) in therapeutic nuclear medicine, the metabolic data assumed in normal dose assessments may not be valid.

239. Since the UNSCEAR 1982 Report [U3], the situation has changed somewhat, at least with respect to the first three reasons: (a) a tentative first estimate of the risk of cancer induction in target organs exists [I4], which facilitates the approximative consideration of beam and target organ doses in effective dose or effective dose equivalent calculations [B19]; (b) cancer therapies are becoming more successful, and the average life-span of surviving cancer patients is increasing, with particularly dramatic improvements for childhood cancers; (c) extensive calculations by Williams et al. [W34] of organ doses outside the beam are available and summarized in ICRP Publication 44 [I4]. Thus, it is now at least feasible to compute effective doses.

240. However, the detriment associated with such effective doses cannot be calculated in the same manner as for healthy workers, nor even as for patients in diagnostic examinations, and it is in any case a by-product of indispensable, life-saving treatment. Furthermore, radiotherapy patients are unique in that deterministic harm constitutes a sizable part of the radiation-induced detriment. Such complications of treatment are discussed in ICRP Publication 44 [I4].

Effective doses are not well suited to describe such effects. Still, effective doses may be useful as supplementary information, to allow for comparisons between treatments and countries.

241. Even with the new data in ICRP Publication 44 [I4], effective dose computations in radiotherapy must be simplifications. For instance, as suggested by Beentjes [B19], it is assumed for the present purpose that all radiotherapy delivers dose distributions similar to those from ^{60}Co sources. Using data from Beentjes [B19], absorbed doses to non-target organs from scattered radiation from ^{60}Co treatments of four major target areas have been calculated (Table 40). It was assumed that these areas are representative of all radiotherapy except skin and female breast radiotherapy, and that the dose to target organs is always 60 Gy. Leakage radiation (a few per cent of the scattered radiation) is disregarded.

242. Cancer mortality following radium treatment for fibrosis with uterine bleeding may illustrate the relevance or otherwise of effective doses in non-target organs. In a study of 4,153 women treated between 1925 and 1965 [I16], average doses were provided for all organs, allowing the calculation of an average effective dose from scattered radiation of 1,070 mSv. To this a correction for target organ doses should be added. Based on the considerations of ICRP [I4] and the interpretation of Beentjes [B19], one may assume at most two fatal second cancers, i.e. less than 0.1% with a cure rate of 50% of 4,153, and a cancer fatality probability coefficient of 0.05 [I8], which corresponds to 40 man Sv, or 10 mSv per woman. The cumulated effective dose, 1,080 mSv, corresponds to a collective effective dose of 4,440 man Sv. With a fatality probability coefficient of 0.05 per man Sv, 222 extra cancer deaths would be expected in the cohort. Actually, after an average observation period of 26.5 years, an excess of 147 cancer deaths was recorded [I16]. Thus, the estimate from effective dose calculations agrees reasonably well with observations.

243. The so-called Bucky, or grenz ray, therapy, which uses 8-17 kV x rays to treat skin disorders, cannot be directly compared to other radiotherapy. Bucky therapy is relatively popular in, for instance, the United States and in Sweden, which has some 15 facilities offering this treatment. The short penetration (half-value layer in tissue: 0.5 mm) precludes any effects in other organs than skin from Bucky therapy. Nevertheless, skin doses of 5-50 Gy are received for a procedure (therapy course) consisting of 10 consecutive treatments; for foot verrucae up to 200 Gy per procedure of 10 treatments are delivered, i.e. 20 Gy per treatment with 4-6 weeks between treatments [L8]. In this particular application, skin surrounding the verrucae is shielded from radiation with vaseline. At least 22 cases of skin cancer following Bucky treatment are known, all with doses higher than 50-200 Gy. For cumulated doses under 100 Gy, no excess cancer risk has been proven [L8].

C. WORLDWIDE EXPOSURES

244. According to the UNSCEAR 1988 Report [U1], about 2.4 persons per 1,000 population were subjected to either teletherapy or brachytherapy annually. Results from the UNSCEAR Survey of Medical Radiation Usage and Exposures show a lower frequency (about 1.4 per 1,000), but this is only a sampling difference. It is expected that treatment frequencies will increase gradually, based on other considerations. The treatment frequency in countries of health-care level II is about 25% of that in level I countries, in conformity with the earlier observation [U1].

245. The UNSCEAR Survey of Medical Radiation Usage and Exposures responses are insufficient to permit analysis for health-care levels III and IV, but there is no particular reason to expect any significant change from the estimates in the UNSCEAR 1988 Report [U1]: 0.1 procedures per 1,000 population for health-care level III and 0.05 per 1,000 population for level IV, i.e. 4% and 2% of the treatment frequency in level I countries.

246. The age- and sex-distributions of tele- and brachytherapy patients appear to agree fairly well with expectations based on age and sex statistics for the corresponding diseases. The doses used for treatment vary, but no particular trend seems to distinguish the different levels of health care. Some new technologies may lead to fewer side effects and/or better results than conventional therapy.

247. The number of radiotherapy patients is suggested as a simple measure that is correlated with the radiological impact associated with therapy (including deterministic treatment complications). Since more reliable numbers are unavailable, the treatment frequencies reported in the UNSCEAR 1988 Report [U1] have been combined with data on populations in the health-care levels, leading to an estimated 4.9 million procedures annually (0.9 per 1,000 population).

248. It may also be of interest to assess the effective dose, using the approach of Beentjes [B19, B36] but modifying it to obtain effective dose rather than somatic effective dose as he did. The collective effective dose equivalent and collective effective dose due to radiotherapy in the Netherlands in 1978-1979 is computed in Table 41 using the normalized organ doses of Table 40 and various further assumptions stated in the Tables. The result is a collective effective

dose equivalent of 19,100 man Sv and a collective effective dose of 10,400 man Sv. The latter value will be used for extrapolation to worldwide exposures. For this purpose, it was assumed that the distribution of different types of cancer is similar in countries of different health-care level. In fact, both distribution and frequency of cancers vary considerably. However, it is believed that variations in distribution do not seriously affect the collective dose estimate, which can indicate only the order of magnitude of the worldwide collective dose. Variations in the frequency of different cancers are to some extent taken into account when therapy frequencies are used as multipliers in the dose calculation.

249. Table 42 lists collective effective doses, estimated on the assumption that they are proportional to the effective doses in the Netherlands [B19], correcting for size of population and for treatment frequency (but, to retain compatibility with effective dose for diagnostic practices as far as possible, not correcting for patient age [B36]). The result is rather imprecise. The estimated annual collective effective dose in Table 42, 1,500,000 man Sv worldwide, does however show that the secondary effects of radiotherapy are not negligible. Probably, they are of the same order of magnitude as those caused by diagnostic practices. It is important, however, to view the secondary effects from therapy in relation to the consequences of no treatment, in which case continuing debilities and early deaths would surely prevail.

D. TRENDS

250. Increasing life-span will make cancer therapy more relevant; increasing affluence will make more equipment available. Radiotherapy is thus likely to become more frequent in most countries [Z11]. Increased awareness of the early symptoms and signs of cancer will presumably also increase demand for radiotherapy. In Peru, 60% of cervical cancer patients now come for treatment in the later stages of the disease, while for instance only 17% of Swedish patients are at the late stages [Z3].

251. The cancer incidence in industrialized countries is roughly 3,500 cases per million population per year. About half of the cases are suitable for radiation therapy. On a global basis, some 10 million new cancer cases occur each year, 6 million of which would be aided by radiotherapy. Since the treatment capacity of one radiotherapy unit is about 500 patients annually [W10], an increase up to about four units per million population could be expected in the long run. In other words, some 3,000 units are probably needed to supplement the 6,000-7,000 units existing worldwide today. However, while more than half of all cases come from developing countries, access to radiotherapy is limited [D16]. In Africa, 45% of the 560 million inhabitants are under 15 years old, so it is almost certain that cancer will become a bigger problem as the population ages. Yet only a third of African countries have any radiotherapy facilities, and in many cases these are ill-equipped and understaffed.

252. Radiotherapy is being developed to achieve higher therapeutic effects and better tolerability, using e.g. hyperfractionation [H11, P8, P24, W27]. Some promising ideas are under consideration. Although their success has so far been limited [H40], some possible advances will be mentioned here. For instance, inverse dose planning means that instead of calculating the dose distribution for a proposed beam configuration, the optimal beam conditions for a desired dose distribution in the patient's body are calculated [A3, B16, K6]. As this technique becomes common, fewer patients will suffer radiation-induced complications after treatment. Another possibility is that target doses could be adjusted to take account of the patient's genetically determined radiation sensitivity [A7, S35]. Such adjustments may be quite important, since genes conferring radiosensitivity may be much more frequent than in the population at large, possibly occurring in as many as 15% of all cancer patients [B3, H3, N2, S20]. Attention to this factor would also reduce the number of complications and thus the radiological insult to the population. The use of whole-body treatment for leukaemia is increasing. The UNSCEAR 1988 Report [U1] considered briefly the doses to fetuses in the radiotherapy of pregnant women. Supplemental information is now available on the use of lead shielding in such cases [L15].

253. Treatment accelerators with higher energies and external beams of fast neutrons have been mentioned as likely new developments [S6], and there is some preliminary experience of fast neutron therapy, which has had, however, only limited success [B8, H13, K11, P16]. Another possible refinement would be photon activation using Mössbauer resonance absorption, in which (for example) an ^{57}Fe compound administered to the patient is induced to produce Auger cascades through photon irradiation. In principle, this technique should permit lethal doses to cancer cells at the expense of only very low doses to normal cell. There are, however, still doubts whether the technique will work in humans, at least for other than very superficial tumours, for which many alternative methods already exist [H20].

254. Proton therapy constitutes another advance [C27]. Thus far, some 7,000 patients have been treated. More than 2,000 were treated in the USSR alone, where clinical work started at three centres in the 1960s, and there were a fairly constant number of

patients (a few hundred each year) during the 1980s [G11]. The advantage of protons is that they cause steep dose gradients at the lateral and back sides of the target dose distributions, thus reducing the irradiation of other than target organs, albeit at great investment costs for the complicated facility.

255. External therapy has been used not only for treating cancer but also for treating benign conditions. For instance, 20,012 patients (99% of them younger than 2 years of age) were treated for haemangiomas at Radiumhemmet in Stockholm between 1909 and 1959. While some centres still advocate the radiation therapy of haemangiomas, it has declined rapidly since the early 1960s [F9]. It appears likely that such therapy will in the future be applied only in special cases, such as bony haemangiomas.

256. Alternative and supplementary treatment options will continue to appear, and in some cases they will be preferred in patient groups at high risk. For instance, children with brain tumours are conventionally treated with radiotherapy, but mental retardation is a frequent side effect, occurring in 38% of all long-term survivors in one study, with younger children being more seriously affected [L9]. Therefore, the tendency is to delay radiation therapy and use chemotherapy for children under 2-3 years of age, who are most sensitive to radiation [L9]. It is not known, however, whether delaying irradiation really improves the functional status of the patients [M14].

257. Quality assurance programmes, instigated in particular by the World Health Organization, are even more important (but also more difficult) in therapy use than in diagnostic use. A number of incidents might have been avoided by a more systematic approach to quality assurance. In one United Kingdom centre, more than 200 patients were treated with overdoses of 25% in 1988 [S36]. A listing of reports that contain technical details on quality assurance programmes in radiotherapy has been published [B40]. A particularly important collection of papers [H9] discusses radiotherapy quality assurance from European, North American and Latin American perspectives. Brahme [B17] discussed quality assurance for external beam therapy.

258. There is scope for other errors in a computer-controlled treatment than in a conventional treatment. Not only must all normal quality assurance be performed, but it is also necessary to check the computer control [M20]. Input of data into check-and-confirm systems may actually contribute to systematic errors, if used as an uncontrolled setup system [L3].

259. A joint study in Finland and the USSR [K20] found unacceptable variations in dose distribution between treatment planning systems and suggested that the quality assurance programmes be improved. Zaharia [Z3, Z10] discussed quality assurance in radiotherapy in developing countries, with special emphasis on Latin America, pointing out the limitations imposed by a lack of resources. For instance, accelerators and quality assurance programmes are unlikely to be available, and cobalt units must be used.

E. SUMMARY

260. Treatments by radiotherapy are intended to deliver high doses to target organs to eliminate malignant or benign conditions. All attempts to calculate effective doses from data on non-target organs will inevitably be open to serious criticism. The secondary effects associated with such doses are difficult to estimate and cannot be directly compared with effects of radiation in other situations. They must be assessed bearing in mind that they are a by-product of indispensable life-saving treatment. Thus, the frequency of treatments and the target doses are primary estimators of the impact of radiotherapy. Nevertheless, effective dose calculations may provide valuable supplementary information.

261. The frequency of radiotherapy treatments by teletherapy and brachytherapy is estimated to be 2.4 per 1,000 population in countries of health-care level I and 25%, 4% and 2% of this value in countries of health-care levels II, III and IV, respectively. The total number of procedures performed annually worldwide is estimated to be 4.9 million.

262. Estimates have been made of the collective effective dose from radiotherapy, determined by considering tissues and organs other than gonads outside the target area. The results, summarized in Table 42, indicate an annual collective somatically effective dose of 1,500,000 man Sv worldwide. Some 66% of this collective dose concerns health-care level I countries, which is directly proportional to treatment frequencies.

V. THERAPEUTIC USE OF RADIOPHARMACEUTICALS

263. Relatively few data are available or were submitted to the Committee for the assessment of therapeutic nuclear medicine. The problems of effective dose, discussed for teletherapy and brachytherapy in Chapter IV, are equally evident for therapy with radiopharmaceuticals. As in those other types of radiotherapy, simple information on the number of patients and doses may be the most suitable measure of the secondary effects of therapy with radiopharmaceuticals.

A. FREQUENCIES OF TREATMENTS

264. A number of different radio-pharmaceuticals are used in the treatments of various diseases, but the use of ^{131}I to treat thyroid conditions predominates. Much less frequent procedures include the treatment of polycythaemia vera with ^{32}P and of hepatic tumours as well as arthritis with ^{90}Y. Frequencies of therapeutic treatments using radiopharmaceuticals in countries responding to the UNSCEAR Survey of Medical Radiation Usage and Exposures are listed in Tables 43 and 44. The population-weighted average frequency of all treatments in 1985-1990 for countries of health-care level I is 0.1 per 1,000 population; the unweighted average of reported values is 0.2. Considering statistical fluctuation, these estimates are hardly different from the estimate of the UNSCEAR 1988 Report [U1], which was 0.4 per 1,000 population. In conformity with other observations from the UNSCEAR Survey of Medical Radiation Usage and Exposures, the treatment frequencies at health-care levels II and III are about an order of magnitude lower than at level I. The distributions of the total frequencies of treatments with radiopharmaceuticals and the average annual frequencies of the main types of treatment are illustrated in Figures IX and X.

265. The age- and sex-distributions of patients are given in Table 45. As expected, thyroid disorders occur more frequently in women. No differences in the age or sex ratio of these patients can be detected between health-care levels. As with tele- and brachytherapy, no trends with time in treatment frequencies are obvious.

266. Blaauboer and Vaas [B6] have estimated that the frequency of thyroid therapy courses using ^{131}I in the Netherlands is 0.35 per 1,000 population. This is somewhat higher than the value of 0.097 per 1,000 population given in Table 44. There are no doubt large uncertainties in estimates depending on the reliability of the underlying samples.

B. DOSES IN TREATMENTS

267. The average activities administered in the therapeutic use of radiopharmaceuticals are listed in Table 46. The amounts used for similar treatments are comparable in most cases, although a 20-fold difference between the extreme values of activity can be identified for thyroid tumour treatment using ^{131}I.

268. While this conventional treatment and its properties are well known, some attention is being given to potential problems with other therapeutic uses of radiopharmaceuticals. Thus, since around 1980, monoclonal antibodies labelled with ^{90}Y or ^{125}I, for example, have been used for radioimmunotherapy (albeit apparently in few cases). In the present context, the question has been raised whether better estimates of bremsstrahlung organ doses are needed when high-energy beta sources such as ^{90}Y are used for radiotherapy [W8]. In the case of ^{90}Y, measurements indicate that the bremsstrahlung doses are usually less than 1% of the beta doses, but Williams et al. [W8] conclude that bremsstrahlung doses are not negligible.

269. Table 47 gives the absorbed doses to non-target organs from ^{131}I thyroid therapy in Japan in 1982, using Maruyama's data on activity and patient number [M10] and the dose conversion factors for adults given in ICRP Publication 53 [I5]. Using these data and an approach similar to that of Beentjes [B19], it is possible to calculate the effective dose equivalent and effective dose. In this case, there is a marked difference between H_E (180 mSv) and E (23 mSv), since the higher absorbed doses appear in remainder organs. The H_E value corresponds to about 530 man Sv, or a per caput effective dose equivalent in Japan from thyroid radionuclide therapy of about 4.4 μSv. This demonstrates that radionuclide therapy contributes but a small part of the per caput dose to the population.

270. Cox et al. [C18] state that radionuclide therapy on pregnant women, particularly in unsuspected early pregnancy, may be associated with much higher fetal doses than would be expected from current methods for dose estimation.

C. WORLDWIDE EXPOSURES

271. The data in Table 43 indicate somewhat lower frequencies of treatments with radiopharmaceuticals than were estimated in the UNSCEAR 1988 Report. However, the data are broader-based than the earlier data. The population-weighted average for 1985-1990 is 0.10 per 1,000 population in countries of health-care

level I, 0.02 per 1,000 population for level II and 0.025 per 1,000 population for level III. The 1988 values [U1] were 0.4, 0.1 and 0.016 per 1,000 population, respectively, and for level IV, 0.008 per 1,000 population, mostly based on extrapolation from diagnostic nuclear medicine frequencies.

272. As in the evaluation of tele- and brachytherapy in Section IV.C, an extrapolated collective effective dose was estimated analogous to that used by Beentjes [B19] and based on the dose data for Japan given in Table 47. This amounts to about 9,300 man Sv worldwide, of which some 6,000 man Sv arise in countries of health-care level I (Table 48). Thus, the estimated secondary effects from therapy with radiopharmaceuticals are negligible in comparison with those from other medical radiation usage.

D. TRENDS

273. Indications are that ^{131}I continues to be used in 99% of therapies [U1]. In the early 1980s, radioimmunotherapy using monoclonal antibodies, which concentrate selectively in tumours, was regarded as "the magic bullet", but the technique still seems to be in development [G1]. A possible refinement is the increased potential for and use of boron neutron capture therapy [A4, F11]. In this technique a compound or monoclonal antibody is tagged with ^{10}B. Neutron-irradiation of this target produces ^{11}B, which fissions instantaneously, yielding alpha particles. The technique will presumably affect only a few patients in the near future, but it could lead to exposures of staff [S6].

E. SUMMARY

274. In therapy using radiopharmaceuticals, the treatment of thyroid conditions with ^{131}I is by far the most common procedure. Polycythaemia vera is treated with ^{32}P, and some benign diseases are sometimes treated with radiopharmaceuticals. Although new procedures may be introduced, they are unlikely to significantly alter current use patterns in the near future.

275. The estimated frequency of treatments with radiopharmaceuticals in countries of health-care level I is 0.1 per 1,000 population. The frequencies are 20% and 10% of this value in countries of health-care levels II-III and IV, respectively. The total number of procedures performed worldwide is estimated to be 210,000 (Table 48). The collective effective dose from such treatments (9,300 man Sv) corresponds to a per caput effective dose of 1.8 μSv; it is a minor component of the total effective dose from all uses of medical radiation.

VI. EXPOSURES OF THE GENERAL PUBLIC

276. Inevitably, medical radiation procedures, like other practices involving radiation, will cause some inadvertent exposure of members of the general public. There are difficulties in putting these exposures into perspective, expressing the exposures per unit practice, for example. There may be some merit in continuing to consider the levels of health care in countries. Most data are available only for countries of health-care level I. Hence, to the extent that information is at all available, the discussion below is limited to doses to exposed persons, numbers of exposed persons, and per caput doses obtained by averaging over populations.

A. DIAGNOSTIC X-RAY EXAMINATIONS

277. It appears very rare that unintentional irradiation of the general public from x-ray facilities occurs, with the possible exception of certain uses of mobile equipment. Use of portable equipment under field conditions could cause some inadvertent exposures, if proper shielding has not been provided. Because of these difficulties, the Basic Radiology System of the World Health Organization has been devised as non-mobile equipment [W3].

278. Some exposure is possible of parents who are requested to hold and/or calm children subjected to x-ray examinations. Few publications address this problem specifically, but it seems reasonable to assume that the doses per examination would be similar to those encountered occupationally. Parents would not be involved as frequently, nor for as long times, as medical staff, so in most cases the integral doses over longer periods of time should be lower than those sustained by exposed medical staff.

B. RADIOPHARMACEUTICALS

279. There are few data on exposures of the public from use of radiopharmaceuticals, but the problem could be larger than that corresponding to use of

x rays, since the sources can be brought outside of the clinic and beyond the radiation protection measures present there. There are, in principle, two routes of such exposure: family members (or some other individuals or visitors) could be exposed to radiation from radiopharmaceuticals in the patient's body, and radioactive wastes released into sewage systems or deposited at refuse dumps could increase background exposures. Excretion of radionuclides from patients, as well as radioactive waste from hospitals and exposures due to radioisotope production, are evaluated in Annex B, "Exposures from man-made sources of radiation". However, exposures of members of the public from radioisotopes present in the bodies of patients are considered in this Annex. The contamination of restroom facilities in hospitals, is reviewed by Ho and Shearer [H16].

280. The problem of radiation from radiopharmaceuticals present in patients is not trivial if the patient is a small child or a parent to a small child. In such cases, family members are likely to be moderately exposed. However, estimated doses to family members are low, usually below 1 mSv, in diagnostic practice, even if the persons involved are in close bodily contact more or less continuously [M3, M28]. Leucocyte scans with ^{111}In constitute a possible exception where special actions may be necessary, if doses exceeding about 1 mSv are to be avoided [M27]. Equivalent dose rates from patients undergoing some typical examinations are given in Table 49 [N6]. The dose rates are of course higher, and the problem can be much more difficult in therapy cases (see Section C below).

281. A study concerning diagnostic nuclear medicine referred to the situation in the United States [B12]. Patients were equipped with dosimeters in order to estimate the effective dose equivalents to critical groups (family members and co-workers) as well as to the entire population. For practical reasons, the dosimeters were put on the patients rather than on the members of the critical groups themselves, and then doses to critical groups were computed using suitable models. The average effective dose equivalents to members of critical groups were 7-20 μSv annually, and the per caput effective dose equivalent to a member of the general public was 0.4 μSv annually [B12]. Since the population of the United States is about 250 million, even this very low individual figure corresponds to a not negligible collective effective dose equivalent of some 100 man Sv (the estimate is, of course, not very precise).

282. Often, patients have to wait between injection and imaging. In some countries, such as the United States, separate waiting rooms are recommended for injected patients, but in other countries this is not the case. Harding et al. [H26] studied doses incurred by relatives, other staff and accompanying nurses in the waiting room at a hospital in the United Kingdom. Median doses were about 2 μSv or less, with a maximum (for a relative) of 33 μSv. Similar conclusions were drawn by Siewert [S4] for the Federal Republic of Germany.

283. One aspect of inadvertent exposures is that breast-fed infants may be exposed via excretion of radiopharmaceuticals in milk of examined mothers. Many studies have been made of this subject (e.g. [T4]). A number of references appear in reports of NCRP and UNSCEAR [N1, U1]. Table 50 shows that in some cases, the effective dose equivalent to a breast-feeding child could be two orders of magnitude higher than that to the mother [I5, J1]. On the other hand, the concentrations of a radiopharmaceuticals in milk usually decrease very rapidly to insignificant levels. Discarding the first, or the first few, milk fractions during the day of administration, thus, usually renders the dose to the infant negligible (a small fraction of a mSv) [J1]. Fibrinogen tagged with ^{125}I is a rare exception, where breast-feeding within three weeks can lead to effective dose equivalents to infants of 10-15 mSv, with a concurrent effective dose equivalent to the mother of about 0.5 mSv [J1]. Inadvertent exposure of the fetus is possible in cases of undeclared early pregnancy. Uterine doses, relevant in such circumstances, are available in ICRP Publication 53 [I5].

284. Little is known about the geographic variations of exposures of the general public from diagnostic nuclear medicine practice. The number of examinations are higher in developed countries, and it seems safe to assume that the doses incurred in the United States due to radiation from radiopharmaceuticals in patients (0.4 μSv per caput annually [B12]) represent the upper end of the possible dose range.

C. RADIATION THERAPY

285. If potential exposures due to accidents or incorrect shielding of facilities are disregarded, the main exposures to the general public may be due to radiation from patients undergoing brachytherapy. Approximate dose rates around the beds of such patients have been computed, for example 0.3 mSv h^{-1} at 1 m and 0.1 mSv h^{-1} at 2 m from a patient containing 3,700 MBq ^{137}Cs or 5,500 MBq ^{131}I [S14]. It is worth noting that afterloading is probably very uncommon in countries of health-care levels II to IV, which means that doses to the public (and to staff) may be higher per treatment than in countries of health-care level I. Dose rates of 0.01 mSv h^{-1} have been observed in rooms above or below a brachy-

therapy patient's room in a hospital in the United States [B14]. Proper shielding reduced this dose rate by some 20%-45%. Although the authors primarily deal with doses to staff, members of the public (other patients, visitors, staff not involved in radiation work) could also be exposed to these radiation fields.

286. Thus, given a suitable set of conditions, public exposure could be modelled. In the United States study just discussed [B14], the model chosen suggested that shielding reduced inadvertent exposure of staff and public by 0.0006 man Sv per average brachytherapy. Of this exposure reduction, 0.00025 man Sv was occupational, so the public exposure without extra shielding should be at most (total minus occupational)/(remaining fraction of dose rate) = (0.0006 - 0.00025)/(1 - 0.45) = 0.0006 man Sv. On the very approximate assumption that all brachytherapy causes doses similar to the doses in ^{137}Cs gynaecological treatments at the specific hospital in the United States, and that the average frequency of brachytherapy for treatment of malignancies in countries of health-care level I is 0.08 per 1,000 population (see Table 42, assuming one third of total treatments are brachytherapy), the per caput dose to the general public due to brachytherapy in countries of health-care level I would be some 0.05 μSv.

287. The problem of radiation from radiopharmaceuticals in the bodies of patients undergoing therapy is more complicated than in diagnostic nuclear medicine. Relatively few patients are involved, but the activities are high enough to cause doses that could exceed a few mSv to exposed members of the public. Hence, various precautions against inadvertent exposure of fellow patients or family members are common [C21]. As an example, Koshida et al. [K18] suggest that ^{131}I therapy patients should not be discharged from the hospital unless the maximum residual activity is less than 510 MBq, the patient's children are aged over 1 year and they keep at a distance of at least 50 cm. In a later paper, they reduced this value to less than 100 MBq [K28]. For the patient to return to the general ward, or for the patient to be discharged from the hospital when children are younger and/or will be closer than 50 cm, stricter recommendations apply.

288. Approximate dose rates around the beds of such patients are similar to those given above. Further illustrations showing how such dose rates change due to radioactive decay after ^{131}I administration can be found in Orito et al. [O5, O6]. Family members may wish to ignore radiation exposure in order to be able to spend as much time as possible with the patient [H18]. Other problems in the therapeutic use of radiopharmaceuticals are the same as those for diagnostic uses.

D. VOLUNTEERS IN MEDICAL RESEARCH

289. The Committee has not previously been able to evaluate the doses to healthy volunteers in medical research. Such volunteers might be considered a small subgroup of the general public. Data on these exposures are not readily available, but some statistics for the Federal Republic of Germany and for the United Kingdom are presented in Table 51. German regulations are somewhat different for three types of research (general medical research using labelled compounds, clinical trials of pharmaceuticals labelled for some specific purpose during the trial, and trials of radiopharmaceuticals), hence the separation of the corresponding volunteer groups in Table 51. This Table clearly shows that the number of volunteers is small enough not to dominate the collective dose to the general population, but it is theoretically possible that some individual doses could be relatively high (i.e. comparable to the dose limit for radiation workers of 50 mSv in a single year). It should be remembered that radioactive labelling in research projects may differ from that normally encountered in radiopharmaceuticals, and can include long-lived nuclides such as ^{14}C [L26]. One difficulty may be to identify the volunteers. In diagnostic use of x rays, extra exposures may be given to patients for research purposes, thus making it difficult to distinguish patients and volunteers.

290. Some factors act towards reducing doses to volunteers. Ethics committees that exist in many countries, albeit with varying regulatory status, usually attempt to prevent unnecessary exposure of volunteers. The 1990 recommendations of the ICRP [I8] suggest that appropriate national bodies might consider dose constraints for volunteers. Such constraints would truncate the upper end of the dose range, thus reducing the average dose to volunteers. Even formal limits have been discussed (Canada [C7]) or implemented (the Federal Republic of Germany [K9] and the United States [U16]), in spite of objections [P6] that dose limits are inappropriate in medical research. To the extent that such limits are used, they can be expected to reduce the average of doses to volunteers, by cutting off the upper tail of the dose distribution.

E. SUMMARY

291. While x-ray examinations are more frequent, examinations and therapy with radiopharmaceuticals constitute the more important route of exposure of the general public. The annual per caput effective dose equivalent caused to members of the public by patients with radionuclides in their bodies is estimated to be 0.4 μSv or less.

VII. EXPOSURES FROM ACCIDENTS IN MEDICAL RADIATION USAGE

292. Most of the available reports on accidents are case studies of particular events. So far, the material permits little in the way of estimating of the accident frequency per unit population or per unit of practice. It must be emphasized that all of the frequency estimates given below are highly imprecise and, owing to erratic reporting, are very likely to be underestimates.

293. Accidents in diagnostic x-ray examinations are not likely to have grave individual consequences. Of the 38 incidents of patient overexposure due to faulty radiation equipment that were reported to the United Kingdom Health and Safety Executive between 1986 and 1990, 30 involved diagnostic x-ray equipment. In these incidents, about 760 patients (about 0.003 per 1,000 population annually, corresponding to about 6 per million x-ray examinations in the United Kingdom) were overexposed, with effective dose equivalents from 0.5 to 13 mSv and a collective effective dose equivalent of some 5 man Sv [G10].

294. In nuclear medicine misadministrations occur, sometimes with fatal results [M29]. The extravasation of correctly measured but incorrectly injected radiopharmaceuticals can also lead to radiation injury [S50]. In the United States about 75 misadministrations in therapy and about 1,300 misadministrations in diagnostic nuclear medicine are reported annually (in all, about 0.006 per 1,000 population annually, or about 140 per million nuclear medicine examinations in the United States). Some 40 of these concern ^{131}I, which can easily be injected in therapeutic quantity [N13]. About 95% of all diagnostic misadministrations involve the correct prescribed activity but the wrong radiopharmaceutical or the wrong patient.

295. While various accidents in teletherapy have caused lethal damage, the serious underexposure of cancer patients may also well have led to fatal results [S51]. It is very difficult to assess the frequency of these accidents. Apart from the general problem of underreporting, these particular accidents are so rare that it is a problem to establish a baseline population or time period. Arias [A14] discusses three teletherapy accidents: Texas, United States, 1986, where two patients died of overexposures from a linear accelerator; Maryland, United States, 1987-1988, where 33 patients were overexposed by up to 75%; Zaragoza, Spain, 1990, where 27 patients 14 of whom died, were overexposed from a linear accelerator. Distributing these 62 patients over the combined population of Spain and the United States and, rather arbitrarily, over 10 years, there would be some 0.00002 victims annually per 1,000 population, or about 10 per million therapy procedures. A separate kind of accident can occur if a disused teletherapy source is removed from the hospital and the public is exposed. A well-known example, the Goiania accident, is discussed in Annex B, "Exposures from man-made sources of radiation".

296. The European Federation of Medical Physicists has initiated a scheme to share information about accidents to patients. So far, only radiotherapy accidents have been reported. Reports obtained to date from Czechoslovakia, the Federal Republic of Germany, Norway, Poland, Russia, Spain, Turkey and the United Kingdom indicate that 1,344 patients in these countries were exposed to higher than prescribed doses and 989 patients to lower than prescribed doses between 1982 and 1991 [H19]. These 134.4 patients annually would correspond to some 0.0003 victims per 1,000 population (the number is of course higher than that given in the preceding paragraph, which deals exclusively with grave accidents).

297. A total of 91 incidents concerning ionizing radiation were reported in the Federal Republic of Germany in 1990 [B7]. Of these, 21 had some connection to medical uses of radiation. Radiopharmaceuticals for diagnostic purposes were lost or stolen in eight cases. There were various failures of remote afterloading equipment for brachytherapy in nine cases, failure of linear accelerators in two cases, failure of one gamma teletherapy device and leakage of faeces contaminated with 131I from the drain of a therapy ward in one case. There were minor exposures of staff in five of the afterloading events. No exposure of patients took place in any of the 21 events.

CONCLUSIONS

298. The use of ionizing radiation in medical diagnostic and therapeutic examinations and treatments convey radiation doses to the individuals involved along with direct benefits in health care. Because of widespread usage of radiation and radioactive materials in medical procedures, the collective dose to the world population is significant. With additional information available on radiation exposures of patients, particularly that received in response to the UNSCEAR Survey of Medical Radiation Usage and

Exposures, improved estimates of worldwide exposures can be made.

299. The Committee has previously extrapolated available data on medical radiation usage to the entire world on the basis of the number of physicians per 1,000 population, a statistic that is available for all countries. This procedure has been maintained for the analysis of this Annex. Four levels of health care are defined to characterize medical radiation usage. Relatively complete data are available on examination and treatment frequencies for countries of health-care levels I and II. At health-care levels III and, in particular, IV, information is still insufficient in many respects, although the contribution to the worldwide collective dose from these countries is small.

300. There are indications that exposures of populations from the diagnostic and therapeutic uses of ionizing radiation are increasing worldwide. Much of this increase can be justified on clinical grounds, particularly in developing countries, where medical services are obviously not yet sufficiently available. The general trends observed with time and between levels of health care cannot be used to anticipate particular conditions in individual countries. Circumstances vary widely, and national trends may differ greatly from the average trends. Nevertheless, the averages for several countries of each level of health care and for five-year time periods should be reasonably representative, i.e. the conclusions drawn here about worldwide exposures should be generally valid.

301. For countries of health-care level I, the population-weighted estimate of the frequency of diagnostic medical x-ray examinations (890 per 1,000 population) is slightly higher than the estimate in the UNSCEAR 1988 Report (800 per 1,000 population), although it seems unlikely that the difference would be statistically significant. Thus, at health-care level I, the total frequency of all x-ray examination was relatively constant during the 1980s. Reduced rates of increase or, in a few countries, decreases are due to the introduction of alternative methods, such as ultrasound and endoscopy. For countries of health-care levels II-IV, examination frequencies appear to be increasing, as expected on the basis of needs for the services and on demographic trends.

302. The estimated per caput effective dose equivalent from x-ray examinations at health-care level I is 1.0 mSv, unchanged from the estimate in the UNSCEAR 1988 Report [U1]. Some examinations with higher doses, such as computed tomography, are becoming more frequent. At the same time, however, better equipment and techniques are allowing doses in other examinations to be reduced. From the wider database available, the per caput effective dose equivalents at levels II and III-IV are estimated to be 0.1 and 0.04 mSv (previously 0.2, 0.07 and 0.03 mSv at levels II-IV, respectively [U1]). The use of fluoroscopy for chest examinations has been clarified for China (level II), but the prevalence of this procedure, which gives higher doses, cannot be certain for other countries at health-care levels II-IV.

303. The estimated effective dose equivalent from diagnostic nuclear medicine examinations increased in countries of health-care level I (0.09 mSv compared with 0.05 mSv previously [U1]) and also in countries of health-care levels II-IV (0.008 mSv compared with less than 0.004 mSv previously [U1]). The estimate for developing countries is higher, since it has become clear that the main radionuclides being used there are long-lived ones. However, the radiological impact of diagnostic nuclear medicine remains small in comparison with that of diagnostic x-ray examinations.

304. For tele- and brachytherapy, the treatment frequencies reported in the UNSCEAR Survey of Medical Radiation Usage and Exposures are lower than those obtained in 1988. This is interpreted as sampling variation as the treatment frequencies are no doubt continuing to increase. The primary measure of the impact of therapy on the population used here is simply the number of patients treated. In addition, estimates of the effective dose and the collective effective dose are shown for illustrative purposes. Therapy with radiopharmaceuticals appears to be slightly less frequent than had previously been estimated [U1]. The frequencies of treatments world-wide are estimated and the effective doses calculated.

305. The estimated doses to the world population from all medical uses of radiation are summarized in Table 52. The per caput effective dose equivalent from diagnostic examinations ranges from 1.1 mSv at level I to 0.05 mSv at levels III-IV. The worldwide per caput effective dose equivalent is 0.3 mSv. From therapy treatments, the per caput effective dose equivalents computed from scattered radiation in non-target organs are estimated to be 0.7, 0.2, 0.03 and 0.02 at levels I-IV, respectively and 0.3 mSv worldwide. The collective effective dose equivalent from diagnostic examinations is estimated to be 1,800,000 man Sv, with nearly 90% from x-ray examinations and the remainder from nuclear medicine and dental examinations. The collective effective dose from therapeutic treatments is estimated to be 1,500,000 man Sv, but this is not strictly comparable to other doses.

306. Effective doses to patients from medical uses of radiation cannot, in general, be used directly in calculations to infer detriment. In Section I.B, various

problems with the estimation of detriment from doses to patients were mentioned. For therapeutic uses of radiation, an added difficulty is that much of the secondary effects are not cancer or hereditary disease but deterministic radiation harm.

307. Much, and optimally most, of the collective dose from medical uses of radiation is offset by direct benefits to the examined or treated patients. There are two basic ways to reduce the risks of radiation detriment to patients: (a) by reducing the collective dose by lowering the number of patients exposed to ionizing radiation or (b) by reducing the individual dose in particular procedures. The number of patients exposed can be lowered by using strict referral criteria. Guidelines on the selection of patients for various x-ray examinations have been given [R26, S2, U11, U12, U13, U14, U15]. Referral criteria that are particularly appropriate for radiology in developing countries are given by WHO [W23, W24, W25, W26]. The use of alternative methods, such as ultrasound and endoscopy, also reduces the number of exposed patients. The dose per procedure can be reduced if the procedure is optimized and if quality assurance programmes are set up to eliminate deviations from the optimum.

Table 1
Medical radiation facilities
Data from UNSCEAR Survey of Medical Radiation Usage and Exposures unless otherwise indicated

Country	Year	Population (thousands)	Number of radio-logists	Diagnostic x-ray units		Teletherapy units			Nuclear medicine clinics
				Medical	Dental	X-ray	^{60}Co, ^{137}Cs	Accelerators	
Health-care level I									
Argentina	1985-1989	33000	2981	5705	18361	235	95	10	390
Australia	1970-1974	12550	420	2107					
	1985-1989	16260	1320	6000	7100	36	15	35	66
Austria	1977	7535							132
Belgium	1986-1990	9921	1021			21	39	20	107
Bulgaria	1980	8862							
Canada	1985-1989	25309	1900	23000	16500	130	31	58	265
Costa Rica	1989	2927					1		
Cuba	1988	10402	632	900			13	1	1
Czechoslovakia	1970-1974	10023	480	1800	2400				
	1981-1985	10320	892	2000	2600	88	46	7	39
	1986-1990	10350	932	2100	2700	78	52	11	43
Denmark	1986-1990	5100	250	1800	4500	10	2	22	30
Ecuador	1985-1989	10500	128	430	640	6	8	0	13
Finland	1970-1974	4610	220						36
	1980-1984	4820	380	2200	3200	31	7	11	51
	1985-1989	4930	400	2100	3900	24	3	21	52
France	1982	54219		13998					
	1987-1990	55632		19548	32438		316	147	548
German Dem. Rep.	1975-1978	16800	700						
	1985-1988	16600	1000	3300	3400	60	9	24	
Germany, Fed. Rep.	1980-1984	59200					196	111	
	1986-1990	62700	3100				185	129	
Greece	1980	9643							
Iceland	1987	245	24	65			1	1	
Ireland	1988	3538							
Italy	1985	57355		17400					
Japan	1970-1974	110044	8742	56607	31612	1113	359		548
	1980-1984	118693	11890	58962	34916		558	108	885
	1985-1989	122264	11754	61345	40005		440	441	1091
Kuwait	1970-1974	1310		172	40	3	2	0	
	1980-1984	1557	61	230	62	2	2	0	
	1985-1989	1856	105	288	95	2	2	1	
Libyan Arab Jamahiriya	1977	2598							
	1986-1990	4000		325			1		
Luxembourg	1988	371	22	144	155	3	1	0	3
Malta	1970-1974	320	4	10	1	2	0	0	
	1980-1984	325	6	16	2	1	2	0	
	1985-1989	344	8	25	3	1	1	0	
Netherlands	1980-1984	14300	650	3000	6000	150	6	35	70
	1985-1989	14600						38	

Table 1 (continued)

Country	*Year*	*Population (thousands)*	*Number of radio-logists*	*Diagnostic x-ray units*		*Teletherapy units*			*Nuclear medicine clinics*
				Medical	*Dental*	*X-ray*	^{60}Co, ^{137}Cs	*Accelerators*	
New Zealand	1970-1974	2920	102	563	789	41	8	2	6
	1980-1984	3202	141	635	930	33	8	6	9
	1985-1989	3320	161	688	987	23	8	7	9
Norway	1970-1974	3900	200	2000	3000	180	1	3	15
	1980-1984	4100	320	2400	4200				36
	1985-1989	4200	350	2200	5000	50	2	13	39
Poland	1985-1989	37572	1500	6793	1289	92	30	21	
Portugal	1988	9778	323						
Romania	1980	22201	975	2746	1100	202	20	2	39
	1985-1989	23000	975	2746	1100	202	20	2	39
Singapore	1985-1989	2647	4	20	6				1
South Africa	1986	32500				13	25	10	
Spain	1985-1989	38558	1645	9000	18000				
Sweden	1970-1974	8129	542	2700	5500	31	23	12	
	1980-1984	8327	645	2400	12500	24	17	27	125
	1985-1989	8414	920	2000	12900	22	14	33	120
Switzerland	1972	6193	92	6000	4000		25	6	
	1982	6335	173	7500	5500	150	26	14	43
	1990	6509		8000	6000	120	19	20	43
USSR	1980	265542							
	1988	283682							
USSR, RSFSR	1976-1980	136528	15860	24760	2880				
	1981-1985	140228	16770	29550	3680				
	1986-1990	146237	17080	31550	4840				
United Kingdom	1981-1985	54600	1600	11000					288
United States	1970-1974	213669	12216	97788	110974	3441			
	1980-1984	234238	12595	129695	187772	3299			
	1985-1989	248630	12381	108903	142699	1324			
Uruguay	1978-1982	2908		33					
Venezuela	1978-1982	15024		150					
Yugoslavia	1970-1974	4776		318	99	7	2		5
	1980-1984	10788		568	239	6	6	1	22
	1985-1989	18681		1624	741	27	14	10	36
Health-care level II									
Algeria	1986-1989	22200				4	3	1	
Barbados	1980-1984	250				2	1	0	1
	1985-1989	250	5	20	1	2	1	0	1
Bolivia	1978-1982	4613		171					
Brazil	1982	127100		13400		230	50	38	68
	1990	150238	12432	10500		1399	99	133	147
Chile	1988	12748					8	2	
China	1970-1974	27056	734	315	315	4	1	0	4
	1981-1985	1010000	81500	68300				37	250
	1986-1990	1080000	120000	120000			600	80	264
China, Taiwan Prov.	1990	20300							
Colombia	1978-1982	25892		1811					
Dominican Republic	1981	5648		71					

Table 1 (continued)

Country	*Year*	*Population (thousands)*	*Number of radio-logists*	*Diagnostic x-ray units*		*Teletherapy units*			*Nuclear medicine clinics*
				Medical	*Dental*	*X-ray*	^{60}Co, ^{137}Cs	*Accelerators*	
Ecuador	1970-1974 1980-1984	6522 8129	30 83	155 305	97 350	2 6	3 7	0 0	5 10
Guatemala	1990	8660				2	4		
Honduras	1990	5049	10	51					
India	1985-1989	776000	4000	45000			151	11	94
Iran (Islamic Rep. of)	1980	38345							
Iraq	1985-1989	17250	1	3			3	3	1
Jamaica	1970-1974 1985-1989	1900 2409							
Mauritius	1986-1989	1040					1		
Mexico	1986-1990	82734					78		102
Nicaragua	1981 1990	2844 3820	 6	 35					
Paraguay	1978-1982	3168		 77					
Peru	1980-1984 1985-1989	18000 20000	 150	1390 2400	1654 1836	20 20	8 11	1 1	20 30
Tunisia	1985-1989	7500	88	740	451	0	3	1	3
Turkey	1986-1990	57000	1077	3500	5000	24	30	10	42
Health-care level III									
Belize	1990	183							
Cape Verde	1985-1989	330	1	1	1	0	0	0	0
Congo	1986-1989	1700				1	1		
Djibouti	1985-1989	383							
Dominica	1990	71	1	4	5				
Egypt	1988	51897	320	72	60	2	22	9	3
Gabon	1986-1989	1000					1		
India	1970-1974	560000					62		34
Kenya	1988	23883				1	2		1
Liberia	1980-1984 1986-1989	1650 2200		24		 1	 1		
Morocco	1986-1989	24300				2	3		
Myanmar	1979-1980 1981-1985	35712 39215	35 43	 328	 15	 3	 6	 1	 1
Nigeria	1977-1983 1986-1989	80556 91200		900		 3	 2		
Philippines	1985-1989	54000	441	1538	25				
Saint Lucia	1990	150	1	9					
Sri Lanka	1979	14647							
Sudan	1984 1986-1990	21215 26000	 38	141 210	 30	 1	 2	 1	 1

Table 1 (continued)

Country	*Year*	*Population* (*thousands*)	*Number of radio-logists*	*Diagnostic x-ray units*		*Teletherapy units*			*Nuclear medicine clinics*
				Medical	*Dental*	*X-ray*	^{60}Co, ^{137}Cs	*Accelerators*	
Thailand	1976-1980 1981-1985 1986-1990	45156 49723 54799	140 290 440	987 1419 1881	159 239 493	50 35 29	10 20 30	0 1 5	
Vanuatu	1985-1989	137	0	6	3	0	0	0	0
Zimbabwe	1986-1989	8600				3	3	1	1
Health-care level IV									
Cameroon	1986-1989	9700				1	3		
Côte d'Ivoire	1977	7088							
Ethiopia	1981-1985 1986-1990	46000 50000							1 1
Ghana	1977	10808		108					
Madagascar	1986-1989	10000					1		
Mozambique	1986-1989	14550					1		
Rwanda	1970-1974 1988-1990	4040 6950	0 2	26 30	2 3				
Senegal	1986-1989	6700				1	1		
Uganda	1986-1989	16600				1			
United Rep. of Tanzania	1986-1989	21700	7				2		
Zaire	1986-1989	32500					1		

The entries in this Table are qualified as follows:

Algeria: Data from IAEA (International Atomic Energy Agency) and from [U1, U17].
Argentina: The number of radiologists excludes 2,149 non-radiologist physicians licensed to use x rays.
Austria: The value given for nuclear medicine clinics is the estimated number of scanners/cameras.
Barbados: Data also from PAHO (Pan American Health Organization).
Brazil: Survey response published as [A11]. Data also from [C14, D4, U1]. Number of radiologists includes 200 radiotherapists and 232 nuclear medicine specialists. Number of nuclear medicine clinics for 1982 is estimated from number of scanners/cameras (207); number for 1990 includes 450 scanners/cameras; 401 further units do *in vitro* work only. Number of ^{60}Co, ^{137}Cs teletherapy units exclude 7 non-operative units; number for accelerators excludes 10 non-operative units.
Cameroon: Data from IAEA (International Atomic Energy Agency) and from [U1, U17].
Canada: The numbers given for ^{60}Co, ^{137}Cs teletherapy units represents licensees, some probably with more than one unit.
Chile: Data from PAHO and from [U17].
Congo: Data from IAEA and from [U1, U17].
Cuba: Data from PAHO and from [U17].
Dominica: Data from PAHO.
Egypt: Numbers of radiologists, diagnostic x-ray units and clinics estimated from Kasr-El Eini Centre, which serves ca. 25% of patients using radiation. Data on therapy units from IAEA.
France: Data from [M40, S17]. The numbers given for diagnostic x-ray units exclude 339 military medical and dental units.
Gabon: Data from IAEA (International Atomic Energy Agency) and from [U1, U17].
German Dem. Rep.: 40% of all x-ray examinations are performed by non-radiologist physicians. The 3300 x-ray units (generators) in 1985-1988 correspond to 5100 tubes.
Germany: 55% of all x-ray examinations are performed by non-radiologist physicians. 75% of diagnostic nuclear medicine is performed outside specialized clinics.
Honduras: Data from PAHO (Pan American Health Organization).
Iceland: Data also from [L16, S14].
India: The number of radiologists excluded 31,000 non-specialist physicians using x rays.
Iraq: Data also from [U1, U17]. Other entries than population size refer to the Institute of Radiology and Nuclear Medicine, Baghdad, which serves an unknown fraction of the population.
Kenya: Data from IAEA and from [U1, U17].
Liberia: Data from IAEA and from [U1, U17].
Libyan Arab Jamahiriya: Data from IAEA and from [U1, U17].
Madagascar: Data from IAEA and from [U1, U17].
Mauritius: Data from [D16, U1, U17].
Morocco: Data from IAEA and from [U1, U17].
Mozambique: Data from [D16, U1, U17].

Table 1 (continued)

New Zealand:	Number of radiologists includes 9, 22 and 28 radiotherapists and 4, 7 and 7 nuclear medicine specialists in 1970-1974, 1980-1984 and 1985-1989, respectively. Number of medical x-ray units includes 9, 5 and 0 mass miniature chest units and 70, 80 and 85 chiropractice units in 1970-1974, 1980-1984 and 1985-1989, respectively.
Nicaragua:	Data from PAHO.
Nigeria:	Data from IAEA and from [U1, U17].
Philippines:	Number given for diagnostic medical and dental x-ray units represent facilities.
Portugal:	Data from [C15].
Saint Lucia:	Data from PAHO.
Senegal:	Data from IAEA and from [U1, U17].
Singapore:	Population size from [U17]. Other entries refer to the National University Hospital, which serves an unknown fraction of the population.
South Africa:	Data from IAEA and from [U1, U17].
Spain:	The number given for diagnostic x-ray units for medical examinations excludes units in which fewer than 1,000 examinations per year are performed.
Sweden:	Data also from [S21]. Number of radiologists includes 82, 120 and 155 radiotherapists in 1970-1974, 1980-1984 and 1985-1989, respectively. X-ray teletherapy units excludes Bucky units.
Switzerland:	Besides radiologists, all generalists, surgeons, internists, paediatricians (sum 1982: 5,970) and dentists (number 1982: 2,728) are licensed to use x rays.
Tunisia:	Data also from [G16]. Number of radiologists includes foreign doctors; of the 76 Tunisian doctors, 4 were radiotherapists, 3 nuclear medicine specialists. Accelerator not taken into use (1990).
Uganda:	Data from [D16, U1, U17].
USSR:	Data also from [U17].
USSR, RSFSR:	Data for one republic, the Russian Soviet Federative Socialist Republic. Radiologists include diagnostic x-ray specialists only.
United Rep. of Tanzania:	Data from IAEA and from [B18, U1, U17].
Yugoslavia:	1970-1974 data include Bosnia and Herzegovina and Slovenia; in 1980-1984, data include Bosnia and Herzegovina, Croatia and Slovenia; 1985-1989 data include all of Yugoslavia except for Montenegro, Kosovo and Vojvodina.
Zimbabwe:	Data from IAEA and from [D16, U1, U17].

Table 2
Average number of medical radiation facilities per 1,000 population by health-care level
Data from UNSCEAR Survey of Medical Radiation Usage and Exposures

Medical radiation staff / facilities	*Year*	*Health-care level*			
		I	*II*	*III*	*IV*
Radiologists	1970-1974	0.062	0.023		
	1980-1984	0.076	0.064	0.004	
	1985-1990	0.072	0.041	0.006	0.0003
Medical x-ray units	1970-1974	0.45	0.014		0.0006
	1980-1984	0.38	0.071	0.016	0.010
	1985-1990	0.35	0.086	0.018	0.004
Dental x-ray units	1970-1974	0.44	0.012		0.00004
	1980-1984	0.46	0.077	0.005	
	1985-1990	0.38	0.086	0.003	0.0004
Therapy x-ray units	1970-1974	0.014	0.0002		
	1980-1984	0.013	0.0017	0.0007	
	1985-1990	0.0048	0.0050	0.0001	0.0001
Cobalt-60 therapy units	1970-1974	0.0031	0.0001	0.0001	
	1980-1984	0.0034	0.0004	0.0004	
	1985-1990	0.0026	0.0004	0.0002	0.00009
Accelerators	1970-1974	0.0010			
	1980-1984	0.0012	0.0001	0.00002	
	1985-1990	0.0020	0.0001	0.00009	
Nuclear medicine clinics	1970-1974	0.0048	0.0003	0.0001	
	1980-1984	0.0066	0.0003		
	1985-1990	0.0078	0.0003	0.00005	0.00002

Table 3
Annual medical radiation examinations and treatments
Data from UNSCEAR Survey of Medical Radiation Usage and Exposures unless otherwise indicated

Country	Year	Diagnostic examinations (thousands)			Therapeutic treatments (thousands)			
		Medical x rays	Dental x rays	Radio-isotopes	X-ray therapy	Tele-therapy	Brachy-therapy	Radio-isotopes
Health-care level I								
Argentina	1985-1989			415		29.0	6.0	5.3
Australia	1970-1974	4634	1000	52	49.9 [a]			
	1985-1989	9149		112	5.4	4.4	17.5	2.4
Belgium	1986-1990	12772	2855	365				3.0
Canada	1970-1974	18880 [b]			432 [a]			
	1985-1986	26563 [b]			519 [a]			
Cuba	1988-1990	6396		10	2.3 [a]		0.5	0.4
Czechoslovakia	1976-1980	11112	720	660	0.9	2.9	0.2	4.9
	1981-1985	10882	883	943	0.6	3.6	0.2	6.2
	1986-1990	9498	884	1183	0.3	3.7	0.3	9.4
Denmark	1985-1989	2600	2400	72	7.0	7.0	0.6	0.1
Ecuador	1985-1989	530	65.4	8.5	0.5	0.9	0.2	0.07
Finland [R16]	1977	5100	955	59				1.5
	1984	4600		85				1.8
	1986-1987	4300	1100	100	0.7 [a]			
France [L20, M40]	1982	45350						
	1988-1990	55060		387				
German Dem. Rep.	1974-1978	19000	2500	115				
	1981-1988	19000	2500	160				
Germany, Fed. Rep. of	1976-1980			1899				
	1981-1990	71600	16600	2450				
Italy	1974			400				
	1983-1985	42700		579				
	1989			551				
Japan	1970-1974	73064	91500	168	132	1656	15.5	4.4
	1980-1984	96300	99040	541	13	1762	13.6	3.0
	1985-1989	141500	95768	989				
Kuwait	1985-1989	1137	190	24.3	0.3	0.9	0.02	0.03
Luxembourg	1988	294	69.1	9.2	3.4	4.0	0.03	0.07
Malta	1970-1974	33.2	0.9		0.1	0.2	0.01	
	1980-1984	84.7	2.3		0.1	0.4	0.01	
	1985-1989	110	3.2		0.1	0.5	0.01	0.03
Netherlands	1980-1984	7900	5700	200	2.5	23	1.1	1.5
New Zealand	1970-1974	1790	~1000	18.9	3.9	3.2	0.3	0.5
	1980-1984	2263		25.9	1.5	6.0	0.3	0.6
	1985-1989	2114	913	24.5	1.1	8.6	0.2	0.5
Norway	1970-1974	1600	2500	16.0	1.0			0.08
	1980-1984	2200	3300	36.0				0.3
	1985-1989	2200	3500	39.0	0.04			0.6
Poland	1985-1989	24949	2300					
Portugal [C15, S52]	1988-1989	5900						
Romania	1980	13205	706	66.9	33.9	3.8	0.1	
	1985-1989				9.1	4.8	1.5	1.2
	1990	10688	704	55.8	111	46		
Spain	1986-1990	22290	9000					

Table 3 (continued)

Country	*Year*	*Diagnostic examinations (thousands)*			*Therapeutic treatments (thousands)*			
		Medical x rays	*Dental x rays*	*Radio-isotopes*	*X-ray therapy*	*Tele-therapy*	*Brachy-therapy*	*Radio-isotopes*
Sweden	1970-1974	4800	3600	77.0	6.8	9.2	2.0	2.7
	1980-1984	4700	7000	128	2.2	11.4	1.6	3.3
	1985-1989	4400	7000	122	1.6	13.3	1.5	3.6
Switzerland	1972-1976	6446	1834	284				9.8
	1982	6582	2059					
USSR	1981	254400						
USSR, RSFSR	1976-1985	136800	8570					
	1986-1990	144250	11740					
United Kingdom	1976-1980	22700	6055					
	1981-1989	25230	9000	369		150		11
United States	1985-1989	200000	100000	6783				
Yugoslavia	1985-1989	3350	83000	140	15.1	50.2	2.0	2.4
Health-care level II								
Barbados	1980-1984			0.2	0.1	0.3	0.04	0.02
	1985-1989	54.2		0.3	0.1	0.3	0.05	0.04
Brazil [A11,C14,U1]	1982	22750						
	1990	15037		256				
Chile	1982	1911						
China [Z6]	1985	152087	2233	615		96		44
Ecuador	1970-1974	167	10.0	3.1	0.3	0.2	0.04	0.05
	1980-1984	385	35.7	7.4	0.5	0.5	0.09	0.05
Honduras	1990	106						
India	1985-1989	81480		169		106	20.6	2.8
Iran (Islamic Rep.of) [U1]	1981	7221						
Nicaragua	1990	191						
Peru	1985-1989	300		4.8	0.3	2.7	0.9	0.3
Tunisia	1985-1989		100	7.0		6.5	3.0	0.3
Turkey	1981-1985	16663				50		
	1986-1990	29840		174		33		0.5
Health-care level III								
Belize	1990	15.1						
Cape Verde	1985-1989	22.7		0	0	0	0	0
Dominica	1990	12.9						
Egypt	1976-1980	11.0	<0.1	2.6				2.6
	1981-1985			9.4				2.8
	1986-1990			25	2.2 [c]		0.02	3.2
India	1970-1974	19600				40.9	11.4	
Myanmar	1986-1990	397	64					
Nigeria [U1]	1977	2014		<0.01				
Philippines	1985-1989	6148	0.6					
Saint Lucia	1990	19.0						
Sudan	1976-1980			2.1				0.02
	1981-1985			5.7				0.06
	1986-1990	1380		7.1	0.2	1.7	0.04	0.1

Table 3 (continued)

Country	Year	*Diagnostic examinations (thousands)*			*Therapeutic treatments (thousands)*			
		Medical x rays	*Dental x rays*	*Radio-isotopes*	*X-ray therapy*	*Tele-therapy*	*Brachy-therapy*	*Radio-isotopes*
Thailand	1976-1980	2276	64	11				0.008
	1981-1985	3749	115	9.1			0.04	0.011
	1986-1990	4318	115	14	0.09 [a]		0.04	0.013
Vanuatu	1985-1989	11.1		0	0	0	0	0
Health-care level IV								
Ethiopia	1981-1985			0.6				
	1986-1990			4.8				
Rwanda	1970-1974	28.0 [b]						
	1988-1989	61.1 [b]						

The entries in this Table are qualified as follows:

Barbados: The value given for medical x-ray examinations is estimated from the number examined in the public sector (35,200) and the number of pieces of equipment in the public sector (13 of 20 in Barbados).
Belize: Data from PAHO. Number of patients: 13,036.
Canada: Therapy numbers refer to treatments, not patients.
Chile: Data also from [U1].
Cuba: Data from PAHO (Pan American Health Organization). X-ray examinations refer to 5.7 million patients.
Czechoslovakia: The values given for x-ray therapy, teletherapy and brachytherapy for the years 1976-1980, 1981-1985 and 1986-1990 exclude treatment of benign conditions (39,000 patients annually 1976-1985, 24,000 patients annually 1986-1991).
Denmark: The value given for medical x-ray examinations includes 7,000 interventional radiology.
Dominica: Data from PAHO. Number of patients: 10,816.
Ecuador: The value given for medical x-ray examinations for the years 1980-1984 includes 19 interventional radiology; for the years 1985-1989 27,000 interventional radiology.
Finland: The value given for dental x rays includes 400,000 pantomographic examinations; the value of 0.7 given for x-ray therapy, tele- and brachytherapy represents primary stage radiotherapy only; the value of 2.2 represents total number of patients.
France: The value given for radioisotope examinations is estimated from Hôpital Henri Mondor, which serves about 2% of the population of France.
German Dem. Rep.: Total number of therapeutic treatments in 1985 = 40,000 of which 20,000 for cancer.
Germany, Fed.Rep.: The number of diagnostic examinations with radioisotopes is estimated from data covering 7% of the population for the years 1976-1980 and from data covering 21% of the population for the years 1981-1985 and 1986-1990. Total number of therapeutic treatments in East Germany 1985 = 40,000 of which 20,000 for cancer.
Honduras: Data from PAHO.
Italy: Data also from [U1].
Japan: Dental examinations include 1,650,000, 9,640,000 and 11,229,000 pantomographic examinations in the years 1970-1974, 1980-1984 and 1985-1989. Numbers for x-ray therapy and teletherapy refer to treatments, not patients.
Kuwait: The value for medical x-ray examinations includes 3,000 interventional radiology examinations.
Luxembourg: Numbers for x-ray therapy and teletherapy refer to treatments, not patients.
Malta: The value for medical x-ray examinations in the years 1985-1989 includes 150 interventional radiology examinations.
New Zealand: The value for medical x-ray examinations includes 359, 129 and 67 mass miniature chest examinations and 30, 41 and 47 chiropractic examinations in the years 1970-1974, 1980-1984 and 1985-1989, respectively.
Nicaragua: Data from PAHO.
Norway: The values given for x-ray therapy are from one hospital only, to indicate trend.
Romania: The values given for medical and dental x rays as well as for x-ray therapy and teletherapy are estimated from data comprising 60%-65% of the population. Numbers for 1990 x-ray therapy and teletherapy refer to treatments, not patients.
Spain: The value given for medical x-rays excludes military, legal and pre-employment examinations.
Saint Lucia: Data from PAHO. Number of patients: 16,300.
Sweden: The value for medical x-ray examinations includes 6,000 interventional radiology examinations.
Switzerland: The values given for radioisotope examinations and treatments are estimated from data covering 4% of the population.
Turkey: The values given for diagnostic examinations and therapeutic treatments with radioisotopes are estimated from data covering 1% of the population; the values for therapeutic treatments from data covering 2% of the population.
USSR: Data also from [U1].
Yugoslavia: Value for medical x-ray examinations includes 1,700 interventional radiology. Values given for therapeutic treatments are for Bosnia and Herzegovina, Croatia, Slovenia and Serbia, excluding Kosovo and Vojvodina (73% of the population of Yugoslavia).

[a] Value is for all therapeutic treatments.
[b] Value is for both medical and dental x rays.

Table 4
Medical radiation services worldwide, 1985-1990
Normalized quantities determined from UNSCEAR Survey of Medical Radiation Usage and Exposures

Quantity	Level of health care				World
	I	II	III	IV	
Normalized values					
Physicians per 1,000 population	2.6	0.55	0.18	0.053	0.98
Radiologists per physician	0.028	0.075	0.032	0.006	0.04
Radiologists per 1,000 population	0.072	0.041	0.006	0.0003	0.04
X-ray units per 1,000 population	0.35	0.086	0.018	0.0042	0.14
X-ray units per radiologist	4.9	2.1	3.1	14	3.4
X-ray examinations per x-ray unit [a]	2400	1600	3900	2000	2100
X-ray examinations per 1,000 population [a]	860	140	70	9	300
Nuclear medicine examinations per 1,000 population [b]	16	0.5	0.3	0.1	4.5
Tele- and brachytherapy patients per million population [c]	2.4	0.6	0.1	0.05	0.9
Radiopharmaceuticals therapy patients per million population [d]	0.4	0.02	0.02		<0.13
Absolute values [e]					
Population (millions)	1350	2630	850	460	5290
Physicians (thousands)	3600	1400	150	24	5200
Radiologists (thousands)	97	108	5.2	0.13	210
X-ray units (thousands)	470	230	15	1.9	720
X-ray examinations (millions) [a]	1160	360	60	4.0	1600
Nuclear medicine examinations (millions) [b]	22	1.4	0.3	0.05	24
Tele- and brachytherapy patients (thousands) [c]	3200	1600	85	23	4900
Radiopharmaceuticals therapy patients (thousands) [d]	600	65	21		~700

[a] Diagnostic medical x-ray examinations (does not include dental x-ray examinations); number of countries and population in sample: level I: 25 (935 million = 68% of entire level I population); level II: 8 (2,062 million = 78%); level III: 9 (175 million = 21%); level IV: 1 (7.1 million = 1.5%).

[b] Number of countries and population in sample: level I: 19 (634 million = 47% of entire population of level I countries); level II: 10 (2065 million = 79%); level III: 4 (171 million = 20%); level IV: 1 (50 million = 11%).

[c] Because of inconsistencies in data reported in Table 3 (i.e. number of separate treatments or of treated patients), the data of the UNSCEAR 1988 Report [U1] have been used.

[d] Number of countries and population in sample: level I: 16 (181 million = 13% of entire level population); level II: 6 (1,940 million = 74%); level III: 5 (133 million = 16%). It is assumed that the unknown frequency in level IV countries is lower than the frequency in level III countries.

[e] Absolute values refer to 1990.

Table 5
Comparison of effective dose and effective dose equivalent

Examination		*Ratio of effective dose to effective dose equivalent (E/H_E) as reported by*					
		[H36]	*[L22]*	*[S44]*	*[Z7]*	*[L2]*	*[W28]*
Diagnostic x-ray examinations							
Chest	AP	0.79-0.90			0.51		
	PA	0.85-0.92	0.99	0.83	0.75		0.80
	LAT	0.65-0.76	0.76	0.83			
Skull	AP	0.38-0.43	0.67				
	PA	0.28-0.31	0.59				0.62
	LAT	0.24-0.27	0.55				
Ribs				1.27			
Thoracic spine	AP			0.86-1.15			1.11
	LAT			0.85			
Lumbar spine	AP			1.36-1.40			
	LAT			0.77			1.01
Pelvis		1.00-1.20	0.80				0.86
Abdomen	AP	1.80-2.10	1.00	1.43			
	PA	0.88-1.10					1.00
	LAT			0.94			
G.I. tract	Upper						1.20
	Lower						1.14
Urography (I.V.)							1.05
Mammography						0.33	
CT	Head						0.52
	Chest						0.91
	Abdomen						0.81
	Pelvis						0.77

Examination	*Radiopharmaceutical*	*Ratio of effective dose to effective dose equivalent (E/H_E) as reported by*			
		[H36]	*[G21]*	*[G22]*	*[J8]*
Nuclear medicine examinations					
Brain	Tc-99m gluconate	0.62			0.61
Cerebral blood flow	Tc-99m HMPAO		0.91		0.73
	Tc-99m ECD		0.78		
	Tc-99m MRP 20		1.01		
Bone	Tc-99m pyrophosphate	0.74			0.74
Liver/spleen	Tc-99m sulphur colloid	0.56			0.65
Biliary	Tc-99m HIDA	0.63			0.76
Blood pool, multigated	Tc-99m erythrocytes	0.72			0.94
Myocardial	Tc-99m pyrophosphate	0.74			0.74
	Tc-99m MIBI			0.73	
	Tc-99m teboroxime			0.83	
	Tl-201 chloride	0.83			0.81
Lung	Tc-99m MAA	1.0			0.92
Kidney	Tc-99m gluconate	0.62			0.61
Inflammation	Ga-67 citrate	0.83			0.86
Thyroid scan	Tc-99m pertechnetate	1.1			1.1
Thyroid uptake/25%	I-131 sodium iodide	1.6			1.7
	I-123 sodium iodide	1.6			1.6

Table 6
Total annual number of diagnostic x-ray examinations per 1,000 population [a]
Data from UNSCEAR Survey of Medical Radiation Usage and Exposures

Country	*1970-1979*	*1980-1984*	*1985-1990*	*Country*	*1970-1979*	*1980-1984*	*1985-1990*
Health-care level I							
Australia	490		560	Malta	100		320
Belgium			1290	Netherlands	570	550	530
Canada	860	1020	1050	New Zealand	610	710	640
Cuba		140	620	Norway		640	620
Czechoslovakia	1110	1050	920	Poland			660
Denmark			510	Portugal			700
Finland	1080		870	Romania	790	600	470
France		840	990	Spain			570
German Dem. Rep.	1100	1100	1100	Sweden	590		520
Germany, Fed. Rep. of	860		1030	Switzerland	1040	1040	
Italy		740		USSR, RSFSR	950	1020	990
Japan	830		1160	United Kingdom	420	460	
Kuwait			720	United States		790	800
Luxembourg			810				
				Average	820	810	890
Health-care level II							
Barbados			160	Ecuador	26		53
Brazil		180	93	India			110
Chile		170		Iran (Islamic Rep. of)		180	
China		110	150	Mexico		70	
Colombia		210		Nicaragua		57	13
Costa Rica		270		Peru			15
Dominican Republic		20		Turkey			524
				Average	26	140	120
Health-care level III							
Belize			83	Philippines			110
Cape Verde			69	Saint Lucia			130
Dominica			180	Sri Lanka [U1]	21		
Ghana [U1]	22			Sudan			53
India [U1]	23			Thailand	50	75	79
Liberia [U1]	80			Vanuatu			100
Myanmar			10				
				Average	23	75	67
Health-care level IV							
Cote d'Ivoire [U1]	40			Nigeria	25		
Kenya [U1]	36			Rwanda	8.0		8.8
				Average	27		8.8

[a] Dental x-ray examinations not included.

Table 7
Average annual number of diagnostic x-ray examinations per 1,000 population [a]
Data from UNSCEAR Survey of Medical Radiation Usage and Exposures unless otherwise indicated

Country	Year	Chest examinations			Extremities	Spine	Pelvis	Skull	Abdomen	GI tract		Cholecystography	Urography	Angiography	Mammography	CT	Other (except dental)
		Radiography	Mass miniature	Fluoroscopy						Upper	Lower						
Health-care level I																	
Australia	1970-1974		150	120	79	24	16	41	14	19	6.8	9.4	12	1.6	0.30		
	1985-1990	120		0.14	130	39	30	32	18	23	13	4.7	18	10	12	30	78
Belgium	1985-1990	240			250	84	84	91	44	21	12	3.8	13	8.5	32	50	360
Canada	1980-1984	330			260	75	38			88	44		32		2.7		150
	1985-1990	310			240	91	47	60		72	36		26		6.0	22	130
Czechoslovakia	1975-1979	250	420		79	24	15	51	11	37	9.0	17	13	3.2			174
	1980-1984	200	310		86	20	22	40	10	35	8	14	11	3.5		2.8	293
	1985-1990	200	110		92	17	26	29	10	24	5.8	7.1	9.1	3.6	2.8	4.3	375
Finland	1975-1979	260	330		190	19	32	35	18	22	17	9.0	9.0	6.4	2.6	0.7	132
	1985-1990	320			220	24		18		8.4	11	1.4	6.6	5.2	27	14	215
France	1980-1984	290			190	87	62	74	29	21	15	12	36	9.6	4.8		13
	1985-1990	340			210	92	59	75	37	10	13	3.0	16	8.6	34		99
German Dem. Rep.	1975-1985	180	270	<4	710	27	21	-	-	30	4.2	22	21	1.8	2.4	0.7	50
Germany, Fed. Rep.	1975-1979	330			170	58	49	108	4.1	45	23		42		28		
	1985-1990	210			270	130	88	73	35	29	14	13	32	18	54	35	24
Italy	1980-1984	240	81		140	76	40	42	22	31	15	13	13		6.7	10.4	14
Japan	1970-1974	280	300		53	1.1	23	27	22	100	6.2		6.1				
	1975-1979	340	130		70	51	20	34	34	124	8.1		14	0.49	1.2	13	
	1985-1990	440	95		99	66	33	56	82	156	15		13	2.7	1.1	97	
Kuwait	1985-1990	220	51	62	150	60	13	65	58	6.9	2.1	1.5	12	1.7	1.0	9.9	3.4
Luxembourg	1985-1990	99		23	160	160	110	143	8.6	17	15	1.3	20	11	32	25	
Malta	1970-1974	47			27	4.6	2.3	6.0	2.5	6.2	1.1	1.5	2.9				2.9
	1985-1990	110			71	18	8.9	11	20	7.6	3.1	1.0	7.6	1.0	0.9	6.4	58
Netherlands	1970-1974	100	190	8	88	23	18	34	8.7	29	11	15	15	0.5	3.0		27
	1980-1984	160	14	13	160	29	27	41	12	19	10	4.8	14	4.8	12.4	9.7	31
	1985-1990	160	0	1.1	170	30	29	36	18	14	8.0	2.6	11	3.3	13	14	26

Table 7 (continued)

Country	*Year*	*Chest examinations*			*Extrem-ities*	*Spine*	*Pelvis*	*Skull*	*Abdomen*	*GI tract*		*Chole-cysto-graphy*	*Uro-graphy*	*Angio-graphy*	*Mammo-graphy*	*CT*	*Other (except dental)*
		Radio-graphy	*Mass miniature*	*Fluoro-scopy*						*Upper*	*Lower*						
New Zealand	1980-1984	130	40	0	120	40	30	25	15			5.0	35				270
Norway	1980-1984	120	84	5.2	150	38	46	6.3	8.0	22	111	3.0	20	0.0	2.5	10.0	16
	1985-1990	140	44	26	150	35	55	4.0	7.5	13	9.2	0.40	12	5.8	18	24	80
Poland	1985-1990	130	160	5.8	79	67	12	43	33	35	19	11	9.2	0	0.37	1.0	61
Romania	1970-1974		410	242	36	27	9.3	24	2.0	11	4.8	12	5.3				
	1980-1984	20	210	191	36	8.1	9.2	12	4.9	57	16	5.0	3.1				20
	1985-1990	24	140	115	44	10	13	21	6.6	51	12	4	8.2	1.7	1.7	0.46	16
Spain	1985-1990	150			88	120	18	18	52	29	15		14		21	13	41
Sweden	1970-1974	120		111	65	22	35	44	12	30	16	18	23	1.2	3.1		94
	1985-1990	120			55	21	43	15	7.7	12	13	5	14	0.24	46	11	158
Switzerland	1970-1974	180	160	226	210	42	36	69	12	46	13	28	30				
	1980-1984	340	150	64	210	41	57	77	21	25	13	19	25				
USSR, RSFSR	1975-1979	51	510	165	84	8.1	9.1	24	2.3	40	4.9	5.5	4.4		1.0		46
	1980-1984	60	590	110	87	8.8	11	27	3.6	44	5.4	8.6	7.5		1.8		57
	1985-1990	69	570	45	96	9.2	11	26	5.5	40	5.5	16	13		1.3		79
United Kingdom	1975-1979	130	26		110	18	32	31	17	10	5.9	6.1	6.9	3.6	0.9	1.3	27
	1980-1984	150	12		110	20	36	35	19	12	6.8	5.9	10	2.5	4.0	4.7	38
United States	1980-1984	280			200	93	21	36	35	33	22	15	18		5.7	14.5	19
Health-care level II																	
Barbados	1985-1990	30			47	18	9.5	11	23	4.4	2.0	0.31	7.7	0.12	1.2	1.4	
Brazil	1985-1990	25			29	9.3		8.9		4.2	2.0		3.7				
China	1980-1984	5.9	0	74	7.7	1.7	0.4	1.5	14	2.217	0.453	0.292	0.057		0.08		6.2
	1985-1990	12	26	64	11	1.9	1.3	0	11	4.6	1.4	0.40	0.30	0.30			10
Ecuador	1970-1974	5.9	3.2	1.5	3.3	1.7	2.7	2.3	4.1	0.58	0.34	0.14	0.21		0.07		
	1985-1990	15	0	3.6	5.6	2.9	4.6	3.9	7.1	2.2	1.2	0.8	1.3	2.5	0.55		
India	1985-1990	54	0	0	17	6	4.3	5.3	3.0	2.3	1.1		5.0				7
Health-care level III																	
Belize	1985-1990	24	0	0	26	10	5.3	6.2	7.4	0.4	0.2	1.4	1.3	0	0	0	0.39

Table 7 (continued)

Country	Year	*Chest examinations*			*Extremities*	*Spine*	*Pelvis*	*Skull*	*Abdomen*	*GI tract*		*Cholecystography*	*Urography*	*Angiography*	*Mammography*	*CT*	*Other (except dental)*
		Radiography	*Mass miniature*	*Fluoroscopy*						*Upper*	*Lower*						
Myanmar	1985-1990	4.4	2.4		0.55	0.32	0.29	0.42	0.50	0.38	0.10	0.10	0.56			0.12	
Philippines	1985-1990	67	1.2	10	11	3.0	3.6	6.3	5.5	1.5	1.4	1.6	1.9	0.16	0.08		
Thailand	1975-1979	29			4.7	3.2	0.9	3.0	4.7	1.4	0.51	0.81	1.2				
	1980-1984	45			7.4	5.0	1.5	3.4	6.5	1.9	0.74	0.93	1.7	0.30	0.20	1.3	
	1985-1990	48			6.6	4.9	1.5	3.1	7.0	1.6	0.73	0.52	1.9	0.37	0.37	2.4	
Vanuatu	1985-1990			44	40	2.5	2.8	4.2	4.7	0.44	0.22		0.62				
Health-care level IV																	
Rwanda	1970-1974	5.2			1.4	0.15	0.15	0.20		0.70		0.03	0.20				
	1985-1990	4.2			2.4	0.30	0.30	1.5	0.70	0.001	0.01	0.003	0.03	0.00010			

The entries in this Table are qualified as follows:

Australia: The value of 30 given for CT includes 14.6 for CT of the skull.
Barbados: Independent estimate for 1990 for total number of examinations (last column): 60.
Belize: Data from PAHO.
Brazil: Values given under lumbosacral are for all spine examinations.
Canada: Data also from [U1]. Value for mass miniature may include a few fluoroscopies. Values given under 1985-1986 for mammography and computed tomography are for the years 1987-1988; for CT, estimated from sample covering 90% of the population.
China: Data also from [U1]. Values given under lumbosacral are for all spine examinations. Value for abdomen is estimated from sample covering 1% of the population.
Cuba: Data from PAHO and also from [U1].
France: Values given under lumbosacral are for all spine examinations.
German Dem. Rep.: Value for extremities includes skull and spine films. Value for other examinations includes abdomen.
India: Data also from [U1].
Italy: Data are for the north-east of Italy. Values given under lumbosacral are for all spine examinations.
Myanmar: Values estimated from a sample covering 33% of the population.
Netherlands: Value for mammography for the period 1984-1985 includes 3.1 screening.
New Zealand: Values exclude all fluoroscopy.
Norway: Data also from [U1]. Values given under lumbosacral are for all spine examinations.
Poland: Value for pelvis/hip excludes pelvis; for abdomen includes fluoroscopy only; and for mammography is for screening.
Rwanda: Data also from [U1]. Values estimated from figures from Kigali Hospital, serving assumedly one third of the population.
Spain: Data also from [U1]. Values given under lumbosacral are for all spine examinations.
Sweden: Value for lumbosacral examinations include the lumbar spine; value for angiography is for cerebral angiography; frequency of all angiography combined is 7 per 1,000 population for the entire period, 2 of which are peripheral venography, which is usually not performed with special angiography equipment.
Turkey: Value given for total (last column) is estimated from a sample covering 1% of the population.
USSR: Values for 1980 are for RSFSR only. Total value for 1987: the range for different republics is 498-1,127. Values given under lumbosacral are for all spine examinations.
United States: Data also from [U1]. Values given under lumbosacral are for all spine examinations. Value for chest radiography is for PA projection.
Vanuatu: Value given for abdomen includes cholecystography.
Yugoslavia: Value for mammography includes 0.1 screening.

[a] Dental x-ray examinations not included.

Table 8
Average annual number of diagnostic x-ray examinations per 1,000 population by health-care level
Data from UNSCEAR Survey of Medical Radiation Usage and Exposures

Examination	Year	Average [a]			Mean ± SD [b]			Median [c]		
		Level I	Level II	Levels III-IV	Level I	Level II	Levels III-IV	Level I	Level II	Levels III-IV
Chest	1970-1979	588	11	18	413 ± 234	11 [c]	17 ± 17	429	11	17
	1980-1984	588	80	45	348 ± 183	80 [d]	45 [e]	305	80	45
	1985-1990	527	118	51	261 ± 149	46 ± 34	21 ± 27	240	30	5.4
Extremities	1970-1979	87	3.3	3.2	99 ± 59	3.3 [c]	3.0 ± 2.3	82	3.3	3
	1980-1984	151	7.8	7.4	143 ± 61	7.7 [d]	7.4 [e]	142	7.7	7.4
	1985-1990	137	15	6.2	143 ± 71	22 ± 17	8.7 ± 14	138	17	1.5
Spine	1970-1979	25	1.7	1.9	25 ± 14	1.7 [c]	1.7 ± 2.2	23	1.7	1.7
	1980-1984	58	1.7	5	45 ± 30	1.7 [d]	5.0 [e]	39	1.7	5
	1985-1990	61	3.9	2	59 ± 45	7.6 ± 6.5	2.1 ± 3.3	50	5.7	0.3
Pelvis/hip	1970-1979	22	2.7	0.57	23 ± 14	2.7 [c]	0.5 ± 0.5	20	2.7	0.5
	1980-1984	31	0.44	1.5	41 ± 28	0.4 [d]	1.5 [e]	38	0.4	1.5
	1985-1990	38	3.4	2	40 ± 30	3.9 ± 3.7	1.4 ± 1.9	30	4.3	0.3
Skull	1970-1979	13	2.3	1.8	42 ± 26	2.3 [c]	1.6 ± 2.0	35	2.3	1.6
	1980-1984	37	1.5	3.4	38 ± 22	1.46 [d]	3.4 [e]	36	1.46	3.4
	1985-1990	46	5.8	3.7	45 ± 35	5.9 ± 4.4	2.2 ± 2.6	34	5.3	1
Abdomen	1970-1979	15	4.1	4.7	11 ± 7.8	4.1 [c]	2.3 ± 3.3	12	4.1	2.3
	1980-1984	22	14	6.5	16 ± 9.9	14 [d]	6.5 [e]	15	14	6.5
	1985-1990	36	7.9	3.4	28 ± 22	8.9 ± 9.1	2.6 ± 3.2	19	7.1	0.6
G.I. tract	1970-1979	73	0.92	1.6	44 ± 30	0.9 [c]	1.3 ± 0.9	42	0.9	1.3
	1980-1984	51	2.7	2.6	59 ± 39	2.7 [d]	2.6 [e]	46	2.7	2.6
	1985-1990	72	5	1.8	44 ± 39	5.1 ± 1.5	0.7 ± 1.1	33	6	0.3
Urography, cholecysto-graphy	1970-1979	19	0.48	1.2	25 ± 16	0.5 [c]	1.1 ± 1.3	20	0.4	1.1
	1980-1984	28	0.35	2.6	28 ± 12	0.3 [d]	2.6 [e]	26	0.3	2.6
	1985-1990	26	2.7	2.2	18 ± 9	3.9 ± 2.8	1.0 ± 1.4	16	3.7	0.3
Angiography	1970-1979	1.6	0	0.3	2.1 ± 2.2	0 [c]	0.2 ± 0.2	1.4	0	0.2
	1980-1984	5.7	0	0.3	5.1 ± 3.1	0 [d]	0.3 [e]	4.2	0	0.3
	1985-1990	7.1	0.27	0.11	5.8 ± 4.9	0.7 ± 1.0	0.06 ± 0.12	4.4	0.3	0
Mammography	1970-1979	5.2	0.07	0.12	4.4 ± 8.9	0.07 [c]	0.06 ± 0.09	1	0.07	0.06
	1980-1984	4.6	0.09	0.2	5.1 ± 3.4	0.08 [d]	0.2 [e]	4.4	0.08	0.2
	1985-1990	14	0.57	0.07	17 ± 17	0.3 ± 0.5	0.04 ± 0.12	12	0	0
Computed tomography	1970-1979	6.1	0	0.14	2.8 ± 3.1	0 [c]	0.07 ± 0.10	1.3	0	0.07
	1980-1984	11	0	1.3	8.7 ± 4.2	0 [d]	1.3 [e]	9.9	0	1.3
	1985-1990	44	0.42	0.42	22 ± 23	0.9 ± 0.9	0.3 ± 0.8	14	0.4	0
Total	1970-1980	814	26	29	737 ± 286	26 [d]	36 ± 22	806	26	32
	1980-1985	804	141	75	738 ± 267	151 ± 80	75 [e]	744	173	75
	1985-1990	887	124	64	755 ± 247	136 ± 167	82 ± 52	696	99	81

[a] Overall average: total number of examinations divided by the total population of countries (thousands).
[b] Mean or median of individual values of countries.
[c] Data from Ecuador only.
[d] Data from China only (except total).
[e] Data from Thailand only.

Table 9
Age- and sex-distribution of patients undergoing x-ray examinations, 1985-1990
Data from UNSCEAR Survey of Medical Radiation Usage and Exposures

Health-care level	*Country*	*Age distribution (%)*			*Sex distribution (%)*	
		0-15 years	*16-40 years*	*>40 years*	*Male*	*Female*
	Chest radiography					
I	Australia	10	22	68	51	49
	Czechoslovakia	11	31	58	55	45
	Germany, Fed. Rep. of	5	21	74	53	47
	Japan	6	22	72	52	48
	Kuwait	6.9	37	57	52	48
	Netherlands	5.6	16	78	54	46
	New Zealand	13	24	63	56	44
	Poland				55	45
	Romania	34	31	35	57	43
	Spain	8.5	21	69	57	43
	Sweden	4.6	16	80	49	51
	Switzerland	8	31	61	57	43
	USSR, RSFSR	13	24	63		
	United Kingdom	6	24	70	52	48
	Average	8%	23%	69%	53%	47%
II	China	13	45	43	63	37
	Ecuador	8.2	57	35	59	41
	India	28	38	34	63	37
	Jamaica	7.6	50	43	49	51
	Turkey	30	30	40	60	40
	Average	20%	42%	39%	63%	37%
III	Djibouti	32	35	33	52	48
	Myanmar	10	40	50	60	40
	Philippines	12	50	37	57	44
	Average	11%	46%	42%	58%	42%
	Chest photofluorography					
I	Australia	9.5	14	76	53	47
	Japan	7.7	47	45	51	49
	Kuwait	19	46	35	55	45
	Poland				56	44
	Romania	5.6	71	23	55	45
	USSR (RSFSR)	6	50	44		
	Yugoslavia	0	35	65	55	45
	Average	7%	48%	46%	53%	47%
III	Myanmar	3	37	60	54	46
	Philippines	4	58	38	45	55
	Average	4%	49%	47%	49%	51%
	Chest fluoroscopy					
I	Netherlands	3.9	14	82	57	43
	Poland				59	41
	Romania	15	38	47	53	47
	Switzerland	10	34	56	52	48
	USSR, RSFSR	2	34	64		
	Yugoslavia	17	33	50	50	50
	Average	5%	33%	62%	55%	45%
II	China	20	53	27	57	43
	Turkey	5	65	30	50	50
	Average	19%	54%	27%	57%	43%
III	Philippines	35	23	46	56	44
	Vanuatu	27	45	28	59	41
	Average	35%	23%	46%	56%	44%

Table 9 (continued)

Health-care level	*Country*	*Age distribution (%)*			*Sex distribution (%)*	
		0-15 years	*16-40 years*	*>40 years*	*Male*	*Female*
Extremities						
I	Australia	22	37	41	50	50
	Czechoslovakia	17	46	37	59	41
	Germany, Fed. Rep. of	11	33	56	50	50
	Japan	22	19	69	50	50
	Kuwait	23	45	32	51	49
	Netherlands	20	43	37	52	48
	New Zealand	26	47	27	56	44
	Poland				53	47
	Romania	25	37	38	58	42
	Sweden	15	27	57	46	54
	Switzerlnd	22	39	38	58	42
	USSR, RSFSR	15	33	52		
	United Kingdom	21	50	29	53	47
	Yugoslavia	17	33	50	50	50
	Average	18%	32%	52%	52%	48%
II	China	19	50	32	64	36
	Ecuador	6.5	50	43	76	24
	India	25	48	28	71	29
	Jamaica				52	48
	Turkey	25	55	20	65	45
	Average	22%	49%	30%	67%	33%
III	Myanmar	22	40	38	68	32
	Philippines	27	47	25	69	32
	Vanuatu	26	60	13	70	30
	Average	25%	44%	30%	69%	32%
Skull						
I	Australia	22	41	37	49	51
	Czechoslovakia	17	50	33	53	47
	Germany, Fed. Rep. of	18	33	49	52	48
	Japan	24	30	46	49	51
	Kuwait	22	44	34	52	48
	Netherlands	22	41	38	48	52
	New Zealand	24	41	35	56	44
	Norway	16	44	40	58	42
	Poland				51	49
	Romania	16	42	42	54	46
	Spain	19	35	46	52	48
	Sweden	8.4	38	53	45	55
	Switzerland	19	43	38	54	46
	USSR, RSFSR	15	44	41		
	United Kingdom	21	40	39	52	48
	Yugoslavia	6.3	25	69	60	40
	Average	19%	37%	44%	51%	49%
II	Ecuador	2.9	56	41	56	44
	India	22	59	19	68	32
	Turkey	20	40	40	60	40
	Average	22%	58%	21%	67%	33%
III	Djibouti	19	44	37	52	48
	Myanmar	39	42	19	70	30
	Philippines	24	50	27	63	37
	Vanuatu	16	54	30	62	38
	Average	30%	47%	24%	66%	34%
Lumbosacral spine						
I	Australia	3.3	36	61	44	56
	Czechoslovakia	3.9	31	65	50	50
	Germany, Fed. Rep. of	4	32	64	46	54
	Japan	1.2	35	64	56	44

Table 9 (continued)

Health-care level	*Country*	*Age distribution (%)*			*Sex distribution (%)*	
		0-15 years	*16-40 years*	*>40 years*	*Male*	*Female*
I (continued)	Kuwait	8.4	44	47	44	56
	Netherlands	5.9	40	54	49	51
	New Zealand	5.4	40	55	51	49
	Norway	1.5	39	59	47	53
	Poland				50	50
	Romania	4.2	41	55	50	50
	Sweden	3.2	30	67	43	57
	Switzerland	4	47	49	50	50
	USSR, RSFSR	9	39	62		
	United Kingdom	8	38	54	46	54
	Yugoslavia	13	25	63	40	60
	Average	6%	36%	61%	50%	50%
II	China	7.2	46	47	58	42
	Ecuador	4	56	40	64	36
	India	5.3	48	47	62	38
	Turkey	15	50	35	60	40
	Average	7%	47%	47%	60%	40%
III	Djibouti	12	38	50	44	56
	Myanmar	7.2	39	53	55	45
	Philippines	15	42	43	62	38
	Vanuatu	7.4	52	41	59	41
	Average	12%	41%	47%	59%	41%
Pelvis						
I	Australia	14	26	61	38	62
	Czechoslovakia	11	29	60	52	48
	Germany, Fed. Rep. of	5	15	80	49	51
	Japan	3.5	17	79	46	54
	Kuwait	15	31	54	40	60
	Netherlands	17	17	66	38	62
	New Zealand	19	25	55	42	58
	Romania	33	34	34	43	57
	Spain	15	25	61	47	53
	Sweden	3.6	11	85	35	65
	Switzerland	20	25	55	50	50
	USSR, RSFSR	7	41	52		
	United Kingdom	14	30	56	40	60
	Yugoslavia	2.5	38	60	20	80
	Average	9%	27%	64%	44%	56%
II	China				58	42
	Ecuador	10	65	25	40	60
	India	16	50	34	68	32
	Turkey	15	50	35	50	50
	Average	16%	50%	34%	62%	38%
III	Myanmar	9.4	30	61	52	48
	Philippines	17	46	37	52	48
	Vanuatu	20	60	20	48	52
	Average	14%	39%	47%	52%	48%
Hip/femur						
I	Australia	11	14	75	38	62
	Czechoslovakia	87	4	9	43	57
	Germany, Fed. Rep. of	4	9	87	52	48
	Japan	24	25	51	43	57
	Kuwait	14	23	63	41	59
	Netherlands	17	17	66	38	62
	New Zealand	19	23	58	54	46
	Romania	21	37	42	57	43
	Sweden	12	7.7	81	35	65
	Switzerland	8	33	58	53	47

Table 9 (continued)

Health-care level	*Country*	*Age distribution (%)*			*Sex distribution (%)*	
		0-15 years	*16-40 years*	*>40 years*	*Male*	*Female*
I (continued)	USSR, RSFSR	28	23	49		
	United Kingdom	15	32	53	42	58
	Yugoslavia	17	33	50	50	50
	Average	21%	23%	56%	45%	55%
II	Ecuador	16	58	26	42	58
	India	16	50	34	68	32
	Turkey	15	40	45	55	45
	Average	16%	49%	35%	67%	33%
III	Djibouti	30	45	25	51	49
	Myanmar	16	30	54	53	47
	Philippines	19	45	37	61	39
	Vanuatu	29	47	24	66	34
	Average	18%	39%	44%	58%	42%
Abdomen						
I	Australia	10	24	66	53	47
	Czechoslovakia	8.6	27	64	53	47
	Germany, Fed. Rep. of	8	24	68	41	59
	Japan	8.2	24	68	54	46
	Kuwait	11	38	51	43	57
	Netherlands	6.1	23	71	53	47
	New Zealand	13	28	59	49	51
	Norway	17	31	53	47	53
	Poland				54	46
	Romania	15	36	48	54	46
	Spain	11	39	51	52	48
	Sweden	11	17	72	47	53
	Switzerland	4	31	65	54	46
	USSR, RSFSR	17	20	63		
	United Kingdom	10	27	63	44	56
	Yugoslavia	5.9	35	59	50	50
	Average	11%	25%	63%	50%	50%
II	Ecuador	4.9	39	56	55	45
	India	16	45	39	64	36
	Jamaica				48	52
	Turkey	30	30	40	50	50
	Average	17%	44%	39%	63%	37%
III	Djibouti	25	40	35	42	58
	Myanmar	17	39	44	51	49
	Philippines	19	45	36	50	50
	Vanuatu	10	66	23	35	65
	Average	18%	43%	39%	50%	50%
Upper GI tract						
I	Australia	1.4	20	79	40	60
	Czechoslovakia	1.2	35	64	52	48
	Germany, Fed. Rep. of	4	21	75	41	59
	Japan	0.7	24	76	53	47
	Kuwait	1.6	43	56	49	51
	Netherlands	3	29	69	51	49
	New Zealand	5.1	30	66	50	50
	Norway	0.5	33	66	45	55
	Poland				47	53
	Romania	8.9	39	52	52	48
	Spain	5	28	67	51	49
	Sweden	1.8	17	81	45	55
	Switzerland	2	40	58	58	42
	USSR, RSFSR	4	28	68		
	United Kingdom	2	30	68	49	51
	Yugoslavia	0	33	67	50	50
	Average	3%	27%	70%	49%	51%

Table 9 (continued)

Health-care level	*Country*	*Age distribution (%)*			*Sex distribution (%)*	
		0-15 years	*16-40 years*	*>40 years*	*Male*	*Female*
II	China	5.4	46	49	57	43
	Ecuador	10	60	30	33	67
	India	11	45	45	69	31
	Jamaica				45	55
	Turkey	15	50	35	60	40
	Average	8%	46%	47%	62%	38%
III	Myanmar	5.5	41	54	54	46
	Philippines	10	46	44	60	40
	Vanuatu	9.1	36	55	52	48
	Average	8%	44%	48%	57%	43%
Lower GI tract						
I	Australia	4	30	66		
	Czechoslovakia	2.5	16	81	42	58
	Germany, Fed. Rep. of	0.5	6	94	44	56
	Japan	1.9	13	85	52	48
	Kuwait	7.2	28	65	46	54
	Netherlands	2.2	24	74	40	60
	New Zealand	0.6	22	78	41	59
	Norway	0.2	24	76	38	62
	Poland				46	54
	Romania	16	33	51	48	52
	Spain	4	25	71	42	58
	Sweden	3.4	15	82	40	60
	Switzerland	1	23	76	50	50
	USSR, RSFSR	1	25	74		
	United Kingdom	1	14	85	39	61
	Yugoslavia	0	22	78	50	50
	Average	2%	19%	79%	46%	54%
II	China	5.4	46	49	57	43
	Ecuador	9.9	60	30	43	57
	India	7.2	28	65	76	24
	Jamaica				36	64
	Turkey	10	40	50	50	50
	Average	6%	39%	55%	64%	36%
III	Myanmar	3	48	49	58	42
	Philippines	13	29	59	55	45
	Vanuatu	17	50	33	60	40
	Average	9%	37%	55%	56%	44%
Cholecystography						
I	Australia	0.5	33	67		
	Czechoslovakia	0.7	29	70	24	76
	Germany, Fed. Rep.	1	12	87	34	66
	Japan	0	21	79	59	41
	Kuwait	0.4	44	55	30	70
	Netherlands	0	20	80	37	63
	New Zealand	1.7	38	61	33	67
	Norway	0	22	78	35	65
	Poland				29	71
	Romania	0.8	40	59	38	62
	Sweden	0.3	24	76	37	63
	Switzerland	1	36	63	38	62
	USSR, RSFSR	3	30	67		
	United Kingdom	0.5	19	81	30	70
	Yugoslavia	0	20	80	90	10
	Average	1%	24%	75%	44%	56%
II	Ecuador	1	80	19	66	34
	India	14	18	68	60	40
	Turkey	2	28	70	30	70
	Average	13%	19%	68%	58%	42%

Table 9 (continued)

Health-care level	*Country*	*Age distribution (%)*			*Sex distribution (%)*	
		0-15 years	*16-40 years*	*>40 years*	*Male*	*Female*
III	Myanmar	0.9	55	44	50	50
	Philippines	7.6	61	32	53	47
	Average	5%	58%	37%	52%	48%
			Urography			
I	Australia	9	29	62	51	49
	Czechoslovakia	4.3	30	66	51	49
	Germany, Fed. Rep. of	5	19	76	54	46
	Japan	8.3	24	67	55	45
	Kuwait	15	41	44	55	45
	Netherlands	11	27	63	50	50
	New Zealand	17	31	52	49	51
	Norway	3.5	31	65	51	49
	Poland				46	54
	Romania	5.2	37	58	47	53
	Spain	3.1	35	62	56	44
	Sweden	9.7	20	70	57	43
	Switzerland	27	38	35	79	21
	USSR, RSFSR	7	35	58		
	United Kingdom	9	21	70	68	32
	Yugoslavia	0	13	87	100	0
	Average	7%	28%	65%	57%	43%
II	Ecuador	18	45	36	45	55
	India	19	48	33	84	16
	Jamaica				47	53
	Turkey	10	50	40	55	45
	Average	18%	48%	34%	81%	19%
III	Myanmar	2	46	52	52	48
	Philippines	13	39	48	64	36
	Vanuatu	5.9	59	35	65	35
	Average	8%	42%	50%	59%	41%
			Angiography			
I	Australia	1.7	8.9	89	58	42
	Czechoslovakia	1.6	18	81	58	42
	Germany, Fed. Rep. of	4	9	87	59	41
	Japan	0.2	27	73	47	53
	Kuwait	1.9	36	62	53	47
	Netherlands	0	5.9	94	63	37
	New Zealand	0	21	79	54	46
	Poland				48	52
	Romania	2.9	46	51	67	33
	Sweden	2.9	20	77	49	51
	USSR, RSFSR	4	22	74		
	Average	2%	21%	77%	53%	47%
II	Ecuador	15	50	35	72	28
	India	17	33	50	90	10
	Turkey	5	35	60	55	45
	Average	16%	33%	50%	87%	13%
III	Myanmar	11	45	44	60	40
	Philippines	21	34	45	68	32
	Average	17%	39%	45%	65%	35%
			Mammography			
I	Australia	0.1	30	70		
	Czechoslovakia	0	35	65	0	100
	Germany, Fed. Rep. of	0	27	75	1.7	98.3
	Japan	0	51	49	0	100
	Kuwait	0	44	56	0	100

Table 9 (continued)

Health-care level	*Country*	*Age distribution (%)*			*Sex distribution (%)*	
		0-15 years	*16-40 years*	*>40 years*	*Male*	*Female*
I (continued)	Netherlands	0	28	72	1	99
	New Zealand	0	25	75	0	100
	Norway	0	25	75	0.3	99.7
	Romania	0.3	58	42	0	100
	Spain	1.2	37	62	0.6	99.4
	Sweden	0	8.9	91	0.2	99.8
	USSR, RSFSR	0	25	75		
	United Kingdom	0	0	100	0	100
	Yugoslavia	0	44	56	0	100
	Average	0.10%	32%	68%	0.41%	99.59%
III	Myanmar	0	40	60	0	100
	Philippines	0	11	89	0.5	99.5
	Average	0%	23%	77%	0.29%	99.71%
Computed tomography						
I	Australia	4.5	30	66	46	54
	Czechoslovakia	8.9	33	58	52	48
	Germany, Fed. Rep. of	7	14	79	48	52
	Japan	5	15	80	55	45
	Kuwait	5.4	45	49	51	49
	Netherlands	5.8	25	69	53	47
	New Zealand	12	26	62	53	47
	Norway	6.1	27	67	53	47
	Poland				56	44
	Romania	7.4	39	54	67	33
	Sweden	6.8	21	73	53	47
	United Kingdom					
	Head	6	27	67	50	50
	Body	1	23	76	52	48
	Yugoslavia	10	30	60	40	60
	Average	6%	22%	73%	52%	48%
II	Turkey	30	30	40	50	50
III	Myanmar	4	40	56	52	48

The entries in this Table are qualified as follows:

China: Data are for Beijing area only (about 3% of the population).
Djibouti: Data from Institute P. Pascal only.
Germany, Fed. Rep. of: Data are from hospitals only.
Jamaica: Data are from Kingston Hospital only.
Myanmar: Data are from Gyangon General Hospital only.
Romania: Data are for 1990.
Sweden: Data are for Stockholm county only (about 20% of the population); age distribution: 0-14 years, 15-39 years, >40 years.
Switzerland: Data are for 1982.
Turkey: Values are estimated from sample of 1% of the population.
United Kingdom: Data are for 1981-1985, except for mammography and computed tomography.
Yugoslavia: Data are for Serbia only (about 40% of the population).

Table 10
Entrance surface doses and effective dose equivalents to patients undergoing diagnostic x-ray examinations [a]
Data from UNSCEAR Survey of Medical Radiation Usage and Exposures unless otherwise indicated

Country	Dose quantity	Year	Chest examinations			Extremities	Skull	Lumbosacral spine	Pelvis / hips	Abdomen	GI tract		Cholecystography	Urography	Angiography	Mammography Screening /clinical	CT (slice doses) [b]
			Radiography	Photofluorography	Fluoroscopy						Upper	Lower					
Health-care level I																	
Argentina	ESD	1985-1989		0.65 (0.3-1.5)	6.5 (4-12)	3 (1-5)	2 (1-3)	30 (20-45)	1.3 / 8 (0.8-15)	4 (3-7)	8 (1.5-20)	8 (1.5-20)	5.5 (4-10)	6.5 (4-10)	5 (3-8)	-/22 (7-35)	30 (15-55)
Australia	ESD	1970-1974 1985-1989	0.4 (0.1-1.5)	2.6	1.4 (0.1-16)	3 (0.2-41) 2.3 (0.6-4.2)	17 (0.1-92) 3.6 (2-5)	63 (0.7-348) 28 (10-90)	9.8 / 11 (0.1-99) 4.0 / 4.4 (0.7-14)	11 (0.2-88) 7.0 (1.2-25)	25 (5.3-60) 24	9.4 (8.7-101)	28 (8.3-109) 18	57 (4-671) 40 (8-126)		-/14 (0.4-58)	60 (20-560)
Canada	ESD	1985-1989	0.13 (± 0.10)			0.14 (± 0.07)	0.84 (± 0.40)	12 (± 5.5)	3.6 / 1.6	3.1 (± 2.1)	2.2	3.0 (± 2.1)	15	2.3 (± 1.0)			
Czechoslovakia	ESD	1970-1974 1986-1990	0.5 (0.5-29) 0.45 (0.05-28)	6.1 (0.7-39) 6 (0.6-38)		2.5 (0.2-40) 1.5 (0.2-35)	9 (3-46) 8 (3-45)	31 (5-150) 26 (4-130)	13 / 12 (2.8-76) 10/10 (3-59)	9 (4-30) 8 (4-29)	14 (3-280) 12 (3-260)	20 (3-100) 18 (3-98)	11 (2-30) 10 (2-30)	14 (3-100) 12 (3-97)	300 (100-800) 400 (120-800)	60/37 (-/1-45)	
	H_E	1976-1980 1986-1990	0.07 0.07	0.7 0.7			0.4 0.5	2.9 3.1	1.9 1.9	2.9 2.8	4.5 2.5	12.7 7.7	1.9 1.9	3 3		9.5/ 9.5/-	
Finland	ESD	1978 1988	1.2 [c] (0.3-5.7) 0.27 (0.04-0.8)	1.7 (0.9-3.6)			3.1 [d] (1.0-8.0)	60 [e] (8-90) 8 (3-30)		5 [d] (1-20)	290 (55-1400)			42 (8-80)		20 (1-200) 6.3/- (2-14)	
	H_E	1978 1988	0.21 0.05				0.01	7.6 1.0		0.91						1.0/-	
France [U1]	H_E	1982	0.3				1.4	4.7	1.6	2.6	6.7	10	7.2	10			
Germany, Fed. Rep. of	ESD	1989-1991	0.18 (0.09-20)			0.12 (0.06-1.8)	3.7 (1.9-18)	18 (9.0-130)	3.7 (2.0-36)	4.0 (2.0-61)	2.4 (1.3-35)	2.0 (0.8-33)	5.0 (3.0-82)	2.4 (2.0-73)			
Italy (north-east) [P19, U1]	ESD [c] ESD [d] ESD [e]	1983 1983 1983	0.5 (± 0.7) 1.3 (± 1.7) 2.7 (± 2.8)	2.6 (± 0.9)			4.6 (± 2.9) 4.1 (± 2.9) 2.6 (± 1.9)	9.5 (± 8.3) 28.3 (± 24.9)	10.6/3.7 (± 12.4/2.7) -/4.3 (± -/3.7)	6.6 (± 3.1) 8.1 (± 4.7)				5.5-5.8 (± 2.6-1.7) 6.9-9.2 (± 4.6-6.6)			

Table 10 (continued)

Country	Dose quantity	Year	Chest examinations			Extre-mities	Skull	Lumbo-sacral spine	Pelvis / hips	Abdomen	GI tract		Chole-cysto-graphy	Uro-graphy	Angio-graphy	Mammo-graphy Screening /clinical	CT (slice doses) [b]
			Radio-graphy	Photo-fluorography	Fluoro-scopy						Upper	Lower					
Italy (continued)	H_E	1983	0.18	0.25			0.22	2.5	2.3/0.9	1.9	9.3	9.0		7.1			
Japan	ESD	1970-1974 1985-1989 1989	 0.52	2.3 [f] (± 0.38) 1.7 [f]			 3.5 10	 5.3		 3.6	 3.5 46	 4.3 72		 3.0	 1.6		 23-32
	H_E	1976-1980 1986 1989	0.10 0.05 0.06	0.30	0.12		0.3-0.9 0.09 0.05	1.5-1.6 0.60	 0.25	 0.29	13-14 1.2 2.7	1.0-1.2 2.0 3.0	 0.55	0.6 0.70			 0.5-6.9
Kuwait	ESD	1985-1989	0.43 (0.07-1.0)	0.033 (0.03-0.04)	2.4 (1.8-2.5)	0.15 (0.01-0.25)	2.2 (0.7-4.7)	4.2 (2.1-5.7)	3.0 / 2.8 (1.4-3.9)	3.8 (2.0-4.3)	2.3 (0.8-3.0)	2.3 (0.8-3.0)	2.8 (1.6-3.8)	2.9 (1.4-3.8)	2.1 (1.0-4.3)	3 (1.5-19)	70 (32-128)
New Zealand	ESD	1983-1984	0.83 (0.02-47)	0.6 (0.2-1.8)		0.62 (0.01-23)	5.6 (0.13-39)	33 (0.01-391)	9.5 / 5.9 (0.01-242)	9.0 (0.07-158)	36	41	9.6 (0.01-39)	10 (0.51-71)	291	9 (0.4-26)	32-78 (28-48)
	H_E	1981-1985	0.11	0.10		<0.001	0.3	1.4	1.1/0.8	0.7	7.2	13	0.4	1.8	0.5	0.5	2, 12
Norway	H_E	1988	0.15		0.23			1.6	0.7 / 0.4	0.9	2.5/5	6.4/ 10		2.6			
Poland	ESD	1985-1989	1.5	6.0	10	1.0	15	22	/ 5.9	42	8.0		28	11			
Portugal [C25, S52]	ESD [f]	1989-1990	0.41 (0.08-4.2)			0.82 (0.98-14)	9.6 (0.65-28)	7.9 (1.8-31)		6.1 (0.80-14)				7.0 (0.76-31)			70 (12-231)
Romania	ESD	1980 1990	6.3 2.4 (1.1-5.8)	8.3 5.9 (3.9-15)	9.7 13 (6.6-27)	- -	24 20 (6.4-35)	62 53 (21-82)	30/26 25/19 (4.3-60)	18 19 (11-36)	46 55 (18-162)	 77 (26-92)	35 40 (20-58)	71 48 (28-91)	- 21 (13-33)	- -	12 18 (11-27)
	H_E	1980 1990	0.50 0.23	0.72 0.66	0.74 1.0	- -	0.11 0.12	2.4 1.9	3.1/1.6 2.7/1.3	1.1 1.4	3.0 3.4	 5.2	1.3 1.4	4.3 3.5	 0.15		1.3 1.9
Spain	ESD	1986-1990	1.0 (0.2-3.0)			0.9 (0.1-1.8)	6.7 (2-15)	39 (15-50)	19 (7-40)	12 (6-20)							
	H_E		0.29			0.10	0.14	2.1	2.0	1.2	5.5	9.7		6.7		/1.2	3.8
Sweden	H_E [g]	1970-1974 1985-1989	0.30 (0.19-0.40) 0.14 (0.01-1.0)		1.0 (0.51-3.1) -	0.29 - 0.08 (0.03-0.20)	0.97 - 0.19 (0.17-0.20)	5.9 (3.0-11) 2.4 (0.39-6.4)	1.2/1.7 (0.57-2.0) 0.64/0.86 (0.20-4.3)	2.9 - 1.8 (0.47-3.9)	4.4 (1.3-6.6) 4.6 (0.86-17)	8.6 (5.3-13) 6.1 (1.0-27)	1.3 (0.57-1.4) 0.86 (0.26-2.1)	7.3 (5.1-7.3) 3.6 (0.21-14)	9.7 - -		 5

Table 10 (continued)

Country	Dose quantity	Year	Chest examinations			Extremities	Skull	Lumbo-sacral spine	Pelvis / hips	Abdomen	GI tract		Cholecystography	Urography	Angiography	Mammography Screening /clinical	CT (slice doses) [b]
			Radiography	Photofluorography	Fluoroscopy						Upper	Lower					
Switzerland	ESD	1982	0.5 (0.1-1.3)	5.0 (3.9-9)	-		5.2 (1-14)	14 (0.8-30)	7.1/6.5 (0.6-15)	5.9 (1-11)	3.6 (0.5-8)	3.1 (0.5-9)	6.9 (1-13)	6.7 (5-10)			
	H_E	1982	0.06	0.6			0.6	0.8	0.85/0.2	1.4	0.4	0.4	0.4	2.1			
USSR [U1]	H_E	1982	0.36		1.2	0.01	0.17	4.4	1.5	1.5	1.5, 9.5	3.6, 14	2.0	2.5			
USSR, RSFSR	H_E	1976-1980 1981-1985 1986-1990	0.35 0.30 0.30	0.65 0.60 0.60	1.2 1.15 1.0	0.002 0.002 0.002	0.2 0.2 0.2	2.3 2.4 2.5	2.0 / 1.4 2.0 / 1.5 2.0 / 1.5	1.9 1.8 1.8	8.0 7.7 7.3	16.0 15.5 15.0	2.0 2.0 2.0	4.5 4.5 4.5	1.2 / - 0.5 / 0.4 /		
United Kingdom	ESD [h]	1983	0.23 (0.03-1.4)	1.2 -			4.4 (1.8-13)	20 (3.8-107)	6.6/ (0.9-32)	8.4 (0.7-62)							
	H_E	1981-1985 1986-1990	0.05			0.05	0.15	2.2	1.2/1.4	1.4	3.8	7.7	0.95	4.4	9.0	0.15-1.0	3.5, 8.0
United States	ESD	1984-1989	0.18 (0.01-0.94)					4.9 (0.70-25)		4.2 (0.58-19)						1.8 (0.4-12)	(33-63)
	H_E	1980	0.07			0.1	0.13	1.3	0.6	0.56	2.4	4.6	1.9	1.6			
Health-care level II																	
Brazil [D4]	ESD	1987	0.39 [c] (0.05-1.5)	6.5 [d] (1.5-24)			5.9 [e] (1.5-17)			8.7 [h] (1.5-25)							
China	ESD	1986-1990	1.1 (0.10-15)		10 (1-143)	2.3	13	33 (2-286)	11	8.5 (0.8-135)	52 (0.5-800)	58	27 (0.2-238)		26	/ 2.5	
	H_E	1986-1990	0.06		0.29	0.06		2.7	1.6	0.13	7.5		1.6				
Ecuador	ESD	1985-1989	0.81 (0.77-0.89)			0.77 (0.66-0.88)	2.5 (2.4-2.6)	9.8 (9.5-10)	2.1 / 1.0 (0.9-26)	4.6 (2.5-6.7)	3.3 (0.82-5.7)	2.6 (1.2-3.9)	2.6 (1.7-3.6)	3.7 (3.2-4.2)	1.2 (0.4-8.2)	7.9 (7.0-8.7)	14 (13.5-14.4)
India	ESD	1985-1989	0.2			0.19	9.5	50	50	5.5	34	25		29			
	H_E	1985-1989	0.016			0.0001	0.13	2.5	2.5	0.35	1.4	1.6		1.7			
Jamaica	ESD	1985-1989		0.25 (0.2-0.3)			1.2 (1.2-1.3)			1.2 (1.2-1.3)			1.2	1.7 (1.6-1.8)			

Table 10 (continued)

Country	*Dose quantity*	*Year*	*Chest examinations*			*Extre-mities*	*Skull*	*Lumbo-sacral spine*	*Pelvis / hips*	*Abdomen*	*GI tract*		*Chole-cysto-graphy*	*Uro-graphy*	*Angio-graphy*	*Mammo-graphy Screening /clinical*	*CT (slice doses)* [b]
			Radio-graphy	*Photo-fluorography*	*Fluoro-scopy*						*Upper*	*Lower*					
Health-care level III																	
Myanmar	ESD	1970-1980	0.7	3.6		0.26	3.7	4.7	3.8 / 3.8	4.7	3.4	4.0	3.4	4.2	4.2	/ 0.65	
		1981-1985	0.80	3.5		0.24	3.5	4.0	3.3 / 3.5	3.7	3.3	3.4	3.3	3.7	3.9	/ 0.60	
		1986-1990	0.32	2.9		0.23	2.9	3.9	2.9 / 3.0	3.3	2.8	3.0	3.0	3.3	3.8	/ 0.55	
	H_E	1976-1980	0.039	0.18		0.003	0.035	0.045	0.036	0.23	0.41	0.43	0.17	0.22	0.21	/ 0.03	
		1981-1985	0.040	0.18		0.002	0.035	0.040	0.035	0.19	0.40	0.41	0.17	0.19	0.20	/ 0.03	
		1986-1990	0.016	0.14		0.002	0.029	0.039	0.029/0.030	0.16	0.34	0.35	0.15	0.17	0.19	/ 0.03	
Thailand	ESD	1976-1980	0.29 (0.26-0.33)				4.1 (3.5-3.7)			4.2 (3.9-4.5)				4.9 (4.7-5.1)			
		1986-1990	0.21 (0.17-0.25)	0.09 (0.08-0.09)	6.5 (3.4-9.5)	0.07 (0.04-0.1)	2.4 (2.2-2.5)	2.8 (2.4-3.1)	3.2 / 2.5 (2.3-3.5)	2.6 (2.5-2.6)	3.4 (3.1-3.6)		3.1 (2.7-3.5)	2.9 (2.8-3.0)	2.6 (2.2-2.9)		

The entries in this Table are qualified as follows:

Australia: Value under CT is for skull CT only.
Canada: Data are for one Ottawa hospital only.
China: Data for Beijing area represent 3% of the population; data for entire nation are for 1986-1990.
Denmark: Data are also from [J11].
Ecuador: Value for chest radiography includes fluoroscopy (20% of examinations.)
Finland: Data are also from [H32, R25].
Japan: Data are also from [M4, U1].
New Zealand: Value under lumbosacral is for lumbar spine. Gastrointestinal tract ESDs refer to fluoroscopy only. When serial and follow-up films are added, total ESD is 75 mGy for upper GI and 99 mGy for lower GI tract. Value under angiography is for coronary catheterization. H_E for mammography 1976-1980: 1.6 mSv, 1986-1990: 0.6 mSv. ESD value under CT is multiple average dose to head for average years 1983-1984, to body for range. H_E value for CT is 2 for head, 12 for abdomen.
Norway: Values under GI tract are for barium/double contrast.
Peru: Data are from Instituto Peruano de Energia Nuclear only (bout 60% of all examinations).
Poland: Value under abdomen is for fluoroscopy.
Romania: Values under CT are, with the exception of the last entry (E, 1990), for chest.
Spain: Values under lumbosacral are for all spine examinations.
Sweden: Value under lumbosacral includes lumbar spine; value under angiography is for cerebral examination.
Thailand: Data are from National Cancer Institute and from the Rajavithi Hospital only.
USSR (RSFSR): Values under GI tract are for fluoroscopy examinations.
United Kingdom: Data also from [W22]. Entry under angiography is for lymphangiography only. Values under CT: first value refers to head; second value to body.
United States: Data also from [U1]. Value under mammography is for mostly screening; range under CT is multiple-scan absorbed doses in a sample and is not considered statistically representative.
Yugoslavia: Data are for Serbia only (about 40% of the population).

[a] The entrance surface dose (ESD) is given in mGy and the effective dose equivalent (H_E) is given in mSv. Average for years as indicated and range in parentheses.
[b] Doses are computed tomography dose index (CTDI) or multiple-scan average dose (MSAD).
[c] PA projection.
[d] LAT projection.
[e] AP projection.
[f] Converted from entrance surface exposure assuming that 1 mR = 0.0087/0.75 mGy ESD. Applies also for ranges where given.
[g] All but CT: Converted from energy imparted assuming that 1 mJ corresponds to 0.0143 mSv. CT data from [S58].
[h] For most frequent projections.

Table 11
Average effective dose equivalent from diagnostic medical x-ray examinations
Data from UNSCEAR Survey of Medical Radiation Usage and Exposures

Examination/site	*Average effective dose equivalent (mSv)*		
	Level I		*Level II*
	1970-1979	*1980-1990*	*1980-1990*
Chest radiography	0.25	0.14	0.04
Chest miniature	0.52	0.52	
Chest fluoroscopy	0.72	0.98	0.29
Extremities	0.02	0.06	0.03
Lumbosacral spine	2.2	1.7	2.6
Pelvis	2.1	1.2	2.0
Hip/femur	1.5	0.92	2.0
Skull	0.50	0.16	0.13
Abdomen	1.9	1.1	0.22
Lower GI tract	9.8	4.1	5.0
Upper GI tract	8.9	7.2	1.6
Cholecystography	1.9	1.5	1.6
Urography	3.0	3.1	1.7
Angiography	9.2	6.8	
Mammography	1.8	1.0	
Computed tomography	1.3	4.3	

Table 12
Factors of technique affecting doses to patients from x-ray examinations
[C26, D8, J12, L10, M21, N5, R4, R18, S13, S31, S53, S56, S57, W14]

Factor	*Effect*
Procedure-related	
Referral criteria	Stricter criteria reduce per caput doses by removing clinically unhelpful examinations
Availability of previously taken films	May eliminate some retakes and thus reduce per caput doses
Number of radiographs per examination	Positively correlated with dose
Fluoroscopy time and current	Positively correlated with dose
Quality assurance programmes, including repeat/reject rate assessments and patient dose surveys	May reduce per caput doses
X-ray beam collimation	Area positively correlated with dose
Shielding of sensitive organs	May reduce doses
Choice of projection	Dose depends on projection
Optical density of radiographs	Positively correlated with dose
Compression of attenuating tissue	Reduces dose and scatter and improves image quality
Matching exposure factors to patient stature	May reduce doses
Equipment-related	
Exposure time	Long time, low current combinations may increase dose due to reciprocity law failure
Kilovoltage	Higher kilovoltage may reduce dose and contrast
X-ray tube voltage wave-form	Three-phase and constant potential x-ray beams reduce dose and contrast
X-ray tube target metal	Molybdenum may increase dose and contrast compared to tungsten
Filter type	Rare-earth K-edge filters or other filters producing a beam of higher half-value layer reduce dose and contrast
Anti-scatter grids	Increase dose and image quality
Distance (air gap)	Adjustment for increased magnification nominally increases dose but may also obviate need for a grid
Attenuation between patient and image receptor	Low attenuation (e.g. carbon fibre couch top) reduces dose
Screen/film combination	Faster rare earth screens reduce dose, sometimes also image quality
Film processing	Long processing time or chemicals and temperature that increase speed of development reduce dose
Image intensifier	Sensitive (e.g. CsI) photocathodes and digital image processing may reduce dose
Recording method	Video recorder reduces fluoroscopy dose compared to cine camera
Pulsed fluoroscopy with image storage device	Reduces fluoroscopy dose
Spot film fluorography	With modern equipment, may reduce dose compared to radiography
Computed radiography	Potential for reduction of dose and of image quality

Table 13
Doses to patients from angiography examinations
[S37, V14]

Examination		Entrance surface dose (mGy)	Organ absorbed dose (mGy)							
			Eye lens	*Red bone marrow*	*Lung*	*Thyroid*	*Breast*	*Bladder*	*Testis*	*Ovary*
Cerebral	Conventional	282-482	-	7-52	0.2-14	10-73	0.1-7	-	0.02-0.2	0.2-1
	Conventional, PA	-	-	-	-	-	-	-	0.1	0.01
	Digital, PA	-	-	-	-	-	-	-	0.01	0.03
Neck	Conventional	142-230	32-107	5-12	-	5-87	-	-	0.03	0.04
	Subtraction, analog	502	2	12	-	4	1	-	0.02	<0.01
	Subtraction, digital	37	0.2	0.6	-	7	-	-	-	-
Thorax	Conventional	24-502	0.2	0.5-54	2-32	0.1-73	0.8-73	-	0.02-11	0.07-12
	Conventional, AP	-	-	0.9	6	20	20	0.05	-	0.05
	Conventional, PA	-	-	-	-	-	-	-	0.2	0.07
	Subtraction, analog	21-232	0.03	0.4	1	0.8-4	0.9	-	<0.01-0.3	<0.01-0.1
	Subtaction, digital, PA	-	-	0.4	1	4	0.9	<0.01	0.2	<0.01
Angiocardiography	Conventional	482	-	79	27	6	80	-	2	5
	Subtraction, analog	86-111	0.2-0.3	3-10	20-23	0.3-3	2-4	-	<0.01-2	<0.01-5
Abdomen	Conventional	482-523	-	33-41	27-32	0.9-1	60-89	-	0.2-0.3	3-9
	Conventional, PA	-	-	-	-	-	-	-	1.9	2
	Subtraction, digital, PA	-	-	-	-	-	-	-	1.5	1.6
Renovasography	Conventional	101-533	<0.01	0.5-36	0.2-19	0.04-0.9	0.2-29	-	0.08-1	0.2-29
	Conventional, AP	-	-	1	0.2	0.07	0.3	0.1	-	0.2
	Subtraction, digital, AP	-	-	2	0.2	1	2	1	-	2
	Subtraction, digital, PA	-	-	29	0.04	0.9	0.2	0.08	-	2
Pelvis	Conventional	78-402	<0.01	0.6-10	0.2-1	<0.01-0.08	0.2-0.5	-	3-29	1-29
	Conventional, PA	-	-	-	-	-	-	-	13	33
	Subtraction, analog	577	<0.01	9	-	0.07	-	-	227	19
	Subtraction, digital, PA	-	-	-	-	-	-	-	26	57

Table 14
Doses to patients from computed tomography examinations in the United Kingdom, 1989
[S42, S43]

Examination		*Effective dose equivalent* [a] *(mSv)*	*Effective dose* [b] *(mSv)*	*Collective effective dose equivalent* [a] *(man Sv)*	*Collective effective dose* [b] *(man Sv)*
Type	*Number*				
Head, routine	296650 (35%)	3.49	1.80	1035 (23%)	534 (16%)
Posterior fossa	68850 (8.1%)	1.22	0.71	84.0 (1.9%)	48.9 (1.5%)
Pituitary	17850 (2.1%)	1.10	0.59	19.6 (0.4%)	10.5 (0.3%)
Internal auditory meatus	18700 (2.2%)	0.43	0.34	8.0 (0.2%)	6.4 (0.2%)
Orbits	16150 (1.9%)	1.13	0.60	18.2 (0.4%)	9.7 (0.3%)
Facial bones	8500 (1.0%)	0.69	0.61	5.9 (0.1%)	5.2 (0.2%)
Cervical spine	15300 (1.8%)	1.94	2.89	29.7 (0.7%)	44.2 (1.3%)
Thoracic spine	5950 (0.7%)	7.76	5.82	46.2 (1.0%)	34.6 (1.1%)
Chest, routine	67150 (7.9%)	9.13	8.33	613 (14%)	559 (17%)
Mediastinum	34000 (4.0%)	7.39	7.09	251 (5.5%)	241 (7.3%)
Abdomen, routine	98600 (11.6%)	8.82	7.16	870 (19%)	706 (21%)
Liver	29750 (3.5%)	10.20	7.18	303 (6.7%)	214 (6.5%)
Pancreas	22950 (2.7%)	6.71	4.57	154 (3.4%)	105 (3.2%)
Kidneys	14450 (1.7%)	8.62	5.81	125 (2.8%)	84.0 (2.6%)
Adrenals	8500 (1.0%)	3.74	3.04	31.8 (0.7%)	25.8 (0.8%)
Lumbar spine	59500 (7.0%)	5.98	3.60	356 (7.9%)	214 (6.5%)
Pelvis, routine	47600 (5.6%)	9.38	7.26	446 (9.9%)	345 (10%)
Other	19550 (2.3%)			108 (2.4%)	100 (3.0%)
Total	850000 (100%)	5.3	3.9	4500 (100%)	3300 (100%)

a Using ICRP 1977 weighting factors.
b Using ICRP 1990 weighting factors.

Table 15
Doses to patients from computed tomography examinations in Japan
[N8]

Examination	*Dose quantity*	*Dose to*	*Dose*		
			Minimum	*Maximum*	*Average*
Head	Absorbed dose (mGy)	Bone marrow	0.7	2.1	1.5
		Thyroid	0.2	0.8	0.5
		Eye	8.7	47.2	22.4
	Effective dose equivalent (mSv)		0.2	0.7	0.5
Chest	Absorbed dose (mGy)	Breast	8.7	39.6	15.9
		Lungs	12.6	35.0	19.6
		Bone marrow	3.9	11.5	5.7
		Thyroid	1.2	3.0	1.9
	Effective dose equivalent (mSv)		4.3	14.1	6.9
Upper abdomen	Absorbed dose (mGy)	Large intestine	0.7	1.7	1.0
		Ovary/testis	0.4 / 0.04	1.0 / 0.2	0.6 / 0.1
		Bone marrow	1.4	3.7	2.2
	Effective dose equivalent (mSv)	Female	2.6	7.4	3.8
		Male	2.5	7.2	3.7
Lower abdomen	Absorbed dose (mGy)	Large intestine	11.3	34.5	19.2
		Ovary/testis	8.7 / 0.5	27.1 / 1.6	15.1 / 1.0
		Bone marrow	3.5	9.5	5.6
	Effective dose equivalent (mSv)	Female	4.1	12.5	7.1
		Male	2.0	6.2	3.6

Table 16
Doses from mammography examinations

Country and year	*Technique*	*Absorbed dose in breast (mGy)* [a]		*Effective dose equivalent (mSv)*	
		Per film	*Per patient*	*Per patient*	*Per caput*
Australia, 1989 [H37]	Patients				
	All with grid, screen/film	1.3 ± 0.4 (0.5-2.3)			
Australia 1989-1990 [T19]	48 mm phantom				
	Xeroradiograph [b]	2.3			
	Screen/film:				
	With grid [c]	1.8 ± 0.8	3.6		
	No grid	0.8 ± 0.5	1.6		
	Overall	1.7 ± 0.8 (0.1-6.8)	3.4		
Canada, Manitoba 1988 [H31]	47 mm phantom				
	Xeroradiograph	3.3		0.82	
	Screen/film	1.4 (0.8-1.9)		0.30	
	Overall		4.0	0.60	0.014
Italy, 1987-1990 [R19]	50 mm phantom				
	39% with grid		1.5 (63%)		
			1.0 (39%)		
Ireland, 1989 [H43]	60 mm phantom				
	Screen/film	1.5 (0.9-2.3)			
New Zealand 1988-1989 [W11] and UNSCEAR Survey	All screen/film:				
	30 mm phantom				
	No grid	0.6 ± 0.3			
	Overall	1.0 ± 0.6		0.30	
	Magnification	2.5 (0.7-7.2)			
	45 mm phantom				
	No grid	1.1 ± 0.4			
	With grid	2.3 ± 1.0			
	Overall	2.0 ± 1.1 (0.5-4.8)		0.60	
Poland, 1988 [D7]	30 mm phantom				
	Xeroradiograph	4.8	6.4		
Portugal 1988-1989 [C15]	All screen/film:				
	40 mm phantom				
	No grid	0.8			
	Stationary grid	1.0			
	Moving grid	2.0			
	Overall	1.4			
Sweden 1989-1990 [L10]	All screen/film:				
	45 mm phantom				
	No grid	0.7 (0.5-1.1)			
	Moving grid	1.5 (1.2-1.9)			

[a] ± SD; range in parentheses.
[b] 2% of all centres.
[c] 80% of all centres.

Table 17
Average annual number of dental x-ray examinations per 1,000 population
Data from UNSCEAR Survey of Medical Radiation Usage and Exposures unless otherwise indicated

Country	*1970-1979*	*1980-1984*	*1985-1990*	*Country*	*1970-1979*	*1980-1984*	*1985-1990*
Health-care level I							
Australia	80			Netherlands	150	399	411
Belgium			288	New Zealand	321		275
Cuba				Norway	641	805	833
Czechoslovakia	72	86	85	Poland			61
Denmark			471	Portugal			86
Finland			223	Romania	20	32	42
France		540		Spain			232
Germany, Fed. Rep. of			264	Sweden	443	841	832
Italy		119		Switzerland	296	325	
Japan	831	834	783	USSR, RSFSR	50	74	80
Kuwait			219	United Kingdom	112	165	
Luxembourg			186	United States	350	456	402
Malta	3	6.2	8.2				
				Average	320	390	350
Health-care level II							
Brazil			4.7	Ecuador	1.5	4.4	6.2
Chile		3.9		Tunisia			1.3
China		0.8	2.1				
				Average		0.8	2.5
Health-care level III							
Egypt	0.7			Sri Lanka	0.8		
Myanmar			1.6	Thailand	1.4	2.3	2.1
				Average		0.8	1.7

The entries in this Table are qualified as follows:

France: Value represents number of films.
Germany, Fed. Rep. of: Pantomograms not included.
Italy: Value is for north-east of Italy.
Japan: Data also from [U1].
Netherlands: Data also from [V2, V10].
New Zealand: Data also from [W12].
Sweden: Data also from [S1, S3].

Table 18
Estimates of effective dose equivalent from dental x-ray examinations
Data from UNSCEAR Survey of Medical Radiation Usage and Exposures, unless otherwise indicated

Country	*Year*	*Entrance surface dose (mGy)*	*Effective dose equivalent (mSv)*	*Country*	*Year*	*Entrance surface dose (mGy)*	*Effective dose equivalent (mSv)*
Health-care level I							
Argentina	1985-1989	4 (1.5-40)		New Zealand	1975-1979	5.2 (1.2-19)	
Australia	1970-1974	7.4			1985-1989	4.9 (1.2-22)	0.11
Czechoslovakia	1970-1979	25 (0.1-30)	0.15	Poland	1985-1989	3	
	1986-1990	18 (0.1-25)	0.15	Romania	1980-1984	10.7	0.004
France [B5]	1984	(3.9-13.5)	0.07		1985-1990	28 (3.3-46)	0.01
Japan	1970-1974	5.8 (3.5-8.7)		Spain	1986-1990	6.0 (0.9-12)	
	1980-1984	3.1	0.03, 0.04	Sweden	1980-1984	5	0.03
Kuwait	1985-1989	3.2 (0.76-9.7)		USSR, RSFSR	1985-1990		0.02
Netherlands	1974-1985	(0.9-31)	0.02-0.28	United Kingdom	1981-1985		0.02, 0.03
Health-care level II				**Health-care level III**			
Brazil	1987		0.2	Myanmar	1985-1990	6.4	0.32
Ecuador	1985-1989	1.9 (1.3-2.7)					

The entries in this Table are qualified as follows:

Australia: ESD given is per film.

France: The range of the ESD is the average for different projections. The value given for the effective dose equivalent is per film, the effective dose equivalent per caput is 0.037 mSv.

Japan: Data also from [U1]. The ESD has been estimated from exposure (mR) multiplied by 0.0087/0.75. The first value for effective dose equivalent for 1985-1989 is for intraoral, the second value for extraoral examinations. The per caput effective dose equivalent for Japan is 0.027 mSv [I12]. For 1989, H_E: 0.024 mSv; E: 0.052 mSv [M44].

Netherlands: Data also from [V2, V10]. Range of ESD: on average, 2.4 films are used per examination. Effective dose equivalent is for complete mouth survey; for pantomogram it is 0.13 mSv.

New Zealand: Data also from [W12]. The ESD values are per film. The ESD value for the period 1985-1989 is qualified by the fact that on average 1.6 films were used per examination.

Romania: Effective dose equivalent is per caput.

Spain: The values for ESD (and range) are for intraoral examinations.

Sweden: Data also from [S1, S3]. On average, 1.25 films were used per examination; 1985-1989: on average, 2.4 films were used per examination. The effective dose equivalent per caput is 0.01 mSv, for the complete mouth survey it is 0.14-0.23 mSv.

USSR: The value for effective dose equivalent is given for intraoral examinations.

United Kingdom: The first value of the effective dose equivalent is for intraoral, the second one for extraoral examinations. On average 2.4 films were used per examination (1981-1985).

Table 19
Mean absorbed doses from dental x-ray examinations in France [a]
[B5]

Organ	*Mean absorbed dose (mGy)*							
	Periapical incisor		*Periapical molar*		*Panoramic projections*			
	Upper	*Lower*	*Upper*	*Lower*	*Maxillary occlusal*	*Circular: 2 centers of rotation*	*Circular: 3 centers of rotation*	*Elliptical*
Lens	0.10	0.07	0.05	0.02	3.60	0.03	0.03	0.08
Thyroid	0.14	0.08	0.04	0.08	0.07	0.01	0.05	0.06
Parotids	0.01	0.02	0.40	0.41	0.04	0.90	1.40	0.08
Tongue	0.12	0.27	0.05	0.06	0.12	0.40	3.10	0.59
Sublinguals	0.03	0.03	0.10	0.13	0.04	-	-	-
Pharynx	<0.01	0.01	0.06	0.04	0.01	0.19	0.80	0.40
Sinuses	0.08	0.06	0.28	0.04	4.35	-	-	-
Back of neck	0.04	0.02	0.04	0.03	0.04	-	-	-
Brain	<0.01	<0.01	0.01	<0.01	0.01	-	-	-
Bone surface	0.07	0.09	0.65	0.74	0.10	0.10	0.15	0.15

[a] Underlined values are doses >0.2 mGy.

Table 20
Collective dose from diagnostic x-ray examinations worldwide, 1985-1990

Examination/site	*Number of examinations per 1,000 population*				*Effective dose equivalent per examination (mSv)*				*Annual collective effective dose equivalent (man Sv)*			
	Level I	*Level II*	*Levels III-IV*	*World*	*Level I*	*Level II*	*Levels III-IV*	*World*	*Level I*	*Level II*	*Levels III-IV*	*World*
Chest radiography	171	22	34	63	0.14	0.14	0.14	0.14	31500	8130	6240	45900
Chest miniature	260	20	1.5	77	0.52	0.52	0.52	0.52	182000	27100	1040	210000
Chest fluoroscopy	33	48	9.0	34	0.98	0.98	0.98	0.98	43100	124000	11500	178000
Extremities	121	11	5.6	38	0.06	0.06	0.06	0.06	10600	1800	440	12800
Lumbosacral spine	54	3.0	1.8	16	1.7	2.6	2.6	1.8	122000	20400	6130	148000
Pelvis	21	1.5	0.89	6	1.2	2.0	2.0	1.3	32800	7710	2320	42900
Hip/femur	12	1.1	0.89	4	0.92	2.0	2.0	1.1	15300	5740	2320	23300
Skull	40	4.4	3.3	13	0.16	0.16	0.16	0.16	8560	1860	690	11100
Abdomen	32	6.0	3.0	12	1.1	1.1	1.1	1.1	44700	16600	4180	65500
Upper GI tract	52	2.8	0.89	15	4.1	5.0	5.0	4.2	285000	36700	5800	328000
Lower GI tract	11	0.99	0.69	4	7.2	7.2	7.2	7.2	112000	18800	6520	137000
Cholecystography	9	0.21	0.78	3	1.5	1.6	1.6	1.5	18100	900	1630	20600
Urography	14	1.8	1.2	5	3.1	3.1	3.1	3.1	58200	14700	4660	77500
Angiography	6	0.21	0.10	2	6.8	6.8	6.8	6.8	57300	3670	880	61900
Mammography	12	0.43	0.06	3	1.0	1.0	1.0	1.0	17000	1170	84	18300
CT	39	0.32	0.38	10	4.3	4.3	4.3	4.3	224000	3610	2110	230000
Total	887	124	64	304					1262000	292000	56500	1610000
Average per examination (mSv)					1.05	0.90	0.67	1.0				
Average dose per caput (mSv)					0.93	0.11	0.043	0.30				

Table 21
Contribution of different types of diagnostic examinations to the collective dose

Examination/site	*Contribution to total collective dose (%)*			
	Level I	*Level II*	*Levels III-IV*	*World*
Upper GI tract	23	13	10	20
Computed tomography	18	1	4	14
Chest mass miniature	14	9	2	13
Chest fluoroscopy	3	42	20	11
Lumbosacral spine	10	7	11	9
Lower GI tract	9	6	12	9
Urography	5	5	8	5
Angiography	5	1	2	4
Abdomen	4	6	7	4
Pelvis	3	3	4	3
Chest radiography	2	3	11	3
Hip/femur	1	2	4	1
Cholecystography	1	0.3	3	1
Mammography	1	0.4	0.1	1
Extremities	0.8	0.6	0.8	0.8
Skull	0.7	0.6	1	0.7

Table 22
Annual individual and collective effective dose from diagnostic x-ray examinations
Data from UNSCEAR Survey of Medical Radiation Usage and Exposures unless otherwise indicated

Country	Year	*Effective dose equivalent (mSv)*		Collective effective dose equivalent (man Sv)	Reference
		Per individual patient	*Per caput*		
Health-care level I					
Canada	1980	0.8 [a]	1.0 [a]	24000 [a]	[U1]
Czechoslovakia	1980	0.9	0.6	8600	[K17]
Denmark	1986-1990	1.4	0.7	3600	
Finland	1978 1987	0.6 0.8	0.7 0.7	3300 3500	[U1] [R9]
France	1982	2.0	1.6	89000	[U1]
Germany, Fed. Rep. of	1979 1983 1988	2.0 [a] 1.0	1.7 [a] 1.5 1.0	102000 90000 61000	[U1] [B7] [S17]
Italy	1983	1.1	0.8	48000	[P19, U1]
Japan	1979 1989	 1.9	1.3 2.2	151000 266000	[U1] [M32]
New Zealand	1981-1985	0.67	0.4	1400	
Netherlands	1980 1987	0.57 0.56	0.34 0.31	4800 4500	[B6] [B6]
Norway	1988	0.9	0.6	2500	[S22]
Poland	1976 1988	 1.2	1.7 0.8	58700 30000	[U1] [L21]
Portugal	1988-1989	0.76	0.53	5400	[S52]
Romania	1980 1990	1.1 1.1	0.6 0.5	14100 12300	
Spain	1985-1986	1.4	0.8	31100	[V5]
Sweden	1985	1.1	0.6	4600	[V4]
Switzerland	1985-1990	0.4	0.4	2700	
USSR	1980 1986-1987	1.1 1.15	1.1 1.15	292000 326000	[N4] [N4, S18]
USSR, RSFSR	1976-1980 1981-1985 1986-1990	1.18 1.14 1.14	1.13 1.16 1.10	153700 163300 161000	
United Kingdom	1983 1989	0.7	0.3 0.35	16000 20000	[H10] [S43]
United States	1980	0.5	0.4	92000	[N1, U1]
Health-care level II					
China Beijing area Entire nation	 1983 1985	 0.6 0.6	 0.4 0.09	 3600 94000	 [Z1, Z4] [Z6]
India [b]	1989	0.2	0.02	16800	[S40]
Iran (Islamic Rep. of) [b]	1980	0.5	0.09	3500	[U1]
Iraq [b]	1972	0.7 [a]	0.2 [a]	1700 [a]	[U1]
Turkey [b]	1977		0.2 [a]	7000 [a]	[U1]
Health-care level III					
Myanmar	1986-1990	5	0.05	2000	
Thailand [b]	1970		0.2 [a]		[U1]

Table 22 (continued)

The entries in this Table are qualified as follows:

Italy: Data for the north-east of country have been extrapolated to the entire country.

Japan: Collective effective dose equivalent includes 16,100 man Sv from stomach mass screening; 69,000 man Sv from chest mass screening; 5,600 man Sv from computed tomography; 2,900 man Sv from dental radiography.

Spain: Excluding military and pre-employment screening.

---

[a] Estimated from genetically significant dose, GSD [0.3 mSv and average ratio GSD/H_E for health-care level I (0.3/1; range of level I ratios: 0.14/1-0.5/1)].

[b] Apparently excludes fluoroscopy. For approximate adjustment, it could be assumed that 50% of all examinations are fluoroscopic and that these cause, on average, 15 times higher absorbed doses per examination [U1].

Table 23
Estimated doses to the world population from diagnostic medical and dental x-ray examinations

Health-care level	*Population (millions)*	*Annual per caput effective dose equivalent (mSv)*		*Annual collective effective dose equivalent (10^3 man Sv)*	
		Medical	*Dental*	*Medical*	*Dental*
I	1350	1	0.01	1300	14
II	2630	0.1	0.001	290	3
III	850	0.04	0.0003	40	0.3
IV	460	0.04	0.0003	20	0.1
Total	5290	-	-	1600	17
Average	-	0.3	0.003	-	-

Table 24
Regulations or recommendations on quality assurance
Data from UNSCEAR Survey of Medical Radiation Usage and Exposures, unless otherwise indicated

Country	*X-ray diagnostics*			*Radiation therapy*			*Nuclear medicine*		
	Legal regulations	*Recommendations*	*No QA rules*	*Legal regulations*	*Recommendations*	*No QA rules*	*Legal regulations*	*Recommendations*	*No QA rules*
Health-care level I									
Argentina		*			*			*	
Australia	*			*			*		
Belgium			*			*			*
Canada [a]	*	*			*	*		*	
Czechoslovakia		*				*		*	
Denmark	*			*			*		
Ecuador	*				*			*	
Finland		*		*				*	
France	*			*			*		
Germany, Fed. Rep. of	*			*			*		
Japan [b]			*			*			*
Kuwait	*			*			*		
Luxembourg	*			*			*		
Malta		*				*			*
New Zealand			*	*				*	
Norway			*			*			*
Poland		*			*			*	
Romania		*			*			*	
Singapore		*						*	
Spain	*			*			*		
Sweden	*			*			*		
Switzerland		*		*				*	
USSR, RSFSR		*			*		*		
United Kingdom		*			*			*	
United States [c]	*	*			*			*	
Yugoslavia	*			*			*		
Total	12	12	4	12	8	6	10	12	4

Table 24 (continued)

Country	*X-ray diagnostics*			*Radiation therapy*			*Nuclear medicine*		
	Legal regula-tions	*Recom-menda-tions*	*No QA rules*	*Legal regula-tions*	*Recom-menda-tions*	*No QA rules*	*Legal regula-tions*	*Recom-menda-tions*	*No QA rules*
Health-care level II									
Barbados	*				*			*	
China	*			*			*		*
Honduras [d]		*							
India		*		*				*	
Iraq	*			*			*		
Jamaica			*			*			*
Nicaragua [d]			*						
Peru [e]			*			*			*
Turkey		*			*			*	
Total	3	3	3	3	2	2	2	3	3
Health-care level III									
Cape Verde		*							
Djibouti			*			*			*
Dominica [d]			*						
Egypt	*			*			*		
Myanmar		*							
Philippines		*							
Saint Lucia [d]			*						
Sudan		*			*			*	
Thailand		*			*			*	
Total	1	5	3	1	2	1	1	2	1
Health-care level IV									
Ethiopia					*			*	
Rwanda		*				*			*
Total		1			1	1		1	1

[a] For x-ray diagnostics, legal provincial regulations prevail and federal recommendations have been made. For radiation therapy, recommendations exist in some provinces. In practice, recommendations on nuclear medicine are enforced as legal regulations.
[b] The Japanese Industrial Standards are used as technical guides for x-ray diagnostics and radiation therapy.
[c] For x-ray diagnostics, a few states have legal regulations and federal recommendations have been made.
[d] Data from PAHO.
[e] Regulations in preparation.

Table 25
Total annual number of nuclear medicine examinations per 1,000 population
Data from UNSCEAR Survey of Medical Radiation Usage and Exposures unless otherwise indicated

Country	*1970-1979*	*1980-1984*	*1985-1990*	*Country*	*1970-1979*	*1980-1984*	*1985-1990*
Health-care level I							
Argentina			11.5	Kuwait			13.1
Australia	3.8	8.9	8.3	Luxembourg			23.5
Austria [U1]	18.0			Netherlands			11.6
Belgium			36.8	New Zealand	5.6	7.3	7.5
Bulgaria [U1]		13.0		Norway	3.9		9.3
Canada			12.6	Romania		3.0	3.5
Czechoslovakia	13.6	18.3	22.9	Sweden	9.8		12.6
Denmark	14.0	14.2	13.4	Switzerland	44.9		
Finland [A12, L18]	12.6	17.7		USSR [N4]		3.9	
France [L20, U1]		9.0	6.9	United Kingdom		6.8	
Germany, Fed.Rep.	31.1	39.7	39.8	United States			25.7
Italy	6.0		7.3	Yugoslavia			6.1
Japan			8.3				
				Average	11	6.9	16
Health-care level II							
Barbados			1.0	Iraq			1.2
Brazil [C14]			1.7	Jamaica	2.8		2.0
China			0.6	Peru			0.2
Cuba [U1]	0.8			Tunisia			1.0
Ecuador	0.5		0.8	Turkey			2.5
India		0.1	0.2				
				Average	0.9	0.1	0.5
Health-care level III							
Egypt	0.07	0.21	0.48	Sudan	0.12	0.28	0.28
Myanmar	0.54	0.36	0.11	Thailand	0.25	0.18	0.26
				Average	0.25	0.25	0.30
Health-care level IV							
Ethiopia		0.014	0.10				

Table 26
Average annual number of diagnostic nuclear medicine examinations per 1,000 population
Data from UNSCEAR Survey of Medical Radiation Usage and Exposures, unless otherwise indicated

Country	Year	Bone	Brain	Cardiovascular	Liver/spleen	Lung		Kidney	Thyroid		Other
						Ventilation	Perfusion		Scan	Uptake	
Health-care level I											
Argentina	1985-1989	2.8	0.4	1.6	1.1	0.24		0.8	4.5		
Australia	1970	0.05	1.0		0.6	0.001	0.5	0.1	1.5 [b]		
	1980	2.0	1.5	0.2	1.7	0.3	0.9	0.1	0.8	0.05	0.3
	1984	2.6	0.3	1.0	1.2	0.6	0.9	0.5	0.8	0.07	0.9
	1991	3.4	-	1.5	0.2	1.5 [a]		0.8	0.6	0.01	0.3
Canada	1985-1989	16.8	4.0	0.8	1.0	0.2	0.4	0.3	0.9	0.8	0.5
Czechoslovakia	1970-1974	0.09	1.3	0.02	3.6	0.05	0.1	6.1	1.7	1.0	
	1976-1980	2.1	0.4	0.2	2.6	0.2	0.4	4.3	1.8	0.5	0.6 [c]
	1981-1985	3.4	0.5	0.5	1.9	0.4	1.1	6.7	1.9	0.2	1.6 [c]
	1986-1990	4.6	0.6	1.2	2.2	0.6	1.8	8.4	1.8	0.2	1.6 [c]
Denmark	1977-1980	2.2	2.4	0.6	1.2	0.1	0.5	3.9	1.3	0.7	1.1
	1981-1989	2.7	1.4	1.0	0.7	0.4	0.7	4.5	1.0	0.5	1.3
	1986-1990	2.5	0.8	1.1	0.1	0.4	0.7	4.8	1.6	0.3	1.1
Finland [A12]	1975	0.6	3.4	0.3	1.9	0.06	0.6	3.3	1.3	0.6	0.5
	1982	3.1	4.9	0.6	2.2	0.05	1.1	3.0	1.8	0.2	0.7
France [L20, U1]	1990	2.6		0.7		1.4			1.9		0.4
Germany, Fed. Rep. of	1976-1980	4.4	4.0	0.2	4.0	0.05	2.2	3.9	9.3	1.8	1.2
	1981-1985	9.6	1.4	2.4	1.3	0.2	2.9	2.7	18.2	0.2	0.9
	1986-1990	10.3	1.1	2.8	0.9	0.2	3.1	2.5	17.7	0.2	0.9
Italy	1974	0.06	0.6	0.09	1.2 [d]	0.06	0.04	0.7	0.2	3.0	0.2
	1985	2.0	0.2	0.3	1.5	0.02	0.2	0.3	2.0	0.7	0.1
Japan	1985-1989	2.1	0.3	0.9	0.9	0.3		1.8	0.4	0.4	1.4
Kuwait	1985-1989	1.7	0.2	1.8	1.1	0.4	0.8	3.9	3.2	0.03	
Netherlands	1985-1989	3.6	1.2	1.5	1.5	0.4	0.7	0.8	1.1	0.3	0.4
New Zealand	1970-1974	0.3	1.2	0.3	0.7		0.3	0.06	0.4	1.2	0.2
	1975-1979	1.5	2.4	0.1	1.3	0.1	0.6	0.2	0.7	0.7 [e]	
	1980-1984	2.2	1.3	0.4	1.2	0.4	0.5	0.5	0.7	0.3 [f]	
	1985-1989	2.8	1.0	0.4	0.6		0.6	0.8	0.7	0.3	

Table 26 (continued)

Country	*Year*	*Bone*	*Brain*	*Cardiovascular*	*Liver/spleen*	*Lung*		*Kidney*	*Thyroid*		*Other*
						Ventilation	*Perfusion*		*Scan*	*Uptake*	
Norway	1970-1974 1985-1989	0.2 3.4	0.7 0.2	 1.5	0.8 0.5	0.01 0.2	0.1 0.6	0.5 1.0	0.7 1.1	0.8 0.6	0.2 0.3
Romania	1980 1985-1989	0.06 0.05	0.2 0.2	0.04 0.03	1.0 1.1	0.06 0.06		0.3 0.3	1.4 [g] 0.7	 0.7	0.02 0.4
Sweden	1974 1985-1987	0.5 4.2	1.5 0.4	0.004 0.7	1.4 0.7	0.3 0.2	0.3 1.2	2.7 3.0	1.7 1.6	1.5 0.5	
Switzerland	1976	5.8	5.1	7.0	4.3	1.1	1.4	0.4	4.5	5.0	10.3
United Kingdom	1981-1985	1.7	0.9	0.2	0.9	0.3	0.5	0.5	0.4	0.1	1.2
United States	1985-1989	8.3	0.4	5.4	1.9	2.3	3.0	1.2	1.6	0.7	0.8
Yugoslavia	1985-1989	0.7	0.3	0.2	0.7	0.005	0.1	2.5	1.3	0.2	0.1
Health-care level II											
Barbados	1985-1988	0	0.4	0	0.09	0	0.1	0.08	0.4	0	
China	1985	0.002	0.003	0.0003	0.02			0.15	0.06	0.25	0.11
Ecuador	1970-1974 1985-1989	0 0.1	0.0003 0.01	0 0.05	0.01 0.1	0 0	0 0.03	0.01 0.01	0.21 0.2	0.25 0.3	
India	1985-1989	0.03	0.006	0.02	0.03	0.001	0.001	0.03	0.04	0.06	0.006
Iraq	1985-1989	0.1	0.08	0	0.08	0	0	0.02	0.9	0	0.006
Jamaica	1970-1974 1985-1989	0 0.2	1.0 0.7	0 0.001	0.3 0.1	0 0	0.1 0.2	0.1 0.04	1.0 0.7	 0	0.1 <0.01
Peru	1985-1989	0.09	0.02	0.001	0.05	0	0.002	0.01	0.03	0.009	
Tunisia	1985-1989	0.2	0.004	0.02	0.05		0.04	0.008	0.3	0.3	0.01
Turkey	1991	0.35	0.008	0.35	0.17		0.04	0.18	1.4		0.05
Health-care level III											
Myanmar	1975-1979 1978-1984 1985-1990	0.0009 0.002 0.0002	0.03 0.02 0.00003	0.001 0.001 0.00005	0.15 0.08 0.0002		0.0001 0.0008 0.00003	0.008 0.001 0.00005	0.12 0.07 0.0003	0.12 0.07 0.0003	0.23 0.19 0.11

Table 26 (continued)

Country	Year	Bone	Brain	Cardiovascular	Liver/spleen	Lung		Kidney	Thyroid		Other
						Ventilation	Perfusion		Scan	Uptake	
Egypt	1975-1979		0.01	0.001				0.1	0.02	0.02	
	1980-1984	0.1	0.03	0.005	0.01		0.004	0.03	0.03	0.0009	
	1985-1990	0.2	0.003	0.03	0.02	0.02	0.02	0.09	0.06	0.0008	0.008
Sudan	1985-1990	0.01	0.02		0.0007		0.0001	0.01	0.25	0.02	
Thailand	1976-1980	0.001	0.03	0.0007	0.04	0.00006	0.0002	0.002	0.07	0.10	0.0009
	1981-1985	0.01	0.01	0.002	0.005	0.0001	0.0005	0.005	0.05	0.001	0.0001
	1986-1990	0.04	0.003	0.007	0.024	0.002	0.002	0.006	0.08	0.09	0.001
Health-care level IV											
Ethiopia	1981-1985	-	0.001	-	0.004	-	-	0.0003	0.004	0.004	-
	1985-1989	-	0.02	-	0.03	-	-	0.0009	0.03	0.03	-

The entries in this Table are qualified as follows:

Australia: Administration of Tl-201 in cardiovascular examinations: 1980, −70%; 1984, −30%, 1991, −70%. Administration of Tc-99m in cardiovascular examinations: 1980, −30%; 1984, −70%; 1991, −30%.
Canada: Data are for Nova Scotia Province only (about 3.5% of the population). Data for 1985-1989 are weighted annual averages for Nova Scotia and Prince Edward Island, together comprising 4% of the population of Canada.
Egypt: Estimated from Kaar-El-Eini Centre Hospital, serving 25% of patients examined with radiation.
France: Values for 1990 are estimated from one hospital serving about 2% of the population.
India: Data also from [U1].
Iraq: Value given under "Other": Tc-99m.
Italy: Values given under "Other" are for oncology (Ga-67.)
Jamaica: Values given under "Other": placenta, Meckel's, Tc-99m.
Japan: Value given under "Other" is for Ga-67 examinations.
New Zealand: Value given under "Other" is for placental blood pool, In-113m.
Norway: Values given under "Other" are for full range of textbook procedures.
Romania: Values given under "Other" are for 1980 and 1990 for pancreas.
Sweden: Lung ventilation value for 1974: all Xe-133 gas; for 1985-1987: −70% Tc-99m aerosol, 20% Xe-133 gas, 10% In-133m. Renal value for 1984: −50% I-131 hipp, 40% I-125 hipp, 10% Cr-51 EDTA, <1% Tc-99m DTPA/DMSA; for 1985-1987: −45% Cr-51 EDTA, 30% I-131 hipp, 20% Tc-99m DTPA/DMSA, 5% I-125 hipp. Thyroid scan value for 1974: −75% I-131 NaI, 25% Tc-99m pertechnetate; for 1985-1987: −70% Tc-99m pertechnetate, 30% I-131 NaI.
Tunisia: Value given under "Other": gastrointestinal studies, colloids.
Thailand: Data are from the National Cancer Institute and the Rajavithi Hospital only.
Yugoslavia: Data are for Serbia only (about 40% of the population).

---

[a] Value is for ventilation and perfusion.
[b] Value is for both thyroid scan and thyroid uptake.
[c] Blood cells, Tc-99m, HMPAO.
[d] About 40% Au-198, 50% Tc-99m.
[e] Iodine-131 intake only.
[f] Iodine-131 uptake: 0.02.
[g] About 60% infection localization (Ga-67; 40% WBC (In-111 oxine).

Table 27
Average annual number of diagnostic nuclear medicine examinations per 1,000 population by health-care level
Data from UNSCEAR Survey of Medical Radiation Usage and Exposures

Examination	*Year*	*Average* [a]			*Mean ± SD* [b]			*Median* [b]		
		Level I	*Level II*	*Level III-IV*	*Level I*	*Level II*	*Levels III-IV*	*Level I*	*Level II*	*Levels III-IV*
Bone	1970-1980	0.84	0	0.001	1.4 ± 2.0	0	0.0005 ± 0.0006	0.60	0	0.0004
	1980-1985	2.6		0.041	2.4 ± 2.7		0.024 ± 0.045	2.1		0.002
	1985-1990	4.8	0.016	0.084	3.3 ± 2.6	0.11 ± 0.11	0.056 ± 0.099	2.8	0.10	0.011
Brain	1970-1980	1.3	0.23	0.022	1.9 ± 1.6	0.34 ± 0.59	0.017 ± 0.014	1.5	0	0.018
	1980-1985	1.1		0.013	1.1 ± 1.3		0.011 ± 0.011	1.0		0.011
	1985-1990	0.42	0.006	0.007	0.63 ± 0.92	0.12 ± 0.24	0.007 ± 0.008	0.36	0.010	0.003
Cardiovascular	1970-1980	0.53	0	0.0007	0.77 ± 2.1	0	0.0005 ± 0.0005	0.11	0	0.0004
	1980-1985	0.58		0.003	0.57 ± 0.74		0.002 ± 0.002	0.28		0.001
	1985-1990	2.6	0.008	0.014	1.3 ± 1.7	0.044 ± 0.11	0.008 ± 0.013	0.99	0.001	0
Liver/spleen	1970-1980	1.7	0.087	0.086	1.8 ± 1.4	0.12 ± 0.19	0.047 ± 0.069	1.2	0.013	0.021
	1980-1985	1.2		0.034	1.0 ± 0.75		0.029 ± 0.035	1.1		0.012
	1985-1990	1.4	0.023	0.016	0.89 ± 0.62	0.076 ± 0.06	0.014 ± 0.012	0.88	0.066	
Lung ventilation	1970-1980	0.13	0	0.0001	0.16 ± 0.32	0	0.00002±0.00003	0.06	0	0
	1980-1985	0.26		0.0001	0.19 ± 0.17		0.00003±0.00006	0.15		0
	1985-1990	1.2	0.001	0.008	0.49 ± 0.62	0.0001±0.0003	0.003 ± 0.007	0.25	0	0
Lung perfusion	1970-1980	0.34	0.024	0.0003	0.58 ± 0.65	0.036 ± 0.062	0.0001±0.0002	0.46	0	0.0001
	1980-1985	0.94		0.002	0.71 ± 0.81		0.001 ± 0.002	0.67		0.001
	1985-1990	2.2	0.002	0.008	0.78 ± 0.98	0.046 ± 0.071	0.005 ± 0.010	0.58	0.018	0
Kidney	1970-1980	1.8	0.041	0.006	1.9 ± 1.9	0.051 ± 0.079	0.0049 ± 0.0047	0.71	0.012	0.005
	1980-1985	1.3		0.009	1.6 ± 2.2		0.007 ± 0.012	0.48		0.001
	1985-1990	1.4	0.096	0.023	1.9 ± 2.1	0.053 ± 0.062	0.020 ± 0.036	0.88	0.27	0.006
Thyroid scan	1970-1980	1.3	0.40	0.066	2.1 ± 2.7	0.42 ± 0.55	0.067 ± 0.042	1.3	0.21	0.063
	1980-1985	2.5		0.048	2.3 ± 5.1		0.059 ± 0.049	0.90		0.056
	1985-1990	1.8	0.062	0.066	2.4 ± 4.0	0.39 ± 0.46	0.079 ± 0.087	1.4	0.25	0.063
Thyroid uptake	1970-1980	2.2	0.25	0.10	1.4 ± 1.5	0.083 ± 0.143	0.104 ± 0.092	0.77	0	0.080
	1980-1985	0.17		0.063	0.15 ± 0.16		0.078 ± 0.085	0.15		0.051
	1985-1990	0.55	0.17	0.052	0.38 ± 0.30	0.091 ± 0.13	0.051 ± 0.049	0.32	0.52	0.028
Total	1970-1980	10.9	0.86	0.25	15 ± 13	1.35 ± 1.23	0.24 ± 0.21	12.6	0.80	0.18
	1980-1985	6.9	0.10	0.19	12.7 ± 9.8	0.10 [c]	0.21 ± 0.13	10.3	0.10	0.21
	1985-1990	16.2	0.54	0.25	15 ± 10	1.1 ± 0.76	0.25 ± 0.15	12.0	1.0	0.26

[a] Overall average: total number of examinations divided by the total population of countries (thousands).
[b] Mean or median of individual values of countries.
[c] Data from India only.

Table 28
Age- and sex-distribution of patients undergoing diagnostic nuclear medicine examinations, 1985-1990
Data from UNSCEAR Survey of Medical Radiation Usage and Exposures

Health-care level	Country	Age distribution (%)			Sex distribution (%)	
		0-15 years	16-40 years	>40 years	Male	Female
	Bone					
I	Australia	6	25	69	47	53
	Canada	3.4	10	87	36	64
	Czechoslovakia	1.9	49	49	48	52
	Germany, Fed.Rep.	2	4	94	48	52
	Italy	0.8	8.2	91	34	66
	Kuwait	45	30	25	60	40
	Netherlands	3.9	24	72	53	47
	New Zealand	5.8	13	81	44	56
	Norway	2.6	11	86	52	48
	Romania	3.5	19	78	65	35
	Sweden	2.7	13	85	46	54
	Yugoslavia	3.4	30	67	41	59
	Average	3%	14%	83%	45%	55%
II	China	21	35	44	63	37
	Ecuador	5.1	25	70	63	37
	Iraq				30	70
	Peru	20	41	40	40	60
	Average	18%	35%	47%	51%	49%
III	Egypt	4.4	40	56	31	69
	Myanmar	0	40	60	60	40
	Sudan	0	2	98	49	51
	Thailand	0.3	33	67	17	83
	Average	1%	32%	67%	36%	64%
	Brain					
I	Australia [a]	20	22	58	52	48
	Canada	2.6	25	72	49	51
	Czechoslovakia	0	18	82	54	46
	Germany, Fed. Rep. of	0	25	75	25	75
	Italy	0	10	90	53	47
	Kuwait	4.7	76	20	90	10
	Netherlands	3.6	17	80	58	42
	New Zealand	4.5	30	66	53	47
	Norway	1.6	19	80	46	54
	Romania	8.6	48	43	57	43
	Sweden	0.1	26	74	50	50
	Yugoslavia	0	30	70	45	55
	Average	3%	23%	74%	46%	54%
II	China	17	24	59	60	40
	Ecuador	0	14	86	10	90
	Iraq				48	52
	Peru	48	26	26	40	60
	Average	24%	23%	53%	46%	54%
III	Myanmar	0	0	100	50	50
	Sudan	21	18	61	42	58
	Thailand	1.4	26	73	45	55
	Average	5%	16%	79%	46%	54%
IV	Ethiopia	12	64	24	58	42
	Cardiovascular					
I	Australia (thallium)	0.1	9	91	62	38
	Australia (technitium)	2	11	87	62	38
	Canada	6	9.5	85	62	38

Table 28 (continued)

Health-care level	*Country*	*Age distribution (%)*			*Sex distribution (%)*	
		0-15 years	*16-40 years*	*>40 years*	*Male*	*Female*
I (continued)	Czechoslovakia	3.8	52	45	64	36
	Germany, Fed. Rep. of	0	17	83	75	25
	Italy	0	11	89	76	24
	Kuwait	0.8	29	70	55	45
	Netherlands	0.6	9.1	90	66	34
	New Zealand	0.7	13	86	66	34
	Norway	0.1	23	77	58	42
	Romania	0	14	86	50	50
	Sweden (blood pool)	0	46	54	66	34
	Sweden (myocardical)	0	1.4	99	64	36
	Yugoslavia	2	25	73	75	25
	Average	1%	16%	83%	68%	32%
II	China				33	67
	Ecuador	0	10	90	75	25
	Average	0%	10%	90%	43%	57%
III	Egypt	0	0	100	70	30
	Myanmar	0	0	100	75	25
	Sudan	0	2	98	49	51
	Thailand	0.3	33	67	17	83
	Average	0%	11%	89%	51%	49%
Liver/spleen						
I	Australia	10	22	68	45	55
	Canada	5.7	16	79	44	54
	Czechoslovakia	4.7	55	40	58	42
	Italy	37	62	48	52	66
	Kuwait	1.6	25	73	45	55
	Netherlands	1.2	13	86	56	44
	New Zealand	1.2	14	85	50	50
	Norway	0.7	22	77	51	49
	Romania	2.9	34	63	50	50
	Romania	6.6	41	52	79	21
	Sweden	1.7	11	87	44	56
	Yugoslavia	8	30	62	66	34
	Average	5%	27%	67%	56%	44%
II	China	2.4	32	66	71	29
	Ecuador	5.8	32	62	50	50
	Iraq				34	66
	Peru	5.6	47	48	40	60
	Average	3%	34%	63%	62%	38%
III	Egypt	10	33	57	66	34
	Myanmar	0	50	50	50	50
	Sudan	4	45	51	50	49
	Thailand	0.3	27	73	50	50
	Average	4%	37%	60%	55%	45%
Lung ventilation						
I	Australia [b]	1	17	82	42	58
	Canada	1.7	10	88	66	34
	Czechoslovakia	0	63	37	53	47
	Germany, Fed. Rep. of	0	0	100	38	62
	Italy	0	5.6	94	54	46
	Kuwait	0	35	65	50	50
	Netherlands	0.6	14	85	61	39
	New Zealand	0.8	28	72	54	46
	Norway	1.4	15	83	40	60
	Romania [b]	0	37	63	67	33
	Sweden	0	21	79	49	51
	Average	0%	13%	86%	51%	49%
III	Egypt	0	58	42	48	52

Table 28 (continued)

Health-care level	*Country*	*Age distribution (%)*			*Sex distribution (%)*	
		0-15 years	*16-40 years*	*>40 years*	*Male*	*Female*
		Lung perfusion				
I	Canada	0.6	16	84	44	56
	Czechoslovakia	0.5	64	36	50	50
	Kuwait	0	35	65	50	50
	Netherlands	0.4	18	82	56	44
	New Zealand	0.6	24	75	54	46
	Norway	0.5	16	83	44	56
	Sweden	0.1	15	84	42	58
	Yugoslavia	0	33	67	65	35
	Average	0%	26%	73%	52%	48%
II	Ecuador	0	25	75	38	62
	Peru	8.3	33	58	50	50
	Average	5%	30%	64%	46%	54%
III	Myanmar	0	0	100	50	50
	Sudan	0	0	100	100	0
	Average	0%	0%	100%	69%	31%
		Kidney				
I	Australia	31	23	46	54	46
	Canada	25	31	44	30	70
	Czechoslovakia	21	39	40	50	50
	Germany, Fed. Rep. of	10	30	60	60	40
	Italy	14	21	65	54	46
	Kuwait	15	72	13	70	30
	Netherlands	14	38	48	45	55
	New Zealand	15	32	53	55	45
	Norway	3.8	26	70	49	51
	Romania	0.9	36	63	45	55
	Sweden	21	26	53	52	48
	Yugoslavia	5.7	32	62	29	71
	Average	14%	29%	57%	50%	50%
II	China	5.2	49	46	59	41
	Ecuador	0	89	11	10	90
	Iraq				58	42
	Peru	9.9	50	41	50	50
	Average	5%	52%	43%	54%	46%
III	Egypt	18	56	27	62	38
	Myanmar	0	100	0	75	25
	Sudan	15	36	49	52	48
	Thailand	1.7	22	76	14	86
	Average	8%	52%	40%	48%	52%
IV	Ethiopia	7.7	74	18	33	67
		Thyroid scan				
I	Canada	0.8	48	51	14	86
	Czechoslovakia	3.3	64	33	18	82
	Kuwait	5	75	20	20	80
	Netherlands	0.7	31	69	31	69
	New Zealand	1.7	29	69	16	84
	Norway	2.4	29	69	16	84
	Sweden	0.9	24	75	19	81
	Yugoslavia	0.5	30	70	28	72
	Average	1%	40%	59%	21%	79%
II	China	4.5	53	43	22	78
	Ecuador	9	22	69	14	86
	Peru	9.8	39	51	20	80
	Average	6%	49%	46%	21%	79%

Table 28 (continued)

Health-care level	*Country*	*Age distribution (%)*			*Sex distribution (%)*	
		0-15 years	*16-40 years*	*>40 years*	*Male*	*Female*
III	Egypt	9.5	62	33	24	76
	Myanmar	0	18	82	25	75
	Sudan	4	71	25	14	86
	Thailand	1.9	52	46	11	89
	Average	4%	50%	47%	19%	81%
IV	Ethiopia	0.7	80	20	40	60
			Thyroid uptake			
I	Australia	2	36	62	15	85
	Canada	0	42	58	14	86
	Czechoslovakia	0	56	44	24	76
	Germany, Fed. Rep. of	0	16	84	26	74
	Italy	1	37	62	16	84
	Kuwait	0	90	10	30	70
	Netherlands	0.4	37	63	40	60
	New Zealand	0	20	80	20	80
	Norway	1.5	22	77	17	83
	Romania	4.5	37	58	33	67
	Yugoslavia	0	45	55	18	82
	Average	1%	33%	66%	22%	78%
II	China	6.5	60	34	23	77
	Ecuador	9.1	22	69	14	86
	Iraq				24	76
	Peru	12	47	41	20	80
	Average	7%	55%	38%	22%	78%
III	Myanmar	0	35	65	30	70
	Sudan	4	71	25	14	86
	Thailand	1.8	52	46	12	88
	Average	2%	50%	48%	18%	82%
			Other			
I	Canada (Ga-67)	2.1	33	65	50	50
	Canada (In-111)	0	12	88	57	43
	Czechoslovakia, blood cells	6	59	35	52	48
	Italy (Ga-67)	0	26	74	50	50
	Netherlands	4.4	31	64	49	51
	Romania	0	63	37	100	0
	Yugoslavia	0	50	50	50	50
	Average	1%	35%	64%	58%	42%
II	China	2	27	71	64	36
			All organs			
I	Japan	3	7.7	89	54	46

The entries in this Table are as follows:

Canada: Data are for Nova Scotia Province only (about 3.5% of the population).
Peru: Data are from Instituto Peruano de Energia Nuclear only, where about 60% of all examinations are carried out.
Romania: Data are for 1990.
Sweden: Data are for Stockholm county only (about 20% of the population). Age distribution: 0-14 years, 15-39 years, >40 years.
Thailand: Data are from the National Cancer Institute and Rajavithi Hospital only.
Yugoslavia: Data are for Serbia only (about 40% of the population).

[a] Values are meaningful for early part of the period only, since CT and magnetic resonance imaging (MRI) have replaced Tc-99m.
[b] Includes lung perfusion.

Table 29
Average activity administered in diagnostic nuclear medicine examinations
Data from UNSCEAR Survey of Medical Radiation Usage and Exposures unless otherwise indicated

PART I: BONE, BRAIN, CARDIOVASCULAR

Country	Year	*Average activity administered (MBq) (Range in parentheses)*							
		Bone		*Brain*			*Cardiovascular*		
		^{99m}Tc *phosphate*	*Other/unknown*	^{99m}Tc *pertechnetate*	^{99m}Tc *gluconate*	*Other/unknown*	^{99m}Tc *erythrocytes*	^{201}Tl *chloride*	*Other/unknown*
Health-care level I									
Argentina	1985-1989		555			740			740
Australia	1970 1980 1984 1991	730 783 827		456 754 801 -	492 773 -		643 874 878	64 76 82	
Canada	1970-1974 1985-1989	740 (74-925)	3.7 [a]		740	18.5 [b]	740 (555-925)		
Czechoslovakia	1970-1974 1976-1985 1986-1990	450 (400-600) 500 500 (400-600)	180	45 (25-240) 180 240 (25-320)		700 [c]	450 (400-500) 500 500 (400-550)	70 70	700 [d]
Denmark	1989-1990	628		695	615	380 [e], 665 [c]	765	98	880 [d], 370 [f]
Finland [A12]	1975 1982	350 (185-555) 520 (370-800)		460 (370-555) 520 (370-740)			590 (370-740) 600 (370-740)		
Germany, Fed.Rep.	1986-1990	621		614	537	525 [e], 130 [g]	730	74.9	
Italy	1985-1989	614 (370-740)				583 [h] (492-740)	709 (55-925)		
Japan	1985-1989	720				135 [g]		100	
Kuwait	1985-1989	805 (716-894)		740 (626-854)			647 (555-739)		
Netherlands	1985-1989	500		350 (400-750)			750 (400-750)	100 (75-120)	
New Zealand	1970-1974 1985-1989	360 (100-677) 720 (74-1110)		468 (155-900) 730 (74-925)				85 (63-167)	390 (344-574) [i] 731(111-1295)[i]
Norway	1970-1974 1985-1989	507 (± 121 SD) 574 (± 91 SD)		523 (± 130 SD) 615 (± 139 SD)			764 (± 145 SD)	96 (± 56 SD)	

Table 29 (continued)

Country	*Year*	*Average activity administered (MBq) (Range in parentheses)*							
		Bone		*Brain*			*Cardiovascular*		
		^{99m}Tc phosphate	*Other/unknown*	*^{99m}Tc pertechnetate*	*^{99m}Tc gluconate*	*Other/unknown*	*^{99m}Tc erythrocytes*	*^{201}Tl chloride*	*Other/unknown*
Poland [U1]	1981				592				
Romania	1980-1989 1990	370 455	185 [i] 5.3 [j]	370 555		740 [k]			0.4 [l] / 1.9 [m] 460 [k] / 585 [i]
Sweden	1974 1985-1989	330 420 (160-600)		400 530 (350-700)			370 650 (50-900)	55 72 (50-120)	
Switzerland	1976	555				111	555		
United Kingdom	1981-1985	518 (333-740)		491 (333-740)	572 (370-750)	536 [c] (370-740)	658 (296-800)	68 (40-100)	464 [k] / 566 [i] (185-800)
Yugoslavia	1985-1989	555 (350-740)				555 [c] (370-740)	555 (100-740)		
Health-care level II									
China Beijing area Entire nation	 1985-1989 1986-1989	 740 (55-925)	 4.8 [a]	 370 (296-555)		 138 [h]			 370 (222-518) 1.5 [n]
Ecuador	1970-1974 1985-1989	 740 (-925)				7.4 (-9.3) 555 [e] (-740)	 555 (-740)		
India	1985-1989	670 (370-925)		516 (370-925)			659 (407-1110)	74 (56-111)	
Iraq	1985-1989	(650-750)				(650-750) [h]			
Jamaica	1970-1974 1985-1989	 182 (-740)				370 [e] (-740) 182 [e] (-740)	 370 (-740)		
Peru	1985-1989	740 (555-925)				740 [e] (555-925)			
Tunisia	1970-1974 1985-1989	555 370				296 [e] 185 [e]	 259		
Health-care level III									
Egypt	1986-1990	540		270		500 [c]	500	81	270 [d]
Myanmar	1976-1985 1986-1990	370 370		370 370					185 [w] 185 [w]

Table 29 (continued)

Country	Year	Average activity administered (MBq) (Range in parentheses)							
		Bone		Brain			Cardiovascular		
		^{99m}Tc phosphate	Other/unknown	^{99m}Tc pertechnetate	^{99m}Tc gluconate	Other/unknown	^{99m}Tc erythrocytes	^{201}Tl chloride	Other/unknown
Sudan	1986-1990	555			444				
Thailand	1976-1980 1981-1985 1986-1990	275 269 197				312 [e] 350 [e] 359 [e]	740 584 475		
Health-care level IV									
Ethiopia	1970-1989			500 [e] (370-555)		500 (370-555)			

PART II: LIVER/SPLEEN, LUNG, KIDNEY

Country	Year	Average activity administered (MBq) (Range in parentheses)							
		Liver / spleen			Lung			Kidney	
		^{99m}Tc colloid	^{99m}Tc HIDA	Other/unknown	^{99m}Tc MAA	^{99m}Tc microspheres	Other/unknown	^{131}I hippurate	^{123}I hippurate
Health-care level I									
Argentina	1985-1989		111				74		
Australia	1970 1980 1984 1991	61 115 121 128			120 110 174	60 97 102 -	111 [o] 434 [o] 371/222 [p] 252 [o]		
Canada	1970-1974 1985-1989	111 (37-148)		111 [q]	111 (37-148)	185 (148-222)	18.5		
Czechoslovakia	1970-1974 1976-1985 1986-1990	60 (40-120) 240 240 (80-300)	160 160		160 (100-400) 240 280 (200-400)	160 (100-400) 240 (200-400)	80 [p] 80 [p]		
Denmark	1989-1990	65-129	183			102	260 [o] / 10.5 [p]	1-29	108
Finland [A12]	1975 1982	74 (19-300) 120 (40-220)		130 (74-220) 120 (74-200)				0.9 (0.4-3.7) 1.0 (0.4-1.6)	
Germany, Fed. Rep.	1986-1990	135-143	168	141-160 [r]/3.7 [s]	129	148		1.4 [t]/11 [u]	40.4

Table 29 (continued)

Country	Year	Average activity administered (MBq) (Range in parentheses)							
		Liver / spleen			Lung			Kidney	
		^{99m}Tc colloid	^{99m}Tc HIDA	Other/unknown	^{99m}Tc MAA	^{99m}Tc microspheres	Other/unknown	^{131}I hippurate	^{123}I hippurate
Italy	1985-1989			140 [h] (55-448)			116/191 [h] (55-925)		
Japan	1985-1989	196			230				
Kuwait	1985-1989	92 (55-129)	92 (55-129)		155 (118-192)	1042 (908-1176)			
Netherlands	1985-1989	75 (75-110)	100		75 (75-150)			2	20 (2-20)
New Zealand	1970-1974 1985-1989	101 (26-259) 162 (37-370)			146 (33-370) 151 (30-750)				
Norway	1970-1974 1985-1989	118 (± 47 SD) 125 (± 40 SD)			95 (± 39 SD) 98 (± 29 SD)			4.2 (± 3 SD) 4.9 (± 1.1 SD)	
Poland [U1]	1981	148						1.2	
Romania	1980 1990	55.5		9.3 [v]/11.1 [n]/111 [q] 84 [h]/8.8 [v]	74 148		9.3 [v]/74 [w] 11.1 [v]	9.3 3.5	
Sweden	1974 1985-1989	70 125 (70-400)			66 87 (35-120)	440 (30-1900)	5.1 [o] 420 [o] (10-800)	0.9 0.9 (0.1-4.5)	
Switzerland	1976			74	37		185 [o]		
United Kingdom	1981-1985	91/57 (37-200)	144 (40-370)	56 [h] (8-150)	88 (37-222)	88 (37-222)	243 [o] / 1724 [w] (74-3700)	2.5 (0.4-3.7)	28 (10-185)
Yugoslavia	1970-1974 1985-1989			10 (8-12) 74 (60-150)			3.7 (3-5) 74 (60-150)	6 (5-8) 6 (5-8)	
Health-care level II									
China Beijing area Entire nation	1970-1974 1985-1989 1986-1990	222 (185-370)		74 (37-100) 97 [h] / 22 [v]				0.37 (0.26-0.56) 0.37	
Ecuador	1970-1974 1985-1989	296 (-444)		9.3 (-13)	296 (-444)			1.1 (-1.9)	
India	1985-1989	140 (74-189)				128 (74-277)		1.5 (0.3-2.6)	
Iraq	1985-1989	(80-120)							

Table 29 (continued)

Country	Year	Average activity administered (MBq) (Range in parentheses)							
		Liver / spleen			Lung			Kidney	
		^{99m}Tc colloid	^{99m}Tc HIDA	Other/unknown	^{99m}Tc MAA	^{99m}Tc microspheres	Other/unknown	^{131}I hippurate	^{123}I hippurate
Jamaica	1970-1989	37 (-111)			12 (-111)				
Peru	1985-1989	185 (111-259)			110 (74-148)				
Tunisia	1970-1974 1985-1989	 74		19 [v]		111 74			
Health-care level III									
Egypt	1986-1990	135	135		135		270 [e]	9	
Myanmar	1976-1990	74			74				
Sudan	1986-1990	148	148		148				
Thailand	1986-1980 1981-1985 1986-1990	101 104 137			260 269 118		1152 [h]		
Health-care level IV									
Ethiopia	1970-1974 1986-1990	37 (37-74) 111		74 (37-74)					

PART III: KIDNEY, THYROID

Country	Year	Average activity administered (MBq) (Range in parentheses)							
		Kidney			Thyroid				
		^{99m}Tc gluconate	^{99m}Tc other	Other/unknown	^{99m}Tc pertechnetate	^{131}I uptake	^{131}I scan	^{123}I uptake	^{123}I scan
Health-care level I									
Argentina	1985-1989		555 [e]						
Australia	1970 1980 1984 1991	109 279 513 234	 490 [e] 427 [e] 415 [e]		61 145 156 178	1.4 0.5 0.7 1.0			

Table 29 (continued)

Country	Year	Average activity administered (MBq) (Range in parentheses)							
		Kidney			Thyroid				
		^{99m}Tc gluconate	^{99m}Tc other	Other/unknown	^{99m}Tc pertechnetate	^{131}I uptake	^{131}I scan	^{123}I uptake	^{123}I scan
Canada	1970-1974 1985-1989		 296 [e] (74-370)	11.1 [x]	 260 (185-370)	0.6 0.6 (0.4-0.6)	0.9		
Czechoslovakia	1970-1974 1976-1985 1986-1990		80 [e] [y](60-120) 180 [e] / 150 [y] 180 [e] / 150 [y]		60 (40-160) 240 240 (60-300)	1.5 (1-2) 1 1 (1-2)			
Denmark	1989-1990		150 [e] / 98 [z]		140		6.9		72
Finland [A12]	1975 1982				90 (37-185) 140 (48-370)	1.0 (0.4-2.0) 1.3 (0.4-1.9)	2.2 (0.7-3.7) 2.1 (1.1-3.7)		
Germany, Fed.Rep.	1986-1990		282 [e] / 160 [y]	315 [aa]/502 [i]/ 10.2 [bb]	42.1		9.46	4.44	
Italy	1985-1989			1.4 [n]	78	1			
Japan	1985-1989		320 [e z]		360 (males) 450 (females)		6		
Kuwait	1985-1989		259 (148-370)		185 (148-222)	0.3 (-0.7)			
Netherlands	1985-1989				50	0.2 (0.2-7)		2 (2-20)	30
New Zealand	1970-1974 1985-1989	210 (81-592)	116 [y] (74-1110) 340 [e] (20-623)		140 (22-460) 144 (9-370)	0.7 (0.11-3.9) 9.5 (0.7-33)			
Norway	1970-1974 1985-1989		150 113 (± 91 SD)		71 (± 39 SD) 69 (± 40 SD)	1.1 (± 0.5 SD) 1.2 (± 0.7 SD)	1.2 (± 0.3 SD) 1.5 (± 0.4 SD)		
Poland [U1]	1981	136	192 [y]		37	2.7			
Romania	1980 1985-1989 1990		148 [e] / 222 [i] 222 295 [e]	74 [w]	37 37 43.5	1.1	3.0 3.0 2.2		
Sweden	1974 1985-1989		140 115 (1-270)		70 90 (10-200)	0.4 0.9 (0.1-14)	1.8 2.5 (0.3-30)		
Switzerland	1976			185	13			37	
United Kingdom	1981-1985		246[e]/102[y] (37-555)		11-76 (0.6-200)		1.8/108[z] (0.18-500)	45 (0.2-10)	13 (2-100)
Yugoslavia	1970-1974 1985-1989				 74 (60-120)	0.4 (0.3-0.4) 0.4 (0.3-0.5)	3.7 (3-5)		

Table 29 (continued)

Country	Year	Average activity administered (MBq) (Range in parentheses)							
		Kidney			Thyroid				
		^{99m}Tc gluconate	^{99m}Tc other	Other/unknown	^{99m}Tc pertechnetate	^{131}I uptake	^{131}I scan	^{123}I uptake	^{123}I scan
Health-care level II									
China									
Beijing area	1970-1974					0.11 (0.07-0.15)	3.7 (1.5-9.3)		
	1985-1989		260 [y] (222-296)			0.11 (0.07-0.15)	11.1 (7.4-18.5)		
Entire nation	1986-1990				23	0.10	5.9		
Ecuador	1970-1974					3.0 (-5.6)	3.0 (-5.6)		
	1985-1989		296 [e] (-444)			3.0 (4.4)	3.0 (4.4)		
India	1985-1989		194 (74-555)		94 (15-148)	0.74 (0.2-1.9)	1.7 (0.9-3.7)		
Iraq	1985-1989		(200-400) [e, z]						
Jamaica	1970-1974					10 (-25)	10 (-26)		
	1985-1989		74 (-182)		74 (-148)				
Peru	1985-1989		740 (555-925)		185 (111-259)	0.4 (0.2-0.4)			
Tunisia	1970-1974		185 [e]		111	3.7			
	1985-1989		111 [e]		111	1.1			
Health-care level III									
Egypt	1986-1990		81 [e], 135 [y]		81	0.28	2.7		
Myanmar	1976-1980		74 [y]			0.37	1		
	1981-1985		74 [y]			0.37	1		
	1986-1990		74 [y]			0.37	1		
Sudan	1976-1980					1.1	1.1		
	1981-1985					1.1	1.1		
	1986-1990		148 [e], 74 [y]		37	1.3	1.3		
Thailand	1976-1980		12 [e]			0.5	0.45		
	1981-1985		20 [e]			0.35	0.47		
	1986-1990		21 [e]			0.12	0.23		
Health-care level IV									
Ethiopia	1970-1989		74 [y] (37-74)			1.7 (1.7-2.2)	1.7		

Table 29 (continued)

The entries in this Table are qualified as follows:

Australia:	Owing to the substitution of CT and MRI for Tc-99m, the number for brain examinations with Tc-99m pertechnetate and Tc-99mTc-gluconate for 1991 is too small to state average. Information pertaining to Part III of Table: ^{67}Ga citrate tumour/infection, 1980: 166 MBq; 1984: 210 MBq; 1991: 212 MBq.
Czechoslovakia:	Information pertaining to Part III of Table: Tc-99m HMPAO blood cells, 1976-1990: 160 MBq.
Canada:	Data are for Nova Scotia Province only (about 3.5% of the population).
New Zealand:	Almost all ^{131}I uptakes are done on patients receiving large therapeutic ^{131}I doses. In effective dose estimations uptake should be assumed = 0. About one third of ^{99m}Tc thyroid scans are also used to assess uptake.
Yugoslavia:	Data are for Serbia and Macedonia only (about 50% of the population). Data for 1970-1974 are for Serbia only.

---

[a] Radioisotope used is Sr-85.
[b] Radioisotope compound used is I-131 RHSA.
[c] Radioisotope compound used is Tc-99m HMPAO.
[d] Radioisotope compound used is Tc-99m MIBI.
[e] Radioisotope compound used is Tc-99m DTPA.
[f] Radioisotope compound uses is Tc-99m PP.
[g] Radioisotope compound used is I-123 amphetamine.
[h] Radioisotope used is Tc-99m.
[i] Radioisotope used is Tc-99m pertechnetate.
[j] Radioisotope used is Se-75 methionine.
[k] Radioisotope compounds used are Tc-99m phosphate/phosphonate.
[l] Radioisotope compound used is Fe-59 citrate.
[m] Radioisotope compound used is Cr-51 citrate.
[n] Radioisotope used is I-131.
[o] Radioisotope used is Xe-133.
[p] Radioisotope form used is Tc-99m aerosol.
[q] Radioisotope compound used is In-111m colloid.
[r] Radioisotope compounds of Tc-99m are millimicrospheres, denatured erythrocytes and phytate.
[s] Radioisotope form used are Cr-51 denatured erythrocytes.
[t] ING.
[u] Sequence.
[v] Radioisotope used is Au-198.
[w] Radioisotope used is In-113.
[x] Radioisotope used is Hg-197.
[y] Radioisotope compound used is Tc-99m DMSA.
[z] Radioisotope compound used is Tc-99m MAG3.
[aa] Radioisotope compound used is Tc-99m gluconate.
[bb] Radioisotope compound used is Cr-51 EDTA.

Table 30
Effective dose equivalents to patients from diagnostic nuclear medicine examinations (mSv)

Examination	*Health-care level I*			*Health-care level II*
	Czechoslovakia, 1987 [H30]	*Denmark, 1990 [E3]*	*Italy, 1989 [D11]*	*China, 1985 [Z6]*
Bone	4.5	1.1-6.8	0.5	
Brain	3.5-6	0.6-11.3	3.7	1.8
Cardiovascular	4.3-17.2	3.0-22.5	13	
Liver/spleen	1.4-3.5	0.9-2.6	1.9	22, 1.2 [a]
Lung ventilation		0.07-0.25		
Lung perfusion	1.2	1.1	1.4	
Kidney	0.04-2.1	0.01-1.3	1.7	<0.1
Thyroid scan	1-36.3	2.1-13.7	2.1	94, 0.3 [b]
Thyroid uptake	3.1	3		1.5
Average	2-4	3	4.5	15-30

[a] When Tc-99m is available. Standard procedure: Au-198.
[b] When Tc-99m is available. Standard procedure: I-131.

Table 31
Age-dependent analysis of effective dose equivalents to patients from diagnostic nuclear medicine examinations

Organ	*Radiopharmaceutical*	*Dose factor (mSv/MBq)*	*Average activity [a] (MBq)*	*Effective dose equivalent per examination (mSv)*	*Examinations per 1,000 population [a]*	*Effective dose equivalent per caput (μSv)*
Age group: 0-9 years						
Bone	Tc-99m phosphate	0.025	380	9.5	0.17	1.6
Brain	Tc-99m gluconate	0.024	460	11.1	0.05	0.6
Cardiovascular	Tl-201 chloride	2.0	37	73	0.004	0.3
	Tc-99m erythrocytes	0.025	555	13.9	0.006	0.08
Age group: 10-19 years						
Bone	Tc-99m phosphate	0.010	570	5.7	0.20	1.1
Brain	Tc-99m gluconate	0.011	690	7.6	0.19	1.5
Cardiovascular	Tl-201 chloride	0.36	55	19.7	0.004	0.08
	Tc-99m erythrocytes	0.011	830	9.1	0.006	0.05
Age group: adults						
Bone	Tc-99m phosphate	0.008	790	6.3	6.39	40.3
Brain	Tc-99m gluconate	0.009	962	8.7	4.47	38.7
Cardiovascular	Tl-201 chloride	0.23	76	17.5	0.79	13.8
	Tc-99m erythrocytes	0.0085	1156	9.8	1.19	11.7
Liver/spleen	Tc-99m colloid	0.014	117	1.6	4.81	7.9
	Tc-99m HIDA	0.024	226	5.4	0.16	0.9
Lung	Tc-99m MMA	0.012	114	1.4	1.83	2.5
Kidney	Tc-99m gluconate	0.009	523	4.7	0.75	3.5
Thyroid	Tc-99m pertechnetate	0.015	250	3.8	1.12	4.5
	I-131 ionic	6.6 [b]	0.38	2.5	1.36	3.4
Total					23.6	127.2

[a] Activity administered and examination frequency for Manitoba, Canada [H17]. For children, it was assumed here that activities administered were reduced according to Beentjes [B20].

[b] Assumed thyroid uptake: 15%.

Table 32
Collective doses from nuclear medicine examinations, 1985-1990

Examination	*Number of examinations per 1,000 population*				*Effective dose per examination (mSv)*				*Annual collective effective dose (man Sv)*			
	Level I	*Level II*	*Levels III-IV*	*World*	*Level I*	*Level II*	*Levels III-IV*	*World*	*Level I*	*Level II*	*Levels III-IV*	*World*
Bone	4.8	0.016	0.084	1.3	6.3	6.3	6.3	6.3	40700	270	690	41700
Brain	0.42	0.006	0.007	0.11	8.7	8.7	8.7	8.7	4930	140	80	5150
Cardiovascular	2.6	0.008	0.014	0.68	14	14	14	14	49900	300	260	50400
Liver/spleen	1.4	0.023	0.016	0.38	3.5	22	22	4.3	6660	1330	460	8450
Lung ventilation	1.2	0.001	0.008	0.30	0.3	0.3	0.3	0.3	470	1	3	480
Lung perfusion	2.2	0.002	0.008	0.56	1.4	1.4	1.4	1.4	4160	7	15	4180
Kidney	1.4	0.096	0.023	0.41	4.7	4.7	4.7	4.7	8880	1190	140	10200
Thyroid scan	1.8	0.062	0.066	0.51	3.8	94	94	12	9290	15300	8130	32700
Thyroid uptake	0.55	0.167	0.052	0.24	2.5	2.5	2.5	2.5	1860	1100	170	3130
Total	16.4	0.38	0.28	4.4					127000	19600	9900	156000
Average dose per examination (mSv)					5.7	20	27	6.7				
Average dose per caput (mSv)					0.094	0.0075	0.0076	0.030				

Table 33
Contribution of various types of nuclear medicine examinations to the collective dose, 1985-1990
Data from UNSCEAR Survey of Medical Radiation Usage and Exposures

Examination	*Contribution to total collective dose (%)*			
	Level I	*Level II*	*Levels III-IV*	*World*
Cardiovascular	39	1	3	32
Bone	32	1	7	27
Thyroid scan	7	78	82	21
Kidney	7	6	1	7
Liver/spleen	5	7	5	5
Brain	4	1	1	3
Lung perfusion	3	0.4	0.2	3
Thyroid uptake	1	6	2	2
Lung ventilation	0.4	0.004	0.03	0.3

Table 34
Annual individual and collective effective dose from nuclear medicine examinations
Data from UNSCEAR Survey of Medical Radiation Usage and Exposures unless otherwise indicated

Country	Year	Effective dose equivalent H_E (mSv)		Collective effective dose (man Sv)	Reference
		Per individual patient	Per caput		
Health-care level I					
Australia	1980	2.5	0.02	290	[U1]
Bulgaria	1980	8.4	0.11	970	[U1]
Canada	1980	3.8	0.17	4200	[L7]
Manitoba	1985	5.2	0.13	127	[H17]
Quebec	1989	6.4	0.42	2800	[R10]
Czechoslovakia	1983	2.2	0.04	430	[H30]
	1987	2.4	0.06	610	
Denmark	1985	3	0.05	250	[E3]
	1990	3	0.05	250	
Finland	1982			430 [e]	[A12]
German Democratic Republic	1978	3.4	0.03	480	[E5]
	1981	2.2	0.02	340	
Germany, Fed. Rep. of (Bavaria and West Berlin)	1985-1986	2.7-3.2 [a]	0.11-0.12 [a]	7000	[K10]
Greece (northern part)	1984-1988	2.5 [b]			[P20]
Italy	1982	2.9	0.03	1510	[D11]
	1983	3.3	0.03	1890	
	1989	4.5	0.04	2450	
Japan	1982	4.1	0.035	4240 [f]	[M11, M12]
Netherlands	1984	2.9	0.034	480 [g]	[B20]
		2.7 [c]	0.031	450 [e]	[B20]
Poland	1981	25.7 [d]	0.06	2000	[S41, U1]
Sweden	1986	3.5	0.05	420	[V4]
USSR	1981	8.2	0.032	8600	[N4]
United Kingdom	1982	2.5	0.02	1000	[H10]
United States	1982	5.0	0.14	32100	[M41, N1]
Health-care level II					
China	1981-1985	8 [h]	0.005	4980	[U1, Z6]
		15-34 [i]	0.02	21000	
India	1985-1989	7.9 [j]	0.002	1340	

[a] Value for Bavaria and West Berlin extrapolated to the entire country (except new Bundesländer).
[b] Corresponds to 2.0 mSv/examination (some patients had more than one examination).
[c] Estimate accounting for age distribution of population.
[d] High value caused by ubiquitous use of I-131, 47% of all examinations with an average collective dose per patient of 51.5 mSv.
[e] Of this value 51% is due to Tc-99m, 47% to I-131 and 2.1% to all other nuclides.
[f] Collective dose component to women is 1,910 man Sv.
[g] The collective dose due to the somatic part of the effective dose equivalent is reported to be 575 man Sv [B20].
[h] Probably underestimate due to low precision in computation.
[i] Using two different methods to estimate collective dose per examination from [Z6]. High value depends on I-131 thyroid scintigraphy with collective dose per examination being 94 mSv.
[j] Mainly due to use of I-131.

Table 35
Estimated doses to the world population from nuclear medicine examinations

Health-care level	Population (millions)	Annual per caput effective dose equivalent (mSv)	Annual collective effective dose equivalent (10^3 man Sv)
I	1350	0.09	130
II	2630	0.008	20
III	850	0.008	6
IV	460	0.008	4
Total	5290	-	160
Average	-	0.03	-

Table 36
Total annual number of radiotherapy treatments per 1,000 population
Data from UNSCEAR Survey of Medical Radiation Usage and Exposures unless otherwise indicated

Country	*Teletherapy*			*Brachytherapy*		
	1970-1979	*1980-1984*	*1985-1990*	*1970-1979*	*1980-1984*	*1985-1990*
Health-care level I						
Argentina						0.2
Australia	2.0		1.5	0.8		0.2
Canada		1.6	2.9			
Cuba			0.2			0.05
Czechoslovakia	2.9	4.2	2.7	0.2	0.1	0.1
Denmark			1.2			0.1
Finland			1.2			
Iceland [L16]			1.2			
Japan	0.7		0.7	0.2	0.2	
Kuwait			0.2			0.06
Luxembourg						0.07
Malta						0.03
Netherlands			1.8			0.1
New Zealand	0.4	0.4	0.6	0.1	0.08	0.07
Norway	0.5 [a]		3.9	0.2		0.1
Romania		1.7	6.8		0.06	
Sweden	0.6		0.8	0.3	0.2	0.1
Switzerland			1.8			0.1
United Kingdom		2.4 [b]				
United States		2.4 [b]				
Yugoslavia			0.6			0.9
Average	1.0	2.4 [b]	1.2	0.26	0.17	0.24
Health-care level II						
Barbados			0.6			0.2
China			0.2			0.08
Ecuador	0.03		0.08	0.006		0.02
India			0.1			0.03
Iraq			0.1			0.009
Jamaica			0.1			0.07
Peru	0.09		0.1	0.03		0.04
Turkey	0.7	0.9	0.7			
Average	0.1		0.2	0.02		0.06
Health-care level III						
Egypt			0.04			0.0005
India	0.07			0.02		
Myanmar		0.2	0.2	0.01	0.01	0.02
Sudan			0.08			0.0003
Thailand			0.09		0.04	0.04
Average			0.1	0.02	0.03	0.02

[a] Malignant disease only.
[b] Value includes brachytherapy.

Table 37
Average annual number of teletherapy and brachytherapy treatments per 1,000 population
Data from UNSCEAR Survey of Medical Radiation Usage and Exposures, unless otherwise indicated

PART I: TELETHERAPY

Country	*Year*	*Leukaemia*	*Lymphoma*	*Breast tumour*	*Respiratory system*	*Female genital organs*	*Wilms' tumour*	*Neuro-blastoma*	*Benign diseases*
Health-care level I									
Australia	1970-1974	0.010	0.12	0.27	0.16	0.042	0.003	0.041	1.3
	1985-1989	0.021	0.017	0.19	0.29	0.11	0.0006	0.001	0.9
Czechoslovakia	1970-1974	0.004	0.058	0.19	0.19	0.19			1.2
	1976-1980	0.006	0.028	0.15	0.15	0.071	0.001		3.4
	1981-1985	0.006	0.024	0.16	0.17	0.076	0.001		3.8
	1986-1990	0.004	0.017	0.16	0.16	0.075	0.0004	0.0001	2.3
Denmark	1985-1989	0.009	0.058	0.18	0.11	0.14	0.11		
Finland	1987	0.016	0.032	0.29	0.20	0.081	0.004	0.002	
Japan	1970-1974		0.75 [a]	3.33 [a]	2.34 [a]				0.35 [a]
	1975-1979		0.025	0.075	0.093	0.12			0.013
	1985-1990		0.046	0.059	0.17	0.081			0.002
Kuwait	1985-1989	0.016	0.021	0.059	0.029	0.022	0.002	0.002	0.012
Netherlands	1987	0.028	0.076	0.49	0.44	0.11			
	1988-1989	0.045	0.15	0.98	0.85	0.22			
New Zealand	1970-1974	0.003	0.033	0.14	0.13	0.086			
	1975-1979		0.027	0.086	0.014	0.09			
	1980-1984	0.009	0.027	0.077	0.16	0.082			
	1985-1989	0.016	0.053	0.21	0.20	0.078	0.001	0.002	0.007
Norway	1970-1974	0.001	0.044	0.18	0.047	0.27		0.0003	
	1985-1989	0.002	0.074	0.18	0.16	0.17	0.0001	0.001	3.3
Romania	1980	0.043 [b]		0.12	0.12	0.13			1.2
	1990	0.025	0.028	0.53	0.49	1.1			3.8
Sweden	1970-1974	0.029	0.075	0.36	0.054	0.089	0.002	0.007	0.009
	1985-1989	0.024	0.093	0.41	0.077	0.14	0.002	0.001	0.023
Yugoslavia	1985-1989	0.017	0.031	0.12	0.13	0.26	0.010	0.061	0.007
Average	1970-1979	0.010	0.038	0.12	0.11	0.11	0.001		0.40
	1980-1984	0.029	0.025	0.13	0.14	0.11	0.001		2.0
	1985-1990	0.018	0.045	0.16	0.20	0.16	0.008	0.020	0.48
Health-care level II									
Barbados	1985-1989			0.24	0.064	0.24	0.016		
China									
Beijing area	1970-1974	0	0.016	0.019	0.023	0.009	0	0.003	0.001
	1985-1986	<0.0001	0.014	0.021	0.034	0.010	0.0001	0.009	0.004
Entire nation	1986-1990			0.036	0.037	0.045			
Ecuador	1970-1974	0.0005	0.002	0.008	0.002	0.015	0	0	0.002
	1985-1989	0.002	0.007	0.021	0.005	0.042	0.0001	0.001	0.005
India	1985-1989	0.0032	0.0047	0.011	0.0087	0.036	0.0007	0.0004	0.0036
Iraq	1985-1989	0.009	0.005	0.041	0.037	0.015	0.001	0.0009	0
Jamaica	1985-1989		0.004	0.055	0.005	0.002	0.0008		0.064
Peru	1970-1974	0.014		0.013	0.005	0.053	0.0006	0.0003	
	1985-1989	0.012		0.016	0.009	0.068	0.001	0.0004	0.013
Turkey	1976-1979	0.19	0.16	0.10	0.13	0.04	0.04	0.03	
	1980-1984	0.22	0.28	0.10	0.12	0.06	0.07	0.02	
	1985-1990	0.17	0.18	0.10	0.046	0.040	0.042	0.006	
Average	1970-1980	0.016	0.015	0.016	0.011	0.042	0.003	0.002	
	1985-1990	0.004	0.005	0.026	0.025	0.041	0.001		0.004

Table 37 (continued)

Country	*Year*	*Leukaemia*	*Lymphoma*	*Breast tumour*	*Respiratory system*	*Female genital organs*	*Wilms' tumour*	*Neuro-blastoma*	*Benign diseases*
Health-care level III									
Egypt	1985-1990	0.002	0.006	0.026	0.003	0.0005	0.001	0.0005	0.004
India	1970-1974	0.0007	0.0017	0.0047	0.0022	0.020	0.0003	0.0001	0.0035
Myanmar	1980-1984	0.002	0.004	0.012	0.023	0.019	0.0002	0.0001	
	1985-1990	0.001	0.004	0.013	0.024	0.018	0.0001	0.0002	
Sudan	1985-1990	0.005	0.008	0.009	0.003	0.008	0.002	0.002	
Thailand	1986-1990	0.010	0.010	0.019	0.008	0.037	0.001		0.0002
Average	1970-1980	0.0007	0.002	0.005	0.002		0.0003	0.0001	0.004
	1980-1984	0.002	0.004	0.012	0.023	0.019	0.0002	0.0001	
	1985-1990	0.005	0.007	0.018	0.009	0.017	0.0008	0.0006	0.004

PART II: BRACHYTHERAPY

Country	*Year*	*Breast tumour*	*Prostate tumour*	*Female genital organs*		*Brain tumour*	*Other tumours*	*Benign diseases*
				Radium	*Afterloading*			
Health-care level I								
Australia	1970-1974		0.001	0.068 [c]			0.18	0.51
	1985-1989	0.016		0.019 [c]	0.034		0.076	
Czechoslovakia	1970-1974			0.064	0.16			
	1976-1980			0.16	0.031		0.003	0.006
	1981-1985			0.091	0.046			0.002
	1986-1990			0.034	0.10		0.002	0.0003
Denmark	1985-1989	0.020	0.0009	0.073	0.012		0.003	
Japan	1970-1974	0.001		0.082			0.024	
	1975-1979			0.19			0.0007	
	1980-1984			0.025	0.035			
Kuwait	1985-1989				0.006			0.054
Malta	1985-1989				0.028			
Netherlands	1988-1989	0.017	0.001	0.049				
New Zealand	1985-1989				0.066			
Norway	1970-1974	0.001		0.13			0.010	
	1985-1989		0.0005	0.043	0.049	0.0002	0.005	
Romania	1980				0.054		0.005	
Sweden	1970-1974		0.0004	0.037	0.006			0.001
	1985-1989		0.002	0.029 [d]	0.14			0.004
Yugoslavia	1985-1989	0.029	0.015	0.15	0.63	0.022	0.004	
Average	1970-1979	0.0001	0.0005	0.16	0.068		0.016	0.16
	1980-1984			0.034	0.035		0.004	0.002
	1985-1990	0.019	0.005	0.062	0.22	0.010	0.024	0.021
Health-care level II								
Barbados	1985-1989			0.24 [e]				
China	1986-1990	0.02		0.0004	0.007	0.008	0.047	
Ecuador	1970-1974			0.006				
	1985-1989			0.015	0.002			
India	1970-1974			0.008	0.012		0.0006	0.0002
	1985-1989	0.0003	0.00001	0.002	0.022		0.002	0.0007

Table 37 (continued)

Country	*Year*	*Breast tumour*	*Prostate tumour*	*Female genital organs*		*Brain tumour*	*Other tumours*	*Benign diseases*
				Radium	*Afterloading*			
Iraq	1985-1989			0.009 [e]				
Jamaica	1985-1989			0.061				0.012
Peru	1970-1974 1985-1989			0.031 0.044			0.001 0.0004	
Average	1970-1979 1980-1984 1985-1990	 0.012	 0.00001	0.024 0.002	 0.013	 0.008	0.0007 0.028	 0.001
Health-care level III								
Egypt	1985-1990			0.005				
Myanmar	1975-1979 1980-1984 1985-1990			0.011 0.012 0.016				
Sudan	1985-1990				0.0003			
Thailand	1981-1985 1986-1990			0.041 0.016	 0.023			
Average	1970-1979 1980-1984 1985-1990			0.008 0.029 0.010	0.012 0.016		0.0006	0.0002

Qualifications of entries in this Table have been given as follows:

Canada:	Data for 1985-1989 from Nova Scotia and Prince Edward Island, about 4% of the population of the country. Data for earlier periods from Nova Scotia only, about 3.5% of the population of the country.
Cuba:	Data from PAHO.
Denmark:	Data also from [L16].
Finland:	Data also from [L16].
Iraq:	Data from Institute of Radiology and Nuclear Medicine, Baghdad.
Jamaica:	Data from Kingston Hospital only.
Netherlands:	Data also from [B6]. Values for 1988-1989 are number of treatments, not patients.
Norway:	Data also from [L16]. Values include palliative treatments; doses for curative treatments only are about 10% higher. Value given for benign disease is for 1990.
Sweden:	Data also from [L16]. Data for teletherapy are scaled up from non-random sample of 33% of patients (neither afterloading nor head/neck are evenly distributed in the country.) Data for brachytherapy are scaled up from non-random sample of 28% of patients: there were more children than average.
Turkey:	Data from Hacettepe University (2% of the population).
Yugoslavia:	Data for teletherapy exclude Montenegro, Vojvodina and Kosovo. Data for brachytherapy are for Croatia only (about 20% of the population of the former Yugoslavia).

[a] Number of treatments, not patients.
[b] Value is for both leukaemia and lymphoma.
[c] Iridium, not radium.
[d] Radium and caesium.
[e] Manual administration of caesium-137.

Table 38
Age- and sex-distribution of patients undergoing teletherapy and brachytherapy treatments, 1985-1990
Data from UNSCEAR Survey of Medical Radiation Usage and Exposures

PART I: TELETHERAPY

Health-care level	*Country*	*Age distribution (%)*			*Sex distribution (%)*	
		0-15 years	*16-40 years*	*>40 years*	*Male*	*Female*
			Leukaemia			
I	Australia	21	45	34	63	37
	Czechoslovakia	38	9.6	52	60	40
	Kuwait	73	20	6.7	53	47
	New Zealand	47	30	23	60	40
	Norway	25	35	40	70	30
	Romania	22	0	78	71	29
	Sweden	41	30	29	57	43
	Yugoslavia	95	5	0	50	50
	Average	43	17	39	61	39
II	Ecuador	56	33	11	50	50
	India	34	39	27	63	37
	Iraq	60	21	18		zz
	Turkey	87	10	2.9	56	44
	Average	35	38	27	63	37
III	Egypt	19	34	47	66	34
	Myanmar	4.2	46	50	50	50
	Thailand	83	13	4	51	49
	Average	39	29	32	56	44
			Lymphoma			
I	Australia	4	26	70	53	47
	Czechoslovakia	0	39	61	53	47
	Japan	13	23	64	56	44
	Kuwait	24	41	35	69	31
	New Zealand	2.3	28	69	64	36
	Norway	1	31	68	57	43
	Sweden	3.8	18	79	55	45
	Yugoslavia	17	33	50	50	50
	Average	11	25	64	55	45
II	Ecuador	2.8	40	57	78	22
	India	23	38	39	75	25
	Iraq	20	53	27	zz	zz
	Turkey	63	23	13	13	87
	Average	23	38	39	75	25
III	Egypt	18	37	46	62	38
	Myanmar	5.4	21	73	63	37
	Thailand	9.3	26	64	60	40
	Average	11	29	60	62	38
			Breast tumour			
I	Australia	0	11	89	1	99
	Czechoslovakia	0	14	86	1	99
	Kuwait	0.9	39	60	0	100
	New Zealand	0	7.6	92	1	99
	Norway	0.1	11	89	0	100
	Romania	0	7.3	93	0	100
	Sweden	0	5	95	2	98
	Yugoslavia	0	8.3	92	0	100
	Average	0.02	9.7	90.4	0.5	99.5
II	China	3.1	30	67	5	95
	Ecuador	0	29	71	0	100
	India	0	28	72	1	99
	Iraq	0	40	60	0	100
	Turkey	0.1	29	71	0	100
	Average	0.1	28.3	71.5	1.1	98.9

Table 38 (continued)

Health-care level	*Country*	*Age distribution (%)*			*Sex distribution (%)*	
		0-15 years	*16-40 years*	*>40 years*	*Male*	*Female*
III	Egypt	0.7	36	63	1	99
	Myanmar	0	17	83	1	99
	Thailand	0	41	59	0	100
	Average	0.2	32.8	66.9	0.6	99.4
Lung/thorax						
I	Australia	0	1.3	99	75	25
	Czechoslovakia	0	3.2	97	89	11
	Japan	0.2	5	95	81	19
	Kuwait	1.8	3.6	95	85	15
	New Zealand	0	1.5	98	67	33
	Norway	0	1.4	99	75	25
	Romania	0	5.1	95	34	66
	Sweden	0.2	3.4	96	69	31
	Yugoslavia	0	13	87	90	10
	Average	0.1	5.1	94.9	76	24
II	China	1.6	32	67	71	29
	Ecuador	0	12	88	88	12
	India	0	13	87	80	20
	Iraq	1	8.4	91	83	17
	Turkey	0.7	11	88	94	6
	Average	0.2	15.1	84.7	79	21
III	Egypt	0	18	82	81	19
	Myanmar	0	3.3	97	71	29
	Thailand	0	23	77	23	77
	Average	0	16	84	57	43
Gynaecological						
I	Australia	0	12	88	0	100
	Czechoslovakia	0	11	89	0	100
	Japan	0.3	12	87	0	100
	Kuwait	2.5	30	68	0	100
	New Zealand	0	22	78	0	100
	Norway	0.8	7.9	91	0	100
	Romania	0	42	58	0	100
	Sweden	0	5.9	94	0	100
	Yugoslavia	0	14	86	0	100
	Average	0.2	15.4	84.0	0	100
II	China	0.6	10	89	zz	zz
	Ecuador	1.4	14	84	0	100
	India	0	25	75	0	100
	Iraq	1.6	41	58	0	100
	Turkey	11	21	68	0	100
	Average	0.1	23.4	76.4	0	100
III	Egypt	0	33	67	0	100
	Myanmar	0.6	6.4	93	0	100
	Thailand	0.1	30	70	0	100
	Average	0.2	24.7	75.1	0	100
Wilms' tumour						
I	Australia	100	0	0	56	44
	Czechoslovakia	95	5.5	0	55	45
	Kuwait [a]	100	0	0	67	33
	New Zealand [b]	100	0	0	50	50
	Norway [c]	100	0	0	100	0
	Sweden [b]	100	0	0	80	20
	Yugoslavia	100	0	0	50	50
	Average	99	1	0	60	40

Table 38 (continued)

Health-care level	*Country*	*Age distribution (%)*			*Sex distribution (%)*	
		0-15 years	*16-40 years*	*>40 years*	*Male*	*Female*
II	Ecuador [c]	100	0	0	100	0
	India	65	11	24	68	32
	Iraq	100	0	0	50	50
	Turkey	100	0	0	68	32
	Average	66	11	23	68	32
III	Egypt	96	0	4	40	60
	Myanmar [a]	100	0	0	33	67
	Thailand	100	0	0	44	56
	Average	99	0	1	40	60
Neuroblastoma						
I	Australia	50	44	6	56	44
	Czechoslovakia	33	67	0	100	0
	Kuwait [d]	75	25	0	50	50
	New Zealand [e]	100	0	0	50	50
	Norway [e]	16	33	50	71	29
	Sweden [b]	100	0	0	80	20
	Yugoslavia	30	40	30	50	50
	Average	49	37	14	65	35
II	Ecuador	50	50	0	50	50
	India	73	17	10	64	36
	Iraq	100	0	0	67	33
	Turkey	89	11	0	67	33
	Average	73	17	10	64	36
III	Egypt	90	10	0	47	53
	Myanmar [c]	100	0	0	0	100
	Thailand	100	0	0	63	36
	Average	96	4	0	40	59
Benign diseases						
I	Australia	1	9	90	65	35
	Czechoslovakia	0	1.4	99	36	64
	Japan	4.2	38	58	58	42
	Kuwait	4		zz	50	50
	New Zealand	1.6	44	52	55	45
	Sweden		60	39	42	58
	Average	3	34	63	56	44
II	Ecuador	0	8.3	92	98	2.5
	India	3	43	54	51	49
	Average	3	43	55	52	48
All malignant tumours						
I	Japan	2.4	13	85	49	51
	Netherlands	0.2	6.4	93		zz
	Romania	1.3	14	85	37	63
	Average	2	13	86	47	53
II	China	4.3	24	72	44	56
	India	3	25	72	19	81
	Average	3	25	72	22	78

Table 38 (continued)

PART II: BRACHYTHERAPY

Health-care level	*Country*	*Age-distribution ()*			*Sex-distribution ()*	
		0-15 years	*16-40 years*	*>40 years*	*Male*	*Female*
Breast tumour						
I	Australia	0	23	77	0	100
II	China	3.1	30	67	5	95
	India	0	0	100	0	100
	Average	2	17	81	3	97
III	Thailand	0	63	37	0	100
Prostate tumour						
I	Australia	0	0	100	100	0
	Czechoslovakia	0	0	100	100	0
	Norway	0	0	100	100	0
	Average	0	0	100	100	0
II	Turkey	0	0	100	100	0
Gynaecological (radium)						
I	Australia	0	19	81	0	100
	Czechoslovakia	0	0	100	0	100
	Norway	0	10	90	0	100
	Average	0	12	88	0	100
II	China	0.6	10	89	0	100
	Ecuador	0	22	78	0	100
	India	0	40	60	0	100
	Iraq	0	0	100	0	100
	Jamaica	0	16	84	0	100
	Peru	0	12	88	0	100
	Average	0.3	22.2	77.2	0	100
III	Thailand	0	58	41	0	100
Gynaecological (afterloading)						
I	Australia	0	8.9	91	0	100
	Czechoslovakia	0	17	83	0	100
	New Zealand	0	25	74	0	100
	Norway	0	12	88	0	100
	Sweden	0	4.7	95	0	100
	Average	0	12	88	0	100
II	China	0.6	10	90	0	100
	Ecuador	0	42	58	0	100
	India	0	27	73	0	100
	Turkey	0	45	55	0	100
	Average	0.3	17.3	82.7	0	100
III	Egypt	0	33	67	0	100
	Thailand	0	34	66	0	100
	Average	0	34	66	0	100
Brain tumour						
I	Australia	0	100	0	100	0
	Norway [c]	0	0	100	0	100
	Average	0	81	19	81	19
II	China	7.3	37	55	64	3

Table 38 (continued)

Health-care level	*Country*	*Age-distribution ()*			*Sex-distribution ()*	
		0-15 years	*16-40 years*	*>40 years*	*Male*	*Female*
Other tumours						
I	Australia	0	100	0	100	0
	Czechoslovakia	4-5	95-96	0	11-66	34-89
	Norway	0	0	100	58	42
	Sweden [f]	0	0	100	50	50
	Average	1	68	31	60	15
II	India	0	12	88	68	32
III	Thailand	0	46	54	30	70
Benign diseases						
I	Czechoslovakia	0	0	100	0	100
	Kuwait				80	20
	Average	0	0	100	12	88
II	India	7	71	22	48	52
	Jamaica				30	70
	Average	7	71	22	48	52
All malignant tumours						
I	Romania	1.3	14	85	37	63
II	China	4.3	24	72	44	56

The entries in this Table are qualified as follows:

Myanmar: Data from Yangon General Hospital only.
Romania: Data are from a sample of 4 of the population in 1990. For leukaemia, values include lymphoma. For "All malignant tumours", data are for Co-60 only, namely 34 of all patients; most other patients were treated with x rays.
Thailand: Data from Department of Radiology, National Cancer Institute, Bangkok, only.
Turkey: Data are for 1986-1990.
Yugoslavia: Data are for Serbia only (about 40% of the population).

[a] Three patients.
[b] Five patients.
[c] One patient.
[d] Four patients.
[e] Six patients.
[f] Two patients.

Table 39
Doses to patients undergoing radiation teletherapy and brachytherapy, 1985-1989
Data from UNSCEAR Survey of Medical Radiation Usage and Exposures

PART I: TELETHERAPY

Country	Dose region	*Absorbed dose (Gy) (Range in parentheses)*							
		Leukaemia	*Lymphoma*	*Breast tumour*	*Lung/ thorax tumour*	*Gynaeco-logical tumour*	*Wilms' tumour*	*Neuro-blastoma*	*Benign disease*
Health-care level I									
Australia	Target	20 (8-25)	40 (35-45)	50 (30-60)	60 (20-60)	50 (30-55)	(10-25)	(10-40)	
Czechoslovakia	Target Surface	15.5 (2-36) 13.4 (1-43)	35 (9.6-46.8) 40.2 (10.5-50)	49 (8-56) 55.4 (7.2-60)	51 (20-60) 35 (25-40)	53.4 (8-70) 40 (14-60)	(10-40) (10-40)	(10-40) (10-40)	(0.5-10) 6 (1.5-6)
Finland	Target	24, 12 [a]	45	45-60	40-60	44-55	20-30	30	
Germany, F.R.	Target	(18-20)	40	(45-60)	50	(40-50)	40	40	
Kuwait	Target Surface	18 (15-24) 12	36 (30-40) 24	45 (45-50) 37 (26-30)	40 (40-50) 24 (24-30)	40 (40-50) 24 (24-30)	45 (30-45)	45	(30-45) (4-25)
Malta	Target		35 (30-40)	50 (45-60)	45 (30-50)	45 (35-50)	25 (20-35)	30 (12-45)	
Netherlands	Target		40 (33.6-50)	59 (44.3-70)	46 [b], 69 [c] (32-70)	52.5 (40-75)			
New Zealand	Target	19 (18-24)	38 (35-40)	30-55	30-55	42 (33-45)	24 (15-25)	30 (6-35)	12-48 (-50)
Norway	Target Surface	35 (20-40) 21	35 (30-45) 50 (43-60)	32 (20-60) 46 (29-86)	33 (20-50) 47 (29-71)	35 (30-50) 50 (43-71)	11	54 (30-61)	
Sweden	Target Surface	(20-30)	(20-50) (20-35)	(47-70) (30-45)	(20-60)	(30-60) (28-45)			(7-40)
Yugoslavia	Target	20 (20-30)	30 (20-50)	50 (50-70)	45 (43-60)	20 (20-60)	20 (20-40)	20 (20-40)	10 (10-20)
Health-care level II									
Barbados	Target			45 (30-50)	35 (20-45)	35 (20-45)			
China	Surface Target	50 (46-55) 60 (56-65)	40 (36-55) 50 (46-60)	40 (36-45) 50, 46 (46-56)	40 (36-70) 50, 48 (46-87)	50 (46-80) 60, 51 (56-100)	40 (36-41) 50 (46-51)	40 (36-42) 50 (46-52)	30-60 (12-65) 17-70 (14-75)
Ecuador	Target Surface	1.5 (2.5) 1.8 (3.0)	1.5 (2.0) 1.8 (3.0)	2.0 (2.3) 2.4 (2.9)	2.0 (4.0) 2.4 (4.8)	2.0 (2.5) 2.4 (3.0)	1.0 (1.25) 1.2 (1.5)		2.0 (3.0) 2.4 (8.6)
India	Target Surface	22 (10-35) 17 (6-40)	40 (30-60) 36 (7.5-85)	47 (35-70) 44 (9.9-71)	51 (25-70) 41 (11-70)	55 (30-75) 42 (9-86)	30 (15-60) 19 (15-35)	30 (15-60) 20 (5.6-45)	(3-30) (0.9-65)
Iraq	Target	20 (18-24)	35 (35-40)	45 (40-45)	30 (30-40)	50 (45-55)	35 (30-40)	40	
Jamaica	Target Surface		35 40	40 47	40 46	50 56	40 47	40 47	15 18
Peru	Target Surface	18 (18-24) 12.6 (12.6-17)	44 (25-50) 32 (15-30)	60 (50-70) 66 (41-58)	50 (60) 45 (-54)	50 (40-60) 21 (20-30)	30 (20-40) 21 (14-28)	30 (25-35) 20 (17-24)	17 [d] (12-23)
Health-care level III									
Egypt	Target			50	(50-60)	50	24-35	40	
Myanmar	Target Surface	40 (20-40) 40 (20-40)	40 (20-40) 42 (21-42)	50 (40-60) 52 (41.5-62.3	40 (20-40) 42 (21-42)	40 (40-60) 41.9 (41.9-62.8)	30 (20-40) 30.1 (20.1-40.2)		
Sudan	Target Surface	15 20	45	40 (36-40)	30 24	60 26	40 32	30 25	
Thailand	Target Surface	24 (21-24) 14.4 (12.6-14.4)	44 (40-46) 26.4 (24-27.6)	50 (45-50) 30 (27-30)	65 (60-65) 39 (36-39)	45 (40-50) 27 (24-30)	30 (27-30) 18 (16.2-18)	40 (40-50) 24 (24-30)	(9-15) [e]

Table 39 (continued)

PART II: BRACHYTHERAPY

Country	*Target absorbed dose (Gy) (Range in parentheses)*						
	Breast tumour	*Prostate tumour*	*Gynaecological*		*Brain tumour*	*Other tumours*	*Benign disease*
			Radium	*Afterloading*			
Health-care level I							
Australia	20 (10-30)		25 (20-50)			25-40 (20-)	
Czechoslovakia			25 (20-60)	25 (20-60)		(40-60)	(20-25) [f]
Kuwait	20 (20-40)		40 (30-40)	40 (30-40)			20
Malta				70 (65-75)			
Netherlands			29 (14-40				
New Zealand				35 (15-75)			
Norway		160 (160-)	40 (40-)	25 (25-)	54 (54-)	20-30 (20-)	
Sweden		20 (15-20)	60	(20-45)		(30-60)	
Health-care level II							
Barbados			60 (40-80)				
China	26		38	33	20		
Ecuador			30 (40)	30 (32)			
India	15 (10-20)	(30-35)	49 (15-82)	29 (15-75)		(8-75)	20 (10-30)
Iraq			20 [g]				
Jamaica			26 (39)				36
Peru			44 (30-45)			38-60 (30-80)	
Health-care level III							
Egypt				30		24	
Myanmar			40 (30-50)				
Sudan				48			
Thailand	25 (20-30)		30 (25-30)	30 (25-30)			

The entries in this Table are qualified as follows:

China: Under teletherapy, the second values for the surface dose region under breast tumour, lung/thorax tumour and gynaecological tumour are from a nationwide study.
Myanmar: Data from Yangon Hospital only.
Thailand: Data from Department of Radiology, National Cancer Institute, Bangkok, only.
Yugoslavia: Excluding Montenegro, Vojvodina and Kosovo.

---

[a] Whole-body treatments.
[b] Lung proper only.
[c] Other respiratory tract.
[d] The entrance surface dose (Gy) has been estimated from exposure (R) multiplied by 0.0087/0.75. This applies also to range.
[e] Keloid.
[f] Endometrial hyperplasia.
[g] Combined with external beam.

Table 40
Doses from scattered radiation from therapy using cobalt-60
[B19, I4]

Organ	*Normalized dose to tissue (mSv per Gy to target organ)*							
	Target in neck		*Target in bronchus*		*Target in pancreas*		*Target in central pelvis*	
	Female	*Male*	*Female*	*Male*	*Female*	*Male*	*Female*	*Male*
Gonads	0.1	0.1	0.1	0.1	4.0	0.5	[b]	47
Breast	0.3	-	19	-	11	-	0.5	-
Red bone marrow [a]	6.7	6.1	66	62	67	58	65	60
Lung	0.9	0.9	127	95	21	18	0.5	0.5
Thyroid	[a]	[a]	82	78	0.8	0.7	0	0
Bone surface	5.0	4.8	30	31	24	23	13	13
Remainder								
Brain	1.7	1.9	3.3	3.4	0.2	0.1	0.1	0.1
Kidney	0.1	0.1	1.9	1.4	[a]	[a]	4.5	4.0
Pancreas	0.1	0.1	3.6	3.5	[a]	[a]	2.7	1.9
Spleen	0.1	0.1	3.8	3.0	212	183	2.6	1.8
Uterus	0.1	-	0.2	-	8.2	-	•	-
Effective dose equivalent (H_E)	1.8	1.5	37	26	55	32	11	22
Effective dose (E)	1.1	0.95	30	23	16	11	8.3	17

[a] Assuming bone marrow in beam gets 60% of dose to target organ.
[b] Organ in beam.

Table 41
Collective effective dose from radiotherapy in the Netherlands, 1978-1979 [a]
[B19]

Target region [b]	*Number of patients*		*Effective dose equivalent* [c] *(mSv)*		*Effective dose* [c] *(mSv)*	
	Male	*Female*	*Male*	*Female*	*Male*	*Female*
Neck	414	628	108	92	64	57
Thorax	317	331	2210	1540	1790	1370
Pancreas and gall bladder	1635	1856	3320	1910	963	680
Pelvis	4533	4078	671	1300	496	1020
Collective dose (man Sv)			18630		10330	
Addition for target region			420 [d]		105 [e]	
Total			19050		10435	

[a] Breast cancer and skin cancer disregarded because there are no data on scattered radiation; lung cancer disregarded because treatment is in most cases only palliative.
[b] A target dose of 60 Gy is assumed.
[c] Per patient.
[d] 21,000 radiotherapy patients, cure rate 50%, at most 0.1% second cancers in target organs [I4], yield 5.25 deaths from second cancers. With a probability coefficient of 0.0125 per man Sv [I1], 5.25 deaths correspond to 5.25/0.0125 = 420 man Sv.
[e] Cancer fatality probability coefficient is 0.05 per man Sv [I8].

Table 42
Estimated doses to the world population from teletherapy and brachytherapy

Health-care level	*Population (millions)*	*Annual number of procedures per 1,000 population [U1]*	*Number of procedures (millions)*	*Annual collective effective dose (10^3 man Sv)* [a]
I	1350	2.4	3.2	980
II	2630	0.6	1.6	480
III	850	0.1	0.085	26
IV	460	0.05	0.023	7
Total	5290	-	4.9	1500
Average	-	0.9	-	-

[a] Values are based on effective dose, E, assuming 10,400 man Sv per 14.3 million population (figures from the Netherlands [B19]) = 730 man Sv per million population at health-care level I and a treatment frequency of 0.0024, i.e. 730/2.4 = 300 man Sv per 1,000 procedures.

Table 43
Total annual number of treatments with radiopharmaceuticals per 1,000 population
Data from UNSCEAR Survey of Medical Radiation Usage and Exposures

Country	*1970-1979*	*1980-1984*	*1985-1990*	*Country*	*1970-1979*	*1980-1984*	*1985-1990*
Health-care level I							
Argentina			0.16	Malta			0.075
Australia	0.15	0.15	0.14	Netherlands			
Belgium	4		0.31	New Zealand	0.16	0.097	0.17
Canada			0.88	Norway	0.059		0.12
Czechoslovakia	0.073	0.12	0.18	Romania		0.051	0.052
Denmark	0.13	0.18	0.21	Sweden	0.34		0.43
Finland	0.32	0.36		Switzerland	1.55		
Japan	0.049	0.025	0.030	United Kingdom		0.20	
Kuwait			0.018	Yugoslavia			0.11
Luxembourg			0.19				
				Average	0.086	0.093	0.10
Health-care level II							
Barbados			0.15	Iraq			0.013
China			0.035	Jamaica	0.17		0.005
Ecuador	0.007		0.0065	Peru			0.011
India			0.0036	Turkey			0.008
				Average	0.044		0.021
Health-care level III							
Egypt	0.064	0.061	0.062	Thailand	0.008	0.011	0.013
Myanmar	0.014	0.011	0.005	Tunisia	0.035		0.042
Sudan	0.001	0.003	0.006				
				Average	0.025	0.025	0.025

Table 44
Average annual number of therapeutic treatments with radiopharmaceuticals per 1,000 population
Data from UNSCEAR Survey of Medical Radiation Usage and Exposures unless otherwise indicated

Country	*Year*	*Thyroid tumours*	*Hyperthyroidism*	*Polycythaemia vera*	*Other tumours*	*Benign diseases*
Health-care level I						
Argentina	1985-1989	0.16				
Australia	1970	0.001	0.13	0.013		
	1980	0.024	0.12	0.012		
	1984	0.022	0.083	0.024		0.022
	1991	0.11 [a]		0.010		0.011
Belgium	1986-1990					
Canada	1985-1989	0.009	0.57	0.28		0.023
Czechoslovakia	1970-1974	0.016	0.013	0.011	0.007	0
	1976-1980	0.031	0.022	0.007	0.012	0.024
	1981-1985	0.035	0.022	0.008	0.018	0.038
	1986-1990	0.050	0.046	0.009	0.022	0.055
Denmark	1977-1980	0.023	0.097		0.006	
	1981-1985	0.029	0.15		0.005	
	1989-1990	0.023	0.19		0.001	
Finland [A12]	1975	0.005	0.29	0.012		0.008
	1982	0.038	0.28	0.040		0.005
Japan	1985-1989	0.025	0.005			
Kuwait	1985-1989	0.018				
Malta	1985-1989	0.003	0.064	0.008		
Netherlands	1984	0.097				
New Zealand	1970-1974	0.011	0.14	0.014		
	1985-1989	0.018	0.11	0.036		
Norway	1970-1974	0.004	0.033	0.0008	0.022	
	1985-1989	0.019	0.084	0.001	0.012	0.006
Romania	1980	0.041	0.010			
	1985-1989	0.043	0.009			<0.001
	1990	0.038	0.004			0.52
Sweden	1970-1974	0.31		0.032	0.001	0.003
	1985-1989	0.39		0.034	0.003	0.001
Switzerland	1976	1.0		0.022		0.52
United Kingdom	1981-1985	0.015	0.14	0.025	0.013	
Yugoslavia	1985-1989	0.009	0.029	0.005	0.053	0.014
Average	1970-1979	0.059	0.088	0.014	0.009	0.013
	1980-1984	0.033	0.10	0.024	0.013	0.025
	1985-1990	0.063	0.022	0.016	0.028	0.018
Health-care level II						
Barbados	1985-1989	0.15				
China						
Beijing area	1985-1989		0.005			
Entire nation	1986-1990	0.00006	0.0056		0.011	0.018
Ecuador	1970-1974	0.002	0.005			
	1985-1989	0.003	0.004			
India	1985-1989	0.0006	0.0029	0.0001		
Iraq	1985-1989	0.012		0.001		

Table 44 (continued)

Country	*Year*	*Thyroid tumours*	*Hyperthyroidism*	*Polycythaemia vera*	*Other tumours*	*Benign diseases*
Jamaica	1970-1974	0.093	0.077			
	1985-1989		0.005			
Peru	1985-1989	0.002	0.008			
Turkey	1991		0.008			
Average	1970-1979	0.023				
	1980-1984					
	1985-1990	0.0004	0.0004	0.0001	0.011	0.018
Health-care level III						
Egypt	1975-1979	0.024	0.040			
	1980-1984	0.017	0.044			
	1985-1989	0.023	0.039			
Myanmar	1975-1979	0.0006	0.013			
	1980-1984	0.001	0.010			
	1985-1989	0.0002	0.0038			
Sudan	1975-1979	0.001	0.0005			
	1980-1984	0.0001	0.002	0.0006		
	1985-1989	0.0003	0.0038	0.0015		
Thailand	1976-1980	0.008			<0.0001	
	1981-1985	0.011			<0.0001	
	1986-1990	0.013			0	
Tunisia	1970-1974	0.011	0.023	0.0009		
	1985-1989	0.013	0.027	0.002		
Average	1970-1979	0.010	0.023		0.00004	
	1980-1984	0.009	0.024	0.001	0.00003	
	1985-1990	0.011	0.020	0.002		

The entries in this Table are qualified as follows:

Canada: Nova Scotia Province only (about 3.5% of the population).

Turkey: Data are from Gazi University (1% of the population).

Yugoslavia: Data exclude Montenegro, Vojvodina and Kosovo; "other" tumours and benign diseases based on Croatia data only (about 20% of the population).

[a] Value is for both thyroid tumours and hyperthyroidism.

Table 45
Age- and sex-distribution of patients undergoing treatment with radiopharmaceuticals, 1985-1990
Data from UNSCEAR Survey of Medical Radiation Usage and Exposures

Health-care level	*Country*	*Age distribution (%)*			*Sex distribution (%)*	
		0-15 years	*16-40 years*	*>40 years*	*Male*	*Female*
		Thyroid tumours				
I	Canada	0	25	75	10	90
	Czechoslovakia	0	74	26	31	69
	Kuwait				37	63
	Netherlands	2	20	78	33	67
	New Zealand	0	40	60	7	93
	Norway	0	32	68	20	80
	Romania				25	75
	Yugoslavia	0	0	100	50	50
II	Ecuador	0	32	68	10	90
	Iraq				40	60
	Peru				20	80
III	Thailand	0.7	15	84	23	77
		Hyperthyroidism				
I	Canada	0	26	74	25	75
	Czechoslovakia	0	49	51	26	74
	Netherlands	0	32	68	19	81
	New Zealand	0	28	72	25	75
	Norway	0	14	86	22	78
	Romania	0			25	75
	Yugoslavia	0	0	100	10	90
II	China					
	Beijing area	0	67	33	29	71
	Entire nation	1.5	55	43	26	74
	Ecuador	0	33	67	15	85
	Iraq				21	79
	Jamaica	0	58	42	33	67
	Peru				30	70
III	Thailand	0	31	69	17	83
		Polycythaemia vera				
I	Czechoslovakia	0	57	43	51	49
	New Zealand	0	0	100	53	47
	Yugoslavia	0	17	83	90	10
		Other tumours				
I	Czechoslovakia	0	9.8	90	61	39
	Norway	0	23	77	0	100
		Benign diseases				
I	Canada	0	0	100	50	50
	Czechoslovakia	0	0	100	19	81
	Romania				36	64

The entries in this Table are qualified as follows:

Canada: Nova Scotia Province only (about 3.5% of the population).
Romania: Data are for 1990 only.
Thailand: Data are from Department of Radiology, National Cancer Institute, Bangkok, and Rajavithi Hospital only.
Yugoslavia: Data are for Serbia only (about 40% of the population).

Table 46
Average activity administered in therapy treatments with radiopharmaceuticals
Data from UNSCEAR Survey of Medical Radiation Usage and Exposures

Country	*Year*	*Average activity administered (MBq) (Range in parentheses)*						
		Thyroid tumours	*Hyper-thyroidism*	*Polycythaemia vera*	*Other tumours*		*Benign diseases*	
		^{131}I *iodide*	^{131}I *iodide*	^{32}P *phosphate*	^{90}Y *colloid*	*Other*	^{198}Au *colloid*	*Other*
Health-care level I								
Australia	1970 1980 1984 1991	5550 4225 4950 983 [a]	351 310 430	157 160 182 169				 183 [b] 265 [b]
Canada	1970-1974 1985-1989	3700 (-5550) 3700 (-5550)	185 (-1100) 185 (-1110)					111 [c] (-185) 111 [c] (-185)
Czechoslovakia	1970-1974 1985	6500 (5000-12000) 6500 (5500-22000)	200 (150-300) 200 (150-300)	185 (100-250) 185 (100-250)		600-3000 [d] (400-5500) 600-3000 [d] (400-5500)	 185 (150-450)	 185 [b] (150-450)
Japan	1976-1980 1981-1985		180 400					
Kuwait	1985-1989	3630 (1700-7770)	535 (399-671)	176 (152-180)				
Malta	1985-1989	3700	259 (-370)					
Netherlands	1988-1990	5500 (3700-5800)	500 (150-1800)					
New Zealand	1973 1985-1989	3145 (2220-3700) 1632 (370-4200)	400 (74-1480) 425 (150-2700)	154 (111-204) 172 (100-259)				
Norway	1970-1974 1985-1989	3000 (1000-5000) 3600 (2100-5100)	195 (131-259) 310 (152-468)			3700 [e] 300 [f]	 110	 750 [g]
Romania	1980 1985-1989	3700 3700	222 222					
Sweden	1974 1985-1989	1700	344	230 224 (140-335)	185	 2874 [h] (2000-3700)	160 150 (110-185)	150 [b] 187 [b] (150-200)
Switzerland	1976	925		185				74
United Kingdom	1981-1985	3304 (110-5000)	335 (120-1550)	207 (111-444)	191 (55-280)			
Yugoslavia	1970-1974 1985-1989	3700 3700	185 (100-200) 185 (100-200)					
Health-care level II								
Barbados	1985-1989		296 (222-296)	294 (222-370)				
China Beijing area Entire nation	 1970-1974 1985-1989 1986-1990		 296 (148-740) 259 (111-740) 162			 8.7 [g]		

Table 46 (continued)

Country	*Year*	*Average activity administered (MBq) (Range in parentheses)*						
		Thyroid tumours ^{131}I *iodide*	*Hyper-thyroidism* ^{131}I *iodide*	*Polycythaemia vera* ^{32}P *phosphate*	*Other tumours*		*Benign diseases*	
					^{90}Y *colloid*	*Other*	^{198}Au *colloid*	*Other*
Ecuador	1970-1974 1985-1989	3700 (-9250) 3700 (-9250)	296 (-444) 296 (-444)					
India	1985-1989	5330 (3700-7400)	190 (74-226)	127 (74-296)				
Iraq	1985-1989	1850 (-5550)	200 (-1000)	200 (-400)				
Jamaica	1970-1974 1985-1989	370	182 370					
Peru	1985-1989	3700 (2960-4440)	259 (185-370)					
Health-care level III								
Egypt	1976-1980 1981-1985 1986-1990	2700 2500 4000	600 800 1000					
Myanmar	1976-1980 1981-1985 1986-1990	1850 1850 1850	185 185 185					
Sudan	1976-1980 1981-1985 1986-1990	 3700 3700	185 185 222	 185 259				
Thailand	1985-1989	270						

The entries in this Table are qualified as follows:

Canada: Nova Scotia Province only (about 3.5% of the population).
Jamaica: Value for thyroid tumours treated with ^{131}I iodide to be checked.
Yugoslavia: Excluding Montenegro, Vojvodina and Kosovo.

[a] Value is for both thyroid tumours and hyperthyroidism.
[b] Yttrium-90 colloid.
[c] Chromic phosphorus-32.
[d] P-32 $Na_2H\ PO_4$ (600 MBq), Au-198, P-32 colloid (3,000 MBq).
[e] Gold-198.
[f] Phosphorus-32.
[g] Iodine-131.
[h] Iodine-131 MIGB.

Table 47
Absorbed dose to non-target organs from therapy treatments of adult thyroid with iodine-131 iodide in Japan, 1982 [a]

Organ	*Dose factor [I5] (mGy/MBq)*	*Absorbed dose (mGy)*	*Number of therapies [M10]*
Bladder wall	0.52	209	2956
Bone surface	0.047	18.9	2956
Breast	0.043	17.3	2956
Stomach wall	0.46	185	2956
Small intestine	0.28	113	2956
Upper large intestine	0.059	23.7	2956
Kidney	0.06	24.1	2956
Lung	0.053	21.3	2956
Red bone marrow	0.054	21.7	2956
Ovary	0.043	17.3	2328
Testis	0.028	11.3	628

[a] 402 MBq administered [M10]; assumed thyroid uptake: 15%.

Table 48
Estimated doses to the world population from therapeutic treatments by nuclear medicine procedures [a]

Health-care level	*Population (millions)*	*Annual number of procedures per 1,000 population*	*Number of procedures (thousands)*	*Annual collective effective dose (10^3 man Sv) [b]*
I	1350	0.1	135	6.0
II	2630	0.02	53	2.4
III	850	0.02	17	0.8
IV	460	0.01	5	0.2
Total	5290	-	210	9.3
Average		0.04	-	-

[a] Based on extrapolation of data from the Netherlands [B19].
[b] Assuming an effective dose per treated patient of 40 mSv/0.9 (40 mSv calculated for thyroid therapy in Japan; thyroid therapy assumed to be 0.9 of all treatments), as calculated for Japan with the methodology of Beentjes [B19].

Table 49
Equivalent dose rates from adult patients undergoing nuclear medicine examinations [N6]

Examination	*Radiopharmaceutical*	*Amount administered (MBq)*	*Time after administration*	*Distance (cm)*	*Equivalent dose rate ($\mu Sv\ h^{-1}$)*
Bone	Tc-99m MDP	740	0	100	9
			1 h	100	6.3
			2 h	100	4.7
			3 h	100	3.5
Liver	Tc-99m S colloid	150	0	100	2
Blood pool	Tc-99m RBC	740	0	100	14
Tumour	Ga-67 citrate	110	0	100	3.5
CSF	In-111 DTPA	19	0	100	0.8
Heart	Tl-201 chloride	740	0	[a]	20
Heart	Tc-99m HSA	190	0	[a]	15
Bone	Tc-99m MDP	740	0	[a]	25
Heart	Tc-99m RBC	1000	20 min	100	18

[a] Side of stretcher.

Table 50
Effective dose equivalent to mother and breast-feeding child for common nuclear medicine examinations [J1]

Examination	*Radiopharmaceutical*	*Activity administered (MBq)*	*Effective dose equivalent (mSv)*	
			Mother	*Child*
Thyroid scintigraphy	Tc-99m pertechnetate	120	1.3	3.6
Renography	I-131 iodohippurate	0.4	0.02	2.8
Clearance	Cr-51 EDTA	4	0.01	0.006
Thrombosis test	I-125 fibrogen	4	0.44	13

Table 51
Exposures of volunteers in medical research and clinical trials

Country	*Year*	*Radionuclide administered*	*Number of studies*	*Number of volunteers* [a]	*Activity administered per volunteer (MBq)* [b]	*Committed effective dose (mSv)* [c]	*Ref.*
Clinical trials of labelled pharmaceuticals							
Germany, Fed. Rep. of	1978-1988	H-3 C-14 S-35	15 62 2	85 (3-8) 452 (3-30) 14 (7)	3.7 (1.9-16.7) 3.7 (0.37-11) 3.7	0.03-0.3 0.2-6 0.4	[B7]
Total	11 years		79	551			
Use of radioactive substances in medical research							
Germany, Fed. Rep. of	1988	Cr-51 Fe-59 Tc-99m In-111 I-123 Xe-133	2 1 5 1 3 1	18 (6-12) 12 107 (10-32) 80 105 (15-70) 26	3.79 1 350-740 20 150-185 900		[B7]
Clinical trials of radiopharmaceuticals							
Germany, Fed. Rep. of	1988	Tc-99m MAB In-111 MAB I-125 I-131 MAB	32 6 3 2	1286 (15-120) 175 (10-80) 500 (100-200) 35 (15-20)	220-1300 74-75 3.7 185		[B7]
Clinical trials of labelled pharmaceuticals							
United Kingdom	1978-1986	H-3 C-14 S-35	4 55 1	40 (3-15) 201 (2-10) 3	~10.5 ~1-3 2.8	0.03-0.3 0.01-5.5 0.3	[N7]

[a] Number of volunteers per study in parentheses.
[b] Activity administered per study in parentheses.
[c] Estimated to give upper limit values.

Table 52
Estimated doses to the world population from medical uses of radiation

Medical radiation use	*Effective dose equivalent per caput (mSv)*					*Collective effective dose equivalent (10^3 man Sv)*				
	Level I	*Level II*	*Level III*	*Level IV*	*World*	*Level I*	*Level II*	*Level III*	*Level IV*	*World*
Diagnosis										
Medical x-ray examinations	1.0	0.1	0.04	0.04	0.3	1300	290	40	20	1600
Dental x-ray examinations	0.01	0.001	0.0003	0.0003	0.003	14	3	0.3	0.1	17
Nuclear medicine	0.09	0.008	0.008	0.008	0.03	130	20	6	4	160
Total	1.1	0.1	0.05	0.05	0.3	1400	310	46	24	1800
Therapy [a]										
Radiotherapy	0.7	0.2	0.03	0.02	0.3	980	480	26	7	1500
Nuclear medicine	0.004	0.0009	0.0009	0.0004	0.002	6	2	0.8	0.2	9
Total	0.7	0.2	0.03	0.02	0.3	990	480	27	7	1500

[a] Evaluated for effective doses.

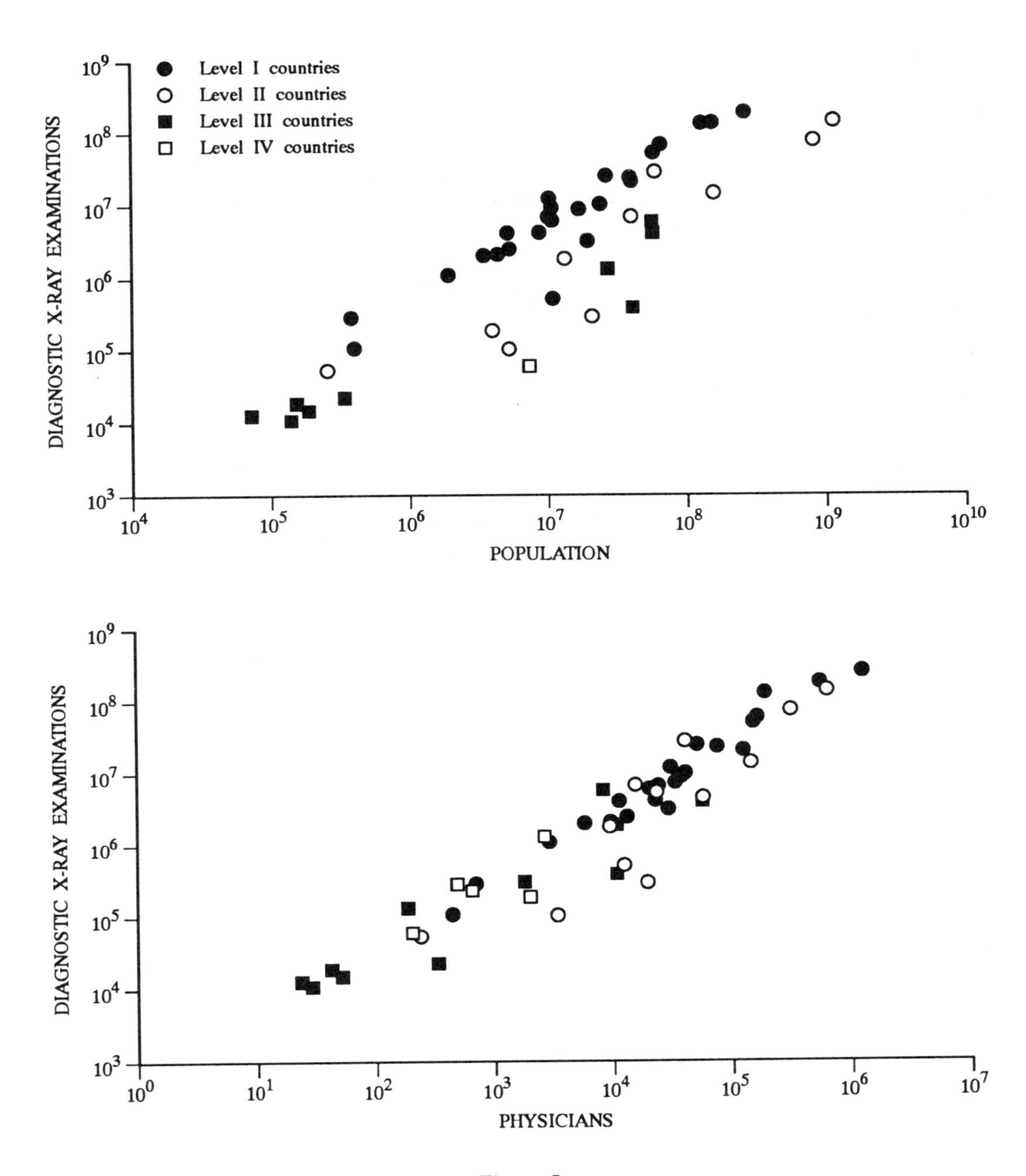

Figure I.
Diagnostic medical x-ray examinations in relation to population and number of physicians.

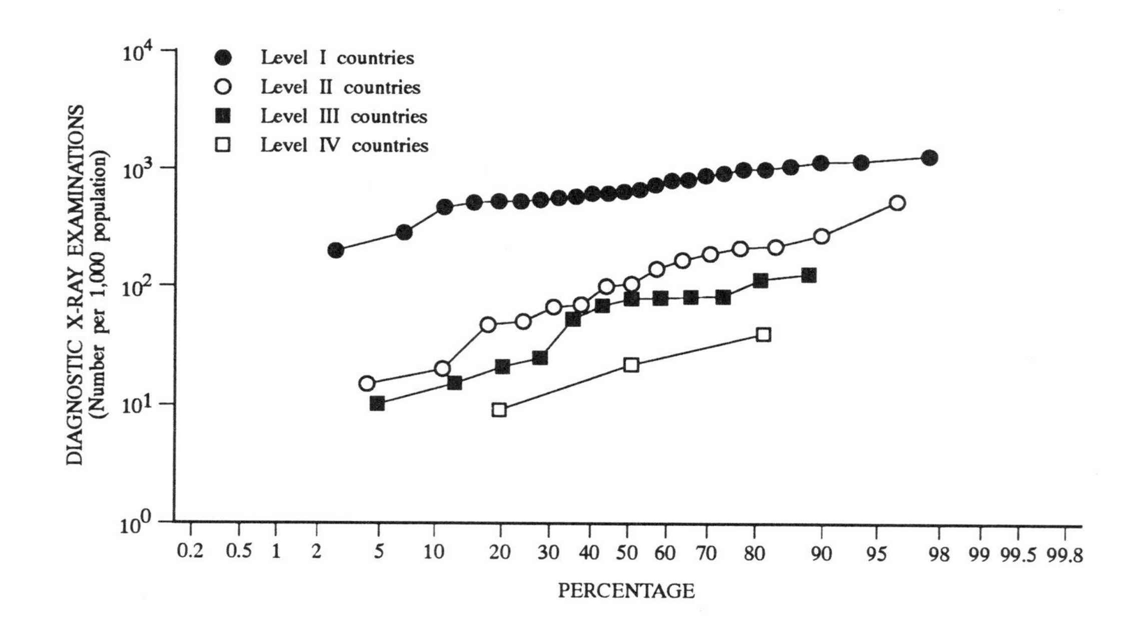

Figure II.
Distribution of total annual frequency of diagnostic medical x-ray examinations.

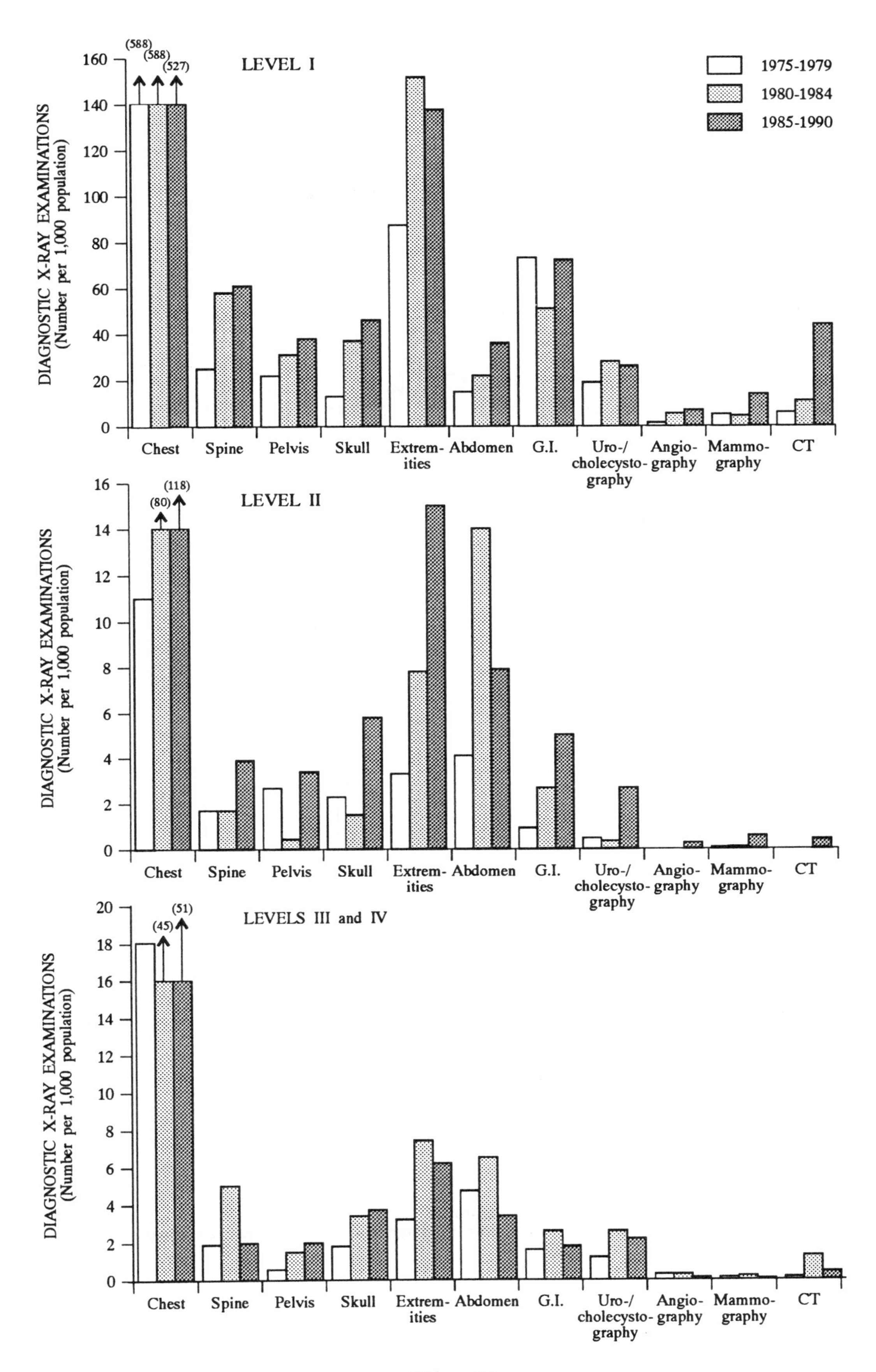

Figure III.
Average annual frequency of diagnostic medical x-ray examinations.

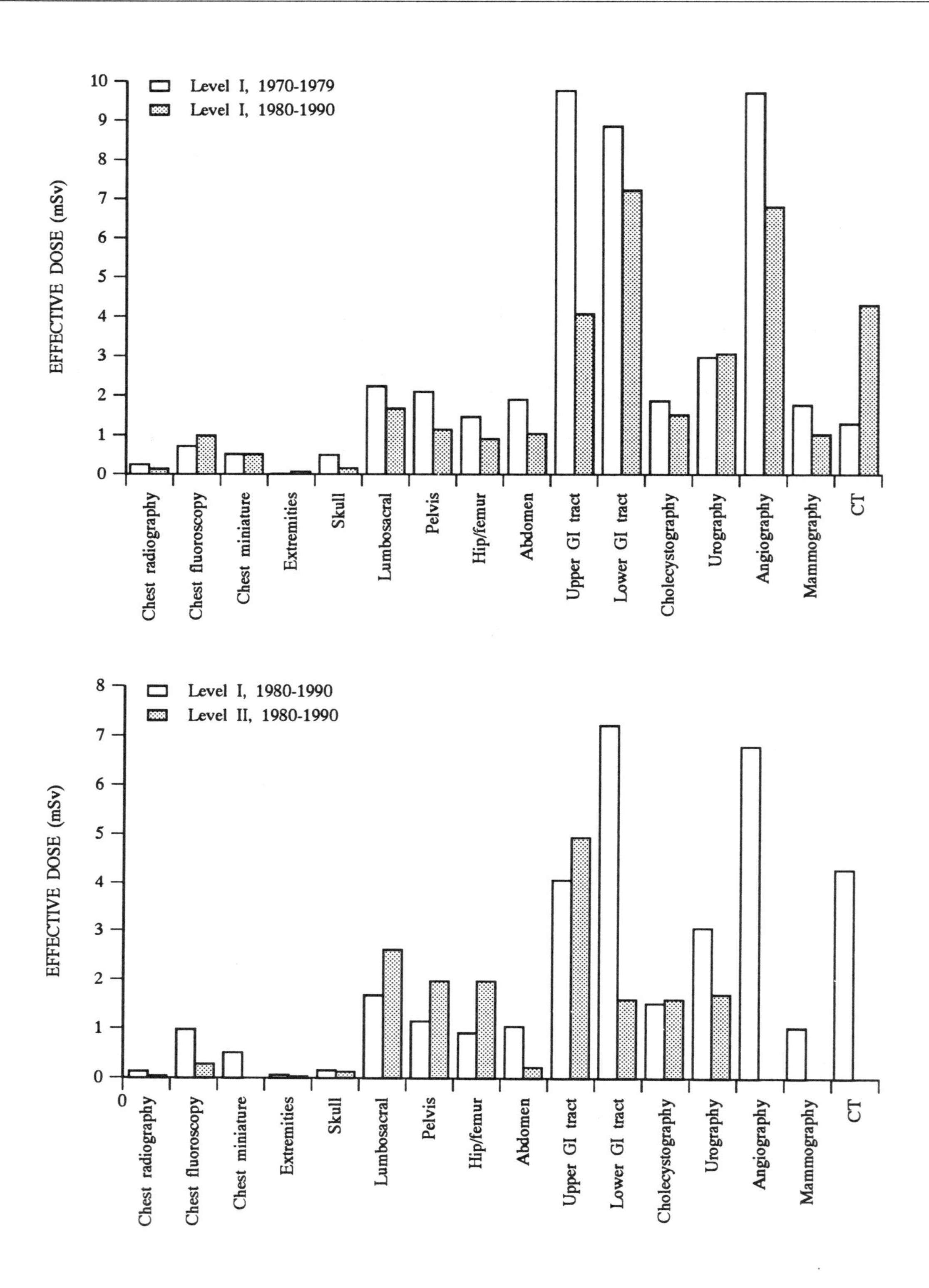

Figure IV.
Population-weighted average effective dose in diagnostic medical x-ray examinations.

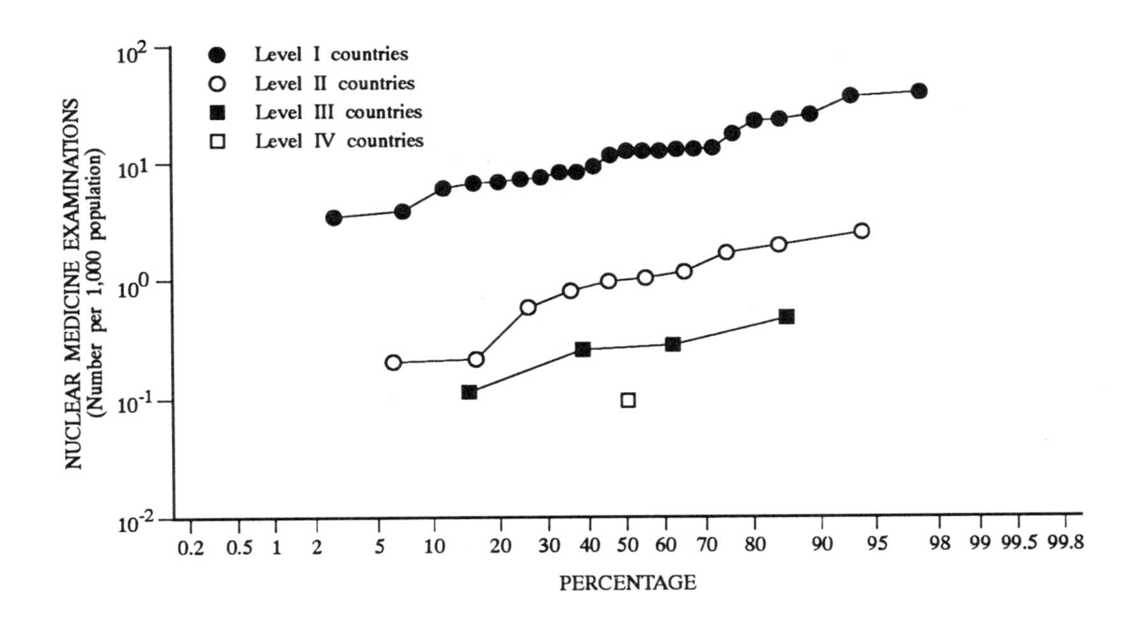

Figure V.
Distribution of total annual frequency of diagnostic nuclear medicine examinations in 1985-1990.

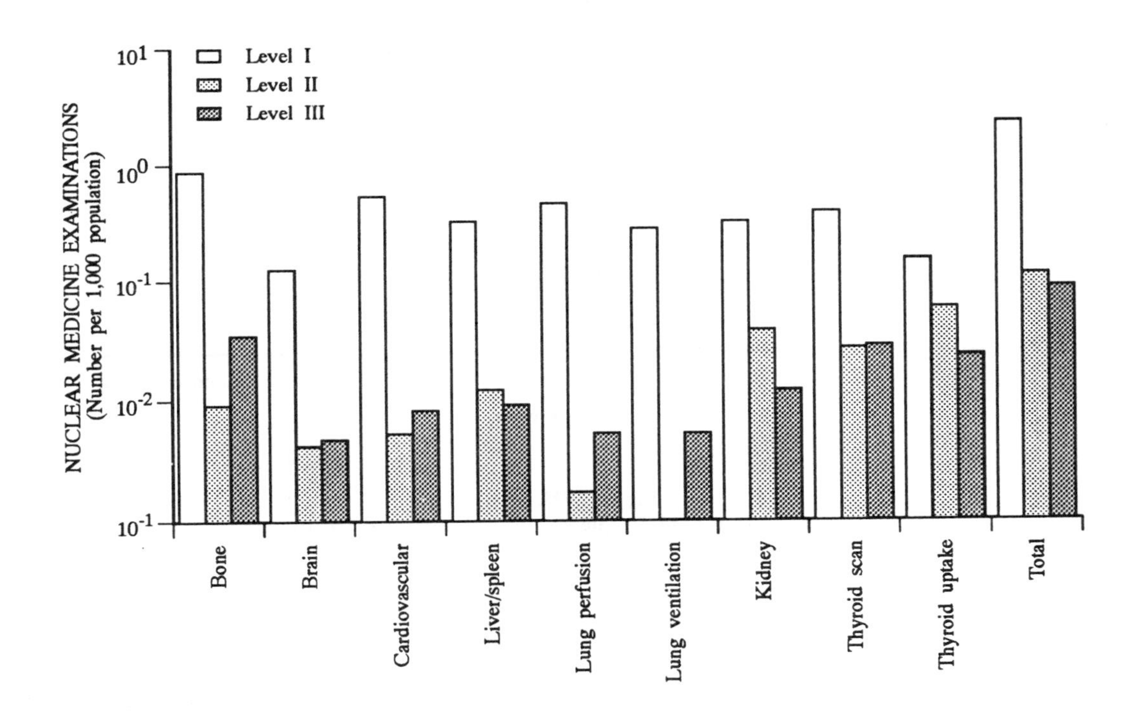

Figure VI.
Average annual frequency of diagnostic nuclear medicine examinations in 1985-1990.

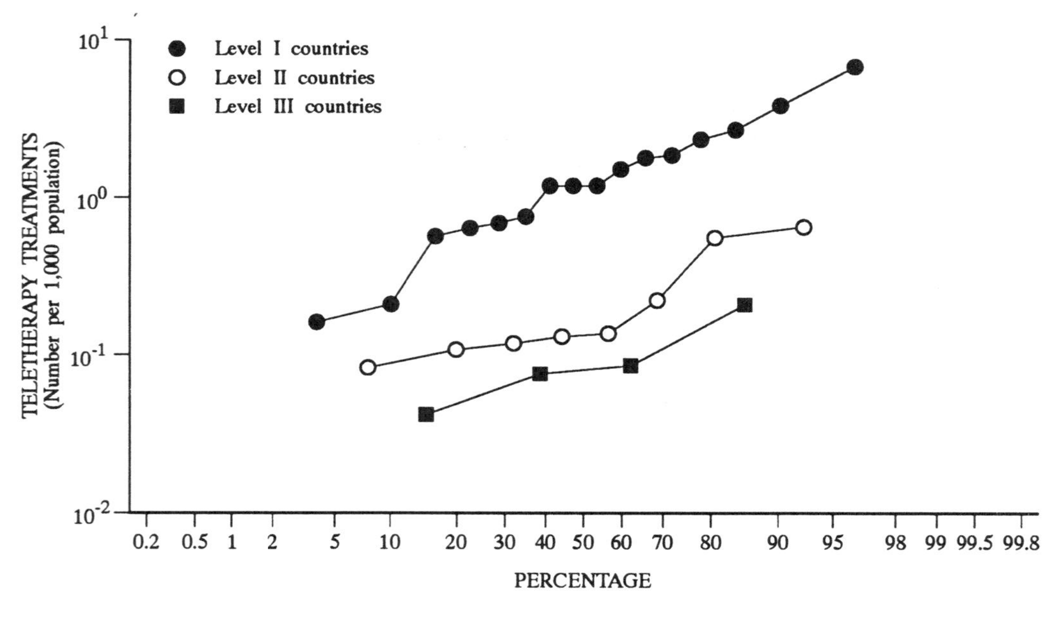

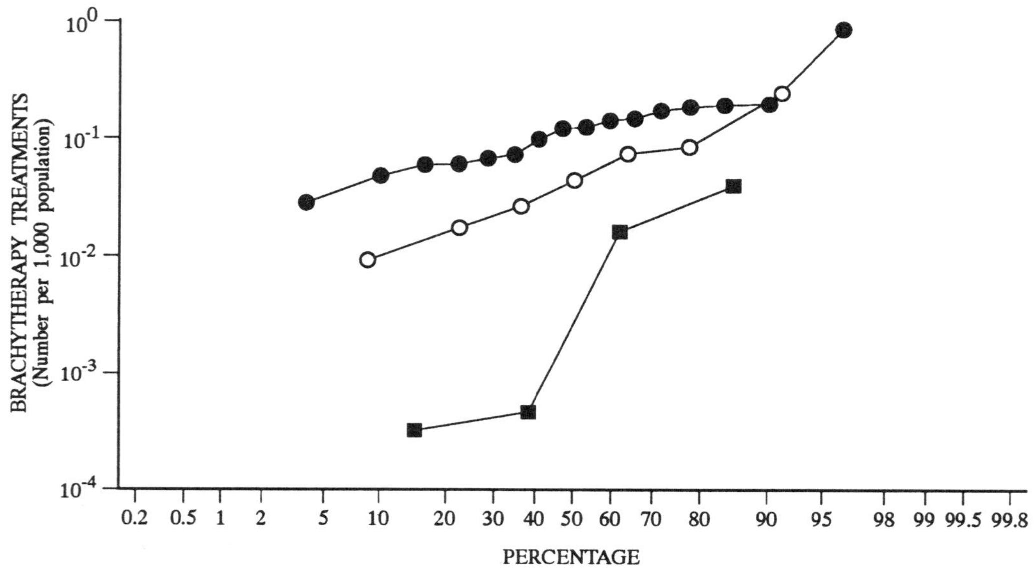

Figure VII.
Distribution of total annual frequency of radiotherapy treatments.

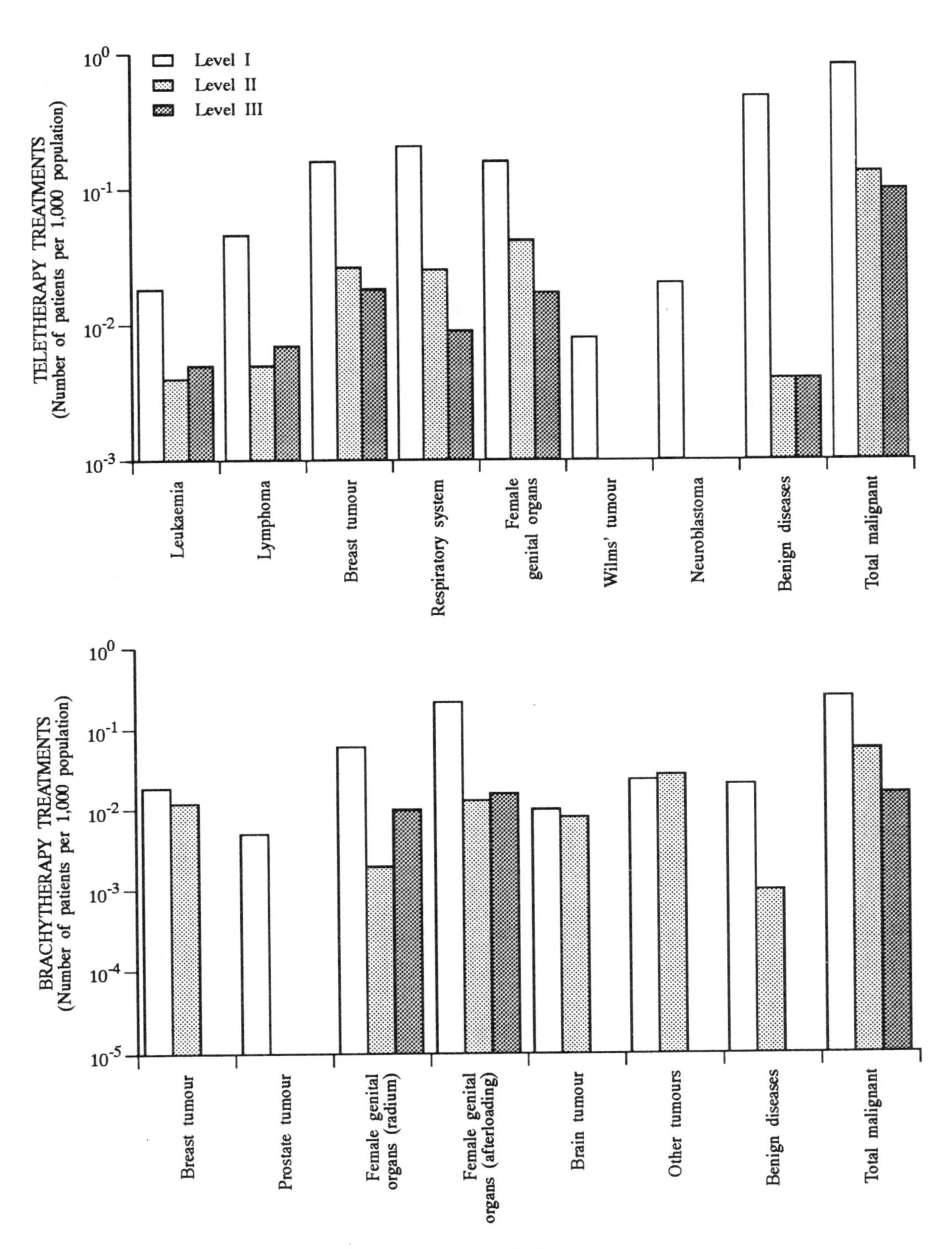

Figure VIII.
Average annual frequency of radiotherapy treatments in 1985-1990.

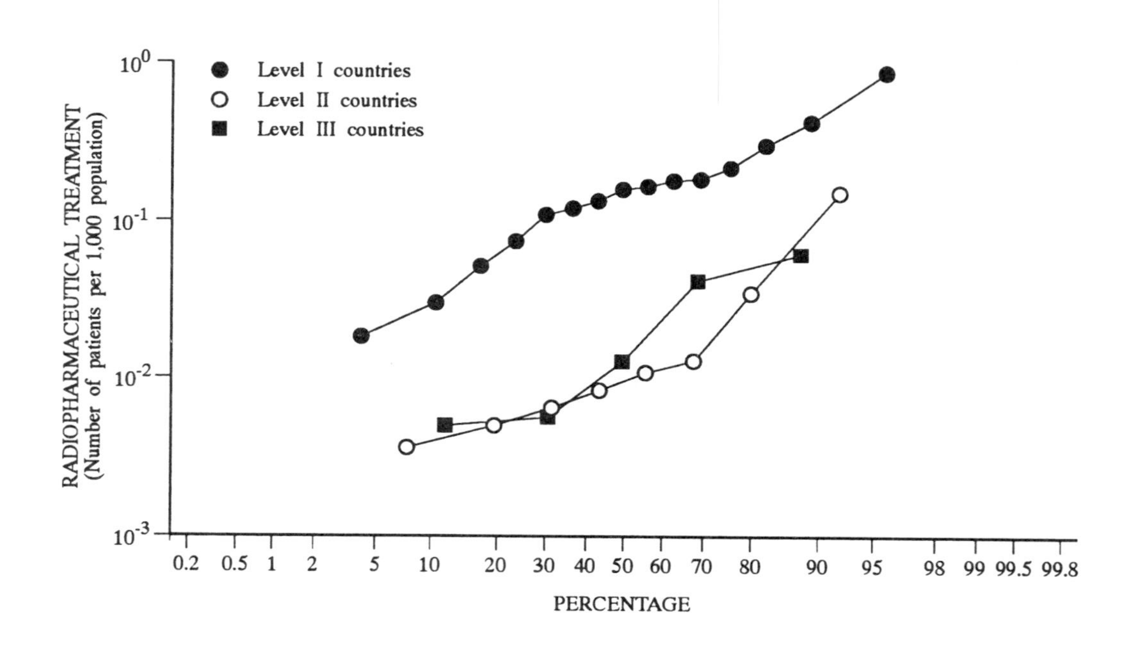

Figure IX.
Distribution of total annual frequency of therapy treatment with radiopharmaceuticals.

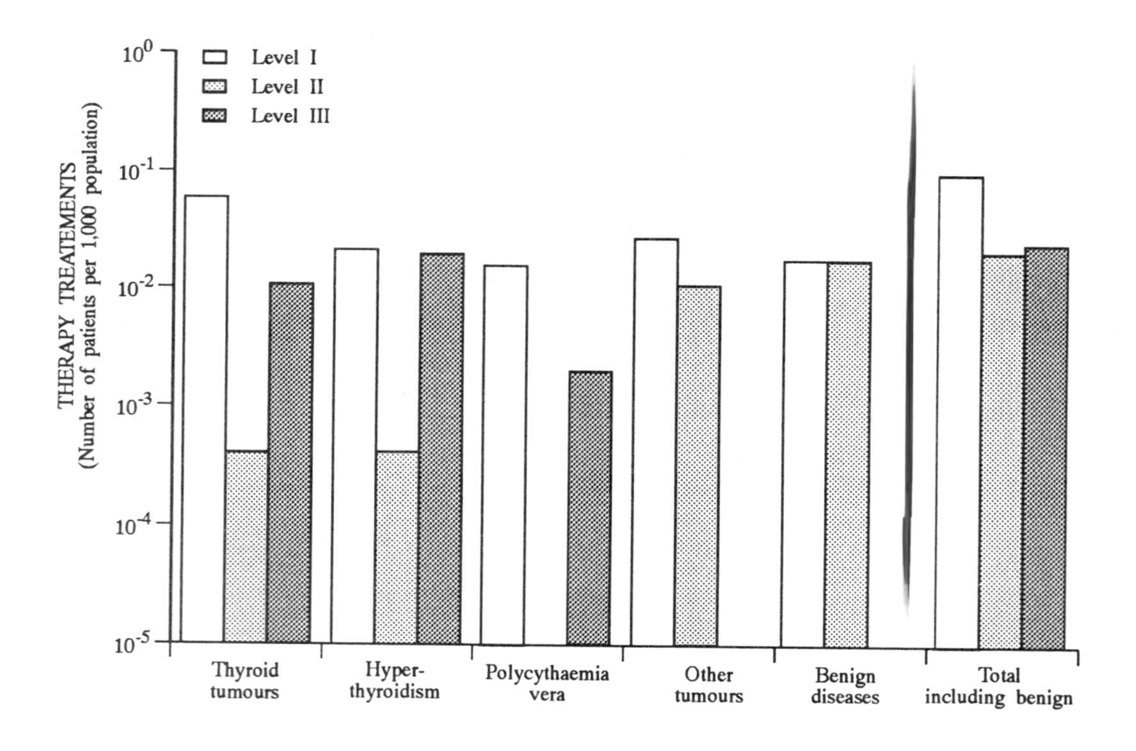

Figure X.
Average annual frequency of therapy treatments with radiopharmaceuticals in 1985-1990.

References

PART A

Responses to UNSCEAR Survey of Medical Radiation Usage and Exposures

Country	*Response from*
Argentina	J. Skvarca. Ministerio de Salud y Acción Social, Departamento de Radiofísica, Buenos Aires, Argentina. (September 1990 and December 1991).
Australia	D. Webb. Medical Radiation Section, Australian Radiation Laboratory, Victoria, Australia. (May 1990, December and April 1991).
Barbados	J. Rajendran. Queen Elizabeth Hospital, St. Michael, Barbados. (February 1990).
Belgium	SPRI-DBIS, Ministère Volksgezondheid & Leefmilieu, Bruxelles, Belgium. (November 1991).
Belize	C. Borrás. Pan-American Health Organization, Washington. (December 1991).
Burma	S. Tun Aung and U. Maung Gyi. Radiotherapy and Radiology Department, Mandalay General Hospital, Myanmar, Burma. (1990). T. Than OO and S. Than Tun Aung. Radiotherapy Department, Yangon General Hospital, Myanmar, Burma. (April 1990).
Canada	P. Dvorak. Bureau of Radiation and Medical Devices, Health and Welfare, Ottawa, Canada. (April, March 1990 and October 1991).
Cape Verde	D. Dantas Dos Reis. Dr. Agostinho Neto Hospital, Ministry of Health, Praia, Cape Verde. (April 1990 and October 1991).
Chile	C. Borrás. Pan-American Health Organization, Washington. (December 1991).
China	Z. Liangan. Institute of Radiation Medicine, Chinese Academy of Medical Sciences, China. (November 1991 and January 1992). Wu Shengcai, Yue Baoreng and Cui Jianguo. Laboratory of Industrial Hygiene, Ministry of Public Health, China. (June 1990).
Costa Rica	C. Borrás. Pan-American Health Organization, Washington. (December 1991).
Cuba	C. Borrás. Pan-American Health Organization, Washington. (December 1991).
Czechoslovakia	E. Kunz. National Institute of Public Health, Centre of Radiation Hygiene, Praha, Czechoslovakia. (April 1990). V. Klener. National Institute of Public Health, Centre of Radiation Hygiene, Praha, Czechoslovakia. (November 1991).
Denmark	K. Ennow and O. Hjardemaal. National Institute of Radiation Hygiene, Brønshøj, Denmark. (June 1990 and January 1992).
Djibouti	Ministry of Public Health and Social Affairs, Djibouti. (April 1990).
Ecuador	M.F. Campaña. Dirección de Ciencias Biofísicas, Comision Ecuatoriana de Energia Atomica, Quito, Ecuador. (February 1990).
Ethiopia	S. Demena. Department of Internal Medicine, Nuclear Medicine Unit, Addis Ababa, Ethiopia. (April 1990 and October 1991).
Finland	S. Rannikko. Finnish Centre for Radiation and Nuclear Safety, Department of Inspection and Metrology, Helsinki, Finland. (April and October 1991).
France	P. Pellerin. Service Central de Protection contre les Rayonnements Ionisants, Le Vésinet, France. (April 1990).

Country	*Response from*
Germany, Fed.Rep.	W. Burkart. Bundesamt für Strahlenschutz, Institut für Strahlenhygiene, Neuherberg, Germany. (October 1991).
Guatemala	C. Borrás. Pan-American Health Organization, Washington. (December 1991).
India	U. Madhvanath. Division of Radiological Protection, Bhabha Atomic Research Centre, Bombay, India. (December 1991).
Iraq	A. Al-Douri. Physics Department, Institute of Radiology and Nuclear Medicine, Baghdad, Iraq. (1991).
Italy	Ministero della Sanità, D.G.S.I.P., Div. VIIa, Rome, Italy. (June 1990). F. Dobici. ENEA, Divisione Radioisotopi e Macchine Radiogene, Rome, Italy. (October 1991).
Jamaica	A. Beach. Radiotherapy Department, Kingston Public Hospital, Kingston, Jamaica. (July 1990).
Japan	T. Maruyama. Division of Physics, National Institute of Radiological Sciences, Chiba-shi, Japan. (1991).
Kuwait	F. Sulaiman. X-ray Office, Ministry of Public Health, Safat, Kuwait. (April 1990 and November 1991).
Luxembourg	P. Kayser. Direction de la Santé, Division de la Radioprotection, Luxembourg. (February 1990).
Malta	M. Gauci. Occupational Health Unit, Department of Health, Valletta, Malta. (April 1990).
Mexico	R. Ortiz Magaña. Comisión Nacional de Seguridad Nuclear y Salvaguardias, Mexico. (October 1991).
Netherlands	L.B. Beentjes. Health Physics Department, University of Nijmegen, Netherlands. (July 1990 and October 1991).
New Zealand	B.D.P. Williamson and V.G. Smyth. National Radiation Laboratory, Christchurch, New Zealand. (July 1990).
Norway	J. Unhjem. National Institute of Radiation Hygiene, Østerås, Norway. (April 1990). G. Saxebøl. National Institute of Radiation Hygiene, Østerås, Norway. (August 1990).
Peru	R. Ramírez Quijada. Instituto Peruano de Energía Nuclear, Lima, Peru. (1990). L. Pinillos Ashton. Ministry of Health, Lima, Peru. (1990).
Philippines	M. Elesango. Radiation Health Service, Department of Health, Manila, Philippines. (April 1990).
Poland	M.A. Staniszewska and J. Jankowski. Institute of Occupational Medicine, Department of Radiation Dosimetry, Łódź, Poland. (April 1990).
Romania	C. Milu. Radiation Hygiene Laboratory, Institute of Hygiene and Public Health, Bucharest, Romania. (April 1990). C. Diaconescu. Radiation Hygiene Laboratory, Institute of Public Health and Medical Researches, Iassy, Romania. (November 1991).
Rwanda	Division Surveillance Epidemiologique, Ministere de la Sante, Kigali, Rwanda. (June 1990).
Singapore	T. Goh. Diagnostic Imaging Services, National University Hospital, Singapore. (1990).
Spain	E. Vañó Carruana. Catedra de Fisica Medica, Facultad de Medicina, Universidad Complutense, Madrid, Spain. (April 1990 and October 1991).
Sweden	W. Leitz, J. Karlberg and P. Hofvander. National Institute of Radiation Protection, Stockholm, Sweden. (May 1990 and October 1991).

Country	*Response from*
Switzerland	J. Marti. Radiation Protection Division, Federal Office of Public Health, Bern, Switzerland. (November 1991).
Thailand	Ministry of Public Health, Bangkok, Thailand. (February 1990).
Tunisia	S. M'Timet. Centre National de Radioprotection, Ministere de la Sante Publique, Tunis Jebbari, Tunisie. (August 1990).
Turkey	A. Gönül Buyan, F. Gözbebek and B. Ceyhan. Turkish Atomic Energy Authority, Ankara, Turkey. (October 1991).
United Kingdom	B.F. Wall. National Radiological Protection Board, Chilton, Great Britain. (March 1990 and October 1991).
United States	R.L. Burkhart. Centre for Devices and Radiological Health, Food and Drug Administration, Maryland, United States. (April 1990).
Vanuatu	R.E. Fey. Ministry and Department of Health, Port Vila, Vanuatu. (April 1990).
Yugoslavia	V. Radmilović. Federal Secretariat for Labor, Health, Veterans Affair and Social Policy of Yugoslavia, Belgrade, Yugoslavia. (October 1990 and November 1991).

PART B

A1 Anisimov, S.I., V.N. Popov, R.V. Chepiga et al. Radiation dose to patients and informativeness of the images obtained during eye examinations using x-ray computed tomography. Med. Tekh. (July/Aug): 38-40 (1987). (in Russian).

A2 Aikenhead, J., J. Triano and J. Baker. Relative efficacy for radiation reducing methods in scoliotic patients. J. Manip. Physiol. Ther. 12: 259-264 (1989).

A3 Arranz, L. Radiation protection implications of developing technologies and practices. in: Radiation Protection Toward the Turn of the Century, Paris, (in press, 1993).

A4 Allen, B.J., D.E. Moore and B.V. Harrington. Progress in Neutron Capture Therapy for Cancer. Plenum Press, New York & London, 1992.

A5 Atkins, H.L., S.R. Thomas, U. Buddemeyer et al. MIRD dose estimate Report No. 14: Radiation absorbed dose from technetium-99m-labeled red blood cells. J. Nucl. Med. 31: 378-380 (1990).

A6 American Cancer Society. Mammography guidelines 1983: Background statement and update of cancer-related checkup guidelines for breast cancer detection in asymptomatic women age 40-49. CA-Cancer J. Clin. 33: 225 (1983).

A7 Ågren, A., A. Brahme and I. Turesson. Optimization of uncomplicated control for head and neck tumors. Int. J. Radiat. Oncol. Biol. Phys. 19: 1077-1085 (1990).

A8 American Cancer Society. Guidelines for the cancer-related checkup - recommendations and rationale: Cancer of the breast. CA-Cancer J. Clin. 30: 224-240 (1980).

A9 Adams, J. The establishment of dose reducing protocols using rare earth filters in paediatric radiography. Radiogr. Today 56: 11-12 (1990).

A10 Axelsson, B., H. Forsberg, B. Hansson et al. Multiple-beam equalization radiography in chest radiology. Acta Radiol. 32: 12-17 (1991).

A11 Araujo, A.M.C., M.T. Carlos, L.R.F. Cruz et al. Fontes de Radiaçao Ionizante Utilizadas em Medicina no Brasil. Comissao Nacional de Energia Nuclear, Rio de Janeiro, Brazil, 1991.

A12 Asikainen, M. Radionuclides used in diagnostic nuclear medicine and doses 1982. STUK-B60 (1984).

A13 Atkins, H.L., D.A. Weber, H. Susskind et al. MIRD dose estimate report no. 16: Radiation absorbed dose from technetium-99m-diethylenetriaminepentaacetic acid aerosol. J. Nucl. Med. 33: 1717-1719 (1992).

A14 Arias, C.F. Potential exposures in radiation medicine. p. 356-359 in: Worldwide Achievement in Public and Occupational Health Protection Against Radiation. Worldwide Achievement in Public and Occupational Health Protection Against Radiation. Proceedings of the 8th International Congress of the International Radiation Protection Association, Montréal, 1992.

A15 Alm Carlsson, G. and D.R. Dance. Breast absorbed doses in mammography: evaluation of experimental and theoretical approaches. Radiat. Prot. Dosim. 43: 197-200 (1992).

B1 Bush, W.H., D. Jones and R.P. Gibbons. Radiation dose to patient and personnel during extracorporeal shock wave lithotripsy. J. Urol. 138: 716-719 (1987).

B2 Bertelli, L., I.E.C. Nascimento and G. Drexler. Influence of tissue weighting factors on risk weighted dose equivalent quantities. Radiat. Prot. Dosim. 37: 85-88 (1991).

B3 Børresen, A.-L. Role of genetic factors in breast cancer susceptibility. Acta Oncol. 31: 151-155 (1992).

B4 Benson, J.S. Patient and physician radiation exposure during fluoroscopy. Radiology 186: 286 (1992).

B5 Benedittini, M., C. Maccia, C. LeFauré et al. Doses to patients from dental radiology in France. Health Phys. 56: 903-910 (1989).

B6 Blaauboer, R.O. and L.H. Vaas. Estimated radiation exposure in the Netherlands in 1987 (Twentieth report). RIVM Report No. 248601002. Dutch National Institute of Public Health and Environmental Protection (1989). (in Dutch).

B7 Bundesminister für Umwelt, Naturschutz und Reaktorsicherheit (BR Deutschland). Berichte der Bundesregierung an den Deutschen Bundestag über Umweltradioaktivität und Strahlenbelastung in den Jahren 1983, 1984, 1985, 1986, 1987, 1988, 1989, 1990 and 1991 an den Deutschen Bundestag. Bonn, 1984-1992.

B8 Budach, V. The role of fast neutrons in radiooncology - a critical appraisal. Strahlenther. Onkol. 167: 677-692 (1991).

B9 Busch, H.P. and M. Georgi (eds.). Digital radiography. Workshop Quality Assurance and Radiation Protection, Mannheim 7-9 May 1992. Schnetztor-Verlag, Konstanz, 1992.

B10 Bansal, S. and J.H. Sunshine. Hospital and office practices of radiology groups. Radiology 183: 729-736 (1992).

B11 Bydder, G.M. Magnetic resonance imaging: present status and future perspectives. Br. J. Radiol. 61: 889-897 (1988).

B12 Benedetto, A.R., T.W. Dziuk and M.L. Nusynowitz. Population exposure from nuclear medicine procedures: measurement data. Health Phys. 57: 725-731 (1989).

B13 Bergström, K., S. Aquilonius, M. Bergström et al. PET, a new imaging technique. Läkartidn 86: 2371-2377 (1989). (in Swedish).

B14 Black, R.E. and K.J. Stehlik. Reducing radiation from brachytherapy patients with a cost-effective bedshield. Health Phys. 56: 939-941 (1989).

B15 Borrman, H. and P. Holmberg. Radiation doses and risks in dento-maxillofacial radiology. Proc. Finn. Dent. Soc. 85: 457-479 (1989).

B16 Brahme, A. Treatment optimization using physical and biological objective functions. in: Radiation Therapy Physics. (A. Smith, ed.) Springer Verlag, Berlin, 1992.

B17 Brahme, A. (ed.). Accuracy requirements and quality assurance of external beam therapy with photons and electrons. Acta Oncol. (Suppl.) 1: (1988).

B18 Baker, M.E. and F.R. Porter. A report on radiology at Muhimbili Medical Center, Dar es Salaam, Tanzania. Am. J. Roentgenol. 159: 195 (1992).

B19 Beentjes, L.B. The risks, expressed in collective doses, from radiotherapy in the Netherlands. Klin. Fysica 3: 116-121 (1987). (in Dutch).

B20 Beentjes, L.B. and C.W.M. Timmermans. Age and sex specific population doses (SED and GSD) due to nuclear medicine procedures in the Netherlands. Nucl. Med. Biol. 17: 261-268 (1990).

B21 Beentjes, L.B. and C.W.M. Timmermans. Annual frequency of diagnostic x-ray examinations in the Netherlands. Health Phys. 59: 357-358 (1990).

B22 Beentjes, L.B. and C.W.M. Timmermans. Age and sex specific radiographic examination frequency in the Netherlands. Br. J. Radiol. 63: 691-697 (1990).

B23 Bouhnik, H., J.J. Bard, J. Chavaudra et al. Évaluation des doses délivrées au cours d'examens radiologiques. J. Radiol. 72: 403-420 (1991).

B24 Bick, U., W. Wiesmann, H. Lenzen et al. Utilizing digital luminescence radiography in pediatric radiology: a report of initial experiences. Electromedica 59: 26-30 (1991).

B25 Byrne, C.M., M.J. Pharoah and R.E. Wood. Skin exposure and thyroid dose distribution using niobium filtration. J. Can. Dent. Assoc. 57: 663-665 (1991).

B26 Bristow, R.G., R.E. Wood and G.M. Clark. Thyroid dose distribution in dental radiography. Oral Surg., Oral Med., Oral Pathol. 68: 482-487 (1989).

B27 Benazzi, A., G. Cucchi and V. D'Arcangelo. Radiazioni ionizzanti assorbite dal paziente. Dent. Cadmos 7: 77-78 (1991).

B28 Beck, T.J. and B.W. Gayler. Image quality and radiation levels in videofluoroscopy for swallowing studies: a review. Dysphagia 5: 118-128 (1990).

B29 Berthelsen, B. and Å. Cederblad. Radiation doses to patients and personnel involved in embolization of intracerebral arteriovenous malformations. Acta Radiol. 32: 492-497 (1991).

B30 Boice J.D., D. Preston, F.G. Davis et al. Frequent chest x-ray fluoroscopy and breast cancer incidence among tuberculosis patients in Massachusetts. Radiat. Res. 125: 214-222 (1991).

B31 Bartels, G. Die Aufzeichnungspflicht der Röntgenverordnung. Dtsch. Krankenpflegez. 43: 22-26 (1990).

B32 Bassey, C.E., O.O. Ojo and I. Akpabio. Repeat profile analysis in an x-ray department. J. Radiol. Prot. 11: 179-183 (1991).

B33 Burkhart, R.L. Quality assurance programs for diagnostic radiology facilities. HEW (FDA) 80-8110 (1980).

B34 Bäuml, A. Qualitätssicherung in der Röntgendiagnostik - eine preiswerte Maßnahme der Strahlenhygiene. Roentgenpraxis 42: 112-114 (1989).

B35 Bäuml, A. Proposed limiting values for performance criteria in acceptance testing of diagnostic X-ray equipment in the Federal Republic of Germany. p. 25-26 in: Technical and Physical Parameters for Quality Assurance in Medical Diagnostic Radiology. (B.M. Moores, F.E. Stieve, H. Eriskat et al., eds.) British Institute of Radiology, Report 18, London, 1989.

B36 Beentjes, L.B. and C.W.M. Timmermans. Patient doses in the Netherlands. Radiat. Prot. Dosim. 36: 265-268 (1991).

B37 Beckman, M. Unpublished statistics from the Stockholm County Council Patient Register (1992).

B38 Baldas, J., J. Bonnyman, S.F. Colmanet et al. Quality assurance of radiopharmaceuticals - specifications and test procedures. ARL/TR093 (1990).

B39 Baldas, J., J. Bonnyman, Z. Ivanov et al. Results of the quality assurance testing programme for radiopharmaceuticals 1989. ARL/TR100 (1991).

B40 Bäuml, A. Qualitätskontrolle und Qualitätssicherung in der Radiologie. Bundesgesundheitsblatt 29/4: 128-132 (1986).

C1 Ciccozzi, A., A. Testa, M. Bultrini et al. Dosimetria clinica in xeromammografia con sistema "low dose". Radiol. Med. 74: 567-568 (1987).

C2 Contento, G., M.R. Malisan, R. Padovani et al. A comparison of diagnostic radiology practice and patient exposure in Britain, France and Italy. Br. J. Radiol. 61: 143-152 (1988).
C3 Commission of the European Communities. Quality criteria for diagnostic radiographic images in paediatrics. Radiation Protection Programme, Document XII/307/91, 1992.
C4 Clifton, J.S. Image quality - a European dimension. Mitt. Dtsch. Ges. Med. Phys. 20/2: 47-54 (1988).
C5 Centre for Devices and Radiological Health. Centre participates in national maternal and infant health survey. Radiol. Health Bull. 23/11: 1-2 (1989).
C6 Colette, H., N. Day, J. Rombach et al. Evaluation of screening for breast cancer in a non-randomized study (the DOM-project) by means of a case-control study. Lancet I: 829 (1985).
C7 Cohen, M. Irradiation of human subjects in medical research: proposal for a Canadian policy. J. Can. Assoc. Radiol. 35: 97 (1984).
C8 Carter, H.B., E.B. Näslund and R.A. Riehle Jr. Variables influencing radiation exposure during extracorporeal shock wave lithotripsy. Urology 30: 546-550 (1987).
C9 Commission of the European Communities. Progress report - radiation protection programme - 1988. EUR-12064 (1989).
C10 Clark, D.E., R.A. Danforth, R.W. Barnes et al. Radiation absorbed from dental implant radiography: a comparison of linear tomography, CT scan, and panoramic and intra-oral techniques. J. Oral Implantol. 16: 156-164 (1990).
C11 Clementz, B.-G., C. Ytterbergh and I. Telenius. Radiation dose in assessment of tibial torsion with a mobile C-arm fluoroscope. Upps. J. Med. Sci. 94: 67-72 (1989).
C12 Cagnon, C.H., S.H. Benedict, N.J. Mankovich et al. Exposure rates in high-level-control fluoroscopy for image enhancement. Radiology 178: 643-646 (1991).
C13 Calzado, A., E. Vañó, P. Morán et al. Estimation of doses to patients from "complex" conventional X-ray examinations. Br. J. Radiol. 64: 539-546 (1991).
C14 Campos de Araujo, A.M., P.G. Cunha, G. Drexler et al. Occupational and medical exposures in Brazil. p. 639-644 in: Strahlenschutz für Mensch und Umwelt. (H. Jacobs and H. Bonka, eds.) Fachverband für Strahlenschutz, FS-91-55-T, 1991.
C15 Carvalho, A.F., M.P. Rocha, J.G. Alves et al. Radiation doses from mammography in Portugal. Radiat. Prot. Dosim. 36: 261-263 (1991).
C16 Conference of Radiation Control Program Directors, Inc. Average patient exposure guide. CRCPD Publication 88(5) (1988).
C17 Commission of the European Communities. Quality criteria for diagnostic radiographic images. Radiation Protection Programme, Document XII/173/90, 1990.
C18 Cox, P.H., J.G.M. Klijn, M. Pillay et al. Uterine radiation dose from open sources: the potential for underestimation. Eur. J. Nucl. Med. 17: 94-95 (1990).
C19 Commission of the European Communities. European guidelines for quality assurance in mammography screening. Europe Against Cancer, Document CEC V/775/92, 1992.
C20 Chen, W.-C., Y.-H. Lee, M.-T. Chen et al. Factors influencing radiation exposure during the extra-corporeal shock wave lithotripsy. Scand. J. Nephrol. 25: 223-226 (1991).
C21 Culver, C.M. and H.J. Dworkin. Radiation safety considerations for post-iodine-131 hyperthyroid therapy. J. Nucl. Med. 32: 169-173 (1991).
C22 Chapple, C.-L., K. Faulkner, R.E.J. Lee et al. Results of a survey of doses to paediatric patients undergoing common radiological examinations. Br. J. Radiol. 65: 225-231 (1992).
C23 Conway, B.J., J.L. McCrohan, R.G. Antonsen et al. Average radiation dose in standard CT examinations of the head: Results of the 1990 NEXT survey. Radiology 184: 135-140 (1992).
C24 Christensen, J.J., L.C. Jensen, K.A. Jessen et al. Dosimetric investigations in computed tomography. Radiat. Prot. Dosim. 43: 233-236 (1992).
C25 Carvalho, A.F., A.D. Oliveira, E.M. Amaral et al. Assessment of patient doses and image quality in computed tomography. Laboratorio Nacional de Engenharia e Tecnologia Industrial, Departamento de Protecção e Segurança Radiológica, Portugal, 1991.
C26 Cranage, R.W., C.J. Howard and A.D. Welsh. Dose reduction by the use of erbium filtration in a general radiographic room. Br. J. Radiol. 65: 232-237 (1992).
C27 Coutrakon, G., M. Bauman, D. Lesyna et al. A prototype beam delivery system for the proton medical accelerator at Loma Linda. Med. Phys. 18: 1093-1099 (1991).
D1 Dienstbier, Z. and Z. Prouza. The radiation burden during nuclear-medicine diagnostic in children in the Czech Socialist Republic. Radiol. Diagn. 29: 181-185 (1988).
D2 Drexler, G., H. Eckerl and M. Zankl. On the influence of the exposure model on organ doses. Radiat. Prot. Dosim. 28: 181-188 (1989).
D3 Dubin, N. Effect of different mammographic radiation exposures on predicted benefits of screening for breast cancer. Stat. Med. 1: 15-24 (1982).
D4 Drexler, G., P. Cunha and J.E. Peixoto. Medical and occupational exposure in Brazil. Radiat. Prot. Dosim. 36: 101-105 (1991).
D5 Drexler, G., H. Eriskat and H. Schibilla (eds.). Criteria and methods for quality assurance in medical x-ray diagnosis. Br. J. Radiol. (Suppl.) 18: (1985).
D6 Dubin, N. Benefits of screening for breast cancer: application of a probabilistic model to a breast cancer detection project. J. Chronic Dis. 32: 145-151 (1979).
D7 Dąbrowski, R., M. Wylezińska, B. Gwiazdowska et al. X-ray doses absorbed by patients during xerox-mammography. Postepy Fiz. Med. 23: 137-147 (1988). (in Polish).
D8 Desponds, L., C. Depeursinge, M. Grecescu et al. Influence of anode and filter material on image quality and glandular dose for screen-film mammography. Phys. Med. Biol. 36: 1165-1182 (1991).
D9 Dawood, R.M. and C.M. Hall. Too much radiation for too many children? Br. Med. J. 296: 1277-1278 (1988).
D10 Dutkowsky, J.P., D. Shearer, B. Schepps et al. Radiation exposure to patients receiving routine

scoliosis radiography measured at depth in an anthropomorphic phantom. J. Pediatr. Orthop. 10: 532-534 (1990).

D11 Dobici, F., A. Susanna and J. Wells. Radiation exposure of the Italian population due to nuclear medicine examinations. in: World Congress on Medical Physics and Biomedical Engineering, Kyoto, Japan, 1991.

D12 Dvorak, P. and C. Lavoie. Exotic filter materials for diagnostic x-ray equipment - are they superior to commonly available materials? p. 211-214 in: Worldwide Achievement in Public and Occupational Health Protection Against Radiation. Worldwide Achievement in Public and Occupational Health Protection Against Radiation. Proceedings of the 8th International Congress of the International Radiation Protection Association, Montréal, 1992.

D13 Drexler, G. Das Konzept der effektiven Dosis in der Röntgendiagnostik. Strahlenschutz Forsch. Prax. 34: 1-14 (1993).

D14 Dahlbom, M., E.J. Hoffman, C.K. Hoh et al. Whole-body positron emission tomography: Part I. Methods and performance characteristics. J. Nucl. Med. 33: 1191-1199 (1992).

D15 Dyet, J.F., W. Hartley, A.R. Cowen et al. Digital cardiac imaging - the death knell of cineangiography? Br. J. Radiol. 65: 818-821 (1992).

D16 Durosinmi-Etti, F.A., M. Nofal and M.M. Mahfouz. Radiotherapy in Africa: Current needs and prospects. Int. At. Energy Agency Bull. 4: 24- 28 (1991).

D17 Dance, D.R., J. Persliden and G. Alm Carlsson. Calculation of dose and contrast for two mammographic grids. Phys. Med. Biol. 37: 235-248 (1992).

D18 Diaz-Romero, F. and J. Hernandez-Armas. Doses and detriment to patients from vascular and interventional radiology. p. 363-366 in: Worldwide Achievement in Public and Occupational Health Protection Against Radiation. Proceedings of the 8th International Congress of the International Radiation Protection Association, Montréal, 1992.

E1 Eilles, C. Strahlenexposition bei der SPECT mit Möglichkeiten der Reduktion der Strahlenexposition bei Patienten und Personal. Strahlenschutz Forsch. Prax. 31: 119-131 (1990).

E2 Eckelman, W.C. The status of radiopharmaceutical research. Nucl. Med. Biol. 18(7): iii-vi (1991).

E3 Ennow, K. Use of radiopharmaceuticals in Denmark in 1990. National Institute for Radiation Hygiene, Denmark, 1991. (in Danish).

E4 Ewen, K. Welche Auswirkungen hat die novellierte Röntgenverordnung auf die Strahlenexposition des Patienten und des Personals in der Medizin? p. 635-638 in: Strahlenschutz für Mensch und Umwelt. (H. Jacobs and H. Bonka, eds.) Fachverband für Strahlenschutz, FS-91-55-T, 1991.

E5 Ertl, S., H. Deckart and M. Tautz. Radiation dose and risk of patients through nuclear medicine procedures in the GDR: A comparison of 1978 and 1981. Eur. J. Nucl. Med. 9: 241-244 (1984).

F1 Fraser, G.M. Patient dose reduction. Clin. Radiol. 44: 212-213 (1991).

F2 Fitzgerald, M. and J.-M. Courades. Medical radiation protection practice within the EEC. British Institute of Radiology, London, 1991.

F3 Feygelman, V.M., W. Huda and K.R. Peters. Effective dose equivalents to patients undergoing cerebral angiography. Am. J. Neuroradiol. 13: 845-849 (1992).

F4 Faulkner, K., J.L. Barry and P. Smalley. Radiation dose to neonates on a special care baby unit. Br. J. Radiol. 62: 230-233 (1989).

F5 Fregene, A.O. Nuclear medicine in Nigeria. p. 575 in: Nuclear Medicine and Related Radionuclide Applications in Developing Countries. IAEA, Vienna, 1986.

F6 Felmlee, J.P., J.E. Gray, M.L. Leetzow et al. Estimated fetal radiation dose from multislice CT studies. Am. J. Roentgenol. 154: 185-190 (1990).

F7 Frost, F., V. Taylor and M. Odlaug. Mammography quality assurance in Washington State. Health Phys. 62: 131-135 (1992).

F8 Fosmark, H. and J.F. Unhjem. Radiation in connection with angiography. National Institute for Radiation Hygiene, Norway. SIS-a-87-2 (1987). (in Norwegian).

F9 Fürst, C.J., M. Lundell and L.-E. Holm. Radiation therapy of hemangiomas, 1909-1959. Acta Oncol. 26: 33-36 (1987).

F10 Farman, A.G. and E.T. Parks. Radiation safety and quality assurance in US dental hygiene programmes, 1990. Dento-Maxillo-Facial Radiol. 20: 152-154 (1991).

F11 Fukuda, H., T. Kobayashi, J. Hiratsuka et al. Estimation of absorbed dose in the covering skin of human melanoma treated by neutron capture therapy. Pigment Cell Res. 2: 365-369 (1989).

F12 Fishman, E.K., B. Drebin, D. Magid et al. Volumetric rendering techniques: applications for three-dimensional imaging of the hip. Radiology 163: 737-738 (1987).

F13 Fishman, E.K., D. Magid, D.R. Ney et al. Three-dimensional imaging and display of musculoskeletal anatomy. J. Comput. Assist. Tomogr. 12: 465-467 (1988).

G1 Goldenberg, D.M. and G.L. Griffiths. Radioimmunotherapy of cancer: Arming the missiles. J. Nucl. Med. 33: 1110-1112 (1992).

G2 Gurwitsch, A.M. Detailerkennbarkeit im Röntgenbild und die Grenzen der möglichen Strahlenbelastungssenkung. Fortschr. Geb. Roentgenstr. Nuklearmed. 148: 444-447 (1988).

G3 Goren, A.D., J.J. Sciubba, R. Friedman et al. Survey of radiologic practices among dental practitioners. Oral Surg., Oral Med., Oral Pathol. 67: 464-468 (1989).

G4 Geterud, K., A. Larsson and S. Mattsson. Radiation dose to patients and personnel during fluoroscopy at percutaneous renal stone extraction. Acta Radiol. 30: 201-206 (1989).

G5 Griffith, D.P., M.J. Gleeson, G. Politis et al. Effectiveness of radiation control programme for Dornier HM3 lithotriptor. Urology 33: 20-25 (1989).

G6 Gilman, E., A.M. Stewart, E.G. Knox et al. Trends in obstetric radiography, 1939-1981. J. Radiol. Prot. 9: 93-101 (1989).

G7 Gudden, F. and H. Kuhn. Reduktion der notwendigen Dosis in der Röntgendiagnostik. Roentgenpraxis 45: 44-48 (1992).

G8 Groner, C. Top 25 most frequently performed radiological and imaging procedures. Healthw. 26: 31 (1990).

G9 Germond, M., S. Raimondi, P. Schnyder et al. Comparison dosimétrique des méthodes de pelvimétrie utilisant la technique radiologique conventionelle et le scanner à rayons X. J. Gynecol. Obstet. Biol. Reprod. 18: 1002-1006 (1989).

G10 Gill, J.R. Overexposure of patients due to malfunctions or defects in radiation equipment. Radiat. Prot. Dosim. 43: 257-260 (1992).

G11 Goldin, L.L., V.S. Khoroshkov, E.I. Minakova et al. Proton therapy in USSR. Strahlenther. Onkol. 165: 885-890 (1989).

G12 Gibbs, S.J., A. Pujol, W.D. McDavid et al. Patient risk from rotational panoramic radiography. Dento-Maxillo-Facial Radiol. 17: 25-32 (1988).

G13 Glaze, S., A.D. LeBlanc, S.C. Bushong et al. Patient and personnel exposure during extracorporeal lithotripsy. Health Phys. 53: 623-629 (1987).

G14 Ghosh, P.R. The international state of PET. J. Nucl. Med. 32(4): 28N-51N (1991).

G15 Gezondheidsraad (Netherlands). Endoscopy - advisory report. Report No. 1989/04 (1989).

G16 Gharbi, H.A., J.C. Vicel, H. Abdesselem et al. La radiologie en Tunisie - Bilan actuel, perspectives d'avenir. J. Radiol. 67: 839-843 (1986).

G17 Gilgenbach, R., U. Schröder and L. Heuser. Strahlenexposition bei der Angiographie der hirnversorgenden Arterien. Fortschr. Röntgenstr. 153: 418-422 (1990).

G18 Gifford, D. Reducing radiation exposure of patients. Br. Med. J. 301: 451-452 (1990).

G19 Grapengiesser, S. and W. Leitz. Optimization of radiation protection in diagnostic radiology. p. 351-364 in: Radiation Protection Infrastructure. IAEA-SM-309/21. IAEA, Vienna, 1990.

G20 Gröndahl, H.-G. Digital radiology in dental diagnosis: a critical view. Dento-Maxillo-Facial Radiol. 21: 198-202 (1992).

G21 Gupta, M.M., S.C. Jain and A. Nagaratnam. The effect of change in tissue weighting factors on effective dose computation due to certain new radiopharmaceuticals in Indian patients. p. 388-391 in: Worldwide Achievement in Public and Occupational Health Protection Against Radiation. Proceedings of the 8th International Congress of the International Radiation Protection Association, Montreal, 1992.

G22 Gupta, M.M. and A. Nagaratnam. Effect of new ICRP recommendations on the effective dose of some new radiopharmaceuticals. p. 392-395 in: Worldwide Achievement in Public and Occupational Health Protection Against Radiation. Proceedings of the 8th International Congress of the International Radiation Protection Association, Montreal, 1992.

G23 Gosch, D. and S. Gursky. Describing the radiation exposure of patients in diagnostic radiology on the basis of absorbed energy. Radiat. Prot. Dosim. 43: 115-117 (1992).

H1 Hagekyriakou, J. and M.A. Chaudhri. Radiation exposures to patients during cardiac angiography and coronary angioplasty. p. 732-735 in: Radiation Protection Practice. Proceedings of the 7th International Congress of the International Radiation Protection Association, Sydney, 1988.

H2 Havukainen, R. Survey of dental radiographic equipment and radiation doses in Finland. Acta Radiol. 29: 481-485 (1988).

H3 Hall, E.J. Review article: The gene as theme in the paradigm of cancer. Br. J. Radiol. 66: 1-11 (1993).

H4 Huda, W., G.A. Sandison and T.Y. Lee. Patient doses from computed tomography in Manitoba from 1977 to 1987. Br. J. Radiol. 62: 138-144 (1989), with corrections in Br. J. Radiol. 65: 91 (1992).

H5 Huda, W., J. Bews and A.P. Saydak. Radiation doses in extracorporeal shock wave lithotripsy. Br. J. Radiol. 62: 921-926 (1989).

H6 Huda, W., G.A. Sandison, R.F. Palser et al. Radiation doses and detriment from chest x-ray examinations. Phys. Med. Biol. 34: 1477-1492 (1989).

H7 Holm, T., G.P. Hanson and S. Sandström. High image quality and low patient dose with WHO-BRS equipment. p. 153-155 in: Optimization of Image Quality and Patient Exposure in Diagnostic Radiology. (B.M. Moores, B.F. Wall, H. Eriskat et al., eds.) British Institute of Radiology, Report 20, London, 1989.

H8 Huda, W. and A.M. Sourkes. Individual and population doses in Manitoba from chiropractic x-ray procedures. J. Radiol. Prot. 9: 241-245 (1989).

H9 Hanks, G.E. (ed.). Quality assurance in radiation therapy: clinical and physical aspects. Int. J. Radiat. Oncol. Biol. Phys. (Suppl. 1) 10: (1984).

H10 Hughes, J.S., K.B. Shaw and M.C. O'Riordan. Radiation exposure of the UK population - 1988 review. NRPB-R227 (1989).

H11 Horiot, J.C., R. Le Fur, T. N'Guyen et al. Hyperfractionation versus conventional fractionation in oropharyngeal carcinoma: final analysis of a randomized trial of the EORTC cooperative group of radiotherapy. Radiother. Oncol. 25: 231-241 (1992).

H12 Hjardemaal, O. Organizing quality control programmes. p. 16-19 in: Technical and Physical Parameters for Quality Assurance in Medical Diagnostic Radiology. (B.M. Moores, F.E. Stieve, H. Eriskat et al., eds.) British Institute of Radiology, Report 18, London, 1989.

H13 Husband, D.J., R.D. Errington, S. Myint et al. Accelerated fast neutron therapy: A pilot study. Br. J. Radiol. 65: 691-696 (1992).

H14 Horton, D., A.M. Cook and A.D. Taylor. Audit in action: Significant reduction of double-contrast barium enema screening time with no loss of examination quality. Br. J. Radiol. 65: 507-509 (1992).

H15 Hart, D. and J.C. Le Heron. The distribution of medical x-ray doses amongst individuals in the British population. Br. J. Radiol. 65: 996-1002 (1992).

H16 Ho, S.-Y. and D.R. Shearer. Radioactive contamination in hospitals from nuclear medicine patients. Health Phys. 62: 462-466 (1992).

H17 Huda, W. and K. Gordon. Nuclear medicine staff and patient doses in Manitoba (1981-1985). Health Phys. 56: 277-285 (1989).

H18 Hellström, G. and P. Hofvander. Personal communication. Swedish Radiation Protection Institute, Stockholm (1989).

H19 Haywood, J.K., South Cleveland Hospital, England. Communication to UNSCEAR Secretariat (1993).

H20 Humm, J. Therapy by photon activation? Nature 336: 710-711 (1988).
H21 Huda, W., B. Lentle and J.B. Sutherland. The effective dose equivalent in radiology. J. Can. Assoc. Radiol. 40: 3-4 (1989).
H22 Hahn, K. and R. Piepenburg. Nuklearmedizinische Nierenfunktionsdiagnostik - aktueller Stand. Nuklearmediziner 14(4): 197-206 (1991).
H23 Holman, B.L. and M.D. Devous, Sr. Functional brain SPECT: The emergence of a powerful clinical method. J. Nucl. Med. 33: 1888-1904 (1992).
H24 Huda, W. and A.M. Sourkes. Radiation doses from chest x rays in Manitoba (1979 and 1987). Radiat. Prot. Dosim. 28: 303-308 (1989).
H25 Howell, R.W. Radiation spectra for Auger-electron emitting radionuclides: Report no. 2 of AAPM nuclear medicine task group 6. Med. Phys. 19: 1371-1383 (1992).
H26 Harding, L.K., N.J. Harding, H. Warren et al. The radiation dose to accompanying nurses, relatives and other patients in a nuclear medicine department waiting room. Nucl. Med. Commun. 11: 17-22 (1990).
H27 Huda, W. and K. Bissessur. Effective dose equivalents, H_E, in diagnostic radiology. Med. Phys. 17: 998-1003 (1990).
H28 Hentschel, F. Risiko und Stellenwert der konventionellen Myelographie unter Berücksichtigung der Strahlenbelastung des Patienten. Psychiatr., Neurol. Med. Psychol. 41: 31-37 (1989).
H29 Huda, W., J. McLellan and Y. McLellan. Reply to letter from Dr. J. C. Le Heron on "Effective dose in diagnostic radiology". J. Radiol. Prot. 12: 113 (1992).
H30 Hušák, V. and H. Říčková. Activities of administered radiopharmaceuticals and population dose from nuclear medicine in Czechoslovakia. Cesk. Radiol. 44: 333-339 (1990). (in Czech).
H31 Huda, W., A.M. Sourkes, J.A. Bews et al. Radiation doses due to breast imaging in Manitoba: 1978-1988. Radiology 177: 813-816 (1990).
H32 Havukainen, R. and M. Pirinen. Patient Doses and Image Quality in some X-ray Examinations in Finland. Nordic Society for Radiation Protection, 1990.
H33 Hart, D. and B.F. Wall. Study of causes of variation in doses to patients from x-ray examinations. NRPB-M212 (1990).
H34 Huda, W. and J. Bews. Population irradiation factors (PIFs) in diagnostic medical dosimetry. Health Phys. 59: 345-347 (1990).
H35 Huda, W., K. Gordon and I.D. Greenberg. Diagnostic thyroid procedures and corresponding radiation doses in Manitoba: 1981-1985. Health Phys. 59: 287-293 (1990).
H36 Huda, W., J. McLellan and Y. McLellan. How will the new definition of "effective dose" modify estimates of dose in diagnostic radiology? J. Radiol. Prot. 11: 241-247 (1991).
H37 Heggie, J.C.P. A survey of doses to patients in a large public hospital resulting from common plain film radiographic procedures. Australas. Phys. Eng. Sci. Med. 13: 71-80 (1990).
H38 Holmberg, P. and H. Borrman. Effective dose equivalent in dento-maxillofacial radiology. Proc. Finn. Dent. Soc. 85: 481-484 (1989).
H39 Hallén, S., K. Martling and S. Mattsson. Dosimetry at x-ray examinations of scoliosis. Radiat. Prot. Dosim. 43: 49-54 (1992).
H40 Hill, C.R. A future for radiological science? Br. J. Radiol. 64: 289-297 (1991).
H41 Hologic, Inc. QDR-1000/W Whole Body X-ray Bone Densitometer. Information Leaflet H-025 4/91, Waltham, MA, 1991.
H42 Hasert, V. Zur Strahlenexposition und zum Strahlenrisiko des Patienten bei der Mammographie. Radiol. Diagn. 29: 605-609 (1988).
H43 Hone, C.P., D. Howett and N. O'Donovan. A Survey of Breast Doses and Image Quality in Mammography in Ireland. Nuclear Energy Board, Dublin, Ireland, 1989.
H44 Horner, K. and P.N. Hirschman. Dose reduction in dental radiography. J. Dent. 18: 171-184 (1990).
H45 Hedgpeth, P.L., A.S. Thurmond, R. Fry et al. Radiographic fallopian tube recanalization: Absorbed ovarian radiation dose. Radiology 180: 121-122 (1991).
H46 Hart, D. and P.C. Shrimpton. The significance of patient weight when comparing X-ray room performance against guideline levels of dose. Br. J. Radiol. 64: 771-772 (1991).
I1 International Commission on Radiological Protection. Recommendations of the ICRP. ICRP Publication 26. Annals of the ICRP 1(3). Pergamon Press, Oxford, 1977.
I2 International Commission on Radiological Protection. Reference Man: Anatomical, physiological and metabolic characteristics. ICRP Publication 23. Pergamon Press, Oxford, 1975.
I3 Isberg, A., P. Julin, Th. Kraepelien et al. Absorbed doses and energy imparted from radiographic examination of velopharyngeal function during speech. Cleft Palate J. 26: 105-109 (1989).
I4 International Commission on Radiological Protection. Protection of the patient in radiation therapy. ICRP Publication 44. Annals of the ICRP 15(2). Pergamon Press, Oxford, 1985.
I5 International Commission on Radiological Protection. Radiation dose to patients from radiopharmaceuticals. ICRP Publication 53. Annals of the ICRP 18 (1-4). Pergamon Press, Oxford, 1987.
I6 International Atomic Energy Agency. Nuclear medicine and related radionuclide applications in developing countries. IAEA, Vienna, 1986.
I7 International Atomic Energy Agency. Dynamic functional studies in nuclear medicine in developing countries. IAEA, Vienna, 1989.
I8 International Commission on Radiological Protection. Recommendations of the ICRP. ICRP Publication 60. Annals of the ICRP 21 (1-3). Pergamon Press, Oxford, 1991.
I9 International Commission on Radiological Protection. Statement from the 1983 Washington Meeting of the ICRP. Annals of the ICRP 14 (1). Pergamon Press, Oxford, 1984.
I10 Iinuma, T.A. and Y. Tateno. Risk-benefit analysis for mass screening of breast cancer utilizing mammography as a screening test. Nippon Acta Radiologica 49: 1091-1095 (1989). (in Japanese).

I11 International Commission on Radiological Protection. Statement from the 1987 Como Meeting of the ICRP. Annals of the ICRP 17(4). Pergamon Press, Oxford, 1987.

I12 Iwai, K., K. Hashimoto, N. Mase et al. Estimation of stochastic risks occured by dental radiographic examination in Japan, 1987. Part 2: Estimation of population doses and stochastic risks. Jpn. Soc. Dent. Radiol. 29: 245-251 (1989).

I13 Ivanov, V.I., L.A. Lebedev, V.P. Sidorin et al. Reduction of radiation exposure of the population due to optimisation of the regimes of fundamental fluoroscopical examinations. TsNIIatominform-ON-1-88. Moscow, Russia, 1988. (in Russian).

I14 International Commission on Radiological Protection. Addendum 1 to ICRP Publication 53: Radiation dose to patients from radiopharmaceuticals. ICRP Publication, 1993. (in press)

I15 International Atomic Energy Agency. Developments in radioimmunoassay and related procedures. IAEA, Vienna, 1992.

I16 Inskip, P.D., R.R. Monson, J.K. Wagoner et al. Cancer mortality following radium treatment for uterine bleeding. Radiat. Res. 123: 331-344 (1990).

J1 Johansson, L. Patient irradiation in diagnostic nuclear medicine. Ph.D. Dissertation, ISBN 91-7222-961-6, Göteborg, 1985.

J2 Jolles, P.R., P.R. Chapman and A. Alavi. PET, CT, and MRI in the evaluation of neuropsychiatric disorders: current applications. J. Nucl. Med. 30: 1589-1606 (1989).

J3 Jones, D.G. and B.F. Wall. Organ doses from medical x-ray examinations calculated using Monte Carlo techniques. NRPB-R186 (1985).

J4 Jangland, L. and B. Axelsson. Niobium filters for dose reduction in pediatric radiology. Acta Radiol. 31: 540-541 (1990).

J5 Jangland, L. and R. Neubeck. A comparison study of radiation doses to patients and personnel from some types of angiography examinations. SSI Report 460-87 (1990). (in Swedish).

J6 Jeans, W.D. The development and use of digital subtraction angiography. Br. J. Radiol. 63: 161-168 (1990).

J7 Jones, D.G. and P.C. Shrimpton. Survey of CT Practice in the UK. Part 3: Normalised organ doses calculated using Monte Carlo techniques. NRPB-R250 (1991).

J8 Johansson, L., S. Mattsson, B. Nosslin et al. Effective dose to the patient from radiopharmaceuticals calculated with the new ICRP tissue weighting factors. p. 41-51 in: Proceedings of the Fifth International Radiopharmaceutical Dosimetry Symposium, Oak Ridge, Tennessee, 1992.

J9 Johansson, L., S. Mattsson, B. Nosslin et al. Effective dose from radiopharmaceuticals. Eur. J. Nucl. Med. 19: 933-938 (1992).

J10 Jennings, P., S.P.G. Padley and D.M. Hansell. Portable chest radiography in intensive care: A comparison of computed and conventional radiography. Br. J. Radiol. 65: 852-856 (1992).

J11 Jessen, K.A., J.J. Christensen, J. Jørgensen et al. Determination of collective effective dose equivalent due to computed tomography in Denmark in 1989. Radiat. Prot. Dosim. 43: 37-40 (1992).

J12 Jadva-Patel, H. The use of thin metal filters to reduce dose to patients. Radiogr. Today 57: 18-22 (1991).

K1 Kicken, P.J., J.H. Janssen, H.R. Michels et al. Radiation exposure during cardiac catheterization procedures. p. 737-740 in: Radiation Protection Practice. Proceedings of the 7th International Congress of the International Radiation Protection Association, Sydney, 1988.

K2 Kimme-Smith, C., L.W. Bassett and R.H. Gold. Evaluation of radiation dose, focal spot, and automatic exposure of newer film-screen mammography units. Am. J. Roentgenol. 149: 913-917 (1987).

K3 Kapa, S.F. and D.A. Tyndall. A clinical comparison of image quality and patient exposure reduction in panoramic radiography with heavy metal filtration. Oral Surg., Oral Med., Oral Pathol. 67: 750-759 (1989).

K4 Kircos, L.T., L.L. Angin and L. Lorton. Order of magnitude dose reduction in intraoral radiography. J. Am. Dent. Assoc. 114: 344-347 (1987).

K5 Kaiser, W.A. Magnetic-Resonance-Mammography (MRM). Springer-Verlag, Berlin, 1992.

K6 Källman, P., B.K. Lind and A. Brahme. An algorithm for maximizing the probability of complication-free tumour control in radiation therapy. Phys. Med. Biol. 37: 871-890 (1992).

K7 Kerr, I.H. Reply to Dr. Fraser. Clin. Radiol. 44: 213 (1991).

K8 Kerr, I.H. Patient dose reduction in diagnostic radiology. Clin. Radiol. 43: 2-3 (1991).

K9 Kaul, A. Institut für Strahlenhygiene des Bundesgesundheitsamtes, Neuherberg, Germany. Communication to UNSCEAR Secretariat. (1989).

K10 Kaul, A., G. Hinz, H.D. Roedler et al. Arten und Häufigkeit nuklearmedizinischer Untersuchungsverfahren und dadurch bedingte Strahlenexposition von Patienten und Gesamtbevölkerung. Forschungsvorhaben Strahlenschutz 1009 des Bundesministers des Innern, Bonn, 1988.

K11 Krüll, A., R. Schwarz, D. Heyer et al. Results of fast neutron therapy of adenoidcystic carcinomas of the head and neck at the neutron facility Hamburg-Eppendorf. Strahlenther. Onkol. 166: 107-110 (1990).

K12 Kogutt, M.S., F.H. Warren and J.A. Kalmar. Low dose imaging of scoliosis: use of a computed radiographic imaging system. Pediatr. Radiol. 20: 85-86 (1989).

K13 Kassebaum, D.K., N.E. Stoller, W.D. McDavid et al. Absorbed dose determination for tomographic implant site assessment techniques. Oral Surg., Oral Med., Oral Pathol. 73: 502-509 (1992).

K14 Kendall, G.M., B.F. Wall and S.C. Darby. X-ray exposures of the foetus. J. Radiol. Prot. 9: 285-287 (1989).

K15 Kalender, W.A. Effective dose values in bone mineral measurements by photon absorptiometry and computed tomography. Osteoporosis Int. 2: 82-87 (1992).

K16 Kimme-Smith, C., L.W. Bassett, R.H. Gold et al. Testing mammography equipment: Evolution over a 4-year period. Med. Phys. 19: 1491-1495 (1992).

K17 Kodl, O., J. Šnobr, E. Kunz et al. Exposure of patients to ionizing radiation in radiodiagnosis. Cesk. Radiol. 42: 54-63 (1988).

K18 Koshida, K., S. Koga, T. Orito et al. Levels for discharge to home and return to general ward of patients who received therapeutic dose of ^{131}I based on external exposure dose. Kaku Igaku 26: 591-599 (1989). (in Japanese).

K19 Kogutt, M.S., J.P. Jones and D.D. Perkins. Low-dose digital computed radiography in pediatric chest imaging. Am. J. Roentgenol. 151: 775-779 (1988).

K20 Kosunen, A., H. Järvinen, S. Vatnitskij et al. Intercomparison of radiotherapy treatment planning systems using calculated and measured dose distributions for external photon and electron beams. STUK-A98 (1991).

K21 Kimme-Smith, C., L.W. Bassett, R.H. Gold et al. Increased radiation dose at mammography due to prolonged exposure, delayed processing, and increased film darkening. Radiology 178: 387-391 (1991).

K22 Kling Jr., T.F., M.J. Cohen, R.E. Lindseth et al. Digital radiography can reduce scoliosis x-ray exposure. Spine 15: 880-885 (1990).

K23 Kheddache, S., L.G. Månsson, D. Schlossman et al. Digital chest radiography with a large-screen image intensifier. Electromedica 55: 21-27 (1987).

K24 Kheddache, S., L.G. Månsson, J.E. Angelhed et al. Effects of optimization and image processing in digital chest radiography: An ROC study with an anthropomorphic phantom. Eur. J. Radiol. 13: 143-150 (1991).

K25 Kapa, S.F. and D.A. Tyndall. Patient exposure reduction in panoramic radiography. Gen. Dentistry May-June: 169-171 (1991).

K26 Kassis, A.I. The MIRD approach: Remembering the limitations. J. Nucl. Med. 33: 781-782 (1992).

K27 Kereiakes, J.G. and D.V. Rao. Auger electron dosimetry: Report of AAPM nuclear medicine committee task group no. 6. Med. Phys. 19: 1359 (1992).

K28 Koga, S., K. Koshida, T. Orito et al. Discharge level of patients who received therapeutic amount of radioactive iodine-131. p. 396-399 in: Worldwide Achievement in Public and Occupational Health Protection Against Radiation. Proceedings of the 8th International Congress of the International Radiation Protection Association, Montréal, 1992.

K29 King, S.B. and J.D. Talley. Coronary arteriography and percutaneous transluminal coronary angioplasty. Circulation 79: 19-23 (1989).

L1 Lin, P.J. and A.F. Hrejso. Patient exposure and radiation environment of an extracorporeal shock wave lithotripsy. J. Urol. 138: 712-715 (1987).

L2 Lokan, K. Australian Radiation Laboratory. Communication to UNSCEAR Secretariat (1993).

L3 Leunens, G., J. Verstraete, W. Van den Bogaert et al. Human errors in data transfer during the preparation and delivery of radiation treatment affecting the final result: "garbage in, garbage out". Radiother. Oncol. 23: 217-222 (1992).

L4 Lam, C. and C.J. Martin. Design of a database with graphical analysis for x-ray quality assurance and dose information to assist in a programme for patient dose reduction. Br. J. Radiol. 64: 831-835 (1991).

L5 Le Heron, J. and B. Williamson. Performance of x-ray facilities in general medical practice. Radiat. Prot. News and Notes 5: 9-12 (1989).

L6 Leitz, W.K., B.R. Hedberg-Vikström, B.J. Conway et al. Assessment and comparison of chest radiography techniques in the United States and Sweden. Br. J. Radiol. 63: 33-40 (1990).

L7 Létourneau, E.G. Bureau of Radiation and Medical Devices, Canada. Communication to UNSCEAR Secretariat. (1989).

L8 Lindelöf, B. Grenz ray therapy in dermatology - an experimental, clinical and epidemiological study. Acta Derm.-Venereol. (Suppl.) 132: Thesis (1987).

L9 Lannering, B. Brain tumours in children. Thesis, ISBN 91-7900-842-9, Göteborg (1989).

L10 Leitz, W. Qualitätssicherung der Mammographie in Schweden. p. 162-163 in: Strahlenschutz im Medizinischen Bereich und an Beschleunigern. (D. Harder, ed.) Fachverband für Strahlenschutz, FS-90-60-T, 1990.

L11 Lindskoug, B.A. Exposure parameters in x ray diagnostics of children, infants and the newborn. Radiat. Prot. Dosim. 43: 289-292 (1992).

L12 Letourneau, E.G. Communication to UNSCEAR Secretariat. Bureau of Radiation and Medical Devices, Canada (1990).

L13 Larsson, S.A., A.-M. Danielsson, H. Jacobsson et al. Quality assurance of gamma camera scintigraphy in Sweden. SSI Report 92-13 (1992). (in Swedish).

L14 Li, D. Communication to UNSCEAR Secretariat (1991).

L15 Lin, F.-J., M.-Y. Leu and J.-J. Hwang. Determination of possible doses to the gonads or fetus in pregnant patients during radiation therapy. J. Formosan Med. Assoc. 88: 462-468 (1989).

L16 Lote, K., T. Möller, E. Nordman et al. Resources and productivity in radiation oncology in Denmark, Finland, Iceland, Norway and Sweden during 1987. Acta Oncol. 30: 555-561 (1991).

L17 Law, J. Patient dose and risk in mammography. Br. J. Radiol. 64: 360-365 (1991).

L18 Länsimies, E., J.T. Kuikka and P. Karjalainen. Radiation absorbed doses from diagnostic thyroid procedures in Finland in 1985. Nucl. Med. Commun. 8: 111-113 (1987).

L19 Leitz, W., B.R.K. Hedberg-Vikström, L.G. Månsson et al. In search of optimal chest radiography techniques. Br. J. Radiol. 66: 314-321 (1993).

L20 Lemaire, G. Centre d'Etudes Nucléaires, France. Communication to UNSCEAR Secretariat (1991).

L21 Liniecki, J. Radiological protection in medicine - current and prospective work of the ICRP. p. 1193-1199 in: Worldwide Achievement in Public and Occupational Health Protection Against Radiation. Proceedings of the 8th International Congress of the International Radiation Protection Association, Montréal, 1992.

L22 Le Heron, J.C. Effective dose in diagnostic radiology. J. Radiol. Prot. 12: 111-112 (1992).

L23 Le Heron, J.C. Estimation of effective dose to the patient during medical x-ray examinations from measurements of the dose-area product. Phys. Med. Biol. 37: 2117-2126 (1992).

L24 Lindskoug, B.A. Reference man in diagnostic radiology dosimetry. Radiat. Prot. Dosim. 43: 111-114 (1992).

L25 Lindskoug, B.A. The Reference Man in diagnostic radiology dosimetry. Br. J. Radiol. 65: 431-437 (1992).

L26 Landau, B.R. and W.W. Shreeve. Radiation exposure from long-lived beta emitters in clinical investigation. Am. J. Physiol. 261 and Endocrinol. Metab. Clin. N. Am. 24: E415-E417 (1991).

M1 Moström, U. and C. Ytterbergh. Spatial distribution of dose in computed tomography with special reference to thin-slice techniques. Acta Radiol. 28: 771-777 (1987).

M2 Mettler, F.A., J.E. Briggs, R. Carchman et al. Use of radiology in United States hospitals: 1980-1990. Radiology (1993, in press).

M3 Mountford, P.J. Estimation of close contact doses to young infants from surface dose rates on radioactive adults. Nucl. Med. Commun. 8: 857-863 (1987).

M4 Maruyama, T., Y. Kumamoto, K. Nishizawa et al. Frequency of x-ray diagnostic examinations in Japan, 1986. Radioisotopes 42: 113-119 (1993). (Japanese).

M5 Manninen, H., O. Kiekara, S. Soimakallio et al. Reduction of radiation dose and imaging costs in scoliosis radiography - application of large-screen image intensifier photofluoroscopy. Spine 13: 409-412 (1988).

M6 MacMahon, B. Prenatal x-ray exposure and twins. N. Engl. J. Med. 312: 576-577 (1985).

M7 Moores, B.M., F.E. Stieve, H. Eriskat et al. (eds). Technical and Physical Parameters for Quality Assurance in Medical Diagnostic Radiology. British Institute of Radiology, Report 18, London, 1989.

M8 Merritt, C.R.B. Ultrasound safety: what are the issues? Radiology 173: 304-306 (1989).

M9 Miller, A.B., G.R. Howe and C. Wall. The national study of breast cancer screening. Protocol for a Canadian randomized controlled trial of screening for breast cancer in women. Clin. Invest. Med. 4: 227-258 (1981).

M10 Maruyama, T., Y. Noda, Y. Kumamoto et al. Estimation of frequency, population doses and stochastic risks in medical uses of radiopharma-ceuticals in Japan, 1982. 1. The number of medical examinations using radiopharmaceuticals. Nippon Acta Radiologica 48: 911-920 (1988). (in Japanese).

M11 Maruyama, T., H. Yamaguchi, Y. Noda et al. Estimation of frequency, population doses and stochastic risks in medical uses of radiopharmaceuticals in Japan, 1982. 2. Determination of organ or tissue doses and effective dose equvalents. Nippon Acta Radiologica 48: 1536-1543 (1988), with corrections in Nippon Acta Radiologica 50: 111 (1990). (in Japanese).

M12 Maruyama, T., H. Yamaguchi, Y. Noda et al. Estimation of frequency, population doses and stochastic risks in medical uses of radio-pharmaceuticals in Japan, 1982. 3. Population doses and risk estimates. Nippon Acta Radiologica 48: 1544-1552 (1988). (in Japanese).

M13 Mtimet, S., A. Kraiem, H. Essabah et al. Etat actuel de la medecine nucleaire en Tunisie. p. 576 in: Nuclear Medicine and Related Radionuclide Applications in Developing Countries. IAEA, Vienna, 1986.

M14 Mulhern, R.K., M.E. Horowitz, E.H. Kovnar et al. Neurodevelopmental status of infants and young children treated for brain tumors with preirradiation chemotherapy. J. Clin. Oncol. 7: 1660-1666 (1989).

M15 Menzel, B. and W. Kraus. Strahlenexposition im Kindes- und Jugendalter durch röntgendiagnostische Maßnahmen - Erfahrungen und Schlußfolgerungen. Radiol. Diagn. 29: 157-167 (1988).

M16 Månsson, L.G., S. Kheddache, D. Schlossman et al. Digital chest radiography with a large image intensifier - evaluation of diagnostic performance and patient exposure. Acta Radiol. 30: 337-342 (1989).

M17 Manny, E.F., H. Rudolph and M.A. Wollerton. Pre-employment low back x rays - an overview. HHS (FDA) 81-8173 (1981).

M18 McClean, P.M. and L.P. Joseph. Plain skull film radiography in the management of head trauma: an overview. HHS (FDA) 81-8172 (1981).

M19 Moores, B.M., B.F. Wall, H. Eriskat et al. (eds.). Optimization of Image Quality and Patient Exposure in Diagnostic Radiology. British Institute of Radiology, Report 20, London, 1989.

M20 Morgan, H.M. Quality assurance of computer controlled radiotherapy treatments. Br. J. Radiol. 65: 409-416 (1992).

M21 McDonnell, D. and C. Price. Effects of additional filtration on image quality in dental radiography: comparison of niobium with aluminium. Dento-Maxillo-Facial Radiol. 21: 73-76 (1992).

M22 Moores, B.M. European standards in diagnostic radiology: the Euro x ray. p. 219-221 in: Optimization of Image Quality and Patient Exposure in Diagnostic Radiology. (B.M. Moores, B.F. Wall, H. Eriskat et al., eds.) British Institute of Radiology, Report 20, London, 1989.

M23 Maccia, C., B.F. Wall, R. Padovani et al. Results of a trial set up by a study group of the Radiation Protection Programme of the CEC. p. 242-246 in: Optimization of Image Quality and Patient Exposure in Diagnostic Radiology. (B.M. Moores, B.F. Wall, H. Eriskat et al., eds.) British Institute of Radiology, Report 20, London, 1989.

M24 McGurk, M., R.W. Whitehouse, P.M. Taylor et al. Orbital volume measured by a low-dose CT scanning technique. Dento-Maxillo-Facial Radiol. 21: 70-72 (1992).

M25 Mathiesen, T. and H. Flensburg. Breast cancer mortality reduction in three current randomized mammographic screening trials. Breast Dis. 5: 91-104 (1992).

M26 Maccia, C. La dose reçue par les patients au cours des examens de radiodiagnostic et son optimisation. Radioprotection 25: 43-62 (1990).

M27 Mountford, P.J., M.J. O'Doherty, N.I. Forge et al. Radiation dose rates from adult patients undergoing nuclear medicine investigations. Nucl. Med. Commun. 12: 767-777 (1991).

M28 Mountford, P.J., M.J. O'Doherty, L.K. Harding et al. Radiation dose rates from paediatric patients undergoing $^{99}Tc^{m}$ investigations. Nucl. Med. Commun. 12: 709-718 (1991).

M29 Mettler, F.A. Jr. and R.C. Ricks. Historical aspects of radiation accidents. p. 17-30 in: Medical Management of Radiation Accidents. (F.A. Mettler, Jr., C.A. Kelsey and R.C. Ricks, eds.) CRC Press, Boca Raton, 1991.

M30 Moroni, J.P., A. Biau and J. Durgeat. Measurement of doses to workers and patients during specialized catheterism examinations. SCPRI Presentation to ICRP Committee 3, 1984.

M31 Maruyama, T., K. Iwai, N. Mase et al. Estimation of frequency and population doses from dental radiographic examinations in Japan. Jpn. Soc. Dent. Radiol. 31: 7-17 (1991).

M32 Maruyama, T., Y. Kumamoto, Y. Noda et al. Determinations of organ or tissue doses and collective effective dose equivalent from diagnostic x-ray examinations in Japan. Radiat. Prot. Dosim. 43: 213-216 (1992).

M33 Maglinte, D.D.T., R. Graffis, L. Jordan et al. Extracorporeal shock wave lithotripsy of gallbladder stones: a pessimistic view. Radiology 178: 29-32 (1991).

M34 Månsson, L.-G., S. Kheddache, J. Börjesson et al. Digital chest radiography with a large image intensifier. An ROC study with an anthropomorphic phantom. Eur. J. Radiol. 9: 208-213 (1989).

M35 MacDonald-Jankowski, D.S. and C.P. Lawinski. The reduction in radiation dose for intra-oral radiographs by the use of thin K-edge filters. Br. J. Radiol. 64: 524-528 (1991).

M36 Morse, M.H. CT scan radiation dosage. Br. Dent. J. 170: 366 (1991).

M37 Mini, R., P. Schneeberger and J. Feuz. Die Strahlenbelastung der Organe bei Schirmbildaufnahmen. Schweiz. Med. Wochenschr. 121: 938-942 (1991).

M38 Maccia, C., B.M. Moores, U. Nahrstedt et al. CEC Quality Criteria for Diagnostic Radiographic Images and Patient Exposure Trial. EUR-12952 (1990).

M39 Mikušová, M. and A. Drábková. Evaluation of irradiation of patients during x-ray examinations on examination plates. Cesk. Radiol. 45: 159-165 (1991).

M40 Maccia, C. Trends in medical diagnostic radiology in France: Comparison of patient age distribution between 1982 and 1988. Radiat. Prot. Dosim. 36: 253-256 (1991).

M41 Mettler Jr., F.A., J.H. Christie, A.G. Williams Jr. et al. Population characteristics and absorbed dose to the population from nuclear medicine: United States - 1982. Health Phys. 50: 619-628 (1986).

M42 MacDonald-Jankowski, D.S. and C.P. Lawinski. The effect of thin K-edge filters on radiation dose in dental radiography. Br. J. Radiol. 65: 990-995 (1992).

M43 Mejia, A.A., T. Nakamura, M. Itoh et al. Absorbed dose estimates in positron emission tomography studies based on the administration of ^{18}F-labeled radiopharmaceuticals. J. Radiat. Res. 32: 243-261 (1991).

M44 Maruyama, T., Y. Kumamoto, Y. Noda et al. Estimation of frequency, collective effective dose and population doses from radiographic dental examinations in Japan, 1989. National Institute of Radiological Sciences, NIRS-30 (1991).

N1 National Council on Radiation Protection and Measurements. Exposure of the U.S. population from diagnostic medical radiation. NCRP Report No. 100 (1989).

N2 Norman, A., A.R. Kagan and S.L. Chan. The importance of genetics for the optimization of radiation therapy. Am. J. Clin. Oncol. 11: 84-88 (1988).

N3 National Council on Radiation Protection and Measurements. Quality assurance for diagnostic imaging equipment. NCRP Report No. 99 (1988).

N4 Nikitin, V.V., Y.O. Yakubovskij-Lipskij, S.A. Kalnickij et al. Statistics of medical exposure in the U.S.S.R. Radiat. Prot. Dosim. 36: 243-246 (1991).

N5 National Radiological Protection Board. Patient dose reduction in diagnostic radiology. Documents of the NRPB, Volume 1(3) (1990).

N6 National Council on Radiation Protection and Measurements. Radiation protection for medical and allied health personnel. NCRP Report No. 105 (1989).

N7 National Radiological Protection Board. Unpublished statistics (1990).

N8 Nishizawa, K., T. Maruyama, M. Takayama et al. Determinations of organ doses and effective dose equivalents from computed tomographic examination. Br. J. Radiol. 64: 20-28 (1991).

N9 Naidich, D.P., C.H. Marshall, C. Gribbin et al. Low-dose CT of the lungs: preliminary observations. Radiology 175: 729-731 (1990).

N10 Nemiro, E.A., M. Viderman, D.Ia. Gubatova et al. Comparative assessment of doses that patients are exposed to radiodiagnosis of urinary disorders. Vestn. Rentgenol. Radiol. 4: 36-39 (1989). (in Russian).

N11 National Radiological Protection Board. Protection of the patient in x-ray computed tomography. Documents of the NRPB, Volume 3(4) (1992).

N12 Noël, A., Bonnefoux, I., J. Stines et al. Exemple d'application d'un protocole de contrôle de qualité en mammographie. Feuill. Radiol. 31: 403-412 (1991).

N13 National Council on Radiation Protection and Measurements. Misadministration of radioactive material in medicine - scientific background. NCRP Commentary No. 7 (1991).

N14 National Council on Radiation Protection and Measurements. Mammography - a user's guide. NCRP Report No. 85 (1986).

O1 Oyama, Y., K. Imamura, H. Ashida et al. What is the clinical disadvantage of discarding old radiographs? Survey of patients not re-examined for a long time. Br. J. Radiol. 65: 668-671 (1992).

O2 Ohta, K., M. Kai and K. Kusama. Estimation of embryonic doses in radiological examination on upper GI-tract in Japan. p. 352-355 in: Worldwide Achievement in Public and Occupational Health Protection Against Radiation. Proceedings of the 8th International Congress of the International Radiation Protection Association, Montréal, 1992.

O3 Olsson, S. and S. Svahn. Radiologists link up with PACS. Medicinsk Teknik 4: 28-34 (1989). (in Swedish).

O4 Ott, R.J. Nuclear medicine in the 1990s: a quantitative physiological approach. Br. J. Radiol. 62: 421-432 (1989).

O5 Orito, T., S. Koga, A. Takeuchi et al. An analysis of the spatial dose distribution around the patient with therapeutic dose of ^{131}I. Hoken Butsuri 19: 3-11 (1984). (in Japanese).

O6 Orito, T., S. Koga, A. Takeuchi et al. An analysis of the spatial dose distribution around the patient with therapeutic dose of I-131. p. 202-205 in: Worldwide Achievement in Public and Occupational Health Protection Against Radiation. Proceedings of the 8th International Congress of the International Radiation Protection Association, Montreal, 1992.

O7 Oliveira, S.M.V., A.M.C. Araujo and G. Drexler. Ionizing radiation sources used in medical applications in Brazil. p. 228-231 in: Worldwide Achievement in Public and Occupational Health Protection Against Radiation. Proceedings of the 8th International Congress of the International Radiation Protection Association, Montréal, 1992.

P1 Prado, K.L., J.T. Rakowski, F. Barragan et al. Breast radiation dose in film/screen mammography. Health Phys. 55: 81-83 (1988).

P2 Pond, G.D., G.W. Seeley, T.W. Ovitt et al. Intraoperative arteriography: comparison of conventional screen-film with photostimulable imaging plate radiographs. Radiology 170: 367-370 (1989).

P3 Panzer, W., C. Scheurer, G. Drexler et al. Feldstudie zur Ermittlung von Dosiswerten bei der Computertomographie. Fortschr. Geb. Roentgenstr. Nuklearmed. 149: 534-538 (1988).

P4 Peixoto, J.E., M.C. Campos and R.Q. Chaves. A database for the national radiation control programme in medical and dental radiography. International Atomic Energy Agency: Radiation Protection Infrastructure. IAEA-SM-309/50, Vienna, 1990.

P5 Properzio, W.S., R.L. Burkhart and R.E. Gross. Quality assurance in diagnostic radiology: the economic and radiation protection impact of a nationwide voluntary programme. p. 50-57 in: Radiation Protection: Patient Exposure to Radiation in Medical X-ray Diagnosis. (G. Drexler, H. Eriskat and H. Schibilla, eds.) CEC, Brussels, 1981.

P6 Patterson, J. and D. Summer. Irradiation of volunteers in nuclear medicine. J. Nucl. Med. 30: 2062-2063 (1989).

P7 Petoussi, N., M. Zankl, F.-E. Stieve et al. Patient organ doses for proposed technical parameters and their variations. p. 246-249 in: Optimization of Image Quality and Patient Exposure in Diagnostic Radiology. (B.M. Moores et al., eds.) British Institute of Radiology, Report 20, London, 1989.

P8 Plowman, P.N. and A.N. Harnett (eds.). Megavoltage radiotherapy 1937-1987. Br. J. Radiol. (Suppl.) 22: (1988).

P9 Panzer, W. and M. Zankl. A method for estimating embryo doses resulting from computed tomographic examinations. Br. J. Radiol. 62: 936-939 (1989).

P10 Panzer, W., C. Scheurer and M. Zankl. Dose to patients in computed tomographic examinations: results and consequences from a field study in the Federal Republic of Germany. p. 185-188 in: Optimization of Image Quality and Patient Exposure in Diagnostic Radiology. (B.M. Moores et al. eds.) British Institute of Radiology, Report 20, London, 1989.

P11 Poletti, J.L. Radiation dose and image quality of CT scanners: Summary of NRL surveys 1980-1987. NRL 1988/1 (1988).

P12 Pukkila, O. and K. Karila. Interventional Radiology - A New Challenge for Radiation Protection. Nordic Society for Radiation Protection, Ronneby, 1990.

P13 Peters, A.M. Recent advances and future projections in clinical radionuclide imaging. Br. J. Radiol. 63: 411-429 (1990).

P14 Pellerin, Y. and J.P. Moroni. Dose measurements on phantom and patient in dental radiography. SCPRI (1983).

P15 Pugin, J.M., J. Stines, A. Noël et al. Les contrôles de qualité en mammographie. Feuill. Radiol. 31: 307-321 (1991).

P16 Pötter, R., A. Naszály, A. Hemprich et al. Neutron radiotherapy in adenoidcystic carcinoma: preliminary experience at the Münster neutron facility. Strahlenther. Onkol. 166: 78-85 (1990).

P17 Parker, B.R., S.G. Moore, C.J. Bergin et al. Dose reduction in pediatric body CT with ceramic detectors. Radiology 173 (Suppl.): 374 (1989).

P18 Preston-Martin, S., D.C. Thomas, S.C. White et al. Prior exposure to medical and dental x-rays related to tumors of the parotid gland. J. Natl. Cancer Inst. 80: 943-949 (1988).

P19 Padovani, R., G. Contento, M. Fabretto et al. Patient doses and risks from diagnostic radiology in north-east Italy. Br. J. Radiol. 60: 155-165 (1987).

P20 Papadopoulos, G. and D. Okkalides. Dose to patients through nuclear medicine procedures in a department in northern Greece. Eur. J. Nucl. Med. 17: 212-215 (1990).

P21 Peene, P., G. Wilms, A.L. Baert et al. Low dose digital peripheral angiography with continuous C-arm movement. Electromedica 59: 110-114 (1991).

P22 Podoloff, D.A., E.E. Kim and T.P. Haynie. SPECT in the evaluation of cancer patients: Not Quo Vadis; rather, Ibi Fere Summus. Radiology 183: 305-317 (1992).

P23 Piyasena, R.D., A. Cuarón and M. Nofal. Nuclear techniques in the detection and management of cancer. Int. At. Energy Agency Bull. 1: 4-8 (1991).

P24 Pinillos Ashton, L. Analisis del valor de la radioterapia no convencional en cancer localmente avanzado de la mama (estadio clinico III). M.D. Thesis, Universidad Peruana Cayetano Heredia, Lima, 1990.

R1 Rowley, K.A., S.J. Hill, R.A. Watkins et al. An investigation into the levels of radiation exposure in diagnostic examinations involving fluoroscopy. Br. J. Radiol. 60: 167-173 (1987).

R2 Rosenkranz, G., L. Berndt, S. Geissler et al. Die Strahlenbelastung von Linse und Gonaden bei ausgewahlten CT-Untersuchungen. Digit. Bilddiagn. 7: 177-182 (1987).

R3 Rao, P.N., K. Faulkner, J.K. Sweeney et al. Radiation dose to patient and staff during percutaneous nephrostolithotomy. Br. J. Urol. 59: 508-512 (1987).

R4 Regano, L.J. and R.A. Sutton. Radiation dose reduction in diagnostic x-ray exposures. Phys. Med. Biol. 37: 1773-1778 (1992).

R5 Rainbow, A.J., P. Roginski and W. McGeen. Radiation risk to the patient: A case study involving multiple diagnostic x ray exposures given over a period of 25 years. Radiat. Prot. Dosim. 43: 221-224 (1992).
R6 Roberts, M.M., F.E. Alexander, T.J. Andersson et al. The Edinburgh randomized screening for breast cancer: description of method. Br. J. Cancer 50: 77 (1984).
R7 Racoveanu, N.T. Radiotherapy in developing countries: constraints and possible solutions. p. 381-402 in: Radiotherapy in Developing Countries. IAEA, Vienna, 1987.
R8 Romner, B., B. Ljunggren, L. Brandt et al. Transcranial doppler sonography in the first 12 hours after subarachnoid hemorrhage. J. Neurosurg. 70: 732-736 (1989).
R9 Ranniko, S., A. Servomaa, I. Ermakov et al. Calculation of the estimated collective effective dose equivalent (SE) due to x-ray diagnostic examinations - estimate of the SE in Finland. Health Phys. 53: 31-36 (1987).
R10 Renaud, L. and J. Blanchette. Radiological impact of diagnostic nuclear medicine technology on the Québec population (patients and workers) in 1989. p. 194-197 in: Worldwide Achievement in Public and Occupational Health Protection Against Radiation. Proceedings of the 8th International Congress of the International Radiation Protection Association, Montreal, 1992.
R11 Royal, H.D. Clinical applications of positron emission tomography in cancer: The good, the bad and the ugly. J. Nucl. Med. 33: 330-332 (1992).
R12 Rueter, F.G., B.J. Conway, J.L. McCrohan et al. Assessment of skin entrance kerma in the United States: The nationwide evaluation of x ray trends (NEXT). Radiat. Prot. Dosim. 43: 71-73 (1992).
R13 Rudin, S. and D.R. Bednarek. Minimizing radiation dose to patient and staff during fluoroscopic, nasoenteral tube insertions. Br. J. Radiol. 65: 162-166 (1992).
R14 Rueter, F.G., B.J. Conway, J.L. McCrohan et al. Average radiation exposure values for three diagnostic radiographic examinations. Radiology 177: 341-345 (1990).
R15 Roedler, H.D. and E. Pittelkow. Strahlenexposition des Patienten bei der nuklearmedizinischen Anwendung markierter monoklonaler Antikörper. ISH-143/90 (1990).
R16 Rannikko, S. Communication to UNSCEAR Secretariat. Finland (1990).
R17 Roehrig, H., T.W. Ovitt, G.W. Seeley et al. A new method to determine the lower limits in patient exposure: stacked computed radiography (CR) image detectors. SPIE Semin. Proc. 1231: 479-491 (1990).
R18 Rothenberg, L.N. Patient dose in mammography. Radiographics 10: 739-746 (1990).
R19 Rimondi, O., M. Gambaccini, M. Marziani et al. Il programma DQM e la garanzia della qualità nella mammografia. Radiol. Med. 81: 69-72 (1991).
R20 Rudin, S., D.R. Bednarek and J.A. Miller. Dose reduction during fluoroscopic placement of feeding tubes. Radiology 178: 647-651 (1991).
R21 Robertson, J.S., M.D. Ezekowitz, M.K. Dewanjee et al. MIRD dose estimate no. 15: Radiation absorbed dose estimates for radioindium-labeled autologous platelets. J. Nucl. Med. 33: 777-780 (1992).
R22 Ruiz, M.J., L. González, E. Vañó et al. Measurement of radiation doses in the most frequent simple examinations in paediatric radiology and its dependence on patient age. Br. J. Radiol. 64: 929-933 (1991).
R23 Rosenstein, M., T.J. Beck and G.G. Warner. Handbook of selected organ doses for projections common in pediatric radiology. HEW (FDA) 79-8079 (1979).
R24 Rosenstein, M., O.H. Suleiman, R.L. Burkhart et al. Handbook of selected tissue doses for the upper gastrointestinal fluoroscopic examination. HHS (FDA) 92-8282 (1992).
R25 Rannikko, S. Problems concerning the assessment of the radiation dose to a population as a result of x-ray examinations. Institute of Radiation Protection, Report STL-A37, Helsinki (1981).
R26 Royal College of Radiologists. Making the Best Use of a Department of Radiology - Guidelines for Doctors. RCR, London, United Kingdom, 1988.
R27 Roberts, P.J. Patient dosimetry in diagnostic radiology. ICRU News (Dec.): 10-13 (1992).
R28 Rosenstein, M. Handbook of selected tissue doses for projections common in diagnostic radiology. HEW (FDA) 89-8031 (1988).
S1 Stenström, B., K. Bergman, P.G. Blomgren et al. Collective dose to the Swedish population from intraoral radiography. Swed. Dent. J. 12: 17-25 (1988).
S2 South East Thames Regional Health Authority. Making the best of an imaging department. SETRHA, United Kingdom (1990).
S3 Stenström, B., C.O. Henrikson, L. Karlsson et al. Effective dose equivalent from intraoral radiography. Swed. Dent. J. 11: 71-77 (1987).
S4 Siewert, H. Strahlenschutzprobleme bei der Betreuung von stationären Patienten nach nuklearmedizinischer Diagnostik. Med. Nucl. 1: 29-36 (1989).
S5 Schulman, S. Contrast sharpens MR images. Medicinsk Teknik 6-7: 6-10 (1989). (in Swedish).
S6 Smathers, J.B. Uses of ionizing radiation and medical-care-related problems. Health Phys. 55: 165-167 (1988).
S7 Stieve, F.E. Strahlenexposition von Patienten bei röntgendiagnostischen Massnahmen. p. 37-78 in: Strahlenschutz in Forschung und Praxis 23. G. Thieme Verlag, Stuttgart, New York, 1982.
S8 Strand, S.E. Communication to UNSCEAR Secretariat. University of Lund, Sweden (1989).
S9 Scott Jr., W.W., E.K. Fishman and D. Magid. Acetabular fractures: optimal imaging. Radiology 165: 537-539 (1987).
S10 Skoczylas, L.J., J.W. Preece, R.P. Langlais et al. Comparison of x-radiation doses between conventional and rare earth panoramic techniques. Oral Surg., Oral Med., Oral Pathol. 68: 776-781 (1989).
S11 Sewerin, I. Radiation doses from x-ray examinations in fitting bone-integrated implants for missing teeth. Tandlaegebl. 93: 657-660 (1989). (in Danish).
S12 Sjukvårdens Planerings- och Rationaliseringsinstitut. Magnetic resonance tomography - use and distribution in Nordic countries. SPRI-Report 279 (1990). (in Swedish).

S13 Skubic, S.E., R. Yagan, A. Oravec et al. Value of increasing film processing time to reduce radiation dose during mammography. Am. J. Roentgenol. 155: 1189-1193 (1990).

S14 Sjukvårdens Planerings- och Rationaliseringsinstitut. Radiologists in Nordic countries - summary report. SPRI-Report 275 (1989). (in Swedish).

S15 Stather, J.W., J.D. Harrison and G.M. Kendall. Radiation doses to the embryo and fetus following intakes of radionuclides by the mother. Radiat. Prot. Dosim. 41: 111-118 (1992).

S16 Stieve, F.-E. Institute for Radiation Hygiene, Neuherberg, Germany. Communication to the UNSCEAR Secretariat (1993).

S17 Schibilla, H. Reduction of Patient Exposure in Diagnostic Radiology; A Task of the CEC Radiation Protection Research Programme. Nordic Society for Radiation Protection, Ronneby, 1990.

S18 Stavitsky, R.V., F.M. Lyass, I.E. Kagan et al. Radiodiagnostic dose exposure of the USSR population and measures to reduce it. Med. Radiol. 35: 5-7 (1990). (in Russian).

S19 Schneider, K., H. Fendel, C. Bakowski et al. Results of a dosimetry study in the European Community on frequent x-ray examinations in infants. Radiat. Prot. Dosim. 43: 31-36 (1992).

S20 Swift, M., D. Morrell, R.B. Massey et al. Incidence of cancer in 161 families affected by ataxia-telangiectasia. N. Engl. J. Med. 325: 1831-1836 (1991).

S21 Statistiska Centralbyrån. Statistical abstract of Sweden 1990. Statistics Sweden, Stockholm, 1989.

S22 Saxeboel, G., H.M. Olerud and L.E. Lundgren. Radiation hygiene analysis of radiological activities in Norway. p. 139-147 in: Radiation and Cancer Risk. (T. Brustad, F. Langmark and J.B. Reitan, eds.) Hemisphere Publishing Co., New York, 1989.

S23 Shrimpton, P.C., B.F. Wall, D.G. Jones et al. A national survey of doses to patients undergoing a selection of routine x-ray examinations in English hospitals. NRPB-R200 (1986).

S24 Schaefer, C.M., R.E. Greene, J.W. Oestmann et al. Improved control of image optical density with low-dose digital and conventional radiography in bedside imaging. Radiology 173: 713-716 (1989).

S25 Sakurai, K., J. Hachiya, T. Korenaga et al. Digital radiography of the chest - evaluation of normal anatomical structure and low dose radiography. Nippon Acta Radiol. 44: 11-22 (1984).

S26 Shin, J.H., J. Oestmann, D. Hall et al. Subtle gastric abnormalities in a canine model: detection with low-dose imaging with storage phosphors and its equivalence to conventional radiography. Radiology 172: 399-401 (1989).

S27 Sorenson, J.A. Relationship between patient exposure and measurement precision in dual-photon absorptiometry of the spine. Phys. Med. Biol. 36: 169-176 (1991).

S28 Segal, P. and D.R. Hamilton. Recommendations for Quality Assurance Programs in Nuclear Medicine Facilities. HHS (FDA) 85-8227 (1984).

S29 Siddle, K.J., L.H. Sim and C.C. Case. Radiation doses to the lens of the eye during computerised tomography of the orbit; a comparison of four modern computerised tomography units. Australas. Radiol. 34: 323-325 (1990).

S30 Siddle, K.J. and L. Sim. Radiation dose to the lens of the eye during computerised tomography examinations of the orbit, the pituitary fossa and the brain on a general electric 9800 quick C.T. scanner. Australas. Radiol. 34: 326-330 (1990).

S31 Servomaa, A. and M. Tapiovaara. Radiation quality in assessing glandular dose in film-screen mammography. Phys. Med. Biol. 36: 1247-1248 (1991).

S32 Scher, E.L.C. CT scan radiation dosage. Br. Dent. J. 170: 254 (1991).

S33 Sewerin, I. Radiation doses from x-ray examinations with panorama techniques and with intraoral dental film - an overview. Tandlaegebl. 93: 351-356 (1989). (in Danish).

S34 Suleiman, O.H., J. Anderson, B. Jones et al. Tissue doses in the upper gastrointestinal fluoroscopy examination. Radiology 178: 653-658 (1991).

S35 Suit, H., S. Skates, A. Taghian et al. Clinical implications of heterogeneity of tumor response to radiation therapy. Radiother. Oncol. 25: 251-260 (1992).

S36 Shrimpton, P.C. Quality assurance in radiotherapy. Radiol. Prot. Bull. 127: 4-7 (1991).

S37 Schaberg, J. Strahlenexpositionen bei angiographischen Röntgenuntersuchungen und ein Verglich zwischen der digitalen Technik und konventionellen Methoden. M.D. Dissertation, University of Düsseldorf, Germany, 1987.

S38 Shrimpton, P.C., B.F. Wall and M.C. Hillier. Suggested guideline doses for medical examinations. p. 85-88 in: Radiation Protection - Theory and Practice. (E.P. Goldfinch, ed.) IOPP, Bristol, 1989.

S39 Shrimpton, P.C., D.G. Jones and B.F. Wall. The influence of tube filtration and potential on patient dose during x-ray examinations. Phys. Med. Biol. 33: 1205-1212 (1988).

S40 Supe, S.J., P.S. Iyer, J.B. Sasane et al. Estimation and significance of patient doses from diagnostic x-ray practices in India. Radiat. Prot. Dosim. 43: 209-211 (1992).

S41 Staniszewska, M.A. Radiation risk to patients from nuclear medicine in Poland (1981). Eur. J. Nucl. Med. 13: 307-310 (1987).

S42 Shrimpton, P.C., D. Hart, M.C. Hillier et al. Survey of CT practice in the UK. Part 1: Aspects of examination frequency and quality assurance. NRPB-R248 (1991).

S43 Shrimpton, P.C., D.G. Jones, M.C. Hillier et al. Survey of CT practice in the UK. Part 2: Dosimetric aspects. NRPB-R249 (1991).

S44 Servomaa, A., S. Rannikko and I. Ermakov. Assessment of effective dose in x ray imaging in view of the proposed ICRP risk factors. Radiat. Prot. Dosim. 43: 225-227 (1992).

S45 Stavitskij, R.V., I.A. Ermakov, L.A. Lebedev et al. Equivalent doses to organs and tissues in x-ray examinations - an inquiry. Energoatomizdat, Moscow, 1989. (in Russian).

S46 Stieve, F.-E., M. Zankl, U. Nahrstedt et al. Entrance dose measurements on patients and their relation to organ doses. Radiat. Prot. Dosim. 43: 161-163 (1992).

S47 Shields, R.A. and R.S. Lawson. Effective dose equivalent. Nucl. Med. Commun. 8: 851-855 (1987).

S48 Sastry, K.S.R. Biological effects of the Auger emitter iodine-125: A review. Report no. 1 of AAPM nuclear medicine task group no. 6. Med. Phys. 19: 1361-1370 (1992).
S49 Stubbs, J.B. and L.A. Wilson. Nuclear medicine: A state-of-the-art review. Nuclear News (May): 50-54 (1991).
S50 Shapiro, B., M. Pillay and P.H. Cox. Dosimetric consequences of interstitial extravasation following IV administration of a radiopharmaceutical. Eur. J. Nucl. Med. 12: 522-523 (1987).
S51 Smyth, V.G. A new code of safe practice for the use of irradiating apparatus in radiotherapy. Radiat. Prot. News and Notes 18: 9-13 (1992).
S52 Serro, R., J.V. Carreiro, J.P. Galvào et al. Population dose assessment from radiodiagnosis in Portugal. Radiat. Prot. Dosim. 43: 65-68 (1992).
S53 Suleiman, O.H., B.J. Conway, F.G. Rueter et al. Automatic film processing: Analysis of 9 years of observations. Radiology 185: 25-28 (1992).
S54 Suleiman, O.H., R. Antonsen, B. Conway et al. Assessing patient exposure in fluoroscopy. Radiat. Prot. Dosim. 43: 251-252 (1992).
S55 Schüller, H., O. Köster and K. Ewen. Untersuchung zur Strahlenbelastung von Augenlinse und Schilddrüse bei der hochauflösenden Computertomographie der Zähne. Fortschr. Geb. Roentgenstr. Nuklearmed. 156: 189-192 (1992).
S56 Stines, J., A. Noël, P. Troufleau et al. Facteurs de qualité et mesures de dose en mammographie. Feuill. Radiol. 31: 247-259 (1991).
S57 Schueler, B.A., J.E. Gray and J.J. Gisvold. A comparison of mammography screen-film combinations. Radiology 184: 629-634 (1992).
T1 Tabar, L., C.J. Fagerberg, A. Gad et al. Reduction in mortality from breast cancer after mass screening with mammography. Lancet I: 829-832 (1985).
T2 Tyndall, D.A., S.R. Matteson, R.E. Soltmann et al. Exposure reduction in cephalometric radiology: a comprehensive approach. Am. J. Orthod. Dentofacial Orthop. 93: 400-412 (1988).
T3 Taylor, T.S., R.J. Ackerman and P.K. Hardman. Exposure reduction and image quality in orthodontic radiology: a review of the literature. Am. J. Orthod. Dentofacial Orthop. 93: 68-77 (1988).
T4 Taylor, D.M., G.B. Gerber and J.W. Stather (eds.). Age-dependent factors in the biokinetics and dosimetry of radionuclides. Radiat. Prot. Dosim. 41 (2-4) (1992).
T5 Tanaka, G. Reference Japanese, Vol. 1: Anatomical data. National Institute of Radiological Sciences, NIRS-M-85, 1992.
T6 Taylor, D.M. Why is age-dependent dosimetry important? Radiat. Prot. Dosim. 41: 51-54 (1992).
T7 Tyndall, D.A. Order of magnitude absorbed dose reductions in cephalometric radiography. Health Phys. 56: 533-538 (1989).
T8 Tole, N.M. Studies of patient dose during x-ray diagnosis in Kenya. Radiography 54: 29-31 (1988).
T9 Taylor, C., A.R. Cowen and I.J. Wilson. Patient absorbed doses in digital subtraction angiography. p. 200-202 in: Optimization of Image Quality and Patient Exposure in Diagnostic Radiology. (B.M. Moores, B.F. Wall, H. Eriskat et al., eds.) British Institute of Radiology, Report 20, London, 1989.
T10 Tateno, Y., T. Iinuma and M. Takano (eds.). Computed Radiography. Springer-Verlag, Tokyo, 1987.
T11 Thijssen, M.A., K.R. Bijkerk and J.H. Hendriks. The Dutch protocol for quality assurance in mammography screening. Radiat. Prot. Dosim. 43: 273-275 (1992).
T12 Tautz, M. and G.-A. Brandt. Abschätzung von Organdosen bei standardisierten Röntgenuntersuchungen im Kindesalter. Radiol. Diagn. 29: 169-179 (1988).
T13 Torabinejad, M., R. Danforth and K. Andrews. Absorbed radiation by various tissues during simulated endodontic radiography. J. Endod. 15: 249-253 (1989).
T14 Thoeni, R.F. and R.G. Gould. Enteroclysis and small bowel series: comparison of radiation dose and examination time. Radiology 178: 659-662 (1991).
T15 Thomas, S.R., M.G. Stabin, C.-T. Chen et al. MIRD pamphlet no. 14: A dynamic urinary bladder model for radiation dose calculations. J. Nucl. Med. 33: 783-802 (1992).
T16 Tilyou, S.M. The evolution of positron emission tomography. J. Nucl. Med. 32(4): 15N-26N (1991).
T17 Townsend, D. and M. Defrise (eds.) Fully three-dimensional image reconstruction in nuclear medicine and radiology. Proceedings of an international meeting. Phys. Med. Biol. 37(3): (1992).
T18 Trott, N.G. Radionuclides in brachytherapy: Radium and after. Br. J. Radiol. (Suppl.) 21: (1987).
T19 Thomson, J.E.M., B.F. Young, J.G. Young et al. Radiation doses from mammography in Australia. ARL/TR101 (1991).
T20 Thilander, A., S. Eklund, W. Leitz et al. Special problems of patient dosimetry in mammography. Radiat. Prot. Dosim. 43: 217-220 (1992).
U1 United Nations. Sources, Effects and Risks of Ionizing Radiation. United Nations Scientific Committee on the Effects of Atomic Radiation, 1988 Report to the General Assembly, with annexes. United Nations sales publication E.88.IX.7. United Nations, New York, 1988.
U3 United Nations. Ionizing Radiation: Sources and Biological Effects. United Nations Scientific Committee on the Effects of Atomic Radiation, 1982 Report to the General Assembly, with annexes. United Nations sales publication E.82.IX.8. United Nations, New York, 1982.
U4 United Nations. Sources and Effects of Ionizing Radiation. United Nations Scientific Committee on the Effects of Atomic Radiation, 1977 report to the General Assembly, with annexes. United Nations sales publication E.77.IX.1. United Nations, New York, 1977.
U5 United Nations. Ionizing Radiation: Levels and Effects. Report of the United Nations Scientific Committee on the Effects of Atomic Radiation, with annexes. United Nations sales publication E.72.IX.17 and 18. United Nations, New York, 1972.
U9 United Nations. Report of the United Nations Scientific Committee on the Effects of Atomic Radiation. Official Records of the General Assembly, Seventeenth Session, Supplement No. 16 (A/5216). New York, 1962.

U10 United Nations. Report of the United Nations Scientific Committee on the Effects of Atomic Radiation. Official Records of the General Assembly, Thirteenth Session, Supplement No. 17 (A/3838). New York, 1958.

U11 United States Public Health Service. The selection of patients for X-ray examinations; pelvimetry examination. Centre for Devices and Radiological Health. Department of Health and Human Services, 1980.

U12 United States Public Health Service. The selection of patients for X-ray examinations; presurgical chest X-ray screening examinations. Centre for Devices and Radiological Health. Deptartment of Health and Human Services, 1986.

U13 United States Public Health Service. The selection of patients for X-ray examinations; skull X-ray examination for trauma. Centre for Devices and Radiological Health. Department of Health and Human Services, 1986.

U14 United States Public Health Service. The selection of patients for X-ray examinations; dental radiographic examinations. Centre for Devices and Radiological Health. Department of Health and Human Services, 1987.

U15 United States Public Health Service. The selection of patients for X-ray examinations. Bureau of Radiological Health. Department of Health, Education and Welfare, 1980.

U16 United States Food and Drug Administration. Prescription drugs for human use generally recognized as safe and effective and not misbranded: drugs used in research. Part 361, Title 10, Code of Federal Regulations (1975).

U17 United Nations. Demographic Yearbook 1989. United Nations, New York, 1991.

U18 United Nations. Statistical Yearbook. United Nations, New York, 1987.

V1 Valentin, J. and W. Leitz. Mass screening for breast cancer: benefits, risks, costs. Med. Oncol. & Tumour Pharmacother. 5: 77-83 (1988).

V2 van der Stelt, P.F. and A. Zwigt. Dose distribution in oral radiography. p. 760-763 in: Radiation Protection Practice. Proceedings of the 7th International Congress of the International Radiation Protection Association, Sydney, 1988.

V3 Veit, R. and M. Zankl. Influence of patient size on organ doses in diagnostic radiology. Radiat. Prot. Dosim. 43: 241-244 (1992).

V4 Valentin, J., P.G. Blomgren, G. Hellström et al. New trends affecting Swedish patient doses from diagnostic procedures. p. 720-723 in: Radiation Protection Practice. Proceedings of the 7th International Congress of the International Radiation Protection Association, Sydney, 1988.

V5 Vañó, E., L. González, A. Calzado et al. Some indicative parameters on diagnostic radiology in Spain: first dose estimations. Br. J. Radiol. 62: 20-26 (1989).

V6 Verbeek, A., J. Hendriks, R. Holland et al. Reduction of breast cancer mortality through mass screening with modern mammography. First results of the Nijmegen project, 1975-1981. Lancet I: 1222-1224 (1984).

V7 Veit, R., W. Panzer, M. Zankl et al. Vergleich berechneter und gemessener Dosen an einem antropomorphen Phantom. Z. Med. Phys. 2: 123-126 (1992).

V8 Vetter, R.J., J.E. Gray and J.M. Kofler. Patient radiation doses at a large tertiary care medical center. Radiat. Prot. Dosim. 36: 247-251 (1991).

V9 Valentin, J. and G.A.M. Webb. Medical uses of radiation: Retaining the benefit but recognising the harm. in: Radiation Protection Toward the Turn of the Century, Paris, 1993. (in press)

V10 Velders, X.L. and P.F. van der Stelt. Patient exposure in general dental practice in the Netherlands. p. 208-209 in: Optimization of Image Quality and Patient Exposure in Diagnostic Radiology. (B.M. Moores et al., eds.) British Institute of Radiology, Report 20, London, 1989.

V11 Veit, R. and M. Zankl. Influence of patient size on organ doses in diagnostic radiology. Radiat. Prot. Dosim. 43: 241-243 (1992).

V12 Velders, X.L., J. van Aken and P.F. van der Stelt. Risk assessment from bitewing radiography. Dento-Maxillo-Facial Radiol. 19: 209-213 (1991).

V13 Vehmas, T., R. Havukainen, M. Tapiovaara et al. Radiation exposure during percutaneous nephrostomy. Fortschr. Roentgenstr. 154: 238-241 (1991).

V14 Vogel, H. Strahlendosis und Strahlenrisiko in der bildgebenden Diagnostik. Ecomed Verlagsgesellschaft, Landsberg, Germany, 1989.

V15 Vasisht, C.M. and Y.Y. Bakir. Radiation protection surveys - as an optimising procedure in diagnostic radiology. p. 775-778 in: Radiation Protection Practice. Proceedings of the 7th International Congress of the International Radiation Protection Association, Sydney, 1988.

V16 van Kempen, R.J. Pattern of diagnostic procedures in radiology in the Netherlands. Radiat. Prot Dosim. 36: 257-259 (1991).

V17 Vessey, M. Breast Cancer Screening 1991: Evidence and Experience since the Forrest Report. NHSBSP Publications, Sheffield, United Kingdom, 1991.

V18 Vañó, E., L. González, A. Calzado et al. Some results of a patient dose survey in the area of Madrid. p. 180-185 in: Optimization of Image Quality and Patient Exposure in Diagnostic Radiology. (B.M. Moores, B.F. Wall, H. Eriskat et al., eds.) British Institute of Radiology, Report 20, London, 1989.

V19 Vetter, R.J., J.E. Gray and J.M. Kofler. Patient radiation doses at a large tertiary care medical centre. Radiat. Prot. Dosim. 36: 247-251 (1991).

W1 World Health Organization. World Health Statistics Annual. WHO, Geneva, 1980.

W2 Weingärtner, R., V. Schuchardt, H.H. Thiemann et al. Strahlenbelastung Frühgeborener durch Röntgenaufnahmen des Thorax. Kinderärztl. Prax. 57: 33-35 (1989).

W3 World Health Organization. WHO/BRS Basic Radiology System. WHO, Geneva, 1986.

W4 Williamson, B.D.P. Review of the results of routine radiation protection surveys of radiography-only diagnostic x-ray machines, February 1987 - May 1991. NRL 1991/1 (1991).

W5 Workman, A. and A.R. Cowen. Exposure monitoring in photostimulable phosphor computed radiography. Radiat. Prot. Dosim. 43: 135-138 (1992).

W6 Weber, D.A., P.T. Makler, E.E. Watson et al. Radiation absorbed dose from Technetium-99m-labeled bone imaging agents. J. Nucl. Med. 30: 1117-1122 (1989).

W7 Wang, S. and X. Liu. Nuclear medicine in China. p. 555 in: Nuclear Medicine and Related Radionuclide Applications in Developing Countries. IAEA, Vienna, 1986.

W8 Williams, L.E., J.Y.C. Wong, D.O. Findley et al. Measurement and estimation of organ bremsstrahlung radiation dose. J. Nucl. Med. 30: 1373-1377 (1989).

W9 Wall, B.F., M.C. Hillier and G.M. Kendall. An update on the frequency of medical and dental x-ray examinations in Great Britain, 1983. NRPB-R201 (1986).

W10 Walstam, R. Karolinska Institute, Stockholm, Sweden. Communication to the UNSCEAR Secretariat (1990).

W11 Williamson, B.D.P. and J.L. Poletti. Radiation doses and some aspects of image quality in mammography facilities in New Zealand. NRL 1990/1 (1990).

W12 Williamson, B.D.P. Radiation doses to patients from dental radiography in New Zealand. NRL 1990/6 (1990).

W13 Wahner, H.W., W.L. Dunn, M.L. Brown et al. Comparison of dual-energy x-ray absorptiometry and dual-photon absorptiometry for bone mineral measurements of the lumbar spine. Mayo Clin. Proc. 63: 1075-1084 (1988).

W14 Wu, X., G.T. Barnes and D.M. Tucker. Spectral dependence of glandular tissue dose in screen-film mammography. Radiology 179: 143-148 (1991).

W15 Williamson, B.D.P. Rare earth metal filters in diagnostic radiography. Radiat. Prot. News and Notes 6: 10-13 (1989).

W16 Wu, J.-R., T.-Y. Huang, D.-K. Wu et al. Radiation exposure of pediatric patients and physicians during cardiac catheterization and balloon pulmonary valvuloplasty. Am. J. Cardiol. 68: 221-225 (1991).

W17 Wallis, J.W. and T.R. Miller. Three-dimensional display in nuclear medicine and radiology. J. Nucl. Med. 32: 534-546 (1991).

W18 Walker, A., K. Horner, J. Czajka et al. Quantitative assessment of a new dental imaging system. Br. J. Radiol. 64: 529-536 (1991).

W19 Wenzel, A. Radiographic screening for identification of children in need of orthodontic treatment? Dento-Maxillo-Facial Radiol. 20: 115-116 (1991).

W20 Wall, B.F. and P.C. Shrimpton. Patient exposure criteria. p. 239-241 in: Optimization of Image Quality and Patient Exposure in Diagnostic Radiology. (B.M. Moores, B.F. Wall, H. Eriskat et al., eds.) British Institute of Radiology, Report 20, London, 1989.

W21 Westmore, D.D. Relative radiation dosage in renal diagnostic modalities. Med. J. Aust. 3: 422-423 (1989).

W22 Wall, B.F. and J.G.B. Russell. The application of cost-utility analysis to radiological protection in diagnostic radiology. J. Radiol. Prot. 8: 221-229 (1988).

W23 World Health Organization. A rational approach to radiodiagnostic investigations. WHO, Report TRS 689, Geneva, 1983.

W24 World Health Organization. Future use of new imaging technologies in developing countries. WHO, Report TRS 723, Geneva, 1985.

W25 World Health Organization. Rational use of diagnostic imaging in paediatrics. WHO, Report TRS 757, Geneva, 1987.

W26 World Health Organization. Effective choices for diagnostic imaging in clinical practice. WHO, Report TRS 795, Geneva, 1990.

W27 Withers, H.R. The EORTC hyperfractionation trial. Radiother. Oncol. 25: 229-230 (1992).

W28 Wall, B.F. Radiation exposure of the patient in diagnostic radiology. Paper submitted at a Workshop: European School of Radiological Protection, Radiation Protection of the Patient. Neuherberg, 1992.

W29 Wackers, F.J.T. Planar, SPECT, PET: The quest to predict the unpredictable? J. Nucl. Med. 31: 1906-1908 (1990).

W30 White, S.C. 1992 assessment of radiation risk from dental radiography. Dento-Maxillo-Facial Radiol. 21: 118-126 (1992).

W31 White, S.C. and B.M. Gratt. Evaluation of Niobi-X filtration in intraoral radiology. Oral Surg., Oral Med., Oral Pathol. 72: 746-755 (1991).

W32 Whall, M.A. and P.J. Roberts. Radiation dose in relation to compressed breast thickness for screening mammography. Radiat. Prot. Dosim. 253-255 (1992).

W33 Wade, J.P. Accuracy of pelvimetry measurements on CT scanners. Br. J. Radiol. 65: 261-263 (1992).

W34 Williams, G., M. Zankl and G. Drexler. The calculation of dose from external photon exposures using reference human phantoms and Monte-Carlo methods. 4. Organ doses in radiotherapy. GSF-S-1054 (1984).

Y1 Yu, X., X. He, Y. Yuan et al. Body surface exposure from diagnostic chest x-ray examinations in population of Hunan Province. Chin. J. Radiol. Med. Prot. 8: 244-246 (1988). (in Chinese).

Y2 Yoshizumi, T.T. and C.A. Chuprinko. Accidental CT scanning without Al filtration and its dosimetry. Health Phys. 56: 253-254 (1989).

Z1 Zheng, J., F. Sun, D. Jia et al. Estimation and assessment of population doses from diagnostic x-ray procedures in Beijing. Proc. CAMS and PUMC 3: 12-19 (1988).

Z2 Zankl, M., R. Veit, G. Williams et al. The construction of computer tomographic phantoms and their application in radiology and radiation protection. Radiat. Environ. Biophys. 27: 153-164 (1988).

Z3 Zaharia, M. Latin American experience. Int. J. Radiat. Oncol. Biol. Phys. 10 (Suppl. 1): 161-162 (1984).

Z4 Zheng, J.-Z. Annual per caput effective dose equivalent of Beijing inhabitants from diagnostic x-ray procedures. Health Phys. 59: 939-940 (1990).

Z5 Zeman, R.K., F. Al-Kawas and S.B. Benjamin. Gallstone lithotripsy: is there still cause for optimism? Radiology 178: 33-35 (1991).

Z6 Zhang, L., J. Zhang, D. Jia et al. The frequencies and doses of medical exposure in China. Proc. CAMS and PUMC 5: 200-206 (1990).

Z7 Zankl, M., N. Petoussi and G. Drexler. Effective dose and effective dose equivalent - the impact of the new ICRP definition for external photon irradiation. Health Phys. 62: 395-399 (1992).

Z8 Zoetelief, J., J.J. Broerse and M.A.O. Thijssen. A Dutch protocol for quality control in mammography screening: dosimetric aspects. Radiat. Prot. Dosim. 43: 261-264 (1992).

Z9 Zoeller, G., G. May, R. Vosshenrich et al. Digital radiography in urologic imaging: Radiation dose reduction on urethrocystography. Urol. Radiol. 14: 56-58 (1992).

Z10 Zaharia, M. Experiencia en America Latina. p. 211-213 in: Control de Calidad en Radioterapia, Aspectos Clínicos y Físicos. Pan American Health Organization Scientific Publication No. 499 (1984).

Z11 Zaharia, M. Development of radiotherapy in Peru related to Quality Assurance. p. 141-149 in: Proceedings of a Workshop, 2-7 December 1984, Schloß Reisensburg, Germany. BGA-Schriften 5/1986 (1986).

Z12 Zaharia, M., E. Caceres, S. Valdivia et al. Radiotherapy in the management of locally advanced breast cancer. Int. J. Radiat. Oncol. Biol. Phys. 13: 1179-1182 (1987).

Z13 Zaharia, M., E. Caceres, S. Valdivia et al. Postoperative whole lung irradiation with or without adriamycin in osteogenic sarcoma. Int. J. Radiat. Oncol. Biol. Phys. 12: 907-910 (1986).

Z14 Zaharia, M., L.E. Salem, R. Travezan et al. Postoperative radiotherapy in the management of cancer of the maxillary sinus. Int. J. Radiat. Oncol. Biol. Phys. 17: 967-971 (1989).

Z15 Zankl, M., N. Petoussi, R. Veit et al. Organ doses for a child in diagnostic radiology: comparison of a realistic and a MIRD-type phantom. p. 196-198 in: Optimization of Image Quality and Patient Exposure in Diagnostic Radiology. (B.M. Moores et al., eds.) British Institute of Radiology, Report 20, London, 1989.

Z16 Zankl, M. and W. Panzer. The calculation of dose from external photon exposures using reference human phantoms and Monte Carlo methods. Part VI: Organ doses from computer tomographic examinations. GSF-Report 30/91, München, 1991.

ANNEX D

Occupational radiation exposures

CONTENTS

INTRODUCTION

1. Many individuals are exposed to radioactive materials or radiation sources in the course of their work. The Committee has been interested in evaluating occupational radiation exposures to determine the annual collective dose to workers in various sectors of industry. For purposes of comparison, the doses have often been expressed in terms of some normalized measure of the practice. The total collective dose has been assessed as a measure of the radiation-induced detriment to these individuals.

2. Occupational radiation exposures are monitored in the workplace for the purposes of controlling doses to individuals and demonstrating compliance with occupational exposure limits. Differences exist among countries, however, in the procedures adopted for the monitoring and reporting of occupational exposures; these reflect, inter alia, differences in regulatory systems, in regulatory requirements, in the size of the country, in the uses made of ionizing radiations and in the nature and scale of the radiation protection problems anticipated [D6, G4, G5]. As a result, monitoring data are not always collected and reported in a comparable fashion. This has implications in making valid comparisons between data reported by different countries and, to a lesser extent, between data for different uses of ionizing radiation within a given country. The Committee has adopted a number of assumptions and developed a number methodological approaches for data evaluation to overcome, or at least minimize the impact of, differences in the monitoring and reporting of occupational exposures. This, in turn, has had some effect on data collection and reporting practices.

3. Much progress has been made in the assessment and evaluation of occupational exposures since the Committee's first comprehensive treatment of the topic in the UNSCEAR 1977 Report [U4]. Improvements in the quality of reporting and collation of data have largely been responsible for the progress. There remain, however, areas where adequate data and analyses are lacking and where further investigations are needed to elucidate trends. In the UNSCEAR 1982 Report [U3], occupational exposures were reviewed and a number of recommendations were made for analyses of data that would give much clearer indications of the occupational exposures in all areas of work. Particular attention was drawn to the need for data on the pattern of dose accumulation over a working lifetime, especially for those occupations where higher levels of exposure are encountered, and to the benefits, in terms of facilitating a reliable estimate of collective dose, of reporting monitoring data in narrower bands of individual dose, especially at high doses. A more limited analysis of occupational exposures was undertaken in the UNSCEAR 1988 Report [U1] with updating of the levels of exposure in the nuclear power industry, in the medical uses of radiation and in selected groups exposed to natural radiation.

4. The analysis of occupational exposures in this Annex represents a continuation of the earlier work of the Committee. The main objectives of this continuing analysis are:

(a) to assess annual external and committed internal doses and cumulative doses to workers (both the average dose and the distribution of doses within the workforce) for each major practice involving the use of ionizing radiation. This provides a basis for estimating the average individual risk and distribution of risks in a workforce and for subgroups within it;

(b) to assess the annual collective doses to workers for each of the major practices involving the use of ionizing radiation. This provides a measure of the contribution made by occupational exposures to the overall impact of that use and the impact per unit practice (the contributions made by exposures of members of the public are assessed in other Annexes);

(c) to analyse trends with time in occupational exposures in order to evaluate the effects of changes in regulatory standards or requirements (e.g. changes in dose limits, increased attention given to reducing doses to as low as reasonably achievable), new technological developments, modified working practices and radiation protection programmes more generally;

(d) to compare exposures in different countries and to estimate the worldwide levels of exposure for each major use of ionizing radiation;

(e) to evaluate data on accidents involving the exposure of workers to levels of radiation that have caused clinical effects.

Within this context, the purpose of this Annex is to provide a comprehensive and structured analysis of the levels and trends in occupational exposures over the period 1975-1989. Consideration is given to annual and cumulative individual doses, to annual collective doses and their magnitudes per unit practice and to accidents involving high exposures and clinical effects. Particular emphasis is given to those occupations not considered in the UNSCEAR 1988 Report [U1], to those where the need for more information was identified by the Committee in the UNSCEAR 1982 Report [U3] and to those occupational subgroups which, in general, are exposed significantly in excess of the average. There is no intention to evaluate the totality of radiation exposures that may be received by people while at work of any nature. Consideration is limited to those occupations where the nature or circumstances of the work undertaken may lead to significant additional exposure, at least to some members of the workforce.

5. This analysis enables broad comparisons to be made between occupational exposures arising in various industrial and medical activities and between countries. From longer-term monitoring, trends in average individual doses and collective doses from particular practices or entire industries can be assessed and changes in underlying dose distributions can be examined. Trends in doses with time can be assessed in terms of a wide variety of quantities of potential interest (e.g. changes in regulatory standards, technological advances etc.).

6. To obtain the data needed for this review, the Committee has undertaken a survey of occupational radiation exposures worldwide by means of a questionnaire to countries with significant numbers of workers involved in radiation-related activities. This questionnaire specifically requested data on annual individual and collective occupational exposures incurred in operations of the nuclear fuel cycle, in other industrial uses of radiation, in medical uses of radiation and data on accidents with the potential to cause clinical effects. From the extensive and detailed annual data submitted, the Committee computed averages for the five-year periods 1975-1979, 1980-1984 and 1985-1989 to indicate representative average annual values and the basic trends. The assessment has benefited from the substantial database that has been provided, for which the Committee gratefully acknowledges the collaboration of so many countries. Those countries responding to the UNSCEAR Survey of Occupational Exposures are listed in Part A of the References.

I. ANALYSIS OF OCCUPATIONAL DOSE DISTRIBUTIONS

A. DOSE MONITORING DATA

7. The main function of monitoring in the workplace is to provide information for the control and further reduction, where appropriate, of exposures and to ensure satisfactory working conditions. This entails providing the information necessary for estimating the exposure of workers in terms of those quantities in which the basic limits, either primary or secondary, are expressed. However, none of these quantities (e.g. the effective dose, the equivalent dose in a tissue or organ and the intake of a radionuclide) can, in practice, be measured directly, so they must be estimated on the basis of other measured or assessed quantities. Individuals are monitored using equipment carried on their person (e.g. film badge, personal air sampler etc.) or by measuring the quantities of radioactive materials in their bodies or in excreta. Models appropriate for the exposure conditions of interest are used to estimate the relevant dosimetric quantities from these measurements; in general, the modelling approach is chosen cautiously to ensure that the risk of underestimating the exposure of an individual is acceptably small. In some cases exposures are assessed from monitoring of the working environment and knowledge of the habits and location of the workforce.

8. The nature and type of the measurements made and the realism and complexity of the model or models used to interpret them may vary considerably with the exposure conditions and their potential significance. Differences in these inevitably lead to different levels of conservatism in the doses reported or recorded in monitoring programmes. Such differences place limitations on the extent to which direct comparisons can be fairly made between reported data. Where these limitations may be of practical significance for the data included in this Annex, they are identified.

1. Quantities measured

9. ***External exposure.*** Film, thermoluminescent and other personal dosimeters are used for monitoring individual exposures to external radiation. The choice of dosimeter in any particular circumstances will be influenced by the nature of the radiations likely to be encountered. Dosimeters normally provide a measure of the equivalent dose in the skin in the immediate vicinity of the dosimeter and to immediately underlying tissue in this region. They do not, in general, provide an estimate of the absorbed dose or equivalent dose in other organs or tissues, which in principle need to be assessed to determine the effective dose. The relationship between the dosimeter measurement and the doses in particular organs and tissues of the body is influenced by many factors, such as the type, quality and spatial extent of the radiation, the orientation of the worker relative to the radiation field, the position and composition of the organs in the body etc. Several of these factors will be functions of both time and position in the workplace.

10. Practical guidance on measurement quantities that could be related to the effective dose equivalent and to the dose equivalent in the skin was issued by ICRU in 1985 [I14]. For environmental or area monitoring, the ambient dose equivalent, $H^*(d)$, for strongly penetrating radiation and the directional dose equivalent, H(d), for weakly penetrating radiation were introduced. For individual monitoring, the individual dose, penetrating, $H_p(d)$, and the individual dose, superficial, $H_s(d)$ were introduced. The relationships between these quantities and the effective dose equivalent, H_E, were discussed by ICRP [I3] and ICRU [I14, I15].

11. Some further alterations in radiation quantities have been made. The ICRU recommended in 1992 use of the personal dose equivalent, $H_p(d)$, for individual monitoring, which combines the concepts of the individual dose, penetrating and the individual dose, superficial [I16]. The ICRP introduced in 1991 the effective dose, E, which incorporates tissue weighting factors as in the effective dose equivalent, H_E, albeit for additional tissues specified and with revised numerical values [I7]. The adjustment of the absorbed dose required to reflect radiation quality has been changed by the introduction of radiation weighting factors. An analysis of the relationships between these radiation quantities will be issued by a joint task group of ICRP and ICRU. It can be assumed that the quantities introduced by ICRU provide reasonable approximations of the effective dose and equivalent dose in the skin when these quantities are calculated using the relationships between quality factors and linear energy transfer given in ICRP Publication 60 [I7].

12. In most practical situations, dosimeters provide reasonable approximations to the personal dose equivalent $H_p(d)$ at least at the location of the dosimeter. In situations where the exposure of the body is relatively uniform, it is common practice to enter the dosimeter reading, suitably calibrated, directly into the dose records as a surrogate for the effective dose. However, because the personal dose equivalent generally provides an overestimate of the effective dose, this practice results in an overestimation of recorded and reported doses, with the degree of overestimation depending on the energy of the radiation and the nature of the radiation field. For many practical situations involving relatively uniform exposure to fairly high-energy gamma radiation, the degree of overestimation is modest; for exposure to low-energy gamma- or x-radiation, the overestimation could be substantial. For photon energies below ~50 keV it can exceed a factor of 2, depending on the orientation of the body.

13. For exposure to spatially variable radiation fields or where there is partial shielding of the body or extreme variations in the distances of parts of the body from the source, the relationships between the dosimeter measurement and the effective dose are more variable and complex. Where the circumstances so justify, additional measurements or theoretical analyses may be used to establish reliable relationships on a case-by-case basis for the exposure conditions of interest. The direct entry of dosimeter measurements into dose records in these more complex situations (or the use of very simple and deliberately cautious assumptions to establish the relationships between the two quantities) lead, in general, to overestimates in the recorded exposures. Where such practice has been adopted in the recording of doses, care is needed in their interpretation, in particular when comparisons are made with doses arising elsewhere.

14. For its previous assessments the Committee adopted the convention that all quantitative results reported by monitoring services represent the average absorbed dose in the whole body (or the effective dose). It further assumed that the dose from natural background radiation has been subtracted from the reported results and that medical radiation exposures have not been included. The Committee also recognized that it is almost always the reading from the dosimeter, suitably modified by calibration factors, that is reported, without consideration of its relationship to the absorbed doses in the various organs and tissues of the body or to the effective dose. This is still regarded as a reasonable convention to adopt, in particular as most data are for external exposure of the whole body to relatively uniform photon radiation of moderately high energy. In situations where exposure of the body is very non-uniform (especially in medical practice) or where exposure is mainly to low energy radiation, the use of this convention will result in an overestimate of effective doses, which then need appropriate qualification. Because the relationship between the reported dosimeter reading and the average absorbed dose in the whole body (or the effective dose) varies with the circumstances of the exposure, caution needs to be exercised when aggregating or directly comparing data from very dissimilar types of work. Appropriate qualifications of the reported data are made in those cases where the adoption of the above convention may lead to significant misrepresentation of the actual doses.

15. ***Internal exposure***. The assessment of internal doses from the intake of radioactive material into the body is, in general, more difficult than the measurement of external doses. It is impossible to measure directly the internal dose received by an individual. Instead, it must be calculated based on the quantity and distribution of radioactive material in, or estimated to be taken into, the body, metabolic data, the type and energy of radiation emitted, the fraction

of the emitted energy absorbed by various organs and tissues etc. Various types of monitoring are undertaken to aid the evaluation of internal exposures, depending on the radionuclide concerned and the mode of exposure. These include the use of personal air samplers and/or area monitoring to assess intakes by inhalation, the biological monitoring of excreta and the external counting of the whole or parts of the body.

16. The level of internal contamination, and subsequently dose, is easy to determine by biological monitoring for some radionuclides (e.g. tritium, at least in inorganic form) but very difficult for others (e.g. ^{239}Pu), especially at long times after intake or in cases of multiple intake. In general, the uncertainty associated with the estimation of effective doses from the intake of radionuclides into the body is much larger than that associated with external dosimetry; however, it very much depends on the nuclide in question, the techniques used and the level of contamination.

17. In practice there are few occupations for which exposures from internal contamination are significant. The costs and practical difficulties of providing a personal monitoring service produce strong pressures for designs that reduce internal exposures below levels where continuous personal monitoring is necessary. Historically, in most organizations where internal exposures were potentially significant, estimates were made of the body (or organ) content of a radionuclide, or groups of radionuclides, as a fraction of the Maximum Permissible Body Burden, and the results of the monitoring were usually expressed in these terms. The situation is changing, however, in particular in those countries that have given regulatory effect to the recommendations of the ICRP in its Publication 26 [I1]. In these countries, the results of monitoring internal exposures are now being reported in terms of the committed effective dose from intakes within the year of interest; in general, however, the contribution made by internal exposure is small. These aspects are addressed further in paragraph 27.

18. The few occupations for which internal exposure is potentially significant are uranium mining and milling (inhalation of radon daughters and ore dust); underground work in general, and in particular other forms of mining (inhalation of radon daughters and dust), the luminizing industry (tritium), the operation of heavy water reactors (tritium), fuel fabrication (uranium), fuel reprocessing (actinides), nuclear weapons production (tritium, uranium and plutonium). Quantitative data, albeit limited in some cases, on internal exposures in each of these areas are included in this Annex. Internal exposures could also be significant during the decommissioning of nuclear installations and in nuclear medicine; however, data are unavailable for these activities.

2. Monitoring practice

19. Decisions on who is to be monitored in a workforce, and to what degree, are influenced by the likelihood of exposures at or above different levels. However, as other considerations, (e.g. practicability and industrial relations) are also relevant, the decisions made by operational managements may differ. The outcome is the lack of a consistent approach to monitoring between industries or between countries or even within an industry or within a country. In Publication 26 and in its earlier publications, the ICRP recommended [I1, I2] that in cases where it is very unlikely that annual doses will exceed three tenths of the dose limit, individual monitoring is not necessary, although it may sometimes be carried out to confirm that conditions are satisfactory.

20. The ICRP recommendations have had, and continue to have, a major influence on monitoring practice. However, the relative ease, low cost and sensitivity of monitoring devices for external radiation means that these are much more widely issued than would be expected from the suggested criteria. The devices having been issued, even trivial doses are often reported, despite the ICRP having recommended a recording level of one tenth of the annual limit. The situation for internal exposures is, however, quite different, with monitoring being undertaken only in those few circumstances where there is a clear need.

21. In Publication 60 [I7], the ICRP has recommended that external radiation should be monitored for all those who are occupationally exposed, unless it is clear that their doses will be consistently low or, as in the case of aircrew, that the circumstances prevent the doses from exceeding an identified value.

22. Different approaches are adopted in designating which workers in a workforce are to be monitored. This is to be expected for the reasons previously addressed (e.g. see paragraph 2). However, such differences, if substantial, could limit the extent to which direct and valid comparisons can be made between reported monitoring data for different occupations or industries and/or between data for the same occupation or industry carried out in different locations. This difficulty can, to some extent, be overcome by making comparisons between data for those measurably exposed [i.e. those for which any dosimeter issued during the year in question recorded a dose in excess of the minimum detectable level (MDL) or, alternatively, in excess of some administratively established reporting level] as opposed to those monitored. Even this, however, does not completely circumvent the problem because there are differences in MDLs (or reporting levels) for different sets of

data. The potential magnitude of this problem can be readily appreciated by reference to the variability in the ratio of the number of persons monitored and those measurably exposed in various occupations. This ratio was found to vary from about 1 to 10 for different occupations in the United States [N1] and over an even greater range in Canada [F2]; a value of about 2 was typical of the nuclear industry in the United States.

23. Because of these difficulties, a distinction is made throughout this Annex between average doses estimated for monitored and measurably exposed workers. When appropriate, indications are given of how data expressed in the different ways can be modified to enable direct and more valid comparison. The implications of these difficulties are largely confined to the evaluation and comparison of the size of the exposed workforce and average levels of individual dose. In general, they do not unduly influence the estimation of the collective dose apart from those cases where individual exposures are mostly very low and the ratio of monitored to measurably exposed workers very high.

3. Recording and reporting practice

24. The way in which occupational exposures are recorded and reported differs significantly between occupations and countries. The more important of these include the recording of doses that are less than the MDL, the assignment of notional doses, the protocol for determining who in the workforce is to be monitored (visitors, administrative staff etc.), the inclusion of contract workers in addition to employees, the recording and reporting of internal exposures and the general way in which occupational exposure distributions are reported.

25. MDLs may differ between occupations and certainly differ between countries. When doses are determined to be less than the MDL, the value recorded in the records may be zero, some pre-designated level or the MDL value itself. These differences affect the comparability of results. It is therefore important that reported data on occupational exposures be accompanied by information on the MDL and how doses less than it were recorded.

26. When dosimeters are lost, or the readings are otherwise not available, notional doses are assigned to an individual dose record. A variety of procedures are used in determining the notional dose. These include the assignment of the appropriate proportion of the annual authorized limit for the period for which the dosimeter was lost; the assignment of the average dose received by the worker in the previous 12 months; the assignment of the average dose received by co-workers in the same period etc. Some of these procedures can distort records significantly, particularly if large numbers of dosimeters are lost within a particular occupational group. Where this is the case, direct comparisons with other data may be invalid or at least need qualification. Such potential difficulties could be overcome if, in these cases, modified data sets were available in which the notional doses were substituted by doses calculated from the average dose over the remainder of the year for each individual or by the average dose received by co-workers during the period in question. This procedure would only be appropriate for dosimeters lost in routine situations; when high exposures are suspected, such as in accidents, individual dose reconstruction would be a more appropriate basis for determining the dose to be recorded.

27. In the past, internal and external exposures were generally recorded separately and often in different ways, with little or no attempt made to present distributions of the summed exposures. Significant variations also occurred in the reporting levels for internal contamination, and this further enhanced the difficulties of compilation and comparison of statistics on internal exposure. This situation is changing, however, and internal exposures are increasingly being recorded in terms of committed doses from intakes within the year of interest and, moreover, added to any dose received from external sources. The generation of these more complete dose records will enable more valid and reliable comparisons to be made of doses in various occupations and industries. These changes in recording procedures have two implications, however. First, in the transitional period not all dose distributions are likely to be based on the sum of internal and external doses, and due provision will need to be made for this in any comparisons. Secondly, previous estimates of occupational exposures will need to be updated, in particular for those occupations and industries (e.g. fuel fabrication and fuel reprocessing) where internal exposures may have been significant but were not included in the reported data.

28. Two particular features of the way in which occupational dose distributions are reported influence the ease and effectiveness with which the relevant data can be extracted and compared. The first is the categories or types of occupation for which data are commonly reported. Significant differences are apparent in the occupational categories used in different countries. The advantages of reporting data according to a broadly agreed categorization scheme are self-evident, but the difficulties of achieving consensus in this area are not to be underestimated, especially in the light of long-established national

practices, which often will have evolved to accommodate particular national interests and/or concerns. Nevertheless, efforts to achieve greater uniformity in the collection and reporting of data would be of general benefit. The categories used by the Committee for evaluating occupational exposures are given in Table 1. Although the categories are broad, their wider use would simplify and unify the data collection and reporting.

29. The second feature influencing data extraction and comparison is the level of detail or resolution adopted when reporting the distribution of occupational exposures, in particular, at the higher levels of individual dose. Analytical procedures have been developed by the Committee [U3, U4] to enable quantities of interest to be extracted almost irrespective of how the data were reported, but if the data were all reported in a sufficiently detailed and consistent manner, these procedures would be largely unnecessary. Analytical techniques may, however, play a continuing important role in the estimation of future annual and cumulative doses, subject to various assumptions on dose limits or dose constraints in particular occupations. This topic is discussed further in the next Section, where procedures for data reporting are given with a view to achieving greater consistency between the data and facilitating their evaluation and comparison.

30. Finally, two additional points could affect the validity of comparisons between occupational exposures in different groups or within the same group over time: first, whether any administrative changes have occurred in dose recording that may affect the reported doses from one year to another and, secondly, whether the reported doses are complete, in particular whether contract workers as well as employees are included in the statistics. The reported data are not always explicit with regard to these points.

B. CHARACTERISTICS OF DOSE DISTRIBUTIONS

31. Dose distributions are the result of many constraints imposed by the nature of the work itself, by management, by the workers and by legislation. In some job categories it may be unnecessary for workers ever to receive more than very low doses, whereas in other jobs workers may have to be exposed to high doses fairly routinely. Management controls act as feedback mechanisms, especially when individual doses approach the annual dose limit, or some proportion of it, in a shorter period of time.

32. The Committee is principally interested in making comparisons of dose distributions and in evaluating trends. For these purposes, it identified three characteristics of dose distributions as being particularly useful:

(a) the average annual effective dose (i.e. the sum of the annual dose from external irradiation plus the committed dose from intakes in that year), E, which is related to the average level of individual risk;
(b) the annual collective effective dose, S (referred to as M in earlier UNSCEAR Reports), which is related to the impact of the practice;
(c) the ratio, SR, of the annual collective effective dose delivered at annual individual doses exceeding 15 mSv to the total collective dose. SR (referred to as MR in earlier UNSCEAR Reports) provides an indication of the fraction of the collective dose received by workers exposed to higher levels of individual risk. This ratio is termed the collective dose distribution ratio.

33. Another ratio, NR, of the number of workers receiving annual individual doses exceeding 15 mSv to the total monitored or exposed workforce, is reported in many occupational exposure statistics, often when the ratio SR is not provided. The more frequent reporting of the ratio NR is probably due to the ease with which it can be estimated. In the past, this ratio was not used or reported by the Committee because of its potential sensitivity to how the size of the workforce is defined (those monitored, those measurably exposed etc.); consequently, comparisons of values of this ratio reported for different occupations and in different countries would, in general, require some qualification. The ratio SR on the other hand, is relatively insensitive to this parameter and is therefore a better means of affording fair comparisons between exposures arising in different industries or practices. Notwithstanding the limitations of the ratio NR, it is now included in the characteristics reported by the Committee. This change is largely a reflection of the more frequent reporting of the ratio NR in occupational exposure statistics, but it also reflects its potential for use in more limited circumstances (e.g. when analysing trends with time in a given workforce or making comparisons between workforces that have been defined in comparable ways). The ratio SR, however, remains the most appropriate basis for comparing data generally.

34. The annual collective effective dose, S, is given by

$$S = \sum_{i=1}^{N} E_i \qquad (1)$$

where E_i is the annual effective dose received by the ith worker and N is the total number of workers. In practice, S is often calculated from collated dosimetry results using the alternative definition

$$S = \sum_{j=1}^{r} N_j E_j \qquad (2)$$

where r is the number of effective dose ranges into which the dosimetry results have been collated and N_j is the number of individuals in the effective dose ranges for which E_j is the mean annual effective dose. The average annual effective dose, $\bar{E}$, is equal to S/N. The number distribution ratio, NR, is given by

$$NR_{15} = \frac{N(>15)}{N} \qquad (3)$$

where N(>15) is the number of workers receiving annual doses exceeding 15 mSv. The annual collective dose distribution ratio, SR, is given by

$$SR_{15} = \frac{S(>15)}{S} \qquad (4)$$

where S(>15) is the annual collective effective dose delivered at annual individual doses exceeding 15 mSv.

35. The total number of workers, N, warrants further comment, as it has implications for the various quantities estimated. Depending on the nature of the data reported and subject to the evaluation (or the topic of interest), the number of workers may be those monitored, those classified, those measurably exposed, the total workforce or some subset of this. These quantities, therefore, will always be specific to the nature and composition of the workforce included in the estimation; when making comparisons, caution should be exercised to ensure that like is being compared with like. These aspects were discussed in Section I.A, where the implications of different monitoring and reporting practices for the assessed average individual and collective doses were identified. In this Annex consideration is, to the extent practicable, limited to the estimation of the above quantities for the monitored and measurably exposed workforces; however, lack of uniformity between employers and countries in determining who should be monitored and/or what constitutes measurably exposed means that even these comparisons between ostensibly the same quantities are less rigorous than might appear. Where necessary, quantities estimated for a subset of the workforce (e.g. those measurably exposed) can be transformed to apply to the whole workforce; methods of achieving this, based on characteristics of the dose distributions, are discussed below.

36. The three quantities used in the past by the Committee have provided a useful basis for summarizing and comparing occupational exposures. One of the quantities, the collective dose distribution ratio SR, may, however, become increasingly less useful or informative. In the event that regulatory dose limits are reduced by a significant amount, the fraction of the collective dose arising from annual individual doses in excess of 15 mSv is likely to decrease. The quantity may then cease to serve the purpose intended for it. The Committee believes, therefore, that it would be useful to estimate and report additional values of the collective dose distribution ratio, but for the fraction of the collective dose arising from levels of annual individual dose lower than the previously adopted value of 15 mSv. These collective dose distribution ratios are designated, SR_E, where the subscript E signifies the level of annual individual dose to which the ratio refers. These comments apply equally to the ratio NR.

37. In summary, the following characteristics of dose distributions will be considered by the Committee in its reviews of occupational exposure:

(a) the average annual effective dose (i.e. the sum of the annual dose from external irradiation and the committed dose from intakes in that year), $\bar{E}$;
(b) the annual collective effective dose (i.e. the sum of the annual collective dose from external irradiation and the committed collective dose from intakes in that year), S;
(c) the collective dose distribution ratio, SR_E, for a value of E of 15 mSv in this Annex and additionally for lower values in the future;
(d) the number distribution ratio, NR_E (the fraction of the workforce exposed to annual doses in excess of E) for a value of E of 15 mSv in this Annex and additionally for lower values in the future;

To facilitate the task of extracting data from dose distributions, persons reporting data are encouraged to include these characteristics explicitly in their dose distributions. In addition to the annual collective dose, it would also be very useful to have information provided so that normalized forms of this quantity can be derived, i.e. expressed in terms of unit practice, for example per reactor or per unit energy generated. This facilitates comparison between practices.

38. Ideally, these characteristics of dose distributions would be evaluated by those reporting the data from the complete, detailed recording of doses to workers within a particular workforce, and they would be presented in the requisite form. In practice, however, this does not always occur. Data on occupational exposures are completed in a variety of forms, some of which do not lead to the explicit presentation of all those quantities of interest to the Committee. In these cases the quantities must be calculated from the data presented, and the Committee has developed analytical

procedures for this purpose. These are summarized below. Further details of the procedures are presented in the UNSCEAR 1982 Report [U3]. The need for the Committee to use such procedures has, however, diminished with time, owing to improvements in and more comprehensive reporting of occupational exposures.

39. In the UNSCEAR 1977 Report [U4] (Annex E), it was noted that many dose distributions exhibit a log-normal character, especially at doses well below the annual dose limit. This property can be readily identified by plotting the cumulative frequency of the number of individuals with doses less than a given level on a probability axis against the logarithm of dose. Where the required information cannot be extracted directly from the reported results, a log-normal fit to the appropriate part of the distribution can be used to extract the collective dose and the fraction of the collective dose delivered in different individual dose ranges. This procedure can also be used, where necessary, to assess collective doses to the large numbers of workers in the lowest dose band, who may receive very low or zero doses but nonetheless are given dosimeters.

40. A variable x is said to be distributed log-normally if the values of $y = \ln x$ are distributed normally. The mean, median and mode of the distribution of y is μ; the variance of the distribution of y is σ^2. The probability that a value of x will lie between x and x + dx is

$$P(x)\,dx = \frac{1}{\sigma\sqrt{2\pi}}\,\frac{1}{x}\,e^{-\frac{(\ln x - \mu)^2}{2\sigma^2}}\,dx \qquad (5)$$

Since the data rarely fit a log-normal distribution over the whole range, the quantity of use is the collective dose S_E, up to a certain annual effective dose E. This is given by

$$S_E = N\int_0^E x\,P(x)\,dx \qquad (6)$$

This can be expressed as

$$S_E = \frac{N}{\sqrt{2\pi}}\,e^{\mu+\frac{\sigma^2}{2}}\int_{-\infty}^{T} e^{-\frac{t^2}{2}}\,dt \qquad (7)$$

where the substitution variable $t = (\ln x - \mu - \sigma^2)/\sigma$. The substitution using t is made to render S_E in the form shown, since tabulations of the cumulative normal distribution function are readily available. The choice of the appropriate value of E for each distribution is made by inspecting the data plotted on log probability graph paper; very often 10 or 15 mSv is a convenient value.

41. Graphical techniques are often of sufficient accuracy for analyses of dose distributions and are described both in standard texts [F1] and in the context of occupational dose distribution analysis [B1]. If a straight line is fitted to the plot of the cumulative frequency versus ln E, then the value of E is $(\mu - \sigma)$ at a cumulative frequency of 15.87% and $(\mu + \sigma)$ at a cumulative frequency of 84.13%. S_E can then be obtained from standard tabulations.

42. Alternatively, a wide variety of numerical and/or analytical techniques can be used to evaluate the quantities of interest from the dose distributions. For example, when sufficient data are available, the methods of maximum likelihood or of least squares can be used to obtain the equation for the best-fit line up to an annual dose E, chosen from inspection of the plot; the collective dose up to that value of dose can then be obtained by numerical integration. To estimate the collective dose in the ranges above E, where the dose distribution deviates from log-normal, it may be sufficient to multiply the number of individuals in each dose range by the mid-point dose of the range, if this information is available with adequate resolution. Equally, graphical or various curve-fitting techniques can be employed to evaluate the integral and other quantities of the dose distribution.

43. Investigations by Kumazawa et al. [K1] have shown that the control exercised over doses approaching the dose limit results in a normal distribution of doses in the higher dose ranges, and that a combination of a log-normal and a normal distribution (but not a mixed distribution of them) may provide a more generally applicable means of representing occupational dose distributions. Such hybrid log-normal distributions have been shown to provide a good representation of observed data in many circumstances [E1].

44. The distribution function of a variable x is hybrid log-normal if the values of $y = \ln(\rho x) + \rho x$ ($\rho > 0$) are distributed normally. The mean, median and mode of the distribution of y is μ and the variance of the distribution of y is σ^2. The probability that a value of x will lie between x and x + dx is given by

$$P(x)\,dx = \frac{1}{\sigma\sqrt{2\pi}}\left(\rho + \frac{1}{x}\right) e^{-\frac{[\ln(\rho x) + \rho x - \mu]^2}{2\sigma^2}}\,dx \qquad (8)$$

where ρ, μ and σ are parameters of the hybrid log-normal distribution. It should be noted that μ and σ^2 do not have the usual meanings of mean and variance for variate x that they have for the normal distribution. The parameter ρ is a measure of the degree of control exercised to avoid approaching or exceeding some level of exposure. As $\rho \rightarrow 0$, the distribution tends to the log-normal distribution; as $\rho \to \infty$, it tends to the normal distribution (defined only above zero).

45. For a hybrid log-normal distribution, the ratios NR_E and SR_E, are given by

$$NR_E = \frac{\int_E^\infty P(x)\,dx}{\int_0^\infty P(x)\,dx} \quad \text{and} \quad SR_E = \frac{\int_E^\infty x\,P(x)\,dx}{\int_0^\infty x\,P(x)\,dx} \qquad (9)$$

All of these integrals have to be evaluated numerically. Graphical and computational methods for deriving the parameters ρ, μ and σ of the hybrid log-normal distribution that provides the best fit to a given set of data are described in the literature [K1, S1]. Computational techniques for evaluating the above integrals are also available [K2].

46. The hybrid log-normal distribution is finding increasing use in the analysis and reporting of occupational exposures, particularly in the United States, where it has been used by several agencies in their most recent compilations of annual statistics [E3, R2, M3]. One of its uses has been to re-evaluate statistics compiled previously on a simpler basis; its use in this context led the United States Department of Energy [M3] to conclude that collective doses reported in previous years were probably overestimates by, on average, 15%-20%. More importantly, it provides a means to assess the degree of active control used in different occupations to reduce the frequency of annual doses approaching dose limits or other constraints. Similarly, it can be used to predict future trends in dose subject to assumptions on the degree of control exercised over the occurrence of higher individual doses.

47. The hybrid log-normal distribution may also provide a useful means of reporting dose distribution data succinctly. If dose distributions are generally well fitted by the hybrid log-normal form, it would be possible to describe a complete distribution of exposures by specifying the three parameters of the hybrid log-normal distribution function. It would then be possible to generate from these three parameters any characteristic of the dose distribution that may be considered useful now or in the future. Given the flexibility offered by this approach, the merits of reporting occupational exposures in terms of the three parameters of the hybrid log-normal distribution warrants further consideration. The additional computational effort involved in deriving these parameters may impede the wide-scale adoption of this approach.

48. The need for succinct reporting of dose distributions has, however, diminished with the growth and ease of use of computer databases. Vast amounts of data can now be readily stored in an accessible form. Provided occupational exposure databases are created with sufficient resolution, it will be possible, using simple arithmetic techniques, to estimate with adequate precision all of the characteristics presently of interest to the Committee; any other characteristics that might eventually be of interest could likewise be readily evaluated. Access to such databases in the future is likely to reduce the use made by the Committee of empirical fits to dose distributions to extract required quantities. In these circumstances, the future use of empirical fitting by the Committee is likely to be limited to the extraction of quantities of interest from data compiled with inadequate resolution in the past; additionally, the techniques will continue to be used to provide insights into matters such as the influence of dose limits or constraints on the characteristics of dose distributions and for purposes of estimating the magnitude of, and trends in, future annual and cumulative doses.

C. ESTIMATION OF WORLDWIDE EXPOSURES

49. Inevitably, the data provided in response to the UNSCEAR Survey of Occupational Exposures will remain incomplete in terms of estimating worldwide levels of dose. Procedures have therefore been developed by the Committee to derive worldwide doses from the data available for particular occupational categories. Two procedures have been developed, one for application to occupational exposures arising at most stages in the commercial nuclear fuel cycle and the other for general application to other occupational categories.

50. In general, the reporting of exposures arising in the commercial nuclear fuel cycle is more complete than that of exposures arising from other uses of radiation. The degree of extrapolation from reported to worldwide doses is, therefore, less and can be achieved with greater reliability than for other occupational categories. Moreover, worldwide statistics are generally available on capacity and production in various stages of the commercial nuclear fuel cycle. Such data provide a convenient and reliable basis for extrapolating to worldwide levels of exposure. Thus, the worldwide annual collective effective dose, S_w, from a given part of the nuclear fuel cycle (e.g. uranium mining, fuel fabrication or reactor operation) is estimated to be the total of annual collective effective doses from reporting countries times the reciprocal of the fraction, f, of world production (uranium mined, fuel fabricated, energy generated etc.)

accounted for by these countries, namely,

$$S_w = \frac{1}{f}\sum_{c=1}^{n} S_c \qquad (10)$$

where S_c is the annual collective dose from country c and n is the number of countries for which occupational exposure data have been reported. The fraction of total production can be expressed as

$$f = \sum_{c=1}^{n} P_c / P_w \qquad (11)$$

with P_c and P_w the productions in country c and in the world, w, respectively.

51. The annual number of monitored workers worldwide, N_w, is estimated by a similar extrapolation. Because of more limited data, the worldwide distribution ratios, $NR_{E,w}$ and $SR_{E,w}$, are simply estimated as weighted averages of the reported data. The extrapolations to worldwide collective effective doses and numbers of monitored workers and the estimation of worldwide average distribution ratios are performed on an annual basis. Values of these quantities have been averaged over five-year periods, and the average annual values are reported in this Annex.

52. For exposures to radiation other than in operations of the nuclear fuel cycle, statistics are not so readily available on the worldwide level of the practices or their distribution among countries. In these cases a simpler and, inevitably, less reliable method of extrapolation has to be used. A variety of approaches are possible (e.g. scaling by size of population, by employment in industrial or medical professions or by some measure of industrial output). In the end, it has seemed to be most practical and reasonable to extrapolate on the basis of gross national product (GNP) of countries. Several considerations influence the choice of this quantity in preference to others, notably the availability of reliable worldwide statistics on gross national products and their potential for general application; the latter is a consequence of the expectation that the gross national product is reasonably correlated with both the level of industrial activity and medical care in a country, characteristics unlikely to be found in any other single quantity. To make the extrapolation more reliable, it is applied not globally but separately over particular geographic or economic regions, followed by summation over these regions. This results in extrapolations of available data within groups of countries with broadly similar levels of economic activity and allows for general geographical comparisons.

53. The worldwide annual collective effective dose for other uses of radiation, is estimated as

$$S_w = \sum_{r=1}^{m} S_r \qquad (12)$$

where

$$S_r = \frac{1}{g_r}\sum_{c=1}^{n_r} S_c \qquad (13)$$

where S_r is the annual collective effective dose in geographic or economic region r, n_r is the number of countries in region r, for which occupational exposure data have been reported, m is the number of regions and g_r is the fraction of the GNP of region r, represented by those countries for which occupational exposure data are available and is given by

$$g_r = \sum_{c=1}^{n_r} G_c / G_r \qquad (14)$$

where G_c and G_r are the GNPs of country c and region r, respectively, and are expressed in United States dollars.

54. The above equations are applied to estimate collective doses for those regions for which occupational exposure data are available for at least one country within the region. For those regions for which no data for any country were reported, a modified approach is adopted. In these cases the regional collective dose is estimated as

$$S_r = G_r \sum_{c=1}^{n} S_c / \sum_{c=1}^{n} G_c \qquad (15)$$

For the purposes of this analysis the world was divided into nine geographic or economic regions comprising: countries of the Organization for Economic Cooperation and Development (OECD), comprising 24 countries; Eastern Europe, including the former USSR; Latin America; Africa, excluding South Africa; the Indian subcontinent; south and south-west Asia; centrally planned economies in east and south-east Asia; non-centrally planned economies in east and south-east Asia and Oceania.

55. The annual number of monitored workers worldwide, N_w, is estimated by the same procedure. The worldwide distribution ratios are estimated as for operations of the nuclear fuel cycle, but where the averaging was performed first on a regional basis prior to summing over all regions. For selected occupational categories, estimates are also made of the number of measurably exposed workers worldwide, M_w. These are estimated on a regional basis from the quotient of annual collective effective dose and the average annual dose to measurably exposed workers.

56. Given the approximate nature of this form of extrapolation, it has been applied not to annual data but to data averaged over five-year periods. Representative data on the gross national product were used for each of the three periods (specifically, 1977, 1983 and 1989) [I17, U11]. The particular years used are of no absolute importance, as it is only the relative values of gross national products within a given period that are relevant to the extrapolation.

D. CUMULATIVE DOSE DISTRIBUTIONS

57. The subject of cumulative and lifetime occupational doses to workers and their distribution for particular workforces is an important one that needs to be addressed. There are, however, few data available in the open literature that either report values directly or allow estimates to be made. Of particular interest are the cumulative or lifetime doses among those groups of workers who regularly experience high average annual effective doses.

58. The Committee has made no assessment of cumulative lifetime doses since the UNSCEAR 1977 Report [U4], when simple linear extrapolation was used to estimate doses for a few categories of workers for whom data on average doses and years of employment were available. The deficiencies in such a simple extrapolation were well recognized, but there was hope that this simple treatment would stimulate more rigorous investigations of the relationship between the rate of accumulation over the years of employment and the total dose received. This hope has not been realized to any great extent, and there still remain few published analyses of cumulative or lifetime doses that the Committee can use as a basis for a thorough assessment.

59. The progress the Committee can make in this area will inevitably be constrained by published data or data made available by national authorities. The published data are reviewed in this Annex, and the distributions of cumulative and lifetime doses in particular occupations are assessed. Given the importance of the topic, it would be useful if national authorities and some large employers would make available other relevant, but so far unpublished, data and could undertake further analyses in this area. It is evident that much progress will be made in this regard in support of epidemiological studies that have been, or are in the process of being, carried out for particular occupational groups. The temporal patterns of individual exposures are essential components of such studies, and it should be possible to extract the required data and report them in a suitably anonymous fashion so that the privacy of the records of individual workers is safeguarded. The protocols under which data were collected for epidemiological studies may, however, in some cases inhibit the use of the data for the purposes of interest to the Committee.

II. THE NUCLEAR FUEL CYCLE

60. The fuel cycle that serves nuclear power reactors used for the generation of electrical energy is a major identified practice giving rise to occupational exposures. Exposures arising from this practice were discussed and quantified in the UNSCEAR 1972 [U5], 1977 [U4], 1982 [U3] and 1988 [U1] Reports, with comprehensive treatment in the 1977 and 1982 Reports. In comparison with many other sources of exposure, this practice is well documented, and considerable quantities of data on occupational dose distributions are available, in particular for more recent years. Consideration is given in this Annex to occupational exposures arising at each major stage of the fuel cycle. As the final stage of treatment and disposal of the main solid wastes is not yet sufficiently developed to warrant a detailed examination of potential exposures, it is given only very limited consideration. However, occupational exposures from waste disposal are not expected to significantly increase the sum of the doses from the other stages in the fuel cycle. For similar reasons, no attempt is made to estimate occupational exposures during the decommissioning of nuclear installations, although this will become an increasingly important source.

61. For each stage of the fuel cycle estimates are made of the magnitude and temporal trends in the annual collective and average individual doses, the numbers of monitored workers and the distribution ratios. The collective doses are also expressed in normalized terms, that is per unit practice relevant to the particular stage of the cycle. For uranium mining and milling, fuel enrichment, fuel fabrication and fuel reprocessing, the normalization is initially presented in terms of unit mass of uranium or fuel produced or processed; these quantities can be re-normalized in terms of the equivalent amount of energy that can be (or has been) generated by the fabricated (or enriched) fuel. The bases for the normalizations, namely, the amounts of mined uranium, separative work during

enrichment and the amount of fuel required to generate a unit of electrical energy in various reactor types, are given in Annex B, "Exposures from man-made sources of radiation". For reactors, several ways of normalizing the data may be appropriate, depending on how the data are used. In this Annex, normalized collective doses are given per reactor and per unit electrical energy generated.

62. To allow proper comparison between the doses arising at different stages of the fuel cycle, all the data are ultimately presented in the same normalized form, in terms of the electrical energy generated (or the amount of uranium mined or fuel fabricated or reprocessed, corresponding to a unit of energy subsequently generated in the reactor), which is the output from the nuclear power industry. This form of normalization is both valid and useful when treating data accumulated over a large number of facilities or over a long time period. It can, however, be misleading when applied to data for a single facility for a short time period; this is because a large fraction of the total occupational exposure at a facility arises during periodic maintenance operations when the plant is shut down and not in production. Such difficulties are, however, largely circumvented in this Annex, since the data are presented in an aggregated form for individual countries and averaged over five-year periods.

63. In addition to the annual dose, the rate at which dose is accumulated during the career of an individual (cumulative or lifetime dose) is an important statistic in judging the significance of occupational exposures. As mentioned above, however, there are as yet few data available on cumulative or lifetime doses. Accordingly, the subject is not treated separately for each stage of the fuel cycle, but it is addressed in Section II.G for the nuclear fuel cycle as a whole.

64. Various national authorities or institutions have used different methods to measure, record and report the occupational data included in this Annex. The main features of the procedures used by each country that responded to the UNSCEAR Survey of Occupational Exposures are summarized in Table 2. The potential for such differences to compromise or invalidate comparisons between data is discussed in Section I.A.3. The reported collective doses and the collective dose distribution ratios are largely insensitive to the differences that have been identified in Table 2, and the quantities can generally be compared without further qualification. The average doses to monitored workers and the number distribution ratios are, however, sensitive to decisions and practice on who in a workforce is to be monitored. Differences in these areas could not be discerned from responses to the UNSCEAR Survey of Occupational Exposures nor, consequently, can they be discerned from Table 2. However, because the monitoring of workers in the nuclear power industry is in general fairly comprehensive, comparisons of the average individual doses (and number distribution ratios) reported here are judged to be broadly valid. Nonetheless, it must be recognized that differences in monitoring and reporting practices do exist, and they may, in particular cases, affect the validity of comparisons between reported data; to the extent practicable, where such differences are likely to be important they are identified.

A. URANIUM MINING AND MILLING

65. Uranium is obtained from ore mined in several countries, with the largest producers within WOCA (World Outside Centrally planned economies Area) being Australia, Canada, France, Namibia, Niger, South Africa and the United States; in addition, uranium exploration and/or production is being undertaken on a smaller scale in several other countries. Data on the annual production of uranium are given in Annex B, "Exposures from man-made sources of radiation". Uranium mining operations involve the removal from the ground of large quantities of ore containing uranium and its decay products at concentrations up to several thousand times the concentrations of these nuclides in the natural terrestrial environment. The concentration of uranium in mined ores is typically between 0.1%-3% U_3O_8 but in exceptional cases may be as high as a few tens of per cent. Mining is carried out by either underground or open-pit methods, which account for most of the uranium produced; in recent years *in situ* solution mining has also been carried out, although this makes only a small contribution to overall uranium production. In some cases uranium is obtained as a by-product of the mining of gold or other metals.

66. Uranium milling operations involve the processing of large quantities of ore to extract partially refined uranium. The process of extraction involves the following steps: crushing, grinding, chemical leaching, separation of the uranium from the leach solution, precipitation, drying and packing of the extracted material. Most mills use an acid leach extraction process, although other processes are in use. The uranium concentrate, often referred to as yellowcake, is used as feed for fuel fabrication plants, where it is further refined, converted and, if necessary, enriched.

67. Both internal exposure and external irradiation may be significant contributors to occupational exposure during uranium mining. Internal exposure

may arise from the inhalation of radon and its decay products and the inhalation of ore dust containing long-lived alpha emitters of the uranium chain. A number of factors will influence the relative contribution of each source, including, among others, the type of mining undertaken (i.e. deep mining or open-pit) and the efficacy of ventilation underground. The main source of internal exposure in underground mines is, in general, the inhalation of radon and its decay products; where these have been reduced to a low level, the inhalation of ore dust may be a significant contributor. In open-pit mines, particularly in dry climates, inhalation of ore dust is likely to be the main source of internal exposure. Because of the confined space underground and practical limitations to the degree of ventilation that can be achieved, internal exposure is of greater significance in underground mines than in open pit mines. Occupational exposure from the inhalation of radon decay products in underground mines was recognized as a major radiological protection problem in the 1960s and early 1970s. In the intervening period much has been done to reduce airborne concentrations of radon and its decay products in mines and, consequently, exposures from this source. Improvements continue but with increasing cost and difficulty as the concentrations are reduced.

68. Occupational exposures from uranium mining in 14 countries, averaged over 1975-1979, 1980-1984 and 1985-1989, are summarized in Table 3; data are reported separately for underground and open-pit mining. The contributions to the totals, where available, of external exposure and internal exposure from inhalation of radon progeny and ore dust are indicated. Some comments on the tabulated doses are necessary however, in particular on the doses from inhalation of radon progeny. In general, in the data reported to the Committee (or published elsewhere), doses from inhalation of radon progeny were estimated on the basis of a conversion factor of 10 mSv WLM^{-1}. In Annex A the annual effective dose from radon progeny for members of the public has been taken to be 1 mSv from indoor exposure (7,000 hours per year) to a radon concentration of 40 Bq m^{-3} or an equilibrium equivalent concentration (EEC) of 16 Bq m^{-3}. Assuming the same numerical relationship between dose and concentration applies to occupational exposures, the value of the conversion factor expressed in units of dose per working level month (WLM) is: 1 mSv ÷ 7,000 hours ÷ 16 Bq m^{-3} × 6.3 10^5 Bq h m^{-3} WLM^{-1} = 5.6 mSv WLM^{-1}. This is consistent with the value of 5 mSv WLM^{-1} suggested in a consultative document issued by ICRP [I13]. While it has been possible to modify reported doses for this change in conversion factor, insufficient data were available to enable the reported data on distribution ratios to be modified. The tabulated values of NR_{15} and SR_{15}, while valid within the context within which they were reported, are strictly applicable to a value of E somewhat less than 15 mSv; the exact value to which they refer will depend on the particular data set, in particular on the relative contribution of radon progeny to the total dose.

69. Estimates of worldwide levels of exposure from uranium mining, also given in Table 3, have been derived by extrapolating the reported production to total world uranium production. The numbers of monitored workers and the annual collective and individual doses, averaged over the same five-year periods, are illustrated in Figure I. The normalized collective dose and the dose distribution ratios are presented in Figure II.

70. Data on national uranium production have been obtained from responses to the UNSCEAR Survey on Occupational Exposures or, in their absence, from OECD [O2]. Worldwide levels of production were obtained as the sum of data reported by OECD [O2], which was limited to WOCA (World Outside Centrally planned economies Area) countries; data reported to UNSCEAR for Czechoslovakia and the German Democratic Republic; and estimates for China and the former USSR. Production in China was estimated from reported collective doses [I10], assuming that the collective dose per unit mass of uranium mined was equal to the average in those countries for which data were available for underground mines in 1985-1989. This rough estimate of annual production in China was assumed, in the absence of better data, to apply throughout the period 1975-1989. The mining of uranium in the former USSR was nominally assumed equal to that estimated for China.

71. The annual amount of uranium mined worldwide, averaged over five-year periods, was 50-60 kt. The production was highest in 1980-1984 and 10%-15% lower in 1975-1979 and 1985-1989. By far the majority of uranium (about 80%) was mined underground in this period, although the contribution from open-pit mining increased with time. About a quarter of a million workers were involved in uranium mining worldwide; 99% of them, on average, were employed in underground mines, with about one third of these in gold mines in South Africa in which uranium is also extracted. The worldwide annual collective effective dose, averaged over 1975-1989, is estimated to have been about 1,300 man Sv, although there is evidence that levels were about 20% lower than this average in the most recent five-year period; open-pit mining made only a minimal contribution to the total (about 1% on average). The average annual effective dose to monitored workers (or more strictly to those workers whose doses were assessed, either from personal or environmental monitoring) in underground mines has declined from about 5.5 to about

4.5 mSv between the first and third five-year periods. In open-pit mining the corresponding doses were lower, declining from about 2.0 mSv to about 1.6 mSv over the same period (Figure I). The normalized collective effective dose from underground mining decreased from about 30 to about 26 man Sv kt^{-1} uranium [6.6 to 5.7 man Sv $(GW\ a)^{-1}$] between the first and third five-year periods; in open-pit mining, the normalized doses were much lower, having decreased from about 1.1 to about 0.3 man Sv kt^{-1} uranium [0.24 to 0.06 man Sv $(GW\ a)^{-1}$] over the same period (Figure II). For uranium mining as a whole, the normalized collective dose decreased from 26 to 20 man Sv kt^{-1} uranium [5.7 to 4.3 man Sv $(GW\ a)^{-1}$].

72. The reporting of data on distribution ratios is less comprehensive than that on other quantities of interest. Moreover, the situation is further complicated by the modification of reported data to take account of the adoption here of a conversion factor of 5.6 mSv WLM^{-1} for exposure to radon progeny compared with a value of 10 mSv WLM^{-1} generally used in the reported data. While reported doses can be readily modified to account for this change, this cannot be done for the reported distribution ratios. In these circumstances consideration is limited here to an analysis of trends in the reported distribution ratios, while recognizing that the ratios strictly are applicable to values of E somewhat less than 15 mSv (moreover, with the value of E differing between countries depending on the relative contribution of inhalation of radon progeny with total dose). For those countries reporting data on distribution ratios, the fraction of the monitored workforce in underground mines in these countries receiving reported annual effective doses greater than 15 mSv declined from 0.39 in 1975-1979 to 0.26 in 1985-1989; the fraction of the reported collective effective dose arising from reported individual doses above the same level also declined, from 0.69 to 0.53 over the same period. It is not possible to be precise with regard to the level of dose to which these ratios apply when using a dose conversion factor of 5.6 mSv WLM^{-1}, but it is of the order of 10 mSv. The distribution ratios in open-pit mining were much smaller; over the same period the reported number distribution ratio, averaged over those countries providing data on this quantity, declined from about 0.005 to 0.0004 and the reported collective dose distribution ratio from 0.026 to 0.006 (Figure II); for the dose conversion factor adopted in this Annex the value of dose to which these ratios apply is within a range of about 10 to 12 mSv. These values for the reported distribution ratios, averaged over the countries which provided such data, can be considered indicative of worldwide levels.

73. The data for individual countries and their trends with time vary considerably about the average worldwide values (see Table 3). For underground mining the average annual effective dose, averaged over the five-year periods, typically varied within a range of 3-20 mSv; Bulgaria was a notable exception. For open-pit mining the corresponding range of variation was typically about 1-5 mSv. The variation in normalized collective effective doses was even greater, between about 1 and 110 man Sv kt^{-1} uranium [0.25 to 25 man Sv $(GW\ a)^{-1}$] for underground mines; doses in Canada, France and the United States were at the lower end of this range and those in Argentina, India and South Africa at the upper end. For open-pit mines the range of variation was about 0.04-16 man Sv kt^{-1} uranium [0.01-4 man Sv $(GW\ a)^{-1}$]. The range of variation between countries for the reported distribution ratios was somewhat smaller than the range for other quantities.

74. Internal exposure makes by far the greatest contribution to the total exposures in underground mining. Averaging over those countries (Australia, Canada, China, Czechoslovakia, France, the German Democratic Republic, India and South Africa) reporting data on at least two of the three main contributors to exposure (in those cases where only two pathways were quantified the contribution of the third was assumed to be zero), about 70% of exposures arose on average from the inhalation of radon daughters, about 3% from the inhalation of ore dust and about 27% from external irradiation. For open-pit mining there was much greater variation reported in the contribution of the respective exposure pathways. In Argentina, external irradiation contributed about 80% and inhalation of radon daughters about 20% to total exposures; the contribution of ore dust was small by comparison. In Canada in 1985-1989 (doses from milling were included in the data for earlier periods), external irradiation and the inhalation of radon daughters were also the main contributors to total exposure (about 50% and 43%, respectively), with a contribution of about 6% from the inhalation of ore dust. The Australian data showed a somewhat different distribution, with the largest contribution from ore dust (about 75%) and external irradiation and radon daughters contributing about 22% and 2%, respectively. Averaging over these three countries during the 1980s, external exposure has contributed about 70% of the total dose and inhalation of radon progeny about 30%; about 4% of the total has arisen from inhalation of dust.

75. Occupational exposures from uranium milling in nine countries, averaged over 1975-1979, 1980-1984 and 1985-1989, are summarized in Table 4. The reported data for milling were modified in the same way as those for mining (see paragraph 68) in respect of exposure from inhalation of radon progeny (i.e.

conversion factor of 5.6 mSv WLM^{-1} adopted, compared with 10 mSv WLM^{-1} used in reported data. The qualifications made in paragraph 68 with respect to the tabulated distribution ratios apply equally here. Estimates of worldwide levels of exposure are also given in Table 4; they were derived by extrapolating to the total world production of milled uranium. Data on the amounts of uranium milled in individual countries were obtained from responses to the UNSCEAR questionnaire or, in their absence, from OECD [O2], subject to the simplifying assumption that the amount of uranium milled in any year was equal to that mined. This same assumption was used in estimating the amount of uranium milled worldwide. The numbers of monitored workers, the annual collective and individual doses, averaged over the five-year periods, the normalized collective dose and the dose distribution ratios are illustrated in Figures I and II.

76. The average number of workers in uranium milling worldwide is much smaller than the number in mining. It increased from about 12,000 in 1975-1979 to about 20,000 since then. The worldwide annual collective effective dose, averaged over the whole period, 1975-1989, is estimated to have been about 120 man Sv. A small downward trend with time is evident, with a decrease of about 10 man Sv between the first five-year period and the subsequent periods. The worldwide average annual effective dose to monitored (or more strictly, assessed) workers in milling decreased from about 10 mSv in 1975-1979 to about 6 mSv subsequently and is somewhat greater than that experienced in underground mining. The normalized collective effective dose from milling has decreased from about 2.4 in 1975-1979 to about 2.0 man Sv kt^{-1} uranium [about 0.5-0.4 man Sv $(GW\ a)^{-1}$] after that time. In comparison, the normalized collective dose from open-pit mining was smaller on average by a factor of about 2 and that for underground mining was more than an order of magnitude greater.

77. Relatively few data have been reported on distribution ratios for milling and, as for mining, interpretation of the data that do exist is complicated by the revision of reported doses to conform with the dose convention used in this Annex for exposure from inhalation of radon progeny. For the reasons set out above (see paragraph 72) consideration is limited to an analysis of the trends in the reported distribution ratios. Averaging over the available data, the fraction of the monitored workforce receiving reported annual effective doses greater than 15 mSv declined, from about 0.4 in 1975-1979 to about 0.2 in 1985-1989; the fraction of the collective effective dose arising from individual doses above that level declined, from about 0.8 to about 0.4 over the same period. It is impossible to be precise with regard to the level of dose to which these ratios refer when using a dose conversion factor of 5.6 mSv WLM^{-1} for inhalation of radon progeny, but it is of the order of 12 mSv. In the absence of more comprehensive data, these values of the distribution ratios can be considered indicative of worldwide levels.

78. The data for individual countries and their trends with time vary considerably about the average worldwide values (see Table 4). The average annual effective dose to monitored (or more strictly, assessed) workers, averaged over the five-year periods, varied within the range of about 0.1-13 mSv. The variation in the normalized collective effective doses was even greater, from less than 0.1 to about 30 man Sv kt^{-1} uranium [less than 0.02 to about 6 man Sv $(GW\ a)^{-1}$]; doses in Canada, South Africa and the United States were towards the lower end of this range and those in Czechoslovakia, the German Democratic Republic and India towards the upper end.

79. Internal exposure makes by far the greatest contribution to total exposures in milling. Averaging over those countries (Australia, Canada, Czechoslovakia, German Democratic Republic and India) reporting data on each of the three main contributors to exposure in the 1980s, about 38% of exposures arose from the inhalation of radon daughters, about 47% from inhalation of ore dust and about 15% from external irradiation. Considerable variation is, however, evident between countries in the contributions of the respective exposure pathways. The data for the German Democratic Republic are comparable with the average values; those for Australia and Czechoslovakia indicate much greater contributions from the inhalation of ore dust, while for India, the contribution of ore dust was reported as negligible in comparison with the other exposure pathways.

B. URANIUM ENRICHMENT AND CONVERSION

80. Most thermal reactors use enriched uranium with a level of enrichment of, typically, about 3%; the major exceptions are the Magnox reactors and the pressurized heavy-water-cooled and heavy-water-moderated reactors (HWRs), which use natural uranium. Uranium is converted to uranium hexafluoride before being enriched, generally in gaseous diffusion or centrifuge plants. Most enrichment was historically undertaken by gaseous diffusion, but increasingly the centrifuge process is being used because of its much lower cost; laser enrichment is currently under development and may make a significant contribution to the annual supply of enriched material by the end of the century. At present most enrichment services come from five suppliers:

Department of Energy (United States), Eurodif (France), Techsnabexport (Russian Federation), Urenco (Germany, Netherlands and the United Kingdom) and China. The enrichment capacity of these and a few other small producers was projected to be about 40 million separative work units (MSWU) in 1990 [I4] compared with a demand for about 26 MSWU. After enrichment the uranium is reconverted into a form, generally an oxide, appropriate for fuel fabrication. The depleted uranium, or tails, from the enrichment process are generally stored pending decisions on their future use (e.g. in a fast reactor fuel cycle, further enrichment later or disposal). Occupational exposures occur during both the conversion stages and enrichment. Consideration here is limited to exposures during enrichment.

81. Occupational exposures to workers employed in the enrichment of uranium in six countries are summarized in Table 5. With two exceptions the data are for enrichment by the diffusion process; the exceptions are South Africa, where the jet nozzle process is used, and one of the two entries for the United Kingdom, which is for centrifuge enrichment. Sums or averages of reported data are given in Table 5; however, because of incomplete data on the separative work used in uranium enrichment, an extrapolation based on size of the practice to estimate worldwide doses cannot be applied. The alternative extrapolation, based on gross national product, is also inappropriate in this case, because enrichment is carried out in only a very few countries. In these circumstances, only an approximate estimate of worldwide doses can be made.

82. The annual effective dose to monitored workers, averaged over five-year periods and over all reported data, decreased progressively, from about 0.5 mSv in the first period to about 0.1 mSv in the third. The annual collective effective dose, averaged similarly, also decreased progressively, from about 5 man Sv in the first period to about 0.8 man Sv in the second and 0.4 man Sv in the third; these trends largely reflect trends in the United States, which contributes by far the greater part of the reported collective dose. These doses are from external irradiation. Although the potential exists for internal exposure in enrichment plants, its contribution was reported as negligible in comparison with external irradiation by those few countries reporting data on this aspect. In all countries reporting data, the distribution ratios are all zero, reflecting the relatively low levels of exposure encountered in enrichment compared with other stages of the fuel cycle.

83. Only the United Kingdom has reported data on separative work for enrichment by both the diffusion and centrifuge processes. These data provide the only reliable basis on which to estimate normalized collective doses from enrichment. For enrichment by diffusion, the normalized collective dose was about 0.5 man Sv MSWU^{-1} [0.07 man Sv (GW a)$^{-1}$]; a comparable dose was experienced in the early stages of centrifuge enrichment, but this has since been reduced greatly to about 0.04 man Sv MSWU^{-1} [0.005 man Sv (GW a)$^{-1}$] in the most recent five-year period. The use of much larger centrifuges and the greater throughput of enriched material with time have been the main contributors to these decreases. The normalized collective doses, in terms of energy generated, were estimated assuming that 0.13 MSWU were required to enrich the uranium needed to generate 1 GW a of electrical energy in a light-water-cooled, light-water moderated reactor (LWR).

84. The sums of the reported collective doses (and the average individual doses) in Table 5 are assumed, in the absence of better data, to be representative of worldwide exposures from the enrichment of uranium for use in the commercial nuclear fuel cycle. These data do not include contributions from several countries, most notably China and the former USSR; any underestimate resulting from this omission is, however, likely to be small compared with the overestimate resulting from the fact that the United States data include exposures arising during the enrichment of uranium for both civilian and defence purposes.

85. To estimate the normalized dose that is representative of this stage of the fuel cycle, it is assumed that the reported collective doses in 1975-1989 can be associated with the enrichment of that quantity of uranium needed for the generation of electrical energy by LWRs worldwide during the same period. Based on this assumption, the normalized collective dose, averaged over the whole period, is about 0.17 man Sv MSWU^{-1} [0.022 man Sv (GW a)$^{-1}$]; this is broadly comparable with experience in the United Kingdom for enrichment by the diffusion process. In practice, because a fraction of the reported doses is likely to have arisen during the enrichment of uranium used in defence, the normalized collective dose is likely to be an overestimate.

86. In summary, the individual and collective doses from enrichment are small. Consequently, notwithstanding the major uncertainties in estimating worldwide exposures from this source, they will have little impact on the reliability of the estimated exposure from the whole of the nuclear fuel cycle.

C. FUEL FABRICATION

87. Many types of fuel are fabricated according to the reactor type in which they are used. The characteristics of fuels that are relevant here are the degree of

enrichment and the form, either metallic or oxide. The great majority of reactors use low enriched (typically a few per cent) uranium oxide fuel; the main exceptions are Magnox reactors, which use unenriched metal fuel, and HWRs, which use unenriched oxide fuel. The characteristics of the fuel and the reactor environment in which it is used influence the amount of energy that can be extracted from it per unit mass, and significant differences are to be expected between the various types of fuel. About 95% of fuel is currently fabricated for use in water-cooled reactors of various types, with about 85% for use in LWRs. The capacity for water reactor fuel fabrication in 1990 was estimated to be about 13 kt uranium, and the expected requirement for fuel was about 9 kt [I4].

88. The exposures from fuel fabrication have, in previous UNSCEAR Reports, been considered together with those from uranium enrichment. In this Annex they are evaluated separately in order to provide estimates of the doses arising at each main stage of the fuel cycle. Separate estimates are also made in this Annex for each of the main types of fuel. The purpose of this is to enable more realistic estimates to be derived of the normalized collective dose per unit energy generated for the different fuel cycles based on the various reactor types. The four types of uranium fuel to be considered are unenriched metal fuel, used in Magnox reactors; low enriched oxide fuel, used in advanced gas-cooled, graphite-moderated reactors (AGRs) and in LWRs; unenriched oxide fuel, used in HWRs; and mixed oxide fuels, used in fast breeder reactors (FBRs). Mixed oxide fuels (uranium-plutonium) are increasingly being developed for use in LWRs, but occupational exposures arising during their fabrication have yet to be reported.

89. There are two main sources of exposure in the fabrication of uranium fuels: external exposure to gamma-radiation emitted by the uranium isotopes of concern and their decay products and internal exposure from the inhalation of uranium and its decay products. The relative importance of these two routes of exposure varies with the type of fuel fabricated and the manufacturing process. Data reported from the United Kingdom, where significant resources have been allocated to limit internal exposure, indicate that external exposure is the major source; this, however, may not always be so. Individual monitoring for internal exposure, with formal entry of the results in dose records, is usually carried out for only a fraction of the workforce; monitoring of the working environment is often sufficient.

90. Occupational exposures to workers employed in the fabrication of each type of uranium fuel are summarized in Table 6. The number of monitored workers and the annual collective and individual doses, all averaged over successive five-year periods, are illustrated in Figure III for each fuel type. The normalized collective effective doses and the dose distribution ratios are illustrated in Figure IV.

91. ***LWR fuel.*** LWR fuel is fabricated in several countries and is used in pressurized light-water-moderated, light-water-cooled reactors (PWRs) and in boiling light-water-moderated, light-water-cooled reactors (BWRs). The fuel is uranium oxide with an average enrichment of about 3% and is clad in a zirconium alloy. Mixed oxide (uranium and plutonium) fuels are being fabricated for use in LWRs, but as their contribution is small and few occupational exposure data are available, they are not considered further. The normalized collective effective doses in Table 6 have been estimated assuming that 37 t of LWR fuel is needed, on average, to generate 1 GW a of electrical energy.

92. The data for LWR fuel are incomplete in two respects: first, no data have been obtained from some countries that are major fuel producers and, secondly, some of the reported data did not contain estimates of the amounts of fuel fabricated. Worldwide estimates of the annual collective dose and the number of monitored workers have been obtained by scaling the sum of reported data by the ratio of LWR fuel fabricated worldwide to that fabricated in those countries reporting data. A number of approximations had to be made in this extrapolation process, owing to the absence of adequate data on the production of LWR fuel worldwide and in some of the major producing countries. Annual fuel production in these cases was assumed to be equal to that which would have been needed for the generation of electrical energy by LWRs in those particular countries or the world in that particular year. This approximation was used to estimate fuel production in the United States as well as worldwide. Because the United States also supplies fuel to other countries, the amounts predicted in this way are likely to be underestimates of actual production; the normalized collective doses given for the United States are, by the same token, likely to be overestimates. Similar degrees of under- or overestimation can be expected in the respective worldwide data owing to the major contribution made by the United States to the total fuel production.

93. The worldwide annual amounts of LWR fuel fabricated, averaged over five-year periods, increased from 1.6 kt to about 7.0 kt between the first and third periods. The average number of workers also increased in the same period, but by about 50%, a much smaller increase than in the amount of fuel produced. The worldwide annual effective dose to monitored workers, averaged over five-year periods, decreased progressively, from 1.7 mSv in the first

period to about 0.5 mSv in the third period. Notwithstanding the fourfold increase in fuel produced, the worldwide annual collective dose decreased, from 29 to 11 man Sv. These changes are reflected in a decrease, by an order of magnitude, in the worldwide normalized collective effective dose over the same period, from 18 to 1.6 man Sv kt^{-1} [0.7-0.07 man Sv $(GW\ a)^{-1}$]. The average fraction of the workforce receiving annual doses in excess of 15 mSv, NR_{15}, declined over the period, from 0.013 to 0.0003; the corresponding fraction of the collective dose arising from individual doses in excess of that level, SR_{15}, decreased, from about 0.4 to 0.02.

94. The data for individual countries and their trends with time vary considerably about the average worldwide values. Because of the major contribution made by the United States to worldwide fuel production, the doses for that country are broadly comparable with the worldwide averages, albeit slightly greater in general. The average annual doses to monitored workers in other countries are, in general, smaller than the worldwide averages, often by a significant factor. In Japan, the normalized collective doses are substantially less than the worldwide averages, particularly in earlier times; the values in other countries are broadly comparable with the worldwide averages.

95. Only Spain and Japan have explicitly included the data on internal exposures. In Spain, the annual contribution of internal exposure reported since 1988 varied from 20% to 40%; its explicit inclusion may be one reason why the doses in Spain are, in general, greater than those reported elsewhere. In the absence of further information, the doses reported for those countries not explicitly including internal exposures must be considered to be underestimates by indeterminate amounts. Data on the contribution of internal exposure to the doses in fuel fabrication are an essential requirement if valid comparisons are to be made. The potential importance of neglecting internal exposures can be gauged from a review by the National Council on Radiation Protection and Measurements (NCRP) of occupational exposure in the United States [N1]. In that review it was suggested that when account was taken of internal exposures, the average effective dose to fuel fabrication workers in the United States would increase (from a level of about 1.3 mSv for measurably exposed workers for external exposure alone) to a level comparable with that experienced by nuclear power plant personnel (see Section II.D).

96. ***HWR fuel.*** Fuel for HWRs is fabricated in Argentina, Canada, India and the Republic of Korea, which are the main countries where this reactor type is used. The total of the reported data can, therefore, be assumed to be representative of worldwide exposure arising from the fabrication of this fuel type. The fuel is unenriched uranium oxide. The normalized collective effective doses in Table 6 have been estimated assuming that 180 t of HWR fuel is needed, on average, to generate 1 GW a of electrical energy, except when more specific data on equivalent energy generation were provided in response to the UNSCEAR Survey on Occupational Exposures.

97. The worldwide annual production of fuel, averaged over five-year periods, increased progressively, from about 0.6 kt (about 3 GW a equivalent) in the first period to about 1.6 kt (about 9 GW a equivalent) in the third period. By far the greater part (about 95% averaged over the whole period) of the fuel was fabricated in Canada. The worldwide number of monitored workers has increased over the three periods, from about 500 to about 1,100. The worldwide average effective dose to monitored workers, which was about 1.3 mSv in the first period, declined to about 1 mSv in the second but increased to about 1.7 mSv in the third period. The same doses in Canada increased progressively over this time, from about 1.3 mSv to about 2.4 mSv, with most of the increase occurring in 1985-1989; some of this increase may be attributable to increasing fuel production with a decreasing workforce (at least a monitored workforce). The average doses in the other countries are, in general, less than the worldwide averages. The contribution of internal exposure is not significant; these exposures are included only in Canada and are reported to be negligible. Doses to measurably exposed workers have been reported for three of the countries and are significantly greater than those to monitored workers. The annual dose to measurably exposed workers in Canada, averaged over five-year periods, increased progressively, from about 2 to about 3.6 mSv (i.e. doses were about 50% greater than those to monitored workers).

98. The worldwide annual collective effective dose, averaged over five-year periods, increased from about 0.7 man Sv to about 1.9 man Sv. The worldwide average normalized collective dose decreased from about 1.1 to about 0.9 man Sv kt^{-1} [0.2-0.16 man Sv $(GW\ a)^{-1}$] between the first two periods but increased in the third period to about 1.2 man Sv kt^{-1} [0.22 man Sv $(GW\ a)^{-1}$]. During those 15 years, the normalized dose in Canada decreased progressively from about 1.1 to about 0.7 man Sv kt^{-1} [0.2-0.13 man Sv $(GW\ a)^{-1}$]. The worldwide normalized dose increased in the last five-year period, because much higher than average normalized doses arose during fuel fabrication in India. Significant variation is apparent in the distribution ratios between countries but, in general, the values are small. The fraction of the worldwide workforce receiving annual doses in excess of 15 mSv was about 0.003, averaged over all three periods, with

a significantly lower value in 1980-1984. The fraction of the worldwide collective dose arising from annual doses in excess of the same level was about 0.005, averaged over the same period, again with a much lower value in 1980-1984.

99. ***Magnox fuel.*** Magnox fuel is fabricated mainly in the United Kingdom and is used there and in Japan and Italy in this reactor type. The fuel is natural uranium clad in a Magnox alloy. Metal fuel was also fabricated in France for use in gas-cooled, graphite-moderated reactors (GCR)s in that country. The normalized collective effective doses in Table 6 have been estimated assuming that 330 t of Magnox fuel is needed on average to generate 1 GW a of electrical energy. In the absence of reported data from France, the data for Magnox fuel fabricated in the United Kingdom are assumed to be representative of worldwide levels.

100. The annual amount of fuel fabricated, averaged over five-year periods, remained relatively constant with time at about 850 t. The number of workers has increased from about 900 to about 1,100 over the same period. The annual normalized collective effective dose, averaged over successive five-year periods, increased from about 2 man Sv kt^{-1} [0.7 man Sv $(GW\ a)^{-1}$] in the first period to about 4.3 man Sv kt^{-1} [1.4 man Sv $(GW\ a)^{-1}$] in the last. This increase is largely due to the inclusion, since 1986, of internal exposures in the reported data. The average contribution of internal exposure to the total exposure in 1986-1990 was about 35%; the doses reported for years before 1986 are underestimates by at least a comparable amount and need to be adjusted accordingly. Because of this underestimation in earlier years, the increase with time in the normalized collective doses is more apparent than real.

101. The average annual effective dose to the monitored workforce has varied considerably from year to year but with some indication of a declining trend. The annual dose from external exposure alone was about 2 mSv in the period 1985-1989; taking into account of internal exposure, the average annual dose in the period can be estimated to have been about 3 mSv. The fraction of the workforce receiving annual doses in excess of 15 mSv was low, about 0.002 over the first two five-year periods. Because no account was taken of internal exposure during this period, these values are doubtless underestimates. In 1986, when internal exposure was first included, the fraction increased significantly, to about 0.04 (about 0.018 averaged over the five-year period) but thereafter declined to essentially zero.

102. ***AGR fuel.*** AGR fuel is fabricated only in the United Kingdom and used in reactors there; the reported data can, therefore, be taken as the worldwide level for this type of fuel. The fuel is uranium oxide with an average enrichment of about 2.7% and is clad in stainless steel. The data in Table 6 are predominantly for the fabrication of AGR fuel but include a small component (about 10%) of PWR fuel. The simplifying assumption is made here that the data are solely for AGR fuel, and the normalized collective effective doses have been estimated on the basis that 38 t of AGR fuel is needed, on average, to generate 1 GW a of electrical energy. The data also include the workforce involved in, and the collective dose arising from, fuel fabrication and conversion (and reconversion) of uranium to uranium hexafluoride for enrichment. Only about 5% of the collective dose is attributable to the conversion processes; data are not, however, available on the size of the respective workforces to enable the combined data to be presented separately for conversion and fabrication. The average individual doses to workers involved in conversion and fabrication are, however, similar.

103. The annual amount of fuel produced, averaged over five-year periods, remained relatively constant, at about 400 t. Over the whole period, the number of monitored workers, averaged about 1,800, with evidence of a small increase in the two later five-year periods. The normalized collective effective dose, averaged over five-year periods, changed little between the first two periods and was about 8 man Sv kt^{-1} [0.3 man Sv $(GW\ a)^{-1}$]. In the third period it increased to about 12 man Sv kt^{-1} [0.45 man Sv $(GW\ a)^{-1}$]. Much of this increase may be more apparent than real for the reasons set out above in connection with Magnox fuel, in particular the inclusion of internal exposures in the reported data from 1986 onwards. The contribution from internal exposure was about 35% averaged over the period 1986-1990; accordingly, the doses reported before 1986 are likely to be underestimates by a similar or greater factor and need to be adjusted accordingly.

104. The average annual effective dose to monitored workers varied considerably from year to year, with a slight decline being noticeable. The average annual dose (external exposure only) in the first five-year period declined from about 2.3 to about 2 mSv in the second; to take account of the contribution of internal exposure, these doses should be increased by 30% or more. In the last five-year period the average annual dose (external exposure only) remained about 2 mSv, with a total dose (internal and external exposures) of about 3 mSv. The fraction of the workforce receiving annual doses in excess of 15 mSv was low, about 0.001 over the first two five-year periods. Because no account was taken of internal exposure during this period, these values are doubtless underestimates. In 1986, when internal exposure was first included, the

fraction increased significantly to about 0.05 (about 0.014 averaged over the five-year period) but thereafter declined to essentially zero.

105. ***FBR fuel.*** Data on FBR fuel fabrication have been reported only from Japan and are insufficient to make a reliable estimate of worldwide dose from this type of fuel. It can be noted, however, that the average individual doses are broadly comparable with those arising in Japan during the fabrication of LWR fuel. The normalized collective doses per unit mass of fuel fabricated are, however, very much greater; this difference would decrease if the doses were normalized in terms of potential energy generation, owing to the much greater burn-up achieved by FBR fuels. One probable contributor to the larger normalized doses is the small or pilot scale of fuel production.

106. ***Summary.*** Worldwide exposures from fuel fabrication are summarized in Table 7. The annual amount of fuel fabricated worldwide, averaged over five-year periods, increased threefold (in terms of potential energy that could be generated from it) over the period of interest, during which the monitored workforce has increased by about 40%. Notwithstanding this increase in production, the worldwide annual collective dose has decreased, from 36 to 22 man Sv; an even more striking decrease occurred in the normalized collective dose, from about 0.6 man Sv $(GW\ a)^{-1}$ to about 0.1 man Sv $(GW\ a)^{-1}$. A decrease by a factor of more than 2 occurred in the average dose to monitored workers. The data on distribution ratios are somewhat less complete than those for other statistics of interest. Notwithstanding this, the available data overall indicate a generally downward trend with the ratio NR_{15} decreasing more than a factor of 5 from about 0.01 in the first period to 0.002 in the third; over the same period the ratio SR_{15} decreased by a factor of 20 from about 0.4 to about 0.02.

107. Most of the fuel fabricated was for use in LWRs. About 80% of the total collective dose arose from the fabrication of LWR fuel in the first five-year period; this contribution decreased to about 50% in the latest period, with about 40% from GCR fuel and about 10% from HWR fuel. The normalized collective dose (expressed in terms of potential energy that could be generated by the fuel) is significantly greater for Magnox than for other fuels; the much lower burn-up achieved by Magnox fuel is perhaps the main reason for this difference. Somewhat greater individual doses (approaching a factor of two when averaged over the whole period) are associated with both types of GCR fuel compared with fuel for other reactor types. Some of these comparisons need qualification, however, because internal exposures were not, in general, included in the data reported for LWR fuels. As a consequence, some of the differences between GCR and LWR fuels that are identified here may be more apparent than real. Better quantification is needed of the contribution of internal exposure in LWR fuel fabrication; pending this, the data reported here for this fuel type must be regarded as underestimates.

D. REACTOR OPERATION

108. Within the nuclear fuel cycle, reactors are the most common facility. About 430 reactors were in operation at the end of the 1980s. Consequently, there are more occupational data for reactors than for any other type of nuclear installation. Several reactor types have been developed to the commercial stage, in particular PWRs, BWRs, GCRs (comprising, among others, Magnox and AGRs), HWRs and light-water-cooled, graphite-moderated reactors (LWGRs). Detailed consideration is given to each of these with more limited consideration of liquid metal fast breeder reactors (FBRs) and high-temperature gas-cooled, graphite-moderated reactors (HTGRs), which are still largely at a prototype stage of development.

109. Data on occupational exposures at reactors of each type are summarized in Table 8. Worldwide levels of exposure have been estimated from reported data; the extrapolation is based on the total energy generated by the reactor type relative to the energy generated in countries reporting data. The degree of extrapolation necessary was small, as the reported data were substantially complete (about 90% for PWRs and BWRs, 95% for HWRs, 80% for GCRs and 70% for FBRs).

110. The annual data reported in response to the UNSCEAR Survey of Occupational Exposures have been averaged over five-year periods and only the average values are given in Table 8. The variations in annual values are presented in Figures V and VI to illustrate temporal trends in more detail. Data, where available, are also presented on the main activities that give rise to occupational exposures in the different reactor types and on typical levels of dose that occur when undertaking a number of common tasks.

111. Since relatively few data are available on average doses to measurably exposed workers compared with those to the monitored workers, no attempt has been made to estimate a worldwide average dose. The data that are available indicate that the average dose to measurably exposed workers is typically up to about twice that for the monitored workforce, although there is much variation between countries and with time (see Table 8). More data on average doses to measurably exposed workers would be useful; for the reasons previously identified, comparisons made in these terms would, in general, be more reliable than those made on the basis of the dose to monitored workers.

112. Several factors have influenced the trends in reported exposures. These include the commissioning of a large number of new PWRs in the early 1980s, the lower annual collective doses achieved in new reactors because of additional and improved design provisions, and the large reductions in dose achieved in reactors in the United States once the safety modifications required after the accident at Three Mile Island had been completed. Significant reductions in doses in existing reactors have also been achieved, in particular from the greater attention given to reducing circuit activity levels, the reduction of unscheduled maintenance and the greater emphasis on keeping doses "as low as reasonably achievable" (ALARA).

113. Considerable improvements have taken place in the recording and documentation of occupational exposures in recent years, and the creation of national and international databases has greatly facilitated the reliable extraction of relevant statistics. The use of information from these databases will inevitably lead to some, albeit small, differences between the statistics presented in this Annex and those given in earlier UNSCEAR Reports for the same time periods, but an overriding aim is to treat all data included in a consistent manner.

114. There remain some difficulties in interpreting and ensuring fair comparisons between the various statistics. These difficulties were discussed in general terms in Section I.A, where a number of cautionary remarks were made. Four more specific observations need to be made in the present context. First, differences exist in the protocols adopted in various countries as to the fraction of the workforce that is included when evaluating average annual individual doses; in some cases, only measurably exposed individuals are included, whereas generally, the whole of the monitored workforce is taken into account. To the extent practicable, a clear distinction is maintained throughout this Annex between the average individual doses evaluated in the different ways. The use of different protocols for determining who in the workforce should be monitored is, however, a further confounding factor. Particular care must therefore be exercised when comparing average individual doses to ensure that the comparisons are made on equal grounds. These differences do not, however, materially affect the estimation or the comparison of collective doses, at least not within the inherent uncertainties associated with their evaluation.

115. Secondly, the procedures for the recording and inclusion of doses received by transient or contract workers may differ between utilities and between countries, and this may influence the respective statistics in different ways. In some cases, transient workers may appear in the annual statistics for a given reactor several times in one year (as opposed, ideally, to only once, with the summed dose being recorded); if appropriate corrections are not made, then statistics so compiled will inevitably overestimate the size of the exposed workforce and underestimate the average individual dose and also the fractions of the workforce and the collective dose arising from individual doses greater than the prescribed levels. This will only be important in those cases where extensive use is made of transient workers.

116. Thirdly, different approaches are apparent between countries in how they report the exposures of workers at nuclear installations. The majority present statistics for the whole workforce, i.e. employees of the utility and contract workers, often with separate data for each category; some report data for utility employees only, whereas others present the collective dose for the total workforce but individual doses for the utility workers only. Where necessary and practicable, reported data have been modified to enable them to be fairly compared with other data; these changes are indicated in the respective Tables. Attention is also drawn to any unmodified data for which doubts may exist on whether or to what extent they can be compared fairly with the other data.

117. Fourthly, no undue significance should be attached to normalized collective doses that have been derived on the basis of a small number of reactors operating for a short period. Because much of the exposure arises from maintenance carried out during periodic reactor shutdowns, the normalized doses (and particularly those normalized in terms of energy generated) are useful only when derived as an average of a large number of reactors or over a long operating period.

1. Light-water reactors

118. LWRs comprise by far the majority of the installed nuclear generating capacity. About 70% of them are PWRs and about 30% are BWRs. About 40% the LWRs are installed in the United States and about 20% in France, with the remainder distributed among some 20 countries. With respect to occupational exposures, experience has shown significant differences at PWRs and BWRs. Each type is therefore considered separately.

(a) Average annual doses

119. *PWRs.* External gamma-radiation is the main source of exposure in PWRs. Since there is, in general, only a small contribution from internal exposure, it is only rarely monitored. In general, the contribution of neutrons to the overall level of external exposure is

insignificant. Most occupational exposures occur during scheduled plant shut-downs, when planned maintenance and other tasks are undertaken, and during unplanned maintenance and safety modifications. Activation products, and to a lesser extent fission products, within the primary circuit and coolant are the main source of external exposure. The materials used in the primary circuit, the primary coolant chemistry, the design and operational features of the reactor, the extent of unplanned maintenance etc. all have an important influence on the magnitude of the exposure from this source; significant changes have occurred with time in many of these areas, which have affected the levels of exposure.

120. The worldwide installed capacity of PWRs, averaged over five-year periods, increased from about 50 GW in 1975-1979 to about 180 GW in 1985-1989; the corresponding increase in the average annual energy generated worldwide was somewhat greater, from about 30 to 120 GW a. On average, 40% of this energy was generated by PWRs in the United States and about 20% in France. The number of monitored workers in PWRs worldwide has increased from about 60,000 to about 230,000 over the period (Figure V). The average annual collective effective dose increased by a factor of about 2 (from about 220 to about 450 man Sv) between the first two five-year periods; the increase in the third period to about 500 man Sv was small when compared with the doubling of energy generated in the same period. The normalized collective dose changed little over the first two five-year periods, when it was about 8 man Sv $(GW\ a)^{-1}$; in the third period it decreased substantially, to about 4 man Sv $(GW\ a)^{-1}$ (Figure VI).

121. The annual effective dose to monitored workers, averaged over five-year periods, fell from about 3.5 mSv in the first period to about 2.2 mSv in the third; most of this decrease occurred between the second and third periods. The fraction of the monitored workforce receiving annual doses in excess of 15 mSv decreased progressively, falling from about 0.09 to about 0.03 over the entire period; the corresponding decrease in the fraction of the collective effective dose arising from annual doses in excess of the same level was from about 0.6 to about 0.3. These fractions were estimated from a smaller set of data than was used to estimate doses, as not all countries reported these quantities.

122. There are considerable variations about the worldwide average values in both the trends and levels of dose in individual countries. Average values of individual and normalized collective dose are illustrated in Figure VII for geographical groupings. The regions are Asia, Eastern Europe (including the former USSR), Western Europe and the United States. The normalized collective doses in Western European and Asian reactors are generally significantly lower than the worldwide averages, while those in the United States and Eastern European reactors are higher than the average. The variations in the average individual doses to monitored workers about the average values are less pronounced: only in Asian reactors are the doses consistently less than the average. Considerable variation between countries remains, however, even within these narrower regional groupings (e.g. in Eastern Europe the normalized collective doses in Czechoslovakia and in Hungary were, on average, less by a factor of about 5 than those in the German Democratic Republic and the former USSR).

123. The largest normalized collective effective doses occurred at PWRs in the German Democratic Republic, Spain, the former USSR and United States; in Czechoslovakia, Finland, France, Hungary, South Africa and Sweden, the normalized doses were consistently and significantly less than the worldwide averages. These differences in normalized collective doses are largely, but not entirely, reflected in differences between the average individual doses in the respective countries. Downward trends are apparent in the normalized doses in most countries, in particular between the second and third five-year period; the decrease was most pronounced for the Federal Republic of Germany, Japan, the Republic of Korea, Spain, Sweden, the former USSR and the United States. The data for France show an upward trend, having increased by about 20% over the period; the absolute level of the normalized collective dose is, however, still lower than the average for PWRs overall. A few countries that only recently introduced reactors for generating electrical energy [e.g. South Africa and China (Taiwan)] exhibit comparatively low, albeit increasing, normalized collective doses; this is typical of the trends experienced elsewhere.

124. Variations in the doses between reactors within a country are also of interest. Data for PWRs in the United States are illustrated in Figure VIII, in particular the median, the 25th and 75th percentiles and the minimum and maximum values of the collective effective dose per reactor. A wide range of variation is evident and is to be expected, given that much of the exposure arises during repair and maintenance activities and while making safety modifications, all of which are carried out periodically and at different times and to different degrees on each reactor. The various statistics, however, show the same general trends indicated in Table 8 for the normalized collective effective doses averaged over all PWRs in the United States, in particular the higher doses in the first half of the 1980s, which resulted from safety modifications made in response to the accident at Three Mile Island.

125. ***BWRs***. External irradiation is also the major source of occupational exposure in BWRs, with most exposures arising during scheduled shutdowns, when planned maintenance is undertaken, and during unplanned maintenance and safety modifications. By far the largest number of BWRs are located in the United States and Japan.

126. The worldwide installed capacity of BWRs, averaged over five-year periods, increased from about 29 GW in 1975-1979 to about 67 GW in 1985-1989; the corresponding increase in the average annual energy generated worldwide was somewhat greater, from about 15 to 42 GW a. On average, 40% of this energy was generated by BWRs in the United States and 25% in Japan. The number of monitored workers in BWRs worldwide increased from about 60,000 to about 140,000 over the period (Figure V). The average annual collective effective dose increased from about 280 to about 450 man Sv between the first two five-year periods; it subsequently decreased in the third period, to about 330 man Sv, notwithstanding an increase by more than 60% in the energy generated over the same period. The normalized collective dose, averaged over five-year periods, changed little over the first two periods and was about 18 man Sv $(GW\ a)^{-1}$; in the third period it decreased substantially, to about 8 man Sv $(GW\ a)^{-1}$ (Figure VI).

127. The annual effective dose to monitored workers, averaged over five-year periods, fell from about 4.7 mSv in the first period to about 2.4 mSv in the third; most of this decrease occurred between the second and third periods. The fraction of the monitored workforce receiving annual doses in excess of 15 mSv increased from about 0.07 to about 0.08 between the first two five-year periods and decreased subsequently to about 0.03 in the third period; the fraction of the collective effective dose arising from annual doses in excess of 15 mSv was about 0.6 in each of the first two five-year periods, decreasing to about 0.4 in the third period. These fractions were estimated from a smaller set of data than used to estimate doses, as not all countries reported these quantities.

128. There are considerable variations about the worldwide average values in both the trends and levels of dose in individual countries. Some regional variations are illustrated in Figure VII. The normalized collective doses in Western Europe are significantly less than those elsewhere and are typically smaller by a factor of about 2 than the worldwide averages over the whole period. Those in the United States are, apart from the first period, some three to four times greater than those in Western Europe. For BWRs in Japan and China (Taiwan), the normalized dose, averaged over both countries, in the first period was about twice the worldwide average, but in subsequent periods it was less than the average. The variations in the average annual individual doses to monitored workers exhibit trends similar to those for the normalized doses, but the magnitude of the variations about the average are much smaller.

129. Normalized collective effective doses that are consistently and significantly less than the worldwide averages were reported for BWRs in Finland and Sweden. The largest normalized collective doses occurred in India and were about a factor of 10 greater than the worldwide averages for the corresponding periods. Relatively large normalized doses also occurred in the Netherlands, but these data should not be given undue significance, as they apply only to one small reactor. In most other countries there is considerable variation in the normalized doses about the average values, with little evidence of consistent trends between respective time periods. These differences in normalized collective doses are largely, but not completely, reflected in differences between the average individual doses in the respective countries. Major downward trends with time are apparent in the normalized doses in most countries, in particular between the second and third five-year period analysed; the decrease was most pronounced for the Federal Republic of Germany, Japan, Spain and the United States. In the United States there was a large increase in the normalized collective dose in the second period; the safety modifications made in response to the accident at Three Mile Island were the main reason for this increase. The trend in collective dose per reactor to workers at BWRs in the United States is illustrated in Figure VIII. The wide range of variation between reactors is, in general, greater than the variation for PWRs.

(b) Dose distribution ratios for LWRs

130. Comprehensive statistics have been compiled in the United States on the distributions of individual doses making up the collective effective doses [B2, B4]. These enable reliable estimates to be made of the collective dose distribution ratio, SR, and also of the fraction of the workforce exposed above any prescribed level of individual dose, NR. In Figure IX the distribution ratios NR_E and SR_E are given for selected years as a function of the annual effective dose, E. These distributions are summarized in Table 9. Large reductions with time are evident in the fraction of measurably exposed workers receiving an annual effective dose in excess of 15 mSv. Between 1973 and 1989, this fraction, NR_{15}, decreased from 0.24 to 0.03, with much of the reduction occurring in the 1980s. Over the same period there was a 60-fold decrease (from 0.06 to 0.001) in the fraction of workers exposed to annual doses in excess of 30 mSv, a threefold decrease (from 0.34 to 0.09) in those exposed in

excess of 10 mSv, and a twofold decrease (from 0.43 to 0.22) in those exposed in excess of 5 mSv.

131. The reductions in the percentages of the collective effective dose arising from individual annual doses in excess of particular values are also substantial. The fraction of the collective dose arising from annual individual doses in excess of 15 mSv has decreased fourfold (from 0.71 to 0.19) over the period 1973-1989. Over the same period there was a 30-fold decrease (from 0.30 to 0.009) from annual doses in excess of 30 mSv, a twofold decrease (from 0.85 to 0.43) from doses in excess of 10 mSv and a reduction by a factor of about 1.3 (from 0.93 to 0.70) from annual doses in excess of 5 mSv.

(c) Doses for specific tasks and occupational subgroups

132. Detailed statistics are gathered by the United States Nuclear Regulatory Commission on the collective dose for several general categories of work, job functions and types of personnel [B2, B4, R2]. The distribution of the collective dose between various work functions is shown in Figure X for LWRs during 1975-1989. By far the greater part of the collective dose arises in routine and special maintenance, with the contribution of other categories being small by comparison. Throughout the early 1980s, the contribution of special maintenance was greatest, a consequence of the safety-related modifications made after the accident at Three Mile Island. In the most recent period, the collective dose from routine maintenance exceeded that from special maintenance.

133. The distributions of doses between contract workers and utility personnel for separate work functions at LWRs in the United States [B2] has also been analysed. Most of the collective dose is received by contract worker personnel, in particular during special maintenance. Overall, the collective dose to contract workers is greater by a factor of about 2 than that to utility workers. Data reported for some other countries using LWRs (in particular Finland, France, the German Democratic Republic, the Federal Republic of Germany, Spain and Switzerland) show that contract workers typically receive 60%-90% of the total collective dose [L2].

134. The distribution of collective doses among five occupational groups, averaged over 1987-1989, is summarized in Table 10 for workers at LWRs in the United States. Most of the dose is received by maintenance personnel (66%). The largest individual doses are also received by maintenance personnel (about 30% greater than the average to workers in all other occupational groups), but those to health physicists are of a comparable magnitude.

2. Heavy-water reactors

135. HWRs are used in several countries but most extensively in Canada, where the CANDU reactor was developed and since exported to a number of countries. The main source of occupational exposure in these reactors is, in general, external irradiation, mainly from activation products in the coolant and coolant circuits. As in LWRs, most of the exposures arise during maintenance activities. Internal exposure, however, can also be a significant component of exposure, principally from intakes of tritium produced by activation of the heavy-water moderator.

136. The worldwide installed capacity of HWRs, averaged over five-year periods, increased from 5 GW in 1975-1979 to 14 GW in 1985-1989; the corresponding increase in the average annual energy generated worldwide was somewhat greater, from about 3 to 10 GW a. On average, 85% of this energy was generated by HWRs in Canada. The number of monitored workers in HWRs worldwide increased from about 7,000 to about 18,000 over the period. The average annual collective effective dose increased from about 30 man Sv in the first five-year period to about 45 man Sv in the second period and 60 man Sv in the third. Internal exposure made a significant contribution to the overall dose; the contribution varied from year to year and between countries but on average was 30%, varying typically from 15% to 50%. The normalized collective dose decreased from about 20 to about 8 man Sv $(GW\ a)^{-1}$ between 1975 and 1979 and increased again to about 16 man Sv $(GW\ a)^{-1}$ in 1982 (Figure VI); subsequently the dose decreased to about 6 man Sv on average over the remainder of the 1980s. Averaged over five-year periods, the normalized collective dose was 11 man Sv $(GW\ a)^{-1}$ in the first period, decreasing to 8 man Sv $(GW\ a)^{-1}$ in the second period and to about 6 man Sv $(GW\ a)^{-1}$ in the third.

137. The annual effective dose to monitored workers worldwide showed similar variations, but averaged over five-year periods, it has decreased from 4.8 mSv in the first period to an average of 3.3 mSv over the second and third periods. Data on the average annual effective dose to measurably exposed workers are less complete than other data. The average dose to such workers exceeded that for monitored workers by factors ranging up to about 3, with considerable variation between countries. The fraction of the worldwide monitored workforce receiving annual doses in excess of 15 mSv decreased from 0.12 in the first period to about 0.07 in each of the following periods; the corresponding decrease in the fraction of the collective effective dose arising from annual doses in excess of that level was from about 0.7 to about 0.5. Both fractions show considerable variations from year

to year (Figure VI). They were estimated from a smaller set of data than was used to estimate doses, as not all countries reported this data.

138. There is wide variation in both the trends and levels of the doses in individual countries. In the first period the greater part (about 75%) of the worldwide collective dose occurred in Canada; averaged over the last two periods about 42% of the collective dose occurred in India with about 34% in Canada. The normalized collective dose in Canada was considerably less than the worldwide average, declining progressively from about 10 to about 2 man Sv $(GW\ a)^{-1}$ over the three periods. In Argentina and India the normalized doses have exceeded the worldwide averages and in India substantially so [about 80 man Sv $(GW\ a)^{-1}$, averaged over the period 1980-1989]. The decrease in the average annual individual dose to monitored workers in Canada was far greater than that of the worldwide average, decreasing from about 4.2 to 1.5 mSv over the period (over the same time the average dose to measurably exposed workers decreased from about 9 to about 4 mSv). The annual doses to monitored workers, averaged over the whole periods for which data were reported, were about 11 mSv in Argentina and about 6 mSv in India with considerable year to year variation about these average values.

3. Gas-cooled reactors

139. There are three main types of GCRs: Magnox reactors, including those with steel pressure vessels (SPVs) and those with prestressed concrete pressure vessels (CPVs); advanced gas-cooled reactors (AGRs); and high-temperature gas-cooled reactors (HTGRs). Only the Magnox and AGRs have, as yet, reached commercial application; HTGRs exist only in prototype forms. Most of the experience with GCRs has been obtained in the United Kingdom, where they have been installed and operated for many years. Initially, all GCRs were of the Magnox type; throughout the 1980s, the contribution of AGRs, both in terms of their installed capacity and energy generated, became more important. The relative importance of AGRs will increase as Magnox reactors are decommissioned.

140. ***Magnox and AGRs.*** In previous UNSCEAR Reports the data for Magnox reactors and AGRs have been combined, despite potentially large differences in both the individual and normalized collective effective dose for these reactor types (and also between Magnox reactors with different types of pressure vessel). These differences arise mainly from the use of concrete as opposed to steel pressure vessels in AGRs (and in the later Magnox reactors) and the increased shielding that they provide against external radiation, the dominant source of occupational exposure from this reactor type. In this Annex separate estimates are made for each reactor type.

141. The worldwide installed capacity of GCRs, averaged over five-year periods, increased from about 9 GW in 1975-1979 to about 13 GW in 1985-1989; the corresponding increase in the average annual energy generated worldwide was comparable, from about 5 to 7 GW a. On average, 75% of this energy was generated by GCRs in the United Kingdom. The number of monitored workers in GCRs increased worldwide from about 13,000 to 31,000 over the period. The average annual collective effective dose decreased from 36 man Sv in the first five-year period to 24 man Sv in the third, with much of the decrease occurring between the last two periods. The normalized collective dose, averaged over five-year periods, decreased from about 7 to about 3 man Sv $(GW\ a)^{-1}$ over the period, with most of the decrease again occurring between the last two periods.

142. The annual effective dose to monitored workers worldwide, averaged over five-year periods, fell progressively from 2.8 mSv in the first period to about 0.8 mSv in the third. The fraction of the worldwide monitored workforce receiving annual doses in excess of 15 mSv is small: it decreased from 0.02 to 0.0002 over the period; the data are incomplete on the fraction of the collective effective dose arising from annual doses in excess of that level, but in the third period the fraction was 0.008. The substantial decreases in the average individual and normalized collective doses largely resulted from the gradual introduction of AGRs in the United Kingdom; the doses in these reactors are significantly lower than those in Magnox reactors, at least those with steel pressure vessels.

143. There are major differences in the occupational exposures at different types of GCRs. Data for different generations of Magnox reactors, in particular those with steel pressure vessels and those with concrete pressure vessels, and for AGRs are summarized in Table 11. A distinction is also drawn between exposures in the first-generation Magnox-SPV reactors constructed with the dual purpose of producing weapons-grade plutonium and electrical energy and those later built solely for the generation of electrical energy. The normalized collective effective doses, averaged over the whole period, varied considerably from about 30 man Sv $(GW\ a)^{-1}$ for first-generation Magnox-SPV reactors to about 1 man Sv $(GW\ a)^{-1}$ for both AGR and Magnox-CPV reactors; for second-generation Magnox-SPV reactors the dose was, on average, about 8 man Sv $(GW\ a)^{-1}$. Similar trends are evident in the annual individual doses. The average

annual dose to monitored workers in first-generation Magnox-SPV reactors has remained relatively uniform at about 8 mSv, whereas that in Magnox-CPV reactors declined from about 1 to 0.2 mSv over the period; the average annual dose in the second generation of Magnox-SPV reactors has declined over the same period from about 3 to about 1 mSv.

144. The scale of these differences demonstrates the importance of disaggregating occupational exposures reported for GCRs, in particular if the objective is to estimate normalized collective doses for fuel cycles based on different reactor types. Earlier estimates, based on combined data for GCRs, are largely representative of experience with Magnox-SPV reactors. Much lower doses occur during the operation of both Magnox-CPV reactors and AGRs.

145. ***HTGRs.*** A number of prototype HTGRs have been operated, but this reactor type has yet to be adopted for commercial operation. Occupational exposure data have been reported for only one of these reactors, Fort St. Vrain in the United States [R2]. These data are summarized in Table 8, but they are insufficient to estimate worldwide exposures from this reactor type; the contribution compared with other reactors would, however, be minimal. The data indicate that exposures in HTGRs would be much lower than those encountered in LWRs and about the same or less than those experienced in AGRs.

4. Light-water-cooled, graphite-moderated reactors

146. LWGRs were developed in the former USSR and have only been installed there. Occupational exposure data have been reported in [B11] for LWGRs, but the data are incomplete, both in terms of the number of reactors and the period over which they operated. Overall (worldwide) levels of exposure from this reactor type have been estimated by scaling the reported data to the total energy generated by LWGRs. Data on energy generation were largely obtained from information submitted [B11, I8, I9]; data for missing periods were estimated from the installed capacity and the average load factor for the years when data were available.

147. The worldwide installed capacity of LWGRs, averaged over five-year periods, increased from about 6 GW in 1975-1979 to about 15 GW in 1985-1989 (it should be noted that all doses quoted for the last period are averages over 1985-1987 because no data were available for 1988 and 1989); the corresponding increase in the average annual energy generated worldwide was comparable, from about 4 to 10 GW a. The number of monitored workers in LWGRs worldwide increased from about 5,000 to about 13,000 over this period. The average annual collective effective dose increased from about 36 man Sv in the first five-year period to about 170 man Sv in the third, with much of the increase occurring between the last two periods. The normalized collective dose, averaged over five-year periods, was comparable in the first two periods, about 8 man Sv $(GW\ a)^{-1}$, but doubled to about 17 man Sv $(GW\ a)^{-1}$ in the third period. The annual effective dose to monitored workers worldwide, averaged over five-year periods, was about 6 mSv in each of the first two periods, increasing to about 13 mSv in the third period. No data have been reported on the fraction of the monitored workforce receiving annual doses in excess of 15 mSv or on the fraction of the collective effective dose arising from annual doses in excess of that level.

148. The large increases in both the average individual and normalized collective doses in the third period resulted from the accident at Chernobyl. The effect of the accident on these doses is illustrated in Figures V and VI. In 1986, both the average annual individual and normalized collective doses increased by a factor of about 4 relative to those in the immediately preceding years. In 1987, both doses decreased by a factor of about 2; no data are currently available on how they varied in subsequent years. Increases in exposures were reported [B11] for Chernobyl and other LWGRs during 1986. For the other LWGRs the increases are largely artificial, at least in so far as they have been associated with a particular reactor (exposures received while undertaking temporary work at Chernobyl were included in the records at the LWGR where the workers were normally employed). It may be questioned whether the additional exposures received by operational staff at LWGRs generally (because of time spent at Chernobyl following the accident) should be included here, as opposed to being categorized under exposures from accidents. The doses attributed are, however, strictly limited to those received by operational staff and do not include the much larger collective doses received by those involved with mitigating the consequences of the accident and with subsequent clean-up operations. In this context the attribution is judged appropriate.

5. Fast breeder reactors

149. A number of prototype FBRs with a wide range of installed capacities have been developed and operated over the past three decades. It is unlikely, however, that this type of reactor will see significant commercial use, except possibly in a few countries, before the early decades of the next century. The less-than-expected growth in the use of nuclear energy, the

continuing relatively low cost of uranium and the economic risks of developing a complete fast reactor fuel cycle are the main factors delaying the commercial introduction of FBRs.

150. The worldwide installed capacity of FBRs, averaged over five-year periods, has increased from about 1 GW in 1980-1984 to about 2 GW in 1985-1989; over the same period the average annual energy generated worldwide increased from about 0.5 to about 0.7 GW a. The number of monitored workers in prototype FBRs worldwide is estimated to have increased from about 1,400 to about 2,000 between these two periods. The average annual collective effective dose increased from about 0.6 man Sv to about 1 man Sv during the same time. The normalized collective effective dose, averaged over five-year periods was broadly the same in both periods at about 1.3 man Sv $(GW\ a)^{-1}$. The annual effective dose to monitored workers worldwide, averaged over five-year periods, was about 0.5 mSv in both periods.

151. While these data need to be qualified because they apply specifically to prototype facilities, they do indicate that the levels of occupational exposure in FBRs are likely to be much lower than those experienced at reactors of most other types currently in commercial operation.

6. Summary

152. Data on occupational exposures at reactors worldwide are summarized in Table 12. The worldwide installed capacity of all reactors, averaged over five-year periods, increased from about 100 GW in 1975-1979 to 290 GW in 1985-1989; the increase over the corresponding period in the average annual energy generated was from 55 to about 190 GW a. Averaged over the whole period, about 80% of the total energy was generated in LWRs (of this, about 70% was from PWRs and 30% from BWRs), with contributions of about 7% each from HWRs, GCRs and LWGRs. The number of monitored workers increased from about 150 to 430 thousand over the same period.

153. The annual collective effective dose, averaged over five-year periods, increased from about 600 man Sv in the first five-year period to about 1,000 man Sv in the second, with a further increase to about 1,100 man Sv in the third. The trend in annual values is indicated in Figure V. About 80% of the collective dose occurred at LWRs, with broadly similar contributions from PWRs and BWRs. Averaged over the whole period the contribution of HWRs has been about 5%, that of GCRs about 3% and that of LWGRs about 10% (about 6% prior to the Chernobyl accident).

154. The normalized collective effective dose, averaged over all reactors, varied little before 1984, when it was about 11 man Sv $(GW\ a)^{-1}$; thereafter it declined steadily to about 5 man Sv $(GW\ a)^{-1}$ in 1989 (see Figure VI). A generally decreasing trend is apparent in the normalized collective doses for most reactor types. The values for PWRs, LWGRs (before the Chernobyl accident) and GCRs overall (values for AGRs and Magnox-CPV reactors are much smaller) are broadly comparable; the values for HWRs and BWRs are somewhat larger, the latter substantially so in the earlier years.

155. The annual effective dose to monitored workers, averaged over all reactors, fell steadily from more than 4 mSv in 1975 to about 2 mSv in 1989. With the exception of LWGRs, a downward trend is evident in the average annual dose in each reactor type. There are, however, considerable differences between reactors, both in the absolute magnitudes of these doses and in their rate of decline.

156. Data on the dose distribution ratios NR_{15} and SR_{15} are less complete than data for other quantities (e.g. no data for LWGRs, FBRs, HTGRs and incomplete data for other reactor types). Values of these ratios, averaged over all reported data, are given in Table 12. Until more complete data are obtained, these averages can only be said to be indicative of worldwide values. Averaging over all reported data, the fraction of monitored workers receiving annual effective doses in excess of 15 mSv was about 0.09 in 1975 decreasing to about 0.03 by 1989; over the same period the fraction of the collective dose, arising from annual doses in excess of the same level, decreased from about 0.6 to about 0.3.

E. FUEL REPROCESSING

1. Average annual doses

157. Spent irradiated fuel from nuclear reactors used to generate electrical energy was reprocessed on a commercial scale, for much of the 1970s and all of the 1980s, in only two countries, France and the United Kingdom. The facilities in those two countries have, however, also been used to reprocess irradiated fuel from other countries. In the United Kingdom only uranium metal fuel from Magnox reactors has to date been reprocessed on a commercial scale; a new plant for the reprocessing of oxide fuel is, however, scheduled to begin operation in the early 1990s. In France, before 1976, only metallic fuel was reprocessed on a commercial scale; oxide fuel reprocessing began in 1976 and is now by far the largest constituent of fuel reprocessed.

158. In previous UNSCEAR Reports occupational exposures at the commercial reprocessing facilities in

France and the United Kingdom were discussed. In addition, data were presented for a number of small-scale and/or prototype reprocessing plants. In this Annex consideration is largely directed towards the commercial-scale facilities, because it is these which determine the overall levels of both past and current exposures from this stage of the fuel cycle; data on prototype facilities are, however, provided for completeness.

159. External irradiation is the main contributor to occupational exposure in fuel reprocessing, although internal exposure may be significant in some operations, in particular those that involve actinides. Where internal exposures may be significant, personal monitoring is carried out, using methods appropriate to the circumstances of the exposure; these may include the wearing of personal air samplers, biological monitoring and whole body or lung counting. The contributions from internal exposure have in general, however, only recently been included in reported data on occupational exposure.

160. In previous UNSCEAR Reports a single estimate was reported for the normalized collective effective dose for reprocessing. The estimate was derived from the normalized collective doses estimated for each reprocessing facility and the respective amounts of fuel (in terms of energy equivalence) processed by them. In this Annex separate estimates are made of the normalized collective dose for the reprocessing of uranium metal and oxide fuels. There are several reasons for this. First, the fuels themselves have very different characteristics, as do the plants in which they are processed. Secondly, the normalized collective doses (normalized in terms of energy generation) for reprocessing the two types of fuel have differed by more than an order of magnitude in recent years. Any average value of normalized collective dose is, therefore, very sensitive to the respective amounts of fuel reprocessed and would probably not be valid for other periods or for projecting doses in the future. Thirdly, separate values are necessary in this analysis to provide normalized collective doses for each of the fuel cycles using different reactor, and consequently fuel, types.

161. Data on occupational exposures in reprocessing plants are summarized in Table 13, and some of the main features are illustrated in Figure XI. Few of the reported data contain estimates of the amount of fuel reprocessed or the energy generated from the fuel during its irradiation. In making estimates of worldwide levels of exposure from reprocessing and of average normalized collective doses, consideration has been limited to the commercial reprocessing of fuel at Cap de La Hague in France and Sellafield in the United Kingdom. Both metal and oxide fuels have been reprocessed at Cap de La Hague as well as small amounts of mixed oxide fuels; the relative amounts of each reprocessed in the three five-year periods are indicated in a footnote to Table 13. The doses reported for the reprocessing of Magnox fuels at Sellafield are probably overestimates. These doses are, with the exception of reactor operations, for the Sellafield site as a whole and will, therefore, include exposures from operations unconnected with Magnox reprocessing.

162. Worldwide levels of exposure from reprocessing metal fuels have been estimated by adding the data for the United Kingdom to that fraction of the total exposures occurring at Cap de La Hague attributable to the reprocessing of metal fuels. The normalized collective dose for each fuel type reprocessed at Cap de La Hague was estimated from the reported total collective dose arising in each five-year period and the amounts of each type of fuel reprocessed (the contribution of the small amount of mixed oxide fuel that was reprocessed was neglected). The normalized collective dose for metal fuel was estimated to be about 18 man Sv $(kt)^{-1}$ [6.7 man Sv $(GW\ a)^{-1}$] and for oxide fuel about 14 man Sv $(kt)^{-1}$ [0.7 man Sv $(GW\ a)^{-1}$]. The collective dose attributed to each type of fuel reprocessing in each five-year period was then derived as the product of the respective normalized collective dose and the amount of fuel processed. The numbers of workers attributed to the reprocessing of each fuel type were estimated from the collective doses, assuming that the average individual dose in each group was equal to that for the workforce as a whole.

163. The annual amount of metal fuel reprocessed worldwide, averaged over five-year periods, remained relatively uniform within a range of about 1,000-1,200 t (3-3.6 GW a). The number of monitored workers was typically 7,000-8,000. The average annual collective effective dose has decreased from about 50 man Sv in the first period to about 30 man Sv in the third. The normalized collective dose has declined similarly from about 50 to about 33 man Sv $(kt)^{-1}$ [17-11 man Sv $(GW\ a)^{-1}$], with a comparable decrease in the average annual effective dose to monitored workers from about 7 to about 4 mSv. The average fraction of monitored workers receiving annual doses in excess of 15 mSv decreased from about 0.16 to about 0.009 over the period analysed. These data are illustrated in Figure XI.

164. Over the period as a whole, about 80% of worldwide metal fuel reprocessing took place at Sellafield, with about 90% of the total collective dose arising there. The normalized collective doses for reprocessing metal fuel at Sellafield are typically greater than those at Cap de La Hague by a factor of about 2, apart from in the first five-year period, when the difference was greater. The respective average annual individual doses differ by a similar amount. A large fraction of the exposures at Sellafield has histori-

cally arisen during the decanning of fuel and in other operations conducted near the fuel storage ponds. This situation arose following significant contamination of the pond water from fuel corrosion in the early 1970s and is probably the main source of differences in exposures at Sellafield and at Cap de La Hague. Several factors have contributed to the reduction in exposures at Sellafield since the early 1970s, in particular the allocation of greater resources to ensure that doses were kept as low as reasonably achievable, measures taken to reduce the levels of contamination in pond cooling water and, more recently, the commissioning of a new facility for the receipt, storage and decanning of Magnox fuel.

165. The annual amount of oxide fuel reprocessed in France (and essentially worldwide), averaged over five-year periods, has increased from about 30 t in the first period to about 400 t in the last (about 0.5 to about 9 GW a). The number of monitored workers has increased over the same period from about 100 to about 4,000. The average annual collective effective dose has increased from about 0.4 man Sv in the first period to about 6 man Sv in the third. The normalized collective dose remained fairly uniform at about 14 man Sv $(kt)^{-1}$ [about 0.7 man Sv $(GW\ a)^{-1}$]. Another further reprocessing plant (UP3) was brought into operation at Cap de La Hague in 1990, and following this there was a significant decrease in the normalized collective effective dose, to about 5 man Sv kt^{-1} [0.19 man Sv $(GW\ a)^{-1}$]; on this evidence, somewhat lower normalized doses than reported in Table 13 can be expected in the future. The average fraction of monitored workers receiving annual doses in excess of 15 mSv decreased from about 0.06 to about 0.008 over the period analysed; the corresponding decrease in the fraction of the collective dose arising from individual doses in excess of that level was from about 0.3 to about 0.1.

166. With two exceptions, the doses reported in Table 13 include only exposures from external irradiation. Internal exposures are included in all of the data for Japan and for the United Kingdom from 1986 onwards. The reported doses in all other cases may, therefore, be underestimates, and caution should be exercised when comparing data that have been compiled in different ways. The contribution of internal exposure in the United Kingdom is estimated to be less than 10%.

2. Doses for specific tasks and occupational subgroups

167. The distribution of doses within the workforce involved in the reprocessing of nuclear fuel is, as in other occupations, not uniform, and doses somewhat higher than the average for the workforce as a whole will be received by groups of workers undertaking certain tasks. Statistics have been compiled for several groups of workers employed in the reprocessing of spent nuclear fuel and associated activities at the Sellafield reprocessing plant in the United Kingdom [S5]. The doses to these workers are illustrated in Figures XII and XIII. Annual doses from external irradiation are given in these Figures for the following six groups of workers for the period 1968-1988:

(a) fuel storage and decanning: process workers engaged in the storage under water of spent Magnox fuel and the subsequent removal of the magnesium alloy cladding before chemical dissolution of the fuel element;
(b) chemical separation: process workers engaged in the chemical dissolution of spent fuel to separate reusable uranium and plutonium from the fission product waste;
(c) maintenance: skilled and semi-skilled tradesmen engaged in the routine and breakdown maintenance of mechanical plant items;
(d) maintenance of new plant: skilled and semi-skilled tradesmen engaged in the installation of new mechanical plant items associated with operating facilities;
(e) plutonium finishing: process workers engaged in the conversion of the separated plutonium in the nitrate form into the final metal or dioxide product;
(f) waste processing: process workers engaged in the evaporation (i.e. concentration) and storage of the fission product waste stream separated from the actinides by the chemical reprocessing.

168. A generally downward trend in the average annual effective doses for each of the six groups has been maintained since the early 1970s, and substantial reductions have been achieved. The doses declined from several tens of millisievert in the early 1970s to levels in the range 4-10 mSv (Figure XII). For comparison, the annual effective dose, averaged over the whole workforce employed in reprocessing operations, fell from about 10 to about 3 mSv from 1975 to 1988. Several factors contributed to these reductions: the introduction of annual as opposed to age-related dose limits was influential, but the most important factor was the increased emphasis given, from the late 1970s onwards, by the regulatory authorities and the operator on keeping doses as low as reasonably achievable. ALARA became a central consideration in day-to-day plant operations and in the design of new facilities and the modification of the old plant. The introduction of a design standard for new facilities contributed further to the downward trends in dose, in particular through the 1980s, when a large number of new facilities were commissioned; this standard sought to ensure an average annual dose to the workforce of less than 5 mSv.

169. The reductions in collective effective dose (Figure XIII) are, in general, less pronounced. The trends in the collective dose are, however, generally downwards. Substantial reductions in the collective dose have been achieved in the two subgroups of reprocessing workers contributing most to exposures during reprocessing operations: workers associated with fuel storage and decanning and those associated with maintenance. In the former case the decrease reversed an increasing trend throughout the 1970s, which had resulted from the corrosion of fuel cladding and the contamination of storage ponds. Improvements in the condition of the storage pond and, more significantly, the commissioning of new fuel storage and decanning facilities were responsible for the reversal and for the sharp decline in the exposure of this occupational group. With one exception, the collective doses in the other subgroups exhibited a small decrease. The exception is the collective dose arising from the installation of new plant items; the increase here was associated with the almost twofold increase in the number of workers in this occupational category and doubtless also reflected an increased level of plant modifications and improvements.

F. RESEARCH AND DEVELOPMENT

170. In the UNSCEAR 1977 Report [U4], Annex E, it was estimated that the largest single contribution to the collective dose per unit energy generated came from research and development. A value of 14 man Sv $(GW\ a)^{-1}$ was estimated. This was subsequently judged to have been an overestimate, and in the UNSCEAR 1982 Report [U3], a value of 5 man Sv $(GW\ a)^{-1}$ was suggested as a more reasonable global average.

171. It is difficult to estimate the levels of occupational exposure that can unequivocally be attributed to research and development in the commercial nuclear fuel cycle. Few data are reported separately under this category, and even when they are, uncertainties remain over their proper interpretation. The main difficulties of interpretation are as follows:

(a) data are often compiled for research establishments whose main, but not sole, function is to undertake research and development associated with the commercial nuclear fuel cycle. The fraction devoted to this function is rarely given;
(b) some of the occupational exposures attributed in the preceding Sections to particular parts of the fuel cycle contain a contribution from research and development, but the magnitude of this fraction is difficult to estimate;
(c) normalization of collective doses from research have been made in terms of the nuclear energy generated in the year in which the research was performed. While this convention has the benefit of simplicity, practicability and convenience, the validity of equating the current levels of collective dose and energy generation is open to criticism. The benefits of research inherently accrue over a period quite different from that in which the research was performed. Actually, the normalization should take account of the total energy generated in the period in which the benefits are deemed to accrue. In a rapidly developing industry, it is evident that normalization based on current energy generation is likely to lead to a large overestimate in the early years, followed by an underestimate later as the industry matures and the amount of research declines. Such considerations were at least partially responsible for the large downward revision in the normalized collective dose referred to in the preceding paragraph.

172. Occupational exposures arising in nuclear research, averaged over five-year periods, are summarized in Table 14. There is considerable variation in the levels of collective dose associated with research activities in each country, reflecting, among other matters, the relative role of nuclear energy in the national energy supply and the extent to which nuclear technology was developed domestically or imported from elsewhere. The reported annual collective effective doses range from a very small fraction of a man sievert (e.g. in Finland) to about 40 man Sv in the United Kingdom. Country-to-country differences are to be expected in the occupational exposures associated with this category; however, these differences may have been exaggerated significantly by different reporting approaches. The collective doses attributed to research in the United States and the United Kingdom are by far the largest of those reported (typically, annual doses range between 20 and 30 man Sv in the United States and 20 and 40 man Sv in the United Kingdom). The only other countries reporting annual doses of a few man sievert or greater are Canada, France, Germany and Japan, each of which has a significant nuclear research and development programme.

173. The data given for the United States need to be qualified because of the way in which they have been estimated. They have been extracted from data reported for all employees and contract workers of the Department of Energy [M3]; however, only a fraction of these exposures is associated with research related to the commercial nuclear fuel cycle (much is defence-related). In the absence of definitive data on the magnitude of this fraction, it has been approximately estimated from the total data of the Department of Energy by excluding those categories that are clearly

unrelated to commercial fuel cycle research. The data comprise the sum of exposures reported to arise in fusion, waste management and processing, plus one half of the exposures arising in the following categories: reactors, general research, offices, maintenance and support and other. The somewhat arbitrary inclusion of one half of the exposures attributed to these latter categories (which could not be excluded unequivocally), was intended to minimize the likelihood of underestimating the collective dose that should properly be attributed to commercial nuclear fuel cycle research. The doses given in Table 14 for the United States comprise about one third of the total doses reported by the Department of Energy but are still considered to be overestimates. In previous UNSCEAR evaluations, the total exposures reported by the Department of Energy were attributed to research associated with the nuclear fuel cycle; as a consequence, earlier worldwide predictions of exposures from this source may have been significantly overestimated.

174. Worldwide levels of occupational exposure associated with research are also given in Table 14. They were estimated from the reported data with extrapolation based on gross national product. This method was adopted in preference to the extrapolation used for other parts of the nuclear fuel cycle, which were based on fuel fabricated, energy generated etc.; the difficulties, identified previously, of using energy generation as the basis for normalizing research were responsible for the change to gross national product. The regional groupings of countries were as specified in Section I.C, except that the former USSR was treated separately from the rest of Eastern Europe and, for the purposes of the extrapolation, grouped with those other regions for which no data had been reported or no data were available. The net effect of this change is that the doses for the former USSR were extrapolated on the basis of the normalized collective dose averaged over all reporting countries rather than over just those countries reporting data in Eastern Europe. The former was judged to be a more appropriate basis of extrapolation for a country with a large nuclear industry and research and development programme. The sum of gross national products for those countries reporting data was about 60% of the worldwide total. On average, therefore, the reported data have been scaled upwards by a factor of about 2; there is, however, considerable variation about this average for particular regions.

175. The annual number of monitored workers in research worldwide, averaged over five-year periods, remained fairly uniform, about 130,000. The average annual worldwide collective effective dose has decreased from 170 to 100 man Sv between the first and third five-year periods. The annual effective dose to monitored workers worldwide, averaged over five-year periods, fell from 1.4 mSv in the first period to about 0.8 mSv in the third. For those countries reporting data on this quantity, the fraction of the monitored workforce receiving annual doses in excess of 15 mSv decreased, falling from about 0.04 to about 0.01 over the period; the corresponding decrease in the fraction of the collective effective dose arising from annual doses in excess of that level was from about 0.4 to 0.3. These fractions were estimated from a set of data that was smaller than the set used to estimate doses, as not all countries reported data on these quantities; moreover, in some countries data on only one of the fractions were reported. Fewer data are available on the average doses to measurably exposed workers than on those to monitored workers; consequently no attempt has been made to estimate a worldwide average dose for this quantity. Those data that are available exhibit wide variations, with the average dose to measurably exposed workers varying from marginally in excess of that for the monitored workforce to many times greater.

176. It is of interest to compare the normalized collective doses (normalized in terms of gross national product, the unit for which is 10^{12} US dollars) for the different geographic or economic regions. For 1985-1989, the normalized collective dose averaged over all countries reporting data was about 5.8 man Sv per GNP unit (1989 prices). In comparison, the value for the OECD was about 5.7 man Sv per GNP unit; the values for Latin America, Eastern Europe (excluding the former USSR) and east and south-east Asia (non-centrally planned economies) were all within the range 0.8-1.4 man Sv per GNP unit. The value for India was considerably higher, about 20 man Sv per GNP unit. Considerable variation is, however, evident between countries within these broader regional groupings. For example, within the OECD, values were in the range 0.8-40 man Sv per GNP unit, the larger values being associated with those countries having large nuclear development programmes. The largest of these values was for the United Kingdom, where about half the total collective dose attributed to research arose from the operation and maintenance of a prototype steam-generating heavy water reactor (SGHWR); much of the remainder arose during the operation of reactors for material testing and radioisotope production and the operation of a prototype fast reactor and associated reprocessing and waste management facilities. Whether these exposures should be attributed to research is debatable, in particular those arising from operation of the SGHWR, where one of the considerations influencing its continued operation was the commercial revenue obtained from sales of electrical energy. This is another example of the difficulties encountered in trying to ensure comparability in the data reported for different countries.

177. Estimates have been made of the worldwide normalized collective dose expressed in terms of the nuclear energy generated during the same period as the research was undertaken. The deficiencies of this quantity were noted in paragraph 171, and it has been estimated mainly to provide a basis for comparison with estimates made on this basis in previous UNSCEAR Reports. The present analysis indicates that the global average of 5 man Sv $(GW\ a)^{-1}$ [U3], which was a major downward revision of the previous estimate, may still be a significant overestimate. It yields global average normalized collective doses of about 3, 1.5 and 0.6 man Sv $(GW\ a)^{-1}$ for the three five-year periods; even these values are considered to be overestimates. The sixfold decline in the normalized collective dose over the period analysed is largely an artefact of the normalization procedure, i.e. most of the reduction is a consequence of an increase in the rate of energy generation rather than of a decrease in the exposures associated with research.

178. An alternative, but perhaps more meaningful estimate of the normalized collective dose from research, albeit subject to several important simplifying assumptions, may be made by associating the total collective dose from research carried out in 1955-1989 with the energy generated during the same period plus that likely to be generated, largely with existing reactors, over the next 30 years, i.e. from 1990 to 2019. The total collective dose can be estimated from the worldwide data in Table 14, assuming that the worldwide average annual collective dose in five-year periods before 1975-1979 increased by 35 man Sv per period (i.e. the approximate increase per period between 1975-1979 and 1985-1989). The total energy generated may be estimated as the sum of the total nuclear energy generated up to 1989 plus that assumed to be generated over the next 30 years; the latter estimate assumed that the average rate of energy generation over this time would remain the same as that in 1985-1989. On this basis the normalized collective effective dose from research is estimated, in round terms, to be about 1 man Sv $(GW\ a)^{-1}$ and is considered to be applicable to research carried out in support of the commercial nuclear fuel cycle up to 1989. This value is judged to be a conservative estimate for a number of reasons, not least the probable overestimation of doses that should be associated with research in the period 1975-1989, the probable overestimation of doses attributable to research prior to 1975 and the probable underestimate of the energy generation that should be associated with the research already conducted. For the purpose of assessing overall values of normalized collective doses for the whole fuel cycle, this value of 1 man Sv $(GW\ a)^{-1}$ is assumed to be generally applicable for research, irrespective of when it was undertaken in the past, and to be independent of the fuel cycle considered.

G. CUMULATIVE DOSES

179. The estimation of cumulative occupational doses and their distributions in different workforces is a topic of some importance to those concerned with radiological protection. The cumulative dose received by a worker and its rate of accumulation provide a measure of the additional risk that may result from occupational radiation exposures. The absolute value of this risk and its distribution with time can be compared with risks in other occupations as an input to establishing occupational dose limits. There are, however, few published data on cumulative or lifetime doses, and it is therefore possible to provide only very indicative estimates of cumulative or lifetime doses for a limited number of occupations in particular countries. The increasing use of computerized databases for recording occupational exposures should result in more and better statistics on cumulative dose.

180. The most extensive analysis of cumulative or lifetime doses so far undertaken by the Committee was that for the UNSCEAR 1977 Report [U4]. Those dose estimates need to be revised to take account of subsequent developments in radiological protection standards and practice and of the simplifications that were used in the analysis. The more significant estimates of cumulative doses for nuclear fuel cycle facilities are summarized in this Section. Inevitably, differences exist in how the data on cumulative doses have been compiled and reported, and these limit the extent to which they can be directly compared.

181. ***Summary of cumulative doses reported in previous UNSCEAR Reports.*** Estimates of mean lifetime doses have been made in the United States for various groups of workers (employees of licensees of the Nuclear Regulatory Commission, the Department of Energy and the Navy) [E1]. Since these initial estimates were based on historical data on cumulative doses to workers whose employment had been terminated, no assumptions had to be made about the length of their working lifetimes. For most groups of workers analysed, the mean cumulative effective dose was estimated to be about 10 mSv. The estimates were not very sensitive to the year in which employment was terminated and showed only a small increase in the mean cumulative dose with increasing mean duration of employment (for mean periods in the range 1-10 years). The mean cumulative doses derived from such data may, however, be underestimates, because the data contain records for both permanently and temporarily terminated workers, and probably not all doses from previous periods of employment or with different employers will have been included. Estimates were also made of the maximum cumulative doses among the groups of workers analysed. Based on an analysis of trends in the data for workers in the

nuclear fuel cycle and for industrial radiographers, a maximum cumulative effective dose was estimated in both cases to be about 1.1 Sv; this was in accord with the maximum dose actually recorded in the data.

182. Sont et al. [S3] made estimates of lifetime doses for radiation workers in Canada based on data (up to 1983) contained in the National Dose Registry. The lifetime doses were estimated by linear extrapolation of each individual dose record for an assumed working lifetime of 40 years (i.e. the simplifying assumption adopted in the UNSCEAR 1977 Report). Lifetime doses predicted to be less than 10 mSv (equivalent, on average, to annual doses of 0.25 mSv) were excluded from the analysis. Estimates were made for each occupational category included in the registry.

183. Selected characteristics of the distributions of lifetime doses predicted for workers in the nuclear fuel cycle and industrial radiographers are given in Table 15. The mean lifetime effective dose for workers in the nuclear fuel cycle was predicted to be about 240 mSv, with the median being lower by a factor of about 2. Mean doses greater by a factor of 2 were predicted for particular occupations in the nuclear fuel cycle, i.e. chemical and radiation control, reactor operations and mechanical maintenance. The estimates need, however, to be qualified in the following respects:

(a) the assumption of 40 years for the period of exposure of all workers is very unlikely;
(b) because of the linear extrapolation of doses, no account is taken of how the dose profile may vary with the duration and starting date of employment;
(c) no account is taken of possible changes in dose limits or regulatory requirements over the period.

184. ***Workers at uranium mines in the United States.*** The distribution of cumulative doses received by uranium miners in the United States has been evaluated for the period 1967-1985 [B12]. The doses included only exposure by the inhalation of radon decay products and were derived assuming a conversion of 10 mSv WLM^{-1}; the values have been modified here using a conversion factor of 5.6 mSv WLM^{-1}. During this period, 50% of the miners had cumulative doses greater than 8.4 mSv. The percentage decreased steadily with dose, to 25% of the workforce greater than 28 mSv, 10% greater than 73 mSv, 1% greater than 240 mSv, and 0.1% greater than 380 mSv.

185. ***Workers at reactors in the United States.*** In its recent annual compilations of occupational exposures at commercial reactors and other facilities [R2], the Nuclear Regulatory Commission has explicitly addressed career or cumulative doses among reactor workers. The analysis was based on termination dose records, i.e. records of the cumulative dose at the time an individual terminated work at a reactor facility licensed by the Nuclear Regulatory Commission. It was limited to individuals who terminated their careers between 1977 and 1989 and to those working at reactors at the time of termination. The individual career or cumulative dose was estimated as the sum of all exposures received while working at reactors licensed by the Nuclear Regulatory Commission (but excluding doses that may have been received elsewhere). Data compiled in this way have a number of limitations that need to be recognized in order to be interpreted correctly. Two in particular are worthy of note: first, the data only include exposures that occurred at licensed reactors; and, secondly and perhaps more importantly, a large number of individuals may not have completed their careers on termination and may receive additional exposures during future work involving radiation. Since the mean age at which employment terminated was 36-38 years, there is considerable potential for further exposure at some future time. This consideration is, however, likely to be important only for employment that was terminated in more recent years. The likelihood of a return to radiation work would be expected to decrease with time since the employment terminated.

186. Data have been analysed for over half a million monitored workers, of whom about 300,000 had received a measurable dose (taken as any recorded dose during the period equal to or greater than 0.01 mSv), and statistics compiled on the variation of career or cumulative dose with length of employment, age and sex. Selected data from these statistics are summarized in Table 16 for those terminating employment between 1977 and 1989. For employment periods in the range of a few years to about 20 years, the average career dose increased fairly linearly with the duration of employment, with an average annual increment of about 3.5 mSv. For employment periods in the range of 20 to 25 years, the average annual increment was greater and typically about 5 to 6 mSv. This greater rate of dose accumulation, however, did not persist for even longer periods of employment. For employment periods greater than 25 years (average duration of about 40 years) the average career dose was about 70 mSv, that is an average annual increment of about 1.8 mSv. For career lengths in the range 20-25 years, about 3% of workers received career doses in excess of 500 mSv, with about 20% in excess of 200 mSv and about 40% in excess of 100 mSv. For those with career lengths of 10-15 years, the corresponding percentages were much reduced: about 0.1%, 3.6% and 14%, respectively. The corresponding percentages for other career durations can be found in Table 16.

187. The average career length for those terminating employment in 1977 was about 1 year, increasing to about 5 years in 1989. A less than proportional increase occurred in the average career dose over the same period; the increase was from about 10 mSv in 1977 to about 17 mSv in 1988 with evidence of a more substantial increase to about 26 mSv for those terminating employment in 1989. Data for subsequent years will be of interest to determine whether the latter is a statistical fluctuation or a reflection of an underlying trend. The average age at which employment was terminated changed slightly over this period, from 36 to 38 years.

188. Before the above-mentioned statistics were available from the Nuclear Regulatory Commission, Goldsmith et al. [G1] reported results from a more limited analysis of the cumulative doses for about 9,000 workers who at one time or another were employed at the Calvert Cliffs nuclear power plant in the United States. Two PWRs with a generating capacity of 825 MW each at Calvert Cliffs began operating commercially in 1975 and 1977, respectively. Workers were followed from their time of employment at the plant (including the period of construction) to the end of 1986. The mean follow-up period was 5.4 years, the mean duration of employment at the plant was 1.9 years and overall in the nuclear industry, 3.1 years.

189. For measurably exposed workers (about 80% of those monitored) the average career dose was 21 mSv; the average cumulative dose to contract workers, who comprised about one half of those measurably exposed, was 31 mSv and that to utility workers, 13 mSv. The cumulative collective effective dose to those workers was about 150 man Sv, of which only about one third (about 54 man Sv [B2]) was actually received at the Calvert Cliffs plant; the remainder was received at other licensed facilities. This mean cumulative effective dose of 21 mSv is somewhat greater than the overall average of about 14 mSv reported by the Nuclear Regulatory Commission for all reactor workers who terminated employment between 1977 and 1989. The cumulative dose for workers at the Calvert Cliffs nuclear power plant would be expected to continue to increase for those who had not yet terminated employment.

190. The data on cumulative doses were analysed in terms of the duration of employment at Calvert Cliffs, the duration of employment within the nuclear industry, the age at which employment began in the industry, the number of utilities at which an employee has worked, job category etc. [G1]. Selected characteristics of the distributions of cumulative dose for various employment durations are summarized in Table 17. The mean and median cumulative doses increase with increasing duration of employment in a broadly linear fashion. For contract workers, the average annual increment in dose was about 7 mSv and that for utility employees, about 3.5 mSv. The rate of accumulation of dose by utility workers was similar to that reported by the Nuclear Regulatory Commission for workers with career durations from 5 to 20 years; the rate of dose accumulation by contract workers was two times higher.

191. About 18% of contract workers and 6% of utility workers had received cumulative effective doses in excess of 50 mSv; the corresponding percentages for cumulative doses in excess of 100 mSv were 8.3% and 1.6%. The maximum cumulative dose reported was 470 mSv. The percentages of workers exceeding particular levels of cumulative dose after specified lengths of employment do not support any simple basis for extrapolation, but they nevertheless provide at least a rough indication of the levels of cumulative dose that may be experienced in the future, (or were already experienced in the past), by workers who were employed for longer periods in the industry.

192. The data also show a relationship between the cumulative dose and the number of utilities for which an employee has worked; this, perhaps, is not so surprising, since to at least some extent there must be a correlation between duration of employment and the number of utilities at which an employee has worked. The mean cumulative dose increases from about 8 mSv for contract workers who have been employed by only one utility to >100 mSv for those employed by 15 or more utilities. Cumulative doses were also estimated for selected job categories, and average values are summarized in Table 18. The higher doses received by contract workers compared with utility workers are apparent. By far the highest mean cumulative doses (in excess of twice the mean cumulative dose for the workforce as a whole) are received by workers in health physics.

193. In general, the cumulative doses and other related statistics reported for workers who, at one time or another, had been employed at the Calvert Cliffs reactor exceed those reported by the Nuclear Regulatory Commission for workers whose employment at reactors terminated in 1977-1989. These differences call into question the representativeness of career doses derived from termination records; one interpretation of the differences observed could be that career doses for workers terminating employment may be underestimates of those for workers having the same career duration but remaining in employment. Data in future years will help to elucidate this issue. The Calvert Cliffs data also highlight the significant differences in cumulative doses between utility and contract workers and between occupational categories. Further data on such differences would be useful.

194. ***Workers at a Department of Energy facility in the United States.*** An analysis is being undertaken of lifetime doses received at a large facility operated by the Department of Energy; research and development in support of both the commercial and defence nuclear fuel cycles are undertaken at such facilities. The analysis is still under way, but preliminary results have been presented in [M3]. The study includes more than 300,000 dose histories from more than 30,000 individuals who were employed at the particular facility at some time from 1944 to 1984. Only doses received at that facility are included in the analysis (i.e. doses received before or after to employment at the facility are not included). Data were collected on external and internal exposure, but the preliminary results are concerned solely with external exposure. These data show, for example, that no worker employed 20 years at the facility accumulated a dose greater than 500 mSv, and 10% of them accumulated a dose equal to or greater than 150 mSv. These data, while preliminary, show the magnitude of cumulative exposures over a 40-year period. When the analysis is complete, in particular when both internal and external exposures are included, it should provide further insight into the rate of accumulation of dose during working lifetimes.

195. ***Workers at the Sellafield reprocessing plant in the United Kingdom.*** An analysis [B9] has been made of the cumulative external radiation exposure, up to 1988, of male workers employed at the BNFL site at Sellafield, where various nuclear activities are undertaken in addition to the main one of fuel reprocessing. The trends in the cumulative dose as a function of follow-up time and as a function of the year in which the monitoring of a worker first took place are illustrated in Figure XIV; a subset of the data is given in Table 19. The data clearly indicate that the average cumulative dose in a group of workers followed for a given period decreases from earlier years to more recent years in which the group was first monitored; the effect becomes more pronounced for longer follow-up periods. For a 20-year follow-up period, the average cumulative dose for those who were first monitored in 1950 is about 400 mSv; this is greater by a factor of almost 2 than the average cumulative dose received by those first monitored in the mid- to late 1960s. For a 38-year follow-up period (the maximum), the average cumulative dose for those first monitored in 1950 is about 750 mSv; the cumulative doses for the same follow-up period for those first monitored in 1960 can, at this stage, only be speculative, but by extrapolating existing data and taking into account the effect of a reduction in dose limits, the average cumulative dose for this group of workers appears unlikely to exceed 350 mSv. The decreasing rate of increase in the average cumulative dose with length of follow-up period (for a given year of first monitoring) illustrates the considerable potential for overestimating cumulative doses, if derived on the basis of linear extrapolation of past experience.

196. Further useful insights could be obtained from these data if they could be reported in various disaggregated forms, for example, the distribution of cumulative doses (in addition to the mean) for particular choices of the year of first monitoring and follow-up period, age at first monitoring and main type of work undertaken etc.

197. ***Workers at nuclear establishments in the United Kingdom.*** As part of an analysis of the National Registry for Radiation Workers in the United Kingdom [K5], data were reported on the cumulative doses from external irradiation of workers. These external doses are summarized in Table 20 in three different formats: for each of the major employers of radiation workers included in the study, for year of birth of the workers and for the year in which radiation work began. Since the data include cumulative doses for both current and past employees in each of the organizations up to about 1988, they comprise individual doses accumulated over a wide range of different working periods and at different times.

198. While the data are of general interest, they are particular to the composition of the past and current workforce and their employment characteristics; they cannot (at least in the form in which they have been reported) be used to estimate cumulative doses for different durations of employment for either the past or current workforce. To enable such estimates to be made, the data would need to be disaggregated, at least into the form in which the data for workers at BNFL Sellafield are presented in Table 19. Equally, it would be inappropriate, indeed potentially misleading, to attempt, in the absence of additional information, to draw any firm conclusions about the levels of cumulative dose in different industries based on direct comparisons between the data in Table 20. The respective data may comprise workforces having very different sizes, age structures and employment durations, and these characteristics may, moreover, have varied considerably over time. For example, a major change in the size of a workforce in the recent past could considerably distort the estimated cumulative dose relative to that for an industry having a relatively uniform or even declining workforce.

199. Notwithstanding these qualifications, the data exhibit a number of interesting features. The average cumulative dose at sites of BNFL was greater by a factor of more than 2 than that at research establishments of the Atomic Energy Authority and at

reactors operated by Nuclear Electric. This is to be expected given the somewhat higher doses experienced during reprocessing and at the older reactors operated by BNFL. Smaller average cumulative doses occurred at Ministry of Defence establishments, in particular at the Atomic Weapons Establishment; this reflects the much smaller levels of external dose experienced in the processing of materials for nuclear weapons. The cumulative doses to those monitored by the Defence Radiation Protection Service (activities largely connected with the nuclear submarine programme) are for both civilian and naval personnel; one contributory factor to the lower levels in this group is the relatively short periods, compared with a working lifetime, that naval personnel spend in this role.

200. Cumulative dose as a function of the year of birth of the worker generally decreased, as would be expected, with time; this trend reversed for the earliest years analysed because these workers, on average, had spent a smaller part of their working lives in radiation-related work. Disaggregation of the data according to duration of employment in radiation work would yield statistics of somewhat greater interest and value. The cumulative dose as a function of the year radiation work started shows, apart from the early years, an expected decrease with time. Two factors contribute to this decrease: first, the greater period of time, on average, spent on radiation-related work and, secondly, the generally downward trend in annual doses. The rate of decrease in the average cumulative dose between the periods for which the data are reported is not uniform, indicating that there are factors operating that cannot be discerned from the data in its aggregated form. Again, disaggregation of these data in terms of year and age at which work with radiation began, follow-up period, type of work undertaken etc. is needed for the full potential of these data to be realized.

201. ***Summary.*** In the past few years significantly more data have been reported on cumulative doses during working lifetimes. This was to have been expected from the increasing development and use of computerized databases for occupational exposures. While such data are sparse in comparison with data on annual doses, the imbalance is likely to be reduced in the future. To facilitate the comparison and/or aggregation of cumulative doses for different occupational categories and countries, much more attention should be given to the development and use of common approaches for the compilation and reporting of these data. If data could be presented in sufficient detail to allow their analysis as a function of the year and age of starting radiation-related work, employment duration and type of work undertaken, much greater uniformity in reported cumulative doses and their comparison could be achieved.

H. SUMMARY

202. Worldwide occupational exposures from each stage of the commercial nuclear fuel cycle are summarized in Table 21 and illustrated in Figure XV. The data are annual values averaged over five-year periods. The number of workers in the commercial nuclear fuel cycle rose from an average of about 560,000 in the first five-year period to about 880,000 in the third. About a quarter of a million of these workers were involved in uranium mining and about 130,000 in research and development; the remainder were largely employed in reactor operations (about 150,000 on average in the first five-year period increasing to about 430,000 in the third period). The annual collective effective dose, averaged over five-year periods, increased from about 2,300 man Sv in the first period to about 3,000 man Sv in the second but decreasing in the third period to about 2,500 man Sv. By far the largest contributors to the total collective dose were uranium mining and reactor operation (about 50% and 35%, respectively, averaged over the period 1975-1989).

203. The average annual effective dose to monitored workers in the whole fuel cycle decreased progressively, from an average of 4.1 mSv in the period 1975-1979 to an average of 2.9 mSv in the period 1985-1989. There is, however, considerable variation about these average values for different stages of the fuel cycle (see Figure XV). Downward trends in dose with time are evident for all stages of the fuel cycle; the magnitude of the decrease varies, however, with the stage of the fuel cycle, and there were also considerable year to year variations that are not apparent in the five-year averages. The dose distribution ratios are illustrated in Figure XVI. The fraction, averaged over five-year periods, of monitored workers receiving annual doses in excess of 15 mSv has decreased from about 0.20 to about 0.10 between the first and third periods; the corresponding decrease in the fraction of the collective effective dose has been from about 0.63 to about 0.42. Workers in mining and reactor operation are the main contributors to these two fractions.

204. The normalized collective effective doses for each stage of the fuel cycle are shown in Figure XVI. The collective dose from mining, milling, fuel fabrication and fuel reprocessing have been normalized to the energy equivalent of uranium mined or milled or the fuel fabricated or reprocessed in the respective periods. The estimate of 1 man Sv $(GW\ a)^{-1}$ for research associated with the fuel cycle has been assumed in each period. The overall normalized collective effective dose (i.e. averaging over all stages in all fuel cycles, taking account of their relative magnitudes) is estimated to be 18, 17 and 12 man Sv $(GW\ a)^{-1}$ in 1975-1979, 1980-1984 and 1985-1989,

respectively. These normalized doses exclude fuel reprocessing, which would add about 0.7 man Sv $(GW\ a)^{-1}$ for oxide reprocessing, and 10-15 man Sv $(GW\ a)^{-1}$ for Magnox fuel reprocessing, with the larger value appropriate for earlier times.

205. The components of normalized collective effective doses for the separate fuel cycles based on the various reactor types are summarized in Table 22; the results are illustrated in Figure XVII. For ease of comparison and completeness, a contribution from reprocessing is indicated in each case, whether or not reprocessing of that fuel type has occurred or indeed is even foreseen. With the exception of the fuel cycles based on GCRs, reactor operation makes the largest contribution to the normalized collective effective dose, with the only other large contribution coming from mining. For fuel cycles based on other than GCRs, the normalized collective dose varied within a range of 17-27 man Sv $(GW\ a)^{-1}$ in the first five-year period and 10-14 man Sv $(GW\ a)^{-1}$ in the third period; the decrease was mainly due to decreases in the doses arising during reactor operation.

206. The normalized collective doses for the fuel cycle based on AGRs remained relatively uniform over the whole period, about 9 man Sv $(GW\ a)^{-1}$. This is significantly less than for fuel cycles of other reactor types because of the lower collective doses for the reactors. Uranium mining is the largest contributor to the normalized collective dose for this fuel cycle accounting for 60% or more. For the fuel cycle based on the Magnox reactor, the normalized collective effective dose declined from 36 man Sv $(GW\ a)^{-1}$ in the first period to 27 man Sv $(GW\ a)^{-1}$ in the third. The reprocessing of Magnox fuel makes by far the greatest contribution to the total normalized dose (40%-50%). Reactor operation and mining are the only other significant contributors, with similar contributions. Two factors have been largely responsible for the greater normalized doses associated with the fuel cycle based on Magnox reactors. First, because of its much lower irradiation, the generation of unit electrical energy with Magnox fuel requires larger amounts of uranium to be mined, fuel to be fabricated and fuel to be reprocessed than with fuel cycles based on other reactor types; secondly, the doses from Magnox reprocessing have been greater than anticipated because of major contamination of pond cooling water from fuel corrosion that occurred in the first half of the 1970s at the Sellafield plant in the United Kingdom.

207. Insufficient data are available on cumulative or lifetime doses to enable reliable estimates of worldwide levels or of trends in their values; this situation, however, is changing through the increasing use of computerized databases for occupational exposures and the compilation of data for epidemiological studies on workers. Much improved estimates of cumulative doses can, therefore, be expected over the next few years. To facilitate the comparison and/or aggregation of cumulative doses for different occupational groups and/or countries, it would be useful if data could be reported in a manner which enabled them to be evaluated in terms of the following quantities: the year and age of starting radiation-related work, employment duration and type of work undertaken.

III. DEFENCE ACTIVITIES

208. Radiation exposures to workers in defence activities can be grouped into three broad categories: those arising from the production and testing of nuclear weapons and associated activities; those arising from the use of nuclear energy as a source of propulsion for naval vessels; and those arising from the use of ionizing radiation for the same wide range of purposes for which it is used in civilian spheres (e.g. research, transport and non-destructive testing). The levels of exposure in the first two of these categories are assessed separately and then the overall levels of exposure from defence activities are assessed. It must be recognized that there will be some lack of rigour and/or uniformity in the attribution of exposures to particular defence activities and in the separation of exposures between defence activities and the commercial nuclear fuel cycle. This is inevitable, given differences in how data have been categorized and reported in different countries. In this Annex, for example, all exposures occurring in the mining, milling and enrichment of uranium have been attributed to the commercial nuclear fuel cycle; at least a fraction of these exposures should, however, have been attributed to defence activities. Similarly, some of the exposures attributed to reprocessing and to research and development in the commercial nuclear fuel cycle should also be attributed to defence activities. For these reasons, the doses reported in the remainder of this section are likely to be underestimates of those that should properly be associated with defence activities. The data are not complete for radiation-related defence activities in all countries.

A. NUCLEAR WEAPONS

209. Nuclear weapons have been developed, tested and deployed in the military services of five countries: China, France, the former USSR, the United Kingdom and the United States. The main potential sources of occupational exposure in the development and production of nuclear weapons are the two radioactive fissile materials, plutonium and uranium, and tritium. Exposures may arise by two main routes; the intake of these materials into the body by inhalation or ingestion (or absorption through the skin in the case of tritium) and external irradiation from gamma rays and, to a lesser extent, neutrons. Intake of these elements into the body is minimized by avoiding direct contact and providing containment for the materials during their fabrication into weapons. Some small intakes will, however, inevitably occur, and monitoring is generally undertaken to determine their magnitude. The nature and extent of monitoring depend on the potential for exposure. Where material is being processed, the monitoring may include the use of personal air samplers, whole-body monitoring and bioassay; where the potential for intake is much less, area monitoring of airborne levels may suffice. Because of the steps taken to provide confinement for these materials, external irradiation tends to be the dominant source of exposure for those involved in the production, testing and subsequent handling of nuclear weapons. As the energy of the gamma-radiation typically emitted by the more common isotopes of these elements is relatively low, this is one area where the direct recording of the dosimeter measurement as the received whole-body or effective dose, as is common practice, could lead to significant overestimates. Neutron as well as gamma dosimeters may be used where exposures from the former may be significant.

1. Annual doses

210. Data on occupational exposures from the nuclear weapons programmes in the United Kingdom and the United States are summarized in Table 23 and are illustrated in Figure XVIII. The reported doses are for external irradiation only and include exposures arising in the development and production of weapons as well as in their subsequent handling, although the latter makes only a modest contribution to the overall levels of exposure. The total number of monitored workers (i.e. summed over both countries), averaged over five-year periods, remained relatively uniform over the period analysed, at about 21,000. The total annual collective effective dose, averaged over five-year periods, also varied little and was typically about 14 man Sv. This average value, however, disguises somewhat greater year-to-year variations within the range 10-20 man Sv, although there were no significant trends in the values. About 80% of both the total number of monitored workers and the collective dose were in the United States.

211. The annual effective dose to monitored workers, averaged over all workers and over five-year periods, was about 0.7 mSv in all three periods. Average individual doses in the United States were broadly comparable with those for the total workforce; somewhat higher average annual doses, about 1 mSv, were experienced in the United Kingdom up to the middle of the 1980s, but these later decreased by a factor of more than 2. The annual doses to measurably exposed workers (United States data only) were typically greater than those to monitored workers by a factor of about 2. All the individual and collective doses referred to here need, however, to be qualified. They are the doses recorded by the dosimeter. The actual effective doses would be smaller by a factor of at least 2. This discrepancy is due to the relatively low energy of the gamma-radiation emitted by weapons materials. Data (available only for the United Kingdom) on the fraction of workers receiving annual doses in excess of 15 mSv indicate that, in general, this fraction is zero or very small.

212. Fewer data are available on internal exposures. In the United Kingdom, records of internal exposures from the intake of actinides into the body (and, to a lesser extent, tritium) have been kept since 1986. Doses from intakes of actinides have been measured using personal air samplers worn by individual workers, and those from intakes of tritium have been measured by urine monitoring. Each year, about 1,000 workers were monitored for uranium and plutonium. The average committed effective dose from intakes in 1986 was about 0.15 mSv from uranium and plutonium, and by 1989, these doses had decreased to about 0.05 mSv. In each year also about 500 workers were monitored for tritium intake, and the average annual dose declined from about 0.17 mSv to 0.1 mSv between 1986 and 1989. The resulting collective dose from internal exposure is, therefore, small in comparison with that from external irradiation. Indeed, any underestimate as a result of its omission from the doses reported in Table 23 (at least for the United Kingdom data) is negligible in comparison with the overestimate of external dose as a result of including the dosimeter measurement directly into dose records.

213. Comparable data are not available for other countries that have developed nuclear weapons. More limited data [B10, N2] have, however, recently become available on exposures in reactors and chemical reprocessing plants used in the production of weapons-grade materials in the former USSR. Only individual doses are reported, and in the absence of information on the size of the workforce, no estimate

could be made of collective doses. Moreover, data on exposures arising at other stages of weapons production and testing would be needed before these data could be properly compared with the data presented in Table 23. Nonetheless the data provide some perspective on the levels of dose encountered in the weapons programme in the former USSR.

214. The variation in average individual dose (external irradiation only) to workers in reactors and chemical reprocessing plants is illustrated in Figure XIX. In the late 1940s these average doses were substantial (about 1 Sv) in both the reactors and chemical plants. They had declined to about 100 mSv by the late 1950s and to about 10 mSv by the late 1960s. Thereafter the rate of decrease in dose was more modest. The distributions of dose among the respective workforces are also illustrated in Figure XIX. In the late 1940s and early 1950s, annual doses in excess of 1 Sv were received by a few tens of per cent of workers in both the reactors and chemical plants, with 1%-2% receiving annual doses in excess of 4 Sv. In the chemical plants, essentially the whole workforce was exposed to annual doses in excess of 25 mSv before the early 1960s; the percentage of workers exceeding this level of exposure declined rapidly through the 1960s to essentially zero by the end of that decade. In the reactors, the percentage of workers receiving annual doses in excess of 25 mSv decreased during the 1950s, from essentially 100% to a few tens of per cent; this share subsequently varied from a few to a few tens of per cent through the 1960s before decreasing to a low level in the 1970s.

2. Cumulative doses

215. The distribution of cumulative doses among workers employed in the nuclear weapons programme in the United Kingdom at the end of 1989 [D1] is summarized in Table 24. Less than 1% of the workforce in 1989 received cumulative effective doses in excess of 100 mSv and none received in excess of 500 mSv. In practice all the percentages are overestimates because the effective dose and the dosimeter measurement are assumed to be equivalent.

B. NUCLEAR-POWERED SHIPS AND THEIR SUPPORT FACILITIES

1. Annual doses

216. Nuclear-powered ships (submarines and surface vessels) are operated by several navies, in particular China, France, India, the former USSR, the United Kingdom and the United States. Pressurized water-cooled reactors are used as the power source in almost all cases; in the former USSR several reactors are cooled by liquid metal. Radiation exposures arise on board ship and also at shore-based support facilities, where maintenance, refuelling etc. are carried out and personnel are trained. Data are not available from all countries, but compilations have been made of the exposures arising in the United Kingdom [D1, M11] and the United States [M1, M9, M10, N1, S2].

217. Data on occupational exposures from nuclear-powered ships in the United Kingdom and the United States are summarized in Table 23. The total number of ships in the two navies increased from an average of 135 in 1975-1979 to an average of 167 in 1985-1989. Averaged over the whole period, about 90% of these belonged to the United States navy. The total number of monitored workers increased from about 42,000 in 1975-1979 to about 63,000 in 1985-1989. Most of this increase occurred in the United States, as the number of workers in the United Kingdom remained relatively constant, at about 6,000, throughout the period.

218. The total annual collective dose decreased from about 92 man Sv in the first five-year period to about 57 man Sv in the third. Averaged over the whole period, the contribution of the United States to the total collective dose was about 73%; the magnitude of the contribution differed, however, between five-year periods. The annual dose averaged over all monitored workers decreased from about 2.2 mSv in the first five-year period to about 0.9 mSv in the third; the corresponding decreases in the two countries were from about 4.1 to about 1.9 mSv in the United Kingdom and from about 1.9 to about 0.8 mSv in the United States. Over this same period the fraction of all monitored workers receiving annual effective doses in excess of 15 mSv decreased from about 0.5 to about 0.1; in the United Kingdom the values of this quantity were, in general, about 50% larger than the average values.

219. Estimates have been made of the normalized collective effective dose, with the normalization performed in terms of the number of ships. Averaged over both countries, the annual normalized collective dose has decreased by a factor of about 2, from about 0.7 man Sv per ship in 1975-1979 to about 0.34 man Sv per ship in 1985-1989. The corresponding decrease in the annual normalized dose was from about 1.8 to about 0.6 man Sv per ship in the United Kingdom and from about 0.6 to about 0.3 man Sv per ship in the United States. These and previously identified decreases in exposures were achieved despite a significant increase in the number of ships in service and undergoing refit and maintenance during the period.

220. In general, higher exposures were received by shore-based workers, in particular those who were involved in inspection, maintenance (including refitting and refuelling operations) and repair inside the reactor compartment or on components that form the primary cooling circuit. By comparison the exposures of on-board personnel were generally much lower, owing to the shielding provided around the reactor and its associated systems. These differences are illustrated in Figure XVIII.

221. Averaged over the whole period and both countries, about 45% of the total workforce comprised shore-based workers, although there were significant variations about this average value both with time and between countries; for example, in the United Kingdom about 80% of all workers were shore-based. About 70% of the total collective dose over the whole period was received by shore-based workers, again with variation about this average value between countries and with time (e.g. about 85% of the exposure in the United Kingdom was received by shore-based workers).

222. The most noticeable difference between the two groups of workers is in their average annual doses. Averaged over both countries and over five-year periods, the average annual dose to shore-based workers has decreased from about 3.2 mSv to about 1.5 mSv between the first and third periods; the average doses to on-board workers were typically two to three times lower, decreasing from about 1.3 to about 0.5 mSv over the same period. The data for the two countries exhibit the same trends, but the absolute and relative magnitudes of the doses differ, sometimes significantly. Somewhat higher than average doses may be received by particular subgroups within the broader occupational groupings. For example, at civilian dockyards in the United Kingdom, where much of the maintenance and refitting of ships is undertaken, average annual doses were as high as 10 mSv in some years, although they decreased, in general, over the years. Differences are also apparent between the two groups in terms of the fraction of workers receiving annual doses in excess of particular levels (15 mSv for the United Kingdom data and 10 mSv for the United States data), with the fraction being considerably greater for shore-based workers. In the UK the distribution ratio, NR_{15}, for shore-based workers decreased from about 0.09 to about 0.02 between the first and third five-year periods; the corresponding fractions of on-board workers exceeding that dose decreased from about 0.03 to about 0.01 over the same period. In the United States the distribution ratio, NR_{10}, for shore-based workers decreased from about 0.1 to about 0.03 between the first and third five-year periods, while the ratio for on-board workers decreased from about 0.02 to about 0.001.

2. Cumulative doses

223. The distributions of cumulative doses among workers employed in the naval nuclear propulsion programme in the United Kingdom at the end of 1989 and in the United States at the end of 1991 are summarized in Table 24. Data are given separately for on-board and shore-based personnel and for the total workforce in the case of the United Kingdom. Somewhat higher cumulative doses are evident for shore-based personnel than for those on board, because the latter are naval personnel, whose mean time of service in this capacity is much shorter than that of the mainly civilian workforce in the shore-based facilities, where much of the occupational exposure occurs. In general, the percentages of workers exceeding particular levels of dose in the United Kingdom surpass those in the United States, although not by a great amount.

224. In the United Kingdom, the highest cumulative dose recorded among shore-based personnel was about 800 mSv accrued over a 30-year period. The distribution of cumulative doses varies considerably from one shore-based facility to another, with much higher doses at civilian dockyards, where much of the maintenance etc. is undertaken. Cumulative doses at operational naval bases are lower, both because of differences in the nature of the work carried out and the generally greater mobility of naval personnel. For example, about 20% of the civilian dockyard workforce received a cumulative dose in excess of 100 mSv compared with about 8% for all shore-based personnel.

C. ALL DEFENCE ACTIVITIES

1. Annual doses

225. Data on occupational exposures from all defence activities are summarized in Table 23 for the United Kingdom and the United States and for the sum of both sets of data; the data are illustrated in Figure XVIII. The data include exposures from weapons production and testing, from nuclear ships and from a wide range of other uses of radiation that can be attributed to defence-related activities. These uses include all those encountered in civilian occupations, for example non-destructive testing, transport, research, education and medicine. The contribution from these other sources to the overall levels of exposure from defence-related activities in the United Kingdom varied from about 20% in the late 1970s to only a few per cent in the later 1980s. In the United States this contribution, averaged over the whole period, was about 15%, decreasing over time. By far the greater part of both the total defence

workforce and the total collective dose are associated with nuclear ships; this is not surprising, given the large number of nuclear ships operated by these two countries.

226. The total number of monitored workers, averaged over five-year periods, has increased from about 100,000 to about 130,000 between the first and third periods. This increase largely occurred in the United States; the number of monitored workers in the United Kingdom remained relatively constant, about 12,000, over the period analysed. The total annual collective dose, averaged over five-year periods, decreased from about 140 to about 84 man Sv between the first and third periods; averaged over the whole period, about 75% of the total collective dose was received by workers in the United States. The annual dose to monitored workers, averaged over both countries and over five-year periods, has decreased from about 1.3 mSv to about 0.7 mSv between the first and third periods. Given the much larger contribution made by the United States to the overall data, these average individual doses mainly reflect experience in that country; over the same period, the average annual doses to workers in the United Kingdom were somewhat larger, decreasing from about 3 mSv to about 1.2 mSv.

227. The above data need qualifying with regard to their completeness, in particular whether they include all significant occupational exposures associated with defence activities. For example, they do not include occupational exposures incurred in the mining of uranium used in either the nuclear weapons or the nuclear naval programmes; nor is it clear to what extent the reported data include exposures arising during the enrichment of uranium for both the weapons and naval programmes or exposures arising in the chemical separation and subsequent treatment of plutonium. Such omissions, should they exist, are significant only in the context of the proper assignment of exposures to different practices; any omission here is likely to be compensated for by an overestimate of exposures in other practices (e.g. exposures in mining, enrichment and fuel reprocessing attributed to the commercial nuclear fuel cycle).

2. Worldwide annual doses

228. The data presented above for all defence activities include occupational exposures for only two countries, the United Kingdom and the United States. Occupational exposures from defence-related activities in China, France and the former Soviet Union (i.e. the other countries which have developed nuclear weapons and/or that operate nuclear navies) are not available. Any estimate of worldwide occupational exposures from defence activities can, therefore, be made only by extrapolating the available data to these other countries. Inevitably, this can only be done very approximately, and neither of the methods of extrapolation presented in Section I.C is appropriate.

229. It would be most useful if the extrapolation could be based on normalized collective dose, with the normalization performed in terms of unit explosive yield for weapons and per ship or installed nuclear capacity for the naval propulsion programmes. Data sufficient for making these extrapolations could probably be compiled on weapons stockpiles worldwide and their potential yields and on the worldwide capacity of nuclear navies. The validity of such extrapolations would depend, however, on the representativeness of normalized collective doses derived from experience in the United Kingdom and the United States. The limited data for the nuclear weapons programme in the former USSR (see Figure XIX) do not augur well in this respect; in particular, the reported doses in earlier years in that country were far in excess of those experienced elsewhere. These much higher doses largely preclude the use of normalized collective doses derived in one or two countries for estimating worldwide exposures from defence activities.

230. Pending the acquisition of further data, a very simple approach has been adopted for estimating worldwide exposures from this source, namely, that the worldwide collective dose from defence activities is greater by a factor of 3 than the sum of that experienced in the United Kingdom and the United States. Four assumptions underlie the choice of this factor: first, the level of defence activities in the former Soviet Union and the United States were broadly comparable; secondly, the levels of exposure in the former Soviet Union were greater than in the United States by an indeterminate amount that did not exceed a factor of 2 in 1975-1989; thirdly, the levels of exposure in France have been comparable with those in the United Kingdom; and, fourthly, the exposures in China were not large in comparison with either those in the former Soviet Union or in the United States. Based on these assumptions the estimated worldwide average annual collective effective dose from defence activities would have been about 400 man Sv in 1975-1979, falling to about 250 man Sv in 1985-1989. Given the coarseness of the underlying assumptions, it would not be possible to give a precise estimate of the collective dose; perhaps all that can be concluded is that the worldwide average annual collective dose during the period analysed was about 300-400 man Sv. This estimate is inevitably associated with much uncertainty, which can only be reduced by relevant data from China, France and the former Soviet Union.

3. Cumulative doses

231. The cumulative doses to personnel employed in defence activities in 1989 in the United Kingdom are summarized in Table 24, where data are given separately for service and civilian personnel. Estimates of cumulative doses to defence workers in the United Kingdom [D1] have also been made by the NRPB from data held within the Central Index of Dose Information and the National Registry of Radiation Workers, and these are summarized in Table 25. Direct comparisons should not, however, be made between these two sets of data, as the composition of the respective workforces and the time over which data were compiled differ; these differences are summarized in footnotes to Table 25. Data identified under the heading "weapons programme" in Table 25 are specifically for workers at the Atomic Weapons Establishment but can, to a good approximation, be assumed to be representative of exposures associated with the weapons programme as a whole. The data under the heading "other defence activities" are for all defence workers apart from those at the Atomic Weapons Establishment; most of these exposures will, however, be associated with the naval nuclear propulsion programme.

232. The mean cumulative dose to classified radiation workers in all defence activities in the United Kingdom is 29 mSv; for the weapons programme the mean dose is 21 mSv, and for the naval nuclear propulsion programme it is 37 mSv. These averages, however, disguise significant differences between employees of the Ministry of Defence and contract workers. In the naval nuclear programme the cumulative dose to contract workers is greater by a factor of more than 3 than that to employees (58 mSv compared with 18 mSv), whereas in the weapons programme the dose to contract workers is less than half that to employees (9.4 mSv compared with 21.8 mSv). About 7% of all workers received cumulative doses in excess of 100 mSv and about 0.2% received in excess of 400 mSv; for contract workers in the naval nuclear programme, the corresponding values were about 19% and 0.7%.

233. The mean cumulative doses to workers in the National Registry of Radiation Workers are lower (typically by a factor of about 2) than those in the Central Index of Dose Information, because contractor employees are not included but both classified and non-classified employees are. These results are of interest mainly because they provide an opportunity to determine what fraction of the cumulative dose arises over particular periods or age intervals. Data are given for doses accumulated to age 30 years, and the mean cumulative dose over this period is about one third of the mean cumulative dose overall.

IV. INDUSTRIAL USES OF RADIATION

234. Radiation is used for many purposes in industry. Most of these uses involve sealed radioactive sources or equipment that is electronically energized to produce radiation, for example x-ray machines, electron microscopes and particle accelerators. Some of the main industrial uses include industrial radiography, well logging, luminizing, non-destructive testing, thickness gauging, tracer techniques and the use of x rays for a variety of purposes, like crystallographic and fluoroscopic analyses of materials. The levels and trends in occupational exposure from industrial uses of radiation are reviewed in this Chapter together with those arising during the production of radioisotopes for medical and industrial purposes. In addition, exposures from the use of radiation in research (excluding research undertaken in support of the nuclear power industry) are estimated to the extent that they can be separately identified.

235. The compilation of reliable statistics on occupational exposure in industry is complicated by the diversity of uses to which radiation is put and differences in the way data are reported by different countries, in particular the number and nature of the occupations for which data are reported separately. By far the greater number of occupational exposures in general industry are small, and this has doubtless influenced the relative lack of detail, or disaggregation, in their reporting. In general, data have been reported separately only for those few occupations with the potential for higher doses. Since the availability of reported data clearly determines the level of detail that can be included in this review, consideration is limited to the levels of exposure in industry overall and in those few groups where higher doses could arise and/or for which a number of countries have reported data separately. These separate groups comprise industrial radiographers, luminizers, radioisotope producers and well loggers.

236. Differences may exist in the procedures used in various countries to group workers occupationally, and this places limitations on the validity of direct comparisons between data compiled in different

countries. Where these limitations may be important, they are identified. The extent to which valid comparisons can be made between countries is also influenced by differences in the respective approaches used to measure and report occupational exposures, e.g. the type of dosimeter used, its minimum detectable level (MDL), the dose entered into records when the measured dose is less than the MDL and doses assigned for lost dosimeters. These differences and their implications for validity of comparisons between data were discussed in Chapter I. The approaches used in measuring and reporting occupational exposures in each of the countries for which data were reported are summarized in Table 2. Where important differences in approach are apparent, caution should be exercised in making direct comparisons between data.

237. National data on occupational exposures arising from the industrial use of radiation are given in Table 26 for workers in each of the following areas: industrial radiography, luminizing, production and distribution of isotopes, well logging, tertiary education and research institutes, accelerators and all industrial uses of radiation grouped together. Worldwide levels of exposure have been estimated from the reported national data for each industrial use, with extrapolation within particular regions based on gross national product. In general, the collective dose was well correlated with gross national product, but there were exceptions to this for some countries. The degree of extrapolation needed varied with the industrial use considered but typically was about a factor of 2 on average; there was, however, considerable variation about this average value for particular regions or periods. For some industrial uses insufficient data were available to allow reliable extrapolation.

A. INDUSTRIAL RADIOGRAPHY

238. Industrial radiography is carried out in two quite different sets of conditions. First, it may be undertaken at a single location, usually in a permanent facility that has been designed and shielded for this purpose; in this case items to be radiographed are brought to the facility. Secondly, it may be undertaken at multiple locations in the field, in which case the radiographic equipment is transported to the place of interest. The ease and efficacy of exercising control, supervision and protection in the two cases may be different, and this may have implications for the resulting occupational exposures. Few of the reported data, however, distinguish between exposures from the two types of radiographic practice.

239. Worldwide levels of dose have been estimated from national data by extrapolation within regions based on gross national product. The sum of the gross national products for those countries reporting data was about 35% of the worldwide total in the first five-year period, increasing to about 65% in the third. On average, therefore, the reported data have been scaled upwards by a factor of about 2 with considerable variation, however, about this average for particular periods and regions. Estimates of the numbers of workers and doses in industrial radiography worldwide are illustrated in Figure XX. The annual number of monitored workers in industrial radiography, averaged over five-year periods, is estimated to have increased from about 70,000 in the first period to about 110,000 in each of the last two periods. The average annual collective effective dose is estimated to have increased from about 190 man Sv in the first period to about 230 man Sv in the second, then to have decreased significantly to about 160 man Sv in the third. Roughly half of these collective doses are estimated to have occurred in countries comprising the OECD and about one quarter to one third in the countries of Eastern Europe.

240. The annual effective dose to monitored workers, averaged over five-year periods, fell progressively from about 2.6 mSv in the first period to about 1.4 mSv in the third. This same downward trend is evident in the data for most countries and regional groupings, but there is considerable variation between countries in both the level of the dose and extent of the decrease. For example, average doses to monitored workers were as low as 0.2 mSv in some countries (e.g. France and the German Democratic Republic) to as high as 13 mSv in others (the former USSR). From data reported, the fraction of the monitored workforce receiving annual doses in excess of 15 mSv is estimated to have decreased from about 0.04 in the first period to about 0.03 in both the following periods; the fraction of the collective effective dose arising from annual doses in excess of the same level is estimated to have changed little over the period, remaining at about 0.4. These fractions were estimated from a smaller set of data than used to estimate collective and individual doses and, as a consequence, are less reliable indicators of worldwide levels.

241. Relatively few data are available on average doses to measurably exposed workers as opposed to monitored workers, and no attempt has been made to estimate a worldwide average dose for the former quantity. There is considerable variation between countries in both the absolute levels of these doses and in the ratio of these to the average dose to monitored workers. This ratio varies from about 1 to more than 10. While differences in operational practice and standards of protection will account for some of this variation, the more likely causes are differences in how doses are measured and formally recorded, in who in the workforce is to be monitored and the

completeness of the occupations or uses included in the data reported.

242. Data on occupational exposures arising from fixed and mobile radiography are included in Table 26 under "industrial radiography" for those few countries where exposures in the respective practices could be separated. Data are given for the Netherlands, the United Kingdom and the United States; the totals (or averages) of the reported data are dominated by exposures in the United States, because the number of workers and the collective dose are generally much larger than in other countries for which data are available.

243. The annual doses, averaged over five-year periods and over all reported data, for workers undertaking mobile radiography, (where control and supervision are potentially more difficult), exceed those arising in fixed radiography. The average annual dose from mobile radiography remained relatively unchanged over the period, about 3 mSv, whereas that from fixed radiography declined almost fourfold, from about 1.4 to about 0.4 mSv. The values of the ratios SR_{15} and NR_{15} are, likewise, larger for those involved with mobile than with fixed radiography, with the difference being more pronounced in the case of SR_{15}. Exposures in the Netherlands are much lower than average, but they do exhibit the same general trends with respect to the differences between mobile and fixed radiography. In the data for the United Kingdom, however, only small differences are evident in the occupational exposures for the two types of radiography.

244. A further statistic of interest in the present context is the number of workers receiving accidental overexposures. There were indications in the past that radiography workers, because of the nature of their work (particularly in the case of mobile radiography), might be more liable to receive overexposures than workers in most other occupations. Data on the percentage of radiographers receiving doses in excess of an annual effective dose of 50 mSv, together with the percentage of the collective dose arising from individual doses above the same level, are summarized in Table 27. The data are not complete enough to enable any time trends to be determined. Averaged over the whole period and over all countries, the data indicate that about 0.1% of industrial radiographers receive exposures in excess of 50 mSv each year; about 6% of the average annual collective dose from radiography is estimated to result from such exposures. Significant variation is apparent about the weighted average values for particular countries.

245. If these percentages are assumed to be representative globally, about 100 radiographers worldwide receive doses in excess of 50 mSv every year. While in absolute terms this number is not large, the occurrence of overexposures (normalized to the size of the workforce) in industrial radiography exceeds that in most other occupations. By comparison, in 250,000 monitored workers of the United States Nuclear Regulatory Commission licensees not involved in industrial radiography, there were no reported cases of overexposure in 1986.

B. LUMINIZING

246. Radioactive materials have been used in luminizing for decades. The practice is still widespread, although the numbers of workers involved is modest. There has, with time, been a move away from the use of radium to tritium and, to a lesser extent, ^{147}Pm. Tritium is used both mixed with a phosphor in paint and as a gas enclosed in phosphor-lined, glass-walled tubes. The data reported in Table 26 are, in general, for luminizing with tritium gas, and the doses arise via internal exposure; the exceptions to this are the data for India, which include exposures to tritium and ^{147}Pm, and the United Kingdom, for which the two components are presented separately.

247. The reported data shown in Table 26 are not comprehensive enough to enable a reliable estimate of the worldwide levels of dose from the luminizing industry, but sums (or averages) of available data are given. At least for those countries reporting data, the overall number of monitored workers in the luminizing industry is small and of the order of a few hundred. The total average annual collective effective dose decreased from about 4 man Sv in the first five-year period to about 1.4 in each of the following periods. Over the same period the overall average annual dose to monitored workers decreased from about 7.4 mSv to about 2.7 mSv. Large reductions also occurred in both of the distribution ratios over this period, with the value of NR_{15} decreasing from about 0.2 to about 0.03 and that of SR_{15} decreasing from about 0.6 to about 0.3.

248. Considerable variation about these overall average values and trends with time is evident in the data for individual countries. With the exception of India, there has been a substantial decrease in the annual collective effective dose in each country; the factor by which dose decreased differed between countries within a range of about 2-4. The average annual doses varied greatly between countries and over time, from about 1 mSv to more than 11 mSv. The annual effective doses, averaged over five-year periods, in both Switzerland and the United Kingdom fell by a factor of about 3 over the period analysed; the dose in India remained relatively constant, while

that in France increased by about 30%. These five-year averages disguise an even greater decrease in the annual doses in the United Kingdom, which fell from about 15 mSv in 1975 to 2 mSv in the late 1980s.

249. The average individual doses in the luminizing industries have, historically, been much larger than those in other industries; this situation still prevails, notwithstanding the major reductions in dose that have been achieved in several countries. The number of workers in the luminizing industries in those countries reporting data was, however, small (about 500); worldwide, the number may be significantly greater, and this aspect warrants further analysis.

C. RADIOISOTOPE PRODUCTION AND DISTRIBUTION

250. Radioisotopes are produced for a great variety of industrial and medical purposes. The main source of occupational exposure in radioisotope production and distribution is external irradiation; internal exposure may be significant in some cases, and arrangements are then made for personal monitoring. In general, however, internal exposures have not been included in reported statistics for occupational exposure, except in more recent years, and even then the practice is far from universal. Reporting conventions for workers involved in radioisotope production may also vary from country to country (e.g. whether the reported doses include only those arising during the initial production and distribution of radioisotopes or whether they also include those arising in the subsequent processing, encapsulation, packaging and distribution of radionuclides that may have been purchased in bulk from elsewhere), and this may affect the validity of comparisons between reported doses.

251. Worldwide levels of exposure have been estimated from reported national data, with extrapolation within regions based on gross national product. The coverage and scaling of the data were similar to that for industrial radiography. The annual number of monitored workers from worldwide radioisotope production and distribution, averaged over five-year periods, increased from about 60,000 in the first period to about 90,000 in the third period (see Figure XX). This reflects the increasing use of radioisotopes in both industry and medicine. Notwithstanding the increase, the worldwide average annual collective effective dose is estimated to have decreased from about 130 man Sv in the first period to about 100 man Sv in both the second and third periods. About 70% of these collective doses are estimated to have occurred in countries comprising the OECD, with about 20%, at least in the latter two five-year periods, occurring in Eastern Europe.

252. The annual effective dose to monitored workers worldwide, averaged over five-year periods, fell from about 2.3 mSv in the first period to about 1.1 mSv in the third, with most of the decrease occurring between the first and second periods. This same downward trend is evident in the data for most countries and regional groupings, but there is considerable variation between countries in both the level of the dose and the extent of the decrease. The average dose to monitored workers in different countries and for different periods has varied within a range of 1-9 mSv. The decrease in the average dose over time was less by as much as a factor of 3 in some countries, in others there was essentially no change (in exceptional cases there was even an increase over the period, particularly between the first and second periods).

253. The fraction of the monitored workforce receiving annual doses in excess of 15 mSv is estimated to have decreased from about 0.1 in the first period to about 0.03 in the third; the fraction of the collective effective dose arising from annual doses in excess of the same level is estimated to have changed little over the period, remaining at about 0.2. These fractions were estimated from a smaller set of data than used to estimate collective and individual doses and, as a consequence, are less reliable indicators of worldwide levels.

254. Fewer data are available on average doses to measurably exposed workers than on those to monitored workers, and again no attempt has been made to estimate a worldwide average dose to measurably exposed workers. The reported doses lie, in general, within a range of 2-8 mSv and typically exceed the corresponding doses to monitored workers by a few tens of per cent (and, exceptionally, by factors of 2-3).

255. In the manufacture and processing of radionuclides, there is potential for both internal and external exposure. It is not always apparent, however, from the reported data whether the internal component was significant and whether it was included in the dose estimates. The data for the United Kingdom from 1985 and for Finland from 1987 include doses from intakes of radionuclides; in general, the contribution to the total dose was reported to be a few per cent. All other data on radioisotope production and distribution in Table 26 need clarification in this respect.

D. WELL LOGGING

256. Well logging has been identified in some countries as an occupation that can lead to higher levels of dose than other industrial occupations involving the use of radiation. Both gamma and

neutron sources are used in well logging, but the contribution from each to the reported doses is not generally indicated. Consequently, it has not been possible to transform the reported effective dose equivalents to effective doses. The assumption has been made that the effective dose is equal to the reported effective dose equivalent, while recognizing that this is likely to underestimate the effective dose in so far as the contribution from neutrons is concerned.

257. The data on well logging in Table 26 are not complete enough to enable a reliable estimate of the worldwide levels of dose. Averaged values of the dose to monitored workers and the two distribution ratios are presented in the Table, but summed data are not included because the results could give a misleading picture. The annual dose to monitored workers, from reported data averaged over five-year periods, decreased from about 1.3 mSv to about 1.1 mSv over the period. Somewhat greater proportional reductions are apparent in the distribution ratios over this period, with the value of NR_{15} decreasing from about 0.007 to about 0.002 and that for SR_{15} decreasing from about 0.3 to about 0.04.

258. Variation about these overall average values and trends with time is evident in the data for individual countries. The extent of this variation is, however, less than that observed for other occupations involving the industrial use of radiation. With a few exceptions, the average individual dose to monitored workers in most countries falls within a range of 1-2 mSv. For those countries reporting data on measurably exposed workers, the average annual effective doses typically exceeded those to monitored workers by factors of 2-3; a range of 2-5 mSv encompasses most of the variation in the reported average annual doses to measurably exposed workers.

E. EDUCATION AND RESEARCH

259. Radiation is a research tool in a wide range of disciplines and occupations. It is difficult to make reliable estimates of the levels of exposure in this area, because there is no consistent reporting and few data are identified separately for this category. Data that should rightly be attributed to this category are often aggregated in broad practices of radiation use (e.g. radioisotope manufacture). In many nuclear research establishments, radiation is used for many industrial activities other than support of the commercial nuclear fuel cycle; however, the fraction of exposures arising in the separate activities cannot be readily established.

260. In these circumstances the data in this Section are intended to include only exposures arising in tertiary educational establishments (universities, polytechnics and research institutes with an important educational role) but not those associated with the use of accelerators; data for the latter were in the past often included with those for tertiary education. Notwithstanding this intent, it is unlikely that all of the data in this Section will have been compiled and reported on a truly comparable basis. The data should, therefore, be interpreted with care when comparing them for different countries without further evidence as to their comparability.

261. The data reported by countries are given in the relevant part of Table 26. Worldwide levels of exposures have been estimated from national data by extrapolation within regions based on gross national product. The coverage and scaling of data (by a factor of about 2) were similar to that for industrial radiography. The collective effective dose is less well correlated with gross national product than that for the other occupational categories analysed; the greater potential for non-uniform reporting of data in this category has doubtless contributed to this situation.

262. The annual number of monitored workers involved worldwide in the use of radiation in tertiary education, averaged over five-year periods, is estimated to have varied within the range 140,000-180,000 over the whole period (Figure XX). The worldwide average annual collective effective dose is estimated to have decreased from about 70 man Sv in the first five-year period to about 20 man Sv in the third. About 75% of these collective doses are estimated to have occurred in the countries comprising the OECD.

263. The annual effective dose to monitored workers worldwide, averaged over five-year periods, fell from about 0.55 mSv in the first period to about 0.14 mSv in the third, with most of the decrease occurring between the first and second periods. This downward trend is evident in the data for most, but by no means all, of the countries reporting data, but there is considerable variation between countries in both the level of the dose and the extent of the decrease. The average doses were generally a small fraction of a mSv, sometimes a very small fraction, and exceeded 1 mSv only exceptionally. An important reason for this variability is doubtless the adoption of different protocols for who is to be monitored in the respective workforces. The decrease in average dose over time varied by a factor of as much as 3 in some countries; more exceptionally, there were increases in other countries.

264. The fraction of the monitored workforce receiving annual doses in excess of 15 mSv was small and is estimated to have decreased tenfold, from about

0.004 in the first period to about 0.0004 in the third; the fraction of the collective effective dose arising from annual doses in excess of the same level is estimated to have decreased from about 0.2 to about 0.07 over the same period. These fractions were estimated from a smaller set of data than used to estimate collective and individual doses and, as a consequence, are less reliable indicators of worldwide levels.

265. Fewer data are available on average doses to measurably exposed workers than on those to monitored workers, and again no attempt has been made to estimate a worldwide average dose to this group. The average annual doses to measurably exposed workers exhibited much less variability between countries than those to monitored workers and, in general, fell in a range of 0.5-3 mSv.

F. ACCELERATORS

266. Consideration is limited here to occupational exposures arising from accelerators used for nuclear physics research at universities and national and international laboratories. Accelerators (generally of somewhat smaller size) are increasingly being used for medical purpose; however, the exposures arising from them are more appropriately associated with exposures arising from the medical uses of radiation. Most exposures from accelerators result from induced radioactivity and occur mainly during the repair, maintenance and modification of equipment. These exposures come mainly from gamma-radiation from the activation of solid surrounding materials by penetrating radiation. The potential for internal exposure in the normal operation of accelerators is slight, and doses via this route are negligible in comparison with those from external irradiation. Insufficient information was available to enable doses, reported in terms of effective dose equivalent, to be transformed to effective dose; the simplifying assumption was, therefore, made that they were numerically equal.

267. Early high-energy accelerators used internal targets to produce either radioisotopes or secondary beams of normally unstable particles. Very high levels of activation products were produced in the region of the targets, and typical annual collective doses per accelerator were 1-2 man Sv before 1960; this is still true for many of the early cyclotrons that are still in operation. In 1960-1980, improved beam extraction techniques were developed, which led to reduced levels of activation products; these reductions were, however, largely offset by the continuing increases in beam power.

268. In the 1980s two developments had an important influence on occupational exposures at accelerators. The first was the increasing importance of colliding beam techniques for the production of events of interest to the particle physics community. Average beam intensities, as measured by the number of particles accelerated per day, are several orders of magnitude lower than those used in fixed-target physics experiments. Consequently, the production of activation products has been greatly reduced, and this is reflected in the exposures of maintenance personnel. The second development was a move towards heavy-ion operation, where again the accelerated beam intensities are several orders of magnitude lower than those with proton acceleration. This has also led to a decrease in activation products and, consequently, in exposures during maintenance.

269. Following from these technical developments and the greater emphasis given generally to ALARA programmes at accelerators, there were large reductions in the annual collective effective doses at major accelerator laboratories between the mid-1970s and mid-1980s [P4]. Decreases in annual collective dose, from about 0.1 to 0.02 man Sv, were experienced at Deutsches Elektronen Synchrotron; from about 0.2 to about 0.02 man Sv at Daresbury Nuclear Physics Laboratory; from about 5 to 1.5 man Sv at European Organization for Nuclear Research and from about 0.5 to about 0.2 man Sv at Lawrence Berkeley Laboratory.

270. The relevant data shown in Table 26 are not complete enough to enable a reliable estimate of the worldwide levels of dose from accelerators, but the sums (or averages) of the available data are shown. It should be noted that these summed or average data largely reflect experience in the United States, which is by far the largest contributor to them. The total average annual collective effective dose has decreased from about 7 man Sv in the first five-year period to about 3.5 man Sv in the third period. Over the same period the overall average annual dose to monitored workers decreased from about 1.6 to about 0.6 mSv. The data on distribution ratios, averaged over those countries reporting data, do not include data for the United States, where most of the collective dose arose, so it would be inappropriate to associate these ratios with either the total numbers of workers or the total collective doses, as they were determined largely by the doses from the United States.

271. Considerable variation about these overall average values and trends with time is evident in the data for individual countries. With the exception of one country, the average annual effective doses to monitored workers all fell within the range 0.3-2.7 mSv. In the United States this dose decreased fourfold, from about 2 to about 0.5 mSv over the period analysed; increases are apparent in some of the other countries.

272. The average annual effective doses to measurably exposed workers exhibit trends similar to those to the monitored workforce. With the exception of one country, these doses fell within the range 1-7 mSv and were typically some two to three times greater than those to the monitored workforce.

G. OTHER INDUSTRIAL USES

273. There are many other uses of radiation in industry, e.g. soil moisture gauges, thickness gauges and x-ray diffraction, but occupational exposure data for these are not, in general, separately identified or reported. The number of workers potentially exposed in these other uses may substantially exceed those in the few occupations for which data have been separately presented in this Chapter. The average levels of exposure of workers involved in other uses of radiation are, in general, small. However, because of the way in which they are aggregated, they may disguise somewhat higher average doses in particular occupations. The only way to ascertain the existence of occupations, or subgroups within occupations, receiving doses significantly in excess of the average is for those responsible for compiling data to inspect the data periodically. Such inspection is to be encouraged. An indication of occupational exposures from other uses of radiation can be inferred from the difference between the data for all industrial uses worldwide and those for individual occupations for which it was possible to make worldwide estimates.

H. ALL INDUSTRIAL USES OF RADIATION

274. The last section of Table 26 shows the national data on occupational exposures from all industrial uses of radiation grouped together, excluding the nuclear fuel cycle and defence. The data are more complete than for the separate categories of industrial uses of radiation. Worldwide levels have been obtained by regional extrapolation based on gross national product. The sum of gross national products for the countries reporting data was about 50% of the worldwide total in the first five-year period, increasing to about 80% in the third (the countries accounted for about 15% and 30%, respectively, of the world population). On average, therefore, the reported data have been scaled upwards by a factor of about 1.5; there is, however, considerable variation about this average in the scaling for particular regions.

275. The collective effective doses from all industrial uses of radiation in each country reporting data in 1985-1989 are shown in relation to gross national product in Figure XXI. The broad correlation between the two quantities is evident, with the degree of correlation generally increasing when consideration is limited to particular regional or economic groupings of countries. Data on the regional variations of exposures in industrial uses of radiation are summarized in Table 28. The data for the main regions contributing to the collective dose are illustrated in Figure XXII. Direct comparisons should not be made between the normalized doses for the respective periods as they have been derived on different price bases (1977, 1983 and 1989, respectively); appropriate corrections would need to be made to enable direct comparison. Within a given period, a factor of 2-3 encompasses the range of variation in the normalized collective doses between most regions; values for the United States were typically greater by a factor of 2 than those for the rest of the OECD countries.

276. For some countries within a geographical or economic region, the normalized collective dose (normalized in terms of gross national product) differed greatly from the average for that region. In most of these cases the values were much smaller than the average, suggesting that the reported data may have been incomplete, that much less use was being made of radiation in industry or that much higher standards of protection had been adopted in those countries. Notwithstanding these reservations on the completeness of some of the reported data, no attempt has been made to correct for this, and the reported data were all included in the estimation of worldwide levels of exposure. Any errors due to incompleteness of the reported data are unlikely to be significant in comparison with the uncertainty introduced by the extrapolation process itself.

277. The annual number of monitored workers, averaged over five-year periods, involved with the industrial uses of radiation worldwide is estimated to have varied within the range 500,000-700,000 over the period; the great majority of these workers are employed either in the United States (40%-50%) or in the other countries comprising OECD (30%-40%). The number of workers appears to have increased between the first two periods and then declined in the third (Figure XXII). The average annual collective effective dose was about 900 man Sv in each of the two first periods but decreased significantly in the third to about 500 man Sv; in general, the data for later periods are more reliable because of the smaller degree of extrapolation needed. Roughly equal contributions to this collective dose were made by the United States, the rest of the OECD countries, Eastern Europe and the remainder of the world, although the contribution from Eastern Europe was, in general, smaller than that from the other groupings.

278. The annual effective dose to monitored workers, averaged over five-year periods, fell from about

1.6 mSv in the first period to about 0.9 mSv in the third. This same downward trend is evident in the data for most countries and regional groupings, but there is considerable variation between countries in both the level of the dose and extent of the decrease. For example, average doses to monitored workers vary from as low as 0.1 mSv in some countries (e.g. Finland and Ireland) to as high as 16 mSv in others (the former USSR). Not all countries have provided data on the distribution ratios NR_{15} and SR_{15}. The fraction of monitored workers worldwide receiving annual doses in excess of 15 mSv is estimated from these data to have been about 0.01 in the first five-year period and marginally less in the following two periods. The fraction of the collective dose arising from individual doses in excess of the same level is also estimated to have been fairly constant over the period, about 0.3.

279. Far fewer data are available on average doses to measurably exposed workers than to monitored workers. Most fall in the range 1-5 mSv, but values for several countries fall well outside of this range. Based on these data, the worldwide average annual dose to measurably exposed workers is estimated to have decreased from about 3 mSv in the first two periods to about 2 mSv in the third. Large variations between countries are evident in the ratio of the average dose to measurably exposed and monitored workers. This ratio ranges from about 1 to more than 10; differences in monitoring and reporting practice between countries are probably mainly responsible for this variation. The number of measurably exposed workers is estimated, on a worldwide basis, to be lower by a factor of 2-3 than that of monitored workers. More data on average doses to measurably exposed workers would be useful, as comparisons based on these data are, in general, more reliable than those based on the doses to monitored workers.

280. Some of the variations between countries in the reported statistics undoubtedly arise from differences in how doses are measured and formally recorded, in who in the workforce is to be monitored and in the completeness of the occupations or uses included in the data reported; these aspects warrant closer analysis in future in order to validate comparisons between the data and improve the estimate of worldwide levels of exposure.

I. CUMULATIVE DOSES

281. Few data have been published on cumulative exposures to workers involved with the industrial uses of radiation. Data reported in response to the UNSCEAR questionnaire by Hungary for industrial radiographers are summarized in Table 29 [S8]. The data exhibit, in general, the expected increase in cumulative dose with duration of employment. The average annual increment in dose increases, however, with increasing duration of employment. For those employed or exposed over a period of less than 10 years, the average annual dose was about 4 mSv; for those employed for 15 years the average annual dose was about 7 mSv. Various factors may have contributed to this difference, for example, improvements in practice and radiological standards over time and variations in the type and volume of work undertaken as experience is gained, which will at least be partially correlated with employment duration. About 4% of those employed for more than 10 years had received cumulative doses in excess of 200 mSv; just over 40% of those employed for 14 or 15 years had received cumulative doses greater than 100 mSv.

282. These cumulative doses are broadly comparable with those estimated for contract workers at LWRs in the United States who had at some time in their career been employed at the Calvert Cliffs nuclear power station and are larger than those estimated by the United States Nuclear Regulatory Commission (on the basis of termination records) for all workers at LWRs in the United States. Somewhat larger cumulative doses were experienced at the reprocessing plant at Sellafield in the United Kingdom, at least for those who started working there before the 1970s; for those who started working after that time, the cumulative doses are comparable with those reported here for radiographers.

J. SUMMARY

283. Worldwide exposures from industrial uses of radiation are summarized in Table 30. Estimates have been made for industrial uses as a whole and separately for industrial radiography, for radioisotope production and distribution and for tertiary education and research institutes. By subtracting the data for these separate categories from those for "all industrial activities" given in Table 26, estimates have been made of worldwide doses for "other" industrial uses; these other industrial uses also include doses from those occupational categories that were analysed separately in this Chapter but for which it was not possible to make worldwide estimates (i.e. the luminizing industry, well logging and accelerators). The number of workers and average annual individual and collective doses for these categories are illustrated in Figure XX.

284. Of the average annual number of monitored workers involved worldwide with the industrial uses of radiation (ranging from about 550,000 to 700,000 over the period analysed), about 16%, 13% and 27% are

estimated to have been employed in industrial radiography, isotope production and distribution and tertiary education, respectively. Typically, about 40% or more were assigned to the category of "other".

285. The average annual collective effective dose worldwide from all industrial uses has decreased from about 900 to about 500 man Sv over the period analysed. On average about 25% of the total collective dose arose in industrial radiography, about 14% in isotope production and about 6% in tertiary education. On average more than 50% of the total collective dose occurred in other industrial uses of radiation.

286. The average annual doses to monitored workers in industrial radiography exceeded the average doses from all industrial uses by about 50%. Those in isotope production also exceeded the averages for all industrial uses but to a lesser extent and not in all periods; the doses from tertiary education were, in general, smaller than the overall average doses by factors of 3-6, depending on the period. There is much variation between the values of the distribution ratios NR_{15} and SR_{15} for all industrial uses and the particular occupational categories; those for industrial radiography are invariably greater and those for tertiary education smaller than those for all industrial uses. In general, for each occupational category, the ratio, NR_{15}, was observed to decrease with time; the ratios, SR_{15}, however, with the exception of that for tertiary education, varied little over the period analysed.

V. MEDICAL USES OF RADIATION

287. Radiation is used in medicine for both diagnostic and therapeutic purposes. Its wide range of applications and the types of procedures or techniques employed in the context of patient exposure are reviewed in Annex C, "Medical radiation exposures", where changes in practice and possible future trends are also discussed. Consideration is limited here to the occupational exposures that arise from the application of these procedures. Data on occupational exposures are presented for workers in each of the following areas: diagnostic radiography, dental practice, nuclear medicine (diagnostic and therapeutic), radiotherapy and all medical uses of radiation (for human purposes) grouped together. In addition, separate consideration is given to exposures in veterinary medicine.

288. Previous Chapters of this Annex contained cautionary remarks about the accuracy or validity of reported statistics on occupational exposures and the extent to which they can be fairly compared, either between countries for the same occupational group, or between different occupational groups in the same or different countries. It is in the area of medical uses of radiation where these cautionary remarks are most important, and great care must be exercised in interpreting and evaluating the various statistics. There is considerable potential for drawing erroneous conclusions as a result of the direct and unqualified comparison of data in this area. The reasons for this were already pointed out. They include differences in monitoring and recording practice, in defining the workforce to be monitored, in minimum detectable levels and in the recording of doses less than the minimum detectable level. More important in the medical field, however, are differences in where dosimeters are located (in particular, whether they are above or below lead aprons when these are worn). Further complicating factors are the non-uniformity and low energy of the radiation that contributes most to the overall occupational exposures from the medical uses of radiation in such circumstances; the approach used to derive effective doses from dosimeter measurements can have major implications for the comparability of occupational exposures.

289. To assist in the interpretation and/or qualification of the statistics reported in this Chapter, the main features of the dose monitoring and reporting procedures adopted in each of the countries that have responded to the UNSCEAR Survey of Occupational Exposures in Medicine are summarized in Table 31. Significant differences are evident, in particular in the location of the dosimeter (above or below the lead apron) and whether the direct dosimeter reading or some corrected value was entered into the formal dose record. Other important differences that may influence the comparability and/or accuracy of reported statistics are the minimum detectable levels of the various dosimeters and the manner in which doses less than this level or levels are recorded. These differences must be recognized when comparing the data presented in the following Sections.

290. Notwithstanding these qualifications and reservations, it proved impracticable in this analysis to revise or normalize the reported exposures to ensure that fair comparisons could be made between them. Accordingly, when worldwide levels of exposure were estimated from the available data, no distinction was made between doses measured, recorded or reported in

different ways; all reported doses were assumed to be adequate surrogates for effective dose. More attention needs to be given to this matter to afford better comparability between doses arising in different circumstances and to enable more reliable estimates of worldwide levels of occupational exposure.

291. National data on medical uses of radiation, categorized as diagnostic radiography, dental practice, nuclear medicine, radiotherapy, veterinary medicine and all (human) medical uses of radiation grouped together and averaged, where possible, over five-year periods, are given in Table 32. Worldwide levels of exposure have been estimated from these national data by extrapolation within particular regions based on gross national product as described in Section I.C. In general, the collective dose for each practice was well correlated with gross national product, but there were exceptions for some countries. The degree of extrapolation needed varied with the medical use considered but was typically within a range of about 2 to 7 overall; there was, however, considerable variation about these average values for particular regions or periods.

292. The data on exposures from medical uses of radiation for the United States have been considered seprately from the remainder of the OECD region because of the major contribution to worldwide exposures from this country and the much larger collective dose per unit gross national product. Data for the United States have been reported separately for all medical uses of radiation and for dental radiography; the levels of exposure from diagnostic radiography, nuclear medicine and radiotherapy, taken together, can thus be estimated by simple subtraction of exposures from dental radiography from those for all medical uses. Assumptions must be made, however, on the attribution of this residual dose between the respective uses. In the absence of other indications, the distribution between the three uses was assumed to be the same as that on average for OECD countries (or, more strictly, those reporting data).

A. DIAGNOSTIC RADIOGRAPHY

293. The estimation of occupational exposures from diagnostic radiography is complicated by the fact that the radiation comes largely from point sources fairly close to the workers and is in general of very low energy. Exposure is very non-uniform because of the inverse square law and attenuation in the body. Matters are further complicated by the fact that dosimeters are not always worn at the same location, although they are commonly worn at the waist or neck. Consequently, the effective dose is difficult to infer from a single personal dosimeter reading, especially if the dosimeter is not in the primary radiation field striking the body. For a reliable estimate to be made, detailed information on the circumstances of the exposure and the nature of the radiation are needed. Because of these difficulties, the direct dosimeter reading is commonly used in formal dose records as a surrogate for the effective dose. The compilation of reliable statistics in this area is further hampered by the fact that many of the exposures are close to the minimum detectable level of the dosimeter. Differences in MDLs for various dosimeters and in the protocols for recording doses below these may therefore adversely affect the reliability of the data and compromise the validity of direct comparisons between statistics compiled in different ways.

294. It was judged in the UNSCEAR 1988 Report [U1] that for radiation qualities used in diagnostic x-ray procedures, the dosimeter usually gives a reading that is 2 to 4 times higher than the effective dose if no protective apron is worn and if the exposure is relatively uniform. If a protective apron is worn and the personal dosimeter is placed on the outside, then the dosimeter reading could be as much as 10-20 times higher than the effective dose. It can be seen from Table 31 that in most cases, at least where the information is available, the direct dosimeter reading is entered into formal dose records. The data given may thus be considerable overestimates, particularly for those countries where lead aprons are worn and dosimeters placed above them. Significant differences are also evident in Table 31 in the minimum detectable levels of the dosimeters used and in the assignment of doses when dosimeters are lost; these differences must be recognized when comparing data for the respective countries.

295. Countries reporting data on occupational exposures from diagnostic radiology comprised about 13% of the total gross national product worldwide in the first five-year period increasing to about 18% in the third. On average, therefore, the reported data have been scaled upwards by a factor of about 7; there was, however, considerable variation about this average in the scaling for particular regions.

296. The annual number of monitored workers, averaged over five-year periods, involved worldwide in diagnostic radiography approximately doubled, from about 0.63 to 1.4 million over the period analysed (see Figure XXIII); the great majority of these workers (about 70%) were employed in those countries comprising the OECD. The annual worldwide collective effective dose, averaged over five-year periods, was about 600 man Sv in the first period increasing to about 760 man Sv in the third period. About 75% of the worldwide collective dose occurred

in countries of the OECD in the first period; this proportion dropped to about 60% in the third period.

297. The annual effective dose to monitored workers worldwide, averaged over five-year periods, fell from about 0.9 mSv in the first period to about 0.6 mSv in the third. This same downward trend is evident in the data for most countries and regional groupings, but there is considerable variation between countries in both the level of the dose and the extent of the decrease. Most average annual doses fall in the range 0.1-1 mSv, but somewhat higher values are reported for China, Indonesia and, in particular, Peru. In practice, all of the above doses, both individual and collective, may be considerable overestimates, as it was generally assumed that the dosimeter reading could be equated with effective dose.

298. The fraction of the monitored workforce worldwide receiving annual doses in excess of 15 mSv was small and estimated to have been about 0.003 over the first two periods, with an apparent increase to about 0.005 in the third period; the fraction of the worldwide collective effective dose from annual doses in excess of the same level was about 0.1 in the first period, decreasing to about 0.05 in the second period with an apparent increase to about 0.2 in the third period. Undue significance should not, however, be assigned to these apparent increases in the third period. These increases are due to data for China only being reported for the third period and the somewhat higher values of the distribution ratios reported for this country. For those countries reporting data for the whole period analysed there is evidence, overall, of a small downward trend with time in the values of both ratios.

299. Fewer data are available on average annual doses to measurably exposed workers than to monitored workers, so no attempt has been made to estimate a representative worldwide level. Most doses fall in the range 1-5 mSv, but a few fall well outside of this range (e.g. 11 mSv for China in 1985-1989). The percentage of monitored workers who are measurably exposed varies considerably between countries, from about 5% to almost 90%. Large variations between countries are evident in the ratio of the average dose to measurably exposed and monitored workers. This ratio ranges from about 1 to more than 10; differences in monitoring and reporting practice are probably mainly responsible for the variation.

B. DENTAL PRACTICE

300. Worldwide levels of dose and numbers of workers in dental practice have been estimated from national data by extrapolation within particular regions based on gross national product. The sum of the gross national products for those countries reporting data was about 50% of the worldwide total in the first five-year period, increasing to about 60% in the third. On average, therefore, the reported data have been scaled upwards by a factor of about 2 but with considerable variation about this average value for particular regions.

301. The annual number of monitored workers, averaged over five-year periods, in dental practice worldwide is estimated to have increased from about 400,000 to about 500,000 over the period analysed (see Table 32 and Figure XXIII); more than half these workers were employed in the United States. The average annual collective effective dose was about 120 man Sv in the first period, decreasing to about 25 man Sv in the third, with most of the decrease occurring between the second and third periods. The overall trend largely reflects that in the United States, where the annual collective dose is reported to have decreased over the same period, from about 80 to 12 man Sv. In other countries the downward trend was less pronounced, not evident at all or, occasionally, reversed.

302. The annual effective dose to monitored workers worldwide, averaged over five-year periods, fell progressively from about 0.3 mSv in the first period to about 0.05 mSv in the third, again largely reflecting experience in the United States, which makes a dominant contribution to the total reported. While this same downward trend is evident in most, but not all, countries and regions, there is considerable variation in both the level of the dose and the extent of the decrease for particular countries or regions.

303. The fraction of the monitored workforce (summed over the reported data) receiving annual doses in excess of 15 mSv was very small and is estimated to have varied within the range 0.0003-0.0008 over the three periods; the fraction of the collective effective dose (summed over the reported data) estimated to arise from annual doses in excess of that level varied over a range of about 0.08-0.12. Because the data are incomplete (i.e. no data reported for some countries and for limited periods in other cases), these ratios are not reliable indicators of worldwide levels of these quantities nor of trends in their values. The most that can be concluded from them is that, in general, the fraction of dental workers receiving an annual dose in excess of 15 mSv is very small, i.e. significantly less than one in a thousand workers.

304. Fewer data are available on average annual doses to measurably exposed workers than to monitored workers. Most fell within the range 0.2-3 mSv, but there were exceptions. The proportion of monitored

workers who were measurably exposed varied between countries from a few per cent to essentially 100%; this is indicative of differences in practice with regard to who is monitored and in the reporting and recording of doses, which may partially explain some of the wide variation in reported average individual doses to both monitored and measurably exposed workers.

C. NUCLEAR MEDICINE

305. Over the past decade there has been a rapid expansion in the use of nuclear medicine. Many radionuclides are used to label the pharmaceuticals, but the two most important are ^{99m}Tc and ^{131}I. Preparation and administration of pharmaceuticals are significant contributors to overall levels of exposure. Moreover, as they are administered by injection, relatively high doses to the hands of the workers are also possible. Generally, lead shielded syringes are recommended, but they are not always used. Following injection, the patient is another source of exposure for the medical staff. Internal exposures of workers may also occur, but few data have been reported on their relative contribution. Radiopharmaceuticals are also used in therapy, and the main sources of occupational exposure are the same as in diagnostic use. Since the data on occupational exposures arising in nuclear medicine rarely distinguish between diagnostic and therapeutic applications, this analysis is directed to overall levels of exposure in the field. Consideration is limited here to effective doses to which extremity doses do not contribute. Because of the potential for significant extremity doses in nuclear medicine, these would merit attention in any future analysis.

306. Worldwide levels of dose and numbers of workers involved in nuclear medicine have been estimated from national data using the same extrapolation procedures as described previously. The sum of the gross national products for those countries reporting data was about 12% of the worldwide total in the first five-year period increasing to about 18% in the third. On average, therefore, the reported data have been scaled upwards by a factor of about 7 but with considerable variation about this average value for particular regions.

307. The annual number of monitored workers, averaged over five-year periods, in nuclear medicine worldwide is estimated to have increased from about 60,000 to about 90,000 over the period analysed (see Table 32 and Figure XXIII); more than half of these workers were employed in countries of the OECD. The average annual worldwide collective effective dose was about 60 man Sv in the first five-year period, increasing to about 90 man Sv in each of the following two periods. The annual effective dose to monitored workers worldwide, averaged over five-year periods, was about 1 mSv and varied little over the whole period analysed. A downward trend is evident for some countries and regions, but there is considerable variation between countries in both the levels of dose and the trends. Most average annual doses fell in the range 0.2-2 mSv, but there are exceptions to this generalization, in particular for Mexico and Peru, where somewhat higher doses were experienced in some periods.

308. The fraction of the monitored workforce worldwide receiving annual doses in excess of 15 mSv was small and is estimated to have been about 0.002 for the first two five-year periods with an apparent increase to about 0.004 in the third period; the fraction of the worldwide collective effective dose from annual doses in excess of the same level was about 0.09 in the first period, decreasing to about 0.03 in the second period with an apparent increase to about 0.1 in the third period. Undue significance should not, however, be assigned to these apparent increases in the third period. These increases are due to data for China only being reported for the third period and the somewhat higher values of the distribution ratios reported for this country. For those countries reporting data for the whole period analysed there is evidence, overall, of a small downward trend with time in the values of both ratios.

309. Fewer data are available on average annual doses to measurably exposed workers than to monitored workers, so no attempt has been made to estimate worldwide levels for this quantity. Most doses were between 1 and 4 mSv, but some were considerably greater (e.g. 13 mSv in China in one period). The proportion of monitored workers who were measurably exposed varied from a few per cent to essentially 100%; this is indicative of differences in practice with regard to who is monitored and in the reporting and recording of doses, which may partially explain some of the wide variation in reported average individual doses to both monitored and measurably exposed workers.

D. RADIOTHERAPY

310. Occupational exposures during the practice of radiotherapy come from several sources. In general, the rooms in which external beam radiotherapy is practised are very well shielded, and the staff receive little exposure. An exception to this occurs with either neutron beams or electron accelerators operating above 10 MeV. The neutrons activate nearby materials,

which then constitute a source of radiation and exposure to the workers even after the primary beam has been turned off. In such cases, about 75% of the exposure is due to photoactivation products in the treatment head [U1], and the remainder is due to other activation products in the room; induced activity in the patient is not a significant source.

311. An important source of occupational exposure from radiotherapy is brachytherapy, which often involves the insertion or surgical implantation of radio-active wires, needles or seeds. Preloaded surgical applicators are also sometimes used. There has, however, been a trend in countries with a high level of health care towards the use of after-loading devices, whenever possible, to reduce occupational exposures. This involves the prepositioning of an applicator or holder on or in the patient and the insertion of the radioactive material at a later time. The occupational dose from brachytherapy is very dependent on whether the source insertion is manual or automated in some manner. Once the sources have been inserted, the patient becomes a source of exposure to the medical staff. Because brachytherapy contributes significantly to medical occupational exposures, it should be analysed separately. Since, however, few data have been separately reported on brachytherapy, the analysis of exposures has been carried out for radiotherapy as a whole.

312. Worldwide levels of dose and numbers of workers involved in radiotherapy have been estimated from national data using the same extrapolation procedures as described previously. The coverage and scaling of data were similar to that for nuclear medicine.

313. The annual number of monitored workers, averaged over five-year periods, in radiotherapy worldwide is estimated to have increased from about 80,000 to about 110,000 over the period analysed (see Table 32 and Figure XXIII); more than half of these workers were employed in countries of the OECD. The average annual worldwide collective effective dose is estimated to have been reduced by almost half from about 190 man Sv in the first period to about 100 man Sv in the third period, with the decrease occurring mainly between the second and third periods. The annual effective dose to monitored workers worldwide, averaged over five-year periods, fell from about 2.2 mSv in the first period to about 0.9 mSv in the third. This downward trend is evident in many but by no means all countries and regions, and there is considerable variation in both the level of the dose and the extent of the decrease for particular countries or regions. Most average annual doses fell between 0.5 and 2 mSv, but there were exceptions to this generalization, in particular in Finland, where the doses were much lower, and in Mexico and especially Peru, where they were significantly higher.

314. The fraction of monitored workers, averaged over the reported data, receiving annual effective doses in excess of 15 mSv was small and is estimated to have decreased from about 0.012 in the first period to about 0.008 in each of the subsequent periods. The corresponding fractions of the collective effective dose arising from annual doses in excess of that level were about 0.3 in the first period, decreasing to about 0.2 in the subsequent periods. Since the data for most countries generally exhibit the same trends, these average values can be used to provide a rough estimate of worldwide levels for these quantities.

315. Fewer data are available on average annual doses to measurably exposed workers than to monitored workers. Most fell between 1 and 5 mSv, but there were some exceptions, for example in China, where the reported dose for one period was 10 mSv. The proportion of monitored workers who were measurably exposed varied from less than 10% to essentially 100%; the variation reflects differences in practice with regard to who is monitored and in the reporting and recording of doses, which may partially explain some of the wide variation in reported average individual doses to monitored and measurably exposed workers.

E. ALL MEDICAL USES OF RADIATION

316. National data on occupational exposures from all medical uses of radiation, averaged over five-year periods, are given in the last section of Table 32. Worldwide levels of exposure have been estimated from the reported data by extrapolation based on gross national product. In Figure XXI, the collective effective doses from all medical uses of radiation in each country reporting data in 1985-1989 are shown in relation to the gross national product. The broad correlation between the two quantities is evident, with the degree of correlation generally increasing when consideration is limited to particular regional or economic groupings of countries.

317. For some countries in a geographical or economic region, the normalized collective dose (normalized in terms of the gross national product) differed greatly from the average for that region. In most of these cases the values were much smaller than the average, suggesting that the reported data may have been incomplete, that much less use was being made of radiation in medicine or that much higher standards of protection had been adopted in those

countries. Similar observations have been made for the separate practices involving industrial uses of radiation. Notwithstanding these reservations on the completeness of some of the reported data, no attempt has been made to correct for this, and the reported data were all included in the estimation of worldwide levels of exposure. Any errors due to incompleteness of the reported data are unlikely to be significant in comparison with the uncertainty introduced by the extrapolation process itself and by the assumption that all of the reported data are good surrogates for effective dose.

318. The data on occupational exposures from all medical uses of radiation are presented for various geographic regions and economic groupings in Table 33. Because of its much larger normalized collective dose, the United States has been listed separately from the other OECD countries. Since the normalized collective doses for the respective periods were derived on different price bases (1977, 1983 and 1989, respectively), direct comparisons cannot be made without appropriate corrections. Within a given period, the normalized collective doses vary by a factor of about 2 between most regions. The main exceptions to this generalization are the United States, where the normalized collective dose is some two to three times that for the remainder of the OECD, and Latin America and Asia where the normalized collective doses are substantially less.

319. The exposure data for the major regional groupings of countries are illustrated in Figure XXIV. The worldwide annual number of monitored workers, averaged over five-year periods, is estimated to have increased from about 1.3 to about 2.2 million over the period; the majority of these workers are employed in the United States or in countries comprising the rest of the OECD. The average annual collective effective dose was about 1,000 man Sv in the first and third periods with evidence of an increase of about 10% in the intermediate period; in general, the data for later periods are more reliable because of the smaller degree of extrapolation needed. Notwithstanding this relatively unchanged level of worldwide exposure over the period analysed, somewhat greater changes occurred in particular regions. The significant decrease in the average annual collective dose in the United States and the increase in that from the rest of the world, excluding Eastern Europe and the OECD, are apparent. Half or more of the worldwide collective dose occurs in countries of the OECD, although this contribution has decreased with time.

320. The annual effective dose to monitored workers worldwide, averaged over five-year periods, fell from about 0.8 mSv in the first period to about 0.5 mSv in the third. This same downward trend is evident in the data for most countries and regional groupings, but there is considerable variation between countries in both the level of the dose and extent of the decrease. The average annual doses, and their rate of decline, were broadly comparable in Eastern Europe and in the OECD (excluding the United States); somewhat higher levels of average individual dose have been reported for the United States. No undue significance should be attached to the variation in individual doses illustrated for those countries depicted as the "remainder" in Figure XXIV; any trends in these data will have been distorted because different countries were included in this category in the different time periods. The average annual doses reported by individual countries vary over a considerable range, for example from as low as 0.1 mSv in some countries for some periods (e.g. Germany, Ireland and Switzerland) to as high as a few millisievert in others (e.g. China, Mexico and Peru).

321. The fraction of the monitored workforce worldwide receiving annual doses in excess of 15 mSv was small and is estimated to have decreased from about 0.003 in the first period to about 0.002 in the second with an apparent increase to about 0.009 in the third period; the fraction of the worldwide collective effective dose from annual doses in excess of the same level was about 0.14 in the first period, decreasing to about 0.10 in the second period with an apparent increase to about 0.24 in the third period. The apparent increases in the third period are due to the inclusion of the data for China, which had been reported only for this period. For those countries reporting data for the whole period analysed there is evidence, overall, of a small downward trend with time in the values of both ratios.

322. Few data are available on average doses to measurably exposed workers than to monitored workers. Most fell in the range 1-5 mSv, but values for several countries are well outside of this range (10 mSv for China in 1985-1989). Based on these reported data, a worldwide average annual effective dose of about 1.6 mSv has been estimated as generally applicable over the entire period. Large variations between countries are evident in the ratio of the average dose to measurably exposed and monitored workers. This ratio ranges from about 1 to more than 10; differences in monitoring and reporting practices between countries are probably mainly responsible for this variation. More data on average doses to measurably exposed workers would be useful, as comparisons made on this basis are, in general, more reliable than those made on the basis of the dose to monitored workers.

323. Some of the variation between countries in the reported statistics undoubtedly arises from differences

in how doses are measured and formally recorded, in who in the workforce is to be monitored and in the completeness of the occupations or uses included in the data reported; these aspects warrant closer analysis in future in order to validate comparisons between the data and improve the estimate of worldwide levels of exposure. For example, had data been available for China for the entire period, it is likely that the estimated worldwide values of the two distribution ratios would have shown a downward trend with time, but their absolute levels would have been greater than indicated above, at least for the first two periods.

F. VETERINARY PRACTICE

324. Diagnostic radiography is the main source of occupational exposure in veterinary practice. The annual number of monitored workers, averaged over five-year periods, worldwide is estimated to have increased threefold, from about 50,000 to about 160,000 over the period analysed (see Table 32 and Figure XXIII); more than 70% of the workers were employed in OECD countries. The average annual worldwide collective effective dose is estimated to have increased twofold, from about 25 man Sv in both the first and second periods to about 50 man Sv in the third period. The annual effective dose to monitored workers worldwide, averaged over five-year periods, fell progressively from about 0.5 mSv in the first period to about 0.3 mSv in the third, although there was considerable variation about these values in the doses for individual countries (most fell in the range 0.1-0.8 mSv). These trends in dose and in the number of monitored workers are largely a reflection of experience in the United States, given its very large contribution to the sum of the reported data. Indeed, while a downward trend in individual dose is evident in many countries, it is not evident in all, and the extent of the decrease is, in general, less pronounced than that in the United States.

325. The fraction of monitored workers, averaged over the reported data, receiving annual effective doses in excess of 15 mSv was very small and is estimated to have decreased from about 0.001 in the first period to about 0.0001 in each of the subsequent periods. The corresponding fractions of the collective effective dose arising from annual doses in excess of the same level were about 0.1 in the first period decreasing to about 0.02 in the subsequent periods. These average values are based on insufficient data for them to be judged truly representative of worldwide levels; at best they can be considered as indicative of such levels.

326. Fewer data are available on average annual doses to measurably exposed workers than to monitored workers. Most fell in the range 0.5-2 mSv, but there were some exceptions to this. The proportion of monitored workers who were measurably exposed varied from about 10% to about 50%, owing to differences in practice with regard to who is monitored and in the reporting and recording of doses, which may partially explain some of the wide variation in reported average individual doses to both monitored and measurably exposed workers.

F. SUMMARY

327. Worldwide exposures from the medical uses of radiation for treatment of humans (i.e. excluding veterinary practice) are summarized in Table 34. Worldwide estimates have been made for diagnostic radiography, dental practice, nuclear medicine and radiotherapy, and for all medical uses of radiation. The annual number of monitored workers involved worldwide, averaged over five-year periods, increased from about 1.3 million in the first period to about 2.2 million in the third. Averaged over the whole period, approximately 65% of these workers were involved with diagnostic radiography, 25% with dental practice, 4% with nuclear medicine and 6% with radiotherapy.

328. The worldwide annual collective effective dose, averaged over five-year periods, remained relatively uniform over the whole period, at about 1,000 man Sv. There is evidence that the dose was about 10% greater in the second period than in the first and third periods. This estimate of 1,000 man Sv is lower by a factor of 4 to 5 than the estimate in the UNSCEAR 1988 Report [U1], which was 1 man Sv per million population. The present estimate is based on much more extensive reported data. Even so, it may itself be an overestimate of the worldwide collective dose (doses from diagnostic radiography, which makes by far the greatest contribution to the reported collective dose from all medical uses of radiation, are suspected to have been overestimated).

329. Over the three periods, there appear to have been significant changes in the contribution of different practices to the total collective dose. The contribution of diagnostic radiography is estimated to have increased from 60% to 80% between the first and third periods, whereas that from dental practice decreased from 12% to 3%. The contribution from nuclear medicine increased from about 6% to about 9% over the whole period, whereas that from radiotherapy decreased from about 20% to 10%.

330. The average annual effective doses to monitored workers involved in medical uses of radiation and the doses to monitored workers in each of the main

categories of medical use of radiation all decreased with time, even if by differing amounts. This is apparent in Figure XXIII, where the trends in separate practices are indicated. Radiotherapy has, in general, resulted in the largest average annual doses (about 2.2 mSv decreasing to about 0.9 mSv between the first and third periods), typically exceeding the average for all medical uses by a factor of about 2-3. The average annual doses from nuclear medicine (remaining at about 1 mSv over the whole period) also exceeded the overall averages but to a lesser degree. The average annual doses from diagnostic radiography (about 0.9 mSv decreasing to about 0.6 mSv) were broadly comparable with the averages for all medical uses, whereas those for dental radiography (about 0.3 mSv decreasing to about 0.05 mSv) were much lower. The doses from both diagnostic and dental radiography may, however, be significant overestimates because the dosimeter reading is generally used directly as a measure of effective dose.

331. The fraction of monitored workers worldwide exposed to annual effective doses in excess of 15 mSv is small for each medical practice and for medicine overall. Typically, a small fraction of 1% of workers receive annual doses in excess of this level. The values of this quantity (NR_{15}) are somewhat greater for radiotherapy, and those for dental radiography somewhat lower, than the average for all medical practices. The fraction of the collective dose arising from individual doses in excess of that level has varied significantly between practices within an overall range of about 0.03 to about 0.3; the larger values are generally associated with radiotherapy. For all medical uses of radiation the value of NR_{15} decreased from about 0.003 in the first period to about 0.002 in the second, increasing again in the third to about 0.009. The value of SR_{15} followed the same trend, decreasing from about 0.18 to about 0.12 between the first and second periods and then increasing to about 0.24. These increases in the third period, however, are more apparent than real. They are mainly due to the somewhat higher values for China having been reported only for the third period. For those countries reporting data for the whole period analysed there is evidence, overall, of small downward trends with time in both distribution ratios.

332. The variation in occupational exposures from all medical uses of radiation between different geographic or economic regions is summarized in Table 33 and illustrated for selected regions in Figure XXIV. Averaged over the whole period, 33% of monitored workers worldwide are estimated to have been in the United States, with a similar percentage in the rest of the OECD. In Eastern Europe (including the former USSR) the estimated proportion is 20%; based on less complete data, about 4% are estimated to be in Latin America and 4% in countries with centrally planned economies in Asia. About 1% of the total workforce is estimated to be on the Indian subcontinent and a similar proportion in south and south-east Asia (non-centrally planned economies).

333. The contribution of the United States to the worldwide annual collective effective dose almost halved over the period analysed, decreasing from about 46% to 27%. Averaged over the same period, the contribution of the rest of the OECD was about 20% and that of Eastern Europe about 12%. Based on less comprehensive data, Latin America and countries with centrally planned economies in Asia each contributed about 20%, at least in the more recent five-year periods. The Indian subcontinent and south and south-east Asia (non-centrally planned economies) each contributed about 1%, and there is evidence of a significant increase in the contribution of the latter to about 3% in the most recent five-year period.

334. The data on average individual doses to monitored workers indicate that, in general, the doses in the OECD (excluding the United States) and Eastern Europe were less than the worldwide averages for the respective periods. Those for Asia and Latin America were, in general, significantly in excess of the average, while those in the United States and on the Indian subcontinent were, broadly, of the same magnitude.

335. Normalized collective doses (normalized in terms of both gross national product and population) for individual regions, averaged worldwide, are summarized in Table 33. Significant variation is evident between the various values, with the range of variation being far smaller when the normalization is carried out in terms of gross national product as opposed to population size. In terms of population, the normalized collective doses for particular regions vary over more than two orders of magnitude, from about 0.01 to about 2 man Sv per million people, with a worldwide average of about 0.2 man Sv per million people (compared with a representative value of 1 man Sv per million people assumed in the UNSCEAR 1988 Report [U1]). When expressed in terms of gross national product, the collective doses vary over less than an order of magnitude, and with a few exceptions, the variation is much less than this. A number of trends are apparent in these normalized doses: those for the United States are generally greater than those for the rest of the OECD by a factor of 2-3; those for the rest of the OECD, Eastern Europe and the Indian subcontinent are broadly of the same magnitude; and those for Latin America and the centrally planned economies in Asia are substantially in excess of the worldwide averages of this quantity.

VI. NATURAL SOURCES OF RADIATION

336. All workers are inevitably exposed to natural sources of radiation in the course of their work. With the exception of a few occupations, their exposures to natural radiation do not differ significantly from the general background. In the UNSCEAR 1988 Report [U1], a relatively comprehensive assessment was made of available data on exposures in those occupations or industrial practices where enhanced levels of exposure to natural sources of radiation might be experienced. Estimates were made of doses to aircrew, workers at coal-fired power stations, underground miners and workers involved with the industrial and agricultural uses of phosphates (but not with their mining). Underground mining was estimated to make by far the greatest contribution to the overall collective dose from occupational exposure to natural sources of radiation. These estimates are updated here, with emphasis given to those occupations or practices contributing most to the collective dose and to areas where significant new data have since become available. Exposures to natural sources of radiation from the mining and subsequent processing and use of uranium have already been evaluated in the context of the nuclear fuel cycle and are not considered further here.

A. EXTRACTIVE INDUSTRIES

337. The extraction and processing of earth materials increase the exposure of workers to natural sources of radiation. The general public may be somewhat exposed from the subsequent utilization of the products or by the disposal of wastes. The extractive industries include all forms of mining; attention is focused here on underground operations, where radon exposures are greatest.

1. Underground mining

338. Mining is an extensive industry. As can be seen in Table 35, there are about 4.7 million underground miners worldwide, with 84% engaged in coal mining and 16% in the mining of other minerals [C2]. Among the latter group are about 90,000 engaged in the mining of uranium ores (see Table 3). China is the largest employer of workers in coal mines and South Africa in other mines (mainly gold mines). The numbers of workers listed in Table 35 are estimates for 1991. In addition to the inherent uncertainties in the data, such estimates can fluctuate widely from year to year owing to continually changing regional and global economic conditions.

339. Exposures in underground mining may arise from external and internal sources; the main contributors to internal exposure are the inhalation of radon and thoron progeny and the inhalation of dust containing long-lived alpha emitters of the uranium and thorium series. The relative contribution of each will depend on the type of mine, the geology and the working conditions, particularly the degree of ventilation. Exposures to natural sources of radiation arising from mining have received much less attention than those arising from the industrial and medical uses of man-made sources of radiation. Relatively few data are available for the period of interest and, in general, their quality or reliability is much less than that of the data reported elsewhere in this Annex for other occupations. This is a consequence of the paucity of the data as well as the fact that many were derived from environmental, as opposed to personal, dosimetry; considerable errors in dose estimates can occur when they are based on grab samples of air instead of personal air samplers. This situation is, however, changing, and more comprehensive and reliable data can be expected in the future.

340. Data on exposures to radon and its decay products in about 1,200 underground mines are summarized in Table 36; the data are presented separately for coal and other (excluding uranium) mines. Considerable variation is evident in the average levels of exposure reported between countries. There is also considerable variation between doses at mines within a given country. This is indicated in Table 37, where average individual doses are given for mines in the United States and the former USSR; it should be noted that the tabulated doses differ from those reported in the respective references, in particular a conversion factor of 5.6 mSv WLM^{-1} has been assumed in contrast to a value of 10 mSv WLM^{-1} in the data reported. Data have also been reported for coal and other mines in China [P5, X1]; for non-coal mines, the reported average annual doses are typically more than an order of magnitude greater than the average values reported for other countries. These data for non-coal mines [P5, X1] are not, however, thought to be representative of China as a whole for two reasons: first, the reported values are based on a limited number of grab samples which may not be representative of the conditions experienced by the whole workforce and, secondly, the data are for mines in only one province of China [P6].

341. The data in Table 36 refer to various time periods, which limits the extent to which they can be evaluated in a coherent manner. Neither the quality nor the extent of the data are considered adequate enough to allow their use to establish trends in worldwide exposures from underground mining. They have, however, been used to estimate worldwide doses

from the inhalation of radon progeny, which are summarized in Table 38; these doses can be considered broadly representative for the latter half of the 1980s. The doses were estimated as the sum, over all countries, of the products of the number of miners and the reported exposure to radon progeny. The average exposure, for those countries reporting data, has been assumed applicable worldwide. A conversion factor of 5.6 mSv WLM^{-1} has been assumed in estimating effective doses from the exposures reported in Table 36.

342. The worldwide annual collective effective dose from the inhalation of radon progeny in underground mines (excluding uranium mining) is estimated to be about 5,300 man Sv, with about 1,500 man Sv (about 30%) arising in coal mines and about 3,800 man Sv (about 70%) in other mines. About 30% of the worldwide collective dose from coal mining arose in Poland and about 10% in the former USSR. In other mines, excluding uranium mines, about 50% of the worldwide collective dose occurred in South Africa. The worldwide average annual effective dose was estimated to be about 0.4 mSv in coal mines and about 5 mSv in other mines.

343. Exposures may also occur from external irradiation and from the inhalation of thoron progeny and of dust containing long-lived alpha emitters of the uranium and thorium series; consequently, the dose estimates in Table 38 from the inhalation of radon progeny alone are underestimates of the total dose. Few data are available on these other pathways of exposure, and their relative magnitudes will vary from mine to mine depending on the geology and working conditions. Estimates made for a number of mines in the former USSR [P1] suggest that the contribution from other pathways is about 1 mSv per annum which, except in coal mines, is a small fraction of the dose from radon progeny. In the absence of better data, the annual doses given in Table 38 for radon progeny have been increased by 1 mSv to take account of other exposure pathways. When such an allowance is made, the annual collective effective dose from all exposure pathways for coal mining worldwide becomes about 5,400 man Sv and that from other mining (excluding uranium) about 4,500 man Sv. The corresponding average annual effective doses from all pathways are about 1.4 mSv and 6.4 mSv for coal and other mines, respectively.

344. The doses estimated in the above manner represent exposures received while at work in underground mines. They require further correction, however, if they are to be compared directly with exposures arising in other industries, where exposures from natural sources of radiation are not included in the reported doses. Similar correction is needed if the quantity of interest is the additional, rather than the total, dose received while at work. To enable fair comparisons with exposures in other industries and to allow the derivation of a quantity that represents the additional exposure from the work, the above annual dose estimates need to be reduced by about 0.5 mSv; this is the annual dose that the worker would otherwise have received if not at work. This estimate is based on 2,000 hours work per year and a worldwide average dose from external irradiation and inhalation of radon progeny of 2.4 mSv (see Annex A, "Exposures from natural sources of radiation").

345. After correcting for other exposure pathways and for exposures that would have been received irrespective of work, the worldwide annual collective effective dose from underground (non-uranium) mining, during the latter half of the 1980s, is estimated to have been about 7,500 man Sv; about one half of this total collective dose arose in coal mining with the other half arising in other mines (excluding uranium). For comparison, the annual collective dose from uranium mining (see Table 3), averaged over the period 1975-1989, was about 1,300 man Sv. Of those countries identified separately in Table 38, South Africa (about 27%) makes the largest contribution to the total collective dose with significant contributions also from the former USSR (about 11%) and Poland (about 7%). The additional worldwide average annual effective dose received by underground miners from their work is estimated to have been about 0.9 mSv in coal mines and about 6 mSv in other mines (excluding uranium), although there was considerable variation about these averages between countries and between mines in a given country. Somewhat greater individual and collective doses are likely to have been received before the latter half of the 1980s, because less attention was paid to the control and reduction of exposures from this source. Insufficient data are available, however, to make a reliable estimate of how much greater they might have been; the few data in Table 36 suggest that they may have been substantially greater.

346. Very approximate and tentative estimates were made in the UNSCEAR 1988 Report [U1] of collective doses from natural sources of radiation. For coal mining, an upper estimate of 2,000 man Sv was made for the worldwide annual collective effective dose; this was based solely on exposures in mines in the United Kingdom and on the worldwide production of coal. Given the very approximate nature of this earlier estimate and the change adopted here in the conversion factor for exposure to radon progeny, it compares favourably with the current estimate of about 3,400 man Sv. A very rough estimate of 20,000 man Sv was also made in [U1] for the annual collective effective dose from underground mining

apart from coal and uranium; this earlier estimate was based on a very tentative assumption that the arithmetic mean annual individual dose was 10 mSv (from a range of reported values between 0.1 and 200 mSv) and that there were, on average, 500 underground miners (excluding coal and uranium) per million population. This earlier tentative estimate exceeds the present estimate, of about 4,100 man Sv, by a factor of about 5. Differences in the number of miners (about a factor of 3 lower than before) and in the average individual dose (about a factor of 2 lower than before) are responsible for the decrease in the collective dose estimated previously. For all underground mining (but excluding uranium) the collective dose estimated here (about 7,500 man Sv) is about a factor of 3 less than that estimated in the UNSCEAR 1988 Report [U1].

2. Surface mining

347. Mineral sands are mined and processed in several countries. Monazite, an important constituent of the sands, has concentrations of thorium of about 2.5 10^5 Bq kg^{-1} and concentrations of uranium an order of magnitude less. Surface mining is followed by a wet and then a dry processing stage. The important pathways of exposure are external irradiation from gamma-ray emitting radionuclides of the ^{232}Th and ^{238}U decay series and inhalation of ore dust, the latter being quite pronounced at the dry stage. Exposure and employment information are scarce. Data for Western Australia, a major producer of monazite, show that dry-process workers received appreciable doses from the inhalation of dust [H6]. Annual effective doses for 376 dry-process workers averaged 20 mSv for 1983-1988, with 50% of workers above 15 mSv. About 90% of the dose is from internal exposure. For all categories of workers (1,318 in number), the average annual effective doses averaged 7 mSv, with 15% above 15 mSv [H6]. This information is supported by information from other parts of Australia [J1] and from Malaysia [O1], India [M4] and Brazil [C3], but more data are required from such producer countries for a full global assessment.

348. Similar difficulties affect the assessment of occupational exposures from the mining and processing of phosphate ores. Sedimentary phosphate may contain about 1,500 Bq kg^{-1} of uranium. Surface mining is followed by milling and other physical treatment to upgrade the ore, most of which is later digested with acid to produce fertilizers. The main mechanisms of exposure in the early stages are gamma-irradiation and the inhalation of radon progeny, with some inhalation of ore dust. Data for the initial stages in two mines in the Syrian Arab Republic [O5] indicate that exposures overall are unremarkable and that even the maximum values are not very high. The annual effective doses from gamma rays averaged 0.3 mSv in two mines and 0.1 mSv in two processing plants. The doses from radon progeny ranged from 0.1 WLM to a maximum of 0.7 WLM (i.e. about 0.6 mSv to about 4 mSv using a conversion factor of 5.6 mSv WLM^{-1}). The inhalation of dust could have added 0.5-1 mSv to these doses. Limited, but consistent data are available from India [L3], Israel [T1], United States [H9], Tunisia [M13] and Yugoslavia [K7]; more are needed for a better estimate of exposures worldwide.

349. Based on the limited data available for the mining and processing of mineral sands and phosphate ores, it is evident that the collective doses from these operations are small in comparison with those from underground mining. It is unlikely that the collective effective dose from such operations would exceed about 100 man Sv, although further data are needed to confirm such an estimate.

3. Transport, storage and use of phosphates

350. In the UNSCEAR 1988 Report [U1] very approximate estimates were made of the collective doses worldwide arising in the processing and transport of phosphate rocks and in the transport, storage and use of phosphates as fertilizers. Based on the extrapolation of limited experience in Germany, in which account was taken only of exposure by external irradiation, a worldwide annual dose of about 70 man Sv was attributed to these operations. No further data have been obtained that would allow updating this estimate, which remains very approximate.

B. AVIATION

1. Air travel

351. Flight altitude and duration are the principal determinants of cosmic-ray doses to airline crews and passengers. Modern commercial aircraft have optimum operating altitudes near 13 km, but flight paths are assigned according to use and safety requirements. There do not seem to be enough data available to determine average flight patterns [W2]. In the UNSCEAR 1988 Report [U1], a representative operating altitude of 8 km was assumed, because of the predominance of short-distance flights, with an average speed of 600 km h^{-1}. Other studies assume other altitudes and speeds: for example, an altitude of 9 km and a speed of 650 km h^{-1} were used for an assessment in the United Kingdom [H1], and an altitude of 7 km was used for flights by United States carriers lasting less than an hour and 11 km for longer flights [O4]. At 8 km the effective dose equivalent has been estimated to be 2 μSv h^{-1}, this being the sum of the absorbed dose in tissue of the directly and

indirectly ionizing radiations [H4, N5]. A worldwide measurement programme on Lufthansa airplanes indicated that most flight altitudes were in the range of 10 to 11.9 km with effective dose equivalent rates of less than 5 μSv h^{-1} and 8 μSv h^{-1}, respectively, at these altitudes [R7, R8].

352. Computational codes have been developed to calculate the radiation levels throughout the atmosphere (e.g. [O4]), and additional measurement experience is being acquired (e.g. [R8]). Preliminary assessments of cosmic-ray dose accounting for changes in quality factors [I7] are indicating that effective doses are likely to be a few tens of per cent greater than the effective dose equivalents reported above. Pending these revised estimates and given the other uncertainties inherent in the estimation of doses to aircrew, the simplifying assumption is made here that the effective doses are numerically equal to the reported effective dose equivalents. In addition to variations with altitude, the cosmic-ray dose changes with latitude and solar cycle modulation.

353. A limited number of supersonic airplanes operate commercially and cruise at about 15 km. Doses on board are routinely determined with monitoring equipment. Effective dose equivalent rates are generally around 10 μSv h^{-1}, with a maximum around 40 μSv h^{-1} [U1]. In two years from July 1987, the overall average on six French airplanes was 12 μSv h^{-1} with monthly values up to 18 μSv h^{-1} [P2]; in 1990, the average was 11 μSv h^{-1} and the annual dose to aircrew about 3 mSv [M5]. During 1990, the average dose rate for about 2,000 flights by British airplanes was 10 μSv h^{-1}, with a maximum value of 50 μSv h^{-1} [D4]; annual doses to aircrew are around 2.5 mSv on average with a maximum around 17 mSv [H1]. Neutrons contribute about half of the overall effective dose equivalents. The monitoring equipment serves to warn of solar flares so that the airplanes can be brought to lower altitudes. This is a very small sector of the commercial air transport industry.

354. In the UNSCEAR 1988 Report [U1] annual flying time of 600 hours was assumed to be representative for aircrew, which is compatible with experience in the United Kingdom [H1], Germany [R7, R8] and France [M5]; flying times may be 50% higher in the United States [F3]. The annual collective effective dose equivalent to aircrew in the United States was estimated to be about 400 man Sv in 1985, based on an average annual effective dose equivalent of 3.5 mSv to some 114,000 crew members (of which 46,000 and 68,000, respectively, were flight crew and cabin attendants) [E3]. The annual collective effective dose equivalent to Lufthansa aircrew in Germany has been estimated to be about 30 man Sv, based on 12,000 aircrew and average annual individual dose of 2.5 mSv [R7, R8]. Values reported for a number of other European carriers [M5, M6, S9] are consistent with an estimate of annual effective dose equivalents to aircrew of 2.5 mSv. An approximate estimate of the worldwide collective effective dose equivalent can be made by assuming an average annual dose of 3 mSv (i.e. intermediate between European and United States experience) and taking account of the number of aircrew worldwide which, in the late 1980s, was about a quarter of a million [I12]. The resulting estimate of the worldwide annual collective effective dose equivalent is about 800 man Sv. This value is several times higher than previously estimated [U1]. Although still only approximate, it is better substantiated and should be a more accurate estimate.

355. In addition to aircrew, some other persons, such as professional couriers, receive higher exposures in air travel. An analysis of passengers using London airport in 1988 showed that one in four had made 10 or more journeys during the previous year, corresponding to 30 or more hours aloft, but some professional couriers undertook 200 journeys a year, implying 1,200 flying hours [G2]. The number of these individuals is unknown, but it must be some small fraction of the number of aircrew.

2. Space travel

356. Space travel is restricted to a small number of astronauts and cosmonauts. Current space travel from the United States and the former USSR is restricted to low earth orbits at various inclinations [B13]. Doses are strongly dependent on altitude and less so on inclination. Experimental results from six shuttle missions [B13, N3] and seven space-station missions [B13, N4] indicated that daily effective dose equivalents at altitudes from 300 to 520 km were 0.1-0.7 mSv. Low- and high-LET radiations were determined separately; each contributed about half of the total. Because of the complexities of radiation fields in space vehicles, it is not easy to estimate exposure in terms of effective dose; the simple assumption is therefore made that it is numerically equal to the foregoing values. Because so few individuals are involved, the collective dose from this practice is quite low.

357. A comprehensive review of radiation in space has been published by NCRP [N3]. It treats in detail the physical and biological aspects of the subject and projects dose for possible future space missions.

C. OTHER OCCUPATIONS AND PRACTICES

358. In addition to mines, other places of underground work with potentially increased radon levels include natural caves, subway systems and power stations. In

Germany radon levels exceed 1,000 Bq m^{-3} in 40% of all such underground work locations; in 10%, they exceed 5,000 Bq m^{-3} [S10]. Radon levels in caves in the karstic or limestone regions of several countries are similar [H8, R4, S12]. Unlike mines, caves may not have efficient mechanical ventilation, so radon and progeny levels may be quite high. Typical concentrations of potential alpha energy are about 0.3 WL, implying about 5 mSv effective dose in three months or 20 mSv for a full working year (assuming a conversion factor of 5.6 mSv WLM^{-1}). Some caves exceed 2 WL, however, which could imply substantial doses for some guides.

359. In the UNSCEAR 1988 Report [U1] consideration was given to a number of other industrial processes and occupations that could lead to enhanced levels of exposure to natural sources of radiation. In general, the data for these practices and occupations were not sufficient to enable reliable estimates to be made of worldwide collective doses. Their contribution to the total worldwide occupational exposure from natural sources of radiation is, however, unlikely to be significant. Nonetheless, the collective dose to workers at coal-fired power plants was estimated. The main source of exposure in this case is thought to be the inhalation of airborne fly ash, which contains elevated levels of a number of naturally occurring radionuclides. The upper estimate of the worldwide annual collective effective dose was 60 man Sv, subject to the following assumptions: global annual production of electrical energy of 600 GW a; a labour force of 500 to produce 1 GW a per year; and an individual annual committed effective dose per worker of 0.15 mSv. The last value was estimated for the most exposed group of power station workers in the United Kingdom, assuming exposure to dust at concentrations of 0.5 mg m^{-3}; this value, if applied to all workers, gives an overestimate for the collective dose from the practice.

D. SUMMARY

360. A summary of average individual and collective effective doses to workers worldwide involved in occupations or practices that have increased exposures to natural sources of radiation are summarized in Table 39. The worldwide annual collective effective dose is estimated to be 8,600 man Sv. This dose arises mainly (about 90%) from underground mining. About 45% of the collective dose from mining arises from coal mining and about 55% from the mining of other materials. The estimated collective dose to aircrew is about 800 man Sv (about 10% of the total). The contribution from all other activities is small by comparison and appears unlikely to exceed a few hundred man sievert.

VII. ACCIDENTS

361. Accidents that occur in the course of work add to occupational exposures. Accidents with clinical consequences for those exposed that occurred in 1975-1989 are listed in Table 40, separated into accidents occurring in the nuclear fuel cycle and associated research, industrial uses of radiation, tertiary education and research (including accelerators) and medical uses of radiation. Most of the data were obtained in response to the UNSCEAR Survey on Occupational Exposures. Some additional entries have been made from other compilations of accidents [I11, R3] to the extent that dose information was available or clinical consequences could be ascertained. The accidental exposures listed are for those which have occurred in the course of work; accidental exposures from the theft or loss of industrial or medical sources have been excluded as have accidental exposures of patients during diagnosis or therapy.

362. The majority of accidents occurred in industrial uses of radiation, involving radiography sources and irradiation facilities. In most cases either human carelessness or malfunction of the equipment has been the cause. Two accidents resulted in high doses that caused deaths: one death at Brescia, Italy in 1975, and one in El Salvador in 1989. None of the accidents reported to workers involved in medical uses of radiation caused deaths.

363. There have been relatively few accidents involving serious radiation injury to workers in operations of the nuclear fuel cycle. On the other hand, the accident at Chernobyl in 1986 caused high exposures and acute radiation sickness in 237 persons and the deaths of 28 of them. These were workers at the reactor and members of the fire-fighting and emergency crew, who dealt with the accident in its initial stages. Two other workers at the reactor died as a result of the explosions and fire rather than of radiation injuries. An accident at a criticality facility at Buenos Aires in 1983 resulted in the death of one worker.

364. While accidents causing deaths are well known, there is likely to be substantial underreporting of other accidents. Two considerations support this premise. First, for the period 1975-1984, the number of accidents reported here is almost twice as great as the number reported by Rodrigues de Oliveira [R3], which was based on a detailed and comprehensive review of the literature; it would thus appear that many accidental exposures with actual or potential clinical consequences have not been reported in the literature. Secondly, the data reported in response to the UNSCEAR questionnaire are by no means comprehensive, either in terms of the countries reporting data or in the completeness of the data reported for the period of interest. As is apparent from Table 40, either there have been very large variations in the frequency of accidents in some countries in the different five-year periods, or, as is more likely, the reported data are incomplete. It is difficult to assess the extent of any underestimate, but a very rough extrapolation of the data provided in response to the UNSCEAR Survey on Occupational Exposures suggests that the number of accidents with potential or actual clinical consequences may have been two or three times as great as reported here. There is much uncertainty in this estimate, given the few countries reporting data.

365. It would be of interest to know the collective dose to workers caused by accidents, but the data are too incomplete to make other than a very rough estimate. The doses to those acutely exposed in the Chernobyl accident were reported in detail in the UNSCEAR 1988 Report [U1]. The collective dose to the 28 workers who died was 240 man Sv. The remainder of the workers accounted for 370 man Sv, estimated from the distribution of workers according to degree of radiation sickness and using the mid-point doses that characterize these degrees. The three deaths in other radiation accidents may be estimated to account for 30 man Sv. The remaining entries, even assigning up to 0.5 Sv per accident and underreporting by a factor of 2-3 could add at most about 200 man Sv; this is likely to be a major overestimate, because the majority of accidents involve skin or extremity exposures. This makes a total of less than 900 man Sv for all accidents occurring in 1975-1989. About two thirds of the total resulted from the Chernobyl accident, with the remainder adding at most about 15 man Sv per year to occupational radiation exposures; in reality the latter dose may be substantially less.

366. Additional occupational radiation exposure occurs in the aftermath of accidents, in clean-up and decontamination work. The Chernobyl accident alone involved 600,000 workers, many or possibly most of whom were exposed to the maximum permitted dose limit. This represents a very special case, but nevertheless a substantial collective dose. Only if accurate and more complete records are maintained of exposures caused by accidents can estimates of this component of occupational radiation exposures be improved.

367. In summary, the number of accidents to workers worldwide with clinical consequences reported here for the period 1975-1989 is about 90 involving 362 workers; because of underreporting, the actual number of accidents, may have been two or three times greater. The reported data are too incomplete to make any reliable estimate of trends in accidental exposures with time.

CONCLUSIONS

368. Occupational radiation exposures have been evaluated for five broad categories of work, namely the nuclear fuel cycle, defence activities, industrial uses of radiation (excluding the nuclear fuel cycle and defence), medical uses of radiation and occupations where enhanced exposures to natural sources of radiation may occur. Results for 1985-1989 are summarized in Table 41 and, in abbreviated form, for the whole period of interest (1975-1989) in Table 42. The contribution of each category to the overall levels of exposure and the trends with time are illustrated in Figure XXV. The worldwide average individual and collective effective doses have been derived largely from data reported in response to the UNSCEAR Survey of Occupational Exposures, supplemented where appropriate by data from the literature.

369. ***Summary of exposures in the period 1985-1989.*** The average number of monitored workers worldwide involved with man-made uses of radiation in the period 1985-1989 is estimated to be about 4 million. The majority (about 55%) of these are involved with medical uses of radiation, with about 22%, 14% and 10% with the commercial nuclear fuel cycle, industrial uses of radiation and defence activities, respectively. About 5 million workers are estimated to be exposed to natural sources of radiation at levels in excess of average background levels. By far the majority (about

75%) are coal miners; other occupational groups contributing significantly to this total are underground miners in non-coal mines (about 13%) and aircrew (about 5%).

370. The worldwide average annual collective effective dose to workers from man-made sources of radiation in 1985-1989 is estimated to be about 4,300 man Sv. The collective effective dose from exposures to natural sources (in excess of average levels of natural background) is estimated to be about 8,600 man Sv; it arises mainly from underground mining (about 90%), with broadly comparable contributions from coal mining and the mining of other materials (other than uranium). The estimated collective dose from natural sources of radiation is, however, associated with much greater uncertainty than that from man-made sources of radiation.

371. Of the annual collective effective dose from exposure to man-made sources of radiation (4,300 man Sv), about 58% arises from operations in the nuclear fuel cycle (2,500 man Sv), about 23% from medical uses (1,000 man Sv), about 12% from industrial uses of radiation (510 man Sv) and about 6% from defence activities (250 man Sv). The contribution from medical uses of radiation may, however, be an overestimate by a factor of 2 or more; most of the exposures from this source arise from low-energy x rays from diagnostic radiography, and the dosimeter reading, which is generally entered directly into dose records, may overestimate the effective dose by a large factor.

372. The average annual effective dose to monitored workers varies widely between occupations and also between countries for the same occupation. The worldwide average annual effective doses to monitored workers in industry (excluding the nuclear fuel cycle), medicine and defence activities are less than 1 mSv (about 0.9 mSv, 0.5 mSv and 0.7 mSv, respectively); in particular countries, however, the average annual dose for some of these occupations is several millisievert or even, exceptionally, in excess of 10 mSv. The average annual effective doses to workers in the nuclear fuel cycle are, in most cases, larger than those in other occupations; for the fuel cycle overall, the average annual effective dose is about 2.9 mSv. For the mining of uranium the average annual effective dose to monitored workers in countries reporting data was about 4 mSv, and for uranium milling operations it was about 6 mSv; there are, however, very wide variations about these average values, with doses of about 50 mSv being reported in some countries. The average annual effective dose to monitored workers in LWRs is about 2 mSv, with doses about 50% greater, on average, in HWRs and smaller by a factor of about 2, on average, in GCRs. The individual doses in fuel reprocessing are comparable with those in reactors, whereas those in fuel enrichment are much smaller.

373. The percentage of monitored workers worldwide involved with the use of man-made sources of radiation receiving annual effective doses in excess of 15 mSv is estimated, on average, to have been about 3% during the period 1985-1989. There is, however, considerable variation in this value between occupations. Typically, about 0.1% of monitored workers in medicine and industry (excluding the nuclear fuel cycle and defence) are estimated to have received doses in excess of this level. For the nuclear fuel cycle as a whole, about 10% of monitored workers, on average, exceeded this level of annual effective dose. There is, however, considerable variation between different stages of the fuel cycle (i.e. about 20% for uranium mining and milling, about 3% averaged over all reactors but varying within a range of essentially zero to about 7% depending on the reactor type, about 6% for reprocessing, on average, about 0.2% for fuel fabrication and essentially zero for enrichment). It should be noted that the above percentages, where they include a contribution from workers in uranium mining and milling, may be overestimates. This is due to the assumption that the reported distribution ratios for uranium mining and milling are applicable to an effective dose of 15 mSv; strictly they apply to a dose less than 15 mSv because of the change in the conversion factor (compared with that used in the reported data) for exposures to radon progeny adopted in this Annex.

374. The percentage of the worldwide collective effective dose from all uses of man-made sources of radiation (or more strictly for those uses for which data have been reported) which arises from annual individual doses in excess of 15 mSv is estimated to have been about 30% to 40% during the period 1985-1989. There is, however, considerable variation in this value between occupations. Typically, about 25% and 30%, respectively, of the collective dose in medicine and industry (excluding the nuclear fuel cycle and defence) are estimated to have arisen from annual individual doses in excess of this level. For the nuclear fuel cycle as a whole, about 40% of the collective dose arose from annual individual doses in excess of 15 mSv. There is, however, considerable variation between different stages of the fuel cycle (i.e. about 50% for uranium mining and milling, about 35% averaged over all reactors but varying within a range of essentially zero to about 50% depending on the reactor type, about 10% for oxide fuel reprocessing, about 2% for fuel fabrication and essentially zero for enrichment). It should be noted that the above percentages, where they include a contribution from

workers in uranium mining and milling, may be overestimates for the reasons set out above.

375. The average annual effective dose to workers exposed to enhanced levels from natural sources of radiation, in particular in underground mines, varies considerably between mines and between countries. In coal mines, the average annual effective dose is estimated to be about 1 mSv. In other (non-uranium) mines the worldwide average effective dose is estimated to be about 6 mSv. Aircrew are estimated to receive an average annual effective dose of about 3 mSv.

376. ***Trends in exposures over the period 1975-1989.*** Trends in exposure from man-made sources are illustrated in Figure XXV for each of the main occupational categories considered in this Annex. The trends in occupational exposures from natural sources have not been quantified because insufficient data are available to make meaningful estimates; the few data that do exist, however, suggest that exposures (excluding those to aircrew) before the second half of the 1980s were greater than those estimated here, possibly much greater. The latter is due to somewhat less attention being given in the past to control and reduction of exposures in underground mining.

377. The worldwide annual average number of workers involved with man-made uses of radiation is estimated to have increased from about 2.5 to about 4 million between the first and third five-year periods. The greatest increase (from about 1.3 to about 2.2 million) has been in the number of monitored workers in medicine. The number of monitored workers in the nuclear fuel cycle has also increased significantly (by about 50% from about 0.6 to about 0.9 million). Increases in the numbers of the monitored workers in defence activities and other industrial uses of radiation have been modest by comparison.

378. The annual collective effective dose, averaged over five-year periods, for all operations in the nuclear fuel cycle changed little over the period 1975-1989, notwithstanding the large increase (three to fourfold) in electrical energy generated by nuclear means; some changes, however, occurred in particular stages of the fuel cycle. The annual average collective dose from uranium mining increased by about 25% between the first and second five-year periods decreasing again to about its former level in the third period. There was a decrease by a factor of almost 2 for fuel fabrication, reprocessing and research. The collective dose from reactors increased over the period by a factor approaching 2, with almost all of the increase occurring during 1975-1979 and 1980-1985. The increase in dose between the first two five-year periods was largely attributable to the major plant safety modifications carried out in the earlier 1980s in response the accident at Three Mile Island. Indeed, but for the accident at Chernobyl, the annual average collective dose from reactors in 1985-1989 would probably have decreased relative to the preceding five-year period. Average annual individual effective doses to monitored workers in nuclear fuel cycle operations typically decreased by a factor of about 2 in most stages of the fuel cycle between 1975-1979 and 1985-1989; for uranium mining, the decrease with time was only about 20%.

379. The normalized collective effective dose per unit energy generated has decreased with time for the fuel cycle overall and for most of its stages. For the fuel cycle overall, the normalized collective dose has decreased by almost a factor of 2 from about 20 man Sv $(GW\ a)^{-1}$ to about 12 man Sv $(GW\ a)^{-1}$, with most of this decrease occurring between the second and third five-year periods. For reactors, between the first and second five-year periods, the normalized collective doses changed little, but large decreases occurred in the third period; decreases by a factor of about 2 occurred for PWRs, BWRs and HWRs. These decreases in the third period were a consequence of the completion of most of the safety modifications made following the accident at the Three Mile Island reactor and the much greater attention paid by utilities and regulators to the reduction of occupational exposures in both existing and new reactors. Substantial reductions (by about an order of magnitude) occurred in the normalized collective dose for the fabrication of LWR fuel, although these doses may be underestimates because they do not take account of internal exposures. The normalized doses for the fabrication of other fuels did not decrease. Indeed, those for GCRs would appear to have increased with time; much of this increase, however, is more apparent than real, due to the fact that internal exposures were included only for the third period. For uranium mining, the normalized collective dose decreased by about 25% over the period analysed. The normalized dose for reprocessing oxide fuels changed little over the period analysed, whereas that for Magnox fuels decreased by about a third.

380. The worldwide average annual collective effective dose from all industrial uses of radiation, excluding the nuclear fuel cycle and defence activities, was fairly uniform over the period 1975-1984. It decreased, however, by a factor of almost 2 in the second half of the 1980s. This same trend is reflected in estimates of individual dose; the annual effective dose to monitored workers decreased from an average of about 1.5 mSv, over the period 1975-1984, to an average of about 0.9 mSv in the second half of the 1980s. In defence activities both the average individual and collective doses decreased by a factor of nearly

2 over the period analysed. These decreases were largely a consequence of reductions in doses achieved in the operation and maintenance of nuclear navies, notwithstanding the increase both in the number of ships in operation and in those undergoing refit over this time.

381. The worldwide average annual collective effective dose from all medical uses of radiation, about 1,000 man Sv, changed little over the three five-year periods. A clear downward trend is, however, evident in the worldwide average annual effective dose to monitored workers, which decreased from about 0.8 mSv in the first five-year period to about 0.5 mSv in the third; there was, however, considerable variation between countries. The annual average number of monitored workers in medicine increased by about 75% over the three periods, and this is the reason why the collective dose remained relatively uniform with time, notwithstanding the significant decrease in average individual dose. The extent to which some of these decreases in average individual dose are real or are merely artifacts due to changes in monitoring or recording practice, warrants further analysis.

382. The percentage of monitored workers worldwide involved with all uses of man-made sources of radiation receiving annual effective doses in excess of 15 mSv has decreased progressively from an average of about 5% to about 3% between the first and third five-year periods. This same downward trend is evident in the percentages of nuclear fuel cycle and medical workers worldwide receiving annual doses in excess of this same level. The tabulated data for medical workers show an increase in the third period. This increase, however, is more apparent than real and is due to the inclusion in this period only of data for one country with a very high value of this fraction; if this country were excluded, the trend would be downwards for medical workers throughout the period (see Section V.E). For industrial workers (excluding the nuclear fuel cycle and defence) worldwide there is little evidence in support of any clear trend in the percentage of workers receiving annual doses in excess of 15 mSv.

383. The percentage of the worldwide annual collective effective dose from all man-made uses of radiation arising from annual individual doses in excess of 15 mSv has also decreased progressively from about 45% to about 36%, on average, between the first and third five-year periods. The same downward trend is evident for the collective dose from the nuclear fuel cycle and from medical uses of radiation. The tabulated data for medical uses show an increase in the third period; however, for the reasons set out above, this increase is merely an artifact of the data, and the trend has in fact been downwards over the whole period. For industrial workers there is little evidence of any clear trend with time in the fraction of the collective dose arising from annual doses in excess of 15 mSv.

384. *Cumulative exposures.* Cumulative or lifetime exposures of workers have been analysed to only a limited extent. The examination of termination records has given average rates of dose accumulation for various career lengths, but there was no assurance that the records were either complete or accurate. Some indications of lifetime exposures may be provided by estimates of average annual exposures and career lifetimes, but both parameters are extremely variable between individuals within particular occupations, as well as between occupations and from one country to another. To evaluate actual experience, the need exists for more complete records of employment at all locations and complete dosimetry, including external and internal exposures. Improved data on this aspect can be expected in the next few years with the increasing use of computerized databases for occupational exposures and the compilation of data suitable for epidemiological studies on workers.

385. *Accidental exposures.* Occupational exposures to workers caused by accidents give an added component of dose or injury to those involved. The data compiled indicate that most of the accidents occurred in the industrial uses of radiation and that most of them involved industrial radiography sources. By far the majority of accidental exposures of sufficient magnitude to cause clinical effects were associated with localized exposures to the skin or hands. From 1975 to 1989, 31 people died as a result of radiation exposures received in accidents; 28 of these were at Chernobyl. The number of accidents to workers worldwide with actual clinical consequences that has been reported in the period 1975-1989 is about 90. Because of underreporting of non-fatal accidents, the actual number may have been two or three times greater.

386. *Comparison with previous estimates of occupational exposures.* The estimates of occupational radiation exposure in this Annex have benefited from a much more extensive and complete database than was previously available to the Committee. The efforts by countries to record and improve dosimetric data have been reflected in the responses to the UNSCEAR Survey and have led to improved estimates of occupational exposures. The current estimate of the annual collective effective dose during the second half of the 1980s from occupational exposures to man-made sources of radiation (4,300 man Sv) is lower by a factor of 2 than the estimate made by the Committee in the UNSCEAR 1988 Report for the first half of the 1980s [U1]; the current analysis, however,

suggests that the latter was an overestimate by about a factor of 2 and that the actual reduction in collective dose over this period was relatively small, about 15%-20%.

387. The largest change in the estimates of annual collective dose is for medical uses of radiation. The current estimate indicates that the annual collective dose has remained relatively unchanged over the whole period analysed at about 1,000 man Sv. This is lower by a factor of 5 compared with the estimate made in the UNSCEAR 1988 Report [U1] for the first half of the 1980s, indicating that the latter was over-estimated by a large factor; moreover, as has been noted, the current estimate may still be too large by a factor of 2 or more. The annual collective dose from industrial uses of radiation (excluding the nuclear fuel cycle and defence) is estimated in this analysis to have decreased by about a factor of 2 (from about 900 to 500 man Sv) between the first and second halves of the 1980s. The current estimate of the collective dose for the first half of the 1980s is about a factor of 2 lower than that estimated previously in the UNSCEAR 1988 Report [U1], based on data available at that time.

388. For the nuclear fuel cycle the greatest changes, compared with earlier estimates, are for the mining and milling of uranium and reactor operation. The present estimate of the normalized collective dose during the second half of the 1980s from mining and milling of uranium [about 4.8 man Sv $(GW\ a)^{-1}$] is about seven times greater than estimated previously [U1]. This previous estimate would, however, appear to have been an underestimate by an even greater factor. The current analysis indicates that the normalized collective dose in the early 1980s was actually about 20% greater than that for the second half of the 1980s. The present estimate of the normalized collective dose from reactor operation [about 5.8 man Sv $(GW\ a)^{-1}$] for the second half of the 1980s is smaller, by a factor of about 2, than estimated previously [U1] for the first half of the 1980s; this change reflects a real reduction in dose between the first and second halves of the 1980s, due largely to the completion of plant modifications to LWRs following the accident at Three Mile Island and, to a lesser extent, to the commissioning of new reactors in several countries.

389. The present estimate of the collective effective dose from exposures to enhanced natural sources of radiation at work is about two to three times smaller than the estimate made by the Committee in the UNSCEAR 1988 Report [U1]. Significant differences are apparent, however, in the respective estimates depending on the occupation. For coal mining and aircrew, the present estimates are factors of about 2 and 4 times greater, respectively, than those made previously; the present estimate for other mining (excluding uranium) is, however, a factor of about 5 times smaller than that made previously. The estimates of exposures to natural sources of radiation are not, however, as well supported by data as those for man-made sources. Further monitoring and investigation are needed of this important component of occupational exposures.

Table 1
Occupational categories used by UNSCEAR for evaluating exposures

Exposure source	*Occupational categories*
Nuclear fuel cycle	Uranium mining and milling Uranium enrichment and conversion Fuel fabrication Reactor operation PWRs, BWRs, HWRs, GCRs, LWGRs, FBRs Fuel reprocessing Research and development [a]
Defence activities	Nuclear weapons production Naval nuclear propulsion Other [b]
Industrial uses of radiation (excluding the nuclear fuel cycle and defence activities)	All industrial uses Industrial radiography Fixed, mobile Luminizing Radioisotope production and distribution Well logging Accelerator operation [c] Tertiary education and research [d] Other [e]
Medical uses of radiation	All medical uses Diagnostic radiography Dental radiography Nuclear medicine Radiotherapy Veterinary practice
Natural sources	Underground mining coal other (excluding uranium) Surface mining Aircrew Other

[a] Limited, in principle, to activities directly attributed to the commercial nuclear fuel cycle. It is recognized, however, that because of the way data are collected, the data attributed to this category may include exposures arising from other activities.
[b] To include all other uses encountered in civilian occupations (e.g. non-destructive testing, transport, research, education, etc.)
[c] Limited to accelerators used for nuclear physics research at universities and national or international laboratories.
[d] Limited to tertiary educational establishments (e.g. universities, polytechnics, research institutes with an important educational role, etc.).
[e] The sum of all other industrial uses of radiation (e.g. industrial irradiation facilities, etc.). The exposures attributed to this category should be equal to that for all industrial exposures less the sum of the exposures for those uses separately reported.

Table 2
Dose monitoring and recording procedures for occupational exposures in industry
Data from UNSCEAR Survey of Occupational Exposures unless otherwise indicated

Country	*Occupation*	*Monitored workforce*	*Minimum detectable level (MDL) or recording level*	*Dose recorded when less than MDL*	*Dose recorded for lost dosimeters*	*Doses to contractors included*	*Corrections made to avoid multiple entries for the same individual*
Argentina	All	Those in controlled areas	0.1 mSv	0	Mean value of previous 3 months	Yes	No
Australia	All	Those using radiation devices	0.01 mSv (x) 0.07 mSv (γ)	0	0		Yes
Canada [a]	Mining and milling Reactor operation Other		0.01 WLM 0.01-0.2 mSv 0.2 mSv	0 0 0	No fixed policy No fixed policy No fixed policy	Yes Yes Yes	Yes Yes Yes
Chile	All	Category A workers	0.05 mSv	0.05 mSv	Mean value of periods without accident		
China (Taiwan Province)	Reactor operation All other		0.003-0.05 mSv	Reading 0	Pocket dosimeter or average dose 0	Yes	No
Czechoslovakia	Reactor operation Other	Those wearing personal dosimeters	0.1 mSv 0.2 mSv	0 [b] 0	Mean value for previous 12 months Mean value for previous 12 months	No No	No No
Denmark	All		0.1 mSv	0	0	Yes	Yes
Finland [c]	Reactor operation Other	Those who may exceed 1/3 of dose limit plus optional users	0.1 mSv 0.1 mSv	0 0	Estimate based on working conditions 0	Yes Yes	No No
France	Reactor operation Reprocessing Uranium mining Research	Those provided with a personal dosimeter	0.01 mSv 0.15 mSv 0.20 mSv	0.1 mSv 0 Various 0	Based on electronic dosimeter reading Dose reconstruction after enquiry Attributed by local RP officer Attributed by local RP officer	Yes [d] Yes Yes Yes	No No No No
German Dem. Rep.	Mining (other than uranium)	Those in regions where alpha energy concentrations exceed 0.64 µJ/m³	approx. 2 µSv		Attributed by controlling authority	Yes	Not necessary
Germany, Fed. Rep.	Reactor operation Other	As defined by Radiation Protection Ordinance Those in controlled areas	1 µSv (GM) 0.1 mSv (film) 0.1 mSv (>1978) 0.4 mSv (<1979)	 0 0	Redundant system used; if both lost estimate based on working conditions	Yes Yes	No No
Hungary [e]	All	Those who may exceed 1/10 of dose limit	0.1 mSv [d]	0	0	Yes	Not necessary
India			0.05 mSv (x) 0.1 mSv (n,γ)	0	Mean value of previous 12 months	Yes [f]	Yes
Indonesia	All		0.05 mSv	0.05 mSv		Yes	Yes

Table 2 (continued)

Country	*Occupation*	*Monitored workforce*	*Minimum detectable level (MDL) or recording level*	*Dose recorded when less than MDL*	*Dose recorded for lost dosimeters*	*Doses to contractors included*	*Corrections made to avoid multiple entries for the same individual*
Ireland	All		0.2 mSv (<1987) 0.15 mSv (>1987)	0	0	Yes	No (not significant)
Italy	All		0.1 mSv	0	Mean value for remainder of year		
Japan	Reactor operation Other	Those in controlled areas Those in controlled areas	0.1 mSv 0.1 mSv (TLD) 0.2 mSv (film)	0	Maximum individual dose in group	Yes	No
Netherlands	Accelerators		0.01 mSv	0	0	Yes	
Norway	All		0.4 mSv	0	0	Yes	No
Portugal	All		0.2 mSv				
Republic of Korea	Fuel fabrication Reactor operation Research		0.05 mSv 0.001 mSv 0.1 mSv	0.05 mSv 0 0.095 mSv	Pocket dosimeter or average dose Pocket dosimeter or work condition 30 mSv per quarter	Yes Yes No	Yes Yes No
Spain	Reactor operation Mining and fuel fabrication Other		0.1 mSv 0.2 mSv 0.05 mSv	0 0 0	Area or other dosimeter or 4 mSv Area or other dosimeter or 4 mSv Area or other dosimeter or 4 mSv	Yes Yes Yes	No No No
South Africa	Reactor operation Other		0.1 mSv 0.2 mSv	0 0	Based on QFD reading 4 mSv	Yes Yes	Yes No
Sweden	All		0	0.1 mSv	0	No	No
USSR			0.1 mSv	0.1 mSv			
United Kingdom	BNFL sites Weapons	Those in controlled areas	0.1 mSv 0.05 mSv (external) 0.01 mSv (internal)	As assessed 0 [g]	Working conditions or dose limit rate 4.15 mSv	Yes [h] No	Not necessary Partially
United States	USNRC licensees		0.01 mSv	0	Estimated by licensee	Yes	No

[a] A change from film to TLD dosimetry took place over a five-year period from 1977 to 1981 without any significant change observed in the statistics.
[b] Average individual and collective doses estimated from log-normal fits to data and therefore account is taken of doses occurring below MDL and recorded as zero.
[c] The database includes only workers who have exceeded the recording level, which for reactors was 0.1 mSv with dosimeters issued monthly and 0.5 mSv for all other industrial occupations with dosimeters issued quarterly; the latter recording level was reduced to 0.3 mSv in 1989. Before 1990 the database does not contain the numbers of monitored workers.
[d] Only in collective dose estimates.
[e] Doses recorded above the recording level, which is 0.1 mSv per month for reactor workers and 0.2 mSv per two months for workers elsewhere.
[f] For three out of four power stations.
[g] Before 1986 the dose recorded when less than MDL was 0.05 mSv (external) and 0.01 mSv (internal).
[h] In the BNFL (British Nuclear Fuels plc.) data presented in this Annex, contractors are included only for reprocessing operations.

Table 3
Exposures from uranium mining [a]
Data from UNSCEAR Survey of Occupational Exposures unless otherwise indicated

Country and period		Annual amount of uranium mined [c] (kt)	Equivalent amount of energy [d] (GW a)	Monitored workers (thousands)	Measurably exposed workers (thousands)	Annual collective effective dose [b]			Average annual effective dose		Contribution of exposure pathway (%)			Distribution ratio	
						Total (man Sv)	Average per unit uranium extracted (man Sv per kt)	Average per unit energy generated [man Sv $(GW\ a)^{-1}$]	Per monitored worker (mSv)	Per measurably exposed worker (mSv)	External	Radon daughters	Ore dust	NR_E [e]	SR_E [e]
Underground mines															
Argentina [f]	1975-1979	0.041	0.19	0.25		4.59	111	24.5	18.0					0.54	0.95
Australia [g]	1988-1989			0.41	0.41	1.63			3.98	3.98	39	25	36	0.061	0.22
Bulgaria [I10]	1985-1989			0.50		23.1			46.1		0	100	0		
Canada [h i]	1975-1979	4.73	21.5	5.78	5.06	40.2	8.51	1.87	6.96	7.95	37	63	0.25	0.20	0.57
	1980-1984	5.97	27.1	8.06	6.90	49.6	8.30	1.83	6.15	7.18	43	57	0.30	0.23	0.62
	1985-1989	5.10	23.0	5.19	4.36	30.2	5.59	1.23	5.82	6.93	40	60	0.26	0.26	0.67
China [I10]	1985-1989			6.6		114			17.3		35	65	0		
Czechoslovakia [j]															
	1975-1979	1.78	8.11	9.06		60.4	33.9	7.45	6.67		14	86	0		
	1980-1984	2.02	9.19	8.48		50.2	24.8	5.47	5.92		20	80	0	0.16	0.35
	1985-1989	1.96	8.93	7.46		36.9	18.8	4.14	4.95		16	84	0	0.12	0.28
France [k]	1983-1984	1.85	8.42	1.28	1.25	17.0	9.18	2.02	13.3	13.6	28	72	0	0.48	
	1985-1989	2.29	10.4	1.34	1.28	12.4	5.39	1.19	9.22	9.67	29	71	0	0.40	
Gabon [I10]	1985-1989			0.24		5.06			21.0						
German Dem. Rep. [l]															
	1975-1979	6.26	28.5	14.7	14.7	160	25.5	5.61	10.9	10.9	29	57	14	0.46	0.72
	1980-1984	4.73	21.5	15.1	15.1	147	31.0	6.82	9.69	9.69	29	57	14	0.42	0.65
	1985-1989	4.07	18.5	16.1	16.1	133	32.7	7.18	8.24	8.24	29	56	15	0.31	0.57
India [m]	1981-1984	0.13	0.58	1.16		13.8	108	23.7	11.9		24	76	0		
	1985-1989	0.15	0.68	1.35		15.2	101	22.3	11.3		23	77	0		
South Africa [n]	1975-1979	3.27	14.9	79.0		347	107	23.3	4.39		23	75	0		
	1980-1984	5.07	23.0	93.6		399	78.8	17.3	4.27		25	75	0		
	1985-1989	3.53	16.0	82.2		278	78.8	17.3	3.38		25	75	0		
USSR [I10]	1985-1989								16.3						

Table 3 (continued)

Country and period		Annual amount of uranium mined [c] (kt)	Equivalent amount of energy [d] (GW a)	Monitored workers (thousands)	Measurably exposed workers (thousands)	Annual collective effective dose [b]			Average annual effective dose		Contribution of exposure pathway (%)			Distribution ratio	
						Total (man Sv)	Average per unit uranium extracted (man Sv per kt)	Average per unit energy generated [man Sv $(GW\ a)^{-1}$]	Per monitored worker (mSv)	Per measurably exposed worker (mSv)	External	Radon daughters	Ore dust	NR_E [e]	SR_E [e]
United States [o]	1975-1979	5.51	25.1	6.85		30.9	5.60	1.23	4.51			100			
	1980-1984	5.01	22.8	5.89	3.83	19.4	3.86	0.85	3.29	5.05		100			
	1985-1989	2.27	10.3	0.77	0.62	2.68	1.18	0.26	3.46	4.33		100			
Total of reported data [p]															
	1975-1979	21.6	98.2	116		642	29.7	6.54	5.56		26	70	3.8	0.39	0.69
	1980-1984	23.7	107	133		683	28.9	6.36	5.15		27	70	3.2	0.33	0.61
	1985-1989	19.7	89.4	114		507	25.7	5.66	4.44		28	69	3.2	0.26	0.53
World [q]	1975-1979	45	200	240		1330	29.8	6.55	5.54		26	70	3.8		
	1980-1984	55	250	310		1580	29.0	6.37	5.15		27	70	3.2		
	1985-1989	44	200	260		1140	25.9	5.69	4.45		28	69	3.2		
Open-pit mines															
Argentina	1976-1979	0.067	0.302	0.122		0.302	4.54	1.0	2.48		82	18	0	0	0
	1980-1984	0.146	0.664	0.954		2.29	15.7	3.45	2.40		84	17	0	0	0
	1985-1989	0.092	0.418	0.509		1.25	13.5	2.98	2.45		82	18	0	0	0
Australia [g]	1988-1989	6.5	29.5	0.047	0.047	0.251	0.039	0.008	5.33	5.33	22	2.2	76	0	0
Canada [h r]	1978-1979	2.09	9.50	0.444	0.406	0.996	0.476	0.105	2.24	2.46	13	84	2.7	0.008	0.037
	1980-1984	2.28	10.4	0.820	0.520	0.751	0.329	0.072	0.92	1.44	46	47	6.5	0.001	0.021
	1985-1989	6.71	30.5	1.09	0.876	1.16	0.152	0.034	1.07	1.32	35	39	5.6	0.001	0.010
China [I10]	1985-1989			0.78		1.49			1.91		52	48	0		
France [s]	1985-1989	0.7	3.18	0.41	0.41	0.862	1.23	0.271	2.09	2.09				0.005	
Spain [t]	1986-1989	0.360	1.64	0.375	0.226	0.257	0.712	0.157	0.684	1.14	100	0	0		
Total of reported data [u]															
	1975-1979	1.11	5.05	0.34		0.827	0..744	0.164	2.40		29	69	2.1	0.0049	0.026
	1980-1984	2.43	11.0	1.77		3.06	1.26	0.277	1.73		74	24	1.6	0.0003	0.006
	1985-1989	10.3	46.8	1.62		2.53	0.246	0.054	1.57		60	34	6.2	0.0004	0.006
World [q]	1975-1979	7.1	32	3.9		7.76	1.09	0.239	2.01		29	69	2.1		
	1980-1984	9.1	41	8.1		14.5	1.59	0.349	1.79		74	24	1.6		
	1985-1989	14	62	2.5		3.76	0.258	0.057	1.56		60	34	6.2		

Table 3 (continued)

Country and period		Annual amount of uranium mined [c] (kt)	Equivalent amount of energy [d] (GW a)	Monitored workers (thousands)	Measurably exposed workers (thousands)	Annual collective effective dose [b] Total (man Sv)	Average per unit uranium extracted (man Sv per kt)	Average per unit energy generated [man Sv (GW a)$^{-1}$]	Average annual effective dose Per monitored worker (mSv)	Per measurably exposed worker (mSv)	Contribution of exposure pathway (%) External	Radon daughters	Ore dust	Distribution ratio NR_E [e]	SR_E [e]
Total uranium mining															
World	1975-1979	52	240	240		1300	26	5.7	5.5		26	70	3.8	0.37	0.69
	1980-1984	64	290	310		1600	23	5.5	5.1		27	69	3.1	0.30	0.61
	1985-1989	59	270	260		1100	20	4.3	4.4		28	69	3.2	0.25	0.52

[a] The data are annual values averaged over the indicated periods.
[b] Doses from inhalation of radon daughters estimated using a conversion factor of 5.6 mSv WLM^{-1}; this necessitated a revision of most of the data actually reported which were, in general, based on a conversion factor of 10 mSv WLM^{-1}.
[c] Uranium production data are those reported in response to the questionnaire. If nothing was reported, data were taken from [O2].
[d] Estimated on the simplifying assumption that all the mined uranium is used in LWRs. The assumed fuel cycle requirement is 220 t uranium per GW a.
[e] The values of NR and SR are those reported for the monitored workforce for E = 15 mSv, where the component of dose from radon progeny was derived assuming a conversion factor of 10 mSv WLM^{-1}. Because the radon doses have been modified here using a conversion factor of 5.6 mSv WLM^{-1}, the value of E to which the distribution ratios refer will be less than 15 mSv, the exact value varying with the country and period of interest (i.e. depending on the relative contribution of radon progeny to the total dose).
[f] Estimated by subtracting of reported data on open-pit mining from reported data for total mining; underground mining ceased after 1979.
[g] Data reported for exposed workers,which have been assumed to be the same as monitored workers.
[h] For 1975-1983 the reported data contain a contribution from milling.
[i] Reported data from before 1981 did not include external radiation; an external dose of 2.6 mSv (the average external dose to monitored workers in 1982-1983) has been added here to reported doses before 1981. The reported distribution ratios before 1981 did not take account of external exposure and are therefore underestimates.
[j] Exposures from inhalation of dust are not included; measurements have indicated that it would contribute less than 3 mSv to the annual commited effective dose.
[k] The contribution indicated for radon daughters includes the contribution from inhalation of radon daughters and inhalation of dust; in 1989 the contribution of each of these components was comparable [P3].
[l] Doses estimated on basis of grab samples.
[m] The contribution from the dust is very small because of the low grade of the ore and has been ignored.
[n] Data are for gold mines. In 5 mines out of 40, uranium is produced as a by-product. The numbers of workers and total and normalized collective doses are those that can be attributed to uranium mining. Estimates of dose have been made for the whole workforce from measurements and knowledge of working environments. This average dose has been assumed for the period, and the tabulated collective doses are the product of this dose and the reported annual number of workers.
[o] Reported data only include exposures from inhalation of radon daughters.
[p] Tabulated data on uranium mined, number of workers, doses and distribution ratios comprise the sum or averages of data for Argentina, Canada, Czechoslovakia, France, the German Democratic Republic, India, South Africa and the United States (i.e. those countries for which data for at least one period are complete in terms of these quantities); the percentage contributions to exposure pathways are averaged over Australia, Canada, China, Czechoslovakia, the German Democratic Republic, France, India and South Africa, countries for which data are reported on all three contributions. These data should be interpreted with care, particularly when comparisons are made between different periods, as the countries included in the respective summations may differ from one period to another. The distribution ratios are averages of those reported, and the data on these are often less complete than data for the other quantities.
[q] Estimates extrapolated from total of reported data, based on total uranium mined worldwide relative to that mined in reporting countries.
[r] Reported data before 1981 did not include external radiation; an external dose of 0.3 mSv (the average external dose to monitored workers in 1982-1983) has been added here to reported doses before 1981. The reported distribution ratios before 1981 did not take account of external exposure and are therefore underestimates.
[s] Normalized collective dose and number of workers from [P3] as approximate average of French open-pit mines in 1989; total collective dose and individual doses derived here using estimate of amount mined by subtracting that reported for underground mining from total mined given in [O2]. The percentage contributions of each exposure pathway are approximate averages for open-pit mines in France.
[t] Includes only external exposure; contribution from internal exposure judged negligible by comparison.
[u] Tabulated data on uranium mined, number of workers, doses and distribution ratios comprise the sum or averages of data for Argentina, Australia and Canada (i.e. those countries for which data for at least one period are complete in terms of these quantities); the percentage contributions to exposure pathways are averaged over Argentina, Australia Canada and China, countries for which data are reported on all three contributions. These data should be interpreted with care, particularly when comparisons are made between different periods, as the countries included in the respective summations may differ from one period to another. The distribution ratios are averages of those reported, and the data on these are often less complete than data for the other quantities.

Table 4
Exposures from uranium milling and extraction [a]
Data from UNSCEAR Survey of Occupational Exposures unless otherwise indicated

Country and period	Annual amount of uranium milled [c] (kt)	Equivalent amount of energy [d] (GW a)	Monitored workers (thousands)	Measurably exposed workers (thousands)	Annual collective effective dose [b]			Average annual effective dose		Contribution of exposure pathway (%)			Distribution ratio	
					Total (man Sv)	Average per unit uranium extracted (man Sv per kt)	Average per unit energy generated [man Sv $(GW\ a)^{-1}$]	Per monitored worker (mSv)	Per measurably exposed worker (mSv)	External	Radon daughters	Ore dust	NR_E [e]	SR_E [e]
Australia [f]														
1988-1989	4.20	19.1	0.608	0.608	2.04	0.486	0.107	3.36	3.36	16	0.6	83	0	0
Canada [g]														
1975-1979	4.31	19.6	0.668	0.458	0.66	0.153	0.034	0.99	1.44				0.014	0.16
1980-1984	5.50	25.0	0.852	0.356	0.37	0.067	0.015	0.43	1.04	46	53	1.5	0.002	0.064
1985-1989	9.29	42.2	0.833	0.666	1.30	0.140	0.031	1.56	1.95	65	34	1.3	0.008	0.080
China [I10]														
1985-1989			3.05		9.67			3.17		16	43	42		
Czechoslovakia [h]														
1980-1984	1.82	8.27	1.13		11.4	6.28	1.38	10.1		6	14	80		
1985-1989	1.81	8.24	1.19		11.6	6.42	1.41	9.74		6	21	73		
France [i] [R1]														
1988-1989	2.77	12.6	0.34	0.33	2.04	0.737	0.162	5.93	6.28	29	71	0	0.08	
German Dem. Rep. [j]														
1975-1979	5.47	24.9	3.45	3.45	43.8	8.00	1.76	12.7	12.7	14	46	40	0.48	0.78
1980-1984	4.60	20.9	3.24	3.24	34.1	7.40	1.63	10.5	10.5	14	45	41	0.37	0.65
1985-1989	4.07	18.5	2.99	2.99	24.8	6.10	1.34	8.30	8.30	14	46	40	0.25	0.44
India [k]														
1981-1984	0.128	0.58	0.49		3.58	27.9	6.15	7.35		49	51	0		
1985-1989	0.150	0.68	0.58		3.40	22.6	4.97	5.86		49	51	0		
South Africa [l]														
1979	3.60	16.4	0.388	0.085	0.07	0.018	0.004	0.17	0.78	100	0	0		
1980-1984	4.46	20.3	0.648	0.277	1.93	0.432	0.095	2.97	6.95	100	0	0		
1985-1989	3.00	13.7	0.643	0.257	1.08	0.360	0.079	1.68	4.20	100	0	0		
United States [m]														
1975-1979	8.90	40.5	0.30	0.1	0.03	0.004	0.001	0.11	0.34	100	0	0		
1980-1984	16.8	76.4	4.80	3.0	4.48	0.267	0.059	0.93	1.49	100	0	0		
1985-1989	4.30	19.6	1.00	0.6	0.95	0.221	0.049	0.95	1.59	100	0	0		

Table 4 (continued)

Country and period	Annual amount of uranium milled [c] (kt)	Equivalent amount of energy [d] (GW a)	Monitored workers (thousands)	Measurably exposed workers (thousands)	Annual collective effective dose [b]			Average annual effective dose		Contribution of exposure pathway (%)			Distribution ratio	
					Total (man Sv)	Average per unit uranium extracted (man Sv per kt)	Average per unit energy generated [man Sv $(GW\ a)^{-1}$]	Per monitored worker (mSv)	Per measurably exposed worker (mSv)	External	Radon daughters	Ore dust	NR_E [e]	SR_E [e]
Total of reported data [n]														
1975-1979	18.7	84.9	4.41		44.5	2.38	0.52	10.1		14	46	40	0.41	0.76
1980-1984	28.8	131	10.4		53.2	1.85	0.41	5.1		15	39	46	0.30	0.64
1985-1989	22.4	102	6.98		43.7	1.95	0.43	6.3		16	37	47	0.18	0.43
World [o]														
1975-1979	53	240	12		124	2.36	0.52	10.0		14	46	40		
1980-1984	64	290	23		117	1.84	0.41	5.1		15	39	46		
1985-1989	58	260	18		116	2.01	0.44	6.3		16	37	47		

a The data are annual values averaged over the indicated periods.

b Doses from inhalation of radon daughters estimated using a conversion factor of 5.6 mSv WLM^{-1}; this necessitated a revision of most of the data actually reported which were, in general, based on a conversion factor of 10 mSv WLM^{-1}.

c Amounts of uranium milled are those reported in response to the questionnaire. If nothing was reported, data were assumed to be the amounts mined in the corresponding period [O2].

d Estimated on the simplifying assumption that all the milled uranium is used in LWRs. The assumed fuel cycle requirement is 220 t uranium $(GW\ a)^{-1}$.

e The values of NR and SR are those reported for the monitored workforce for E = 15 mSv, where the component of dose from radon progeny was derived assuming a conversion factor of 10 mSv WLM^{-1}. Because the radon doses have been modified here using a conversion factor of 5.6 mSv WLM^{-1}, the value of E to which the distribution ratios refer will be less than 15 mSv, the exact value varying with the country and period of interest (i.e. depending on the relative contribution of radon progeny to the total dose).

f Data reported for exposed workers, which have been assumed here to be the same as monitored workers.

g For 1975-1983, the quoted values are for extraction only; data for milling for this period are reported together with the mining data.

h Contribution from internal exposure is small and has not been explicitly estimated.

i The contribution from radon also includes the contribution from inhalation of ore dust.

j Doses estimated on basis of grab samples.

k The contribution of dust is small because of the low grade of the ore and has been ignored.

l Because of uncertainties in the fraction of the total doses to workers in uranium milling and extraction, these data have not been included in the summation of doses over countries.

m Data from [E1, E2, E3]; some of the data include only workers exposed in excess of 0.1 WLM.

n Tabulated data on uranium milled, number of workers, doses and distribution ratios comprise the sum or averages of data for Argentina, Canada, Czechoslovakia, France, the German Democratic Republic, India and the United States (i.e. those countries for which data for at least one period are complete in terms of these quantities); the percentage contributions to exposure pathways are averaged over Australia, Canada, Czechoslovakia, the German Democratic Republic and India. These data should be interpreted with care, particularly when comparisons are made between different periods, as the countries included in the respective summations may differ from one period to another. The distribution ratios are averages of those reported, and the data on these are often less complete than data for the other quantities.

o Estimates extrapolated from total of reported data, based on total uranium milled (assumed to be the same as the uranium mined in the same period) worldwide relative to that milled in reporting countries.

Table 5
Exposures from uranium enrichment [a]
Data from UNSCEAR Survey of Occupational Exposures unless otherwise indicated

Country and period	Annual amount of separative work (MSWU)	Average enrichment (%)	Equivalent amount of energy [b] (GW a)	Monitored workers (thousands)	Measurably exposed workers (thousands)	Annual collective effective dose			Average annual effective dose		Distribution ratio	
						Total (man Sv)	Average per unit separative work (man Sv $MSWU^{-1}$)	Average per unit energy generated [man Sv $(GW\ a)^{-1}$]	Per monitored worker (mSv)	Per measurably exposed worker (mSv)	NR_{15} [c]	SR_{15}
France [d] [P2]												
1979				2.36	0.068	0.037			0.016	0.54		
1980-1984				2.33	0.050	0.035			0.015	0.69		
1985-1989				1.77	0.008	0.003			0.002	0.37	0	
Japan [d]												
1987-1989	0.2			0.14		0.00			0		0	
Netherlands [d]												
1985-1989		2.8		0.01		0.01			0.69		0	0
South Africa [d e]												
1975-1979				0.05		0.006			0.13		0	0
1980-1984				0.12		0.013			0.11		0	0
1985-1989	0.10	3.25	0.78	0.09		0.035	0.341	0.044	0.38		0	0
United Kingdom [d f] [B8]												
1975-1979	0.33	1.5	2.50	0.35		0.142	0.438	0.057	0.41			
1980-1982	0.18	0.7	1.41	0.25		0.107	0.584	0.076	0.42			
United Kingdom [d f] [B8]												
1975-1979	0.06	2.52	0.47	0.35		0.040	0.665	0.086	0.12			
1980-1984	0.29	2.88	2.23	0.22		0.049	0.170	0.022	0.22			
1985-1989	0.63	3.12	5.11	0.16		0.023	0.037	0.005	0.15			
United States [d] [E1]												
1975-1979				10.3	8.34	5.14			0.50	0.62	0	0
1980-1984				1.45	0.65	0.62			0.42	0.94	0	0
1985-1989				2.92	0.93	0.36			0.12	0.38	0	0
Total of reported data [g]												
1975-1979				11		5.3			0.46		0	0
1980-1984				4.3		0.78			0.18		0	0
1985-1989				5.0		0.43			0.08		0	0

[a] The data are annual values averaged over the indicated periods.
[b] Estimated on the simplifying assumption that all the enriched uranium is used in LWRs. The assumed fuel cycle requirement is 0.13 MSWU $(GW\ a)^{-1}$.
[c] The values of NR_{15} are for the monitored workforce. Values for the exposed workforce can also be estimated where data are given for both monitored and measurably exposed workers.
[d] Enrichment by diffusion process [France, United Kingdom (first entry), United States]; centrifuge process [Japan, Netherlands, United Kingdom (second entry)]; jet nozzle process (South Africa).
[e] Pilot facility operations only before 1988. Data for separative work, energy equivalent and normalized collective doses are averages over the years 1988 and 1989.
[f] Data are for enrichment only and do not include doses from uranium conversion to uranium hexafluoride. From 1986 onwards doses have been formally estimated and are included in the statistics where they exceed the defined recording level; no internal doses above the recording level were received in 1986-1990.
[g] These data should be interpreted with care, particularly when making comparisons between different periods, as the countries included in the respective summations may differ from one period to another. The distribution ratios are averages of those reported, and the data on these are often much less complete than data for the other quantities.

Table 6
Exposures from fuel fabrication [a]
Data from UNSCEAR Survey of Occupational Exposures unless otherwise indicated

Country and period	Annual amount of fuel fabricated (kt)	Equivalent amount of energy [b] (GW a)	Monitored workers (thousands)	Measurably exposed workers (thousands)	Annual collective effective dose: Total (man Sv)	Annual collective effective dose: Average per fuel fabricated (man Sv per kt)	Annual collective effective dose: Average per unit energy generated [man Sv (GW a)$^{-1}$]	Average annual effective dose: Per monitored worker (mSv)	Average annual effective dose: Per measurably exposed worker (mSv)	Distribution ratio: NR_{15} [c]	Distribution ratio: SR_{15}
LWR fuel											
Japan [d]											
1979	0.82	14.5	1.02		0.54	0.66	0.037	0.53		0	
1980-1984	1.06	18.1	1.44		0.86	0.82	0.048	0.60		0	
1985-1989	1.28	20.7	1.67		0.52	0.40	0.025	0.31		0	
Republic of Korea											
1988-1989	0.03	0.87	0.20		0.06	1.83	0.068	0.30		0	0
Spain											
1986-1989	0.16	4.43	0.35	0.25	0.38	2.33	0.086	1.09	1.53		
Sweden											
1986, 1988-1989	0.26	7.01	0.35	0.09	0.21	0.82	0.030	0.61	2.29		
United States [e f]											
1975-1979	0.95	25.8	11.1	5.85	19.0	19.8	0.734	1.71	3.24	0.013	0.39
1980-1984	1.19	32.3	9.45	5.49	8.68	7.26	0.269	0.92	1.58	0.003	0.12
1985-1989	1.92	51.8	9.95	3.88	4.51	2.35	0.087	0.45	1.16	0.0003	0.014
Total of reported data [g]											
1975-1979	1.12	28.7	11.3		19.1	17.0	0.664	1.69		0.013	0.39
1980-1984	2.25	50.4	10.9		9.54	4.23	0.189	0.88		0.003	0.12
1985-1989	3.50	80.6	12.2		5.48	1.57	0.068	0.45		0.0003	0.015
World [h]											
1975-1979	1.6	42	17		29	18	0.69	1.7			
1980-1984	3.7	81	17		15	4.1	0.19	0.87			
1985-1989	6.8	160	24		11	1.6	0.069	0.45			

Table 6 (continued)

Country and period	Annual amount of fuel fabricated (kt)	Equivalent amount of energy [b] (GW a)	Monitored workers (thousands)	Measurably exposed workers (thousands)	Annual collective effective dose			Average annual effective dose		Distribution ratio	
					Total (man Sv)	Average per fuel fabricated (man Sv per kt)	Average per unit energy generated [man Sv $(GW\ a)^{-1}$]	Per monitored worker (mSv)	Per measurably exposed worker (mSv)	NR_{15} [c]	SR_{15}
HWR fuel											
Argentina [i]											
1980-1984	0.030	0.138	0.104		0.025	0.838	0.180	0.24			
1985-1989	0.046	0.218	0.107		0.024	0.513	0.109	0.22			
Canada [j]											
1975-1979	0.61	3.38	0.53	0.34	0.68	1.12	0.202	1.27	1.99	0.005	0.10
1980-1984	1.13	6.30	0.65	0.36	0.95	0.84	0.151	1.48	2.64	0.0003	0.003
1985-1989	1.41	7.81	0.43	0.28	1.02	0.73	0.131	2.37	3.62	0.0009	0.006
India [k]											
1981-1984	0.02	0.13	0.40	0.11	0.11	4.5	0.82	0.28	1.04	0	0
1985-1989	0.06	0.31	0.50	0.44	0.80	14.1	2.54	1.59	1.81	0.004	0.074
Republic of Korea											
1985-1989	0.06	0.33	0.10	0.03	0.06	0.93	0.168	0.58	2.12	0.002	0.22
Total HWR fuel [l]											
1975-1979	0.61	3.38	0.53		0.68	1.12	0.202	1.27		0.005	0.10
1980-1984	1.18	6.54	1.07		1.06	0.90	0.163	1.00		0.0002	0.002
1985-1989	1.57	8.67	1.14		1.90	1.21	0.219	1.67		0.003	0.042
Magnox fuel											
United Kingdom [B8] and total Magnox [m]											
1975-1979	0.95	2.87	0.88		2.03	2.14	0.708	2.30		0.003	
1980-1984	0.80	2.43	1.00		1.96	2.44	0.806	1.95		0.002	
1985-1989	0.81	2.46	1.11		3.48	4.29	1.42	3.12		0.018 [n]	
AGR fuel											
United Kingdom [B8] and total AGR fuel [o]											
1975-1979	0.44	11.6	1.68		3.76	8.57	0.325	2.24		0.002	
1980-1984	0.40	10.5	1.91		3.20	8.03	0.305	1.67		0.001	
1985-1989	0.46	12.2	1.85		5.51	11.9	0.454	2.97		0.014 [n]	

Table 6 (continued)

Country and period	Annual amount of fuel fabricated (kt)	Equivalent amount of energy [b] (GW a)	Monitored workers (thousands)	Measurably exposed workers (thousands)	Annual collective effective dose			Average annual effective dose		Distribution ratio	
					Total (man Sv)	Average per fuel fabricated (man Sv per kt)	Average per unit energy generated [man Sv (GW a)$^{-1}$]	Per monitored worker (mSv)	Per measurably exposed worker (mSv)	NR_{15} [c]	SR_{15}
FBR fuel											
Japan											
1975-1979	0.01		0.42		0.15	30.14		0.36		0	
1980-1984	0.01		0.69		0.52	68.81		0.75		0	
1985-1989	0.01		0.99		0.48	90.53		0.48		0	

[a] The data are annual values averaged over the indicated periods. Contributions of internal exposures to doses are included for Spain (32%), Canada (0%) and United Kingdom (35% average for both types of fuel in 1985-1989). All other doses are from external exposure only.

[b] The amounts of fuel (uranium) required to generate 1 GW a of electrical energy by each reactor type are taken to be as follows: PWR, 37 t; HWR, 180 t; Magnox, 330 t; AGR, 38 t.

[c] The values of NR_{15} are for the monitored workforce. Values for the exposed workforce can also be estimated where data are given for both monitored and measurably exposed workers.

[d] Internal exposure negligible.

[e] Summary data from annual reports of the United States Nuclear Regulatory Commission. The data for 1975-1981 include exposures during fuel reprocessing. The distribution ratios are not reported formally by United States Nuclear Regulatory Commission licensees. They have been estimated as the mean of the distribution ratios for individual doses of 10 and 20 mSv. This approximation will, in general, cause the tabulated distribution ratios to be overestimates because many occupational exposure dose distributions are log-normal.

[f] No data were available for the annual production of fuel. In their absence, annual fuel production was assumed to be equivalent to the energy generated in the respective years by LWRs in the United States. This assumption is likely to underestimate the fuel produced (and overestimate the normalized collective doses) as some of the fuel was used in reactors outside the United States; moreover, fuel production and energy generation are not contemporaneous.

[g] These data should be interpreted with care, particularly when making comparisons between different periods, as the countries included in the respective summations may differ from one period to another. The distribution ratios are averages of those reported, and the data on these are often much less complete than data on the other quantities.

[h] The reported data have been scaled by the ratio of the worldwide production of fuel to that included in the reported data; in the absence of data on worldwide fuel production, this was assumed to be the annual fuel requirement needed to generate the electrical energy produced by LWRs in the same year. In the absence of better data, the values of the ratios NR_{15} and SR_{15}, averaged over the reported data, can be considered indicative of worldwide levels.

[i] Contribution from internal exposure not included but estimated to be less than 10%.

[j] NR distribution ratios reported for measurably exposed workers adjusted for monitored workforce.

[k] No data reported on the amount of fuel fabricated; assumed to be that needed for the actual generation of energy in India in each period by the particular reactor type.

[l] The countries reporting data are assumed to represent the total worldwide production of fuel of this type.

[m] Some GCR fuel has been fabricated in other countries, but the amount is small in comparison with that fabricated in the United Kingdom and has been ignored.

[n] Internal exposures were included in the reported doses for 1985-1989, but not for earlier periods; the increase in the distribution ratio is more apparent than real.

[o] Data include workers associated with and doses incurred in fuel fabrication and the conversion of uranium to and from uranium hexafluoride for enrichment. About 5% of the collective dose arises during conversion but data on the fraction of the workforce involved in the respective activities are not available; the average individual doses in conversion and fabrication are similar. The data are mainly for the fabrication of AGR fuel, but about 10% of the production is PWR fuel.

Table 7
Summary of worldwide exposures from fuel fabrication [a]

Fuel type	*Annual amount of fuel fabricated* (kt)	*Equivalent amount of energy* [b] (GW a)	*Monitored workers* (thousands)	*Average annual collective effective dose* (man Sv)	*Collective effective dose per unit mass of fuel* (man Sv kt^{-1})	*Collective effective dose per unit energy generated* [man Sv (GW a)$^{-1}$]	*Average annual effective dose to monitored workers* (mSv)	*Distribution ratio* NR_{15}	*Distribution ratio* SR_{15}
1975-1979									
LWR	1.6	42	17	29	18	0.69	1.7	0.013	0.39
HWR	0.61	3.4	0.53	0.68	1.1	0.2	1.3	0.005	0.10
Magnox	0.95	2.9	0.88	2.0	2.1	0.71	2.3	0.003	
AGR	0.44	12	1.7	3.8	8.6	0.33	2.2	0.002	
Total		60	20	36		0.59	1.8	0.012	0.38
1980-1984									
LWR	3.7	81	17	15	4.1	0.19	0.87	0.003	0.12
HWR	1.2	6.5	1.1	1.1	0.90	0.16	1.0	0.0002	0.002
Magnox	0.80	2.43	1.0	2.0	2.4	0.81	2.0	0.002	
AGR	0.40	11	1.9	3.2	8.0	0.31	1.7	0.001	
Total		100	21	21		0.21	1.0	0.002	0.11
1985-1989									
LWR	6.8	160	24	11	1.6	0.07	0.45	0.0003	0.015
HWR	1.6	8.7	1.1	1.9	1.2	0.22	1.7	0.003	0.042
Magnox	0.81	2.5	1.1	3.5	4.3	1.4	3.1	0.018 [c]	
AGR	0.46	12	1.9	5.5	12	0.45	3.0	0.014 [c]	
Total		180	28	22		0.12	0.78	0.002	0.019

[a] The data are annual values averaged over the indicated periods.
[b] The amounts of fuel (uranium) required to generate 1 GW a of electrical energy by each reactor type are taken to be as follows: PWR, 37 t; HWR, 180 t; Magnox, 330 t; AGR, 38 t.
[c] The value for NR_{15} for Magnox and AGR fuel for the period 1985-1090 take account of internal exposures which were not included in earlier periods. The increases in the NR in 1985-1989 are therefore apparent rather than real.

Table 8
Exposures at reactors [a]
Data from UNSCEAR Survey of Occupational Exposures unless otherwise indicated

Country and period	Average number of reactors over the period	Installed capacity (GW)	Energy generated [b] (GW a)	Monitored workers (thousands)	Measurably exposed workers (thousands)	Annual collective effective dose: Total (man Sv)	Annual collective effective dose: Average per reactor (man Sv)	Annual collective effective dose: Average per unit energy generated [man Sv (GW a)$^{-1}$]	Average annual effective dose: Per monitored worker (mSv)	Average annual effective dose: Per measurably exposed worker (mSv)	Distribution ratio: NR_{15} [c]	Distribution ratio: SR_{15}
PWRs												
Belgium [d] [B5]												
1975-1979	4.0	1.67	1.14	2.39		5.28	1.32	4.63	2.21			
1980-1984	5.2	2.75	2.01	4.50		10.1	1.94	5.00	2.24			
1985-1989	7.6	5.49	4.26	8.38		17.9	2.36	4.22	2.14			
China (Taiwan Province)												
1984	1.0	0.95	0.34	3.68		0.26	0.26	0.77	0.07			
1985-1989	2.0	1.90	1.06	2.52		1.41	0.71	1.34	0.56			
Czechoslovakia												
1975-1977	1.0	0.41	0.11	0.87	0.08	0.09	0.09	0.79	0.10	1.17	0.001	0.12
1980-1984	2.2	0.90	0.62	1.56	0.80	1.84	0.83	2.97	1.18	2.30	0.010	0.17
1985-1989	7.0	2.94	2.11	4.14	2.43	3.97	0.57	1.88	0.96	1.64	0.005	0.12
Finland												
1977-1979	1.0	0.47	0.34	0.93	0.47	0.79	0.79	2.31	0.84	1.69	0	0
1980-1984	1.8	0.84	0.67	1.26	0.73	1.80	1.00	2.71	1.43	2.48	0.006	0.072
1985-1989	2.0	0.93	0.84	1.09	0.65	1.73	0.87	2.05	1.59	2.66	0.007	0.073
France [e]												
1977-1979	3.5	3.15	1.93	3.40	0.89	4.34	1.24	2.24	1.28	4.87		
1980-1984	17.2	15.5	11.1	14.4	6.40	29.4	1.71	2.65	2.05	4.60	0.032	
1985-1989	41.0	40.1	28.3	29.7	16.8	78.9	1.92	2.79	2.65	4.68	0.047	
German Dem. Rep.												
1975-1979	4.0	1.39	0.60	3.41		5.10	1.28	8.48	1.50		0.036	0.45
1980-1984	5.0	1.83	1.33	3.12		8.65	1.73	6.49	2.77		0.060	0.44
1985-1989	5.0	1.83	1.35	3.80	1.58	9.24	1.85	6.86	2.43	5.85	0.050	0.42
Germany, Fed. Rep. of												
1975-1979	4.8	3.94	2.71	3.91		17.5	3.64	6.45	4.47			
1980-1984	6.6	6.46	5.03	8.54		34.4	5.21	6.83	4.02			
1985-1989	11.4	12.9	9.53	15.2		32.6	2.86	3.43	2.15			

Table 8 (continued)

Country and period	Average number of reactors over the period	Installed capacity (GW)	Energy generated [b] (GW a)	Monitored workers (thousands)	Measurably exposed workers (thousands)	Annual collective effective dose			Average annual effective dose		Distribution ratio	
						Total (man Sv)	Average per reactor (man Sv)	Average per unit energy generated [man Sv $(GW\ a)^{-1}$]	Per monitored worker (mSv)	Per measurably exposed worker (mSv)	NR_{15} [c]	SR_{15}
Hungary												
1983-1984	1.5	0.66	0.36	1.26	0.29	0.32	0.21	0.89	0.25	1.09	0	0
1985-1989	3.4	1.50	1.19	2.81	0.99	1.70	0.50	1.43	0.61	1.72	0.002	0.053
Japan												
1975-1979	7.0	4.76	2.02	7.21	6.11	14.1	2.02	6.99	1.96	2.32	0.020	0.18
1980-1984	11.8	8.69	5.44	13.2	9.22	30.7	2.60	5.65	2.32	3.33	0.020	0.16
1985-1989	16.2	12.6	9.22	18.6	12.1	33.5	2.07	3.63	1.80	2.76	0.012	0.12
Netherlands												
1975-1979	1.0	0.48	0.37	0.60		4.10	4.10	11.0	6.89		0.136	0.44
1980-1984	1.0	0.48	0.39	0.96		3.58	3.58	9.24	3.75		0.057	0.30
1985-1989	1.0	0.48	0.39	1.14		2.83	2.83	7.21	2.48		0.018	0.15
Republic of Korea												
1977-1979	1.0	0.59	0.27	0.48		1.66	1.66	6.09	3.49			
1980-1984	1.4	0.85	0.54	0.96		4.50	3.21	8.32	4.67			
1985-1989	5.8	4.65	3.32	4.67		12.8	2.20	3.85	2.73			
South Africa												
1984	2.0	1.92	0.45	1.72	0.08	0.12	0.06	0.27	0.07	1.45	0.001	0.29
1985-1989	2.0	1.92	0.96	1.72	0.59	1.61	0.81	1.68	0.94	2.75	0.008	0.18
Spain [f]												
1975-1979	1.0	0.16	0.13	0.22		2.60	2.60	20.7	11.7			
1980-1984	2.6	1.65	0.67	1.51		6.76	2.60	10.1	4.21			
1985-1989	5.6	4.51	3.25	5.30	3.81	17.7	3.17	5.45	3.35	4.65		
Sweden [g]												
1975-1979	1.0	0.80	0.47		0.62	1.52	1.52	3.28		2.46	0.027	0.24
1980-1984	2.2	1.88	0.87		0.97	3.58	1.63	4.10		3.68	0.033	0.27
1985-1989	3.0	2.60	1.93		1.82	4.80	1.60	2.49		2.65	0.027	0.19
Switzerland												
1975-1979	2.2	0.89	0.71	0.63		4.16	1.89	5.83	6.64			
1980-1984	3.0	1.64	1.44	1.49		7.46	2.49	5.20	5.01			
1985-1989	3.0	1.64	1.44	1.67		6.60	2.20	4.58	3.95			

Table 8 (continued)

Country and period	Average number of reactors over the period	Installed capacity (GW)	Energy generated [b] (GW a)	Monitored workers (thousands)	Measurably exposed workers (thousands)	Annual collective effective dose: Total (man Sv)	Annual collective effective dose: Average per reactor (man Sv)	Annual collective effective dose: Average per unit energy generated [man Sv (GW a)$^{-1}$]	Average annual effective dose: Per monitored worker (mSv)	Average annual effective dose: Per measurably exposed worker (mSv)	Distribution ratio: NR_{15} [c]	Distribution ratio: SR_{15}
USSR [h] [B11, I9]												
1978-1979	7.5	2.7	1.7	3.2		19.4	2.59	11.2	6.14			
1980-1984	12.8	5.9	3.8	6.6		32.8	2.56	8.66	4.99			
1985-1987	22.0	13.9	8.7	12.3		57.1	2.60	6.55	4.63			
United States [i]												
1975-1979	34.2	25.2	16.2	38.8	22.8	147	4.31	9.13	3.80	6.47	0.089	0.57
1980-1984	46.8	38.7	22.1	83.1	51.0	276	5.89	12.5	3.32	5.41	0.075	0.53
1985-1989	63.0	59.1	37.4	109.2	61.4	225	3.58	6.02	2.06	3.67	0.036	0.36
Total of reported data [j]												
1975-1979	64.4	42.4	26.1	60.9		212	3.29	8.13	3.48		0.085	0.56
1980-1984	121	86.8	56.3	144		451	3.73	8.01	3.14		0.061	0.48
1985-1989	192	159	112	219		487	2.53	4.36	2.22		0.034	0.32
World [k]												
1975-1979	78	49	27	63		220	2.8	8.1	3.5		0.085	0.56
1980-1984	140	98	56	140		450	3.3	8.0	3.1		0.061	0.48
1985-1989	220	180	120	230		500	2.3	4.3	2.2		0.034	0.32
BWRs												
China (Taiwan Province)												
1981-1984	3.8	3.00	1.83	6.32		14.4	3.84	7.85	2.28			
1985-1989	4.0	3.24	2.32	6.69		18.2	4.55	7.84	2.72			
Finland												
1978-1979	1.0	0.68	0.21	1.44	0.29	0.12	0.12	0.55	0.08	0.40	0	0
1980-1984	2.0	1.36	1.02	1.61	0.88	0.87	0.44	0.86	0.54	0.99	0.000	0.004
1985-1989	2.0	1.47	1.33	1.92	1.14	1.80	0.90	1.36	0.94	1.59	0.002	0.033
Germany, Fed. Rep. of												
1975-1979	3.0	1.65	0.72	3.74		19.9	6.64	27.8	5.33			
1980-1984	4.4	3.80	2.12	10.2		33.4	7.59	15.7	3.28			
1985-1989	7.0	7.21	5.68	12.4		19.4	2.78	3.42	1.56			
India												
1980-1984	2.0	0.410	0.201	3.35	3.30	38.0	19.0	189	11.4	11.5	0.241	
1985-1989	2.0	0.304	0.205	2.69	2.56	23.2	11.6	113	8.63	9.06	0.157	

Table 8 (continued)

Country and period	Average number of reactors over the period	Installed capacity (GW)	Energy generated [b] (GW a)	Monitored workers (thousands)	Measurably exposed workers (thousands)	Annual collective effective dose: Total (man Sv)	Annual collective effective dose: Average per reactor (man Sv)	Annual collective effective dose: Average per unit energy generated [man Sv (GW a)$^{-1}$]	Average annual effective dose: Per monitored worker (mSv)	Average annual effective dose: Per measurably exposed worker (mSv)	Distribution ratio: NR_{15} [c]	Distribution ratio: SR_{15}
Japan												
1975-1979	7.8	5.01	2.30	17.7	18.2	72.9	9.35	31.6	4.12	4.01	0.072	0.34
1980-1984	13.0	9.95	6.24	27.4	18.9	91.4	7.03	14.6	3.34	4.83	0.057	0.34
1985-1989	18.4	15.4	10.6	34.8	20.7	63.6	3.46	6.02	1.83	3.07	0.018	0.20
Netherlands												
1975-1979	1.0	0.054	0.047	0.28		2.31	2.31	49.2	8.38		0.202	0.24
1980-1984	1.0	0.054	0.047	0.47		2.24	2.24	48.1	4.81		0.114	0.27
1985-1989	1.0	0.054	0.049	0.56		1.62	1.62	32.9	2.87		0.038	0.19
Spain [f]												
1975-1979	1.0	0.46	0.32	0.62		5.36	5.36	16.8	8.60			
1980-1984	1.2	0.66	0.27	0.97		7.85	6.54	29.2	8.08			
1985-1989	2.0	1.44	1.09	2.66	2.06	10.1	5.05	9.26	3.80	4.90		
Sweden [l]												
1975-1979	4.6	2.66	1.64		2.09	5.98	1.3	3.65		2.86	0.027	0.24
1980-1984	6.6	4.34	3.46		3.13	8.22	1.25	2.38		2.63	0.033	0.27
1985-1989	9.0	7.02	5.64		3.71	10.7	1.19	1.89		2.88	0.027	0.19
United States [i]												
1975-1979	22.8	14.6	9.37	33.3	19.9	156	6.83	16.6	4.68	7.84	0.064	0.65
1980-1984	26.2	17.9	10.4	53.3	35.1	268	10.2	25.7	5.03	7.63	0.084	0.63
1985-1989	32.2	26.5	14.7	77.2	40.5	181	5.63	12.3	2.35	4.48	0.026	0.43
Total of reported data [j]												
1975-1979	40.6	24.7	14.3	55.9		262	6.46	18.1	4.69		0.066	0.61
1980-1984	59.0	40.8	25.2	102		454	7.69	18.0	4.47		0.079	0.55
1985-1989	77.6	62.6	41.6	139		330	4.25	7.93	2.38		0.026	0.36
World [k]												
1975-1979	51.2	29.3	15.3	59.2		279	5.45	18.3	4.71		0.066	0.61
1980-1984	64.6	44.1	25.1	102		454	7.00	18.0	4.47		0.079	0.55
1985-1989	83.8	66.9	41.8	139		331	3.96	7.94	2.38		0.026	0.36
HWRs												
Argentina [m]												
1975-1979	1.0	0.33	0.26	0.43		4.52	4.52	17.2	10.5		0.26	0.73
1980-1984	1.4	0.59	0.32	0.77		8.04	5.74	25.2	10.5		0.27	0.79
1985-1989	2	0.98	0.61	1.06		12.6	6.29	20.8	11.9		0.29	0.80

Table 8 (continued)

Country and period	Average number of reactors over the period	Installed capacity (GW)	Energy generated [b] (GW a)	Monitored workers (thousands)	Measurably exposed workers (thousands)	Annual collective effective dose: Total (man Sv)	Annual collective effective dose: Average per reactor (man Sv)	Annual collective effective dose: Average per unit energy generated [man Sv (GW a)$^{-1}$]	Average annual effective dose: Per monitored worker (mSv)	Average annual effective dose: Per measurably exposed worker (mSv)	Distribution ratio: NR_{15} [c]	Distribution ratio: SR_{15}
Canada												
1975-1979	8.4	4.32	2.45	5.65	2.62	24.0	2.85	9.77	4.24	9.15	0.11	0.70
1980-1984	13	7.41	4.53	9.27	3.54	20.1	1.57	4.43	2.16	5.67	0.046	0.49
1985-1989	18	11.6	8.03	11.0	4.61	16.7	0.94	2.07	1.51	3.61	0.017	0.23
Czechoslovakia [n]												
1975-1979	1			0.85	0.65	4.61	4.61		5.42	7.03	0.11	0.58
1980-1984	1			0.51	0.36	0.77	0.77		1.51	2.13	0.015	0.22
1985-1989	1			0.54	0.31	0.88	0.88		1.62	2.83	0.020	0.24
India												
1981-1984	2.5	0.51	0.15	3.09	2.19	15.7	6.28	103	5.08	7.17	0.11	
1985-1989	4.2	0.83	0.38	4.40	3.88	28.7	6.83	76	6.51	7.39	0.13	
Republic of Korea												
1983-1984	1	0.68	0.41	0.72		0.65	0.65	1.58	0.90			
1985-1989	1	0.68	0.59	0.81		1.13	1.13	1.91	1.40			
Total of reported data [k o]												
1975-1979	9.40	4.65	2.71	6.08		28.5	3.03	10.5	4.68		0.12	0.71
1980-1984	16.6	8.68	5.13	12.8		40.9	2.47	7.97	3.20		0.073	0.58
1985-1989	25.0	14.1	9.61	17.3		59.0	2.36	6.14	3.41		0.066	0.48
World [l]												
1975-1979	12	5.0	3.1	6.8		32	2.6	11	4.8		0.12	0.71
1980-1984	19	9.0	5.7	14		46	2.4	8.0	3.2		0.073	0.58
1985-1989	26	14	9.8	18		60	2.3	6.2	3.4		0.066	0.48
GCRs												
Japan												
1979	1	0.2	0.1	1.59	0.81	1	1	10	0.63	1.23	0.001	
1980-1984	1	0.2	0.1	2.13	0.95	1	1	10	0.47	1.05	0.0014	0.023
1985-1989	1	0.2	0.1	2.01	0.84	1	1	10	0.50	1.19	0.0002	0.008
Spain												
1975-1979	1	0.48	0.37	0.07		0.30	0.30	0.80	3.98			
1980-1984	1	0.48	0.36	0.18		0.37	0.37	1.02	2.08			
1985-1989	1	0.48	0.33	0.25	0.13	0.28	0.28	0.85	1.12	2.18		

Table 8 (continued)

Country and period	Average number of reactors over the period	Installed capacity (GW)	Energy generated [b] (GW a)	Monitored workers (thousands)	Measurably exposed workers (thousands)	Annual collective effective dose			Average annual effective dose		Distribution ratio	
						Total (man Sv)	Average per reactor (man Sv)	Average per unit energy generated [man Sv $(GW\ a)^{-1}$]	Per monitored worker (mSv)	Per measurably exposed worker (mSv)	NR_{15} [c]	SR_{15}
United Kingdom [p]												
1975-1979	30	6.04	3.40	8.56		24.5	0.82	7.20	2.86		0.02	
1980-1984	32	7.40	4.40	18.0		26.4	0.82	6.00	1.46		0.0054	
1985-1989	37	10.4	6.09	25.4		19.5	0.52	3.20	0.77		0.0002	
Total of reported data [k]												
1975-1979	31.2	6.56	3.79	8.95		25.0	0.80	6.59	2.80		0.020	
1980-1984	34.0	8.08	4.86	20.3		27.8	0.82	5.72	1.37		0.005	
1985-1989	39.2	11.1	6.52	27.6		20.8	0.53	3.19	0.75		0.0002	0.008
World [l]												
1975-1979	40	9.1	5.4	13		36	0.90	6.6	2.8			
1980-1984	41	10	6.0	25		34	0.84	5.8	1.4			
1985-1989	44	13.3	7.4	31		24	0.54	3.2	0.75			
Prototype FBRs												
France												
1986-1989	1	1.10	0.094	0.50		0.033	0.033	0.351	0.067			
USSR (BR350) [q] [B11]												
1978-1979	1	0.35 [r]		0.59		0.61	0.61		1.03			
1980-1984	1	0.35		0.60		0.81	0.81		0.35			
1985-1987	1	0.35		0.49		0.98	0.98		2.00			
USSR (BR600) [B11]												
1980-1984	1	0.6	0.34	0.92		0.40	0.40	1.19	0.43			
1985-1987	1	0.6	0.41	1.08		0.83	0.83	2.04	0.77			
Total of reported data [j s]												
1980-1984	1	0.60	0.34	0.92		0.40	0.40	1.19	0.43			
1985-1989	1.4	1.24	0.32	1.04		0.52	0.37	1.64	0.50			
World [k s]												
1980-1984	4.0	1.0	0.50	1.4		0.61	0.15	1.2	0.44			
1985-1989	4.8	1.9	0.73	2.1		1.0	0.21	1.4	0.48			
LWGRs												
World [t]												
1978-1979	12	5.9	4.35	5.37		35.6	2.97	8.18	6.64			
1980-1984	16.2	10.1	7.50	9.80		62.2	3.84	8.30	6.35			
1985-1987	20	14.7	10.4	13.1		173	8.67	16.7	13.2			

Table 8 (continued)

Country and period	Average number of reactors over the period	Installed capacity (GW)	Energy generated [b] (GW a)	Monitored workers (thousands)	Measurably exposed workers (thousands)	Annual collective effective dose			Average annual effective dose		Distribution ratio	
						Total (man Sv)	Average per reactor (man Sv)	Average per unit energy generated [man Sv (GW a)$^{-1}$]	Per monitored worker (mSv)	Per measurably exposed worker (mSv)	NR_{15} [c]	SR_{15}
HTGRs												
World [u]												
1975-1979	1	0.33	0.034	1.15	0.059	0.031	0.031	0.90	0.027	0.52		
1980-1984	1	0.33	0.071	1.16	0.046	0.017	0.017	0.24	0.015	0.37		
1985-1989	1	0.33	0.030	0.78	0.148	0.097	0.097	3.25	0.124	0.65		

[a] The data are annual values averaged over the periods indicated.

[b] Data on energy generated taken, unless otherwise indicated, from responses to questionnaire or from [I8].

[c] The values of NR_{15} are for the monitored workforce. Values for the exposed workforce can also be estimated where data are given for both monitored and measurably exposed workers.

[d] The numbers of workers include utility workers and contractor workers. Data on number of reactors, installed capacity and energy generated from [I8].

[e] Additional data from [B5, B6]. The reported data are for utility workers, except for collective doses, which are for utility and contractor workers. Additional data have been reported on the exposure of about 30%-40% of contractors [L2, P2]. The numbers of workers and average doses tabulated have been estimated from the reported annual collective doses for the whole workforce (i.e. utility workers and contractor workers), subject to the assumption that the exposures reported for a fraction of the contractor workers are representative of the contractor workers as a whole. The average doses to utility workers are significantly lower than those to contractor workers. During the 1980s the average annual dose to monitored utility workers was about 1 mSv and to monitored contractors about 4 mSv; the corresponding doses to measurably exposed workers were about 2 mSv and 7 mSv, respectively.

[f] Data include both utility workers and contractor workers.

[g] Data on numbers of workers are from [B5]. The distribution ratios are averages for Swedish LWRs overall rather than for PWRs.

[h] The data have been scaled, on the basis of energy generated, from those reported, which did not cover all PWRs in the USSR.

[i] Summary data from annual reports of USNRC. Data are uncorrected for the reporting of transient workers. The NR ratios are for the monitored workforce and have been derived from the ratios reported by [R2] for the measurably exposed workforce. The distribution ratios are not reported formally by USNRC licensees. They have been estimated [R2] as the mean of the distribution ratios for individual doses of 10 and 20 mSv. This approximation will, in general, cause the tabulated distribution ratios to be overestimates because many occupational exposure dose distributions are log-normal.

[j] These data should be interpreted with care, particularly when comparisons are made between different periods, as the countries included in the respective summations may differ from one period to another. The distribution ratios are averages of those reported, and the data on these are often much less complete than data on the other quantities.

[k] These data are the sum of reported data above scaled to account for missing data; the numbers of monitored workers and the collective doses have been scaled on the basis of the total energy generated by the respective reactor type and that for the reported data. In the absence of better data, the values of the ratios NR_{15} and SR_{15}, averaged over the reported data, can be considered indicative of worldwide levels.

[l] Data available are averages for LWRs as a whole and not separately for PWRs and BWRs.

[m] During the early 1980s administrative constraints were placed on energy generation by nuclear means; as a consequence, collective doses per unit energy generation are higher than they would have otherwise been.

[n] Data are for a HWGCR (all the other entries in the Table are for water-cooled reactors); data for NR_{15} and SR_{15} are for measurably exposed workers.

[o] Sum of reported data, excluding Czechoslovakia.

[p] Data included for all commercial GCRs in the United Kingdom, including Magnox and AGRs; data for the various types of GCRs differ significantly and are summarizsed in Table 11.

[q] The plant is used for desalination.

[r] Thermal installed capacity.

[s] Excluding the USSR/BR350, which is a desalination plant.

[t] These data have been scaled on the basis of total energy generated compared to that for the reported data, which did not cover all LWGRs in the USSR.

[u] These data are for the Fort St. Vrain prototype reactor; there were not enough data to allow estimating worldwide doses from other prototype HTGRs.

Table 9
Dose distribution ratios for measurably exposed LWR workers in the United States
[B2, R2]

Year	*Percentage of workers receiving annual effective dose above specified values (NR_E × 100)*				
	1 mSv	*5 mSv*	*10 mSv*	*15 mSv*	*30 mSv*
1973	63	43	34	24	6.3
1977	67	40	26	17	4.7
1981	64	37	23	14	3.0
1985	57	29	16	8.4	0.86
1989	55	22	9.2	3.3	0.10
	Percentage of collective dose from annual individual doses above specified values (SR_E × 100)				
	1 mSv	*5 mSv*	*10 mSv*	*15 mSv*	*30 mSv*
1973	98	93	85	71	30
1977	98	88	76	60	25
1981	97	86	71	52	18
1985	96	80	60	39	6.4
1989	94	70	43	19	0.90

Table 10
Collective effective dose among five occupational groups of LWR workers in the United States in 1987-1989
[B2]

Occupational group	*Monitored workers (thousands)*	*Average annual effective dose to monitored workers (mSv)*	*Average annual collective effective dose [a] (man Sv)*
Maintenance	53.8	4.9	263 (66.4)
Health physics	12.5	4.5	55.8 (14)
Operations	10.4	3.2	33.6 (9)
Engineering	10.4	3.1	32.5 (8)
Supervisory	4.56	2.5	11.4 (3)
Total	91.7	4.3	396 (100)

[a] The percentage of the total collective dose is given in parentheses.

Table 11
Exposures to workers in different types of GCRs in the United Kingdom

Type of GCR	*Average annual effective dose per monitored worker (mSv)*			*Average normalized collective effective dose [man Sv $(GW\ a)^{-1}$]*		
	1975-1979	*1980-1984*	*1985-1989*	*1975-1979*	*1980-1984*	*1985-1989*
Magnox SPC [a]	8.3	9.2	8.2	27	31	27
Magnox SPV [b c]	3.0	1.7	1.1	7.0	9.4	5.8
Magnox CPV [d c]	1.2	0.63	0.15	1.9	1.2	0.57
AGR [c]			0.18			1.1
Average [e]	2.9	1.5	0.77	7.2	6.0	3.2

[a] First-generation Magnox reactors with steel pressure vessels (SPVs); used for defence purposes and generation of electrical energy.
[b] Second-generation commercial Magnox reactors with SPVs [B8].
[c] Average values for reactors operated in England and Wales only [M8].
[d] Third-generation Magnox reactors with concrete pressure vessels (CPVs).
[e] Average values for all types of GCRs in the United Kingdom.

Table 12
Summary of worldwide exposures at reactors [a]

Reactor type	Average number of reactors	Average installed capacity (GW)	Average annual energy generated [b] (GW a)	Monitored workers [c] (thousands)	Average annual collective effective dose [d] (man Sv)	Collective effective dose per unit energy genereated [man Sv (GW a)$^{-1}$]	Average annual effective dose to monitored workers (mSv)	Average annual value of NR_{15} [e]	Average annual value of SR_{15}
1975-1979									
PWR	78	49	27 (49%)	63 (43%)	220 (37%)	8.1	3.5	0.085	0.56
BWR	51	29	15 (27%)	59 (39%)	280 (46%)	18	4.7	0.066	0.61
HWR	12	5.0	3.1 (6%)	6.8 (5%)	32 (5%)	11	4.8	0.12	0.71
LWGR [f]	12	5.9	4.4 (8%)	5.4 (4%)	36 (6%)	8.2	6.6	0.020	
GCR	40	9.1	5.4 (10%)	13 (9%)	36 (6%)	6.6	2.8		
HTGR [g]	1	0.33	0.03	1.2	0.03	0.90	0.03		
Total	190	99	55	150	600	11	4.1	0.078	0.60
1980-1984									
PWR	140	98	56 (55%)	140 (47%)	450 (43%)	8.0	3.1	0.061	0.48
BWR	65	44	25 (25%)	100 (34%)	450 (43%)	18	4.5	0.079	0.55
HWR	19	9.0	5.7 (6%)	14 (5%)	46 (4%)	8.0	3.2	0.073	0.58
LWGR	16	10	7.5 (7%)	9.8 (3%)	62 (6%)	8.3	6.4	0.005	
GCR	41	10	6.0 (6%)	25 (8%)	34 (3%)	5.8	1.4		
FBR	4	1.0	0.50	1.4	0.61	1.2	0.44		
HTGR	1	0.33	0.07	1.2	0.02	0.24	0.01		
Total	280	170	100	290	1000	10	3.5	0.069	0.52
1985-1989									
PWR	220	180	120 (65%)	230 (53%)	500 (46%)	4.3	2.2	0.034	0.32
BWR	84	67	42 (23%)	140 (33%)	330 (30%)	7.9	2.4	0.026	0.36
HWR	26	14	10 (5%)	18 (4%)	60 (6%)	6.2	3.4	0.066	0.48
LWGR [h]	20	15	10 (5%)	13 (3%)	170 (16%)	17	13	0.0002	0.01
GCR	44	13	7.4 (4%)	31 (7%)	24 (2%)	3.2	0.75		
FBR [i]	5	1.9	0.73	2.1	1.0	1.4	0.48		
HTGR	1	0.33	0.03	0.78	0.10	3.3	0.12		
Total	400	290	190	430	1100	5.9	2.5	0.033	0.34

[a] The data are annual values averaged over the respective five-year periods and are, in general, quoted to two significant figures.
[b] Values in parentheses are the percentage contributions, rounded to the nearest per cent, made by that reactor type to the total energy generated.
[c] Values in parentheses are the percentage contributions, rounded to the nearest per cent, made by that reactor type to the total number of monitored workers.
[d] Values in parentheses are the percentage contributions, rounded to the nearest per cent, made by that reactor type to the total collective effective dose.
[e] The values of the ratios, NR_{15} and SR_{15}, are only indicative of worldwide levels. Data on these ratios are not available from all countries, and the tabulated values are averages of those data reported.
[f] Averages of 1978 and 1979 tabulated and assumed representative of whole period in absence of data for earlier years.
[g] Includes data for Fort St. Vrain only; insufficient data to extrapolate to other prototype HTGRs.
[h] Averages of 1985-1987 tabulated and assumed representative of whole period in absence of data for later years in period.
[i] Averaged over 1986, 1987 and 1989, as data for other years in period were unavailable.

Table 13
Exposures from fuel reprocessing [a]
Data from UNSCEAR Survey of Occupational Exposure unless otherwise indicated

Country and period	Type of fuel	Annual amount of fuel reprocessed (kt)	Equivalent amount of energy from reprocessed fuel (GW a)	Monitored workers (thousands)	Measurably exposed workers (thousands)	Annual collective effective dose			Average annual effective dose		Distribution ratio	
						Total (man Sv)	Average per unit of fuel reprocessed (man Sv kt^{-1})	Average per unit energy generated [man Sv $(GW\ a)^{-1}$]	Per monitored worker (mSv)	Per measurably exposed worker (mSv)	NR_{15} [b]	SR_{15}
France (Cap de La Hague) [c]												
1975-1979	U/Ox	0.360	1.46	1.61	1.09	6.50	0.018	4.45	4.03	5.98	0.056	0.294
1980-1984	U/Ox/Mox	0.375	3.87	2.80	1.73	6.50	0.017	1.68	2.32	3.77	0.013	0.112
1985-1989	U/Ox	0.434	8.85	4.74	2.09	6.74	0.016	0.76	1.42	3.22	0.008	0.116
France (Marcoule) [d]												
1975-1979				2.74	1.88	6.31			2.30	3.36		
1980-1984				3.90	2.16	7.55			1.94	3.50		
1985-1989				4.54	1.77	5.79			1.28	3.27		
India [e]												
1981-1984				1.48	1.27	6.76			4.57	5.33	0.087	0.459
1985-1989				1.66	1.32	5.53			3.34	4.19	0.046	0.308
Japan [f]												
1975-1979	Ox/Mox	0.010		0.84		0.38	0.03		0.44		0	
1980-1984	Ox/Mox	0.030		1.37		1.23	0.04		0.89		0.000	
1985-1989	Ox/Mox	0.052		1.87		1.83	0.03		0.98		0.010	
United Kingdom [g h]												
1977-1979	U	0.715	2.17	5.61		46.6	65	21.5	8.31		0.193	
1980-1984	U	0.970	2.94	6.62		40.1	41	13.6	6.05		0.143	
1985-1988	U	0.887	2.69	7.22		29.4	33	11.0	4.07		0.101	
United States [i]												
1975-1979				2.65	2.05	10.8			4.06	5.27		
1980-1984				2.95	2.06	7.43			2.51	3.61		
1985-1989				3.21	1.78	4.89			1.52	2.74		
World (metal fuel) [j]												
1975-1979	U	1.1	3.1	7.1		53	50	17	7.4		0.16	
1980-1984	U	1.2	3.6	8.4		44	38	12	5.3		0.12	
1985-1989	U	0.94	2.9	8.0		31	33	11	3.8		0.092	

Table 13 (continued)

Country and period	Type of fuel	Annual amount of fuel reprocessed (kt)	Equivalent amount of energy from reprocessed fuel (GW a)	Monitored workers (thousands)	Measurably exposed workers (thousands)	Annual collective effective dose			Average annual effective dose		Distribution ratio	
						Total (man Sv)	Average per unit of fuel reprocessed (man Sv kt^{-1})	Average per unit energy generated [man Sv $(GW\ a)^{-1}$]	Per monitored worker (mSv)	Per measurably exposed worker (mSv)	NR_{15} [b]	SR_{15}
World (oxide fuel) [j]												
1975-1979	Ox	0.03	0.5	0.1	0.06	0.36	12	0.70	4.0	6.0	0.056	0.29
1980-1984	Ox	0.18	3.2	1.0	0.62	2.4	14	0.75	2.3	3.8	0.013	0.11
1985-1989	Ox	0.38	8.7	4.0	1.8	5.7	15	0.65	1.4	3.2	0.008	0.12

[a] The data are annual values averaged over the respective five-year periods. The doses are from external exposures only, apart from Japan; and the United Kingdom from 1986 onwards.
[b] The values of NR_{15} are for the monitored workforce. Values for the exposed workforce can also be estimated where data are given for both monitored and measurably exposed workers.
[c] Data from [R1] for the UP2 and UP3 plants at Cap de La Hague; reported data identifies amounts of metal, oxide and mixed oxide fuel reprocessed on an annual basis but doses are reported in a combined form for the site as a whole. The total amounts of each type of fuel reprocessed within the respective periods were as follows: 1975-1979, 1,650 t metal, 146 t oxide and 2.2 t mixed oxide; 1980-1984, 1,031 t metal, 836 t oxide and 7.7 t mixed oxide; 1985-1989, 253 t metal and 1,915 t oxide. Reprocessing also undertaken at Marcoule, but data for that site not included here.
[d] Data from [R1]; reprocessing of irradiated fuel from both the commercial and defence fuel cycles.
[e] Data include exposures in reprocessing and waste management.
[f] Data are for a prototype facility; separate data for uranium and mixed oxide fuels unavailable.
[g] The energy generated by reprocessed fuel was estimated from reported ^{85}Kr discharges [B3] on the assumption that 14 PBq of ^{85}Kr are associated with the generation of 1 GW a by Magnox fuel [U1]. The amount of fuel reprocessed was then derived on the basis of 330 t of uranium in Magnox fuel required to generate 1 GW a of electrical energy [O3].
[h] Data from [B8] are for all operations at the Sellafield site apart from the Calder reactors; other activities, unconnected with Magnox reprocessing, are also undertaken at the site and the reported doses will, therefore, be overestimates. Data are for BNFL employees and contractors. Internal doses not explicitly included, but they contribute less than 10% to the total doses. The data for NR_{15} and SR_{15} are taken from [W4] and are for the Sellafield site as a whole (i.e. including the Calder reactors).
[i] Reprocessing at United States Department of Energy facilities and mainly associated with defence activities rather than the commercial nuclear fuel cycle.
[j] Commercial reprocessing has essentially only been carried out in France and the United Kingdom over the period of interest. The data for these countries are combined to provide an overall estimate of the exposures associated with reprocessing metal and oxide fuels. For metal fuel the total comprises the sum of the data from the United Kingdom and that fraction of the data from France that has been estimated as arising from the reprocessing of metal fuel. For oxide fuel the total comprises that fraction of the data for France that can be associated with the reprocessing of oxide fuel.

Table 14
Exposures from commercial nuclear fuel cycle research and development [a] [b]
Data from UNSCEAR Survey of Occupational Exposure unless otherwise indicated

Country and period	Monitored workers (thousands)	Measurably exposed workers (thousands)	Annual collective effective dose (man Sv)	Average annual effective dose		Distribution ratio	
				Per monitored worker (mSv)	Per measurably exposed worker (mSv)	NR_{15} [c]	SR_{15}
Argentina							
1975-1979	0.2	0.01	0.2	1.0	20	0	0
1980-1984	0.2	0.01	0.17	0.85	17	0	0
1985-1989	0.13	0.018	0.07	0.54	3.9	0	0
Canada [d]							
1975-1979	4.49	3.94	13.5	2.95	3.36	0.055	0.44
1980-1984	4.56	4.30	11.1	2.43	2.57	0.043	0.41
1985-1989	4.20	3.97	6.1	1.45	1.54	0.026	0.40
Chile [e]							
1975-1979	0.02	0.02	0.04	2.41	2.41	0.013	0.031
1980-1984	0.03	0.03	0.05	2.00	2.00	0.032	0.11
1985-1989	0.05	0.05	0.06	1.23	1.23	0.017	0.055
Czechoslovakia							
1975-1979	0.36		0.17	0.48		0	0
1980-1984	0.34		0.18	0.52		0	0
1985-1989	0.36		0.13	0.38		0	0
Finland [f]							
1975-1979		0.01	0.01		1.58		0
1980-1984		0.00	0.01		2.58		0
1985-1989		0.01	0.05		3.47		0.25
France							
1975-1979	20.9	3.19	9.32	0.44	2.92	0.005	
1980-1984	21.0	2.86	8.47	0.40	2.97	0.004	
1985-1989	19.6	2.48	6.14	0.31	2.47	0.002	
Germany, Fed. Rep. of [g]							
1975-1979	0.71		3.80	5.37			
1980-1984	0.84		3.04	3.64			
1985-1989	1.66		1.15	0.69			
Hungary [h]							
1977-1979	0.12	0.01	0.01	0.06	1.49	0	0
1980-1984	0.13	0.01	0.00	0.03	0.83	0	0
1985-1989	0.12	0.01	0.01	0.07	0.96	0	0
India							
1980-1984	2.78	1.97	6.36	2.29	3.23	0.034	0.36
1985-1989	3.62	2.38	4.65	1.28	1.96	0.010	0.18
Indonesia [i]							
1975-1979	0.02		0.09	3.87		0.13	0.37
1980-1984	0.03	0.04	0.10	3.10	2.72	0.16	0.72
1985-1989	0.10	0.10	0.09	0.95	0.95	0.025	0.47
Italy							
1985-1989	2.44	0.45	0.26	0.11	0.58	0.000	0.012
Japan [j]							
1978-1979	4.12		2.13	0.52		0.002	
1980-1984	7.01		7.97	1.14		0.017	
1985-1989	9.18		7.72	0.84		0.008	
Norway [k]							
1980-1984	0.68	0.14	0.53	0.77	3.76	0.008	0.34
1985-1989	0.76	0.15	0.58	0.76	3.88	0.012	0.35

Table 14 (continued)

Country and period	*Monitored workers (thousands)*	*Measurably exposed workers (thousands)*	*Annual collective effective dose (man Sv)*	*Average annual effective dose*		*Distribution ratio*	
				Per monitored worker (mSv)	*Per measurably exposed worker (mSv)*	*NR_{15}* [c]	*SR_{15}*
Republic of Korea [l]							
1975-1979	0.25		0.12	0.46		0.004	
1980-1984	0.79	0.14	0.50	0.64	3.58	0.007	
1985-1989	0.99	0.15	0.65	0.65	4.36	0.009	
South Africa							
1975-1979	0.25		0.12	0.46		0.004	0.065
1980-1984	0.24		0.08	0.33		0.004	0.090
1985-1989	0.23		0.07	0.34		0	0
United Kingdom [m]							
1975-1979	8.49		37.4	4.40		0.085	
1980-1984	9.00		28.2	3.13		0.050	
1985-1989	9.40		24.0	2.55		0.033	
United States [n]							
1975-1979	30.3	14.8	33.0	1.09	2.24		
1980-1984	28.8	12.7	24.2	0.84	1.90		
1985-1989	31.7	11.9	19.2	0.60	1.61		
Total of reported data [o]							
1975-1979	63.4		96.3	1.52		0.035	0.42
1980-1984	75.5		89.4	1.18		0.021	0.39
1985-1989	82.6		66.0	0.80		0.011	0.30
World [p]							
1975-1979	120		170	1.4			
1980-1984	130		150	1.1			
1985-1989	130		100	0.82			

[a] The data are annual values averaged over the indicated periods.
[b] Intended to be exposures directly attributable to research and development solely for the commercial nuclear fuel cycle. Because of the way data are collected, there may be contributions from other activities, partial coverage or other inhomogeneities.
[c] The values of NR_{15} are for the monitored workforce. Values for the exposed workforce can also be estimated where data are given for both monitored and measurably exposed workers.
[d] Data are for research activities carried out by Ontario Hydro and AECL; for 1975-1987, the data contain a component arising from isotope production, which was then undertaken by AECL.
[e] Includes data for fuel research, a research reactor and radioisotope production.
[f] Comprises only personnel working at one research reactor.
[g] Comprises only workers at research and prototype reactors.
[h] Includes only workers employed at the research reactor of the Atomic Energy Institute; some other nuclear fuel cycle research may be carried out at other research and university institutes.
[i] Comprises data for workers at research reactors.
[j] Comprises exposures of workers at test and research reactors, the nuclear ship, ATR, critical assemblies, and at research facilities for nuclear fuel materials.
[k] Comprises only workers at the Institute of Energy Technology.
[l] Comprises exposures of workers at TRIGA research reactors and other fuel research facilities.
[m] Additional data from [W4]. Most of the exposures arise at AEA Technology (formerly UKAEA) sites, but the contribution from other organizations conducting research and development associated with the nuclear fuel cycle are also included. Almost half the collective dose arises from the operation of the prototype SGHWR.
[n] These data are the sum of exposures of particular categories of employees and contractors of the United States Department of Energy; they include the total exposures attributed by USDOE to fusion and waste management and processing and one half of the exposures attributed to each of the following categories: reactors, general research, offices, maintenance, support and other. This allocation exercise is an attempt to separate out the nuclear fuel cycle component from the broader range of research activities undertaken by USDOE. Some categories of data were excluded from the summation because they were not considered relevant to nuclear fuel cycle research (e.g. weapons fabrication) or were already included in another UNSCEAR category (e.g. accelerators). The tabulated doses are likely to be an overestimate of the doses from research that can properly be attributed to the commercial nuclear fuel cycle.
[o] These data should be interpreted with care, particularly when making comparisons between different periods, as the countries included in the respective summations may differ from one period to another. The distribution ratios are averages of those reported, and the data on these are often much less complete than data on the other quantities.
[p] In the absence of better data values of the ratios NR_{15} and SR_{15} for the sum of the reported data can be considered indicative of worldwide levels.

Table 15
Predicted cumulative doses for radiation workers in Canada
[S3]

Job classification	*Number of monitored workers*	*Cumulative effective dose (mSv)* [a]	
		Mean	*Median*
Nuclear power station workers			
Chemical and radiation control	240	459	269
Reactor operations	1371	456	321
Mechanical maintenance	1132	454	283
Fuel handling	228	288	152
Control technicians	564	266	173
Training staff	44	240	127
Electrical maintenance	179	222	115
Construction	1008	130	61
Administration/security/janitorial	1339	120	61
General maintenance	1092	116	67
Health physics	60	106	61
Scientific/professional staff	1454	89	54
Total	9391	242	109
Uranium miners	5429	138	90
Nuclear fuel processors	115	166	114
Industrial radiographers	2076	296	131

[a] Cumulative dose over an assumed working lifetime of 40 years.

Table 16
Distribution of cumulative doses to measurably exposed workers at LWRs in the United States who terminated employment between 1977 and 1989
[R2]

Duration of employment (years)		*Average career effective dose (mSv)*	*Percentage of workers with cumulative effective dose above specified values*						
Range	*Average*		*5 mSv*	*10 mSv*	*20 mSv*	*50 mSv*	*100 mSv*	*200 mSv*	*500 mSv*
1-3	1.9	1.02	40.8	29.5	10.6	4.0	0.29	0	0
3-5	4.0	1.63	48.9	37.8	17.9	9.4	2.0	0.07	0.01
5-10	7.2	25.7	60.4	50.2	29.3	18.9	7.1	0.89	0.01
10-15	12.0	43.6	68.0	58.5	39.2	28.2	13.9	3.6	0.09
15-20	16.6	58.0	71.9	62.6	44.4	33.4	18.8	7.1	0.45
20-25	21.8	117	81.3	72.1	59.5	51.8	37.4	19.9	3.1
>25	40.9	74	56.4	47.5	35.9	30.4	20.4	12.2	2.8
All	3.3	14.4	42.1	31.5	13.7	7.7	2.7	0.51	0.02

Table 17
Characteristics of the dose distributions for monitored workers at the Calvert Cliffs nuclear power plant in the United States
[G1]

Parameters	*Contract workers*					*Utility workers*				
	Duration of employment (years)					*Duration of employment (years)*				
	<1	*1-5*	*5-10*	*10-15*	*>15*	*<1*	*1-5*	*5-10*	*10-15*	*>15*
Number of workers	1347	1434	946	146	26	1972	1691	849	203	7
Mean cumulative dose (mSv)	6.5	22	57	78	124	3.4	12	28	37	61 [a]
Percentage of workers with E_c > 50 mSv	0.76	14	42	48	65	0.04	6.1	19	26	57 [a]
Percentage of workers with E_c > 100 mSv	0.53	3.8	23	31	50	0.04	1.6	6.1	9.9	29 [a]
Percentage of workers with E_c > 200 mSv	0.23	0	4.1	11	19	0	0.6	0.6	2.0	0 [a]

[a] Since the estimates are based on only seven workers, the statistical significance is very weak.

Table 18
Number of workers and cumulative doses at the Calvert Cliffs nuclear power plant in the United States
[G1]

Job category	*Number of monitored workers* [a]			*Mean cumulative effective dose (mSv)* [b]		
	Utility workers		*Contract workers*	*Utility workers*		*Contract workers*
	Plant	*Non-plant*		*Plant*	*Non-plant*	
Maintenance	2300	1000	2000	13	13	19
Operation	400	250	440	13	4	18
Health physics	110	220	710	47	4	71
Supervisory	90	53	140	29	7	25
Engineering	110	150	590	17	7	26
All categories	4960		4000	13		31

[a] Rounded to two significant figures.
[b] To measurably exposed workers.

Table 19
Average cumulative effective doses (mSv) from external radiation to workers at Sellafield [B9]

Follow-up period (years)	*Year of first monitoring*									
	1949-1950	*1953-1954*	*1957-1958*	*1961-1962*	*1965-1966*	*1969-1970*	*1973-1974*	*1977-1978*	*1981-1982*	*1985-1986*
1	2.3	10.1	8.8	5.6	5.1	5	7.6	5.3	3	2.3
2	7.3	24.8	24.4	14.8	15	16.6	23.3	15	7.2	5.8
3	30.8	42.9	43.8	22.4	26.5	31.5	41.3	25.4	12.6	
4	59.5	64	61.7	32.3	40.1	46.1	56.8	35.4	19.3	
5	83.8	81.2	78.9	46.5	53.8	58.2	71	44.4	23.4	
6	110	96.1	94.6	63.6	70.1	73.2	84.4	52.9	29.8	
7	144	114	108.8	82.5	85.7	87	97.9	61.5		
8	179	135	125.2	100	101	97.2	112	69.5		
9	201	150	144.1	116	117	109	125	73.4		
10	220	164	161.3	133	132	120	136	76.1		
11	245	174	180.7	147	142	136	148			
12	266	187	201	160	156	147	157			
13	288	202	219	173	166	156	162			
14	300	218	239	185	176	164	147			
15	319	236	258	196	184	171				
16	335	251	275	207	191	176				
17	359	271	291	215	203	179				
18	379	285	302	229	217	149				
19	404	304	314	238	227					
20	429	317	323	243	228					
21	451	335	332	251	234					
22	468	347	346	259	277					
23	485	363	365	266						
24	502	363	381	280						
25	524	376	387	288						
26	553	395	399	329						
27	569	414	408							
28	587	422	430							
29	622	426	443							
30	632	441	460							
31	665	447								
32	667	462								
33	673	467								
34	686	472								
35	704									
36	721									
37	751									
38	750									

Table 20
Cumulative doses to workers at industrial and research establishments in the United Kingdom [K5]

Distribution basis	Number of workers (thousands)	Collective effective dose (man Sv)	Mean cumulative effective dose (mSv)	Number of individuals in cumulative effective dose range (thousands)			
				<10 mSv	10-50 mSv	50-100 mSv	>100 mSv
Distribution by site (employer)							
BNFL	25.6	1805	70.4	10.2	7.46	3.08	4.85
MOD-AWE	10.2	85	8.3	8.6	1.25	0.24	0.15
MOD-DRPS	27.2	381	14.0	20.7	4.64	1.02	0.88
Nuclear Electric	8.2	198	24.1	4.5	2.53	0.7	0.48
UKAEA	23.9	730	30.5	14.9	5.46	1.63	1.91
Total [a]	95.2	3198	33.6	58.9	21.3	6.67	8.27
Distribution by year of birth							
Before 1915	6.40	361	56.4	3.33	1.53	0.57	0.97
1915-1919	3.46	276	79.7	1.47	0.89	0.38	0.72
1920-1924	6.36	437	68.8	2.77	1.71	0.69	1.20
1925-1929	7.30	456	62.4	3.30	1.95	0.83	1.23
1930-1934	7.98	406	50.8	3.86	2.18	0.84	1.10
1935-1939	8.29	309	37.3	4.43	2.30	0.73	0.83
1940-1944	8.97	259	28.9	5.32	2.39	0.61	0.66
1945-1949	11.1	261	23.6	7.09	2.64	0.68	0.67
1950-1954	10.9	211	19.4	7.38	2.34	0.61	0.52
1955-1959	12.7	156	12.3	9.73	2.09	0.53	0.31
1960-1964	9.14	59	6.5	7.75	1.13	0.20	0.06
1965-1969	2.72	7.9	2.9	2.51	0.19	0.01	0.00
After 1970	0.01	0.0	0.1	0.01	0	0	0
Total [a]	95.2	3198	33.6	58.9	21.3	6.67	8.27
Distribution by year in which radiation work began							
1940-1944	0.00	0.0	35.0	0	0.001	0	0
1945-1949	1.64	83.6	50.9	0.76	0.41	0.23	0.25
1950-1954	5.92	664	112	2.05	1.55	0.68	1.64
1955-1959	10.8	752	69.8	4.34	3.02	1.30	2.11
1960-1964	10.6	460	43.3	5.47	2.85	1.00	1.32
1965-1969	8.34	333	39.9	3.72	2.93	0.79	0.90
1970-1974	10.2	363	35.8	4.98	3.28	0.90	1.00
1975-1979	22.5	399	17.7	15.7	4.52	1.31	0.93
1980-1984	17.9	125	7.0	14.9	2.44	0.42	0.12
After 1985	7.39	19.2	2.6	6.98	0.35	0.06	0.00
Total [a]	95.2	3200	33.6	58.9	21.3	6.67	8.27

[a] Minor inconsistencies in totals are due to rounding of values after summation.

Table 21
Worldwide average annual exposures from the commercial nuclear fuel cycle [a]

Practice	Monitored workers (thousands)	Average annual collective effective dose (man Sv)	Average annual effective dose to monitored workers (mSv)	Distribution ratio [b]	
				NR_{15} [c]	SR_{15}
1975-1979					
Mining [d e]	240	1300	5.5	0.37	0.69
Milling [d e]	12	120	10	0.41	0.76
Enrichment [d]	11	5.3	0.5	0	0
Fuel fabrication	20	36	1.8	0.012	0.38 [h]
Reactor operation	150	600	4.1	0.078 [g]	0.60 [i]
Reprocessing [f]	7.2	53	7.3	0.16	0.29 [f]
Research	120	170	1.4	0.035	0.42
Total	560	2300	4.1	0.20	0.63
1980-1984					
Mining [d e]	310	1600	5.1	0.30	0.61
Milling [d e]	23	120	5.1	0.30	0.64
Enrichment [d]	4.3	0.8	0.2	0	0
Fuel fabrication	21	21	1.0	0.002	0.11 [h]
Reactor operation	290	1000	3.6	0.069 [g]	0.52 [i]
Reprocessing [f]	9.4	47	4.9	0.10	0.11 [f]
Research	130	150	1.1	0.021	0.39
Total	800	3000	3.7	0.16	0.55
1985-1989					
Mining [d e]	260	1100	4.4	0.25	0.52
Milling [d e]	18	120	6.3	0.18	0.43
Enrichment [d]	5.0	0.4	0.08	0	0
Fuel fabrication	28	22	0.78	0.002	0.019 [h]
Reactor operation	430	1100	2.5	0.033 [g]	0.34 [i]
Reprocessing [f]	12	36	3.0	0.064	0.12 [f]
Research	130	100	0.82	0.011	0.30
Total	880	2500	2.9	0.10	0.42

[a] The data are annual values averaged over the indicated periods.
[b] The values of the distribution ratios should only be considered indicative of worldwide levels as they are based, in general, on data from far fewer countries than the data for number of workers and collective doses.
[c] This ratio applies to monitored workers.
[d] Also includes uranium obtained or processed for purposes other than the commercial nuclear fuel cycle.
[e] The data for mining and milling (except for NR and SR) have been modified from those reported by using a conversion factor of 5.6 mSv WLM^{-1} for exposure to radon daughters (cf. 10 mSv WLM^{-1} used in the reported data). The ratios NR_{15} and SR_{15} are averages of reported data in which, in general, the previously used conversion factor has been applied. The tabulated ratios are thus strictly for a value of E somewhat less than 15 mSv. The relationship between the reported and revised data is not linear because exposure occurs from other than just inhalation of radon progeny.
[f] Also includes the reprocessing of some fuel from the defence nuclear fuel cycle.
[g] Does not include data for LWGRs, FBRs and HTGRs.
[h] Ratio applies to LWR and HWR fuels only, as data for other fuels are not available; the ratio would be smaller if all fuel types were included.
[i] Does not include data for GCRs, LWGRs, FBRs and HTGRs.

Table 22
Summary of normalized collective effective doses for the fuel cycle based on specific reactor types [a]

Practice	Normalized collective effective dose [man Sv (GW a)$^{-1}$]					
	LWRs			HWRs	GCRs	
	PWRs	BWRs	All		Magnox	AGRs
1975-1979						
Mining [b]	5.7	5.7	5.7	4.7	8.5	5.7
Milling [b]	0.52	0.52	0.52	0.42	0.78	0.52
Enrichment [c]	0.02	0.02	0.02	0	0	0.02
Fuel fabrication	0.69	0.69	0.69	0.20	0.71	0.33
Reactor operation	8.1	18	12	11	7.8	1.1 [e]
Reprocessing	0.7	0.70	0.70		17	0.75
Research [d]	1	1	1	1	1	1
Total without reprocessing	16	26	20	17	19	9.4
Total with reprocessing	17	27	21		36	8.7
1980-1984						
Mining [b]	5.5	5.5	5.5	4.3	8.3	5.5
Milling [b]	0.41	0.41	0.41	0.33	0.61	0.41
Enrichment [c]	0.02	0.02	0.02	0	0	0.02
Fuel fabrication	0.19	0.19	0.19	0.16	0.81	0.31
Reactor operation	8.0	18	11	8.0	8.0	1.1 [e]
Reprocessing	0.75	0.75	0.75		12	0.75
Research [d]	1	1	1	1	1	1
Total without reprocessing	15	25	18	14	19	8.4
Total with reprocessing	16	26	19		31	9.1
1985-1989						
Mining [b]	4.3	4.3	4.3	3.6	6.7	4.3
Milling [b]	0.44	0.44	0.44	0.36	0.66	0.44
Enrichment [c]	0.02	0.02	0.02	0	0	0.02
Fuel fabrication	0.07	0.07	0.07	0.22	1.4	0.45
Reactor operation	4.3	7.9	5.2	6.2	6.7	1.1
Reprocessing	0.65	0.65	0.65		11	0.65
Research [d]	1	1	1	1	1	1
Total without reprocessing	10	14	11	11	16	7.5
Total with reprocessing	11	15	12		27	8.1

[a] The data are annual values averaged over the indicated periods and are, in general, quoted to two significant figures.

[b] The data for mining and milling (except for NR and SR) have been modified from those reported by using a conversion factor of 5.6 mSv WLM^{-1} for exposure to radon daughters (cf. 10 mSv WLM^{-1} used in the reported data). The ratios NR_{15} and SR_{15} are averages of reported data in which, in general, the previously used conversion factor has been applied. The tabulated ratios are thus strictly for a value of E somewhat less than 15 mSv. The relationship between the reported and revised data is not linear because exposure occurs from other than just inhalation of radon progeny.

[c] Probably an overestimate, as the collective doses from which the normalized values were derived contain a contribution from enrichment for purposes other than the commercial nuclear fuel cycle.

[d] This rounded approximate value has been estimated by associating the collective dose received from research carried out in the period 1955-1989 with the sum of the energy generated in the same period plus that likely to be generated by existing reactors over the next 30 years. The value is judged to be an overestimate.

[e] The value for 1985-1989 was assigned in the absence of other data.

Table 23
Exposures to workers from defence activities [a]
Data from UNSCEAR Survey of Occupational Exposures

Country and period	Number of ships [b]	Monitored workers (thousands)	Measurably exposed workers (thousands)	Annual collective effective dose (man Sv)	Annual collective effective dose per ship (man Sv) [b]	Average annual effective dose		Distribution ratio	
						Per monitored worker (mSv)	Per measurably exposed worker (mSv)	NR_{15}	SR_{15}
Weapons fabrication and associated activities									
United Kingdom [c]									
1975-1979 [d]	Not applicable	3.14		2.95	Not applicable	0.94		0	0
1980-1984		3.71		3.56		0.96		0.0002	0
1985-1989		4.20		2.46		0.59		0	0
United States [e]									
1975-1979	Not applicable	17.6	9.31	10.9	Not applicable	0.62	1.17		
1980-1984		18.3	8.26	11.7		0.62	1.41		
1985-1989		15.9	7.54	11.9		0.75	1.58		
Total [f]									
1975-1979	Not applicable	20.8		13.8	Not applicable	0.67			
1980-1984		22.5		15.2		0.68			
1985-1989		20.1		14.4		0.71			
Nuclear ships and their support facilities									
On-board personnel									
United Kingdom [g]									
1975-1979 [d]	15	1.81		5.89	0.39	3.26		0.025	
1980-1984	16	0.89		2.30	0.14	2.57		0.018	
1985-1989	19	0.86		1.44	0.075	1.68		0.011	
United States [h]									
1975-1979	120	20.1		22.9	0.19	1.14		0.017 [i]	
1980-1984	136	26.2		16.3	0.12	0.62		0.002 [i]	
1985-1989	148	34.1		15.4	0.10	0.45		0.001 [i]	
Total [f]									
1975-1979	135	21.9		28.8	0.21	1.31			
1980-1984	153	27.1		18.6	0.12	0.68			
1985-1989	167	34.9		16.8	0.10	0.48			
Shore-based personnel									
United Kingdom [g]									
1975-1979 [d]	15	4.55		20.4	1.4	4.48		0.088	
1980-1984	16	5.54		17.8	1.1	3.21		0.056	
1985-1989	19	5.39		10.2	0.53	1.89		0.021	
United States [h]									
1975-1979	120	15.1		43.0	0.36	2.84		0.096 [i]	
1980-1984	136	19.1		29.5	0.22	1.54		0.027 [i]	
1985-1989	148	22.3		30.2	0.21	1.36		0.029 [i]	
Total [f]									
1975-1979	135	19.7		63.4	0.47	3.22			
1980-1984	153	24.7		47.3	0.31	1.92			
1985-1989	167	27.7		40.4	0.24	1.46			
All personnel									
United Kingdom [g]									
1975-1979 [d]	15	6.36		26.3	1.8	4.13		0.071	
1980-1984	16	6.43		20.1	1.2	3.11		0.050	
1985-1989	19	6.24		11.6	0.61	1.86		0.019	

Table 23 (continued)

Country and period	*Number of ships* [b]	*Monitored workers (thousands)*	*Measurably exposed workers (thousands)*	*Annual collective effective dose (man Sv)*	*Annual collective effective dose per ship (man Sv)* [b]	*Average annual effective dose*		*Distribution ratio*	
						Per monitored worker (mSv)	*Per measurably exposed worker (mSv)*	NR_{15}	SR_{15}
United States [h]									
1975-1979	120	35.2		65.9	0.55	1.87		0.051 [i]	
1980-1984	136	45.3		45.8	0.34	1.01		0.012 [i]	
1985-1989	148	56.4		45.6	0.31	0.81		0.012 [i]	
Total [f]									
1975-1979	135	41.6		92.2	0.69	2.22			
1980-1984	153	51.8		65.8	0.43	1.27			
1985-1989	167	62.6		57.3	0.34	0.91			
All defence activities									
United Kingdom [j]									
1975-1979 [d]	*Not applicable*	11.9		35.8	*Not applicable*	3.00		0.04	
1980-1984		12.8		26.3		2.06		0.028	
1985-1989		12.2		14.6		1.19		0.010	
United States									
1975-1979	*Not applicable*	92.5	55.8	101	*Not applicable*	1.09	1.81		
1980-1984		104	61.5	56		0.54	0.91		
1985-1989		115	73.0	69		0.60	0.95		
Total [f]									
1975-1979	*Not applicable*	104		137	*Not applicable*	1.3			
1980-1984		116		82		0.71			
1985-1989		127		84		0.66			

[a] The data are annual values averaged over the indicated periods.
[b] This column applies only for entries under "Nuclear ships and their support facilities".
[c] Data from [D1]. The actual effective doses are typically less than 50% of the tabulated values, which are those measured by the dosimeter.
[d] The value for this period are averages for the year 1979.
[e] Includes exposures of employees of the United States Department of Energy and contractors engaged in weapons fabrication and testing. Before 1987 the collective doses were evaluated as the sum of the products of the number of workers and the mean dose in each dose interval; subsequently, actual individual doses were used in the summation.
[f] Values derived as the sum or weighted average of the five-year averaged data for the United Kingdom and the United States.
[g] Data from [D1]. The data are reported for on-board and shore personnel. Shore-based personnel may comprise both civilian and service personnel. Since the early 1980s, dosimeters have been issued only to on-board personnel who need it during their duties at sea and to those designated as classified persons on shore.
[h] Data from [N1, M9 and M10]; the data reported for fleet and shipyard personnel are categorized here under "on-board" and "shore based" notwithstanding the lack of direct equivalence between the respective categories.
[i] The values are for the fraction of the workforce receiving annual doses in excess of 10 mSv.
[j] Data from [D1], including exposures from all defence activities.

Table 24
Distribution of cumulative doses from defence activities in the United Kingdom and in the United States

Cumulative effective dose (mSv)	*Percentage of workforce*		
	Nuclear weapons programme		
United Kingdom, 1989			
0- 50	96.4		
50-100	2.34		
100-200	0.90		
200-300	0.25		
300-400	0.05		
400-500	0.03		
>500	0		
Number of personnel in 1989 [a]	3843		
	Nuclear ships (operation and support)		
United Kingdom, 1989	On board	On shore	Total
0- 50	98.0	83.0	87.4
50-100	1.8	9.2	7.0
100-200	0.2	5.2	3.7
200-300	0.0	1.8	1.3
300-400	0.0	0.57	0.40
400-500	0.0	0.18	0.13
>500	0.0	0.03	0.02
Number of personnel in 1989	1929	4627	6556
United States, 1991			
0- 50	99.67	88.85	
50-100	0.32	6.99	
100-150	<0.01	2.23	
150-200	0	1.12	
200-250	0	0.47	
250-300	0	0.26	
300-500	0	0.08	
>500		<0.01	
	Defence workers		
United Kingdom, 1989	Service personnel	Civilian personnel	Total
0- 50	97.3	85.7	89.7
50-100	2.2	7.4	5.6
100-200	0.31	4.4	3.0
200-300	0.03	1.6	1.1
300-400	0.07	0.54	0.37
400-500	0.08	0.25	0.19
>500	0.001	0.04	0.03

[a] Includes about 95% of the workforce involved with the nuclear weapons programme.

Table 25
Cumulative doses in dose registries for defence workers in the United Kingdom

Cumulative effective dose (mSv)	Percentage of workforce										
	Central Index on Dose Information [a]					*National Registry on Radiation Workers* [b]					
	Weapons programme [c]		*Other defence* [d]		*All defence employees*	*All doses* [e]			*Doses to age 30 years* [f]		
	Employees	*Contract workers*	*Employees*	*Contract workers*		*Weapons programme* [c]	*Other defence activities* [d]	*All defence activities*	*Weapons programme* [c]	*Other defence activities* [d]	*All defence activities*
<1	19.9	21.6	28.8	9.6	20.0	18.7	37.7	33.1	61.8	61.0	61.2
1-5	24.9	28.3	20.8	12.7	20.9	33.0	25.5	27.3	21.4	19.9	20.2
5-10	12.7	19.3	13.0	10.7	12.6	16.7	11.5	12.8	8.4	7.5	7.7
10-20	15.7	18.6	13.1	11.7	14.1	14.9	9.9	11.1	5.3	5.5	5.4
20-50	16.0	9.8	14.7	20.1	16.4	11.9	8.4	9.2	2.4	3.8	3.5
50-100	5.7	2.3	6.3	16.5	8.3	3.2	3.8	3.6	0.50	1.4	1.2
100-200	3.9	0	2.5	11.8	5.2	1.2	2.2	1.9	0.18	0.65	0.53
200-300	0.84	0	0.52	4.5	1.6	0.27	0.67	0.57	0.05	0.14	0.12
300-400	0.28	0	0.16	1.7	0.58	0.08	0.26	0.22	0	0.02	0.01
400-600	0.03	0	0.12	0.74	0.22	0.02	0.12	0.09	0.01	0.01	0.01
>600	0.03	0	0	0	0.01	0.01	0.03	0.03	0.01	0.02	0.01
Number of workers	3913	388	2490	2157	8948	10278	32523	42810	10278	32523	42810
Average cumulative dose (mSv)	21.8	9.4	18.3	58.1	29.0	13.0	14.5	14.1	3.5	5.3	4.9

[a] Data from the Central Index on Dose Information (CIDI) are for classified radiation workers only, including employees and contractors of the Ministry of Defence. External and internal doses are included.
[b] Data from the National Registry on Radiation Workers are for classified and non-classified workers up to 1986, including only employees of the Ministry of Defence and not contractor workers. External and internal doses are included.
[c] Data strictly for the Atomic Weapons Establishment only, but can be assumed to be representative of the weapons programme as a whole.
[d] Data are for those monitored by the Defence Radiological Protection Service. They comprise all defence employees and contractors apart from those of the Atomic Weapons Establishment. Most of these exposures are associated with the naval nuclear propulsion programme.
[e] The percentages are for the total cumulative dose received by individual workers on the National Registry on Radiation Workers.
[f] The percentages are for the cumulative dose received by individual workers up to the age of 30 years.

Table 26
Exposures to workers from industrial uses of radiation (excluding the commercial nuclear fuel cycle and defence activities) [a]
Data from UNSCEAR Survey of Occupational Exposures unless otherwise indicated

Country and period	*Monitored workers (thousands)*	*Measurably exposed workers (thousands)*	*Annual collective effective dose (man Sv)*	*Average annual effective dose*		*Distribution ratio*	
				Per monitored worker (mSv)	*Per measurably exposed worker (mSv)*	NR_{15} [b]	SR_{15}
Industrial radiography							
Argentina							
1985-1989	0.046	0.01	0.027	0.59	2.7	0	0
Australia [c d]							
1985-1989	0.40	0.26	0.40	1.01	1.52	0.007	0.11
Brazil							
1985-1989				3.3	14.5		
Canada							
1975-1979	1.07	0.71	4.33	4.05	6.08	0.077	0.51
1980-1984	1.46	0.76	4.88	3.35	6.41	0.056	0.50
1985-1989	1.43	0.84	6.47	4.51	7.75	0.093	0.57
China (Taiwan Province)							
1985-1989	1.01		1.53	1.52			
Czechoslovakia							
1975-1979	0.54		1.24	2.31		0.027	0.31
1980-1984	1.03		2.19	2.12		0.016	0.16
1985-1989	1.32		2.15			0.011	0.14
Denmark							
1975-1979	0.24		0.23	0.98		0.003	0.080
1980-1984	0.33		0.43	1.33		0.009	0.12
1985-1989	0.41		0.48	1.19		0.004	0.076
Finland							
1980-1984		0.03	0.05		1.51		0
1985-1989		0.06	0.11		1.65		0
France [e]							
1975-1979	1.28		1.47	1.15			0.027
1985-1989	1.6	0.09	0.28	0.18	3.11	0.002	
German Dem. Rep.							
1980-1984	2.09	0.43	0.83	0.40	1.93	0.002	0.17
1985-1989	2.15	0.32	0.39	0.18	1.23	0.002	0.22
Germany, Fed. Rep. of							
1985-1989	4.67	1.61	7.10	1.52	4.41	0.023	0.33
Hungary							
1975-1979	1.13	0.41	2.54	2.25	6.13	0.029	0.40
1980-1984	1.24	0.39	1.47	1.19	3.79	0.012	0.22
1985-1989	1.16	0.37	1.15	0.99	3.14	0.005	0.13
India							
1980-1984	2.93	1.39	9.0	3.07	6.50	0.055	0.55
1985-1989	4.23	2.16	13.2	3.12	6.10	0.058	0.54
Indonesia							
1980-1984	0.14	0.02	0.22	1.53	10.8	0.033	0.45
1985-1989	0.43	0.03	0.40	0.95	14.9	0.059	0.10
Ireland							
1980-1984	0.07	0.04	0.05	0.75	1.39	0	0
1985-1989	0.05	0.03	0.06	1.41	2.57	0.010	0.15

Table 26 (continued)

Country and period	*Monitored workers* (*thousands*)	*Measurably exposed workers* (*thousands*)	*Annual collective effective dose* (*man Sv*)	*Average annual effective dose*		*Distribution ratio*	
				Per monitored worker (*mSv*)	*Per measurably exposed worker* (*mSv*)	NR_{15} [b]	SR_{15}
Japan							
1980-1984	3.31	1.58	5.67	1.71	3.59	0.015	
1985-1989	2.83	1.08	3.35	1.19	3.09	0.006	
Mexico							
1985-1989	0.82	0.49	5.10	6.23	10.5	0.102	0.67
Netherlands [f]							
1980-1984	0.97		0.34	0.35		0.002	0.13
1985-1989	1.02		0.48	0.47		0.004	0.20
New Zealand [M2]							
1980-1984	0.15		0.35	2.33			
Norway							
1980-1984	0.80	0.44	0.79	0.99	1.81	0.001	0.038
1985-1989	0.82	0.40	0.62	0.76	1.56	0.003	0.10
South Africa							
1975-1979	0.57	0.31	0.11	0.19	0.35	0	0
1980-1984	0.75	0.45	2.38	3.18	5.30	0.052	0.44
1985-1989	0.72	0.32	1.68	2.33	5.29	0.033	0.36
Spain							
1985-1989	0.82	0.66	1.23	1.50	1.87	0.018	0.32
Sweden							
1975-1979	0.77	0.19	0.49	0.63	2.56	0.005	0.16
1980-1984	0.66	0.17	0.38	0.57	2.27	0.002	0.059
1985-1989	0.64	0.25	0.28	0.43	1.12	0.002	0.15
USSR							
1975-1979	2.27		30.0	13.2			
1980-1984	2.53		20.2	7.98			
1985-1989	2.63		17.2	6.55			
United Kingdom [g]							
1980-1984	1.82		3.60	1.98		0.023	0.43
1985-1989	4.82	4.08	5.67	1.18	1.39	0.009	
United States [h]							
1975-1979	17		50	2.94			
1980-1984	27		80	2.96			
1985-1989	23	12	39	1.70	3.25		
Total of reported data [i]							
1975-1979	24.0		89.5	3.74		0.037	0.39
1980-1984	42.1		125	2.98		0.028	0.42
1985-1989	49.9		98.7	1.98		0.026	0.44
World [j]							
1975-1979	72		190	2.61			
1980-1984	116		230	1.98			
1985-1989	108		160	1.44			
Radiography carried out at fixed locations [k]							
Netherlands							
1980-1984	0.49		0.04	0.07			
1985-1989	0.54		0.06	0.11			
United Kingdom [K3, H2]							
1980-1984	1.29		2.00	1.55		0.026	
United States [l]							
1975-1979	2.07		2.80	1.35		0.009	0.42
1980-1984	3.54		3.90	1.10		0.007	0.17
1985-1989	1.85		0.67	0.36		0.001	0.19

Table 26 (continued)

Country and period	*Monitored workers (thousands)*	*Measurably exposed workers (thousands)*	*Annual collective effective dose (man Sv)*	*Average annual effective dose*		*Distribution ratio*	
				Per monitored worker (mSv)	*Per measurably exposed worker (mSv)*	NR_{15} [b]	SR_{15}
Total of reported data [i]							
1975-1979	2.07		2.80	1.35		0.009	0.42
1980-1984	3.54		3.90	1.10		0.007	0.17
1985-1989	1.85		0.67	0.36		0.001	0.19
Radiography carried out with mobile units [k]							
Netherlands							
1980-1984	0.28		0.24	0.84			
1985-1989	0.30		0.34	1.17			
United Kingdom [K3, H2]							
1980-1984	0.57		0.99	1.75		0.015	
United States [m]							
1975-1979	10.4	5.78	30.9	2.97	5.34	0.033	0.50
1980-1984	7.71	4.93	25.1	3.26	5.10	0.042	0.49
1985-1989	6.13	4.30	20.0	3.27	4.66	0.043	0.44
Total of reported data [i]							
1975-1979	10.4		30.9	2.97		0.033	0.50
1980-1984	8.56		26.4	3.08		0.041	0.47
1985-1989	6.42		20.4	3.17		0.043	0.44
Luminizing industries [k]							
France [P2]							
1975-1979	0.071		0.375	5.30			0.66
1980-1984	0.044		0.242	5.52		0.14	0.55
1985-1989	0.027		0.182	6.84		0.17	0.52
India [n]							
1980-1984	0.067	0.028	0.077	1.16	2.78	0.011	0.16
1985-1989	0.151	0.056	0.190	1.26	3.37	0.021	0.54
Switzerland [S13]							
1975-1979	0.206		2.31	11.2		0.25	0.53
1980-1984	0.130		1.02	7.82		0.14	0.39
1985-1989	0.158		0.68	4.31		0.039	0.18
United Kingdom (paint) [U3]							
1975-1979	0.093		0.40	4.32			0.35
United Kingdom (tritium) [o]							
1975-1979	0.25		1.46	5.89		0.12	0.65
1980-1984	0.33		1.10	3.33		0.057	0.40
Total of reported data [i]							
1975-1979	0.51		3.77	7.44		0.18	0.58
1980-1984	0.27		1.34	5.01		0.081	0.37
1985-1989	0.54		1.45	2.71		0.026	0.31
Radioisotope production and distribution							
Argentina							
1975-1979	0.17		0.67	4.05		0	0
1980-1984	0.22		0.45	2.10		0	0
1985-1989	0.18		0.44	2.47		0	0
Canada [p]							
1975-1979	0.046	0.032	0.12	2.67	3.84	0.017	0.14
1980-1984	0.033	0.027	0.19	5.83	7.28	0.090	0.41
1985-1989	0.295	0.162	0.48	1.61	2.94	0.014	0.18

Table 26 (continued)

Country and period	*Monitored workers (thousands)*	*Measurably exposed workers (thousands)*	*Annual collective effective dose (man Sv)*	*Average annual effective dose*		*Distribution ratio*	
				Per monitored worker (mSv)	*Per measurably exposed worker (mSv)*	NR_{15} [b]	SR_{15}
Czechoslovakia							
1975-1979	0.18		0.50	2.76		0.018	0.19
1980-1984	0.33		0.60	1.80		0.022	0.30
1985-1989	0.40		0.81	2.05		0.035	0.42
Finland [q]							
1975-1979		0.003	0.011		4.23		0
1980-1984		0.005	0.020		3.92		0
1985-1989		0.013	0.052		4.10		0
Hungary							
1975-1979	0.21	0.079	0.27	1.33	3.49	0.014	0.21
1980-1984	0.25	0.090	0.30	1.18	3.35	0.005	0.097
1985-1989	0.24	0.088	0.32	1.31	3.56	0.008	0.16
India							
1980-1984	0.40	0.31	0.67	1.69	2.20	0.010	0.17
1985-1989	0.51	0.35	0.71	1.39	2.02	0.008	0.14
Indonesia							
1975-1979	0.025		0.11	4.34			
1980-1984	0.034	0.030	0.060	1.76	2.03	0	0
1985-1989	0.046	0.040	0.083	1.81	2.10	0	0
Netherlands [f]							
1985-1989	0.18		0.87	4.97		0.040	0.13
Republic of Korea							
1975-1979	0.023	0.020	0.12	5.22	6.00	0.095	0.32
1980-1984	0.020	0.020	0.15	7.43	7.65	0.34	0.64
1985-1989	0.016	0.013	0.086	5.38	6.52	0.063	0.17
South Africa							
1975-1979	0.019		0.16	8.74		0.23	0.71
1980-1984	0.029		0.16	5.27		0.10	0.57
1985-1989	0.031		0.18	5.75		0.12	0.52
United Kingdom [r]							
1975-1979	0.97		6.39	6.59		0.14	
1980-1984	1.26		4.82	3.84		0.067	
1985-1989	1.72		4.63	2.70		0.029	
United States							
1975-1979	20		40	2.00			
1980-1984	29		30	1.03			
1985-1989	30	17	25	0.83	1.47		
Total of reported data [i]							
1975-1979	21.6		48.3	2.23		0.095	0.18
1980-1984	31.5		37.3	1.18		0.045	0.23
1985-1989	33.2		32.7	0.98		0.025	0.23
World [j]							
1975-1979	57		130	2.25			
1980-1984	82		100	1.26			
1985-1989	88		98	1.12			
Well logging [k]							
Canada							
1975-1979	0.45	0.21	0.52	1.16	2.43	0.008	0.17
1980-1984	1.01	0.58	1.28	1.27	2.21	0.005	0.11
1985-1989	1.11	0.74	1.37	1.24	1.85	0.003	0.051
Czechoslovakia [s]							
1975-1979	0.057		0.058	1.02		0	0
1980-1984	0.092		0.15	1.60		0.002	0.032
1985-1989	0.114		0.20	1.72		0.002	0.016

Table 26 (continued)

Country and period	*Monitored workers (thousands)*	*Measurably exposed workers (thousands)*	*Annual collective effective dose (man Sv)*	*Average annual effective dose*		*Distribution ratio*	
				Per monitored worker (mSv)	*Per measurably exposed worker (mSv)*	NR_{15} [b]	SR_{15}
India [t]							
1980-1984	0.19	0.041	0.072	0.38	1.75	0.006	0.39
1985-1989	0.64	0.30	0.38	0.54	1.25	0.002	0.086
Indonesia							
1980-1984	0.14	0.038	0.12	0.82	3.07	0	0
1985-1989	0.56	0.45	0.84	1.51	1.89	0	0
Mexico							
1985-1989	0.36	0.013	0.004	0.012	0.32	0	0
South Africa							
1975-1979	0.043	0.012	0.000	0.007	0.025		
1980-1984	0.040	0.017	0.064	1.61	3.76		
1985-1989	0.035	0.012	0.053	1.49	4.55		
United States [u]							
1975-1979	7.6		10.3	1.36			0.3
Total of reported data [v]							
1975-1979				1.32		0.007	0.27
1980-1984				1.17		0.004	0.10
1985-1989				1.07		0.002	0.039
Tertiary education and research institutes							
Australia [c d]							
1975-1979	0.55		0.055	0.10			
1985-1989	2.22	0.94	0.069	0.03	0.07	0	0
Canada [w]							
1975-1979	5.01	0.89	0.69	0.14	0.78	0.0005	0.090
1980-1984	7.40	1.02	0.80	0.11	0.78	0.0003	0.044
1985-1989	9.51	1.62	1.05	0.11	0.65	0.0003	0.086
China (Taiwan Province)							
1985-1989	0.71		0.04	0.056			
Czechoslovakia							
1975-1979	0.08		0.04	0.45		0.003	0.23
1980-1984	0.18		0.18	0.97		0.017	0.58
1985-1989	0.21		0.12	0.56		0.001	0.030
Finland [x]							
1980-1984	0.95	0.023	0.038	0.040	1.63	0	0.062
1985-1989	1.18	0.032	0.053	0.045	1.68	0.008	0.11
France [P2]							
1985-1989	3.8	0.09	0.20	0.053	2.22	0.001	
German Dem. Rep. [y]							
1975-1979	2.71		0.034	0.013			
1980-1984	3.07		0.056	0.018			
1985-1989	3.25	0.30	0.16	0.048	0.52		
Germany, Fed. Rep. of [z]							
1985-1989	21.1	1.05	1.53	0.072	1.46	0.0004	0.17
Hungary [aa]							
1975-1979	0.22	0.008	0.022	0.104	2.79	0.0009	0.19
1980-1984	0.21	0.003	0.003	0.015	0.93	0	0
1985-1989	0.21	0.005	0.009	0.044	2.02	0	0
India [bb]							
1980-1984	1.01	0.17	0.29	0.29	1.74	0.003	0.24
1985-1989	1.92	0.47	0.45	0.24	0.97	0.0005	0.067

Table 26 (continued)

Country and period	*Monitored workers (thousands)*	*Measurably exposed workers (thousands)*	*Annual collective effective dose (man Sv)*	*Average annual effective dose*		*Distribution ratio*	
				Per monitored worker (mSv)	*Per measurably exposed worker (mSv)*	NR_{15} [b]	SR_{15}
Indonesia							
1980-1984	0.28	0.19	0.25	0.92	1.33	0.018	0.37
1985-1989	0.66	0.64	0.48	0.72	0.75	0.003	0.11
Italy							
1985-1989	0.66	0.085	0.054	0.082	0.634	0.0003	0.001
Japan							
1980-1984	21.4	0.79	0.49	0.023	0.62	0.0002	
1985-1989	27.6	0.69	0.46	0.017	0.67	0.0000	
Norway [cc]							
1980-1984	0.42	0.025	0.014	0.032	0.55	0	0
1985-1989	0.45	0.029	0.026	0.057	0.90	0.001	0.48
Portugal							
1985-1989	0.78	0.37	0.33	0.42	0.88		
South Africa							
1975-1979	0.23	0.042	0.002	0.007	0.04	0	0
1980-1984	0.36	0.091	0.47	1.29	5.12	0.020	0.45
1985-1989	0.43	0.070	0.21	0.49	3.02	0	0.10
Switzerland [dd]							
1975-1979	7.44		5.91	0.79		0.007	
1980-1984	8.48		3.44	0.41		0.0006	
1985-1989	8.83		2.88	0.33		0.0003	
United Kingdom [l]							
1980-1984	12.5		1.3	0.10		0	0
1985-1989	1.17	0.49	0.38	0.32	0.78	0.002	
United States [m]							
1975-1979	25		18	0.72			
1980-1984	26		15	0.58			
1985-1989	17		6	0.35	0.86		
Total of reported data [i]							
1975-1979	38.6		23.5	0.61		0.004	0.19
1980-1984	66.0		20.4	0.31		0.0007	0.11
1985-1989	85.7		13.6	0.16		0.0004	0.072
World [j]							
1975-1979	140		74	0.55			
1980-1984	180		43	0.24			
1985-1989	160		22	0.14			
Accelerators [k]							
Canada							
1975-1979	0.58	0.19	0.17	0.30	0.91	0.0003	0.098
1980-1984	0.88	0.23	0.40	0.45	1.76	0.0009	0.043
1985-1989	1.00	0.53	1.06	1.06	2.00	0.0038	0.067
Finland							
1980-1984		0.008	0.010		1.23		0
1985-1989		0.007	0.013		1.75		0
Netherlands							
1980-1984	0.18	0.009	0.006	0.03	0.67	0	0
1985-1989	0.16	0.010	0.004	0.03	0.46	0	0
South Africa							
1975-1979	0.07	0.03	0.030	0.46	1.00	0	0
1980-1984	0.10	0.04	0.27	2.72	6.59	0.046	0.55
1985-1989	0.22	0.07	0.34	1.56	4.76	0.035	0.61

Table 26 (continued)

Country and period	*Monitored workers (thousands)*	*Measurably exposed workers (thousands)*	*Annual collective effective dose (man Sv)*	*Average annual effective dose*		*Distribution ratio*	
				Per monitored worker (mSv)	*Per measurably exposed worker (mSv)*	NR_{15} [b]	SR_{15}
United Kingdom [H2] [ee]							
1985-1989	0.50		0.25	0.50		0	0
United States [M1] [ff]							
1975-1979	3.96	1.73	7.19	1.82	4.16		
1980-1984	3.92	1.44	3.07	0.78	2.12		
1985-1989	4.25	1.66	2.07	0.49	1.24		
Total of reported data [i]							
1975-1979	4.50		7.38	1.62		0.0004	0.12
1980-1984	4.93		3.73	0.76		0.005	0.26
1985-1989	5.72		3.52	0.62		0.008	0.19
v All industrial activities (excluding nuclear fuel cycle and defence activities)							
Argentina							
1985-1989	0.066	0.031	0.085	1.29	2.74	0.030	0.61
Australia [c d]							
1975-1979	2.21		0.92	0.41			
1985-1989	7.10	3.33	0.78	0.11	0.23	0.001	0.091
Brazil [D2]							
1985-1989	15	3.1	24	1.6	7.69		
Canada							
1975-1979	8.06	3.60	13.2	1.63	3.66	0.022	0.42
1980-1984	11.0	4.36	14.4	1.31	3.30	0.016	0.34
1985-1989	10.7	4.70	16.2	1.52	3.45	0.023	0.39
China (Taiwan Province)							
1980-1984	2.42		1.91	0.79			
1985-1989	3.04		1.97	0.65			
Czechoslovakia							
1975-1979	1.65		2.26	1.38		0.011	0.23
1980-1984	2.92		3.77	1.29		0.010	0.18
1985-1989	3.62		3.77	1.04		0.010	0.21
Denmark							
1975-1979	0.46		0.32	0.68		0.002	0.058
1980-1984	0.64		0.49	0.76		0.005	0.11
1985-1989	0.80		0.52	0.65		0.002	0.071
Finland [gg hh]							
1975-1979	0.67	0.05	0.14	0.21	2.97		0.20
1980-1984	2.09	0.15	0.26	0.12	1.75	0.0000	0.046
1985-1989	2.36	0.17	0.32	0.14	1.94	0.0004	0.063
France [P2]							
1985-1989	9.90		24.0	2.42			
Germany, Fed. Rep. of							
1985-1989	58.6	14.7	25.6	0.44	1.74	0.008	0.29
Hungary [ii]							
1975-1979	3.26	0.58	3.01	0.92	5.14	0.011	0.36
1980-1984	3.36	0.56	1.93	0.58	3.47	0.005	0.19
1985-1989	3.26	0.53	1.57	0.48	2.97	0.003	0.12
Indonesia							
1980-1984	0.02	0.01	0.01	0.75	1.25		
1985-1989	0.03	0.03	0.03	1.12	1.12		
Ireland							
1985-1989	0.74	0.06	0.08	0.11	1.37	0.0003	0.089

Table 26 (continued)

Country and period	*Monitored workers (thousands)*	*Measurably exposed workers (thousands)*	*Annual collective effective dose (man Sv)*	*Average annual effective dose*		*Distribution ratio*	
				Per monitored worker (mSv)	*Per measurably exposed worker (mSv)*	*NR_{15}* [b]	*SR_{15}*
Italy [jj]							
1985-1989	1.98	0.44	0.87	0.44	1.97	0.004	0.35
Japan							
1975-1979	27.6	3.93	8.93	0.32	2.27	0.008	
1980-1984	29.0	4.06	11.0	0.38	2.70	0.005	
1985-1989	32.0	3.06	8.48	0.27	2.77	0.002	
Mexico							
1985-1989	1.63	0.51	5.23	3.21	10.2	0.047	0.66
Netherlands							
1980-1984	1.71		0.63	0.37		0.005	0.34
1985-1989	2.27		0.88	0.39		0	0.15
New Zealand [M2]							
1980-1984	0.28		0.43	1.50			
Norway [kk]							
1980-1984	1.21	0.51	0.85	0.70	1.67	0.002	0.042
1985-1989	1.44	0.51	0.68	0.47	1.35	0.002	0.094
Portugal [C1]							
1985-1989	0.63	0.52	0.18	0.28	0.34		
South Africa							
1975-1979	2.01	0.79	0.21	0.11	0.27	0	0.046
1980-1984	2.90	1.18	6.11	2.11	5.17	0.026	0.41
1985-1989	2.37	0.55	5.71	2.41	10.5	0.004	0.69
Spain							
1985-1989	3.02	2.49	3.98	1.32	1.60	0.009	0.018
Switzerland							
1975-1979	11.7		10.2	0.87		0.010	0.31
1980-1984	12.9		5.92	0.46		0.003	0.14
1985-1989	13.6		4.08	0.30		0.001	0.081
USSR							
1975-1979	7.78		126	16.2			
1980-1984	9.85		122	12.4			
1985-1989	12.8		104	8.15			
United Kingdom							
1980-1984	28.0		26.0	0.93			
1985-1989	18.8	15.1	21.0	1.12	1.39	0.008	
United States [ll]							
1975-1979	202		290	1.44			
1980-1984	305		380	1.25			
1985-1989	274	101	150	0.55	1.49		
Total of reported data [i]							
1975-1979	240		445	1.81		0.014	0.36
1980-1984	386		552	1.43		0.008	0.29
1985-1989	423		343	0.81		0.007	0.34
World [j]							
1975-1979	530	290	870	1.64	3.0	0.010	0.35
1980-1984	690	300	940	1.36	3.2	0.007	0.28
1985-1989	560	250	510	0.90	2.0	0.009	0.31

[a] The data are annual values averaged over the indicated periods. They were derived as averages over the years for which data were reported; in some cases, data were reported for only a limited number of years in the periods of interest here.

[b] The values of NR_{15} are for the monitored workforce. Values for the exposed workforce can also be estimated where data are given for both monitored and measurably exposed workers.

[c] Data also from [M7] and [S6]; numbers of workers and the collective doses reported in questionnaire for about 70% of the exposed workforce have been extrapolated for entire country.

Table 26 (continued)

[d] The method of dose recording was different in the two periods for which data are reported, and this may partly account for the differences in data. Average individual doses for 1975-1979 were calculated from the total of the reported doses for an occupational category divided by the estimated number of workers in that category with the results rounded to the nearest 0.1 mSv. In 1990 the estimates were based directly on the results of individual monitoring; in the absence of data for 1985-1989, the data for 1990 have been assumed to be representative of this period.
[e] Data from [U3] for 1975-1979 and from [P2] for 1985-1989.
[f] The reported data (covering about 80% of the workforce) have been scaled to represent the whole country.
[g] Data for 1980-1984 from [K3] and [H2] include only those workers whose dose records are held within the Dosemeter Issue and Record Keeping (DIRK) service of the NRPB. The total number of radiographers in the United Kingdom is somewhat larger. Data for 1985-1989 from [H7] and [B7] are for classified workers only.
[h] Data from [E1, E2 and E3]; data are for 1975, 1980 and 1985 but assumed here to be representative of the respective five-year periods.
[i] These data should be interpreted with care, particularly because the countries included in the summations for the respective five-year periods may not be the same, depending on whether data were reported for the period in question. Consequently, direct comparison of data for different periods is invalid to the extent that the data comprise contributions from different countries. It should also be noted that the data on NR_{15} and SR_{15} are averages of data reported on these ratios. In general, these data are less complete than those that form the basis of the summated number of workers and collective doses.
[j] The estimates are extrapolations of regional values based on the gross national product (GNP); because of insufficient data, the estimates of NR_{15} and SR_{15} are averages of reported data, but these may be considered representative for worldwide exposure.
[k] Insufficient data are available for these categories to enable a reliable estimate of worldwide exposures.
[l] Data for licencees of the Nuclear Regulatory Commission only.
[m] Data are for licensees of the United States Nuclear Regulatory Commission only.
[n] The doses include exposures from tritium intake and external radiation from promethium-147.
[o] Data for 1980-1984 from [H1] and [H2]. Data for 1985-1989 from [H7] and [B7] include only classified workers.
[p] Before 1989 radioisotope production was undertaken by Atomic Energy of Canada Limited, and separate statistics for this group of workers are not available. The average data tabulated for 1985-1989 are those for 1989, when production was transferred from Atomic Energy of Canada Limited; this accounts for the significant difference compared with the previous period. The contribution of internal exposure is small.
[q] Internal exposure included after 1986; it amounted to about 50%.
[r] Internal exposure included after 1984; its contribution is small.
[s] For 1980-1989, neutron exposure contributed 30%-60% of the total. About one third of the workforce is employed underground and received an internal dose from radon etc, additional to the doses tabulated, in the range of about 5 to 10 mSv a^{-1}.
[t] Neutrons contribute about 15%-25% to the reported doses.
[u] Data are for licensees of the United States Department of Energy only. The effective doses include a neutron component.
[v] Data are only presented for quantities that are averages of the reported data rather than their sums. Summed data would be potentially misleading because of the main contribution that would be made by the data for the United States, for which data for only one period are available. The data should be interpreted with care. In particular, the countries included in the summation for the reporting periods may not be the same.
[w] Data are mainly from universities but exclude exposures at accelerators and in teaching establishments where little research is undertaken.
[x] Includes all research institutes except research reactors and accelerators. No data are available on exposures in tertiary education.
[y] For 1976-1980, the data are for all universities and technical colleges in the non-medical field. For 1981-1989, the data are for all research and education except for that associated with medical and nuclear sciences.
[z] Data include exposures arising in research and training in natural sciences and technology, including research centres.
[aa] Includes technological education only (i.e. not medicine, science, philosophy etc.).
[bb] Includes data from education and research institutes.
[cc] Data are solely for the Univesity of Oslo.
[dd] Data from [O1]; they may include some data on research for the nuclear fuel cycle.
[ee] Data include exposures at the Science and Engineering (SERC) Laboratories at Chilton and Daresbury.
[ff] Data are for accelerators of the United States Department of Energy. Before 1987 collective doses were evaluated as the sum of the products of the number of workers and the mean dose in each dose interval; subsequently, actual individual doses were used in the summation.
[gg] Includes exposures of workers at the research reactor and in research establishments, including tertiary education.
[hh] Reported data for 1975-1979 contained only estimates of the number of exposed workers; the number of monitored workers was estimated assuming the ratio of exposed to monitored workers in the subsequent period.
[ii] Data do not include exposures for workers in the luminizing industry, in well logging and at accelerators.
[jj] The reported number of workers is small compared with numbers in comparable industrialized countries, which suggests that the data are incomplete.
[kk] Educational establishments not included.
[ll] Data from [E1, E2 and E3]. The data are specifically for the years 1975, 1980 and 1985; they are assumed here to be representative, respectively, of the periods 1975-1979, 1980-1984 and 1985-1989.

Table 27
Percentage of workers in industrial radiography receiving annual effective doses in excess of 50 mSv and the percentage of the collective dose arising from doses above that level
Data from UNSCEAR Survey of Occupational Exposures unless otherwise indicated

Country	*Percentage of workers receiving annual effective dose >50 mSv (NR_{50} × 100)*			*Percentage of collective dose from annual individual doses >50 mSv (SR_{50} × 100)*		
	1975-1979	*1980-1984*	*1985-1989*	*1975-1979*	*1980-1984*	*1985-1989*
Canada	0.5	0.5	0.6	7.3	11	8.2
China (Taiwan Province)			0.7			26
Germany, Fed. Rep. of			0.1			2.4
India		0.5	0.4		13	11
Ireland		0	0		0	0
Japan		0.2	0			
Netherlands		0	0		0	2.8
South Africa		0.3	0		8.5	7.0
United Kingdom [a]		0.13	0.11			
United States [b]						
Fixed locations	0	0	0	5.6	2.1	1.4
Mobile equipment	0.1	0	0	5.2	3.3	2.5
Weighted average [c]	0.10	0.14	0.17	5.4	6.1	6.2

[a] Data from [H1, H2, K3, K4]; those for 1980-1984 are averages over the years 1980 and 1982 and those for 1985-1989 are averages over the years 1986-1987. Data are for radiographers whose dose records are held within the Dosemeter Issue and Record Keeping (DIRK) service of the National Radiological Protection Board (NRPB).

[b] Data for licensees of the United States Nuclear Regulatory Commission only.

[c] Weighted according to the average number of workers or collective dose, as appropriate, in each country in each five-year period.

Table 28
Contribution of different regions to the worldwide exposure from all industrial uses of radiation (excluding the nuclear fuel cycle and defence activities) [a]

Country/region	*Monitored workers* (*thousands*)	*Average annual collective effective dose* (*man Sv*)	*Average annual individual dose to monitored workers* (*mSv*)	*Collective effective dose per unit GNP* [b] (*man Sv per* 10^{12} *$US*)	*Collective effective dose per unit population* (*man Sv per* 10^{9})
1975-1979					
East and south-east Asia [c]					
Eastern Europe [d]	17	176	10	150	440
Latin America					
OECD except United States [e]	210	240	1.1	79	430
United States	200	290	1.4	150	1300
Remainder [f]	100	170	1.7	120	55
Total	530	870	1.6	120	200
1980-1984					
East and south-east Asia [c]	12	9	0.79	20	23
Eastern Europe [d]	20	150	7.9	68	370
Latin America					
OECD except United States [e]	240	240	0.99	49	420
United States	310	380	1.3	110	1600
Remainder [f]	110	160	1.4	73	48
Total	690	940	1.4	72	190
1985-1989					
East and south-east Asia [c]	10	7	0.65	13	15
Eastern Europe [d]	26	140	5.6	41	330
Latin America	24	43	1.8	52	95
OECD except United States [e]	180	130	0.69	16	220
United States	270	150	0.55	31	590
Remainder [f]	41	35	0.85	26	11
Total	560	510	0.9	26	94

[a] The data are annual values averaged over the respective five-year periods and are, in general, quoted to two significant figures.
[b] The normalized collective doses per unit GNP for the three five-year periods are expressed, respectively, in terms of 1977, 1983 and 1989 prices; direct comparison between the values for different periods is possible only after correcting for these different price bases.
[c] Non-centrally-planned economies in east and south-east Asia.
[d] Including the whole of the former USSR.
[e] All countries members of the Organization for Economic Co-operation and Development (OECD) except for the United States.
[f] Includes the remainder of the world for which values are not specifically tabulated elsewhere in the Table. Note that the countries or regions comprising the remainder differ in the respective five-year periods.

Table 29
Cumulative doses received by industrial radiographers in Hungary
[S8]

Duration of employment (years)	*Number of workers*	*Average cumulative effective dose (mSv)*	*Average annual effective dose (mSv)*	*Percentage of workers with cumulative effective doses above specified values*			
				>50 mSv	*>100 mSv*	*>150 mSv*	*>200 mSv*
5	69	14.0	2.8	0	0	0	0
6	72	26.5	4.4	11.1	1.4	0	0
7	44	34.6	4.9	15.9	2.3	0	0
8	44	31.5	3.9	18.2	0	0	0
9	38	37.4	4.2	18.4	5.3	0	0
10	41	44.1	4.4	29.3	4.9	2.4	0
11	32	54.1	4.9	28.1	9.4	6.3	3.1
12	30	60.3	5.0	53.3	16.7	0	0
13	21	66.6	5.6	52.4	14.3	4.8	0
14	26	102.9	7.4	88.5	42.3	7.7	3.8
15	27	102.7	6.8	96.3	44.4	11.1	3.7

Table 30
Summary of worldwide exposures from the industrial uses of radiation (excluding nuclear fuel cycle and defence activities) [a]

Practice	*Monitored workers [b] (thousands)*	*Average annual collective effective dose [c] (man Sv)*	*Average annual individual dose to monitored workers (mSv)*	NR_{15} [d]	SR_{15} [d]
1975-1979					
Industrial radiography	72 (14%)	190 (22%)	2.6	0.037	0.39
Isotope production and distribution	57 (11%)	130 (15%)	2.3	0.095	0.18
Tertiary education and research institutes	140 (25%)	74 (8%)	0.55	0.004	0.19
Other [e]	270 (50%)	480 (55%)	1.8		
All industry	530	870	1.6	0.01	0.35
1980-1984					
Industrial radiography	120 (17%)	230 (24%)	2.0	0.028	0.42
Isotope production and distribution	82 (12%)	100 (11%)	1.3	0.045	0.23
Tertiary education and research institutes	180 (26%)	43 (5%)	0.24	0.001	0.11
Other [e]	310 (45%)	570 (60%)	1.8	0.0007	
All industry	690	940	1.4	0.007	0.29
1985-1989					
Industrial radiography	110 (19%)	160 (31%)	1.4	0.026	0.44
Isotope production and distribution	88 (16%)	98 (19%)	1.1	0.025	0.23
Tertiary education and research institutes	160 (29%)	22 (4%)	0.14	0.0004	0.07
Other [e]	200 (36%)	230 (46%)	1.1		
All industry	560	510	0.90	0.009	0.31

[a] The data are annual values averaged over the respective five-year periods and are, in general, quoted to two significant figures.
[b] Values in parentheses are the percentage contribution of that practice to the total number of monitored workers in industry.
[c] The numbers in parentheses are the percentage contribution of that practice to the collective dose from all industrial uses of radiation.
[d] The values of NR_{15} and SR_{15} should only be regarded as indicative of worldwide experience. Reported data on these ratios were far fewer than for other quantities of interest (e.g. collective dose, monitored workers etc.) and were insufficient to form the basis for a more reliable and representative estimate of worldwide levels.
[e] Estimated from the "all industrial activities" data in Table 26 by subtracting the contributions from the three specified practices.

Table 31
Dose monitoring and recording procedures for occupational exposures in medicine

Country	*Minimum detectable level (MDL) or recording level*	*Dose recorded when less than MDL*	*Location of dosimeter (below or above apron)*	*Dose recorded for lost dosimeters*	*Recorded dose (direct measurement or corrected)*	*Multiple entries for the same individual*
Australia	0.01 mSv (x rays) 0.07 mSv (gamma rays)	0	Below	0	Corrected	No
Brazil	0.2 mSv [a]	0	Below	Monthly average		Yes
China	0.03 mSv	0.01 mSv	Above	Estimated		No
China (Taiwan Province)	0.03	0	Below	0		Yes (before 1986) No (after 1986)
Denmark	0.1 mSv	0	Below	0	Direct	Yes
Finland	1.5 mSv (1975-1979) 0.5 mSv (1980-1988) 0.3 mSv (1989-1990)	0	Above	0	Direct [b]	No
German Dem. Rep.	0.2 mSv	0	Above	Average of last 12 months		Yes
Germany, Fed. Rep. of	0.4 mSv (before 1979) 0.1 mSv (after 1979)	0	Below	Determined by controlling authorities	Direct	
India	0.05 mSv (x rays) 0.10 mSv (gamma rays)	0	Above (1975-1988) Below (1989-1990)	Average during the year	Corrected [c]	No
Ireland	0.1 or 0.15 mSv [d]	0	Below	0	Direct	No
Mexico	0.01 mSv	0		4.16 mSv	Direct	Yes
Spain	0.1 mSv	0	Below	Area, other dosimeter or 4 mSv	Direct	No
Sweden	0.1 mSv	0	Below	0	Direct	No
Switzerland	0.1 mSv	0	Below	0 for those exposed to low doses; otherwise based on average dose	Direct	Yes (before 1990) No (after 1990)

[a] Recording level.
[b] Analyses have indicated that recorded doses are overestimates by a factor in the range of 3-30 for diagnostic radiography, which contributes about 60% of the reported doses.
[c] For diagnostic x rays, a factor of 0.5 is used to convert measured quantity to effective dose.
[d] 0.1 mSv for dental and diagnostic radiography and veterinary practice; 0.15 mSv for nuclear medicine and radiotherapy.

Table 32
Exposures to workers from medical uses of radiation
Data from UNSCEAR Survey of Occupational Exposures unless otherwise indicated

Country and period [a]	*Examinations*	*Monitored workers*	*Measurably exposed workers*	*Annual collective effective dose*	*Average annual effective dose*		*Distribution ratio*	
	(millions)	*(thousands)*	*(thousands)*	*(man Sv)*	*Per monitored worker (mSv)*	*Per measurably exposed worker (mSv)*	NR_{15} [b]	SR_{15}
Diagnostic radiography								
Argentina								
1985-1989		2.20	0.83	2.89	1.31	3.46	0.016	0.56
Australia [c d]								
1975-1979	6.1	3.22		1.70	0.53			
1980-1984	7.6							
1985-1989	9.2	6.21	4.42	0.37	0.059	0.083	0	0
Brazil								
1985-1989	15	3.93	1.01	2.99	0.76	2.97	0.009	0.34
Canada								
1975-1979		8.4	4.5	3.23	0.38	0.72	0.0009	0.065
1980-1984		9.5	2.0	1.71	0.18	0.87	0.0001	0.040
1985-1989	27	10.7	2.7	1.75	0.16	0.64	0.0003	0.034
China								
1985-1989	150	78.1	13.3	143	1.84	10.8	0.032	0.45
China (Taiwan Province)								
1985-1989		3.4		1.49	0.44			
Czechoslovakia [e]								
1975-1979	11	5.08	1.27	3.16	0.62	2.50	0.003	0.18
1980-1984	11	6.89	2.22	4.48	0.65	2.02	0.003	0.092
1985-1989	9.5	8.56	2.65	5.84	0.68	2.21	0.003	0.13
Denmark								
1975-1979	2.5	4.28		1.01	0.24		0	0
1980-1984	2.4	4.02		0.64	0.16		0.0002	0.016
1985-1989	2.6	3.82		0.43	0.11		0.0000	0.006
Finland [f g h]								
1975-1979	5.1	3.88	0.084	0.58	0.15	6.93	0.002	0.46
1980-1984	4.6	4.37	0.29	0.71	0.16	2.43	0.001	0.15
1985-1989	4.3	4.82	0.30	0.92	0.19	3.10	0.002	0.28
France [i]								
1975-1979		33.4		39.7	1.19		0.004	
1980-1984	45	49.0	6.05	28.3	0.58	4.67	0.005	
1985-1989	55	61.8	6.35	20.3	0.33	3.19	0.004	
German Dem. Rep.								
1980-1984	19	19.2	3.12	2.05	0.11	0.66		0.08
1985-1989	19	20.4	1.17	1.68	0.083	1.44		0.11
Hungary								
1975-1979		5.96	1.22	2.32	0.39	1.90	0.002	0.11
1980-1984		7.49	1.01	1.61	0.22	1.60	0.0009	0.088
1985-1989		7.26	0.98	1.49	0.21	1.53	0.0007	0.078
India								
1975-1979	41	6.50	3.64	3.75	0.58	1.03	0.004	0.21
1980-1984	61	8.00	3.97	2.76	0.35	0.70	0.001	0.15
1985-1989	82	10.4	5.42	3.54	0.34	0.65	0.001	0.14
Indonesia								
1975-1979		0.98	0.94	1.59	1.62	1.70	0.002	0.022
1980-1984		1.84	1.76	2.94	1.60	1.68	0.0006	0.009
1985-1989		2.30	2.19	3.84	1.67	1.75	0.001	0.015

Table 32 (continued)

Country and period [a]	Examinations (millions)	Monitored workers (thousands)	Measurably exposed workers (thousands)	Annual collective effective dose (man Sv)	Average annual effective dose: Per monitored worker (mSv)	Average annual effective dose: Per measurably exposed worker (mSv)	Distribution ratio: NR_{15} [b]	Distribution ratio: SR_{15}
Ireland								
1985-1989		1.46	0.12	0.55	0.38	4.69	0	0
Peru								
1980-1984		1.37		4.95	3.61			
1985-1989	0.30	1.48		5.10	3.45			
Spain								
1985-1989	23	34.3	30.9	25.9	0.76	0.84	0.004	0.12
Total of reported data [j]								
1975-1979		65.7		54.8	0.84		0.003	0.14
1980-1984		104		48.3	0.47		0.003	0.08
1985-1989		213		194	0.91		0.015	0.40
World [k]								
1975-1979		630		600	0.94		0.003	0.11
1980-1984		1060		720	0.68		0.003	0.05
1985-1989		1350		760	0.56		0.005 [l]	0.22 [l]
Dental practice								
Argentina								
1985-1989		0.070	0.044	0.033	0.46	0.74	0.014	0.42
Australia [c d]								
1975-1979		1.16		0	0			
1985-1989		3.79	1.60	0.021	0.006	0.013	0	0
Canada								
1975-1979		13.1	0.97	0.42	0.032	0.44	0.0001	0.11
1980-1984		19.5	0.94	0.60	0.31	0.64	0.0001	0.13
1985-1989		24.4	0.94	0.64	0.026	0.68	0.0000	0.28
France [i]								
1975-1979		6.17		2.61	0.42		0.0003	
1980-1984		11.2	0.74	2.42	0.22	3.25	0.002	
1985-1989		16.7	0.86	1.97	0.12	2.31	0.001	
Germany, Fed. Rep. of								
1985-1989	17	7.82	0.18	0.39	0.05	2.16	0.0005	0.60
Hungary								
1975-1979		0.24	0.009	0.013	0.055	1.54	0	0
1980-1984		0.32	0.008	0.008	0.026	1.02	0	0
1985-1989		0.24	0.003	0.003	0.012	0.85	0	0
India								
1975-1979		0.37	0.21	0.17	0.45	0.80	0.0008	0.044
1980-1984		0.45	0.21	0.17	0.38	0.80	0.0008	0.060
1985-1989		0.63	0.32	0.24	0.38	0.74	0.003	0.19
Indonesia								
1975-1979		0.019	0.019	0.025	1.31	1.31	0	0
1980-1984		0.15	0.15	0.28	1.84	1.84	0	0
1985-1989		0.099	0.099	0.15	1.50	1.50	0.002	0.024
Ireland								
1985-1989		0.13	0.003	0.001	0.008	0.30		
Italy								
1985-1989		1.01	0.39	0.074	0.073	0.19	0.0005	0.28
Japan								
1975-1979	95	0.35	0.075	0.13	0.36	1.68		
1980-1984	99	1.75	0.20	0.34	0.20	1.69		
1985-1989	96	3.53	0.35	0.56	0.16	1.60		

Table 32 (continued)

Country and period [a]	*Examinations* (*millions*)	*Monitored workers* (*thousands*)	*Measurably exposed workers* (*thousands*)	*Annual collective effective dose* (*man Sv*)	*Average annual effective dose*		*Distribution ratio*	
					Per monitored worker (*mSv*)	*Per measurably exposed worker* (*mSv*)	NR_{15} [b]	SR_{15}
South Africa								
1975-1979		2.27	1.06	0.12	0.051	0.11	0	0
1980-1984		2.82	0.53	1.52	0.54	2.88	0.0007	0.64
1985-1989		3.33	0.37	4.49	1.35	12.2	0.002	0.18
Spain								
1985-1989	9.0	1.29	1.21	1.56	1.21	1.30	0.005	0.1
Switzerland [m]								
1975-1979		7.09		1.21	0.17		0.0009	0.066
1980-1984	2.1	9.13		0.96	0.11		0.0004	0.088
1985-1989		10.7		0.26	0.025		0.0000	0.015
United Kingdom [H1, W4]								
1980-1984	9.0	20		2	0.1			
1985-1989	9.0	20		2	0.1		0	0
United States [n]								
1975-1979		215		80	0.37			
1980-1984		259		60	0.23			
1985-1989	100	307	61	12	0.039	0.20		
Total of reported data [j]								
1975-1979		242		84.5	0.35		0.0004	0.077
1980-1984		322		68.8	0.21		0.0008	0.084
1985-1989		391		18.5	0.047		0.0003	0.12
World [k]								
1975-1979		370		120	0.32			
1980-1984		500		93	0.19			
1985-1989		480		25	0.05			
Nuclear medicine								
Argentina								
1985-1989		0.92	0.25	0.76	0.82	3.08	0.007	0.26
Australia [c d]								
1975-1979		0.67		0.20	0.30			
1985-1989		2.72	1.31	0.44	0.16	0.33	0	0
Brazil								
1985-1989		0.92	0.25	0.76	0.82	3.08	0.007	0.26
Canada								
1975-1979		0.57	0.41	1.08	1.90	2.63	0.012	0.13
1980-1984		0.85	0.55	1.53	1.81	2.80	0.005	0.046
1985-1989		1.14	0.83	2.24	1.96	2.71	0.004	0.039
China								
1985-1989	0.74	6.08	0.71	9.52	1.57	13.3	0.013	0.27
China (Taiwan Province)								
1985-1989		0.38		0.10	0.27			
Czechoslovakia [e]								
1975-1979		0.74	0.22	0.43	0.58	1.83	0.0012	0.035
1980-1984		1.08	0.67	0.99	0.92	1.48	0.0014	0.027
1985-1989		1.46	0.75	1.26	0.87	1.68	0.0006	0.011
Denmark								
1975-1979	0.067	0.45		0.34	0.76		0	0
1980-1984	0.073	0.48		0.30	0.62		0.0004	0.029
1985-1989	0.069	0.50		0.35	0.70		0	0

Table 32 (continued)

Country and period [a]	*Examinations* *(millions)*	*Monitored workers* *(thousands)*	*Measurably exposed workers* *(thousands)*	*Annual collective effective dose* *(man Sv)*	*Average annual effective dose* *Per monitored worker* *(mSv)*	*Per measurably exposed worker* *(mSv)*	*Distribution ratio* NR_{15} [b]	SR_{15}
Finland [f g]								
1975-1979	0.060	0.60	0.018	0.074	0.12	4.11	0.0003	0.044
1980-1984	0.087	0.68	0.080	0.15	0.23	1.93	0.0009	0.072
1985-1989		0.75	0.11	0.17	0.23	1.62	0	0
France [h]								
1975-1979		2.76		3.25	1.18		0.002	
1980-1984		3.37	0.62	1.61	0.48	2.60	0.003	
1985-1989		3.21	0.54	1.03	0.32	1.92	0.003	
German Dem. Rep.								
1980-1984		0.81	0.20	0.54	0.67	2.68		0
1985-1989		0.83	0.15	0.43	0.51	2.84		0.016
Hungary								
1975-1979		0.36	0.029	0.048	0.14	1.66	0.0005	0.086
1980-1984		0.54	0.092	0.18	0.33	1.93	0.002	0.14
1985-1989		0.72	0.14	0.22	0.31	1.62	0.0004	0.014
India								
1975-1979		0.41	0.12	0.22	0.54	1.82	0.003	0.21
1980-1984		0.49	0.22	0.39	0.80	1.82	0.004	0.10
1985-1989	0.17	0.61	0.30	0.52	0.85	1.75	0.005	0.12
Indonesia								
1980-1984		0.009	0.009	0.011	1.23	1.23	0	0
1985-1989		0.013	0.013	0.015	1.20	1.20	0	0
Ireland								
1985-1989			0.023	0.012		0.5		0
Mexico [o]								
1985-1989		0.42	0.26	1.21	2.88	4.63	0.033	0.33
Peru								
1980-1984		0.12		0.43	3.73			
1985-1989		0.13		0.35	2.75			
Spain								
1985-1989		0.92	0.83	1.61	1.74	1.93	0.009	0.11
Total of reported data [j]								
1975-1979		5.66		5.21	0.92		0.003	0.11
1980-1984		7.91		5.72	0.72		0.003	0.048
1985-1989		15.9		16.6	1.04		0.006	0.17
World [k]								
1975-1979		61		62	1.01		0.002	0.087
1980-1984		81		85	1.04		0.002	0.033
1985-1989		90		85	0.95		0.004 [l]	0.096 [l]
Radiotherapy								
Argentina								
1985-1989	0.04	0.27	0.077	0.28	1.04	3.61	0.004	0.097
Australia [c d]								
1975-1979		0.64		1.47	2.30			
1985-1989	0.03	0.78	0.63	0.27	0.34	0.42	0.002	0.17
Brazil								
1985-1989		0.72	0.24	0.90	1.24	3.73	0.018	0.44
Canada								
1975-1979	0.46	0.54	0.35	0.75	1.40	2.14	0.006	0.27
1980-1984	0.49	0.62	0.36	0.63	1.01	1.78	0.003	0.078
1985-1989	0.52	0.72	0.43	0.59	0.82	1.38	0.0008	0.049

Table 32 (continued)

Country and period [a]	*Examinations*	*Monitored workers*	*Measurably exposed workers*	*Annual collective effective dose*	*Average annual effective dose*		*Distribution ratio*	
					Per monitored worker	*Per measurably exposed worker*	NR_{15} [b]	SR_{15}
	(millions)	*(thousands)*	*(thousands)*	*(man Sv)*	*(mSv)*	*(mSv)*		
China								
1985-1989	0.103	2.54	0.35	3.54	1.39	10.0	0.015	0.31
China (Taiwan Province)								
1985-1989		0.36		0.058	0.16			
Czechoslovakia [e]								
1975-1979	0.009	0.76	0.38	1.43	1.89	3.82	0.004	0.049
1980-1984	0.011	1.11	0.69	2.08	1.87	3.01	0.005	0.082
1985-1989	0.014	1.29	0.63	1.83	1.42	2.90	0.004	0.10
Denmark								
1975-1979		0.92		1.95	2.12		0.034	0.37
1980-1984		1.01		1.12	1.11		0.008	0.17
1985-1989	0.015	1.01		0.38	0.38		0.0004	0.022
Finland [f g]								
1980-1984		0.25	0.026	0.054	0.22	2.08	0.0008	0.30
1985-1989		0.24	0.018	0.026	0.095	1.44	0.0007	0.25
France [i]								
1975-1979		4.77		8.77	1.84		0.009	
1980-1984		6.01	1.30	6.08	1.01	4.68	0.008	
1985-1989		6.49	1.23	3.97	0.61	3.22	0.006	
German Dem. Rep.								
1980-1984		1.20	0.31	1.09	0.91	3.57		0.24
1985-1989		1.03	0.17	0.68	0.66	4.00		0.23
Hungary								
1975-1979		0.36	0.14	0.73	2.05	5.15	0.034	0.36
1980-1984		0.45	0.14	0.61	1.36	4.31	0.016	0.24
1985-1989		0.55	0.15	0.61	1.10	3.97	0.012	0.23
India								
1975-1979	0.052	2.49	1.43	3.91	1.57	2.73	0.017	0.39
1980-1984		2.98	1.53	3.39	1.14	2.22	0.009	0.30
1985-1989	0.13	4.17	2.28	3.94	0.95	1.73	0.007	0.23
Indonesia								
1975-1979		0.091	0.086	0.19	2.10	2.20	0	0
1980-1984		0.31	0.30	0.50	1.60	1.68	0.0007	0.017
1985-1989		0.23	0.22	0.35	1.55	1.63	0.003	0.039
Ireland								
1985-1989		0.30	0.14	0.15	0.50	1.05	0	0
Mexico [o]								
1985-1989		0.31	0.26	0.88	2.84	3.41	0.026	0.33
Peru								
1980-1984		0.088		0.54	6.18			
1985-1989	0.004	0.094		0.48	5.17			
Spain								
1985-1989		1.01	0.96	0.88	0.86	0.91	0.001	0.020
Total of reported data [j]								
1975-1979		9.31		16.5	1.78		0.012	0.30
1980-1984		13.3		15.3	1.15		0.008	0.19
1985-1989		18.8		16.6	0.88		0.007	0.21
World [k]								
1975-1979		84		190	2.23			
1980-1984		110		180	1.58			
1985-1989		110		100	0.87			

Table 32 (continued)

Country and period [a]	*Examinations*	*Monitored workers*	*Measurably exposed workers*	*Annual collective effective dose*	*Average annual effective dose*		*Distribution ratio*	
					Per monitored worker	*Per measurably exposed worker*	*NR_{15}* [b]	*SR_{15}*
	(millions)	*(thousands)*	*(thousands)*	*(man Sv)*	*(mSv)*	*(mSv)*		
Veterinary medicine								
Australia [c d]								
1975-1979		0.39		0.055	0.14		0	0
1985-1989		2.07	0.89	0.018	0.009	0.020	0	0
Canada								
1975-1979		0.77	0.24	0.17	0.22	0.73	0.0008	0.11
1980-1984		1.27	0.22	0.16	0.13	0.74	0.0002	0.026
1985-1989		1.52	0.31	0.17	0.11	0.56	0	0
Czechoslovakia [e]								
1975-1979		0.17		0.10	0.59			
1980-1984		0.23		0.14	0.62			
1985-1989		0.25		0.13	0.52			
Denmark								
1975-1979		0.49		0.022	0.045		0	0
1980-1984		0.52		0.030	0.059		0.0004	0.17
1985-1989		0.71		0.024	0.034		0	0
Finland [f g h]								
1980-1984			0.010	0.012		1.20		0
1985-1989			0.018	0.026		1.44		0
France [i]								
1985-1989		1.19	0.087	0.020	0.17	2.30	0.003	
Hungary								
1975-1979		0.081	0.009	0.045	0.55	5.07	0.010	0.42
1980-1984		0.11	0.007	0.006	0.058	0.94	0	0
1985-1989		0.14	0.010	0.028	0.20	2.78	0.003	0.24
India								
1975-1979		0.062	0.021	0.011	0.17	0.51	0	0
1980-1984		0.080	0.026	0.016	0.20	0.61	0	0
1985-1989		0.092	0.035	0.019	0.20	0.53	0.002	0.20
Ireland								
1985-1989		0.04	0.002	0.001	0.017	0.33	0	0
Japan [p] [H10]								
1985-1989		18.0		1.40	0.078			
South Africa								
1975-1979		0.42	0.28	0.013	0.032	0.048	0.001	0.42
1980-1984		0.61	0.20	0.12	0.20	0.60	0.001	0.056
1985-1989		0.75	0.13	0.24	0.32	1.89	0.001	0.068
Switzerland								
1975-1979		0.44		0.12	0.27		0.0006	0.032
1980-1984		0.59		0.13	0.22		0	0
1985-1989		1.03		0.050	0.049		0	0
United Kingdom [W4]								
1985-1989		4		0.4	0.1		0	0
United States [q] [E1]								
1975-1979		18.1	6.2	14	0.77	2.26		
1980-1984		21	12	13	0.62	1.08		
1985-1989		85	38	36	0.42	0.95		
Total of reported data [j]								
1975-1979		19.7		14.4	0.73		0.001	0.12
1980-1984		23.8		13.5	0.57		0.0002	0.027
1985-1989		96.4		37.1	0.39		0.0001	0.016

Table 32 (continued)

Country and period [a]	*Examinations* (*millions*)	*Monitored workers* (*thousands*)	*Measurably exposed workers* (*thousands*)	*Annual collective effective dose* (*man Sv*)	*Average annual effective dose* — *Per monitored worker* (*mSv*)	*Average annual effective dose* — *Per measurably exposed worker* (*mSv*)	*Distribution ratio* — NR_{15} [b]	*Distribution ratio* — SR_{15}
World [k]								
1975-1979		48		25	0.52			
1980-1984		65		26	0.40			
1985-1989		160		52	0.32			
All (human) medical uses of radiation (excluding veterinary medicine)								
Argentina								
1985-1989		3.45	1.20	3.74	1.08	3.12	0.13	0.48
Australia [c d]								
1975-1979		6.23		3.45	0.55			
1985-1989		15.8	8.96	1.11	0.07	0.12	0.0001	0.041
Brazil [D2]								
1985-1989		76	23	115	1.51	4.96		
Canada								
1975-1979		39.6	11.8	10.4	0.26	0.88	0.0005	0.080
1980-1984		51.7	7.88	8.30	0.16	1.05	0.0002	0.044
1985-1989		62.9	10.8	9.18	0.15	0.85	0.0002	0.058
China								
1985-1989		86.8	14.4	156	1.80	10.9	0.030	0.43
China (Taiwan Province)								
1980-1984		3.08		1.77	0.57			
1985-1989		3.98		1.96	0.49			
Czechoslovakia [e]								
1975-1979		6.78	1.89	5.16	0.76	2.73	0.003	0.13
1980-1984		9.38	3.62	7.80	0.83	2.15	0.003	0.079
1985-1989		11.6	4.04	9.12	0.78	2.25	0.003	0.10
Denmark								
1975-1979		6.13		3.32	0.54		0.005	0.22
1980-1984		6.02		2.08	0.35		0.002	0.10
1985-1989		6.04		1.18	0.20		0	0.011
Finland [f]								
1975-1979		4.98	0.18	1.17	0.23	6.55	0.004	0.45
1980-1984		5.60	0.58	1.23	0.21	2.10	0.001	0.12
1985-1989		6.18	0.49	1.22	0.20	2.50	0.001	0.21
France [i]								
1975-1979		40.9		49.3	1.21		0.004	
1980-1984		59.2	8.06	36.0	0.61	4.46	0.006	
1985-1989		73.7	8.19	25.1	0.34	3.06	0.003	
German Dem. Rep.								
1980-1984		24.6		3.34	0.14			
1985-1989		24.9	1.29	2.56	0.10	1.99	0.001	0.18
Germany, Fed. Rep. of								
1980-1984		134	22.2	26.2	0.20	1.18	0.0008	0.14
1985-1989		185	21.9	23.5	0.13	1.07	0.0005	0.16
Hungary								
1975-1979		7.80	1.43	3.19	0.41	2.23	0.003	0.16
1980-1984		9.15	1.26	2.41	0.26	1.91	0.002	0.13
1985-1989		9.07	1.29	2.34	0.26	1.82	0.001	0.11
India								
1975-1979		9.58	5.22	7.89	0.82	1.51	0.007	0.30
1980-1984		11.6	5.74	6.56	0.57	1.14	0.003	0.22
1985-1989		15.2	8.03	8.02	0.53	1.00	0.003	0.17

Table 32 (continued)

Country and period [a]	Examinations (millions)	Monitored workers (thousands)	Measurably exposed workers (thousands)	Annual collective effective dose (man Sv)	Average annual effective dose: Per monitored worker (mSv)	Average annual effective dose: Per measurably exposed worker (mSv)	Distribution ratio: NR_{15} [b]	Distribution ratio: SR_{15}
Indonesia								
1975-1979		1.07	1.02	1.78	1.67	1.75	0.002	0.02
1980-1984		2.16	2.06	3.44	1.60	1.68	0.003	0.01
1985-1989		2.53	2.41	4.24	1.68	1.77	0.003	0.01
Ireland								
1985-1989		1.69	0.28	0.22	0.13	0.78	0	0
Italy								
1985-1989		44.6	12.6	21.0	0.47	1.66	0.004	0.27
Japan								
1975-1979		55.3	21.7	35.7	0.65	1.65		
1980-1984		111	34.2	44.0	0.40	1.29		
1985-1989		142	38.6	46.6	0.33	1.21		
Mexico [e]								
1985-1989		0.73	0.52	2.09	2.86	4.02	0.030	0.24
Peru								
1980-1984		1.58		7.03	4.46			
1985-1989		1.70		7.14	4.20			
Portugal [C1]								
1985-1989		3.83	0.97	2.01	0.52	2.06	0.003	
South Africa								
1975-1979		8.76	5.49	0.57	0.065	0.103	0.000	0.085
1980-1984		10.7	4.13	7.37	0.687	1.79	0.006	0.52
1985-1989		12.1	2.64	9.53	0.787	3.61	0.005	0.23
Spain								
1985-1989		37.7	34.0	29.3	0.78	0.86	0.004	0.12
Sweden [g]								
1975-1979		11.5	1.29	2.84	0.25	2.21	0.006	
1980-1984		12.8	1.38	2.53	0.20	1.83	0.004	
1985-1989		13.2	3.66	3.13	0.24	0.86	0.002	
Switzerland								
1975-1979		21.5		6.20	0.29		0.001	0.12
1980-1984		30.1		4.97	0.17		0.001	0.092
1985-1989		36.1		1.83	0.05		0.000	0.026
United Kingdom [H1, W4]								
1980-1984		39		28	0.71			
1985-1989		40		8.4	0.21			
United States [n]								
1975-1979		485		460	0.95			
1980-1984		584		410	0.70			
1985-1989		734	267	280	0.38	1.05		
Total of reported data								
1975-1979		671		577	0.86		0.003	0.16
1980-1984		1060		588	0.55		0.002	0.11
1985-1989		1520		644	0.42		0.007 [l]	0.34 [l]
World								
1975-1979		1280	650	993	0.78	1.5	0.003	0.14
1980-1984		1890	520	1140	0.60	1.7	0.002	0.10
1985-1989		2220	590	1030	0.47	1.7	0.009 [l]	0.24 [l]

[a] The data are annual values averaged over the indicated periods. They were derived as averages over the years for which data were reported; in some cases, data were reported for only some of the years in the periods of interest here.

[b] The values of NR_{15} are for the monitored workforce. Values for the exposed workforce can also be estimated where data are given for both monitored and measurably exposed workers.

Table 32 (continued)

c The number of workers and the collective dose have been scaled up by a factor of 1.43, since the reported data included only about 70% of the exposed workforce in Australia.

d The method of dose recording was different in the two periods for which data are reported, and this may account partly for the differences in data. Average individual doses for 1975-1979 were calculated from the total of the reported doses for an occupational category divided by the estimated number of workers in that category, with the results rounded to the nearest 0.1 mSv. In 1990 the estimates were based directly on the results of individual monitoring; in the absence of data for 1985-1989, the data for 1990 have been assumed to be representative of that period.

e The number of workers and the collective dose have been scaled up by a factor of 1.5, since the reported data included only workers in that part of the country that was to become the Czech Republic, which contained two thirds of the country's population.

f The numbers of examinations include those in dental practice, which amount to about 1 million per year.

g Some 14% of the total collective dose from all medical uses of radiation has yet to be assigned to one or other of the various categories. Consequently, the reported doses may be small underestimates, particularly in 1975-1985, where most of the doses yet to be assigned exist.

h Reported doses are overestimates because the dosimeter is calibrated in terms of skin surface dose and is worn above aprons when they are used. For diagnostic x-ray radiology preliminary studies indicate that the overestimate may be a factor in the range of 3-30.

i The number of workers and the collective dose have been scaled up by a factor of 1.33, since the reported data covered only 75% of those monitored.

j These data should be interpreted with care, particularly because the countries included in the summations for the respective five-year periods may not be the same, depending on whether data were reported for the period in question, Consequently, direct comparison between data for different periods is invalid to the extent that the data comprise contributions from different countries. It should also be noted that the data on NR_{15} and SR_{15} are averages of data reported on these ratios. In general, these data are less complete than those that form the basis of the summated number of workers and collective doses.

k The estimates are extrapolations of regional values based on the gross national product (GNP); because of insufficient data, the estimates of NR_{15} and SR_{15} are averages of the data reported on these ratios. In general, these data are less complete than those that form the basis of the summated number of workers and collective doses.

l The apparent increase in the ratios in the third period is consequent upon data for China (for which the values of these ratios are much larger than the average) only being included in the period 1985-1989. Excluding China, there is a downward trend in the values over the whole period.

m Data for dentists in private practice only.

n Data from [E1, E2 and E3]. The data are specifically for the years 1975, 1980 and 1985; they are assumed here to be representative, respectively, of 1975-1979, 1980-1984 and 1985-1989.

o In the absence of data for 1985-1989, the data for 1990 have been assumed representative.

p Data are for holding assistants; 1.06 man Sv of the collective dose arose in radiographic examinations and 0.34 man Sv in fluoroscopy. Some 2.4 million radiographs were taken with about 5% on large animals with the remainder on small animals.

q The values for 1985 (the period 1985-1989) are based on extrapolations of earlier data.

r Reported doses are overestimates because the dosimeter is calibrated in terms of the skin surface dose and is worn above aprons where these are used. For x-ray diagnostic radiology, preliminary studies indicate that the overestimate may be by a factor in the range 3-30; about 60% of the occupational exposures reported for all medical uses of radiation are currently reported to arise in diagnostic radiology.

Table 33
Worldwide exposure from all medical uses of radiation [a]

Country/region	Monitored workers [b] (thousands)	Average annual collective effective dose [c] (man Sv)	Average annual individual dose to monitored workers (mSv)	Collective effective dose per unit GNP [d] (man Sv per 10^{12} $US)	Collective effective dose per unit population (man Sv per 10^9)
1975-1979					
East and south-east Asia [e]	4 (0.3%)	7 (0.7%)	1.7	44	21
Eastern Europe [f]	190 (15%)	110 (11%)	0.57	94	280
Indian subcontinent	12 (0.9%)	10 (1%)	0.82	81	12
Latin America					
OECD except United States	360 (28%)	220 (22%)	0.61	74	490
United States	490 (38%)	460 (46%)	0.95	250	2100
Remainder [g]	230 (18%)	190 (19%)	0.84	160	97
Total	1300	990	0.78	130	230
1980-1984					
East and south-east Asia [e]	10 (0.5%)	16 (1%)	1.6	37	41
Eastern Europe [f]	460 (24%)	150 (13%)	0.31	64	350
Indian subcontinent	15 (0.8%)	9 (0.7%)	0.57	33	9
Latin America	60 (3%)	270 (25%)	4.5	350	650
OECD except United States	610 (32%)	210 (18%)	0.35	43	450
United States	580 (31%)	410 (36%)	0.70	120	1700
Remainder [g]	160 (8%)	90 (8%)	0.55	79	48
Total	1900	1100	0.60	87	240
1985-1989					
Asia [h]	96 (4%)	170 (17%)	1.8	440	140
East and south-east Asia [e]	17 (0.8%)	29 (3%)	1.7	56	66
Eastern Europe [f]	430 (19%)	130 (13%)	0.31	38	300
Indian subcontinent	19 (0.9%)	10 (1%)	0.53	30	9
Latin America	110 (5%)	180 (17%)	1.6	220	400
OECD except United States	740 (33%)	190 (19%)	0.27	24	370
United States	730 (33%)	280 (27%)	0.38	58	1100
Remainder [g]	75 (3%)	35 (3%)	0.47	56	42
Total	2200	1000	0.47	54	190

[a] The data are annual values averaged over the respective five-year periods and are, in general, quoted to two significant figures.
[b] Values in parentheses are the percentage contribution of that practice to the total number of monitored workers in medicine.
[c] The numbers in parentheses are the percentage contribution of that practice to the collective dose from all medical uses of radiation.
[d] The normalized collective doses per unit GNP for the three five-year periods are expressed, respectively, in terms of 1977, 1983 and 1989 prices; direct comparison between the values for different periods is possible only after correcting for these different price bases.
[e] Non-centrally-planned economies in east and south-east Asia.
[f] Including the whole of the former USSR.
[g] Includes the remainder of the world for which values are not specifically tabulated elsewhere in the table. Note that the countries or regions comprising the remainder differ in the respective five-year periods.
[h] Centrally-planned economies in east and south-east Asia.

Table 34
Summary of worldwide exposures from medical uses of radiation [a]

Practice	*Monitored workers* [b] *(thousands)*	*Annual average collective effective dose* [c] *(man Sv)*	*Annual average individual dose to monitored workers* *(mSv a^{-1})*	NR_{15} [d]	SR_{15} [d]
1975-1979					
Diagnostic radiology	630 (55%)	600 (62%)	0.94	0.003	0.11
Dental practice	370 (32%)	120 (12%)	0.32	0.0004	0.077
Nuclear medicine	61 (5%)	62 (6%)	1.01	0.002	0.087
Radiotherapy	84 (7%)	190 (20%)	2.23	0.012	0.30
All medicine	1300	990	0.78	0.003	0.14
1980-1984					
Diagnostic radiology	1100 (61%)	720 (67%)	0.68	0.003	0.05
Dental practice	500 (28%)	93 (9%)	0.19	0.0008	0.084
Nuclear medicine	81 (5%)	85 (8%)	1.04	0.002	0.033
Radiotherapy	110 (6%)	180 (17%)	1.58	0.008	0.19
All medicine	1900	1100	0.60	0.002	0.10
1985-1989					
Diagnostic radiology	1400 (67%)	760 (78%)	0.56	0.005	0.22
Dental practice	480 (23%)	25 (3%)	0.05	0.0003	0.12
Nuclear medicine	90 (4%)	85 (9%)	0.95	0.004	0.096
Radiotherapy	110 (5%)	100 (10%)	0.87	0.007	0.21
All medicine	2200	1000	0.47	0.009	0.24

[a] The data are annual values averaged over the respective five-year periods and are, in general, quoted to two significant figures.
[b] Values in parentheses are the percentage contribution of that practice to the total number of monitored workers in medicine.
[c] The numbers in parentheses are the percentage contribution of that practice to the collective dose from all medical uses of radiation.
[d] The values of NR_{15} and SR_{15} should only be regarded as indicative of worldwide experience. Reported data on these ratios were far fewer than for other quantities of interest (e.g. collective dose, monitored workers etc.) and were insufficient to form the basis for more reliable and representative estimate of worldwide levels.

Table 35
Employment in underground mining worldwide
[C20]

Country	Number of miners (thousands)		
	Coal mining	*Other mining*	*Total*
China	1594	64	1658
Czechoslovakia	55	2	57
Germany	105	4	109
India	669	10	679
Poland	251	10	261
South Africa	46	340	386
Spain	38	4	42
USSR	840	40	880
United Kingdom	46	2	48
United States	51	15	66
Other countries	213	265	478
Total	3908 (84%)	756 (16%)	4664 (100%)

Table 36
Exposures to radon and decay products in non-uranium mines

Country	*Year*	*Coal mining*			*Other mining*			*Ref.*
		Number of mines	*Exposure ($WLM\ a^{-1}$)*	*% above 2 $WLM\ a^{-1}$*	*Number of mines*	*Exposure ($WLM\ a^{-1}$)*	*% above 2 $WLM\ a^{-1}$*	
Australia	1991	3	0.2	0	23	0.1	0	[H5]
Canada	1980s				4	0.4	2	[A1]
France	1981	3	0.2	0	5	1.0	8	[B14]
Germany	1990	20	0.1	0				[R5]
	1991				45	1.4	18	[S10]
India	1980s	5	0.02	0				[M12]
	1980s				22	0.8	9	[N6]
Italy	1970s				35	1.2	8	[S11]
Poland	1980s	71	0.3	0.2	26	0.1	0	[D3]
South Africa	1970s				25	1.7	10	[G3]
	1990				40	0.31		[S7]
USSR		47	0.04		26	0.85		[P1]
United Kingdom	1980s	220	0.1	0				[D5]
	1990				41	0.45	7	[B15]
United States	1975	223	0.1	<1	10	0.5	4	[R6]
	1990				99 [a]	1.2		[B12]
	1985				86 [b]	0.12		[E3]
Yugoslavia	1970s	5	0.2	0				[K6]
	1980s				2	1.7	50	[K6]

[a] Metal mines.
[b] Non-metal mines.

Table 37
Doses to non-urnaium miners in the former USSR and in the United States from inhalation of radon and its decay products

Type of mine	*Measurement period*	*Number of mines*	*Number of workers (thousands)*	*Average annual effective dose (mSv)* [a] [b]
Former USSR [P1]				
Coal				0.2 (0.1-0.9)
Other				4.8 (0.02-24)
United States (metal mines) [c]				
Iron	1985		1	6.7
Copper	1985		2.2	0.7
Lead/zinc	1985		3.9	13
Gold	1985		0.58	6.7
Silver	1985		2.9	1.3
Molybdenum	1985		2.2	1.3
Tungsten	1985		0.06	13
Platinum	1985		1	6.7
Total		99	13.8	6.7
United States (non-metal mines) [c]				
Oil shale	1985		0.25	0.07
Limestone	1985		0.85	0.2
Marble	1985		0.08	2
Clay	1985		0.04	4.7
Fluorspar	1985		0.05	0.33
Potash, soda, borate	1985		2.3	0.13
Phosphate	1985		0.1	20
Salt	1985		1.5	0.7
Gypsum	1985		0.08	1.3
Talc	1985		0.2	4.7
Non-metallic minerals	1985		0.04	0.2
Gilsonite	1985		0.11	0.13
Lime	1985		0.01	5.4
Total		86	5.5	0.67

[a] Range of values in parentheses.
[b] The doses reported in [E3, P1] were derived using a conversion factor of 10 mSv WLM^{-1} for exposure to radon progeny. The doses tabulated have been modified from those reported using a conversion factor of 5.6 mSv WLM^{-1}.
[c] Data from [E3]; they are based on measurements at about 40% of mines in the United States.

Table 38
Worldwide collective dose from inhalation of radon and its decay products from underground mining (excluding uranium) and its distribution between countries

Country	*Number of miners* [a] *(thousands)*	*Exposure to radon progeny* [b]	
		Annual collective effective dose (man Sv)	*Average annual effective dose (mSv)*
Coal mines			
Germany	105	59	0.56
India	669	74	0.11
Poland	251	430	1.7
USSR	840	170	0.2
United Kingdom	46	26	0.56
United States	51	29	0.56
Other	1940	740	0.38
Total	3910	1530	0.38
Other mines (excluding uranium) [c]			
Germany	4	31	7.8
India	10	45	4.5
Poland	10	5.6	0.56
South Africa [d]	340	1900	5.6
USSR	40	190	4.8
United Kingdom	2	5	2.5
United States [e]	48 [f]	240	4.9
Other	334	1800	5.4
Total [g]	700	3780	5.4
All underground mines (excluding uranium mines)			
Total	4610	5310	1.2

[a] Unless otherwise indicated, number of miners is taken from Table 35. In the category "Other mines" the number of miners also include uranium miners; corrections are made for this in the totals.
[b] Derived from reported exposures in Table 36 assuming a conversion factor of 5.6 mSv WLM^{-1}.
[c] The numbers of miners include those working in uranium mines and the estimated collective doses are, therefore, overestimates; this is corrected for in the total collective dose but not on a country by country basis. The reported average individual doses are averages over all underground mines excluding coal and uranium mines.
[d] Exposure data taken from [S7] which are representative for 1990; somewhat higher levels were reported in the 1970s [G3] (see Table 36).
[e] Exposure data taken from [E3] (see Table 36).
[f] Value taken from [E3]; it is for all underground miners in the United States except those working in coal and uranium mines.
[g] Uranium miners have been excluded from the total.

Table 39
Summary of occupational exposures to natural radiation (excluding uranium mining) [a]

Occupation or practice	*Number of workers (thousands)*	*Worldwide annual collective effective dose (man Sv)*	*Average annual effective dose (mSv)*
Coal mining	3900	3400	0.9
Other mining [b]	700	4100	6
Aircrew	250	800	3
Other [c]	300	<300	<1
Total	5200	8600	1.7

[a] Estimated doses are appropriate for the latter half of the 1980s. In mining, somewhat higher individual and collective doses are likely to have been experienced previously. Collective doses to aircrew are likely to have been lower previously because air traffic growth over the period.
[b] Excluding uranium mining.
[c] Includes coal-fired power plants (~300,000 workers, collective dose: <60 man Sv) and extraction of mineral sands, phosphate ores and their subsequent use (collective dose: <200 man Sv).

Table 40
Accidents with clinical consequences to occupationally exposed workers
Data from UNSCEAR Survey of Occupational Exposures unless otherwise specified

Country / location	*Year of accident*	*Type of installation or operation*	*Main cause of exposure*	*Persons affected*	*Nature of exposure and health consequences*
Nuclear fuel cycle					
Argentina Atucha	1977	Nuclear reactor	Worker not wearing lead gloves; contamination of a cut caused by edge of the manway plug	1	Wound contaminated with 3800 Bq (surgical removal of a contaminant); mean beta dose of 364 Gy in period 1977-1985 and annual gamma dose of 0.04 Gy in 1 cm^3 of soft tissue; no deterministic effects observed
Argentina Buenos Aires	1983	Critical facility	Failure to follow procedures in removing water from tank containing fissile material	1	Acute whole-body dose of 43 Gy (23 Gy neutron and 21 Gy gamma); death by acute radiation syndrome (neurological) with radiopneumonitis in right lung
France [a]	1979	Nuclear power plant		1	Whole-body dose of 0.34 Gy
German Dem Rep. Rossendorf	1975	Research reactor	Neutron activation of a sample grossly underestimated	1	Dose of 20-30 Gy to right hand; acute and chronic radiodermatitis (2nd and 3rd degree) and oedema
Hungary Paks	1989	Reactor maintenance	Careless handling of detectors from reactor vessel	1	Whole-body dose of 29 mGy; 1 Gy to fingers on the left hand; temporary increase in temperature in left hand; slight increase in chromosomal aberrations
Sweden Nykoping	1978	Research reactor	Instructions for work not followed	1	Dose of 30 Gy to skin of hand; radiation burn to skin
USSR Chernobyl	1986	Reactor accident	Breach of operating rules	237	Whole-body doses of 1-16 Gy and localized doses to skin; 30 deaths; medical treatment including bone marrow transplants
United States Hanford	1976		Intake of ^{241}Am	1	Dose to bone of 8.6 Gy
United Kingdom [b]	1976		Contamination of both hands and feet from mainly beta-emitting radionuclides	1	Skin dose estimated to be about 1.5 Gy; no clinical effects reported
Industrial uses of radiation					
Argentina La Plata, B.A.	1977	X-ray crystallography	Shutter removed from crystallography set	3	Dose of 10 Gy to hands of one operator (radiation burns); doses to others not quoted
Argentina Buenos Aires	1978	^{192}Ir industrial source	Manual handling of source	1	Dose of 12-16 Gy causing radiation burns to two fingers on left hand
Argentina Buenos Aires	1981	^{192}Ir industrial source	Source became detached and lodged in the delivery tube	2	Doses not quoted; radiation burns on finger tips
Argentina Mendoza	1984	^{192}Ir industrial source	Operator pushed source into camera using a finger	1	Dose of 18 Gy to finger (radiation burn on finger tip) and of 0.1 Gy to the whole body

Table 40 (continued)

Country / location	*Year of accident*	*Type of installation or operation*	*Main cause of exposure*	*Persons affected*	*Nature of exposure and health consequences*
Bangladesh [a]	1989	^{192}Ir radiography source		1	Whole-body dose of 2-3 Gy
China [c]	1980	^{60}Co radiography source		1	Whole-body dose of 5 Gy and localized exposure
China Kaifeng City	1986	^{60}Co source	Accidental exposure for about 3 minutes	2	Whole-body doses of 2.6 and 3.5 Gy; moderate haemopoietic type of acute radiation sickness
China Zhengzhou City	1987	^{60}Co irradiation facility	Accidental entry to irradiation room for 10-15 seconds	1	Estimated whole-body dose of 1.35 Gy; anorexia and nausea four hours later; severe damage to haemopoietic system with restoration of WBC was relatively slow
China Zhao Xian	1988	^{60}Co irradiation facility	Accidental entry to irradiation room for about 40 seconds	1	Estimated whole-body dose of 5.2 Gy; acute radiation sickness (bone marrow syndrome); after three years follow-up, condition good
China Beijing	1989	^{60}Co source	Accidental exposure to source for about 4 minutes	2	Whole-body doses of 0.87 and 0.61 Gy; both suffered mild haemopoietic radiation sickness; recovered
China [c]	1989	^{192}Ir radiography source		1	Localized exposure of 18-37 Gy
Czechoslovakia Pardubice	1977	^{192}Ir industrial radiography source	Technical failure of the equipment and improper actions to bring source back under control	1	Whole-body dose of about 5 mSv; data insufficient for estimating local doses; bullous dermatitis of the thumb of the right hand; plastic surgery two years later
Czechoslovakia Sokolov	1979	^{192}Ir industrial radiography source	Technical failure of the equipment and inadequate monitoring during and after work	1	Whole-body dose of about 5 mSv; data insufficient for estimating local doses; bullous dermatitis of the third finger of the left hand and adjacent areas; plastic surgery two years later
Czechoslovakia Prague	1982	^{192}Ir industrial radiography source	Source transport container declared empty on delivery from abroad and handled as if inactive	1	Whole-body dose of about 2 mSv; data insufficient for estimating local doses; bullous dermatitis of thumb of right hand; conservative treatment
Czechoslovakia Petrvald	1985	Dilution, using a needle, of ^{241}Am solution in glove box	Carelessness and inadequate equipment for work with transuranics	1	Intake through wound of ~600 Bq of ^{241}Am; surgical excision of wound and administration of DTPA
Czechoslovakia Prague	1988	Manufacturing of foils containing ^{241}Am for use in fire alarms	New rolling method not tested inactively first; poor radiation protection practice	1	Inhalation of ~50 kBq of dispersed ^{241}Am; hospitalization and administration of DTPA; no clinical manifestations
El Salvador [a]	1989	^{60}Co irradiation facility		3	Whole-body doses of 3-8 Gy; 1 death
France [c] Nancy	1978	X-ray equipment		1	Localized exposure of hand; amputation of finger
France [c] Montpelier	1979	^{192}Ir radiography source		1	Whole-body and localized exposure; amputation of left arm
German Dem. Rep. Freiberg	1979	X-ray fluorescence unit	Carelessness	1	Dose of 10-30 Gy to right hand and whole-body dose of 0.2-0.5 Gy; acute and chronic radio-dermatitis (2nd and 3rd degree)

Table 40 (continued)

Country / location	*Year of accident*	*Type of installation or operation*	*Main cause of exposure*	*Persons affected*	*Nature of exposure and health consequences*
German Dem. Rep. Bohlen	1980	Analytical x-ray unit	Carelessness	1	Dose of 15-30 Sv to left hand; acute and chronic radio-dermatitis (2nd and 3rd degree)
German Dem. Rep. Schwarze Pumpe	1983	^{192}Ir industrial source	Technical defect and inappropriate handling	1	Dose to the right hand of about 5 Gy; acute and chronic radio-dermatitis (1st degree)
Germany, Fed. Rep.	1975	X-ray fluorescence equipment	Carelessness and technical faults during repair	1	Estimate dose of 30 Gy to the fingers; reddening of two fingers after 10 days
Germany, Fed. Rep.	1975	Welding seam test of x-ray equipment	Carelessness and technical defects	1	Estimated dose of ~2 Gy to the stomach region
Germany, Fed. Rep.	1976	X-ray equipment	Inexpert handling of equipment	1	Estimated whole-body dose of 1 Gy; reddening of skin after 24 hours and radiation after-effects
Germany, Fed. Rep.	1980	Radiogram unit	Defective equipment	2	Estimated dose of 23 Gy to the hand and an effective dose of 0.2 Sv
Germany, Fed. Rep.	1981	X-ray fluorescence equipment	Carelessness	1	Partial body exposure with 20-30 Gy dose to the right thumb; extensive tissue damage developing over several months
Germany, Fed. Rep.	1983	X-ray equipment	Defective equipment	1	Partial body exposure to regions of the body of about 6-12 Gy; localized physical changes
Hungary Győr	1977	Industrial defectoscope	Failure of equipment to withdraw source into its container	1	Whole-body dose of 1.2 Gy; slight nausea, changes in blood and increased frequency of chromosomal aberrations; observation and sedative therapy
Hungary Tiszafured	1984	^{192}Ir industrial defectoscope	Failure of equipment and careless handling of source	1	Whole-body dose of 46 mGy; 20-30 Gy estimated for fingers of left hand; radiation burns on fingers of left hand; irreversible necrosis at tip of one finger, surgically removed; slight increase in chromosomal aberrations
Iraq [a]	1975	^{192}Ir radiography source		1	Whole-body dose of 0.3 Gy plus localized exposure of hand
Italy [a] Brescia	1975	^{60}Co industrial radiography source		1	Whole-body dose of 10 Gy; haematopoietic syndrome; death after 13 days
Indonesia Badak, East Borneo	1982	^{192}Ir industrial radiography source	Repair of the source by the operator	1	Estimated doses of 0.77 Gy to the whole body, 0.64 Gy to the gonads and 11.7 Gy to the hands; oedema and suppuration of the hands
Indonesia Cirebon, West Java	1987	Industrial radiography x-ray machine	Repair of shutter while machine was in operation	1	Dose to dorsum of one hand in excess of 10 Gy; oedema and suppuration of the affected hand
India Vikhroli, Bombay	1982	^{192}Ir pencil source	Failure of security during transport of source; source lost and found by a railway worker	1	Dose of 1.5-35 Gy to skin in the region of the groin and whole-body dose of 0.4-0.6 Gy; severe radiation burns in pelvic region with excruciating pain
India Mulund, Bombay	1983	^{192}Ir projector	Operation by untrained personnel	1	Dose to the skin of 20 Gy and to the whole body of 0.6 Gy; severe damage to fingers, four of which were amputated

Table 40 (continued)

Country / location	Year of accident	Type of installation or operation	Main cause of exposure	Persons affected	Nature of exposure and health consequences
India Visakhapatnam	1985	^{60}Co radiography projector	Violation of safe working practices and lack of maintenance	2	Skin dose of 10-20 Gy to operator and 0.18 Gy to an assistant; damage to fingers, one finger amputated
India Yamunanager	1985	^{192}Ir radiography projector	Violation of safe working practices associated with power failure in the workplace	2	Doses of 8-20 Gy to hands of both operators; damage to fingers; two fingers amputated from each individual
India Hazira, Gujarat	1989	^{192}Ir radiography projector	Failure of safety management and improper maintenance	1	Dose of 10 Gy to fingers and whole-body dose of 0.65 Gy; radiation burns on fingers of both hands; fingers amputated
Norway [c] Kjeller	1982	^{60}Co industrial irradiation facility		1	Whole-body dose of 22 Gy; death after 13 days
Peru Zona del Oleoducto	1977	^{192}Ir source	Untrained personnel and lack of supervision; equipment neither registered nor authorized	3	Maximum doses of 164 Gy to hands; 0.9 Gy to lens of the eye; 2 Gy to the whole body; amputation of fingers of two people and effects on left hand of one
South Africa Sasolburg, Tranvaal	1977	^{192}Ir industrial radiography source	Faulty operation of pneumatically operated container and monitor; carelessness of operator	1	Whole-body dose 1.16 Gy; amputation of 2 fingers, rib removal and skin grafts
South Africa Witbank, Transvaal	1989	^{192}Ir industrial radiography source	Detached source; negligence of radiographer (source not properly attached) and failure of portable monitor to register detached source	3	Whole-body doses of three workers: 0.78, 0.09 and 0.1 Gy, all with an uncertainty of about 0.3 Gy; computed effective dose to the most exposed was 2.25 Sv; most exposed worker: amputation of right leg at the hip after 6 months and amputation of 3 fingers after one year
South Africa Sasolburg, Tranvaal	1990	^{60}Co industrial radiography source	Source left behind after radiography work; loss not detected due to inadequate monitoring; source handled by 6 people	6	Cytogenetic analysis indicated that three people received whole-body doses in excess of 0.1 Gy with a maximum of 0.55 Gy; source handled for periods of 5-20 minutes, but local doses could not be estimated with any accuracy; right hand amputated 10 cm above wrist in one case; patches of sensitive skin on fingers of another; blistering of fingers in two other cases
USSR [a]	1975	^{192}Ir irradiation facility		2	Whole-body doses of 3 and 5 Gy; dose to hands over 30 Gy
USSR [c]	1976	^{60}Co irradiation facility		1	Whole-body dose of 4 Gy; radiation sickness, haematopoietic syndrome
USSR [a]	1980	^{60}Co irradiation facility		1	Dose of 50 Gy to lens
United Kingdom	1977	Filling gaseous tritium light sources	Broken inlet manifold led to the release of escape of ~11-15 TBq of tritium	2	Whole-body doses: 0.62 and 0.64 Sv
United Kingdom [b]	1977	^{192}Ir radiography source	Operator working in a confined area held source for 90 seconds while radiographing a weld	1	Cytogenetic dosimetry estimated an equivalent whole-body dose <0.1 Gy; radiation burns on three fingers
United Kingdom [b]	1978	^{192}Ir radiography source	Radiographer deliberately overexposed himself	1	Cytogenetic dosimetry estimated an equivalent whole-body dose of 1.52 Gy; no localized skin reactions
United Kingdom [b]	1983	Gamma radiography source	Inadvertent exposure of radiographer	1	Whole-body dose of 0.56 Gy

Table 40 (continued)

Country / location	*Year of accident*	*Type of installation or operation*	*Main cause of exposure*	*Persons affected*	*Nature of exposure and health consequences*
United States [c] Pittsburgh	1976	^{192}Ir radiography source		1	Dose of 10 Gy to hand
United States [c] Rockaway	1977	^{60}Co industrial irradiation source		1	Whole-body dose of 2 Gy
United States [c] Monroe	1978	^{192}Ir radiography source		1	Localized exposure of hand; amputation of finger
United States [c] Los Angeles	1979	^{192}Ir radiography source	Source found by worker and put in his pocket for 45 minutes	5	Whole-body exposure of 1 Gy and localized exposures of hand to one person; localized exposure of hands of four others
United States [c] Oklahoma	1981	^{192}Ir radiography source		1	Whole-body and localized exposures
Tertiary education and accelerators					
German Dem. Rep. Halle	1975	X-ray fluorescence unit	Carelessness	1	Dose of 1.2-2 Gy to middle finger of left hand; acute radiodermatitis (1st degree)
German Dem. Rep. Rossendorf	1980	Radiochemical laboratory	Defect in protective glove led to contamination with ^{32}P	1	Dose of 100 Gy to the skin of the left hand; no clinical symptoms
German Dem. Rep. Berlin	1981	Analytical x-ray unit	Carelessness	1	Dose of 5 Gy to the left hand; acute radiodermatitis (1st degree)
German Dem. Rep. Berlin	1982	Analytical x-ray unit	Carelessness	1	Dose of 6 to 18 Gy to right forefinger; acute radiodermatitis (2nd degree)
German Dem. Rep. Leipzig	1983	Radiochemical laboratory	Explosion of vial containing a ^{241}Am solution	1	Committed effective dose of 0.076 Gy
German Dem. Rep. Jena	1988	Analytical x-ray unit	Carelessness	1	Dose of 3 Gy to left hand; acute radiodermatitis (1st degree)
German Dem. Rep. Trusetal	1988	Analytical x-ray unit	Technical defect	2	Maximum dose of 4 Gy to the hand of one person; acute radiodermatitis (1st degree) in one person
Germany, Fed. Rep.	1979	X-ray equipment	Defective equipment	1	Estimated dose to part of the hand 20 Gy and effective dose of 0.6 mSv
Peru Lima	1984	X-ray diffraction equipment	Fault of supervision, deliberate exposure from lack of knowledge of risk; equipment not registered with authorities	6	Localized doses of 5-40 Gy to fingers; skin burns and blistering leaving residual scar tissue
USSR [a]	1977	Protein accelerator		1	Localized dose of 10-30 Gy to hands

Table 40 (continued)

Country / location	*Year of accident*	*Type of installation or operation*	*Main cause of exposure*	*Persons affected*	*Nature of exposure and health consequences*
USSR [a]	1978	Electron accelerator		1	Localized dose of 20 Gy to hands
United States [c]	1978	Accelerator		1	Localized exposure of abdomen, hands and thighs
Medical uses of radiation					
Argentina Tucuman	1975	^{60}Co teletherapy	Failure of source's mechanical dispositive	2	Technician and physician both received high doses to fingers; radiation burns on fingers
Argentina Parana	1979	Diagnostic radiology	Faulty wiring led to emission of x rays when the to of the fluoroscope was open	1	Auxiliary nurse received whole-body dose of 0.94 Gy; slight depression of bone marrow
Argentina La Plata, B.A.	1982	X-ray therapy facility	Operator looked through window while changing x-ray tubes without recognizing system was energized	1	Whole-body dose of 0.12 Gy and dose of 5.8 Gy to lens of eye; cataracts in both eyes
Argentina Buenos Aires	1983	^{60}Co teletherapy	Source jammed during transfer	2	Doses of 0.66 and 0.67 Gy, respectively, to the thorax; slight bone marrow depression
Germany, Fed. Rep. of	1975	X-ray equipment	Probably carelessness in maintenance	1	Dose in excess of 1 Gy to head and upper torso
Germany, Fed. Rep. of	1977	^{192}Ir radiogram unit	Defective equipment	1	Estimated dose to hands of about 5 Gy and effective dose of 0.01 mSv; temporary reddening of fingers
India Ludihana	1980	Radiotherapy (telegamma)	Defective equipment (mercury leaked out through shutter)	3 [d]	Doses of 0.25, 0.4 and 0.5 Gy; no adverse health effects observed
United Kingdom [b]	1975	^{60}Co radiotherapy source	Source jammed in an unshielded position during servicing	2	Personal dosimeters recorded doses of 0.52 and 0.4 Sv
United Kingdom [b]	1977	^{125}I	Accidental contamination of laboratory workers	2	Thyroid dose of ~1.7 Gy to one person from an intake of about 1 MBq; a low dose to other person
United Kingdom [b]	1982	X-ray radiography	Inadvertent exposure to x rays	1	Personal dosimeter recorded a dose of 0.32 Sv
United Kingdom [b]	1985	^{125}I	Technician cut his finger while wearing a glove contaminated with iodine-125; sucked cut finger, which resulted in an intake of about 740 MBq	1	Thyroid dose of about 400 Gy
United Kingdom [b]	1986	^{60}Co radiotherapy source	Exposure during source changing	1	Dose of 15 Gy to the hand; erythema and blistering appeared two weeks later

[a] Data from [I11].
[b] Data comprise a summary of cases of accidental exposure for which chromosome aberration analysis have been undertaken [L1].
[c] Data from [R3].
[d] Unclear whether exposed were workers or patients.

Table 41
Worldwide occupational exposures 1985-1989

Occupational category	*Average annual number of monitored workers (thousands)*	*Annual average collective effective dose (man Sv)*	*Annual average effective dose to monitored workers (mSv)*	*Normalized collective effective dose [man Sv (GW a)$^{-1}$]*	*NR_{15}*	*SR_{15}*
Nuclear fuel cycle						
Mining	260	1100	4.4	4.3	0.25 [a]	0.52 [a]
Milling	18	120	6.3	0.44	0.18 [a]	0.43 [a]
Enrichment	5	0.4	0.08	0.02	0	0
Fuel fabrication						
LWRs	24	11	0.45	0.07	0.0003	0.015
HWRs	1.1	1.9	1.7	0.22	0.003	0.042
Magnox	1.1	3.5	3.1	1.4	0.018	
AGRs	1.9	5.5	3.0	0.45	0.014	
Total	28	22	0.78	0.12	0.002	0.019
Reactor operation						
PWRs	230	500	2.2	4.3	0.034	0.328
BWRs	140	310	2.4	7.9	0.026	0.36
HWRs	18	67	3.4	6.2	0.066	0.48
LWGRs	13	170	13	17		
GCRs	31	24	0.75	3.2	0.0002	0.008
Other	3	1	0.4	1.4		
Total	430	1100	2.5	5.9	0.033	0.34
Fuel reprocessing						
Oxide	4	5.7	1.4	0.65	0.008	0.12
Magnox	8	31	3.8	11	0.092	
Total	12	36	3.0	3.2	0.064	0.12
Research	130	100	0.8	1.0	0.011	0.30
Total	880	2500	2.9	12 [b]	0.10 [a]	0.42 [a]
Defence activities						
Weapons	60	43	0.7			
Ships	190	170	0.9			
Other	130	37	0.3			
Total	380	250	0.7			
Industrial uses of radiation						
Total	560	510	0.9		0.009	0.31
Medical uses of radiation						
Total	2200	1000	0.5		0.009	0.24
Natural sources of radiation (excluding uranium mining)						
Coal mining	3900	3400	0.9			
Other mining	700	4100	6			
Air crew	250	800	3			
Other	~300	<300	<1			
Total	5200	8600	1.7			
Total of exposures						
Man-made	4000	4300	1.1		0.03 [a]	0.36 [a]
Natural sources	5200	8600	1.7			
Total	9200	13000	1.4			

[a] Values for mining and milling are averages of reported values and are overestimates for the revised conversion factor of 5.6 mSv WLM^{-1}. The entries for the totals are thus also overestimates. Excluding mining and milling from the averaging, the entries for total of the nuclear fuel cycle would be 0.03 and 0.32 and for total of man-made exposures 0.01 and 0.29 for NR_{15} and SR_{15}, respectively.

[b] Excluding fuel reprocessing.

Table 42
Trends in worldwide occupational exposures from man-made sources of radiation

Source	*Average annual collective effective dose (man Sv)*			*Average annual effective dose to monitored workers (mSv)*		
	1975-1979	*1980-1984*	*1985-1989*	*1975-1979*	*1980-1984*	*1985-1989*
Nuclear fuel cycle	2300	3000	2500	4.1	3.7	2.9
Defence activities	420	250	250	1.3	0.71	0.66
Industrial uses of radiation	870	940	510	1.6	1.4	0.9
Medical uses of radiation	1000	1140	1030	0.78	0.60	0.47
Total	5490	5330	4290	1.9	1.4	1.1
	Average annual number of monitored workers (thousands)			*Normalized collective effective dose [man Sv $(GW\ a)^{-1}$]*		
	1975-1979	*1980-1984*	*1985-1989*	*1975-1979*	*1980-1984*	*1985-1989*
Nuclear fuel cycle	560	800	880	18 [a]	17 [a]	12 [a]
Defence activities	310	350	380			
Industrial uses of radiation	530	690	560			
Medical uses of radiation	1280	1890	2220			
Total	2680	3730	4040			
	NR_{15}			*SR_{15}*		
	1975-1979	*1980-1984*	*1985-1989*	*1975-1979*	*1980-1984*	*1985-1989*
Nuclear fuel cycle [b]	0.20	0.16	0.10	0.63	0.55	0.42
Defence activities						
Industrial uses of radiation	0.010	0.007	0.009	0.35	0.28	0.31
Medical uses of radiation	0.003	0.002	0.009	0.14	0.10	0.24
Total	0.051	0.040	0.030	0.045	0.40	0.36

[a] Values excluding fuel reprocessing; the normalized doses would be greater by about 1 man Sv $(GW\ a)^{-1}$ for reprocessing of oxide fuel and about 10-15 man Sv $(GW\ a)^{-1}$ for reprocessing metal Magnox fuel (with the higher value pertaining to earlier times).

[b] Values are averages including mining and milling as reported and are thus overestimates for the revised conversion factor of 5.6 mSv WLM^{-1}. If mining and milling are excluded from the averaging, the values of NR_{15} would be about a factor of 3 lower and the values of SR_{15} would decreease by an absolute amount of about 0.1.

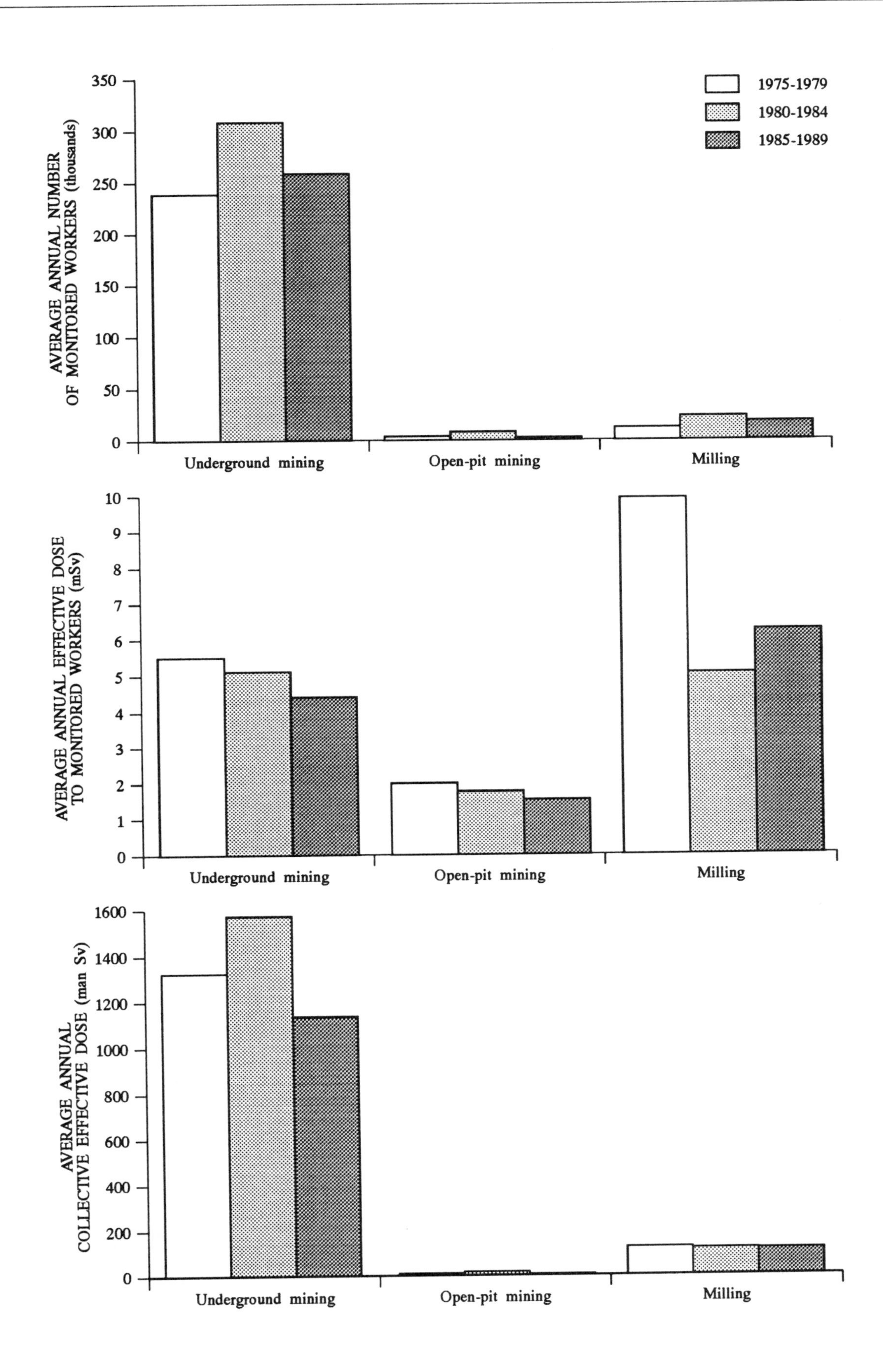

Figure I.
Number of workers and doses to workers in uranium mining and milling.

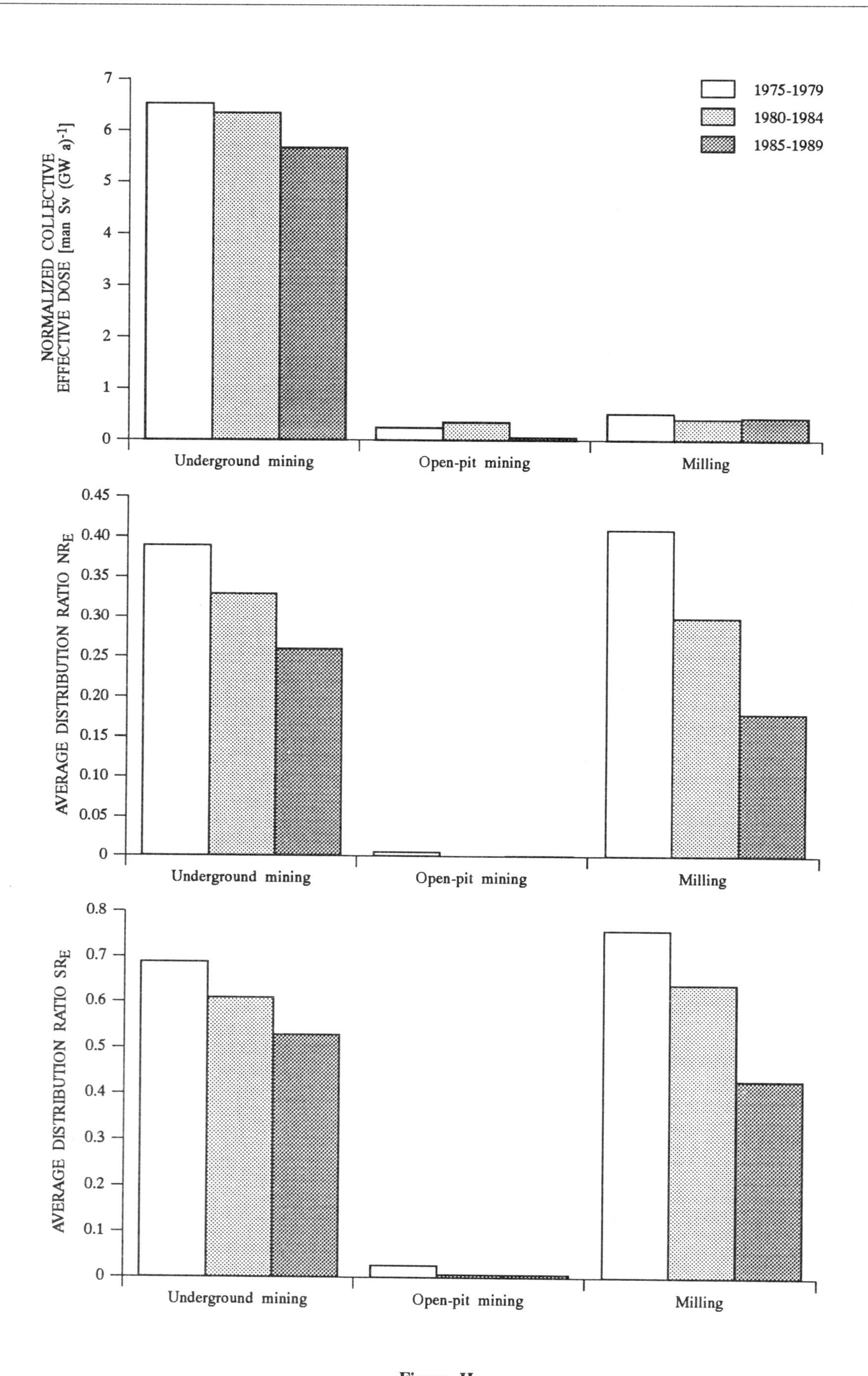

Figure II.
Normalized collective dose and distribution ratios for workers in uranium mining and milling.

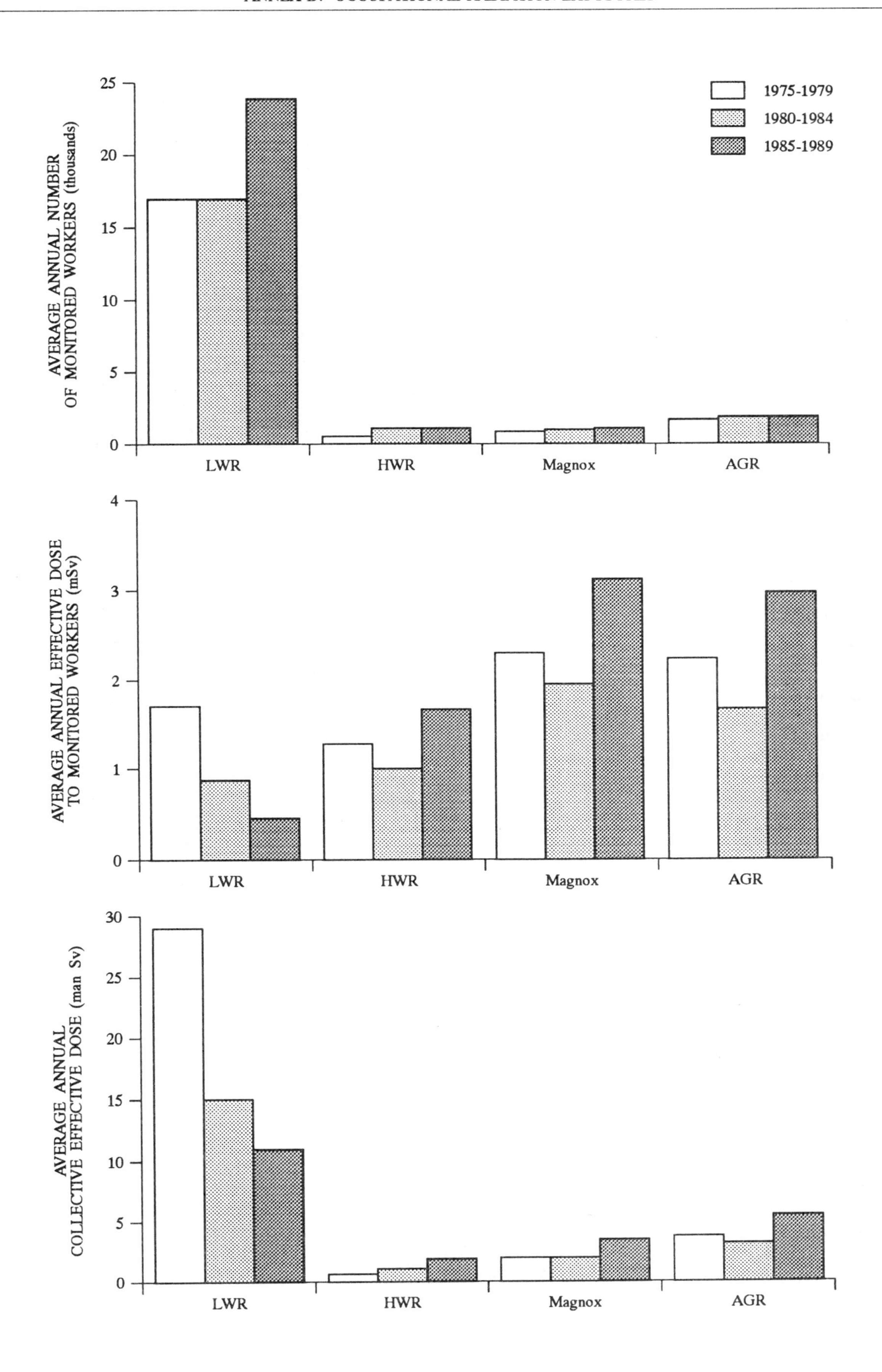

Figure III.
Number of workers and doses to workers in fuel fabrication.

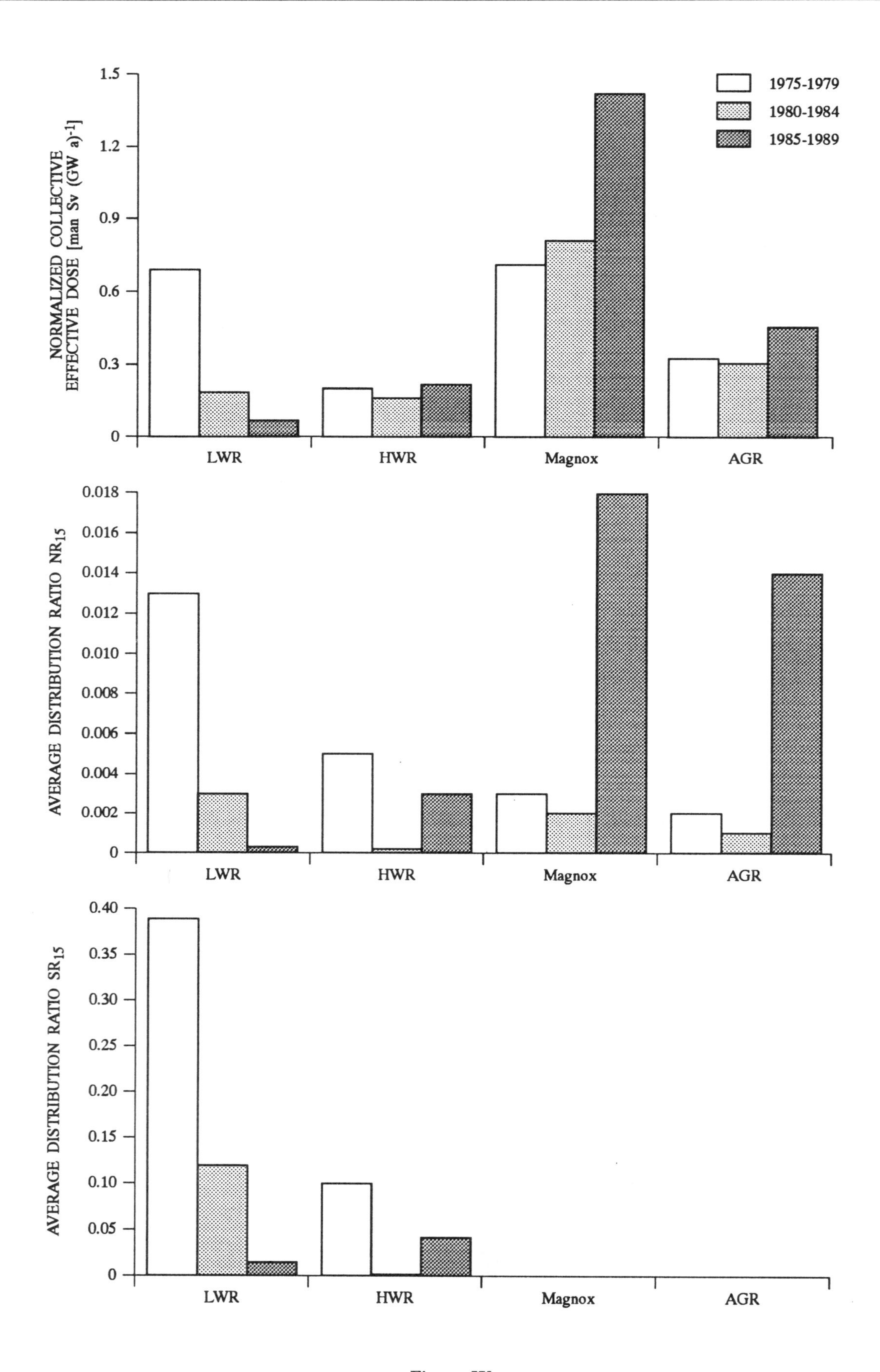

Figure IV.
Normalized collective dose and distribution ratios for workers in fuel fabrication.

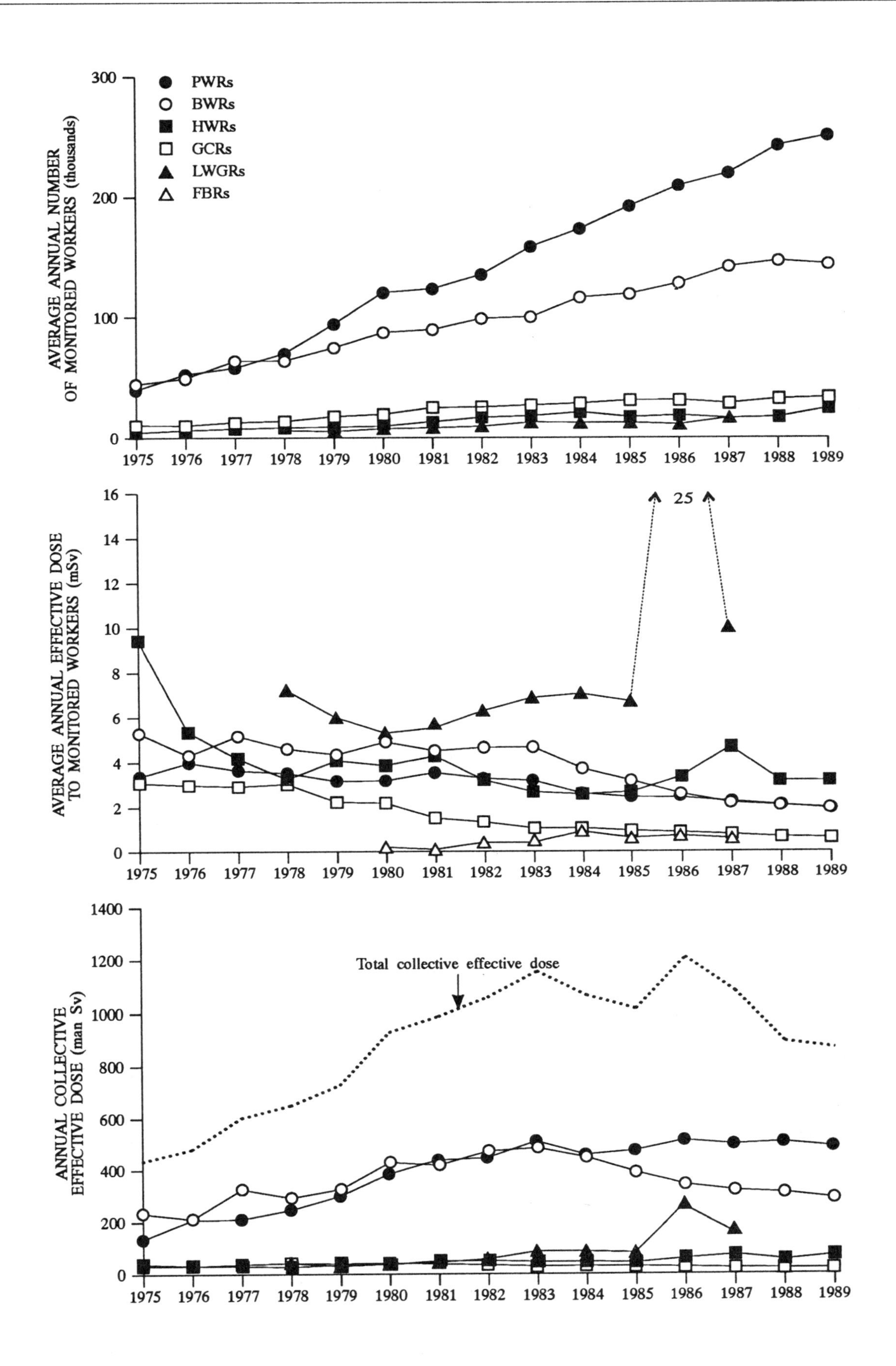

Figure V.
Number of workers and doses to workers in reactors.

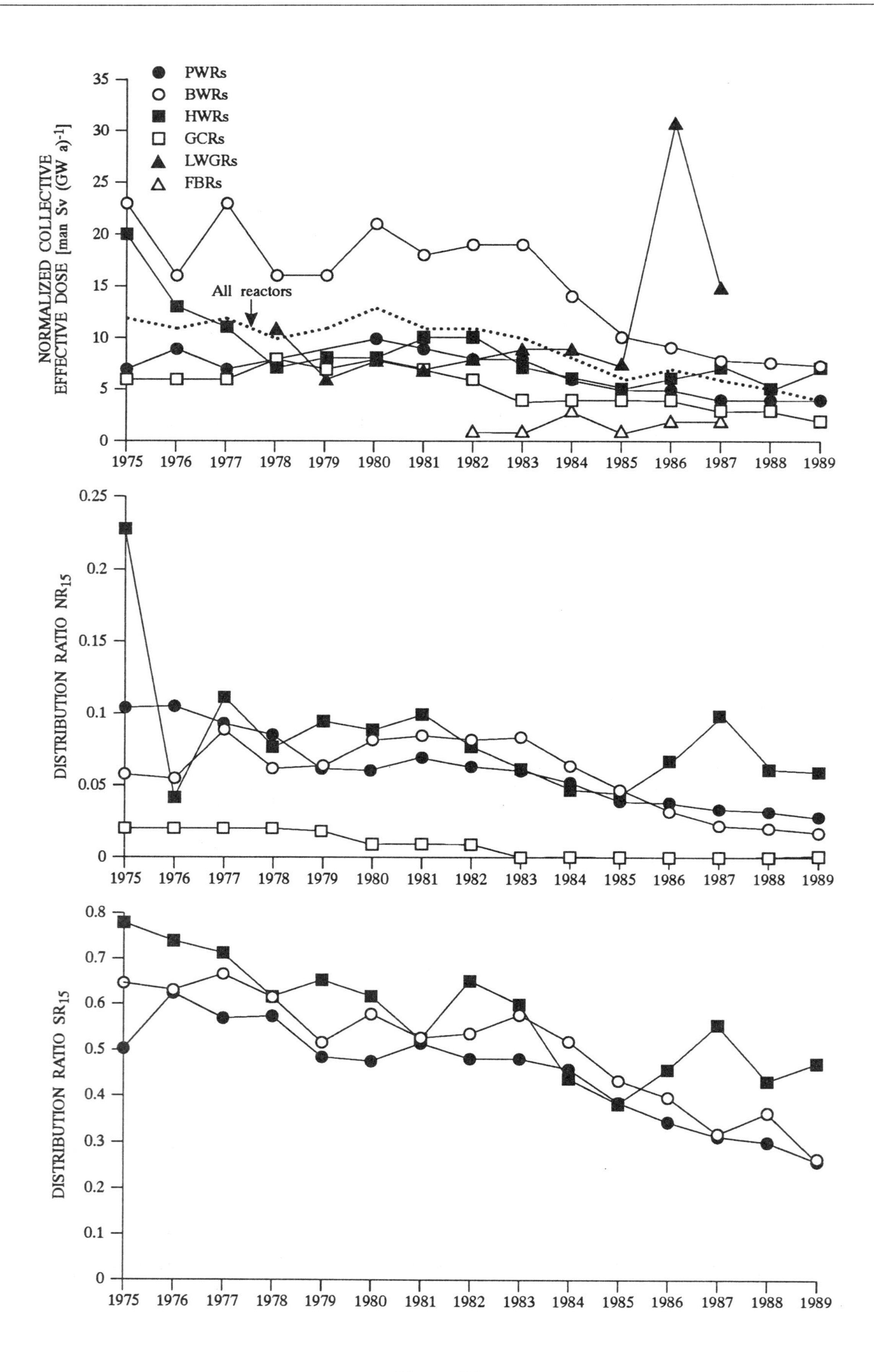

Figure VI.
Normalized collective dose and distribution ratios for reactor workers.

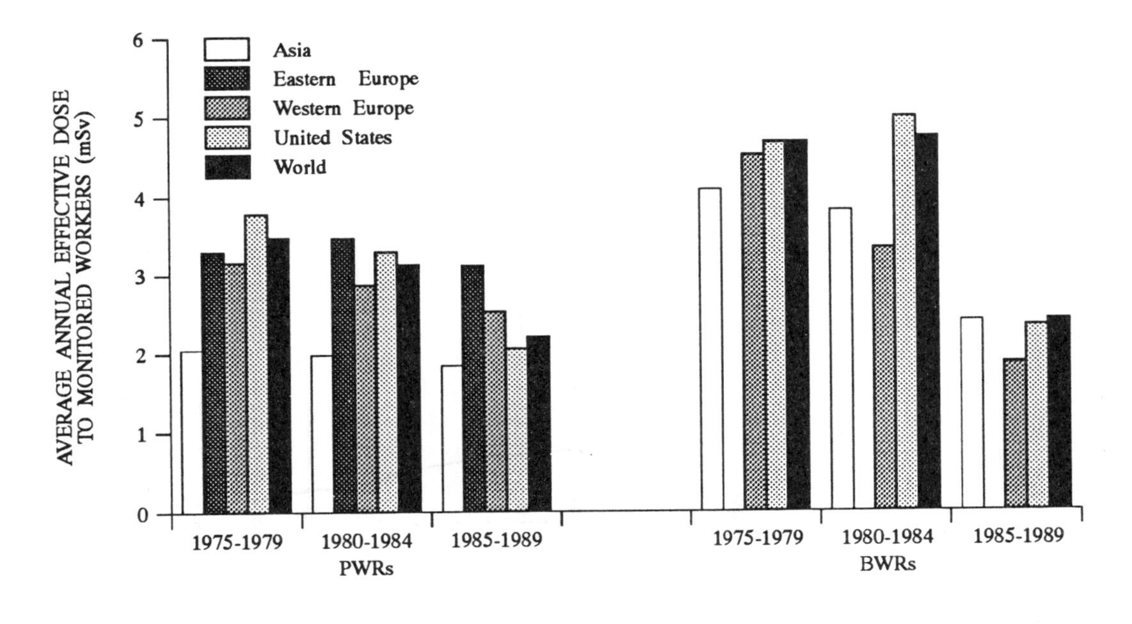

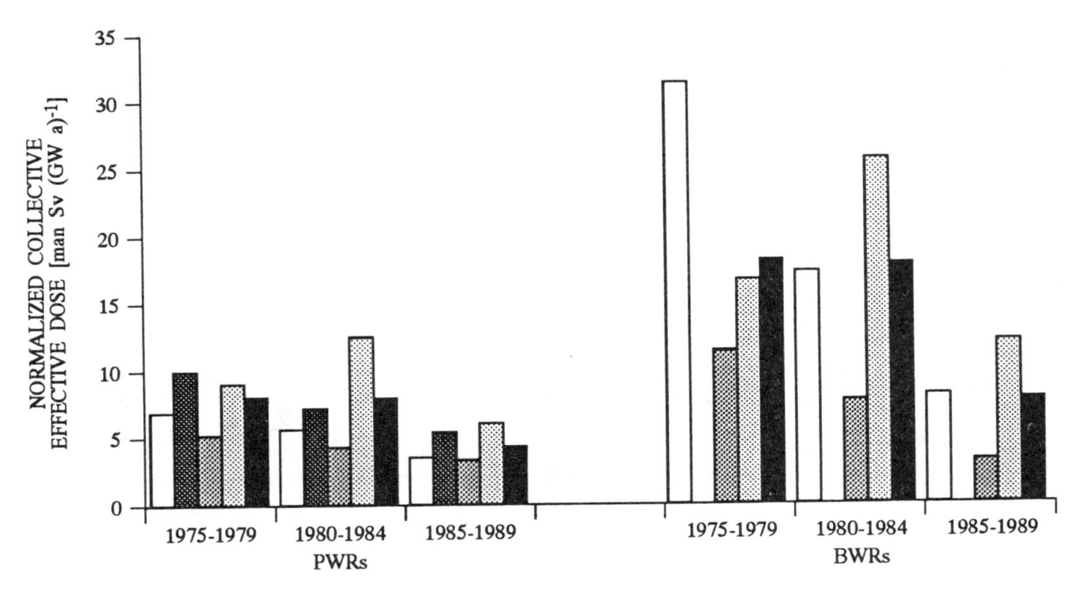

Figure VII.
Regional variations in average annual individual and normalized collective effective doses to workers at LWRs.

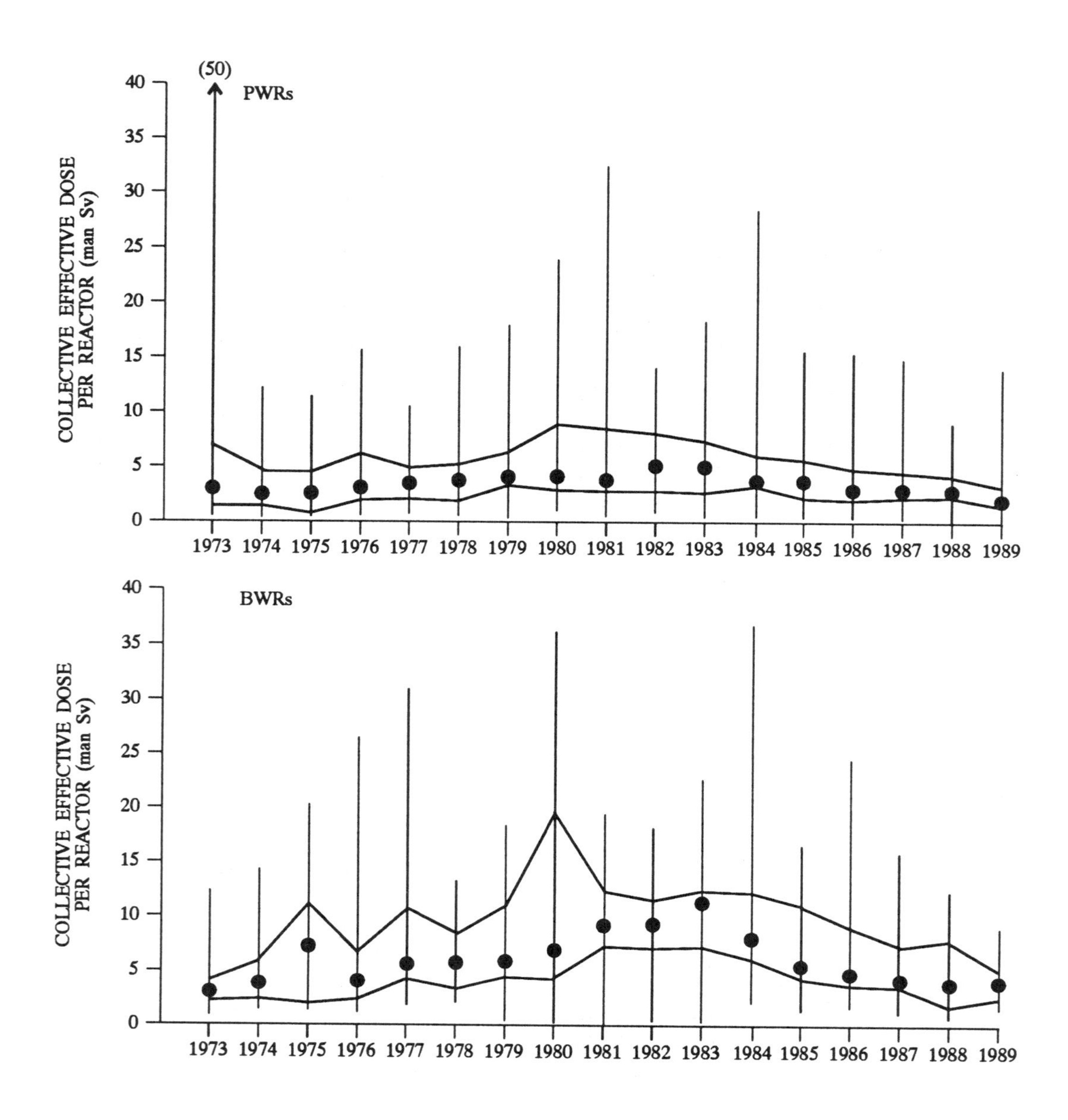

Figure VIII.
Collective dose per reactor to workers in LWRs in the United States.
Median and extreme values with envelope of middle 50% values.
[B3]

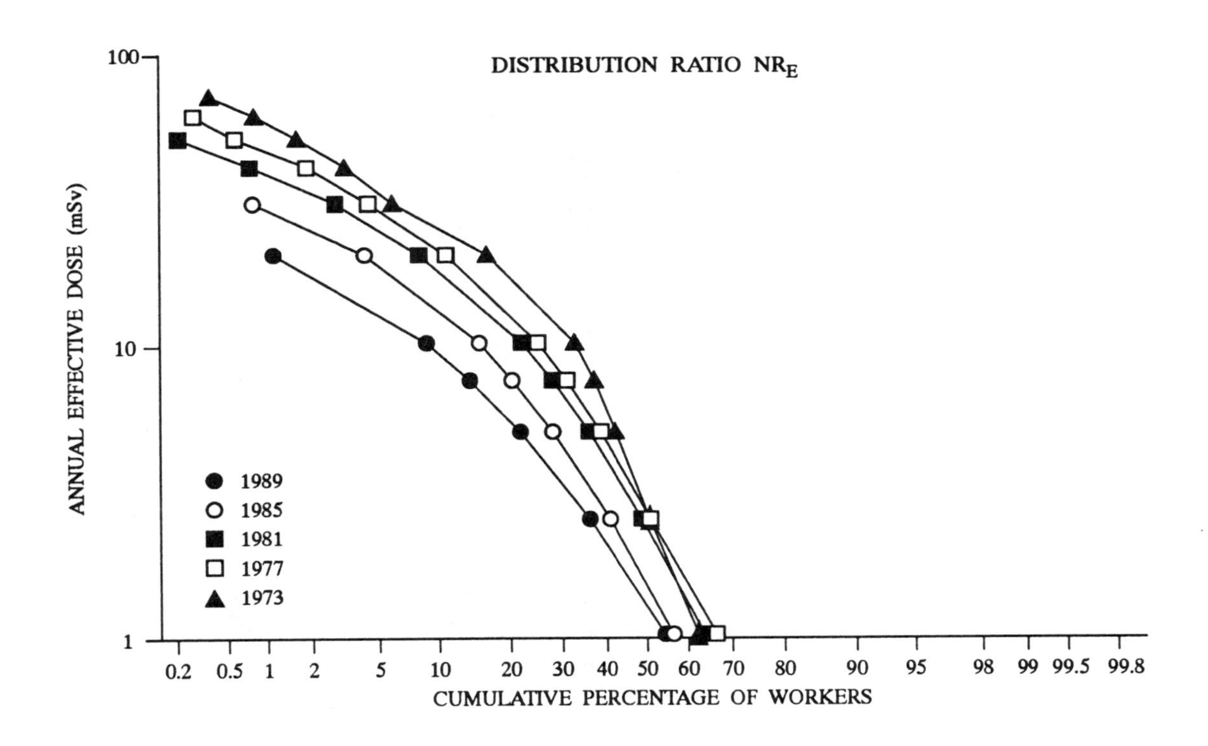

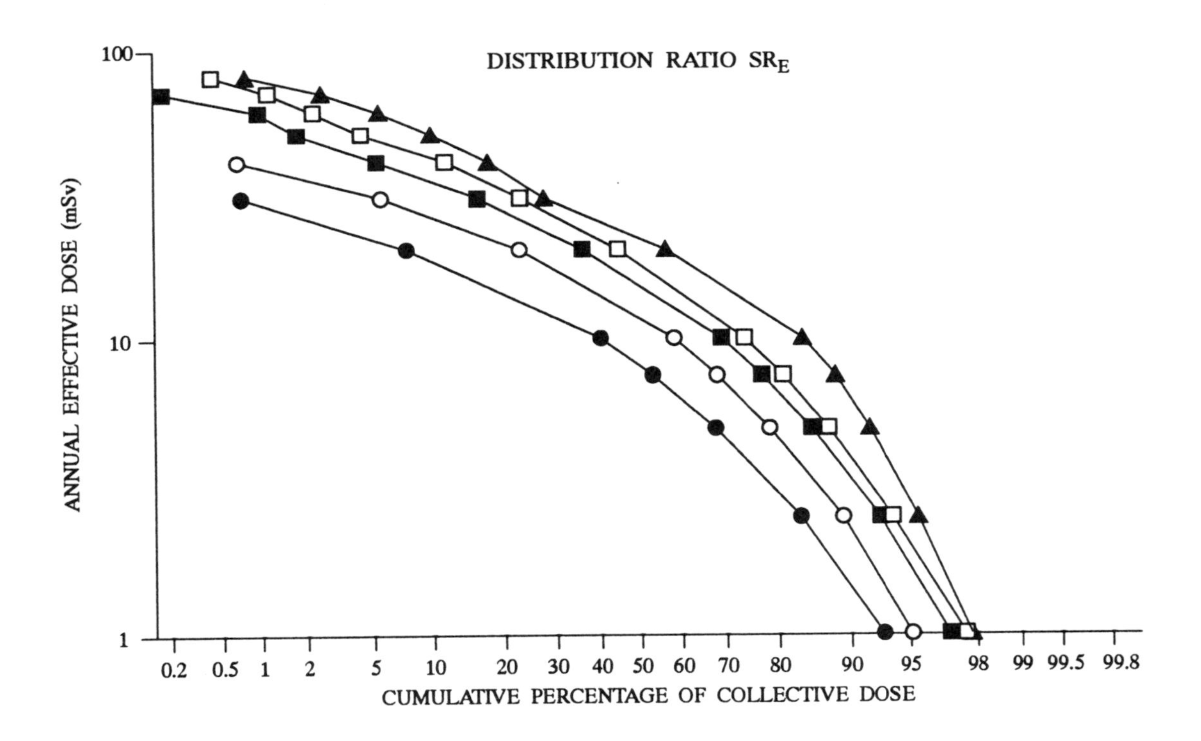

Figure IX.
Cumulative distribution of number of workers and collective dose from workers at LWRs in the United States with doses in excess of the specified values.

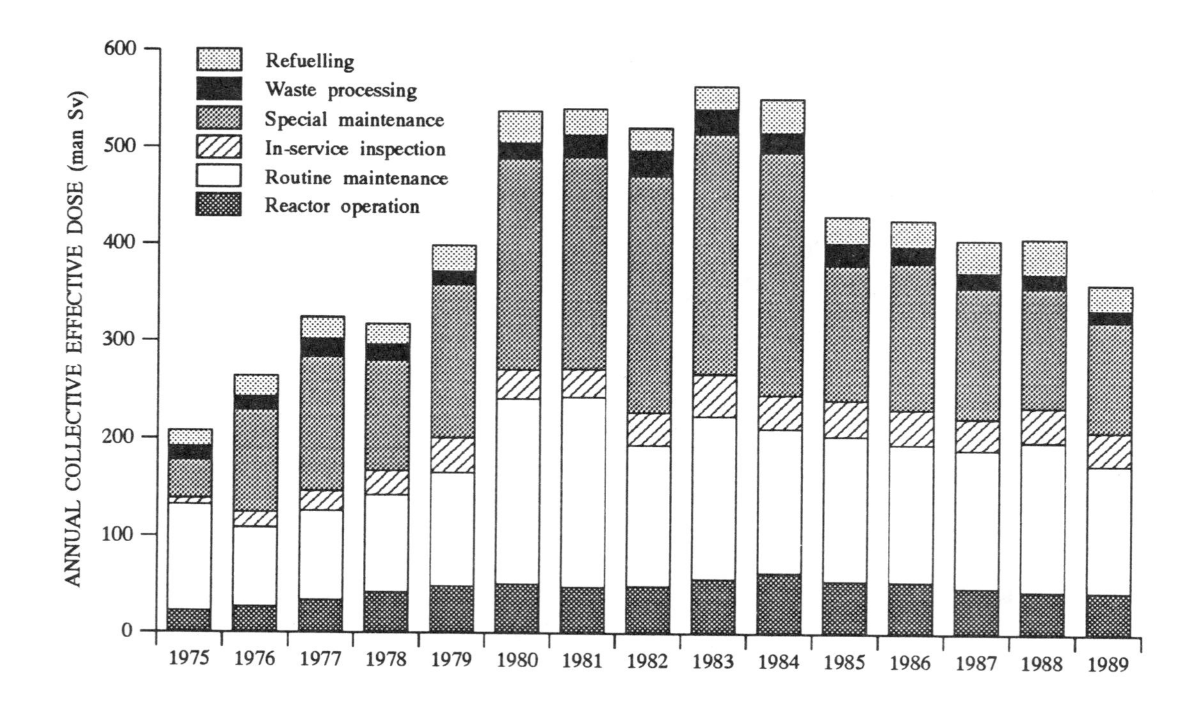

Figure X.
Distribution of collective dose among work functions for workers at LWRs in the United States.

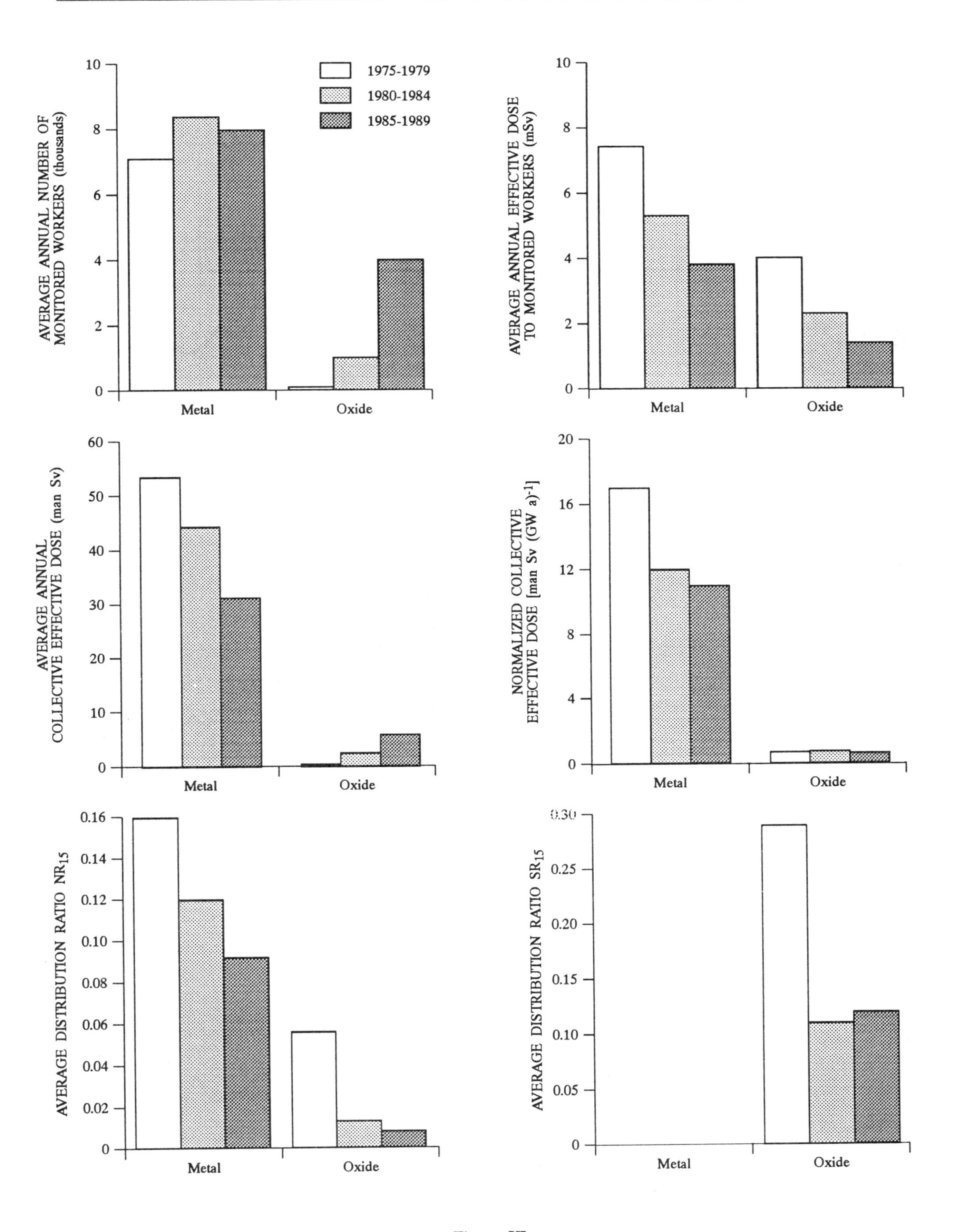

Figure XI.
Number of workers, doses and distribution ratios in fuel reprocessing.

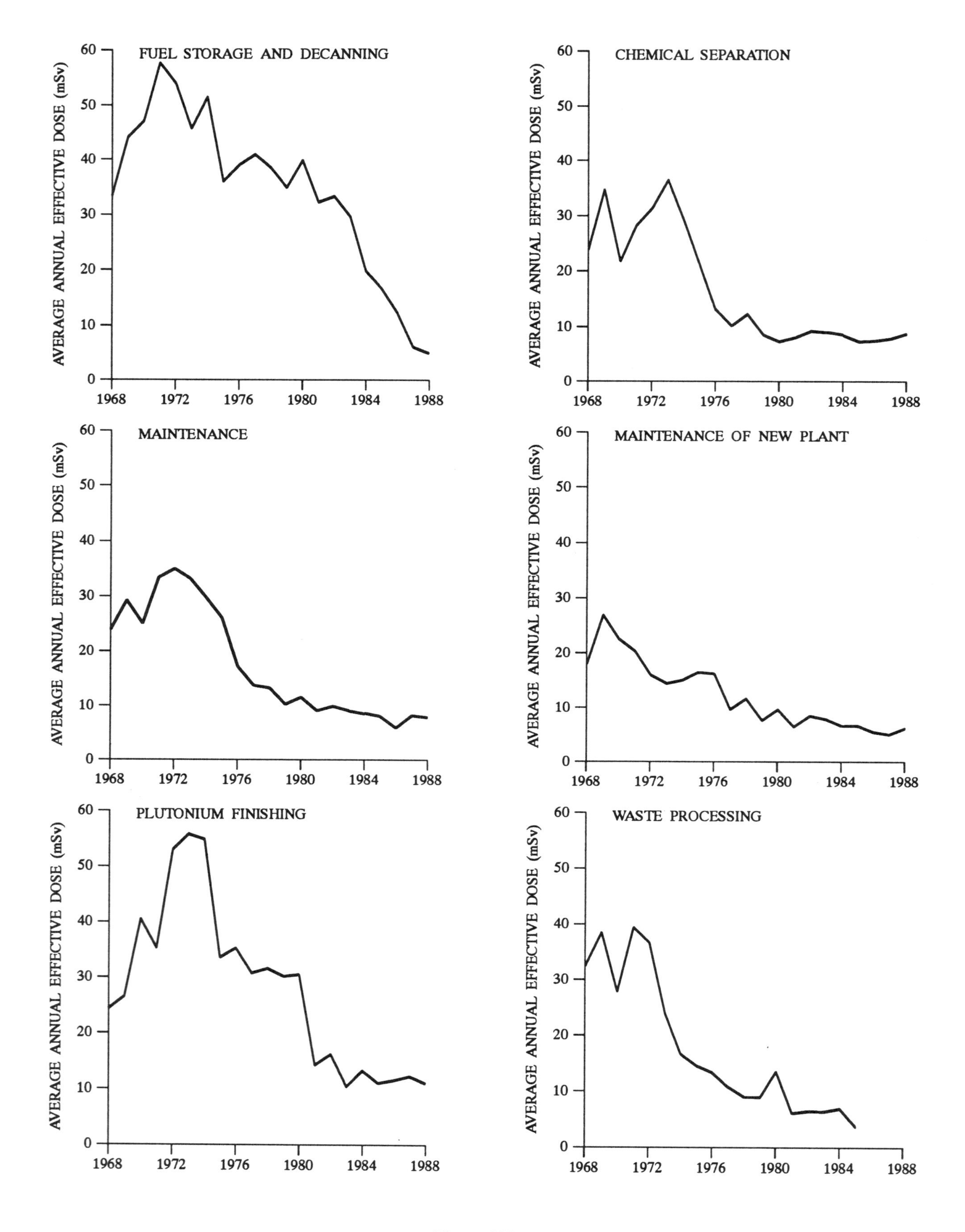

Figure XII.
Variations in average annual effective dose to groups of reprocessing workers at Sellafield, United Kingdom. [S5]

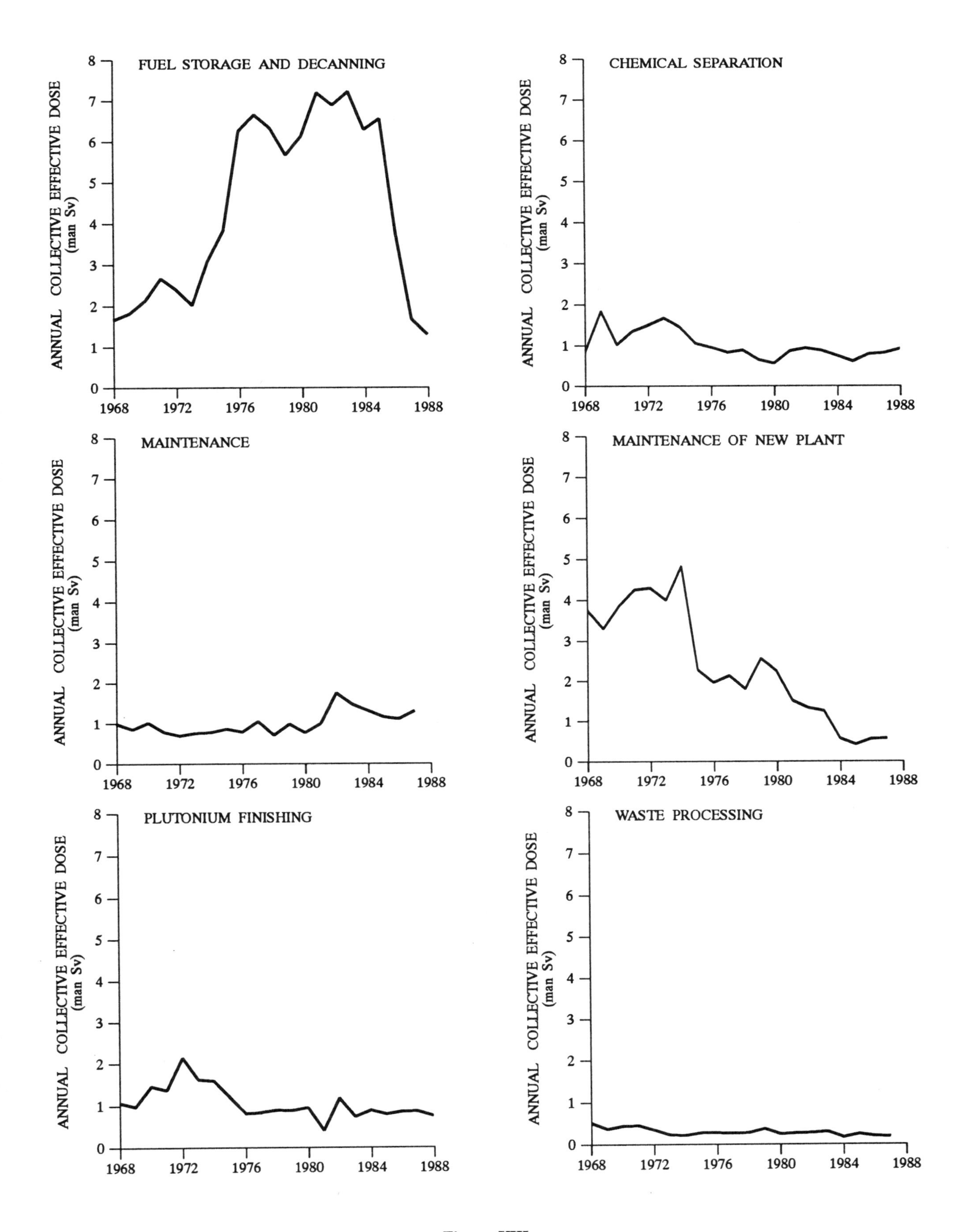

Figure XIII.
Variations in collective effective dose to groups of reprocessing workers at Sellafield, United Kingdom. [S5]

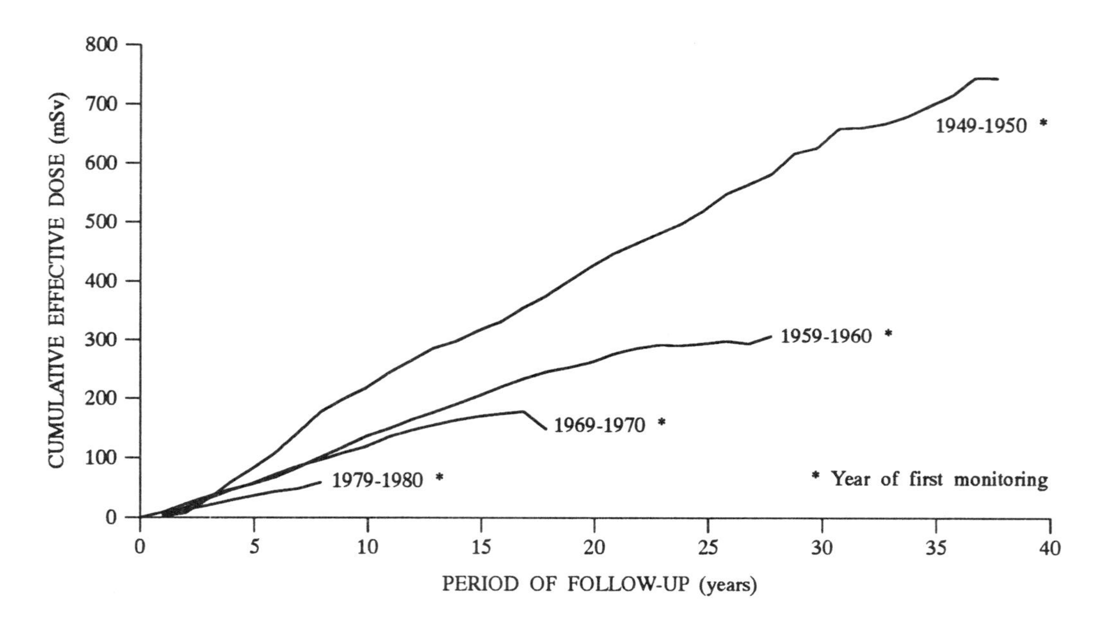

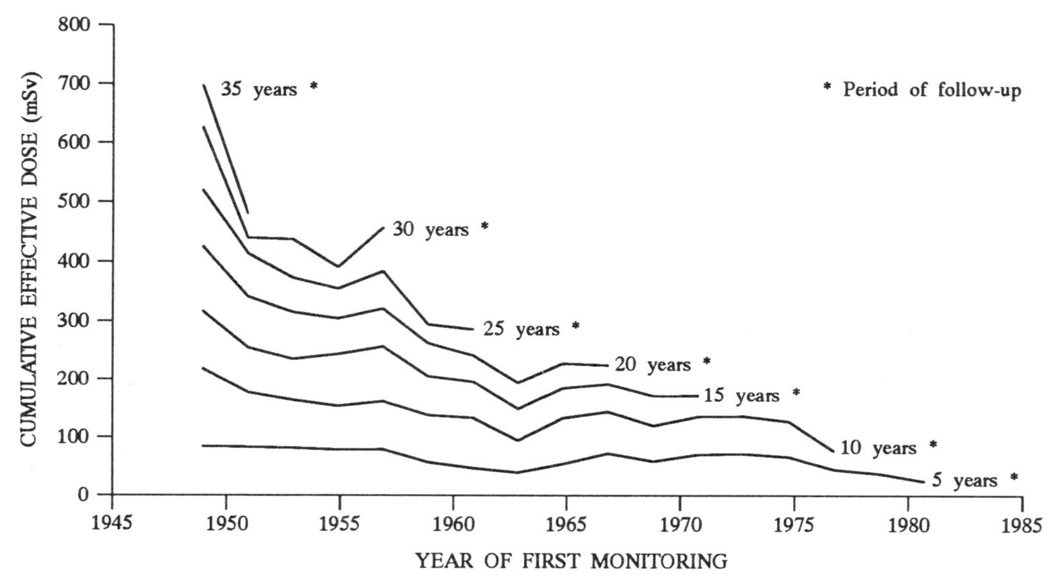

Figure XIV.
Cumulative effective dose to workers at Sellafield reprocessing plant.
[B9]

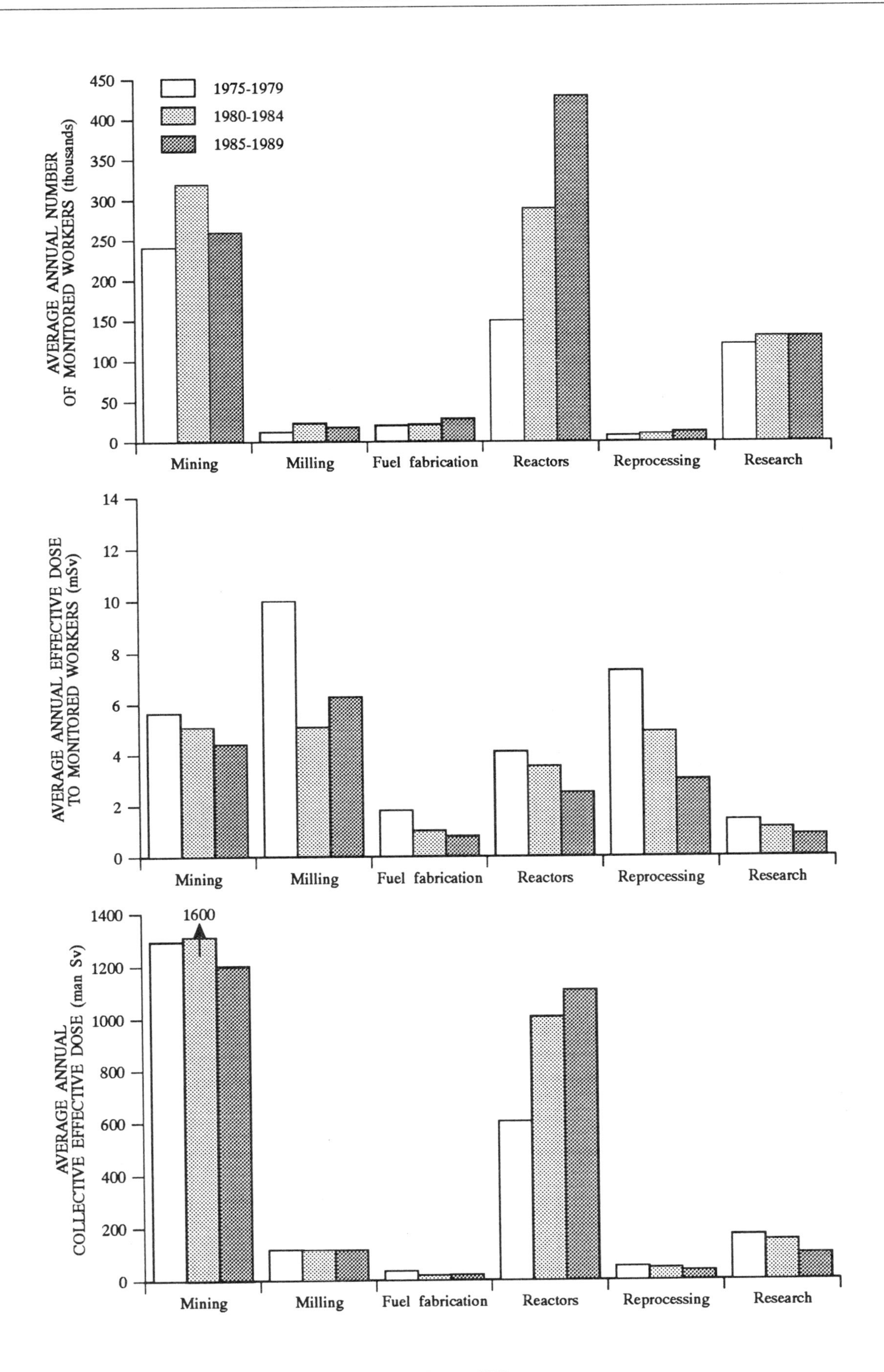

Figure XV.
Number of workers and doses to workers in operations of the nuclear fuel cycle.

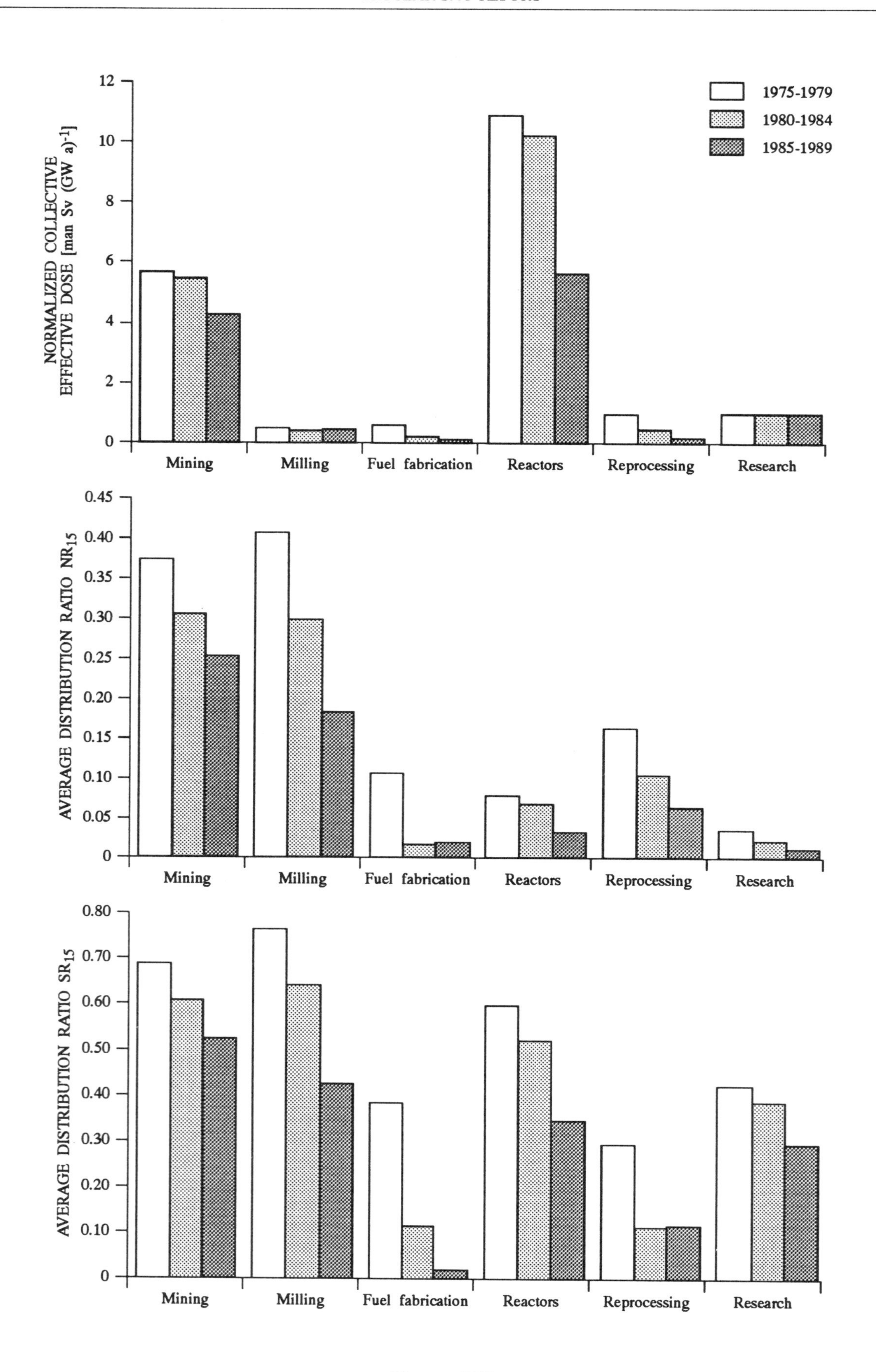

Figure XVI.
Normalized collective dose and distribution ratios for workers in operations of the nuclear fuel cycle.

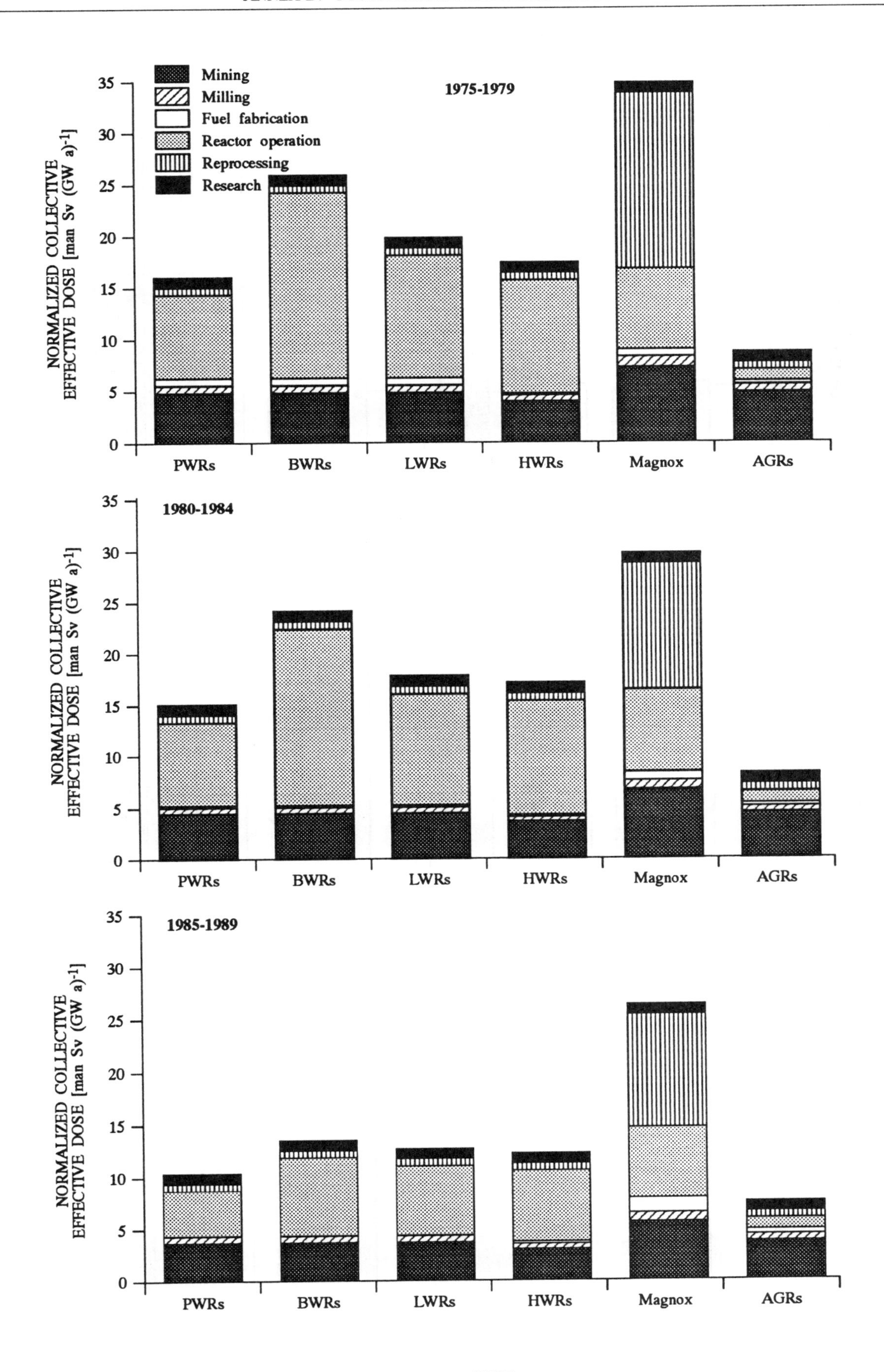

Figure XVII.
Normalized collective doses for workers in operations of the nuclear fuel cycle.

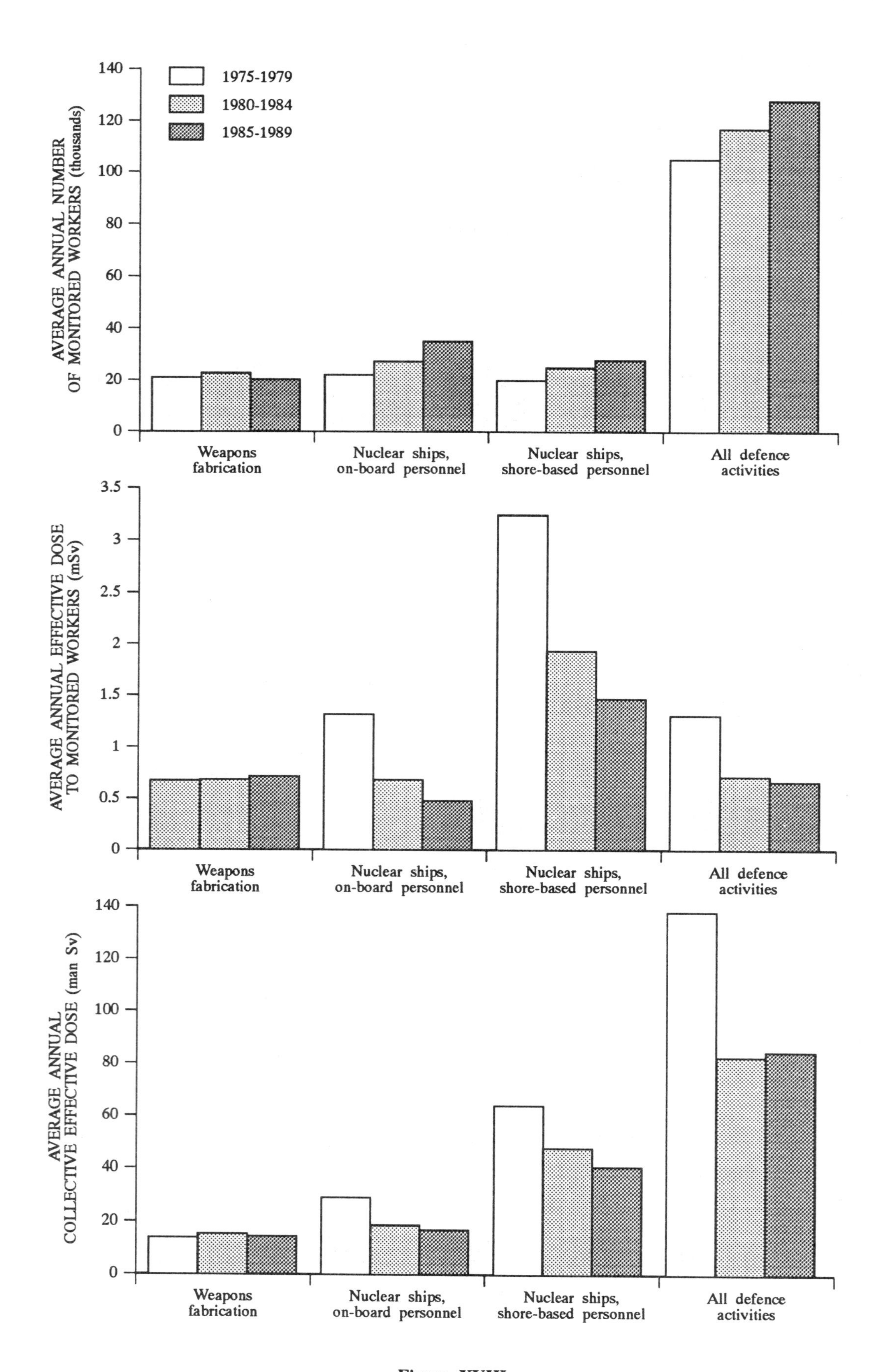

Figure XVIII.
Number of monitored workers and average annual individual and collective doses to workers in occupations involving defence activities (United Kingdom and United States only).

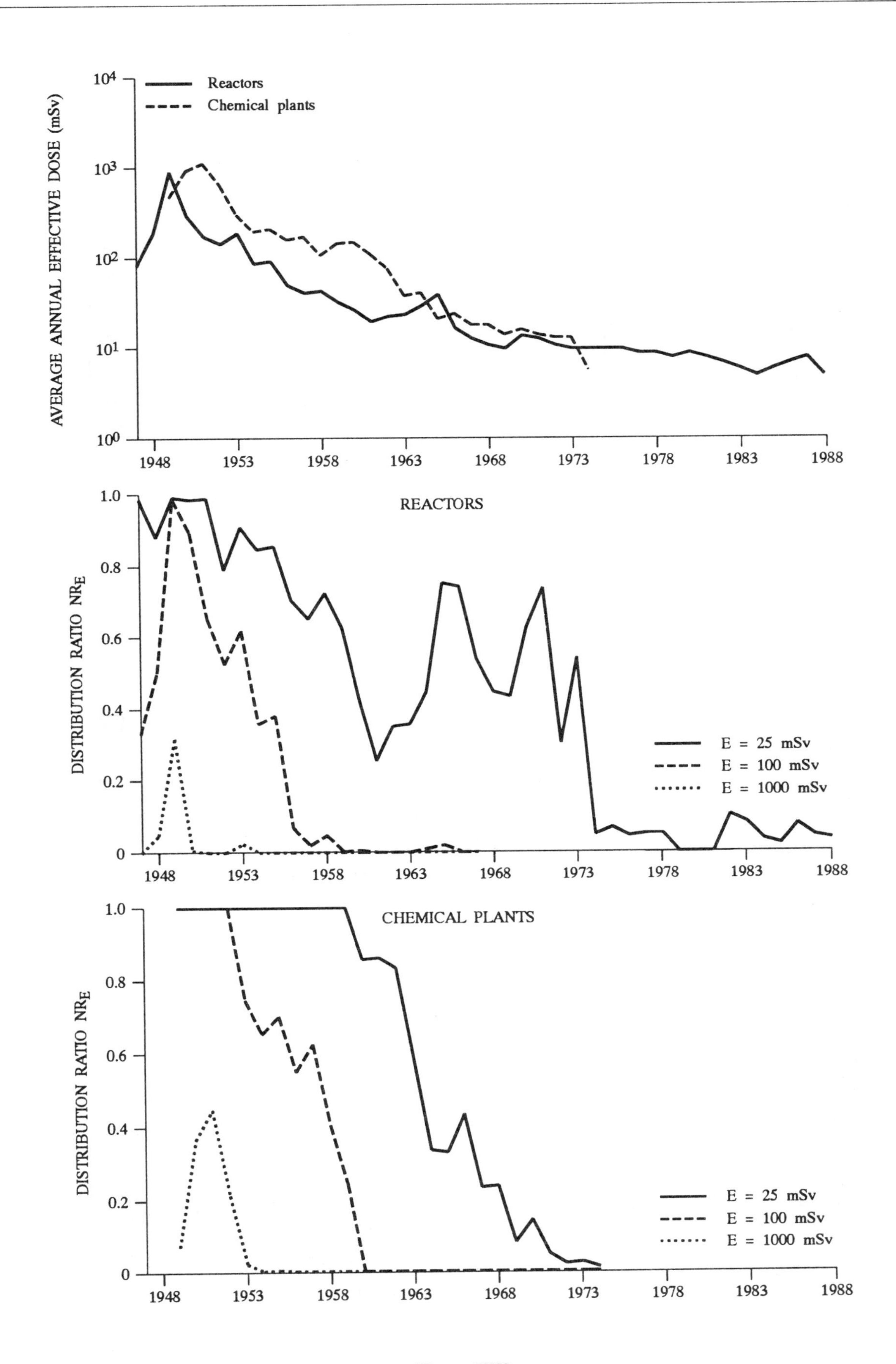

Figure XIX.
Variations in average annual individual doses and distribution ratios for workers involved in the production of weapon materials in the former USSR.

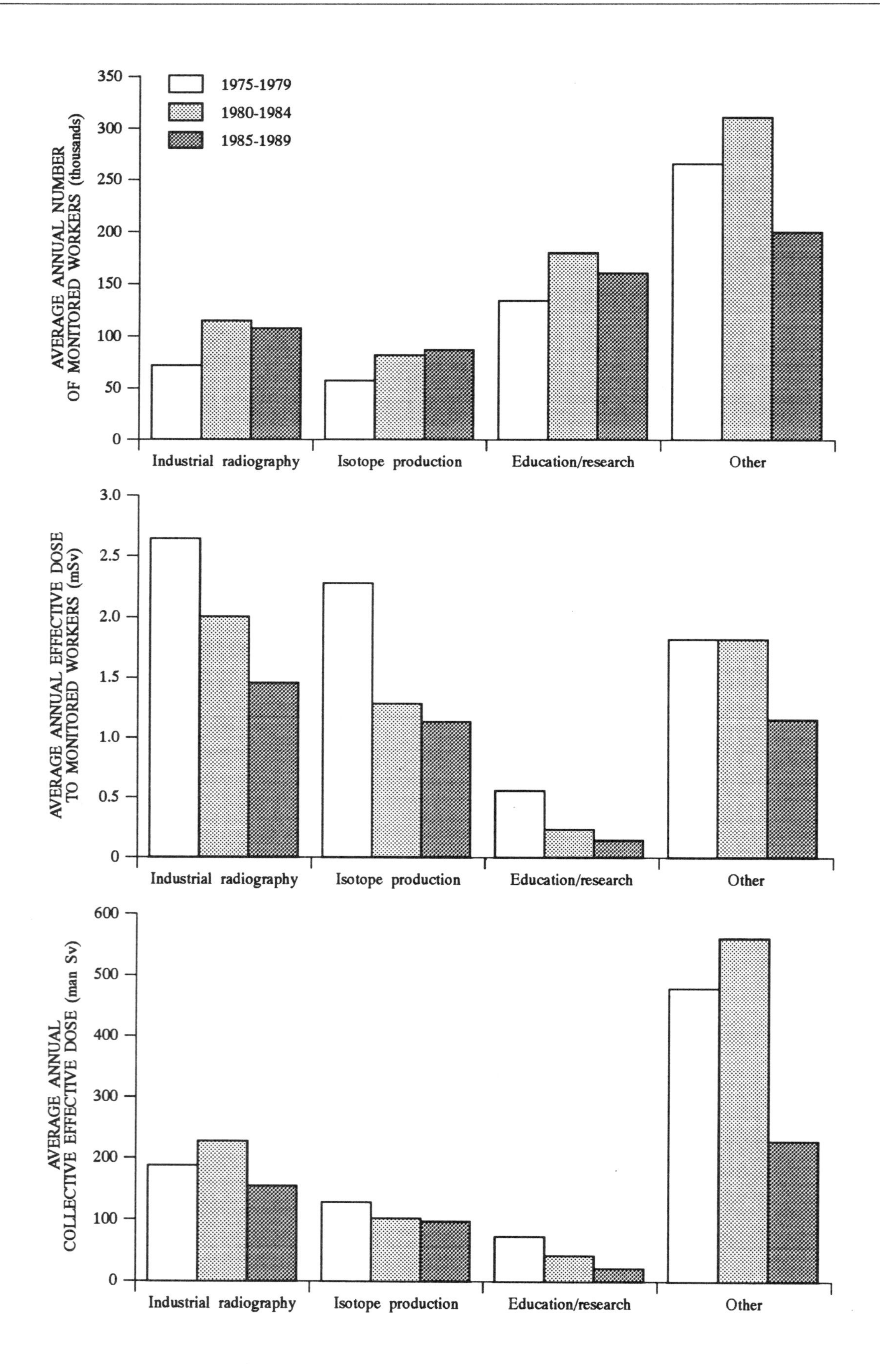

Figure XX.
Number of workers and doses to workers in occupations involving industrial uses of radiation.

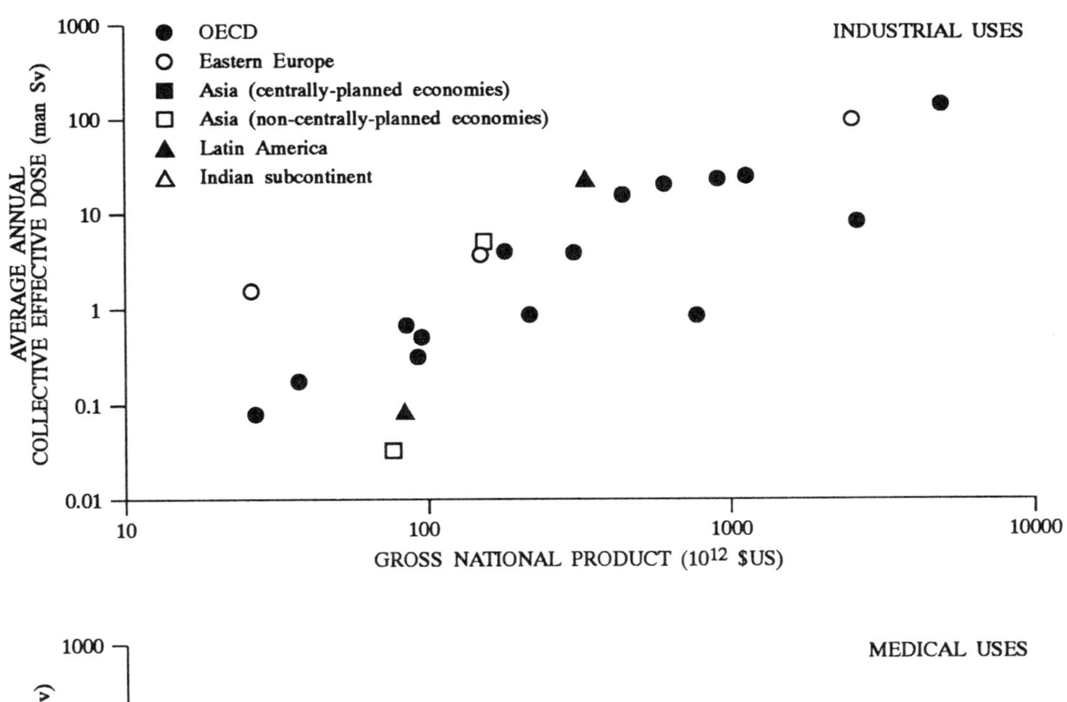

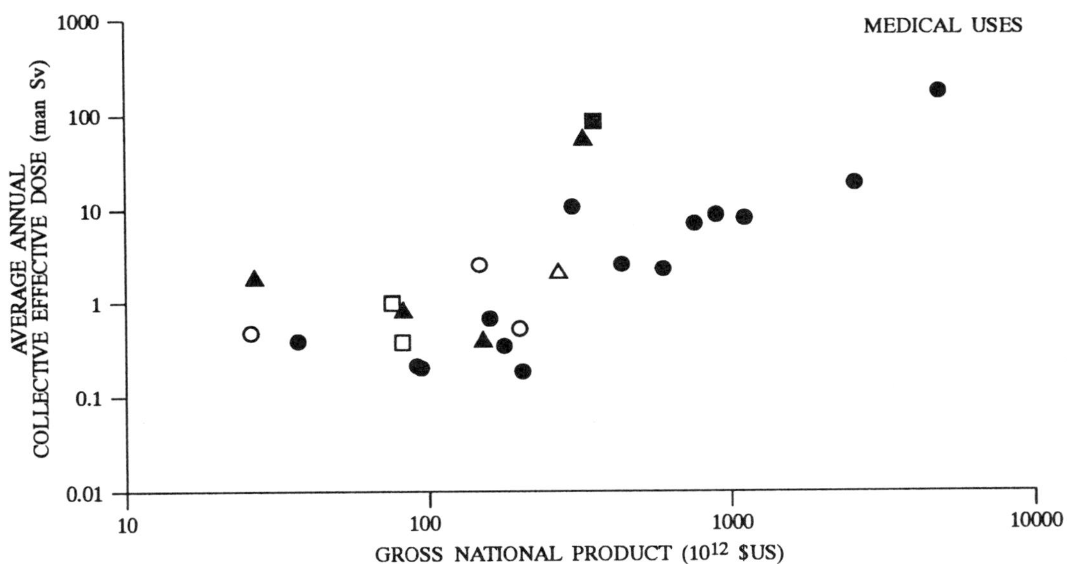

Figure XXI.
Average annual collective dose to workers in occupations involved in industrial and medical uses of radiation during 1985-1989 in relation to gross national product of countries.

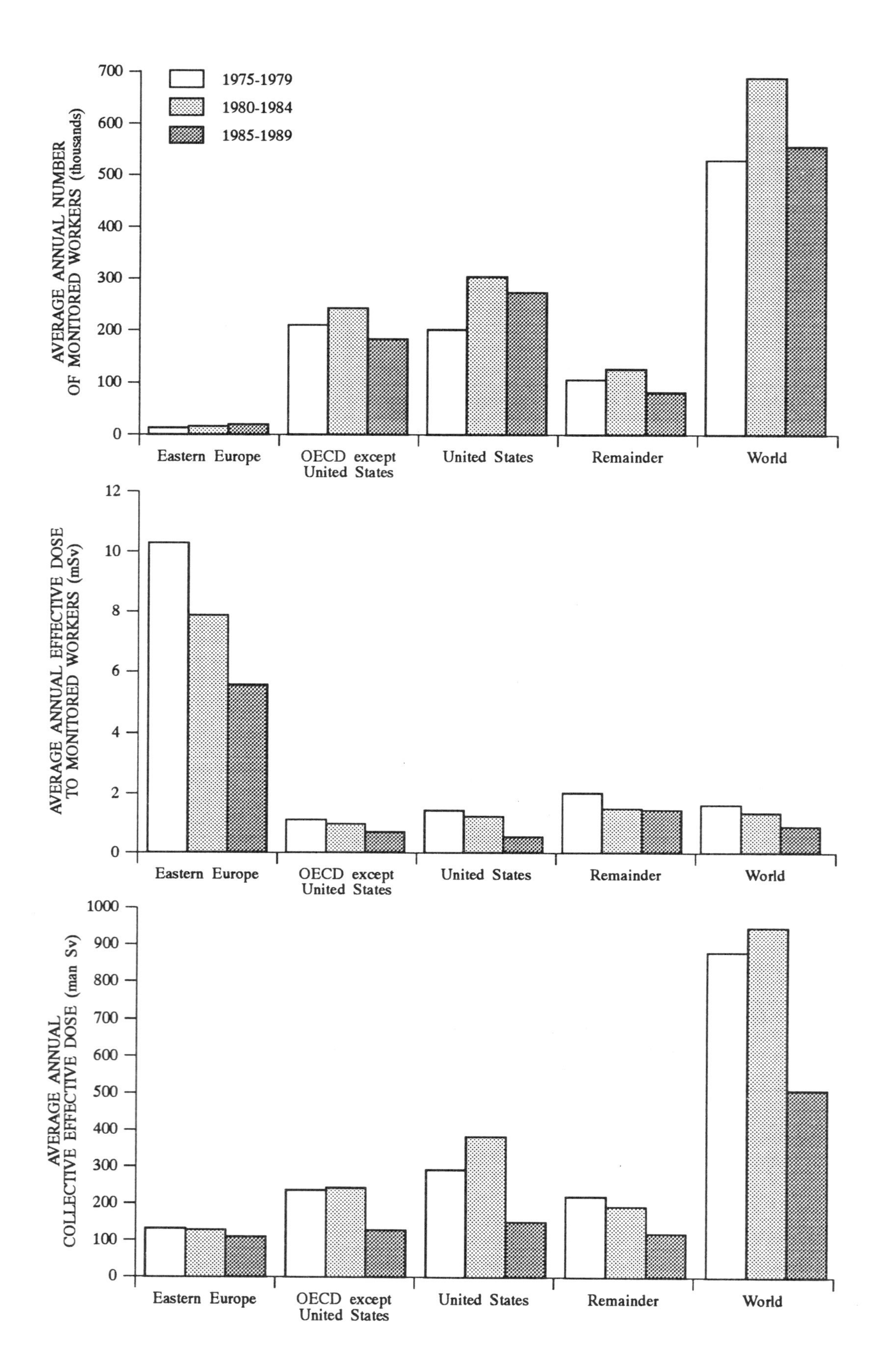

Figure XXII.
Regional data on number and exposure of workers involved in the industrial uses of radiation.

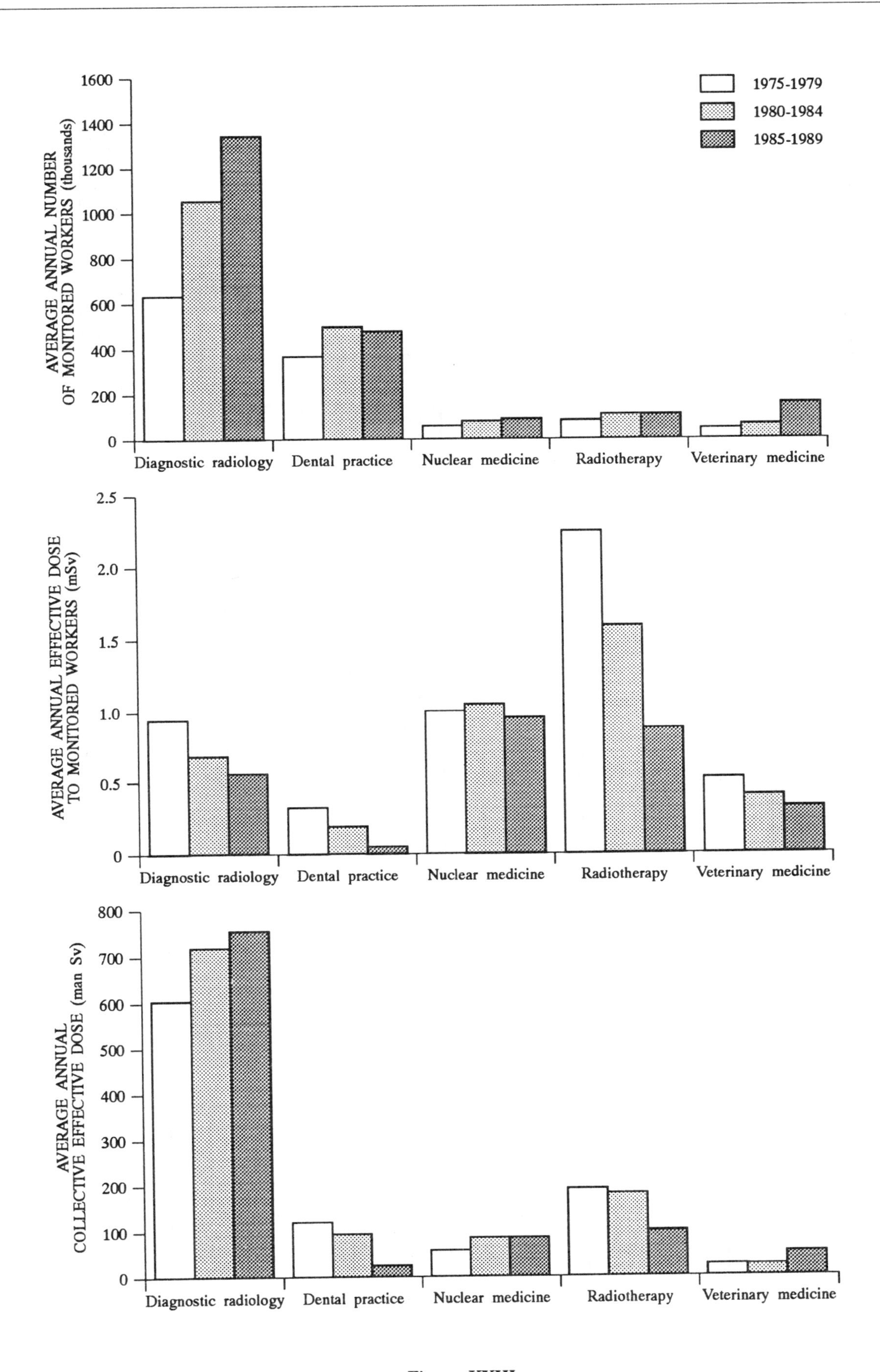

Figure XXIII.
Number of workers and doses in occupations involving medical uses of radiation.

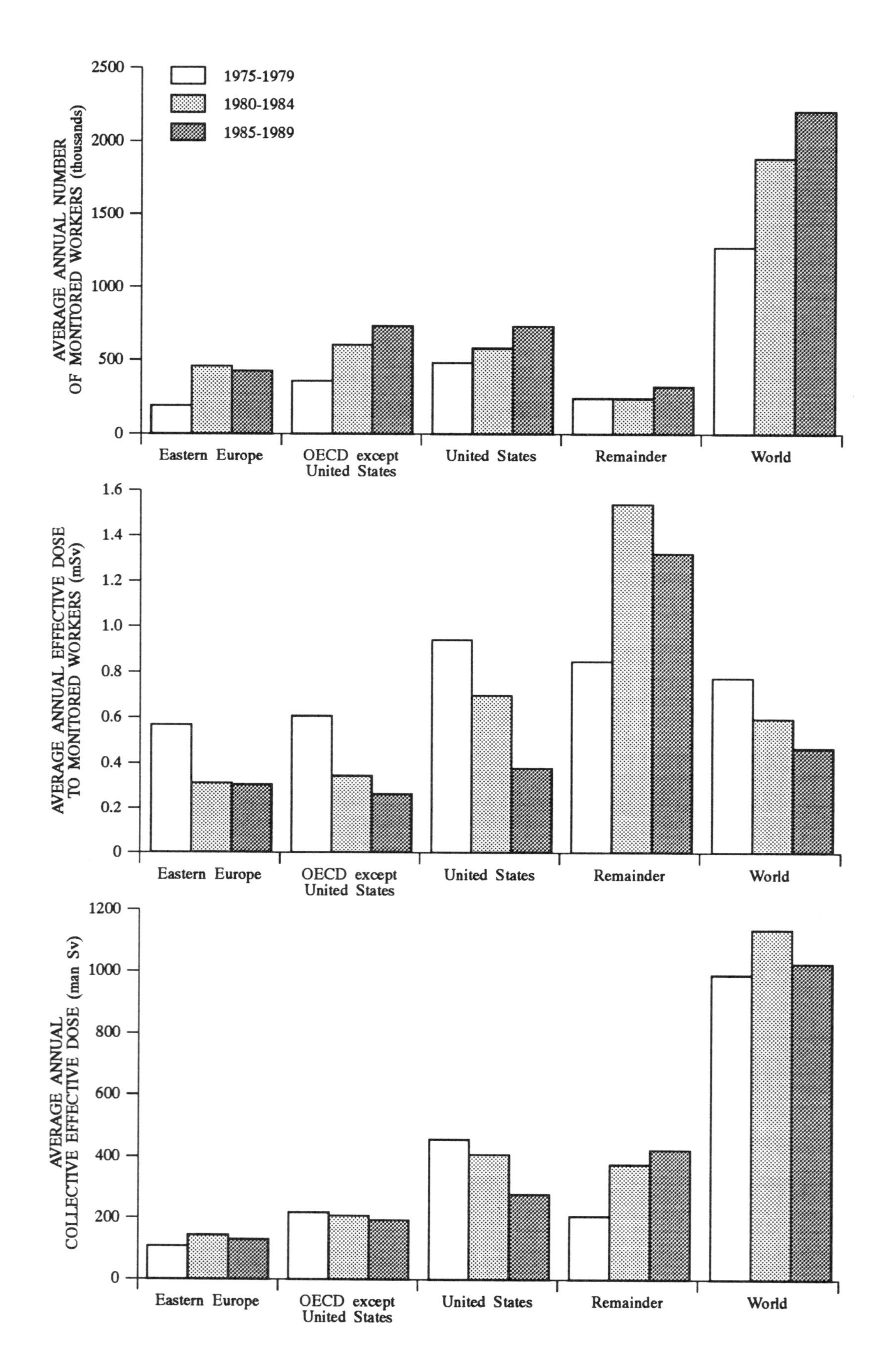

Figure XXIV.
Regional data on number and exposure of workers involved in the medical uses of radiation.

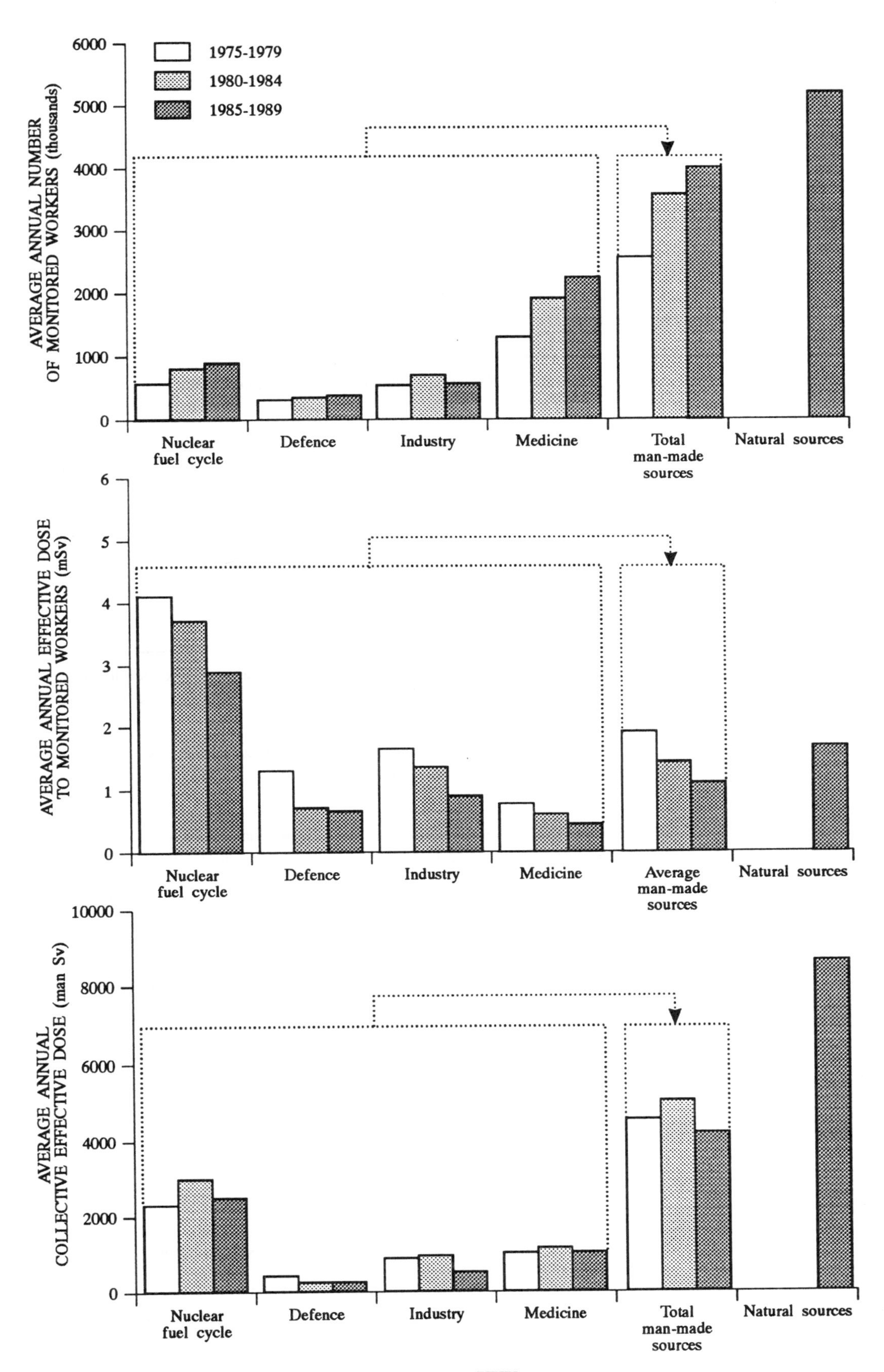

Figure XXV.
Number of workers and doses in all occupational exposures to radiation.

References

PART A

Responses to UNSCEAR Survey of Occupational Exposure

Country	*Response from*
Argentina	E. Palacios. Response to UNSCEAR questionnaire for occupational exposures incurred in industrial uses of radiation. Comisión Nacional de Energía Atómica, Buenos Aires, Argentina. (December 1990 and November 1991). E. Palacios. Response to UNSCEAR questionnaire for occupational exposures incurred in medical uses of radiation. Comisión Nacional de Energía Atómica, Buenos Aires, Argentina. (November 1991). E. Palacios. Response to UNSCEAR questionnaire for occupational exposures resulting from accidents. Comisión Nacional de Energía Atómica, Buenos Aires, Argentina. (October 1991). E. Palacios. Response to UNSCEAR questionnaire for occupational exposures incurred in medical uses of radiation. Comisión Nacional de Energía Atómica, Buenos Aires, Argentina. (February and November 1992). E. Palacios. Response to UNSCEAR questionnaire for occupational exposures incurred in industrial uses of radiation. Comisión Nacional de Energía Atómica, Buenos Aires, Argentina. (November and December 1992).
Australia	N. Morris. Response to UNSCEAR questionnaires for occupational exposures incurred in industrial and medical uses of radiation. Australian Radiation Laboratory, Victoria, Australia. (September 1991). G.C. Mason. Response to UNSCEAR questionnaires for occupational exposures incurred in industrial and medical uses of radiation. Australian Radiation Laboratory, Victoria, Australia. (December 1992).
Brazil	P. Cunha. Response to UNSCEAR questionnaire for occupational exposures incurred in medical uses of radiation. Comissao Nacional de Energía Nuclear, Rio de Janeiro, Brazil. (October 1991).
Canada	J.P. Ashmore. Response to UNSCEAR questionnaire for occupational exposures incurred in industrial uses of radiation. Bureau of Radiation and Medical Devices, Ottawa, Canada. (September 1990, March, July and August 1991). J.P. Ashmore. Response to UNSCEAR questionnaire for occupational exposures incurred in medical uses of radiation. Health and Welfare, Ottawa, Canada. (October 1991). J.P. Ashmore. Response to UNSCEAR questionnaire for occupational exposures resulting from accidents. Health and Welfare, Ottawa, Canada. (November 1991). J.P. Ashmore. Response to UNSCEAR questionnaire for occupational exposures incurred in industrial uses of radiation. Health and Welfare, Ottawa, Canada. (November 1992).
Chile	M. Manuel Echeverria. Response to UNSCEAR questionnaire for occupational exposures incurred in industrial uses of radiation. Comisión Chilena di Energía Nuclear, Chile. (November 1990).
China	Zhang Liangan. Response to UNSCEAR questionnaire for occupational exposures incurred in medical uses of radiation. Institute of Radiation Medicine, Chinese Academy of Sciences, Tianjin, China. (November 1991).
China (Taiwan Province)	Yi-Ching Yang. Response to UNSCEAR questionnaire for occupational exposures incurred in industrial uses of radiation. Atomic Energy Council, Taipei, Taiwan, China. (October 1991). Yi-Ching Yang. Response to UNSCEAR questionnaire for occupational exposures incurred in medical uses of radiation. Atomic Energy Council, Taipei, Taiwan, China. (October 1991).

Country	*Response from*
Czechoslovakia	Z. Melichar. Response to UNSCEAR questionnaire for occupational exposures incurred in industrial uses of radiation. Nuclear Power Plants Research Institute (VUJE), Czechoslovakia. (March 1991). H. Solnická and J. Smetana. Response to UNSCEAR questionnaire for occupational exposures incurred in industrial uses of radiation. Labour Medicine Institute of Uranium Industry and Uranium Mines Management, Pribram, Czechoslovakia. (March 1991). Z. Prouza and V. Klener. Response to UNSCEAR questionnaires for occupational exposures incurred in industrial and medical uses of radiation. Centre for Radiation Hygiene, National Institute for Public Health, Prague, Czechoslovakia. (July 1992). V. Klener. Response to UNSCEAR questionnaire for occupational exposures incurred in industrial uses of radiation. Centre for Radiation Hygiene, National Institute for Public Health, Prague, Czechoslovakia. (November 1992).
Denmark	O. Berg. Response to UNSCEAR questionnaire for occupational exposures incurred in industrial uses of radiation. National Institute of Radiation Hygiene, Bronshoj, Denmark. (April 1991). O. Berg. Response to UNSCEAR questionnaire for occupational exposures incurred in medical uses of radiation. National Institute of Radiation Hygiene, Bronshoj, Denmark. (October 1991).
Finland	H. Hyvönen. Responses to UNSCEAR questionnaire for occupational exposures incurred in industrial uses of radiation. Finnish Centre for Radiation and Nuclear Safety, Helsinki, Finland. (November 1990 and August 1991). H. Hyvönen. Response to UNSCEAR questionnaire for occupational exposures incurred in medical uses of radiation. Finnish Centre for Radiation and Nuclear Safety, Helsinki, Finland. (October 1991).
France	P. Pellerin. Response to UNSCEAR questionnaire for occupational exposures incurred in medical uses of radiation. Service Central de Protection contre les Rayonnements Ionisants, Le Vesinet, France. (April 1992). P. Pellerin. Response to UNSCEAR questionnaire for occupational exposures incurred in industrial uses of radiation. Service Central de Protection contre les Rayonnements Ionisants, Le Vesinet, France. (June 1992). C. Rolland-Piegue and S. Lebar. Response to UNSCEAR questionnaire for occupational exposures incurred in industrial uses of radiation. Compagnie Générale des Matières Nucléaires (COGEMA), Velizy-Villacoublay, France. (July 1992). Ph. Hubert. Response to UNSCEAR questionnaire for occupational exposures incurred in industrial uses of radiation. Institut de Protection et de Sureté Nucléaire (IPSN), Commissariat à l'Energie Atomique (CEA), Fontenay aux Roses, France. (September 1992). C. Rolland-Piegue. Response to UNSCEAR questionnaire for occupational exposures incurred in industrial uses of radiation. Compagnie Générale des Matières Nucléaires (COGEMA), Velizy-Villacoublay, France. (November and December 1992). Ph. Rollin. Response to UNSCEAR questionnaire for occupational exposures incurred in industrial uses of radiation. Electricité de France (EdF), Paris, France. (November 1992).
Germany	M. Grunwald. Responses to UNSCEAR questionnaire for occupational exposures incurred in industrial uses of radiation. Bundesamt für Strahlenschutz (BfS), Salzgitter, Germany. (September 1990 and January 1991). M. Grunwald. Response to UNSCEAR questionnaire for occupational exposures incurred in medical uses of radiation. Bundesamt für Strahlenschutz (BfS), Salzgitter, Germany. (August 1991). A. Kaul. Responses to UNSCEAR questionnaire for occupational exposures incurred in industrial uses of radiation. Bundesamt für Strahlenschutz (BfS), Salzgitter, Germany. (April and August 1991). A. Kaul. Response to UNSCEAR questionnaire for occupational exposures resulting from accidents. Bundesamt für Strahlenschutz (BfS), Salzgitter, Germany. (September 1991). A. Kaul, Arndt and Wolf. Response to UNSCEAR questionnaire for occupational exposures resulting from accidents. Bundesamt für Strahlenschutz (BfS), Salzgitter, Germany. (October 1991).

Country	*Response from*
Germany (continued)	E. Martini. Response to UNSCEAR questionnaire for occupational exposures incurred in medical uses of radiation. Land Mecklenburg-Vorpommern Landesanstalt für Personendosimetrie und Strahlenschutzausbildung-Personendosismeßstelle, Berlin, Germany. (August 1991). J. Schwedt. Response to UNSCEAR questionnaire for occupational exposures incurred in industrial uses of radiation. Bundesamt für Strahlenschutz (Dienststelle Berlin), Berlin, Germany. (May 1991). A. Kaul. Response to UNSCEAR questionnaire for occupational exposures incurred in medical uses of radiation. Bundesamt für Strahlenschutz (BfS), Salzgitter, Germany. (February 1992). A. Kaul. Response to UNSCEAR questionnaire for occupational exposures incurred in industrial uses of radiation. Bundesamt für Strahlenschutz (BfS), Salzgitter, Germany. (December 1992).
Hungary	L.B. Sztanyik and I. Bojtor. Response to UNSCEAR questionnaire for occupational exposures incurred in industrial uses of radiation. National Research Institute for Radiobiology and Radiohygiene, Budapest, Hungary. (January 1991). L.B. Sztanyik and I. Bojtor. Response to UNSCEAR questionnaires for occupational exposures incurred in medical uses of radiation and occupational exposures resulting from accidents. National Research Institute for Radiobiology and Radiohygiene, Budapest, Hungary. (March 1992). I. Bojtor and L.B. Sztanyik. Response to UNSCEAR questionnaire for occupational exposures incurred in medical uses of radiation. National Research Institute for Radiobiology and Radiohygiene, Budapest, Hungary. (June 1992).
India	D.V. Gopinath. Response to UNSCEAR questionnaire for occupational exposures incurred in industrial uses of radiation. Bhabha Atomic Research Centre, Trombay, India. (June 1991 and May 1993). U. Madhvanath. Response to UNSCEAR questionnaires for occupational exposures incurred in industrial and medical uses of radiation. Division of Radiation Protection, Bhabha Atomic Research Centre, Bombay, India. (June 1991). U. Madhvanath. Response to UNSCEAR questionnaires for occupational exposures resulting from accidents and incurred in medical uses of radiation. Division of Radiation Protection, Bhabha Atomic Research Centre, Bombay, India. (December 1991). S. Krishnamony. Response to UNSCEAR questionnaire for occupational exposures incurred in industrial uses of radiation. Health Physics Division, Bhabha Atomic Research Centre, Bombay, India. (November 1992).
Indonesia	I. Rifai. Response to UNSCEAR questionnaire for occupational exposures incurred in medical uses of radiation. Department of Health, Jakarta, Indonesia. (October 1991). S. Soekarno. Responses to UNSCEAR questionnaire for occupational exposures incurred in industrial uses of radiation. National Atomic Energy Agency, Centre for Standardization and Radiological Safety Research, Jakarta, Indonesia. (October 1990, April and September 1991). S. Soekarno. Response to UNSCEAR questionnaire for occupational exposures resulting from accidents. National Atomic Energy Agency, Centre for Standardization and Radiological Safety Research, Jakarta, Indonesia. (November 1991).
Ireland	D. Howett. Responses to UNSCEAR questionnaire for occupational exposures incurred in industrial uses of radiation. Nuclear Energy Board, Dublin, Ireland. (October 1990 and July 1991). D. Howett. Responses to UNSCEAR questionnaire for occupational exposures incurred in medical uses of radiation. Nuclear Energy Board, Dublin, Ireland. (January 1992).
Italy	A. Cavallini and M. Litido. Responses to UNSCEAR questionnaire for occupational exposures incurred in industrial uses of radiation. National Committee for Nuclear and Alternative Energy (ENEA AMB), Bologna, Italy. (January and December 1991). A. Cavallini and M. Litido. Response to UNSCEAR questionnaire for occupational exposures incurred in medical uses of radiation. National Committee for Nuclear and Alternative Energy (ENEA AMB), Bologna, Italy. (December 1991).

Country	*Response from*
Japan	H. Matsudaira. Responses to UNSCEAR questionnaire for occupational exposures incurred in industrial uses of radiation. National Institute for Radiological Sciences, Chiba-shi, Japan. (January and May 1991). T. Yanagi. Response to UNSCEAR questionnaire for occupational exposures incurred in industrial uses of radiation. Nuclear Safety Policy Division, Science and Technology Agency, Tokyo, Japan. (June 1992). T. Maruyama. Response to UNSCEAR questionnaire for occupational exposures incurred in medical uses of radiation. National Institute for Radiological Sciences, Chiba-shi, Japan. (June 1992).
Mexico	J. Raul Ortiz Magaña. Responses to UNSCEAR questionnaire for occupational exposures incurred in industrial uses of radiation. Comisión Nacional de Seguridad Nuclear y Salvaguardias, Mexico. (October 1990 and August 1991). F.V. Rojas. Response to UNSCEAR questionnaire for occupational exposures incurred in medical uses of radiation. Comisión Nacional de Seguridad Nuclear y Salvaguardias, Mexico. (August 1991).
Netherlands	J.W.E. van Dijk. Response to UNSCEAR questionnaire for occupational exposures incurred in industrial uses of radiation. TNO-Gezondheidsonderzoek, Arnhem, Netherlands. (June 1991). P.W.E. Louwrier. Response to UNSCEAR questionnaire for occupational exposures incurred in industrial uses of radiation. National Institute for Nuclear and High Energy Physics (NIKHEF), Amsterdam, Netherlands. (October 1991).
Norway	T. Wøhni. Response to UNSCEAR questionnaire for occupational exposures incurred in industrial uses of radiation. National Institute of Radiation Hygiene, Osteraas, Norway. (October 1990 and October 1991).
Peru	L. Pinillos-Ashton. Response to UNSCEAR questionnaire for occupational exposures incurred in medical uses of radiation. Instituto Nacional de Enfermedades Neoplásicas, Lima, Peru. (December 1991).
Republic of Korea	Chung-Woo Ha. Response to UNSCEAR questionnaire for occupational exposures incurred in industrial uses of radiation. Korea Atomic Energy Research Institute, Daejun, Republic of Korea. (November 1990). Chung-Woo Ha. Response to UNSCEAR questionnaire for occupational exposures incurred in industrial uses of radiation. Korea Atomic Energy Research Institute, Daejum, Republic of Korea. (November 1990). Jae-ho Lim. Response to UNSCEAR questionnaire for occupational exposures incurred in industrial uses of radiation. Korea Electric Power Corporation, Seoul, Republic of Korea. (December 1991). Suing-hyun Yoo. Response to UNSCEAR questionnaire for occupational exposures incurred in industrial uses of radiation. Korea Nuclear Fuel Company Ltd., Daejum, Republic of Korea. (December 1990).
South Africa	I.D. Kruger. Response to UNSCEAR questionnaire for occupational exposures incurred in industrial uses of radiation. Atomic Energy Corporation, Pretoria, Republic of South Africa. (February 1991). T. Volschenk. Response to UNSCEAR questionnaire for occupational exposures incurred in industrial uses of radiation. Radiation Protection Service, South African Bureau of Standards (SABS), Pretoria, Republic of South Africa. (April 1991). D. Woodhall. Response to UNSCEAR questionnaire for occupational exposures incurred in industrial uses of radiation. Koeberg Nuclear Power Station, Kernkrag, Republic of South Africa. (January 1991). K.J. Smit. Response to UNSCEAR questionnaire for occupational exposures incurred in medical uses of radiation. Department of National Health and Population Development, Bellville, Republic of South Africa. (March 1992). I.D. Kruger. Response to UNSCEAR questionnaire for occupational exposures incurred in industrial uses of radiation. Atomic Energy Corporation, Pretoria, Republic of South Africa. (November 1992).

Country	*Response from*
Spain	I.A. Calvo. Response to UNSCEAR questionnaire for occupational exposures incurred in industrial uses of radiation. Consejo de Seguridad Nuclear, Madrid, Spain. (November 1990). M.J. Muñoz. Response to UNSCEAR questionnaire for occupational exposures incurred in industrial uses of radiation. Consejo de Seguridad Nuclear, Madrid, Spain. (December 1991). M.J. Muñoz. Response to UNSCEAR questionnaire for occupational exposures incurred in medical uses of radiation. Consejo de Seguridad Nuclear, Madrid, Spain. (November 1991). M.J. Muñoz. Response to UNSCEAR questionnaire for occupational exposures resulting from accidents. Consejo de Seguridad Nuclear, Madrid, Spain. (November 1991). M.J. Muñoz. Response to UNSCEAR questionnaire for occupational exposures incurred in industrial uses of radiation. Consejo de Seguridad Nuclear, Madrid, Spain. (December 1992).
Sweden	J.C. Lindhé. Response to UNSCEAR questionnaire for occupational exposures incurred in industrial uses of radiation. National Institute for Radiation Protection, Stockholm, Sweden. (October 1990, January and December 1991). G. Szendrö. Response to UNSCEAR questionnaire for occupational exposures incurred in medical uses of radiation. Swedish Radiation Protection Institute, Stockholm, Sweden. (October 1991). G. Szendrö. Response to UNSCEAR questionnaire for occupational exposures resulting from accidents. Swedish Radiation Protection Institute, Stockhlom, Sweden. (October 1991).
Switzerland	M. Moser. Response to UNSCEAR questionnaire for occupational exposures incurred in medical uses of radiation. Federal Office of Public Health, Bern, Switzerland. (October 1991).
USSR	I.P. Korenkov. Response to UNSCEAR questionnaire for occupational exposures incurred in industrial uses of radiation. Central Institute for Advanced Medical Studies, Moscow, USSR. (October 1990).
United Kingdom	J.S. Hughes. Responses to UNSCEAR questionnaire for occupational exposures incurred in industrial uses of radiation. National Radiological Protection Board, Chilton, United Kingdom. (October 1990, August and December 1991). J.S. Hughes. Response to UNSCEAR questionnaire for occupational exposures resulting from accidents. National Radiological Protection Board, Chilton, United Kingdom. (December 1991). Based on a summary from [L5]. R.J. Berry. Response to UNSCEAR questionnaire for occupational exposures incurred in industrial uses of radiation. British Nuclear Fuels plc, Risley, United Kingdom. (March 1992).
United States	B. Millet. Response to UNSCEAR questionnaire for occupational exposures incurred in industrial uses of radiation. Department of Energy, United States. (October 1990). C.T. Raddatz. Response to UNSCEAR questionnaire for occupational exposures incurred in industrial uses of radiation. Summaries from annual reports. NUREG-0713. United States Nuclear Regulatory Commission, United States. (December 1991). C.R. Jones. Response to UNSCEAR questionnaire for occupational exposures incurred in industrial uses of radiation. Department of Energy, United States. (March 1992). R.T. Beckman. Response to UNSCEAR questionnaire for occupational exposures incurred in industrial uses of radiation. Mine Safety and Health Administration (MSHA), Denver, United States. (December 1992). H.S. Gottschalk. Response to UNSCEAR questionnaire for occupational exposures incurred in industrial uses of radiation. Mine Safety and Health Administration (MSHA), Arlington, United States. (January 1993).

PART B

A1 Ashmore, J.P., Bureau of Radiation and Medical Devices, Canada. Communication to the UNSCEAR Secretariat (1991).

B1 Brodsky, A., R.P. Specht, B.G. Brooks et al. Log-normal distributions of occupational exposures in medicine and industry. Ninth Mid-year Topical Symposium on Occupational Health Physics, Denver, Colorado, 1976.

B2 Brooks, B.G. and D. Hagemeyer. Occupational radiation exposure at commercial nuclear power facilities. NUREG-0713, Volumes 3-8 (1982-1989).

B3 British Nuclear Fuels PLC. Annual reports on occupational safety 1984-1987. BNFL (1985-1988).

B4 Brooks, B.G. United States Nuclear Regulatory Commission. Communication to the UNSCEAR Secretariat (1989).

B5 Benedittini, M. Expositions professionelles dans les reacteurs à eau pressurisée: comparaison internationale de quelques indicateurs globeaux entre 1975 et 1989. CEPN No. 178 (1990).

B6 Benedittini, M. Centre d'Etude sur l'Evaluation de la Protection dans le domaine Nucleaire. Communication to the UNSCEAR Secretariat (1990).

B7 Bines, W.P., W.J. Iles, K.A. Fillary et al. Doses to UK radiation workers as recorded at the Central Index of Dose Information. p. 219-224 in: Proceedings of International Conference on Occupational Radiation Protection, Guernsey, April 1991.

B8 British Nuclear Fuels PLC. Communication from R.J. Berry to the UNSCEAR Secretariat (1991 and 1992).

B9 Binks, K., R. Wakeford, R. Strong et al. Cumulative radiation exposure at BNFL Sellafield: a historical perspective. p. 1176-1179 in: Worldwide Achievement in Public and Occupational Health Protection Against Radiation. Proceedings of the 8th International Conference of the International Radiation Protection Association, Montreal, Canada, May 1992.

B10 Buldakov, L.A. et al. Oncological mortality in the workers in the first atomic industrial facility in the USSR. Institute of Biophysics, Russian Federation. Communication to the UNSCEAR Secretariat (1992).

B11 Buldakov, L.A., A.M. Vorobiev, V.V. Kopaev et al. Irradiation of personnel of industrial and power nuclear reactors. Med. Radiol. 3: 38-43 (1991).

B12 Beckman, R.T., Mine Safety and Health Administration, Denver, United States. Communication to the UNSCEAR Secretariat (1992).

B13 Benton, E.V. and T.A. Parnell. Space radiation dosimetry on US and Soviet manned missions. p. 729-794 in: Terrestrial Space Radiation and its Biological Effects. (P.D. McCormack, C.E. Swenberg and H. Bücker, eds.) Plenum Press, New York, 1988.

B14 Bernhard, S., J.A. Le Gac, H. Seguin et al. Radon levels and radon daughter exposures of workers in non-uranium mines of the E.C. p. 625-628 in: Radiation Hazards in Mining - Control, Measurement and Medical Aspects. Society of Mining Engineers, New York, 1981.

B15 Bottom, D.A., D.W. Dixon and T.D. Gooding. Exposure to radon in British mines. in: Proceedings of International Conference on Occupational Radiation Protection, Guernsey, April 1991.

C1 Carreiro, J.V. and R. Avelar. Occupational exposures in medical and paramedical professions in Portugal. Radiat. Prot. Dosim. 36 (2/4): 233-236 (1991).

C2 Churcher, T., A.A.C. Brewis and W.G. Prast. Quantification of Underground Employment. Mining Journal Research Services, London, 1991.

C3 Cunha, K.M.D., S.M. Carvalho, C.V. Barros Leite et al. Particle size distribution in monazite dust. in: The Fourth International Symposium on Radiation Physics, Abstracts. São Paulo, 1988.

D1 Defence Committee. Radiological Protection of Service and Civilian Personnel, Twelfth Report. HMSO, London, 1990.

D2 Drexler, G., P.G. da Cunha and J.E. Peixoto. Medical and occupational exposures in Brazil. Radiat. Prot. Dosim. 36 (2/4): 101-105 (1991).

D3 Domanski, T., W. Chruscielewski, D. Kluszczynski et al. Radiation hazard in Polish mines - measurement and computer simulations. Radiat. Prot. Dosim. 45: 133-135 (1992).

D4 Davies, D.M. Cosmic radiation in Concorde operations and the impact of new ICRP recommendations on commercial aviation. Radiat. Prot. Dosim. 48: 121-124 (1993).

D5 Dixon, D.W., D. Page and D.A. Bottom. Estimates of dose from radon daughters in UK mines. Radiat. Prot. Dosim. 36: 137-141 (1991).

D6 Drexler, G., H.Y. Göksu and T.F. Johns. A comparative study of some aspects of radiation protection and dosimetry procedures. Part I: In the member states of the European Communities. Part II: In the USA and Japan. GSF 13/88 (1988).

E1 Environmental Protection Agency. Occupational exposure to ionizing radiation in the United States: a comprehensive review for the year 1980 and a summary of trends for the years 1960-85. EPA 520/1-84-005 (1984).

E2 Environmental Protection Agency. Occupational exposure to ionizing radiation in the United States: a comprehensive summary for the year 1975. EPA 520/4-80-001 (1980).

E3 Environmental Protection Agency. Occupational exposure to ionizing radiation in the United States: a comprehensive review for the year 1985 and a summary of trends for the years 1960-85. EPA 402-R-93-082 (1993).

F1 Finney, D.J. Probit Analysis (3rd edition). Cambridge University Press, 1971.

F2 Fujimoto, K., J.A. Wilson, J.P. Ashmore et al. Occupational radiation exposures in Canada - 1984. Canadian Department of National Health and Welfare. Report No. 85-EHD-115 (1985).

F3 Friedberg, W., L. Snyder, D.N. Faulkner et al. Radiation exposure of air carrier crew members II. US Department of Transport DOT/FAA/AM-92/2 (1992).

F4 Fernández, P.L., I. Gutierrez, L.S. Quindós et al. Natural ventilation in the paintings room in the Altamira Cave. Nature 321: 586-588 (1986).

G1 Goldsmith, R., J.D. Boice, Z. Hrubec et al. Mortality and career radiation doses for workers at a commercial nuclear power plant: feasibility study. Health Phys. 56: 139-150 (1989).

G2 Gelder, R. Radiological impact of the normal transport of radioactive materials by air. NRPB-M219 (1990).

G3 Guy, M.S.C. Radiation hazard levels prevailing in the South African mining industry. Council for Nuclear Safety, Pretoria. Communication to the UNSCEAR Secretariat (1991).

G4 Göksu, H.Y., D. Regulla and G. Drexler. Present status of practical aspects of individual dosimetry. Part I: European countries member states. GSF 16/93 (1993).

G5 Göksu, H.Y., D. Regulla and G. Drexler. Present status of practical aspects of individual dosimetry.Part II: Eastern European countries. GSF 17/93 (1993).

H1 Hughes, J.S., K.B. Shaw and M.C. O'Riordan. Radiation exposure of the UK population - 1988 review. NRPB-R227 (1989).

H2 Hughes, J.S. and G.C. Roberts. The radiation exposure of the UK population - 1984 review. NRPB-R173 (1984).

H3 Hipkin, J. and C.A. Pereira. Committed dose equivalents to tritium users 1977-1980. J. Soc. Radiol. Prot. 2 (3): 29-30 (1982).

H4 Hajnal, F., J.E. McLaughlin, M.S. Weinstein et al. 1970 sea-level cosmic-ray neutron measurements. HASL-241 (1971).

H5 Hewson, G.S., P.J. Tippet, B.H. O'Connor et al. Preliminary study of radon in underground mines in Western Australia. Report No. 79, MERIWA, Perth (1991).

H6 Hewson, G.S. Radiation exposure status of mineral sands industry workers (1983-1988). Radiat. Prot. Aust. 8: 3-12 (1990).

H7 Health and Safety Executive/National Radiological Protection Board. Central Index of Dose Information. Summary of Statistics for 1986. HMSO, London, 1991.

H8 Hunyadi, I., J. Hakl, L. Lénárt et al. Regular subsurface radon measurements in Hungarian karstic regions. Nucl. Tracks Radiat. Meas. 19: 321-326 (1991).

H9 Horton, T.R., R.L. Blanchard and S.T. Windham. A study of radon and airborne particulates at phosphogypsum stacks in central Florida. EPA 520/5-88-021 (1988).

H10 Hashizume, T., T. Suganuma and T. Shida. Estimation of collective dose equivalent to holding assistants from veterinary X-ray examination in Japan. Hoken Butsuri (Japan) 23: 187-194 (1988).

I1 International Commission on Radiological Protection. Recommendations of the International Commission on Radiological Protection. ICRP Publication 26. Annals of the ICRP 1(3). Pergamon Press, Oxford, 1977.

I2 International Commission on Radiological Protection. Recommendations of the International Commission on Radiological Protection. ICRP Publication 9. Pergamon Press, Oxford, 1966.

I3 International Commission on Radiological Protection. Data for Use in Protection Against External Radiation. ICRP Publication 51. Annals of the ICRP 17 (2/3). Pergamon Press, Oxford, 1987.

I4 International Atomic Energy Agency. Nuclear power, nuclear fuel cycle waste management: status and trends 1990. Part C of the IAEA Yearbook. IAEA, Vienna, 1990.

I5 International Atomic Energy Agency. MicroPRIS - IAEA Power Reactor Information System - a version of the PRIS for PC users. IAEA, Vienna, 1991.

I6 International Atomic Energy Agency. The nuclear fuel cycle information system - a directory of nuclear fuel cycle facilities. IAEA, Vienna, 1988.

I7 International Commission on Radiological Protection. 1990 Recommendations of the International Commission on Radiological Protection. ICRP Publication 60. Annals of the ICRP 21 (1-3). Pergamon Press, Oxford, 1991.

I8 International Atomic Energy Agency. Operating experience with nuclear power in member states in 1991. IAEA, Vienna, 1992.

I9 Ilyin, L.A., Institute of Biophysics, Russian Federation. Communication to the UNSCEAR Secretariat (1992).

I10 International Atomic Energy Agency. Responses to questionnaire on occupational exposures in mining. IAEA, Vienna, 1992.

I11 International Atomic Energy Agency, Division of Nuclear Safety, Vienna. Communication to the UNSCEAR Secretariat (1992).

I12 International Civil Aviation Organization. Civil Aviation Statistics of the World. Doc 9180/12 (1987).

I13 International Commission on Radiological Protection. Protection against radon-222 at home and at work. (Draft, to be published 1993).

I14 International Commission on Radiation Units and Measurements. Determination of dose equivalents from external radiation sources. ICRU Report 39 (1985).

I15 International Commission on Radiation Units and Measurements. Determination of dose equivalents from external radiation sources. Part 2. ICRU Report 43 (1988).

I16 International Commission on Radiation Units and Measurements. Measurement of dose equivalents from external photon and electron radiations. ICRU Report 47 (1992).

I17 Institut National d'Etudes Démographiques, Paris. Population et Sociétés. Bulletin Mensuel d'Informations Demographiques, Economiques, Sociales. Nos. 126 (1979); 193 (1985); 259 (1991).

J1 Johnston, G. An evaluation of radiation and dust hazards at a mineral sand processing plant. Health Phys. 60: 781-787 (1991).

K1 Kumazawa, S. and T. Numakunai. A new theoretical analysis of occupational dose distributions indicating the effect of dose limits. Health Phys. 41: 465-475 (1981).

K2 Kumazawa, S., J. Shimazaki and T. Numakunai. Numerical calculation methods relating to hybrid log-normal distributions. JAERI/M-82-035, Tokai-Mura (1982).

K3 Kendall, G.M., S.C. Darby and E. Greenslade. Patterns of dose incurred by workers on the National Radiological Protection Board's Dose Record Keeping Service. J. Soc. Radiol. Prot. 2 (3): 20-25 (1982).

K4 Kendall, G.M., E. Greenslade, E.A. Pook et al. Distributions of annual doses to some United Kingdom radiation workers. J. Radiol. Prot. 8 (4): 234-238 (1988).

K5 Kendall, G.M., C.R. Muirhead, B.H. MacGibbon et al. First analysis of the National Registry for Radiation Workers: occupational exposure to ionizing radiation and mortality. NRPB-R251 (1992).

K6 Kobal, I., J. Vaupotič, H. Udovč et al. Radon concentrations in the air of Slovenia underground mines. Environ. Int. 16: 171-173 (1990).

K7 Kovač, J., D. Cesar and A. Baumman. Ten years of radiation monitoring at a phosphate fertilizer plant. p. 214-218 in: Proceedings of the Third Italian-Yugoslav Symposium on Low Level Radiation, Plitvice, 1990.

L1 Lloyd, D.C. et al. Doses in radiation accidents investigated by chromosome aberration analysis VI, VII, VIII, IX, XIII, XIV, XVI, XVII: Reviews of cases investigated, 1976-1987. NRPB-R41, R57, R70, R83, R148, R166, R192, R207 (1976-1987).

L2 Lefaure, C. and J. Lochard. La dosimetrie des travailleurs des entreprises exterieures dans les centrales nucléaires. Risque et Prevention. Bulletin d'information du Centre d'Etude sur l'Evaluation de la Protection dans le Domaine Nucléaire, No. 9. CEA/CEPN (1990).

L3 Londhe, V.S. and S.R. Rao. Study of distribution of some natural radionuclides on processing of rock phosphate. Bull. Radiat. Prot. 11: 181-183 (1988).

M1 Mangeno, J.J. and A.E. Tyron. Occupational radiation exposure from U.S. naval nuclear propulsion plants and their support facilities. U.S. Department of the Navy, NT-87-2 (1987).

M2 McEwan, A.C. Occupational radiation exposures in New Zealand. Radiat. Prot. Dosim. 22 (4): 243-251 (1988).

M3 Merwin, S.E., W.H. Millet and R.J. Traub. Twenty-first annual report. Radiation exposures for DOE and DOE contractor employees - 1988. DOE/EH-0171P (1990).

M4 Mishra, U.C. and T.V. Ramachandran. Technologically enhanced natural radiation sources - a review. Bull. Radiat. Prot. 11: 270-280 (1988).

M5 Montagne, C., J.P. Donne, D. Pelcot et al. Inflight radiation measurements aboard French airliners. Radiat. Prot. Dosim. 48: 79-83 (1993).

M6 McAulay, I.R. Radiation exposure of aircrew. Trinity College, Dublin. Communication to the UNSCEAR Secretariat (1991).

M7 Morris, N. Personal radiation monitoring and assessment of doses received by radiation workers in Australia. ARL/TR-107 (1992).

M8 Mullarkey, D.T., Nuclear Electric, United Kingdom. Communication to the UNSCEAR Secretariat (1992).

M9 Mangeno, J.J., Department of the Navy, United States. Communication to the UNSCEAR Secretariat (1992).

M10 Mangeno, J.J. and C.W. Burrows. Occupational radiation exposure from U.S. naval nuclear propulsion plants and their support facilities. U.S. Department of the Navy, NT-92-2 (1992).

M11 McCormick, W.B., British Ministry of Defence. Communication to the UNSCEAR Secretariat (1992).

M12 Mishra, U.C. and M.C. Subba Ramu. Natural radioactivity in houses and mine atmospheres in India. Radiat. Prot. Dosim. 24: 25-28 (1988).

M13 Majoubi, H.C., A. Abbes, A. Aboudi et al. Etude de la radioactivité naturelle dans le sol du sud tunisien, région de Gasfa Tozeur. Radioprotection 26: 537-549 (1991).

N1 National Council on Radiation Protection and Measurements. Exposure of the US population from occupational radiation. NCRP Report No. 101 (1989).

N2 Nikipelov, B., A. Lyslov and H. Koshurnikova. An experience of the first enterprise of the nuclear industry (levels of exposure and health of workers). Priroda 2: 30-38 (1990).

N3 National Council on Radiation Protection and Measurements. Guidance on radiation received in space activities. NCRP Report No. 98 (1989).

N4 Nguyen, V.D., P. Bouisset, N. Parmentier et al. Real-time quality factor and dose equivalent meter "CIRCE" and its use on-board the Soviet orbital station "MIR". p. 1-17 in: Workshop on Implementation of Dose Equivalent Based on Microdosimetric Techniques in Radiation Protection, Schloss Elmau (Germany), 1988.

N5 National Council on Radiation Protection and Measurements. Exposure of the population in the United States and Canada from natural background radiation. NCRP Report No. 94 (1987).

N6 Nair, N.B., C.D. Eapen and C. Rangarajan. High airborne radioactivity levels due to radon in some non-uranium mines in India. Radiat. Prot. Dosim. 11: 193-197 (1985).

O1 Omar, M., M.Y. Ibrahim, A. Hassan et al. Enhanced radium level in tin mining areas in Malaysia. p. 191-196 in: Proceedings of the International Conference on High Levels of Natural Radiation, Ramsar, 1990. IAEA, Vienna, 1993.

O2 Organization for Economic Cooperation and Development, Nuclear Energy Agency, and International Atomic Energy Agency. Uranium - resources, production and demand, 1989. OECD (1990).

O3 Organization for Economic Cooperation and Development, Nuclear Energy Agency, and International Atomic Energy Agency. Nuclear energy and its fuel cycle. Report by an Expert Group, OECD (1987).

O4 O'Brien, K., W. Friedberg, F.E. Duke et al. The exposure of aircraft crews to radiation of extra-terrestrial origin. Radiat. Prot. Dosim. 45: 145-162 (1992).

O5 Othman, I., M. Al-Hushari and G. Raja. Radiation exposure levels in phosphate mining activities. Radiat. Prot. Dosim. 45: 197-201 (1992).

P1 Pavlov, I. and A. Panfilov. The impact of the new ICRP occupational dose limits on the operation of underground mines. Ministry of Atomic Energy, Russian Federation (1992).

P2 Pellerin, P., Service Central de Protection contre les Rayonnements Ionisants (SCPRI), France. Communication to the UNSCEAR Secretariat (1991).

P3 Pradel, J. Consequence of a reduction in radiation protection limits in mines. p. 231-242 in: Proceedings of the IV National Congress of the Spanish Radiation Protection Society - Implications of the New ICRP

Recommendations on Radiation Protection Practices and Interventions, Salamanca, November 1991. Volume 1. CIEMAT, Madrid, 1992.

P4 Perry, D.R. Trends in radiological and environmental protection at high energy accelerator laboratories. p. 17-22 in: Proceedings of International Conference on Occupational Radiation Protection, Guernsey, April 1991.

P5 Pan, Z. A discussion on some problems existing in BSS. Bureau of Safety, Protection and Health, National Nuclear Corporation, China (1992).

P6 Pan Zi Qiang. Bureau of Safety, Protection and Health, CNNC, China. Communication to the UNSCEAR Secretariat (1993).

R1 Rolland-Piegue, C., Compagnie Générale des Matières Nucléaires (COGEMA), Velizy-Villacoublay, France. Communication to the UNSCEAR Secretariat (1992).

R2 Raddatz, C.T. and D. Hagemeyer. Occupational radiation exposure at commercial nuclear power facilities, 1989. NUREG-0713, Volume 11 (1992).

R3 Rodrigues de Oliveira, A. Un répertoire des accidents radiologiques, 1945-1985. Radioprotection 22 (2): 89-135 (1987).

R4 Robé, M.C., A. Rannou and J. Le Bronec. Radon measurement in the environment of France. Radiat. Prot. Dosim. 45: 455-457 (1992).

R5 Rox, A., J. Fahland, R. Freder et al. Bestimmung von Radon und seinen Folgeprodukten im Steinkohleberg-bau. p. 57-73 in: Messung von Radon und Radon-Folgeprodukten. Verlag TüV, Rheinland, 1991.

R6 Rock, R.L., G. Svilar, R.T. Beckman et al. Evaluation of radioactive aerosols in United States underground coal mines. U.S. Department of the Interior, Bureau of mines report MESA-IR1025 (1975).

R7 Regulla, D. and J. David. Radiation measurements in civil aircraft. GSF 41/91 (1991).

R8 Regulla, D. and J. David. Measurements of cosmic radiation on-board Lufthansa aircraft on the major international flight routes. Radiat. Prot. Dosim. 48: 65-72 (1993).

S1 Sont, W.N. and J.P. Ashmore. 1984 Annual radiation doses in Canada: log-normal and hybrid log-normal analysis using maximum likelihood estimation. Health Phys. 54: 211-219 (1988).

S2 Schmitt, C.H. and J.F. Brice. Occupational radiation exposure from U.S. naval nuclear propulsion plants and their support facilities. U.S. Department of the Navy report NT-84-2 (1984).

S3 Sont, W.N. and J.P. Ashmore. Projected whole body career doses for radiation workers in Canada. Health Phys. 47: 693-700 (1984).

S4 Service Central de Protection contre les Rayonnements Ionisants, Le Vesinet, France. Rapport technique (1989).

S5 Strong, R. and C. Partington. Past trends in occupational exposure in nuclear fuel reprocessing at Sellafield. p. 11-16 in: Proceedings of International Conference on Occupational Radiation Protection, Guernsey, April 1991.

S6 Swindon, T.N. and N. Morris. Personal monitoring and assessment of doses received by radiation workers. ARL/TR-035 (1981).

S7 Stewart, J.M., Chamber of Mines of South Africa, Johannesburg, South Africa. Communication to the UNSCEAR Secretariat (1992 and 1993).

S8 Sztanyik, L.B. and I. Bojtor, National Research Institute for Radiobiology and Radiohygiene, Hungary. Communication to the UNSCEAR Secretariat (1991).

S9 Shaw, K.B. Radiation exposure of civil aircrew. Radiol. Prot. Bull. 127: 15-18 (1991).

S10 Schmitz, J. and R. Fritsche. Radon impact at underground workplaces in Western Germany. Radiat. Prot. Dosim. 45: 193-195 (1992).

S11 Schiocchetti, G., F. Scacco and G.F. Clemente. The radiation hazards in Italian non-uranium mines: aspects of radiation protection. p. 69-73 in: Radiation Hazards in Mining - Control, Measurement and Medical Aspects. Society of Mining Engineers, New York, 1981.

S12 Štelcl, J., O. Navrátil, J. Pribyl et al. On the sources of radon in the caves in the northern part of the Moravian karst. Scr. Fac. Sci. Nat. Univ. Park Brun. 17: 233-240 (1987).

S13 Switzerland. Office Federal de la Santé Publique, Suisse. Dosimetrie des personnes exposees aux radiations sans l'exercise de leur profession en Suisse. Rapports de la Commission Federale de la Protection contre les Radiations. Rapports 1-15 (1976-1990).

T1 Talmor, A., Y. Laichter and G. Weiser. Estimation of radiation exposure to the population of Arad following the opening of the Sedeh-Zohar phosphates mine. p. 27-32 in: Program and Abstracts of Lectures at the 1988 Annual Meeting of the Israeli Health Physics Society, Herzliya, 1988.

U1 United Nations. Sources, Effects and Risks of Ionizing Radiation. United Nations Scientific Committee on the Effects of Atomic Radiation, 1988 Report to the General Assembly, with annexes. United Nations sales publication E.88.IX.7. United Nations, New York, 1988.

U3 United Nations. Ionizing Radiation: Sources and Biological Effects. United Nations Scientific Committee on the Effects of Atomic Radiation, 1982 Report to the General Assembly, with annexes. United Nations sales publication E.82.IX.8. United Nations, New York, 1982.

U4 United Nations. Sources and Effects of Ionizing Radiation. United Nations Scientific Committee on the Effects of Atomic Radiation, 1977 Report to the General Assembly, with annexes. United Nations sales publication E.77.IX.1. United Nations, New York, 1977.

U5 United Nations. Ionizing Radiation: Levels and Effects. Report of the United Nations Scientific Committee on the Effects of Atomic Radiation, with annexes. United Nations sales publication E.72.IX.17 and 18. United Nations, New York, 1972.

U9 United Nations. Report of the United Nations Scientific Committee on the Effects of Atomic Radiation. Official Records of the General Assembly, Seventeenth Session, Supplement No. 16 (A/5216). New York, 1962.

U11 United Nations. 1987 Statistical Yearbook. Thirty-sixth issue. Department of International Economic and Social Affairs, Statistical Office. New York, 1990.

V1 Viktorsson, C., J. Lochard, M. Benedittini et al. Occupational dose control in nuclear power plants - an overview. p. 13-25 in: Proceedings of International Workshop on New Developments in Occupational Dose Control and ALARA Implementation at Nuclear Power Plants and Similar Facilities, New York, September 1989. NUREG/CP-0110 and BNL-NUREG-52226 (1990).

W1 Wilson, J.A., J.P. Ashmore and D. Grogan. Occupational radiation exposures in Canada 1987. Canadian Department of National Health and Welfare. Report No. 89-EHD-147 (1989).

W2 Wilson, J.W. and L.W. Townsend. Radiation safety in commercial air traffic: a need for further study. Health Phys. 55: 1001-1003 (1988).

W3 Wang Zuoyuan. Typical radiation accidents happened in China. Laboratory of Industrial Hygiene, Ministry of Public Health, Beijing, China, 1990.

W4 Webb, G.A.M., J.S. Hughes and G. Lawson. Current dose distributions in the UK - implications of ICRP Publication 60. NRPB-M286 (1991).

X1 Xingyuan, Z., L. Hanqin and X. Renyi. Radiation hygiene survey of radon in non-uranium mines. Chin. J. Radiol. Med. Prot. 9: 16-18 (1989).

ANNEX E

Mechanisms of radiation oncogenesis

CONTENTS

INTRODUCTION

1. Basic information on cancer induction (oncogenesis) by radiation comes from epidemiological studies of exposed human populations. These give evidence of the relatively wide range of neoplasms involved and of the latency periods and the dose levels at which they are observed. It may be that the limits of resolution of such data are being reached, and for absorbed doses of less than 0.1-0.5 Gy of low linear energy transfer (LET) radiation, there may be increasing dependence on extrapolation procedures. Since most human exposures to radiation occur at doses substantially below 0.5 Gy, the validity of such extrapolations is a crucial factor in risk estimation.

2. The extrapolation of radiation response to low levels of dose is made with dose-effect models derived from physical and biophysical studies of the action of radiation on biological systems [C1, G1, U2]. The principal appeal of these models is that they attempt to describe dose-effect with simple linear or linear-quadratic equations. While in recent years considerable efforts have been made to validate such models of radiation action with respect to fundamental biological factors, such as the macromolecular structure of cellular targets and the influence of post-irradiation repair processes [C2, G2], the unqualified application of simple biophysical equations to a complex multi-factorial biological process such as cancer induction is problematic. That is not to say that simple extrapolations and approximations from animal and cellular dose-effect data will not be possible, but rather that there is as yet insufficient knowledge to make them with confidence.

3. So that future extrapolation of high-dose epidemiological data may be made with confidence, it is crucial that a much more detailed picture be gained of the cellular and molecular processes that mediate oncogenic change in mammalian cells. Much of the mechanistic knowledge of radiation action is derived from studies on cell inactivation, chromosomal change, mutagenesis and the repair of deoxyribonucleic acid (DNA). These data will all continue to contribute towards a broad solution to the problem, but until they can be placed in the correct context through the identification of specific neoplasia-associated cellular events, their direct relevance to oncogenesis will remain uncertain.

4. There is strong evidence that oncogenesis is a multi-step process involving the accumulation of a series of genetic and epigenetic changes in a clonal population of cells, that different steps characterize different neoplasms and that the whole process is strongly influenced by genetic, physiological and environmental factors. The characterization of mechanisms of radiation oncogenesis is therefore a daunting challenge. Its importance to future estimates of cancer risk is, however, sufficiently great that the challenge must be accepted.

5. It is also important to stress that in addition to its obvious relevance to radiological protection, the further understanding of the mechanisms of radiation oncogenesis would contribute substantially to fundamental cancer research, a very active and rapidly developing field in which breakthroughs are being sought. This Annex outlines some of the principal problems, broad theories and experimental strategies regarding the mechanisms of radiation oncogenesis and attempts to anticipate future studies and their potential application in radiation risk estimation.

I. STRUCTURE AND FUNCTION OF MAMMALIAN CELLS

6. A brief description of the cell, its structure and functioning in the mammalian organism will serve as background information for the discussion to follow. Only those more basic aspects of the cell and of molecular biology that are relevant to this Annex are given here. More detailed information can be found in the references (e.g. [A1, C7, W1, W2, W5]).

A. CELLS AND TISSUES

7. The cell is the basic unit of all organisms. Each mammalian cell is bounded by a complex, semi-permeable lipid and protein membrane, which actively mediates the two-way flow of metabolites and presents protein receptor sites to allow the cell to interact with its environment. Contained within the membrane is a highly organized aqueous milieu, the cytoplasm, which contains numerous organelles, principally the nucleus containing the genetic material of the cell (see below), mitochondria (for the generation of biochemical energy), the endoplasmic reticulum (providing surfaces for biochemical reactions) and protein-nucleic acid complexes termed ribosomes (for protein synthesis). Proteins synthesized on ribosomes may act structurally, as catalysts of biochemical reactions (enzymes), or play a coordinating role in cell physiology (intracellular regulators, growth factors, cytokines and hormones).

8. At certain points in their life history cells are required to reproduce themselves; this is achieved by transit through the cell cycle. Most cells established in culture have cell cycle transit times of 18-24 h; *in vivo* cell cycle times range up to a week, these longer periods reflecting varying periods of quiescence in one phase of the cycle. In this cycle the genetic material of the cell is replicated and shared equally between the two identical daughter cells that result from the cell division that terminates the cycle.

9. Even at the single-cell level, the complexity of the biochemical and biophysical reactions that are required for maintenance of biological function is immense. In multicellular organisms, however, cells are required to act in concert in order to provide specialized tissue functions. Beyond that, tissue function itself is required to be interactive, so that the whole physiology of the organism is coordinated and responses to appropriate environmental conditions are available.

10. Although grossly simplistic, the above outline is sufficient to demonstrate the need for a highly complex network of information transfer, which must have its origins in single-cell function and response. The source of this lies in the cell nucleus, specifically in the nucleoprotein complexes that make up the microscopic bodies termed chromosomes.

B. CHROMOSOMES

11. Chromosomes are basic components in cellular reproduction. Before every somatic cell division, chromosomes are duplicated, and each daughter cell normally receives an identical set of chromosomes. Each mammalian species is characterized by a particular and constant chromosome number, size and morphology.

12. Each chromosome contains a single nucleic acid polymer, deoxyribonucleic acid (DNA), which is complexed along its length by proteins such as those of the histone family and others with roles in the regulation of chromosome structure and DNA metabolism. The DNA forms the crucial structural entity, but the whole nucleoprotein complex has a series of orders of structure progressing through secondary solenoid-like bodies (nucleosomes), which stack together to form tertiary chromatin fibres. The individual chromosome, the quaternary structure, is composed of a complex arrangement of these fibres maintained by matrix and scaffold proteins.

13. Although the maintenance of overall chromosome structure is crucial for DNA metabolic processes such as condensation, transcription, replication, recombination and repair, it is the DNA polymer itself that is the source of cellular information and, thereby, physiological control.

14. The information is encoded in a linear sequence of alternating aromatic (nucleic acid) base pairs. The pairing is achieved by a double-stranded helical arrangement, where the four bases, adenine (A), thymine (T), guanine (G) and cytosine (C), on one strand are covalently linked to a sugar-phosphate backbone and specifically pair (A with T, G with C) with the bases on the opposite strand through hydrogen bonding. The relatively weak hydrogen bonding between base pairs allows unwinding of the DNA duplex, which is necessary for some aspects of DNA processing. In particular, DNA replication through DNA polymerase enzyme activity has to occur with high fidelity each time the cell is preparing to divide. This fidelity is achieved by unwinding the DNA and replicating the base sequence on the two strands.

15. The base pair code in DNA is arranged in subunits of three bases, termed codons. Amino acids, the building blocks of protein, are specified by codons, and a string of codons is able to determine the

structure and thereby the function of a single protein (polypeptide chain). Such a functional string of DNA codons represents the basic unit of cellular information and hereditary, the gene. Three specific codons act as "stop" signals, thereby indicating the point at which the gene code is terminated. While all others specify an amino acid, the code is degenerate in that there is more than one codon for most amino acids, i.e. 61 coding units determine the 20 natural amino acids. Other non-coding DNA sequences associated with a given gene act to regulate its activity. In mammalian cells it may be estimated that there are approximately 100,000 genes, each of which depends for its correct function on maintaining a constant DNA base sequence. Changes in these sequences by base pair substitution, loss or addition can change gene function; such changes are termed genetic mutations. However, damage to the DNA does not always result in mutations, since cellular DNA repair enzymes are often able to restore both damaged DNA base and damaged sugar phosphate backbone.

16. Most cellular DNA does not code for proteins, and even allowing for base sequences that act to control gene expression, there appears to be much functional redundancy in the mammalian genome. This feature implies that DNA damage in certain chromosome regions will have little or no consequence for the cell, while in other regions damage may change the activity of key genes, leading to changes in cellular properties. Gene expression occurs when a single-stranded nucleic acid, ribonucleic acid (RNA), is synthesized (transcribed) from the gene. In mammalian genes only part of the linear base sequence actually codes. The coding segments (exons) are separated by non-coding segments (introns), which often constitute the major portion of the gene. Consequently, the primary RNA transcribed from the whole gene has to be appropriately cut and spliced before it is fully functional. This messenger RNA (mRNA) contains a string of codons complementary to those of the gene, and these are used by cellular ribosomes to construct the specified protein. Transcriptional processes and hence gene product availability are closely coordinated in cells by a series of interacting feedback loops.

17. In a given mammalian species, all cells contain the same genes; these cells may, however, differ in the relative activity of those genes. Developmental processes involve the selective functional activation and inactivation of many genes. While a core function is maintained by so-called housekeeping genes, specialized functions in tissues require the expression of appropriate sets of (luxury) genes in certain cell lineages. This reprogramming of the genome has to be stably maintained, since such specialized functions have to operate throughout the subsequent life-span of the cell. It may therefore be seen that this coordinated programming underlies cellular and tissue differentiation and is hence a central feature of normal organogenesis and tissue maintenance. Gene programming, which must be initiated early in embryogenesis, is believed to have its origins in gene activation/inactivation through secondary biochemical modification to DNA, such as DNA base methylation, changes in chromatin structure and/or stable protein binding [H16, M44]. Growth factors, hormones and cytokines also play a role in the mediation of differentiation in many tissues. Such stable changes in gene expression and cellular properties (phenotypes) in the absence of DNA base pair changes are essentially non-genetic and are often referred to as being epigenetic. The specific rearrangement of immunoglobulin germ-line DNA sequences is known to play a key role in the generation of immunocompetence in white blood cells; DNA rearrangement is not, however, believed to be a major mechanism of cell differentiation.

18. While fundamental knowledge of gene function, control and mutation may be traced back to pioneer work in micro-organisms [H1, J1], higher organisms have progressively more complex biological problems, including cancer development (oncogenesis). In a broad histopathological sense, cancer in mammalian tissues presents itself as a caricature of normal cell and tissue development. In some way, intrinsic biological control at both the cellular and tissue level has been subverted. Chapter II outlines some of the theories relating to oncogenesis, particularly those that are relevant to its induction by the exposure of mammalian cells to ionizing radiation.

II. PRINCIPAL THEORIES OF ONCOGENESIS

19. During the last decade there has been a remarkable increase in knowledge of the roles of chromosomal change, of specific cellular genes and of inherited mutations in human oncogenesis. However, huge gaps remain in the understanding of the problem. In the context of radiation oncogenesis, great uncertainty exists in the nature and consequences of the genetic/epigenetic events that mediate the inductive, promotional and progression processes, in the mechanisms and contribution of human genetic susceptibility and in differences in oncogenic mechanisms following exposure to radiation or chemical carcinogens.

A. INDUCTIVE AND DEVELOPMENTAL PROCESSES

1. DNA as a principal target for radiation action

20. The genetic material (DNA) of the cell is known to be damaged following exposure to ionizing radiation. Many induced DNA base damages have been identified (e.g. [F13]), and the induction of DNA strand breakage in cells has recently been reviewed [W12]. There is compelling evidence from a range of *in vitro* cellular studies that the main detrimental effects of radiation derive from its ability to damage cellular DNA. First, at the cellular level it has been shown through selective radioisotope irradiation that the cell nucleus contains the principal targets determining radiosensitivity (see, e.g. [H2, H3]). Secondly, radiation-induced chromosomal damage may be quantitatively correlated with cell inactivation (see, e.g. [J4, L1]) and, to a lesser extent, mutation [C3]. Thirdly, in highly radiosensitive mutant strains of both micro-organisms and cultured mammalian cells, there is a good correlation between radiosensitivity and genetic deficiency in the cellular processes that act on DNA damage [F1]. It has also been shown that the induction of DNA double-strand breaks (dsb) in cells by the introduction of restriction endonuclease enzymes mimics the chromosomal damage resulting from radiation exposure [N1] and that there is a quantitative correlation between DNA dsb induction/ repair and cellular radiosensitivity [R1]. Although none of these observations exclude the involvement of non-DNA targets in some aspects of cellular response, they provide strong evidence for induced DNA damage as the principal mechanism of radiation action. Most of these data relate, however, to radiation-induced chromosome damage and cell inactivation. While the evidence is less extensive, *in vitro* cell transformation has been shown to be induced by DNA breaks produced in cells by restriction endonucleases [B9]; other evidence, outlined in paragraphs 162-165, provides additional support for a DNA target for *in vitro* cell transformation.

21. Microbial genetic techniques have also established a convincing correlation between the capacity of physical and chemical agents to induce somatic mutations in DNA and their activity as carcinogens (see, e.g. [A2]). This basic somatic mutation theory of cancer induction, although defining the principal macromolecular target for radiation oncogenesis as DNA, leaves unanswered important questions regarding the number of cells that need to be mutated in order to initiate the process, the number of gene mutations that are required, whether specific gene mutations in target cells are needed and whether these mutations are dominant or recessive in their action. In recent years, the application of modern methods of cell and molecular genetics to the characterization of neoplasms has led to a significant increase in the understanding of many of these questions.

2. The single-cell origin of neoplasia

22. In order to understand the molecular mechanisms of oncogenesis and the role of genetic and epigenetic change, it is most important to first consider the cellular derivation of disease. Evidence for the monoclonal origin of neoplasia comes from a number of sources.

23. In female mammals, all of whom are heterozygous for X-chromosome-linked genes, X-chromosome inactivation leads to a mosaic of somatic cells in tissues with cells of different clonal origin expressing different forms of the same gene product (i.e. iso-enzymes), depending on which X-chromosome remains active. Neoplasms in female mammals have, in the vast majority of cases, been shown to have only a single form of the gene product (i.e. a single phenotype), implying that the neoplasm was of monoclonal origin [F1]. Studies utilizing restriction enzyme polymorphisms of characterized and anonymous DNA sequences, chromosomal markers and oncogene and immunoglobulin gene rearrangements have all confirmed the original X-chromosome biochemical studies [T1, W3]. Convincing evidence for the monoclonal origin of human and murine colorectal cancer has been provided by cytogenetic and molecular studies of benign and malignant manifestations of this disease [F8, P7]. Most, if not all, malignant human colorectal carcinomas arise from pre-existing benign adenomas [S17]. Thus, although normal colonic epithelium is polyclonal, adenomas arise within single pockets of epithelium, indicating that they were initiated within a monoclonal population of stem cells [F8, F9]. The characteristic cytogenetic and molecular features of such adenomas fully supports this contention. In addition, early pre-neoplastic haemopoietic cells carrying characteristic chromosomal rearrangements have been shown to convert in a monoclonal fashion to overt malignancy (paragraph 72); in animal studies, the monoclonal origin of chemically induced tumours is further supported by the finding of characteristic point mutations in *ras* proto-oncogenes of rodent skin papillomas/carcinomas and breast tumours (paragraphs 188 and 189). Studies on the *p53* gene in human tumours associated with chemical or sunlight exposure also support the monoclonal origin of neoplasia (paragraph 194).

24. Overall, it may be concluded that neoplasms with double phenotypes are rare and that neoplasia develops infrequently from a mixed population of normal cells. Double phenotypes have been recorded in some

induced animal neoplasms, usually where high doses of a potent carcinogen were employed. This probably reflects the coalescence of adjacent primary neoplasms, but there is some evidence that some double-phenotype polyploid neoplasms may originate through the fusion of two single-phenotype cells [T1].

25. Despite the compelling evidence that single neoplasms arise from single ancestral progenitor cells, some caution needs to be exercised with regard to the implications for oncogenic mechanisms. Since many rounds of cell reproduction and clonal evolution/selection occur between neoplastic initiation and final malignancy, the observations summarized above do not exclude initiation of a number of target cells, polyclonal pre-neoplasia and subsequent predominance of a single successful cancer clone. In these contexts, models of radiation carcinogenesis requiring induced damage in more than one cell have been proposed [M1], and it has been argued that radiation-induced murine acute myeloid leukaemia may not develop, as conventionally viewed, through a series of clonal progressions [M2]. It is inherently difficult to study clonal contributions to pre-neoplasia in most irradiated tissues and the problem is not one that will be easily resolved.

26. However, these qualifying remarks do not in the main detract from the conclusion that the majority of neoplasms originate from damage to single cells. In principle, therefore, the traversal of a single target cell by one ionizing track from radiation has a finite probability, albeit low, of initiating neoplastic change. On this basis, although only a proportion of induced pre-neoplastic cells may convert to malignancy, the initiation process may be expected to show a non-threshold response. This may be contrasted with a hypothetical process whereby neoplasia is initiated through damage accumulation in an adjacent set of target cells, producing, for example, a "field effect" in the tissue, resulting in aberrant differentiation. The predictions arising from this are (a) that a significant proportion of benign and malignant neoplasms will be polyclonal; (b) that the requirement for multi-cell damage will tend to produce a dose-effect relationship having a clear low-dose threshold. The current state of knowledge provides little general support for such hypotheses, and in the case of human bladder cancer, where field effects have been specifically postulated, recent molecular studies show multiple site tumours to be monoclonal in origin [S47]. Against this, some benign neurofibromas have, however, been shown to be of polyclonal origin [W6], and threshold-like responses have been reported for the induction of some animal tumours by radiation (see, e.g. [O5]). Related to this are problems regarding the role of multiple events ("hits"), genomic instability and cellular defense mechanisms in neoplastic development. These receive comment later in the Annex.

3. Genetic changes in oncogenesis

27. During the last decade, investigation of the genes directly involved in neoplasia has been one of the most rapid growth areas in cellular and molecular genetics. Consequently, only a very brief summary is possible (see [B1, B6, B18, H4, H46, S18, S63, W14, W20] for reviews). Although the association between chromosomal change and neoplasia was established in the early years of cancer research, the contribution of specific genetic changes to the neoplastic phenotype had to await the advent of recombinant DNA techniques, which allow the identification, isolation (cloning) and characterization of relatively small DNA sequences from whole genomic complexes.

(a) Proto-oncogene activation

28. In this area of research, a major breakthrough was achieved when it was shown that oncogenic DNA sequences (v-*onc*) in an avian virus had related proto-oncogene sequences (c-*onc*) in normal avian DNA [S1]. This approach initially identified c-*src* but was subsequently extended to other proto-oncogenes, e.g. c-*ras* (v-*ras* of rat sarcoma virus) and c-*abl* (v-*abl* of Abelson murine leukaemia virus). Using v-*onc* molecular probes, it has been possible to isolate and subsequently characterize cellular DNA sequences that encode a range of oncogenes [B1]. These and other cellular oncogenes have been characterized by other experimental approaches:

(a) by transferring DNA purified or cloned from a neoplasm into suitable host mammalian cells and establishing a correlation between the genomic integration of a specific donor DNA sequence and the acquisition of a quasi-neoplastic cellular phenotype (see, e.g. [C4, G3]);
(b) by identifying host DNA sequences that are consistently and specifically activated by the adjacent integration of oncogenic viruses (see, e.g. [M3, N2]);
(c) by isolating and characterizing DNA sequences that are located in the breakpoint region of chromosomal rearrangements consistently associated with specific neoplasms (see, e.g. [D1, H4, S63]);
(d) by using molecular hybridization techniques to identify new oncogenes that have conserved certain DNA sequences and are therefore part of a large gene family, some members of which are already known.

29. The characterization of oncogenes in human and animal neoplasms and in *in vitro* cellular systems initially leads to the following broad conclusions:

(a) altered expression of oncogenes may occur through point mutation [B6, B18], chromosomal translocation and juxtaposition with another DNA sequence [H4, S63], insertion of relatively short and specific viral or genomic sequences [N2] or through gene amplification (generation of multiple oncogene copies) (see, e.g. [N7]); there is also evidence that epigenetic mechanisms, such as changes in the extent of DNA methylation, may also play a role in the expression of genes involved in neoplastic changes [F23, J5, S19];

(b) these mechanisms are often characteristic of particular oncogenes but are by no means mutually exclusive;

(c) the activation of particular oncogenes may characterize histopathologically related neoplasms, but equally, the same oncogene may play different temporal roles in different neoplasms [B6];

(d) a given neoplasm will often contain structural and/or activational changes in a number of known oncogenes, and there is evidence for oncogene cooperation in the development of neoplastic phenotypes [H12]; thus, long latency periods might be explained by the need to accumulate such changes;

(e) oncogene activation often generates a dominant phenotypic trait.

There is an ever-growing list of proto-oncogenes, many of which have known chromosomal locations and functions within the cell (see e.g. Table 1); some of these are referred to at various points in this Annex.

(b) Tumour suppressor gene inactivation

30. It may be argued, however, that despite their clear relevance to oncogenesis, dominantly acting oncogenes probably reflect only one aspect of the whole phenotype, determined in part by early scientific methods. In recent years, this view has received strong support from cytogenetic and molecular studies, which have revealed consistent loss of chromosomal regions and genes in a range of human neoplasms [M4, P1, S18, S19, S34]. Such specific losses during oncogenic development are suggestive of a major role for negative regulatory genes and recessive effects in oncogenesis.

31. The loss of negative regulatory signals from genes has been suspected for some years to be an important aspect of neoplastic development. Such genes, often collectively referred to as tumour suppressor genes, were originally proposed by Knudson to be specifically involved in the hereditary predisposition to certain autosomally determined childhood cancers, in particular retinoblastoma [K1, P12] of which 30%-40% are of the heritable type. Knudson's two hit hypothesis for the induction of such neoplasms requires the sequential mutation/loss of both copies of a specific suppressor gene. According to these proposals, the same mutant gene is involved in both familial and sporadic forms of the neoplasm. In the former case, the first mutation occurs pre-zygotically and is thus present in all somatic cells of the offspring. This is then followed by mutation of the second gene in target somatic cells of the affected organ. In the latter case (sporadic neoplasms), both mutations occur post-zygotically in the same target somatic cell. In general, tumour suppressor genes may be viewed as providing negative cellular effects, for the purposes of maintaining cells in a normal proliferative state and/or regulating normal cellular differentiation programmes.

32. The positive phenotypic role of oncogenes provides strong selection in experimental systems (paragraph 28) and was a major factor in their early identification and characterization. In contrast, such selection is far more difficult to achieve for suppressor functions, and as a consequence, research in this area did not make rapid progress until recently. Nevertheless, there is now persuasive evidence that suppressor genes play a normal role in cell cycle control, cell senescence, signal transduction and differentiation and that their loss can contribute to the development of a broad spectrum of neoplasms.

33. The function of tumour suppressor genes was first experimentally demonstrated in somatic cell hybrids produced from the *in vitro* fusion of normal and tumour cells (NT hybrids) [H29, S18]. In these studies, it was shown that genetic contributions from normal cells suppressed the neoplastic potential of the tumour cells, i.e. the malignant state was recessive and subject to negative regulation. As NT hybrids proliferated, they often lost chromosomes, and the loss of certain chromosomes was accompanied by a reversion to a neoplastic phenotype. Thus, tumour suppression was seen to be specific to certain chromosomes and, by implication, to specific genes. Recent technical advances allow the introduction of single normal chromosomes into tumour cells, and this microcell transfer technique has been used to map putative suppressor genes to specific human chromosomes (see, e.g. [S34, T3]).

34. The genetic pedigree analysis of cancer-prone families has also proved to be a powerful tool in the identification of tumour suppressor genes and their linkage on the human genome. Here it is important to recognize that for autosomal "loss of function" genetic traits associated with tumour suppression, the appearance of tumours in offspring is manifested as a dominant trait. Although the genes function in a recessive fashion at the cellular level, their dominance within family pedigrees reflects the high probability

that, in heterozygous offspring, the normal gene will be lost from a target somatic cell, thus initiating the specific tumour. These losses may, in some tumours, be evidenced by specific chromosome deletion events, and the identification of 13q deletions in retinoblastoma and 11p deletions in Wilms' tumour (see [S18, S19]) provided important early clues as to the location of the respective tumour suppressor genes. This approach has also been extended to familial adenomatous polyposis (FAP) [S20] and multiple endocrine neoplasia type 2 [L8], but here allelic losses do not always occur in the chromosomal region that is associated with the cancer predisposition locus.

35. Molecular approaches to suppressor gene identification in human tumours have centred on the analysis of the loss of specific chromosome regions where parental genetic contributions may be identified by the presence of DNA restriction fragment length polymorphisms (RFLPs); that is, where the two autosomal chromosome regions may be genetically distinguished in normal cells of the patient, it becomes possible to use molecular analysis to distinguish specific DNA losses through the loss of heterozygosity in tumours [M4, S19]. Thus, consistent DNA losses for a set of linked genes in a specific chromosome region may be taken as preliminary evidence for the presence of a tumour-specific suppressor gene in the region. This has proved to be an extremely powerful technique for resolving subchromosomal losses and has provided important information on the position and linkage of putative suppressor genes for a range of human tumour types [S18]. It is becoming increasingly clear that many different tumour types are characterized by specific losses, that the same losses are often apparent in different tumour types and that multiple losses are not uncommon. Parental effects on gene loss have also been observed in some tumours (paragraphs 58-60), and overall, it is now obvious that the loss of suppressor gene function plays a very important role in oncogenesis at both the initiation and progression levels [S18, S19].

36. From these crucial observations on the chromosomal linkage of tumour suppressor genes it has proved possible to obtain molecular clones representing the *RB*, *WT*, *p53* and *K-REV 1* genes (see [S18, S19]) and, more recently, candidate genes for human FAP characterized by colorectal carcinoma associated with chromosome 5q DNA sequence losses [F8, K15, N16]. A putative suppressor gene (*NF-1*) for neurofibromatosis has also been isolated [W6]. Table 2 provides a summary of the suppressor gene loci implicated in human tumorigenesis. For some of these it is now possible to suggest specific cellular functions and link these to oncogenic processes.

37. For *RB* and *p53* genes, a principal role of the protein products appears to be in the control of the cell cycle [C10, N23] (see also paragraphs 43-52). In the case of FAP, the closely linked and structurally related *APC* and *MCC* genes on 5q were candidate determinants of colorectal carcinogenesis, and it has been suggested that they may act in concert to control the proliferation of colonic epithelium. Both genes were found to be somatically mutated in sporadically arising tumours, and *APC* was found to carry point mutations in the germ line of FAP patients [K15, N16]. Moreover, the *APC* gene has been implicated in gastric and pancreatic tumours in man [N17] and, in the mouse, is also a germ line determinant of gastrointestinal tract cancer [S48]. *APC* somatic gene inactivation is principally associated with point mutation or deletion, but in one case of human colon cancer, L1 transposon insertion was detected [M46].

38. While *RB* gene function has provided a relatively straightforward example of recessive suppressor gene function, not only in eye tumours but also in other tumour types (see, e.g. [L21]), other tumour suppressor genes may not operate in such a simple manner, and multiple locus interactions may be a more common feature of such genes. There is evidence that predisposition to and development of Wilms' tumour is genetically complex [D12, F10], and recent studies, noted above, suggest that the phenotypic variation between FAP kindreds might be explained by the interaction between *APC* and *MCC* genes. In addition, some uncertainty still surrounds the genetics of the *p53* gene. This gene has been shown to have the properties of a suppressor gene in colorectal carcinoma [B19], and its germ line function in Li-Fraumeni patients (paragraph 127) supports this contention. However, *p53* in certain forms has also been shown to cooperate with *ras* in transforming primary rodent cells [H17], where it appears to act in a quasi-dominant fashion (see also [D15]).

39. In this context, the interaction between sequential gene losses and gene activation has been most clearly demonstrated in human colorectal cancer. Here mutations in at least four or five genes appear to be required for full malignant conversion, with fewer events being required for benign changes [F8, K15, N16]. There is also evidence that while there may be some degree of preference in the sequence of somatic cell genetic events in colorectal carcinogenesis, the overall accumulation of such changes may be more important [F8, F11]; these changes are illustrated in Figure I. Chromosome 5 genes may be *APC* and/or *MCC*; chromosome 18 losses may involve the *DCC* gene and chromosome 17 losses may involve the *p53* gene.

40. The escape from cellular senescence and the acquisition of cellular immortality is believed to be an important feature of the oncogenic process. Recent

studies suggest that cellular senescence is a process of quasi-differentiation, which results from recessive changes in growth-inhibiting genes [G8]. The *p53* gene has been implicated in the immortalization of some murine cells in culture [H39, R15], and a role for normal suppressor gene function in maintaining the senescence process now seems likely; thus, a loss of such genes could be viewed as an integral part of neoplastic development.

41. The immortalization, or life-span extension, of cells *in vitro* may be achieved by the introduction of viral or cellular oncogenes, and this may be linked with the function of these genes in controlling cytoplasmic signal transduction and/or cell proliferation (paragraphs 43-52). *In vivo*, many oncogenic viruses, while eliciting a chronic proliferative response in tissues, do not induce one-step oncogenesis, and further cellular mutations are needed. In the case of viral hepatocellular carcinoma, *p53* mutation appears to at least partially meet this need (paragraph 117). Similar conclusions may be formed from the observation that many immortalized human cell lines do not form tumours when transplanted into immunodeficient mice (see, e.g. [C17]). Thus while immortalization, or life-span extension, may well involve tumour suppressor gene changes and be an important step in the evolution of most tumours, it is not itself an unambiguous marker of tumorigenic potential.

42. In conclusion, it may be seen that both positive regulatory signals from activated oncogenes and the loss of negative signals from suppressor genes contribute, in an interactive fashion, to the development of neoplasia. As may be anticipated, oncogenes and tumour suppressor genes have a normal role to play in cell physiology, and it is through lack of or inappropriate expression, relatively minor structural change and combined effects that they enable the cell to evade the normal constraints of proliferation, migration and terminal differentiation and enter a phase of neoplastic evolution. The specific role of some oncogene and suppressor gene products is known. These include growth factor, growth factor receptor, transmembrane signalling protein, cytoplasmic message transducer, DNA binding protein and a range of regulatory proteins including transcriptional factors influencing all these functions [A13, B1, B6, B18, H4, H46, S18, S63, W14]. It may be envisaged, therefore, that in combination oncogene activation events, the loss of regulatory gene functions and epigenetic changes affecting gene activity can produce a cascade of inappropriate or defective gene expression, thus generating a metastable and grossly abnormal cellular phenotype. These changes may be brought about by a variety of different changes to DNA, point mutation, chromosome translocation/ insertion, intragenic deletion, chromosomal deletion and non-mutational but stable changes to genes, such as DNA methylation.

(c) Cellular proliferative control and gene transcription

43. Cellular growth and proliferation are controlled through the constraints of the cell cycle [M27, N12]. Quiescent cells in the G_0 phase require a mitogenic stimulus to enter an active phase (G_1), where gene activity is greatly increased. At the end of the G_1 phase, DNA replication is initiated; this replication phase is termed S. Chromosome condensation, initiated at the end of the next (G_2) phase and proceeding through the prophase, is followed by assembly of the replicated chromosome on the mitotic apparatus; this M phase, and indeed the whole cycle, is completed when the mitotic cell divides, providing the two daughter cells with an equal share of cytoplasm and chromosomes. If mitotic stimulation continues, the daughter cells enter a second cycle via G_1; if not, they may fall back into a quiescent state.

44. The cell cycle is a highly conserved and ordered process (see [H50, M47, N23, S62]), which like most complex biological events is subject to both positive and negative regulation. At the single-cell level, mitogenesis and DNA replication/condensation need to occur at optimal points in cell development and be completed "on time", such that chromosomes segregate equally to the two daughter cells. Mistiming of cell cycle events would obviously have adverse physiological consequences for the dividing cell or would create genetic abnormalities in its clonal progeny. Equally, the rate of initiation and progression of neighbouring cells through the cycle must also be closely controlled so that tissue maintenance and development proceed without inappropriate clonal expansion.

45. It may be argued, therefore, that the expression of cell cycle defects may be related to some of the inherent characteristics of oncogenic transformation. While this relationship has been suspected for many years, it is only recently that insights have been gained into the molecular and biochemical control of the cell cycle and, particularly, the crucial roles played by some tumour-associated genes (see [B40, N18, R21]).

46. Studies with yeasts [M27, N12] initially provided evidence that the activity of two classes of proteins, cdc-like protein kinases and cyclins, was central to cell cycle control. Acting in concert as complexes, these proteins catalyse essential steps of cell cycle progression directly via phosphorylation of other nuclear proteins or indirectly via activation of secondary regulators. In general, these controls also apply in the case of animal cells [N23].

47. Cdc-like kinases are believed to act at a number of points in the cell cycle [M27, M28, N23], acting as master switches principally through their ability to interact with different members of the cyclin protein family. Cdc-kinases and cyclins form complexes involving the catalytic protein subunit of cdc2 and the regulatory subunit of cyclin. Such complexes are activated by dephosphorylation-phosphorylation steps and subsequently serve to activate secondary proteins which regulate, for example, chromosome replication and condensation, mitotic structures and nuclear membrane breakdown. According to current proposals (see [M27]), it is the timing of these phosphorylation reactions involving cdc2, together with cyclin complexing and breakdown, that provide biochemical and biophysical coordination. It is also clear that secondary regulators working with these complexes are equally important; it is at this point in the control chain that a strong connection with oncogenic processes has emerged [C10, N18].

48. Current evidence (see [H51, M28, W13]) indicates that, amongst others, the *RB* tumour suppressor gene protein is phosphorylated by cdc2-like kinase but that it is the underphosphorylated form of Rb protein that is bound by viral oncoproteins and is found in quiescent (G_0) cells. The active form has also been shown to complex with various cellular nuclear proteins including a transcriptional regulator termed E2F. The Rb and a related protein termed p107 associate with E2F in different complexes that contain a cdc2 related kinase termed cdk2. Rb/E2F and E2F/p107/cdk2/cyclin E complexes are principally found in G_1 while an E2F/p107/cdk2/cyclin A complex is formed in S. Secondary control of proto-oncogenes (eg. *MYC*), cell cycle regulators (eg. *CDC2* and cyclin A) and genes involved in DNA replication and repair (eg. DNA polymerase α, thymidine kinase and thymidylate synthetase) is believed to be effected through E2F binding sites in their gene promotor regions.

49. Further evidence of the importance of Rb/E2F complexing in cell cycle control comes from studies showing that Rb protein regulates the transcription of *FOS* which, along with *JUN*, plays a crucial role in early mitogenic signal transduction pathways involving growth factors and other proto-oncogenes such as *SRC* and *RAS* [R12]; there is also evidence that Rb and transcription-activating Myc proteins interact directly, perhaps in a fashion parallel to that of Rb and E2F. Finally, and in accord with the above data, it has been shown that *RB* gene functions as both a growth and tumour suppressor in human bladder carcinoma cells [T19].

50. Together, these data indicate that normal Rb and Rb-related protein fulfil multiple roles in the control of the cell cycle, not only in regulating the response to early mitogenic signals to the cell but also in mediating the transitional phases of the cycle itself. The fundamental mechanism through which this is achieved centres on the repression of cell growth and division by the Rb binding of regulatory nuclear proteins, such as E2F and Myc, which drive proliferative responses. Mutational loss or inactivation of Rb in an appropriate target cell may therefore be viewed as a principal means of relaxing these controls, but the same relaxation may also be achieved through the activity of viral oncoproteins that interfere with the binding process.

51. The nuclear phosphoprotein product of the *p53* tumour suppressor gene is also suspected of playing a role in cell cycle regulation [L13]. The normal p53 protein is known to complex with the SV40 virus large T antigen, inhibiting its DNA helicase activity, preventing binding with αDNA polymerase and inhibiting viral DNA replication. These observations suggest that, in normal cells, p53 negatively regulates entry into the S phase of the cell cycle through influencing the assembly of late G_1 protein complexes that initiate DNA replication and/or acting as a transcriptional factor influencing critical gene expression.

52. It has been shown that normal p53 binds to specific DNA sequences in the genome having 2 copies of a 10 base pair repeat motif [E9, K12] and that normal p53 is a transcriptional regulator that is inhibited by SV40 large T antigen and by mutant p53 [F21, R21]. Further to this, it is becoming clear that in its role as a transcriptional regulator normal p53 may act as a damage-response protein providing for the arrest of DNA-damaged cells in the G_1 phase of the cell cycle [K26, L28]. This G_1 checkpoint control is believed to facilitate the repair of DNA damage including that induced by radiation; altered checkpoint control may underly the unusual post-irradiation DNA synthesis response recorded earlier in cells from Li-Fraumeni human patients carrying germ line *p53* mutations [P9]. An additional role for *p53* in the triggering of post-irradiation apoptosis (programmed cell death) has also been demonstrated [C32, L29, Y6]. Here, *p53* may be viewed as a primary regulator of a defence mechanism that acts to remove potentially damaged and abnormal cells before they become established in tissues. A defect in this mechanism would have obvious implications for the initiation and/or progression of neoplasia and the high frequen-cies of *p53* mutation seen in human tumours may testify to importance of this gene in maintaining the normal steady state functions of a range of human tissues.

53. In conclusion, although currently confined to only a few tumour genes, there is now compelling evidence that subversion of the control of the bio-

chemical pathways associated with the cell cycle is a major factor in oncogenic transformation. In view of the tumorigenic consequences of *RB* and *p53* germ-line mutations in man, it may also be argued that, in some cases, the loss of cell cycle control is intrinsic to tumour initiation. Coherent molecular and biochemical models are now emerging that explain how the protein products of some key genes of the tumour suppressor and proto-oncogene types interact with the other components of the cell cycle in order to effect fine control. Current models include tumour suppressor proteins with cyclins and transcription factors as the primary control switches, with proto-oncogenes fulfilling a secondary function. If, for the sake of argument, the loss of cell cycle control altered proliferative response, together with defective damage response, is regarded as a consistently early event in tumorigenesis, then irrespective of the physical or chemical nature of the carcinogenic initiator, it may be that mutational loss or inactivation of suppressor genes, such as *RB* or *p53*, is the most effective route for tumour initiation. While still uncertain, molecular studies on *p53* gene mutations in a variety of human solid tumours (see, e.g. [H30]) provide some support for this, as do the data that link *p53* tumour mutations with environmental exposure to carcinogens (paragraphs 194 and 223-226).

(d) Gene dosage, dominant negative effects and genomic imprinting

54. It may be argued that the sequential mutation of target somatic cells is the most important feature of oncogenesis. These changes must occur within an evolving clone of cells, and in order to arise with a reasonable probability at the early phases of the disease, it may be necessary for that clone to be expanding at an abnormally high rate. It may be expected, therefore, that many neoplasia-initiating events will, in appropriate *in vivo* circumstances, provide target cells with some degree of proliferative or selective advantage. For dominantly acting oncogenes, such as those of the *RAS* family, a specific point mutation may satisfy this requirement [B6, B18]. Similarly, the activation of *MYC* and *ABL* proto-oncogenes through, for example, chromosome-specific translocation [H4, N3, N9] could similarly provide a one-step growth stimulus to appropriate target cells. For autosomal recessive genes (tumour suppressor genes), the loss of function of one gene copy will, in principle, only reduce gene product availability to 50%. Such a moderate reduction of gene product availability as a consequence of this change in gene number (usually termed gene dosage) would not obviously provide the appropriate proliferative stimulus to the cell. In familial neoplasms such as retinoblastoma, the loss of the first *RB* suppressor gene occurs pre-zygotically, thus obviating the need for initial clonal expansion (paragraph 31), but since *RB* gene loss also characterizes non-familial retinoblastoma and osteosarcoma, there remains the considerable problem of explaining apparently recessive "loss of function" genes, which at the cellular level may have some degree of dominance.

55. The problem of single autosomal gene loss and phenotypic effect has persisted for some years, and although it is still to be fully resolved, there are a number of mechanisms that would explain it.

56. For some autosomal loci involved in tumorigenesis, gene dosage (one versus two copies of the gene) may be critical, such that loss of even 50% of the gene product in a mutated cell will give rise to a phenotypic change associated with a degree of proliferative/selective growth advantage [F8]. In some individuals this effect might be emphasized by otherwise minor structural differences between alleles, i.e. germ-line mutations of very low penetrance (paragraph 127). Alternatively, particular forms of structural gene mutations may produce so-called dominant negative effects, whereby an abnormal protein determined by the mutated gene interferes with the function of the normal protein specified by its non-mutant homologue [H18]. It has been suggested that such dominant negative effects underlie the oncogenic functions of *p53* suppressor gene mutations (see [D15, W14]). Although gene transfer studies indicated that in some tumorigenic cells wild type *p53* is dominant to mutated *p53* [C18], more recent investigations show that oncogenic forms of *p53* inhibit *p53*-regulated gene expression, thus providing a basis for the selection of *p53* mutant cells during tumorigenesis [K17]. It may be seen, therefore, that gene dosage or dominant negative effects can underlie the action of some tumour suppressor gene mutations, but considerable uncertainty still surrounds the implications of single allelic mutation for tumour initiation.

57. A further possible solution to the problem has recently emerged from molecular studies on sporadic tumours thought to be initiated through suppressor gene loss. For sporadic tumours associated with *RB* and other putative tumour suppressor genes (retinoblastoma, osteosarcoma, rhabdomyosarcoma, neuroblastoma and Wilms' tumour) it has been observed that major chromosome segment loss events occur preferentially from the maternally inherited chromosome and that mutant paternal loci are usually retained in the neoplasm (see [F23, H16, R7, R8]). These results run counter to the normal expectation that in sporadically arising neoplasms there should be an equal probability that somatic cell gene loss will occur from maternal and paternal chromosomes. A process termed genomic imprinting [H19, M14] has been invoked to explain these findings.

58. Genomic imprinting is a poorly understood epigenetic process by which differential expression of certain autosomal chromosomal regions is imposed in somatic cells of the offspring following some form of differential chromosomal modification of male and female gametes. In such situations the successful embryonic/neonatal development of the offspring is thought to be dependent upon the inheritance of equal parental genetic contributions for that chromosomal region. The molecular mechanisms of such imprinting effects are not well understood, but current proposals [B41, H16, R8] include the differential methylation of DNA in imprinted regions, such that the activity of the hypomethylated genes inherited from one parent significantly exceeds that of the hypermethylated genes inherited from the other. Thus, some developmentally associated autosomal recessive genes do not make equal phenotypic contributions to the cell.

59. On the basis of this hypothesis and for the examples cited in paragraph 57 it may be seen that an inactivating mutation in the more active paternally derived suppressor gene of the target somatic cell could reduce gene product availability to a level that deregulated cellular proliferation/differentiation and resulted in the excessive clonal expansion of pre-neoplastic cells. This expanding clonal population carrying the first suppressor mutation may then complete sufficient cell divisions to allow for the probability of spontaneous loss of the second, less active suppressor gene copy of maternal origin. According to the hypothesis [R7, R8], this second mutational event greatly increases the probability that the cell clone will progress towards malignancy.

60. Although an imprinting effect on gene mutability has also been suggested for the *RB* gene in the initiation of osteosarcoma [T5], the above hypothesis does account for the molecular findings in sporadic tumours, and if it is a more general phenomenon, there may be important implications for radiation oncogenesis. Specifically, an increasing number of potentially imprinted chromosomal regions and genes involved in differentiation and development are being identified in man and the mouse [B41, C19, H19, H52]. The involvement of negative regulatory genes in normal cell differentiation and development may mean that some potential tumour suppressor genes are imprinted in specific tissues and, therefore, the loss of one copy may be sufficient to initiate neoplastic change. This, together with the finding of a DNA deletion mechanism for radiation mutagenesis (paragraph 154), implies that radiation may be an efficient "single event" initiating agent for certain neoplasms associated with the loss of tumour suppressor gene function. However, the whole process of imprinting remains poorly understood. The recent observation of imprinting-like effects on the t(9:22) translocation in human chronic myelogenous leukaemia and *N-MYC* amplification in neuroblastoma indicates that such effects may also extend to certain proto-oncogene activation events [F23, H40, R16].

(e) Chromosomal fragile sites

61. Chromosomal rearrangement and deletion is a major feature of oncogenic development, and there is an ongoing debate as to the significance of specific sites of chromosomal instability (fragile sites, c-*fra*) [H25, H26, L9, M5, S21]. These sites, classified according to their frequency in the human population and their inducibility by different chemical treatments of cells, have been suggested as possible predisposing factors in oncogenesis. Some fragile sites are also believed to be preferential targets for the clastogenic action of DNA-damaging agents, including ionizing radiation [Y1]. Despite statistical analyses showing no overall association between common fragile sites and cancer-associated chromosome breakpoints [M48, S21], an association with rare and distamycin A inducible fragile sites remains, particularly with respect to certain leukaemias [H20, L9, S21]. Overall, it appears that the expression of DNA damage is non-uniformly distributed within the mammalian genome, that certain highly recombinogenic sequences are preferentially involved in induced chromosomal changes and that certain classes of these may contribute towards oncogenesis.

62. The molecular structures of fragile sites are not known, although it seems likely that they represent certain reiterated (repeat) DNA sequences that may recombine at a high frequency. In this context, it has been suggested that interstitial telomere-like repeat sequences may be highly recombinogenic [H21]. These DNA repeat sequences, in their normal terminal position on chromosomes, buffer against chromosomal erosion and instability during DNA replication [M15, M29, S22]. However, in some lower organisms, telomere-like repeat (TLR) sequences are highly recombinogenic; it is this feature, together with limited chromosome aberration and mapping data, that initially prompted the speculation that, when located in interstitial sites, they may represent a subclass of mammalian c-*fra* [H21]. Further support for telomere sequence instability has come from both microbial [K18] and *in vitro* mammalian cell studies [F19], but other investigators [I2] failed to find an association between a specific human c-*fra*, *FRA2B*, and a TLR sequence array located in the same chromosomal region.

63. Cytogenetic evidence of telomere-associated chromosomal instability has been obtained in studies with some human leukaemias (see, e.g. [S35]), and

chromosome break healing mechanisms involving the *de novo* addition of telomeric sequences have been developed from studies with lower eukaryotes (see, e.g. [H31]). Under certain circumstances it appears that these DNA repeat sequences are subject to considerable modification in somatic cells, perhaps reflecting their structure and/or the lack of telomerase enzymes, which can act to extend the repeat arrays [B20]. This apparent instability is not, however, restricted to somatic cells, since studies in the mouse clearly show the arrays to be hypervariable within mouse strains, a feature that might be explained by their capacity to initiate DNA recombination and DNA replication slippage or as a consequence of the repeat sequence modification by telomerase, which is believed to occur during gametogenesis [S36, S37]. A possible factor in telomere-like sequence instability is the unusual secondary structure that these sequences adopt *in vitro* [B20, B42, K19]. Such secondary structures, if they were to occur *in vivo*, might also contribute to the fragile site properties suggested above. The contention that such sites may be particularly prone to radiation-induced breakage and rearrangements and that some such events are involved in radiation oncogenesis is supported by recent studies on the nature of the chromosome 2 deletions and rearrangements that are believed to initiate murine myeloid leukaemogenesis (paragraph 183). Alpha-particle-induced chromosomal instability has recently been demonstrated in murine haemopoietic cells [K25], but this has yet to be specifically linked with fragile site expression or neoplastic change.

64. Telomeric DNA sequences are also believed to play a role in cell senescence [G8], and it has been shown that the ageing of human fibroblasts is accompanied by telomeric shortening [H22]. This may be viewed as increasing inherent chromosomal instability and could be a factor in age-related carcinogenesis. There is no doubt that the current intense interest in the involvement of telomeric and other genomic repeat sequences (see, e.g. [B10, B42, K20, S49]) in chromosomal fragility and rearrangement will yield data of direct relevance to molecular mechanisms of chromosomal instability and their role in oncogenesis.

4. Multistage cellular development in oncogenesis

65. The concept of multistage oncogenesis, originally proposed by Berenblum and Schubik in 1948, has been a most valuable and durable concept. In modern developments of this theory, oncogenesis is divided, albeit imprecisely, into three phases: initiation, promotion and progression.

(a) Tumour initiation and other early events in oncogenesis

66. The initiation of oncogenesis may be most simply viewed as one or more stable cellular events arising spontaneously or induced by exposure to a carcinogen, which predisposes carrier cells to subsequent neoplastic conversion. In the case of neoplasms induced in man or experimental animals by single acute doses of a carcinogen, the agent is assumed to act as an initiator by damaging a specific cellular target in a stable and irreversible fashion [B6, B18, Y2]. Throughout this Annex it is argued, on the basis of animal and human data, that specific somatic mutations in target genes are initiating events for neoplasia.

67. In the preceding Section, cytogenetic and molecular findings on suppressor gene mutations and proto-oncogene activation were discussed in respect of their possible roles in oncogenesis, including initiation. In subsequent Sections, data from experimental studies will be discussed, with an emphasis on the molecular nature of induced initiating events. Here it is sufficient to emphasize that at low doses of ionizing radiation, it is knowledge of the induction of early initiating events that may be most important to the understanding of radiation effects. That is not to say however that radiation plays no part in the other stages of oncogenesis.

68. In principle, it appears that neoplasia may be initiated either through proto-oncogene activation or suppressor gene inactivation. Thus, a multiplicity of induced somatic mutations may contribute towards human radiation oncogenesis, and even for a single histopathological form of neoplasia, there may be a number of possible initiating events, albeit with different probabilities of contributing towards overt malignancy. The necessity for a single clone to accumulate further somatic mutations before malignant conversion must be rate-limiting and implies that only a minority of initiated cells progress beyond the pre-neoplastic phase (paragraph 219).

69. At this early phase, aberrant pre-neoplastic clones may be lost through, for example, metabolic insufficiency, non-specific cell selection, the suppressive effects of neighbouring cells, terminal differentiation, cell senescence, programmed cell death (apoptosis) or cell surveillance mechanisms. Thus, the capacity of an initiated cell clone to expand in a relatively undifferentiated state may be viewed as a crucial aspect of the early phase of the disease (paragraph 54). In this respect, the manifestation of benign tissue dysplasias (e.g. papillomas, adenomas and haemopoietic hyperplasia) may be viewed as clonal expansion, limited perhaps by a combination of the factors noted above.

70. Specific examples of tumour-initiating mutations associated with *RAS*, *RB*, *WT*, *p53*, *NF-1* and *APC* genes are discussed elsewhere in this Annex, and the evidence that mutation of these genes in appropriate normal target cells predisposes to malignant conversion is relatively strong. For other tumour mutations it is not yet possible to conclude that they initiated the tumour, only that they are present at an early pre-neoplastic phase, before full clinical progression of disease is manifested.

71. In human neoplasia, particularly leukaemias and lymphomas, early phases of neoplastic development are frequently associated with consistent chromosomal rearrangements, such as the 9:22 translocation in chronic myeloid leukaemia (CML), the 5q-deletion in myelodysplastic syndrome and the 14:18 translocation in follicular lymphoma [H11, S63]. In such cases the progression of early indolent disease is usually accompanied by the selective clonal expansion of neoplastic subpopulations containing further chromosomal abnormalities. In general, in both haemopoietic and solid tumours, the more advanced and aggressive the disease the greater the degree of chromosomal change. Tables 3 and 4 illustrate consistent chromosomal changes recorded in human leukaemias/lymphomas and solid tumours, respectively (see [S45]). In the case of the 9:22 translocation in CML it has been established that a *BCR-ABL* fused gene is produced at the translocation breakpoint; this has tyrosine kinase activity, which produces a stable mitogenic stimulus to the cell. Of particular note are observations of different forms of *BCR-ABL* fusion in acute and chronic myelogenous leukaemia and a likely correlation between mitogenicity of the *BCR-ABL* gene product and the relative aggression of the two myeloid neoplasms (see [G24, N9]). For the 14:18 translocation in follicular lymphoma, molecular studies show that a newly recognized proto-oncogene *BCL-2* is upregulated by juxtaposition with an active immunoglobulin heavy chain gene (see [N9]). It has recently been established that such overexpression of *BCL-2*, rather than being mitogenic, serves the purpose of blocking programmed cell death [H23] and extending the *in vivo* life-span of B-cells (see also [E11]). Thus, certain gene activation events in tumorigenesis do not simply increase proliferation rates but instead block or prolong the normal differentiation pathway. Other examples of chromosomal translocations in acute B-cell and myeloid neoplasms are the t(15;17) in some acute myelogenous leukaemia (involving the *PML* and retinoic acid receptor genes), the t(1;19) in pre-B ALL (involving the *PBX* and *E2A* genes) and the t(17;19) in B-cell ALL (involving the *HFL* and *E2A* genes) (see [E10]). In addition, the 11q breakpoint gene thought to be involved in t(4;11) and t(9;11) acute leukaemias has significant homology to the *trx* transcription factor gene of *Drosophila* [D13].

72. Characteristic chromosomal rearrangements are also seen in human T-cell leukaemias; many of these involve specific sites on chromosomes 7 and 14. In peripheral lymphocytes of ataxia-telangiectasia, clonal rearrangements of this type have been observed in a number of patients showing no other evidence of malignancy. Although often present at relatively high frequencies, these clones do not usually convert to frank leukaemia; in a few cases, however, malignant progression of these clones has been observed (see [T6]). Molecular studies have now established that many of these rearrangements in T-cell neoplasms involve very specific recombination between T-cell receptor (*TCR*) genes and other chromosomal regions encoding transcription factors such as *HOX 11* (see [H32, R3]). The activation of these factors through *TCR* translocation will tend to alter the developmental programmes of T-cell precursors and could explain the early clonal expansion observed in some ataxia-telangiectasia patients. A more complete discussion of many of the chromosomal events noted here is provided by Solomon et al. [S63].

73. In any consideration of the mechanism of low doses of radiation to initiate oncogenesis it is important to attempt to establish the relative probability with which a single ionizing track will intersect a given DNA target, causing a tumour-initiating mutation. This is considered in the following for gain-of-function and loss-of-function mutations.

74. Activation of proto-oncogenes through gain-of-function mutations appears to occur via two principal mechanisms. For proto-oncogenes such as *RAS*, the DNA base-pair (bp) changes required for activation are very restricted, and hence the molecular target (for direct effects) will be small, perhaps only ~10 bp [B6, B18]. For the gene-specific chromosomal translocations involving the juxtaposition of proto-oncogenes such as *ABL*, *BCL-2* and *HOX 11* with other relatively specific activating genes, the molecular target may be larger, perhaps 10^2-10^4 bp [H4, H32, R3, S63]. However, for these events it may in principle be necessary to damage DNA at two specific sites rather than one, thus effectively reducing overall target size. Relative to the size of the whole genome, ~10^9 bp, such gain-of-function, gene-activating mutations would seem therefore to present very small targets for single-track radiation action. Nevertheless, on a target-size basis it has been proposed that the primary event in human CML can be a radiation-induced *BCR-ABL* translocation [H41].

75. This situation may be contrasted with the loss-of-function mutations characteristic of the tumour suppressor roles of genes such as *RB*, *WT*, *APC* and *p53*. Loss-of-function of tumour suppressor genes may occur through point mutation, small intragenic deletion

or larger deletions spanning whole chromosome segments (~10^7 bp) [H30, S18, W14]. The principal limit to the size of the DNA deletions associated with suppressor gene mutation will be the degree to which the cell can sustain viability following substantial genetic losses. Since this will vary with the location of the target gene in relation to essential DNA sequences and, correspondingly, with the genetic background of the cell itself, it is impossible to predict more precisely the target sizes for these deletions. It should also be noted that in the case of dominant negative effects, such as those postulated for *p53*, deletion of the whole gene may not be effective (paragraph 56).

76. In spite of these uncertainties and qualifications made in paragraphs 158 and 159, this simple biophysical argument would predict that radiation-induced loss-of-function mutations may dominate the spectrum of potential initiating events for carcinogenesis. On the basis of the figures given above, the probabilities between "loss" and "gain" events may differ by perhaps two orders of magnitude. It remains to be seen how realistic these estimates might be, but some support for this argument has come from molecular studies on radiation-induced somatic cell mutation (paragraph 154).

77. It may be concluded that tumour-initiating mutations probably vary in form, but on the basis of relative target sizes, it seems likely that tumour suppressor gene mutations may be the predominant form in radiation oncogenesis. Alone, such initiating events in normal target cells will not be sufficient to produce a malignant phenotype, which would require both clonal expansion of initiated cells (promotion) and the accumulation of further epigenetic and genetic changes (promotion plus progression). The point of malignant commitment in a developing neoplasm is therefore difficult to specify; indeed, there may not be an "all or nothing" transition but rather an increasing probability that pre-neoplastic cells will bypass normal cellular constraints and convert to frank neoplasia. Consequently, while oncogenesis may be operationally subdivided into initiation, promotion and progression, these definitions grossly simplify a genetically complex process of cell development that will vary between neoplasms.

(b) Tumour promotion

78. In experimental animal systems, promoters are identified as agents that, alone, have low oncogenic potential but that are able to greatly enhance the yield of neoplasms induced by prior exposure to a sub-carcinogenic dose of an initiator [C11, S2, Y2]. Agents that strongly promote oncogenesis generally do so at low concentrations, but in contrast to initiators, repeated or chronic exposure is usually necessary. A third distinguishing feature is that, unlike initiation, promotional effects are usually reversible. In these respects promotion has the properties of an epigenetic process, involving metastable changes in gene expression and cellular/tissue responses that have dramatic consequences for the initiated cell and its clonal progeny. In the majority of experimental animal systems, initiation and promotion procedures produce an increase in pre-neoplastic lesions or benign neoplasms, and for most promoters there appear to be no dramatic effects on oncogenic progression. The whole question of carcinogenic interaction between radiation and chemicals, including initiation/promotion, has been discussed in depth by Streffer et al. [S2] and Trosko et al. [T12].

79. Neoplastic promotion following ionizing radiation has been studied in both experimental animal systems and *in vitro* transformation systems [H6, K10, L3, S2, T12]. However, much of the detailed knowledge of mechanisms of promotion has come from chemical initiation/promotion studies with rodent skin carcinomas [C11, Y2], coupled with detailed biochemical investigations on the cellular consequences of promoter exposure [N5, N14, T11, T12, W4].

80. The nature of promoter action has, until recently, been obscure. The term promoter is an operational definition encompassing a diversity of chemical entities ranging from the classical phorbol esters through phenobarbital and bile acids to growth factors, hormones and ill-defined dietary components. However, tissue wounding and stress [S23] should also be included in any broad definition. Clearly, not all these factors will operate in all tissues, and it is likely that a range of biochemical pathways can be involved. It is through studies with the phorbol esters, such as TPA (12-*o*-tetradeconylphorbol-13-acetate), diterpenes, indole alkaloid and polyacetate promoters, that an understanding of certain aspects of promotional mechanisms has emerged. High affinity receptors for these promoters have been identified in mammalian cells [N5, W4]. In the case of TPA, that receptor, or part of it, is the calcium- and lipid-dependent enzyme protein kinase C.

81. Protein kinase C, through its ability to phosphorylate and activate a range of cellular proteins and induce the expression of cellular genes, plays a crucial role both in signal transduction across cell membranes into the cytoplasm and in subsequent cellular responses. In this respect, protein kinase C is at the crossroads of a number of biochemical pathways that are known to mediate cellular proliferative response to hormones, growth factors and cytokines. Promoter-mediated activation of protein kinase C will tend to enhance these pathways through a cascade of protein

phosphorylation and gene expression events, a principal outcome of which will be a disturbance in tissue homeostasis. Although diverse in their structure, most tumour promoters share the basic property of inducing a degree of tissue hyperplasia and inflammation; this histopathological feature probably stems from the disturbance of tissue homeostasis.

82. Endogenous promotion is likely to play a far greater role in human oncogenesis than extrinsic chemical factors, and in this respect it is important to recognize that protein kinase C is normally stimulated by increasing cellular diacyl glycerol (DAG) levels through lipid turnover [N5]. Since DAG levels have been shown to be increased following the action of a variety of cellular growth factors and cytokines (see, e.g. [M16, M17]), it follows that these factors probably play a major role in oncogenic promotion. This view is also consistent with observations indicating that the promotional wounding response in Rous sarcoma virus tumorigenesis is mediated by transforming growth factor-ß [S23].

83. However, it has become increasingly clear that tumour promotional pathways are not solely mediated through the biochemical pathways involving protein kinase C and that changes in cellular communication and oxidative metabolism [C21, T11, T12] may also occur in response to exposure to many tumour promoters.

84. The maintenance of tissue homeostasis, which requires cells to establish a critical balance between proliferation and differentiation, is known to involve not only responses to high molecular weight systemic factors (growth factors and hormones) but also lower molecular weight (≤1,000 daltons) ions and metabolites that are exchanged between neighbouring cells linked by so-called gap junctions at cell membranes [L14]. In facilitating cellular communication and biochemical coupling, these junctions are believed to play an important role in the local coordination of cell proliferation.

85. The establishment of gap junctions is determined by a family of conserved mammalian genes, the activity of which appears to be controlled by both systemic factors and intracellular processes mediated through signal transduction pathways. A critical link between gap junction communication and oncogenesis was established by the observation of the stable loss of coupling in many tumour cells [K13, T12]. However, such losses in tumour cells may often be selective, in that tumour cells remain coupled to each other but lose the ability to communicate with normal cells [N13, Y7]. Thus, it became possible to postulate that the signals exchanged between normal cells (homologous coupling) adequately regulate certain proliferation/ differentiation responses but that the selective loss of heterologous coupling allows tumour cells to become more autonomous and less receptive to tissue regulation.

86. The relevance of cellular communication in tumour promotion became obvious when it was shown that a wide range of tumour promoters had the capacity to induce transient dysfunction in gap-junction-mediated processes [M30, N14, Y7]. Additional studies show such inhibition of coupling to be part of the normal proliferative response in tissues, in that inhibition occurs when cells are drawn from a quiescent phase in order to complete tissue growth or repopulation [P10]. It seems likely, therefore, that in some tissues gap junction formation and loss is a secondary component of the complex cellular machinery that drives the cell cycle (paragraphs 48-50).

87. Thus, albeit in a transient fashion, the inhibition of gap junction communication by promotional stimulation may be viewed as a means whereby one layer of cellular proliferative control is removed; this would tend to elicit a mitogenic response in all undifferentiated stem-like cells in tissue. The magnitude of that response may not, however, be uniform, in that cells carrying tumour-initiating mutations in genes central to cell cycle control, such as *RB*, might be expected to respond most strongly. The involvement of tumour-associated mutations affecting cell adhesion proteins, e.g. DCC (deleted in colon cancer) [F11], in gap-junction mediated processes is also possible.

88. The potential complexity of tumour promotion mechanisms is further increased by the finding that some, but not all, promoting agents induce bursts of oxidative metabolism in exposed cells, which lead to the generation of short-lived, free chemical radicals [C21]. Such radicals are highly reactive within the cell and are able to induce damage in a range of macromolecular structures, including cell membranes and chromosomes.

89. In the case of TPA exposure, it has been established that induced radicals such as superoxides, peroxides and arachidonic acid metabolites are able to attack cellular DNA, inducing a range of cytogenetic abnormalities [C21, D11, P11]. On the basis of these observations it has been proposed that TPA-generated chemical radicals act at an early stage of promotion (stage 1) and convert carcinogen-initiated cells to a state in which they are more sensitive to proliferative stimulation (stage 2 promotion) [F15].

90. In the mouse skin papilloma/carcinoma system, TPA has been shown to be a "complete" promoter in that it fulfils both stage 1 and stage 2 promotional requirements; in contrast, the related phorbol ester

RPA fulfils only stage 2 requirements, i.e. it is not clastogenic. The importance of chromosome damage in the stage 1 conversion phase was further established by studies showing that at low doses the alkylating clastogenic agent, methyl methane sulphonate acted synergistically with RPA to effect complete promotion [F16]. Since the conversion stage of promotion involves chromosomal damage, it may centre on changes in gene activity or chromosomal instability; the specificity of such events has not, however, been established.

91. The cytogenetic observations noted above require that a much broader view be taken of the involvement of genetic changes in the promotional phases of oncogenesis. The boundary between initiation and promotion is becoming increasingly artificial, defined only by the tumour system under consideration, the physico-chemical nature of the insult applied and the cellular mechanism being sought. Here it is sufficient to say that, mechanistically, both initiation and promotion probably involve a combination of genetic and epigenetic cellular events and together they drive a clonal population of cells through a pre-neoplastic phase to a point where malignant conversion is assured. Perhaps they differ most clearly in the temporal requirements for phenotypic change and, on current belief, the larger contribution that stable mutagenic change makes to the initiation process.

92. Ionizing radiation is a powerful clastogen and would certainly induce many of the forms of cytogenetic damage currently associated with the conversion stage of tumour promotion. What may be questioned is the extent to which radiation might induce the epigenetic changes associated with stage 2 promotion. As noted below, it seems that, in general, radiation acts as only a weak promotor of neoplastic change.

93. Through its ability to damage tissues and induce a mitogenic response in repopulating cells, radiation could be regarded as a stage 2 promoting agent. Such effects will, however, only be significant at relatively high doses, where substantial cell inactivation has occurred. Thus, it may be argued that for radiological protection considerations, this form of promotional activity is of minor importance. This view may be tempered, however, by recent evidence of upregulation of protein kinase C and proto-oncogene gene products by relatively low doses of radiation [S50, W7, W21], and it will be important to establish whether such biochemical responses extend to other promotional processes, particularly, perhaps, those determining intercellular communication.

94. Recent experimental studies using the mouse skin papilloma/carcinoma system have highlighted some of the difficulties faced in approaching the question of interaction between radiation and other carcinogenic agents. Here it has been shown that beta irradiation induces resistance to chemically induced papilloma but not carcinoma formation [M31]. These observations may imply that radiation induces a DNA repair process that acts differentially on the chemically induced lesions driving promotion-dependent and -independent skin carcinogenesis. However, given the complexity of the promotional processes described here, other explanations should not be excluded. In the same experimental system, chronic beta irradiation lacked action as a complete or stage 2 tumour promoter but did show weak but positive action in stage 1 promotion [M37].

95. The suppression of cellular transformational processes by so-called anticarcinogens or antipromoters has been studied using *in vitro* transformation systems. Protease inhibitors, such as antipain and chymostatin, appear to strongly inhibit radiation transformation in an irreversible fashion, suggesting that they may act at the level of DNA damage modification [K10]. However, since such inhibitors also suppress the promotional activity of TPA, there may also be involvements in cell surface receptor-promoter binding processes or the subsequent protein-kinase-C-mediated message transduction process. Other chemical factors, such as retinoids, ascorbic acid, lymphotoxin and vitamin E, have also been shown to have anticarcinogenic and/or antipromotional activities (see [C11, K10, T20, Y5]). Some of these factors may also act *in vivo* [C11, C15, C16, L15]. In the case of d-limonene it has been suggested that induced changes in the intracellular location of GTP-binding proteins such as $p21^{ras}$ might underlie the anticarcinogenic action [C27].

96. While no single molecular mechanism of antipromotion may exist, at the cellular level, promotional processes are most consistently characterized by the transient loss of intercellular communication. Relevant to this is recent evidence showing that strongly antipromoting agents such as retinoids markedly increase intercellular communication [H48, M45]. *In vitro* antipromotion by ascorbic acid may, however, involve oxygen radical removal from cells [Y10].

97. In conclusion, the promoter enhancement of appropriate biochemical pathways in carcinogen-initiated cells can be viewed as interacting with the stable biochemical sequelae of the initiating event in a target cell in a manner that elicits a supranormal proliferative response. Such a mechanism, depending on the strength of the promoter and the duration of exposure, would tend to establish initiated clones in their host tissues rapidly and efficiently, thus increasing the frequency and proliferative capacity of

pre-neoplastic lesions. Until these transient changes are stabilized through perhaps further clonal mutations, they are, in principle, reversible. Assuming gap junction dysfunction to be a pivotal feature of promotion [T12], then upregulation of junction formation could be regarded as an important mechanism of antipromotion [H48]. On the basis of current experimental knowledge, this may be achieved using exogenous agents such as retinoids but, *in vivo*, endogenous processes involving the regulation of tumour suppressor genes and other cell cycle control factors may be expected to be of greater importance.

(c) Malignant progression

98. During the life history of a neoplasm there is often a progressive tendency towards increased malignancy. This is most frequently seen as a stepwise change in both tumour histopathology and aggression [F3, N3]. In the case of solid tumours, an extended blood supply may be recruited; subsequently, metastatic properties emerge, allowing the neoplasm to spread to distant sites. Phenotypically, neoplastic progression appears to be the most complex of the three phases, and considerable histopathological, cellular, cytogenetic and molecular variation may be seen, even within a single progressing neoplastic clone. Importantly, progression through clinically defined phases is generally, in the absence of clinical intervention, irreversible. This, together with other features discussed later, is suggestive of sequential somatic mutation and consequent selective clonal proliferation.

99. Although the histopathological manifestations of neoplastic progression have been well-documented [F3], it is only recently that some understanding has been gained of the underlying cellular and molecular mechanisms. The apparently stepwise transitions that characterize the progression from benign preneoplastic lesions to aggressively metastatic neoplasms are thought to represent clonal evolution and selection processes driven by genetic and epigenetic cellular changes [K6, N3, N9, S19].

100. At the cytogenetic level these changes are often evidenced by secondary chromosomal translocations, deletions or duplications. Some of these, particularly those appearing at low clonal frequency, probably represent "cytogenetic noise" and may be regarded as neutral. Others appear more consistently in dominant clones and are likely to involve the activation, amplification or loss of specific genes. These may be viewed as positively contributing towards clonal selection, dominance and, thereby, neoplastic progression. Examples of consistent secondary cytogenetic changes in human neoplasms are the 8:14 translocation in some cases of acute lymphocytic leukaemia (*MYC* oncogene activation), the trisomy of chromosome 7 in advanced melanoma (*ERB B* gene dosage?) and the appearance of homologously staining regions and double-minute chromosomes in neuroblastoma (*N-MYC* amplification) [H11, N3]. Secondary mutations potentially relevant to neoplastic progression do not always involve chromosomal change, and in some neoplasms, *RAS* mutations are believed to occur during progression and contribute towards tumour aggression (see, e.g. [R11, V2]). Such studies have also highlighted the genetic polymorphisms in tumours associated with genomic instability [R11]. The polyclonal evolution of tumours may also be studied using experimental molecular markers; for example, using plasmid-transfected mouse fibrosarcoma cells, it has been possible to identify individual clones that have acquired properties associated with preferential metastasis [E5].

101. Secondary chromosomal changes and oncogene activation events have also been characterized in a number of animal neoplasms induced by ionizing radiation or chemical carcinogens and have received comment elsewhere in this Annex. Animal models of neoplastic induction are also beginning to demonstrate the possible roles of induced DNA damage in oncogenic progression. Neoplastic progression in chemically initiated murine skin has been shown to be enhanced by treatment with radiation [B11]. This observation may be consistent with the specific losses from chromosome 7 that have been shown to contribute to the progression of murine skin carcinomas [B12, B29].

102. Studies of this type should extend the knowledge of differences in the genetic events that mediate neoplastic initiation and progression and should indicate the potential contribution of physical and chemical agents in the two phases. In this respect, it is important to recognize that in the case of protracted or fractionated exposures, ionizing-radiation-induced cellular damage may, in principle, contribute to both neoplastic initiation and progression. Parallel but more complex considerations apply in the case of combined exposure to radiation and chemical carcinogens [S2].

103. There is growing evidence that neoplastic progression may be greatly influenced by the acquisition, at a relatively early stage in the process, of intrinsic genomic instability. Benign lesions usually contain few cells with mitotic abnormalities, but these cells usually increase in frequency as the neoplasm progresses. This is often accompanied by increases in ploidy, chromosomal breakage, non-disjunction and sister chromatid exchange [S13], i.e. all the features of the development of abnormalities in DNA metabolism.

104. While the mechanisms underlying these putative defects are still obscure, the consequences are crucial to the understanding of neoplastic progression. Intrinsic chromosomal instability will greatly increase the frequency of spontaneous and induced genetic and epigenetic change within the evolving neoplastic clone. This provides the dynamic heterogeneity at the cellular level that is the hallmark of clonal neoplastic progression. Loss of cell cycle control, established during earlier phases of the neoplastic process (paragraphs 43-53), may play a role in the genetic instability that characterizes tumour progression. It is also possible that mechanisms of genomic instability involving the expression of recombinogenic sites and telomere-like repeat sequences in DNA may contribute to this process; for some human leukaemias there is some evidence for telomere sequence instability [S35] (paragraphs 61 and 64), and one form of heritable colon cancer is characterized by widespread instability of dinucleotide repeat sequences (see paragraph 122).

105. The principal phenotypic characteristic of the malignant progression of many tumours is the ability to spread (metastasize) from the primary tumour mass and to establish secondary growth foci (metastases) at other sites. Figure II provides a schematic representation of the steps involved in the spread of tumours. Such tumour dissemination requires primary tumour cells to acquire a range of new properties, particularly those that determine the relationship between the tumour and its host tissues (see [A4, D5, D6, F3, F5, H33, H42, K2, K5, L5, L6, N6, S14, V3, V4]). Metastasizing cells are first required to invade normal tissues and penetrate blood and lymphatic systems. Subsequently, penetrating cells need to be able to survive passage in these circulatory systems, exit the systems and then establish themselves in surrounding normal tissue. To what extent have experimental approaches succeeded in resolving the complex cellular and molecular processes involved in metastatic growth?

106. The molecular strategies so successful in identifying proto-oncogene and tumour suppressor gene activities in earlier phases of the neoplastic process have not proved to be wholly satisfactory when applied to metastatic mechanisms. While transfer of activated *ras* oncogenes to cell lines such as C3H10T½ and 3T3 has apparently resulted in one-step metastasis [E6], the complexity of the process *in vivo* makes it highly unlikely that invasive properties could simply emerge through single gene mutations. It may be, therefore, that direct approaches to the identification of metastasis genes using such atypical rodent cell lines will tend to give a misleading impression of the process.

107. Indirect approaches have compared gene activities in primary and metastatic tumours of the same origin or type. Using these strategies some evidence for *RAS* gene activation during metastatic progression has emerged (see, e.g. [V2]), but for tumours *in situ* it has proved difficult to obtain clear correlations between levels of *RAS* gene activity and the invasive capacity of the tumour. Indeed in some studies with human colonic tumours, directly conflicting results have been obtained [H33]. Similar conflict is evident in respect to *FOS* gene activity in some experimental mammary tumours. Overall, with the exception of consistent *MYC* gene amplification in certain solid tumours (small cell lung carcinoma and neuroblastoma) and *HER-2/NEU* gene amplification in many mammary tumours, there is a marked lack of correlation between known oncogene activation events and clinical staging criteria [H33]. There is some evidence that the activity of the protein kinase C gene [G11] is one determinant of the metastatic process, but, again, the available data do not allow simple correlations to be established. However, although general correlations between metastasis and tumour gene activity have yet to be established, some comment is possible on specific aspects of the problem.

108. The initial step in metastasis is the attachment of the primary tumour cell to the extracellular stromal tissue matrices and basement membranes [L10]. Cadherin proteins are believed to play a role in cell adhesion, and an inverse correlation has been suggested between E (epithelial) cadherin expression in tumour cells and the loss of cellular differentiation associated with increased metastatic properties [H42, S51]. In addition, so-called integrin glycoproteins are also believed to act as cell surface receptors for cellular attachment, and it has been shown that many meta-stasizing tumours strongly express these molecules at cell surfaces [C22, W15]; there may also be a relationship between cancer development and the synthesis of certain extracellular matrix proteins such as tenascin [K27]. Following such attachment, tumour cells then use a variety of proteolytic enzymes to digest the matrix in order to penetrate normal tissues; of particular current interest is the involvement of metalloproteinases (MP) in this process. The activity of these enzymes is regulated by a specific tissue inhibitor, TIMP, which has been shown to have anti-metastatic activity [S38], and an important role for TIMP in suppressing malignant phenotypes is now suspected [H33, H42]. A specific protease encoded by the transin gene is also known to be expressed during the skin papilloma to carcinoma progression in the mouse [B11]. The metastatic behaviour of some tumours has been linked to the expression of variant CD44 glycoprotein (see [H42]). The finding that CD44 serves to activate both B and T lymphocytes has led to the suggestion that mimicry of lymphocyte behaviour may be an important aspect of the metastatic process [A8].

109. More recently, the invasive characteristics of human breast carcinoma have been directly linked to the expression of a metalloproteinase termed stromelysin-3 [B21]. Of particular importance is the observation that this matrix-digesting enzyme is expressed in stromal rather than tumour cells, with stromelysin-3 gene expression being confined to tissue surrounding only invasive mammary tumours. Thus, the acquisition of metastatic properties appears to involve the specific local stimulation of normal breast tissue through signals received from the tumour; these data provide one of the clearest examples of the intimate relationship between normal and tumour cells during tumour progression.

110. Such interactions are also a crucial aspect of tumour blood supply recruitment. Once a solid tumour has expanded beyond a few millimetres diameter, it becomes necessary for the tumour mass to be served by new blood vessels. Blood supply recruitment from normal tissues (angiogenesis) is known to be an active process mediated by the secretion of angiogenic factors such as fibroblast growth factor, epidermal growth factor, transforming growth factor and angiogenin from the tumour [F17]. In some cases, other cytokines produced by infiltrating leucocytes are also believed to play a role.

111. Cell to cell communication through the establishment of gap junctions has been shown to be selectively lost in many progressing tumours, and the expression of connexins have been analysed in a rat liver tumour system [S65]. Communication between normal cells is believed to be part of the regulatory mechanism for cell proliferation, and its loss may result in the relaxation of the controls that restrict invasive growth. Since a number of oncogenes have been shown to downregulate gap junction formation [T11], the appearance of activated forms of these genes may enhance tumour progression via the loss of cellular communication.

112. Other phenotypic changes, such as increased cell mobility, may also contribute towards the metastatic spread of tumours. The molecular signals that increase tumour cell mobility and thereby promote invasiveness are poorly understood. Secretion of autocrine mobility stimulating factor has, however, been shown to correlate with the invasive properties of human bladder carcinoma [G12], and a so-called scatter factor involved in epithelial cell motility has been shown to be identical with hepatocyte growth factor, the receptor of which is coded by the *MET* proto-oncogene (see [H42]). Some genes involved in the cellular control of metastasis have been isolated by cDNA procedures based on the over- or underexpression of certain mRNA species in metastasizing tumours. Of particular note is the chromosome 17 encoded gene *NM23*, which appears to function as a metastasis suppressor [L22, S39]; the loss of *NM23* expression has been correlated with poor survival in breast cancer [L23].

113. In conclusion, from a clinical viewpoint, the acquisition of metastatic properties is perhaps the most critical aspect of the neoplastic process. Since much of the lethality of human malignancy derives from secondary metastatic growth, tumour progression is a major determining factor in the judgement of tissue weighting in radiological protection. For example, skin tumours, most of which only rarely metastasize to distant sites, have low lethality, and this is reflected in a much lower tissue weighting than that given to breast or lung where, largely as a consequence of secondary growths, the lethal fraction is very much higher. Clearly, an understanding of the cellular and molecular mechanism of the metastatic process will be of long-term value in making informed judgements on such weighting factors.

114. In spite of the difficulties experienced in resolving the complex mechanisms involved, some specific aspects of the metastatic process are now becoming clearer. DNA and gene transfer studies have yet to provide broad guidance on tumour gene involvement, but the overall approach remains valid: some studies (e.g. [R13]) do show promise; cell hybridization [C23] and cDNA screening procedures are also proving to be valuable [S39]. However, perhaps the most critical aspect of the metastatic cascade is the complex interaction between invasive tumour cells and the surrounding stromal structures and cells. In this area significant progress is being made in understanding the underlying mechanisms; it is to be hoped that this will also contribute to the design of more effective therapeutic procedures.

5. Viral involvement

115. Viruses are believed to influence the appearance of neoplasms in experimental animals and man by a number of different mechanisms [N2, O1, P13, W16, Z3] and, worldwide, may account for around 15% of cancer incidence in man [Z3]. Viral oncogenesis is currently believed to proceed via the following routes:

(a) through suppression of host systems for the elimination of tumour cells (e.g. avian reticuloendotheliosis and feline leukaemia virus);

(b) by stimulating cell proliferation through the specific interaction of viral and cellular proteins, either transiently or in a persistent manner (e.g. human papilloma virus and cytomegalovirus);

(c) through the transduction of acquired and activated viral oncogenes and growth-regulating genes to host cells (e.g. Rous sarcoma and Epstein-Barr viruses);

(d) through site-specific integration into the genome of host cells, resulting in the activation or inactivation (insertional mutagenesis) of critical host genes (e.g. avian leukaemia and hepatitis B viruses).

The molecular mechanisms of some of these processes have been studied in detail, but while both DNA and RNA viruses have been implicated in the aetiology of a number of human and animal neoplasms (e.g. anogenital cancer, skin cancer, liver cancer, leukaemias and lymphomas), the overall extent of viral involvement in human oncogenesis remains uncertain. Also, in many instances it is clear that the viral component of disease represents only part of a more complex picture involving interaction with other risk factors (Table 5).

116. In recent years a close association between certain human viruses and specific host genes has become apparent, and the following examples serve to illustrate some of the mechanisms currently believed to operate in human viral oncogenesis.

117. First, a transforming protein (E7) of human papilloma virus 16 (HPV 16, associated with anal and cervical papillomas) has been shown to bind the Rb suppressor protein; a second HPV 16 protein (E6) complexes with the p53 suppressor protein in the cell. Thus, the transforming potential of this virus may be mediated by dual inhibition of tumour suppressor activity [W9]. Secondly, human cytomegalovirus (HCMV) infection, possibly associated with Kaposi's sarcoma and cervical cancer, has been shown to lead to upregulation of cellular *FOS*, *JUN* and *MYC* proto-oncogenes. This occurs prior to the onset of viral protein synthesis and may be mediated by a hit and run process, whereby the interaction of viral particles with cell surfaces triggers cellular proliferation [B13]. Thirdly, the Epstein-Barr virus (EBV) gene *BCRF1* has been shown to be homologous to the cytokine synthesis inhibitory factor gene *IL-10*, suggesting that this oncogenic herpes virus uses a captured cytokine gene to enhance its survival in the host, thus potentiating its oncogenic properties in respect to Burkitt's lymphoma [M18]. Fourthly, human T-lymphotrophic virus (HTLV) has been shown to be associated with a unique form of adult T-cell leukaemia/lymphoma (ATL), with the two main foci of infection being in Japan and the Caribbean (see [B35]). The mechanisms of T-cell oncogenesis following HTLV infection are uncertain but may involve a combination of immunosuppressive effects [J6, K23] and T-cell proliferative dysregulation elicited by virally encoded proteins such as the products of the *tax* and *rex* genes [Z3]. Finally, hepatitis virus and aflatoxin B1 (a mutagenic food contaminant) appear to be strongly interactive factors in the induction of human hepatocellular carcinoma (HCC), which is prevalent in southern Africa and eastern Asia [B22]. The insertional mutagenesis of host genes by hepatitis B virus has been demonstrated, and recent evidence strongly suggests that the aflatoxin component of risk derives from the induction of target liver cell mutations that inactivate the *p53* tumour suppressor gene [B23, H34]. The still uncertain role of germ-line retroviral elements in human tumorigenesis has been reviewed recently [L24].

118. These observations provide evidence that the oncogenic potential of many human viruses derives from their capacity to provide a chronic growth stimulus to cells, often by the interaction of viral oncoproteins with cell cycle control proteins [N18], but that direct mutational damage may underlie the action of other viruses. The apparent synergy between hepatitis B virus and a specific environmental DNA damaging agent (aflatoxin B1), noted above, together with data on retroviral involvement in some radiation-induced animal neoplasms (see paragraph 180) and the inducibility of virus-like elements in mice by radiation [P14], suggests that viral processes may well synergistically influence a component of human radiation oncogenesis; there is, however, only preliminary evidence for this in respect to laryngeal carcinoma associated with papilloma virus infection (see [W16]).

B. HUMAN SUSCEPTIBILITY TO RADIOGENIC CANCER

1. Homozygous deficiencies in DNA repair, cell inactivation and chromosome breakage

119. There is increasing awareness of the strong influence of germ-line gene mutations in human oncogenesis (paragraphs 31-34). In addition to the familial traits associated with specific DNA sequence loss and organ-specific neoplasms (e.g. retinoblastoma, Wilms-aniridia, multiple endocrine neoplasia and familial adenomatous polyposis), there is, in the context of this Annex, the most important problem of cancer susceptibility through deficiencies in DNA metabolism [C12, F1, H5]. The clearest example of this is found in the genetically complex autosomal recessive trait xeroderma pigmentosum (XP). In this genetic disorder, defects in the repair of DNA photoproducts appear to be causally linked with a high incidence of skin neoplasia in the sun-exposed regions of affected patients [B14, C12]. Human and rodent genes involved in the repair of UV-induced damage have been isolated and characterized (see, e.g. [T13, V7]), and there is much new information on the cellular and molecular mechanisms of UV carcinogenesis (see, e.g. [A6, B36]). A detailed description of these mechanisms is, however, outside the scope of this Annex.

120. For ionizing radiation, direct links between the epidemiological, genetic and mechanistic aspects of oncogenesis are less well established. However, potentially relevant DNA repair genes are now being identified and isolated (see, e.g. [K11, T15]), and studies on the autosomal recessive human genetic disorder ataxia-telangiectasia continue to provide potentially important information on the association between cellular radiosensitivity, DNA repair deficiency and cancer proneness [G7, G13]; a candidate gene for ataxia-telangiectasia group D has recently been isolated [K29].

121. ***Cellular radiosensitivity - cell inactivation.*** Although largely restricted to the inactivation of cultured skin fibroblasts, *in vitro* clonogenic techniques have highlighted the relatively wide range of low-LET cellular radiosensitivity in the normal human population [A3, A12, C13, L11]. These data, for both acute and chronic exposures, show that only cells from ataxia-telangiectasia and Nijmegen break syndrome (NBS) homozygotes clearly fall outside the normal range of radiosensitivity and that patients with a variety of other putative DNA repair deficiencies are contained within the relatively broad normal distribution. Cell inactivation is, however, only a crude surrogate for overall cellular radiosensitivity and obviously fails to reflect the genetic complexity of oncogenic processes. The lack of correlation between intrinsic radiosensitivity in fibroblast and T-lymphocyte cell strains also casts some doubts on the predictive value of studies on cell inactivation [G15]. Consequently, the data cited can only be used to provide comment on a single aspect (DNA damage and repair) of the problem; they should not be used alone as an indicator of the distribution of neoplasia susceptibility in a radiation-exposed human population. In spite of these reservations, the overall approach has yielded much useful information (see [A12, G9]).

122. ***Chromosomal radiosensitivity and fragile sites.*** The quantitative estimation of radiation-induced chromosomal abnormalities also identifies ataxia-telangiectasia and NBS homozygous genetic disorders as being abnormally radiosensitive [T6, T7]. While these data are somewhat more relevant to oncogenesis than cell inactivation, here again it may be argued that they are of limited value to radiological protection. This view may, however, be tempered by recent observations suggesting that a range of human disorders predisposing to cancer are characterized by cell-cycle-dependent chromosomal radiosensitivity [S24]. This is a potentially important observation that demands further study. The potential relevance to oncogenesis of specific chromosomal sites of fragility and enhanced recombination is discussed in paragraphs 61-64. For both ionizing radiation and chemical agent exposure of cells, there is growing evidence for the expression of chromosomal sites of preferential induced breakage; in some studies an association with fragile sites and cancer-specific chromosome breakpoints has also been suggested [D7, M19, S25, S26, Y1]. Of particular note are the proposed mutagen sensitive sites (MSS) of human ch5q, which at the cytogenetic level, appear to correspond to the 5q breakpoints that characterize myelodysplastic syndromes (MDS) [M20, Y1]. Since these myeloid disorders and neoplasms are believed to be significantly radiogenic [M21, R9, V5], confirmation of 5q breakpoint concordance for MSS and MDS would be of some importance. Losses from the 5q region in MDS are now believed to centre on the interferon regulatory factor-1 gene [W24]. Recent studies on site-specific chromosomal breakpoints in radiation-induced murine acute myeloid leukaemias (paragraphs 182 and 183) add support to the contention that heritable predisposition to breakage at fragile sites on certain chromosomes may influence susceptibility to radiation leukaemogenesis. The most striking example of genomic instability associated with human cancer predisposition is, however, provided by hereditary non-polyposis colorectal cancer (HNPCC), which is determined by a 2p15-16 locus [P16]. This is believed to account for 4%-13% of all colorectal cancers in industrial nations and is therefore more common than FAP, which accounts for around 1% of such cancers. Contrary to normal expectations based on the HNPCC locus being a tumour suppressor gene, HNPCC tumours do not show characteristic DNA losses in the 2p15-16 region [A16]. Instead, such tumours exhibit widespread alterations in short dinucleotide $(CA)_n$ repeat sequences suggestive of genomic instability mediated through a dominant defect in a DNA replication factor. Such instability can be viewed as a means whereby mutation rates for $(CA)_n$-associated genes are elevated, thus enhancing tumour development. The finding of an excess of other tumour types in HNPCC kindreds indicates that such mechanisms may not be restricted to colonic neoplasms.

123. Although not associated with oncogenic processes, the recent characterization of the X-linked fragile site (*FRA X*) mutation associated with heritable mental retardation in man allows some comment on the genetics of chromosome fragility. The *FRA X* mutation confers not only X-chromosome fragility in somatic cells but also appears to be unstable in germ cells and subject to structural modification that is dependent on its parental route of inheritance [O2, Y8]. This feature appears to contribute to the bizarre genetics of *FRA X* inheritance and expression [R17, S53] and, if it were to apply to cancer-related fragile sites, would tend to disguise the underlying genetic basis of familial predisposition. These *FRA X* data also

highlight the potential importance of DNA repeat sequences and chromosomal instability for certain disease states [R17], a theme that is echoed elsewhere in this Annex.

2. Heterozygous carriers of genetic traits

124. While the overall picture of human genetic influences on cancer susceptibility is becoming clearer, the information available is based largely on studies with highly penetrating dominant mutations and homozygous mutations at autosomal loci. The frequency of such clearly recognizable disorders in the population is low, and while there are obvious implications for affected individuals and their families, the overall contribution to cancers in the population may be relatively small. In contrast, for autosomal recessive traits, the frequency of carrier heterozygotes will be much higher. In the case of the ataxia-telangiectasia disorder, epidemiological studies point towards increased risk of spontaneous neoplasms, particularly breast cancer [P2, S4, U2], and it is possible that such carriers of the ataxia-telangiectasia mutation represent a human subpopulation at increased risk of radiation-induced neoplasia.

125. Similar considerations may apply to the familial traits associated with organ-specific neoplasia. Cytogenetic and molecular studies with these imply that cancer proneness is often associated with the loss of one germ-line copy of a tumour suppressor gene. The spontaneous loss of the other copy in a target somatic cell would then explain the elevated frequency of organ-specific neoplasia and the apparent phenotypic dominance of these traits. An explanation that demands the reduction of target gene number in cells from two to one also implies that certain tissues of affected individuals would be at a considerably elevated risk of radiation-induced neoplasia. Some aspects of therapy-related neoplasia in familial cancer patients have been discussed [S5, U3]. Although the paucity of data precludes detailed analysis, there is evidence of an increased yield of therapy-related second tumours in familial retinoblastoma patients [E12], an observation that is consistent with the known involvement of the *RB* gene in the initiation of tumours other than retinoblastoma, including osteosarcoma [T5]. With respect to radiogenic neoplasms in dominant familial traits, intriguing observations have also been made with basal cell nevus syndrome (BCNS), where there is unambiguous evidence of radiotherapy-induced multiple skin neoplasms [S5]. Although there is evidence for post-irradiation repair/recovery defects in BCNS cells (see [A3, L11, N21]), the disorder may be heterogenous, and at this stage of knowledge it is not possible to directly link cellular repair observations with the clinical manifestation of radiogenic skin carcinoma.

126. The frequency of known highly penetrating human monogenic diseases that are possibly associated with elevated susceptibility to radiation oncogenesis is low. Examples of the estimated frequencies of occurrence of some of these cancer-prone human mutations are listed in Table 6. Consequently, in terms of the whole population, the highly penetrating mutations do not appear to present a significant problem for risk estimation. However, more frequent mutations, such as ataxia-telangiectasia heterozygotes, (estimated frequency of ~1%), who show increased incidences of breast cancer, with a relative risk of 6.8 claimed in one study [P2, S4, S66], together with a possible but still contentious increase in radio-sensitivity [S64], could make significant contributions to population risks.

127. However, it is most important to recognize that cancer is essentially a multifactorial genetic disease and that genes determining cancer susceptibility will differ markedly in the probability of expression (penetrance), as measured by the appearance of one or more tumours in members of families carrying the appropriate mutations. The often-cited retinoblastoma (*RB*) and Wilms' tumour (*WT*) gene mutations are highly penetrating and express as bilateral childhood tumours in a high proportion of carriers. Mutations of lower penetrance have been suspected for many years. However, since they tend to express, perhaps as single adult tumours, in many fewer carriers, they also would be much more difficult to detect in the population, even if they occurred, overall, at a higher frequency. This view has received some support from the finding of relatively low penetrance *p53* germ-line mutations in rare cancer-prone Li-Fraumeni syndrome (LFS) patients [S41] and mutations associated with predisposition to breast and ovarian cancer [H35, K21, S52]. One of these breast cancer genes, *BRCA1*, encoded on chromosome 17, is strongly associated with early onset disease and appears to act as a tumour suppressor. Such heritable forms of breast cancer may account for around 5% of the total in industrialized countries. Since one in ten women develops breast cancer in her lifetime, perhaps as many as one in 200 carry genes that predispose to this neoplasm [K21]. However, with the exception of *BRCA1* most of these mutations are probably of low penetrance. In the case of *p53*, cancer predisposing germ-line mutations are by no means restricted to LFS families [M38, T17] and include one family showing abnormal expression of wild-type p53 protein [B30].

128. Recent observations on the effects of genomic imprinting on the expression of tumour suppressor genes (paragraphs 57-60) are also relevant to patterns of heritable tumour susceptibility. Genomic imprinting

may be considered to be a process whereby the dominance of mutant gene expression is modified according to whether it is inherited from the mother or the father [H19, H43, S27]. In the case of imprinted cancer-susceptibility genes, the expected Mendelian patterns of tumour incidence in affected families will tend to be distorted, depending critically on parental routes of inheritance. An illustration of the inheritance pattern of a human disease with imprinting effects is shown in Figure III. The term maternal imprinting is used to imply that there will be no phenotypic expression of the abnormal allele when transmitted from the mother, and paternal imprinting is used to imply that there will be no phenotypic expression when transmitted from the father. Because there will be a phenotypic effect only when the gene or the chromosome segment in question is transmitted from one or the other parent, there are a number of unaffected carriers. There are equal numbers of affected males and affected females or of unaffected male and unaffected female carriers in each generation [H19] (see also Annex G, "Hereditary effects of radiation").

129. In addition to the imprinting-like effects seen for the *RB*- and *WT*-related genes in man, it may be that this process influences the expression of other tumour suppressor and growth-factor genes with known or suspected involvement in oncogenesis [C23, F23, H19]. The inheritance pattern for familial glomus tumours in man has been shown to be consistent with imprinting [V6]; clinical manifestations, including neoplasia, in the human Beckwith-Wiedermann syndrome are also believed to involve imprinting effects mediated by paternal inheritance of both copies of a region from the short arm of chromosome 11 (paternal disomy/maternal deficiency) (see [L16]). It may be reasonably predicted that other less-well-defined "cancer families" will, in detailed studies, show pedigree distributions indicative of imprinting-like effects. The observation of parent-of-origin effects on leukaemogenic translocations may also have implications for the genetics of haemopoietic neoplasms [H40].

130. In conclusion, based on the frequency of the known highly penetrating mutations, it might be concluded that genetic susceptibility to cancer is not a major factor in the formulation of radiation risk estimates. However, the increasing appreciation of partial effects in heterozygotes, the variable penetrance of mutations, and epigenetic modifying factors should sound a note of caution on this conclusion.

131. An overall genetic contribution to cancer risk in the human population of around 20% has been suggested (see [B24]). Although considerable uncertainty exists, this suggested value implies that as knowledge accrues it should be possible to begin to consider individual risk. For future epidemiological investigation of possible genetic effects on radiation carcinogenesis it will be important to selectively consider familial history of neoplasia along with other relevant factors, such as age of onset in relation to age at exposure. In this specific context, although other explanations are possible, the recent and unexpected findings of an elevated relative risk of early onset breast cancer among the survivors of the atomic bombings in Japan [L30] might accord with the apparently high genetic component of this disease (see paragraph 127). It should be emphasized, however, that the full establishment of such relationships demands extensive investigations of familial cancer incidences and, where possible, molecular analysis of relevant germ- line DNA sequences in order to ascertain the carrier status of the affected individual. If progress in this most important area of human genetics can be maintained, it may be necessary to modify current views on the expected distribution of induced cancers in human populations.

3. Systemic factors

132. Although there is, at present, a paucity of informative data, the identification of initiating events for the principal radiation-induced neoplasms is of critical importance for the further development of mechanistic models of oncogenesis and the validation of dose-effect relationships. Armed with knowledge of the target cell and the initiating event, it may be possible to make informed judgements on the effects of post-irradiation repair processes, on dose rate and on radiation quality effects. However, since oncogenic processes involve far more than initiation, it is of considerable importance to gain a further understanding of the factors that influence the expression and development of neoplastic change, i.e. age, sex, dietary and hormonal factors. In this context, animal models of radiation oncogenesis can be of great value in gaining a broad understanding of these factors (see, e.g. [F2]), and there is also valuable information to be obtained from human population studies.

133. Hormonal status is known to be a major factor in the appearance of tumours in breast, ovarian, testicular and prostate tissues in man and may also be implicated in the progression of other hormone-sensitive or hormone-producing tumours, such as those arising in adrenal and thyroid tissues [L17, M32]. Since, however, hormones and other cytokines play a ubiquitous role in the development and maintenance of all tissues, their action should not be considered to be restricted to the tumour types noted above. On current knowledge and with few exceptions, the principal oncogenic role of such systemic factors centres on their action as tumour promoters or co-carcinogens [M32].

134. The influence of systemic endocrine factors in human radiation oncogenesis is most strongly evidenced by age- and sex-related effects on breast cancer incidence [U1]. These observations imply that hormonal status is a major determinant of the development of this neoplasm and that initiated cells may remain dormant in breast tissues for long periods. Cellular and molecular studies outlined elsewhere (paragraph 189) support this contention and are also broadly consistent with current views on the mechanisms of neoplastic promotion and progression (paragraphs 78-114) that are believed to mediate oncogenesis. Cellular interactions involving hormones and growth factors are also known to influence neoplastic yield in experimental systems through promotional and selection processes; there can be little doubt that such effects are crucial to neoplastic yields in man and may be determined by physiological changes deriving from both genetic and environmental influences.

135. Diet is thought to be a significant factor in carcinogenesis, with fat intake perhaps the most important determinant of cancer in different human populations [C15]. Promotional mechanisms centred on dietary lipid effects on the activity of endocrine systems, on prostaglandin synthesis, on immune functions and on bile acid production have been proposed for some neoplasms and may be supported by epidemiological and animal studies [C15]. Although cellular and molecular data relating directly to these proposals have yet to be presented, it may be relevant that the promotional pathways involving protein kinase C are known to involve cellular lipid turnover (paragraph 82), and it is possible that their activity is influenced by lipid or lipid metabolite availability in tissues. Non-genotoxic chemicals present in the diet or in the environment have also been proposed as factors in human carcinogenesis [C16]. Through their capacity to elicit a chronic proliferative stimulus to cells, it is possible that many of these may act as relatively non-specific tumour-promoting agents; the role of induced mitogenesis and endogenously induced DNA damage in the initiation of oncogenesis has also been considered (see, e.g. [A10, A11, C16]). Although somewhat outside the scope of this Annex, the rate at which cells are believed to sustain and repair endogenous DNA damage, in relation to that small amount of additional damage induced by a low dose of radiation, has received detailed comment [B43, B44, L27, S66, W27] and is of considerable importance to the relationship between DNA repair and radiation carcinogenesis (see also paragraphs 154-159).

136. The possible cellular mechanisms of anti-tumorigenic agents, such as retinoic acid, have been outlined in paragraphs 95-97. Animal studies, particularly with the mouse skin papilloma/carcinoma system, clearly demonstrate the anti-tumorigenic action of retinoic acid *in vivo* [R14], and recently, the retinoic acid treatment of tumour-sensitive transgenic mice carrying an active germ-line copy of a v-*ras* oncogene has been shown to dramatically delay or even completely inhibit the appearance of promoter-induced papillomas [L15].

137. Hormone promotion (paragraph 80), increasing genomic instability (paragraph 104) and intrinsic progressional processes (paragraphs 98-114) have been mentioned as possible factors in age-related carcinogenesis. Also, for familial tumours such as retinoblastoma and some breast and colon tumours, early onset of induced malignant disease would, for genetic reasons, be anticipated. For the early onset (childhood) acute lymphocytic leukaemia, however, a different mechanism may operate; it has been proposed that this disease results from two sequential mutations in haemopoietic target cells [G6]. The first of these is postulated to occur *in utero*, where rapid cell proliferation is required for haemopoietic development, and the second during the neonatal period, when a clonal population of these cells is expanding in response to a primary antigenic stimulus.

138. Animal models provide the basis for quantitative *in vivo* studies on radiation oncogenesis and dose-effect relationships (see, e.g. [E2, M1, M2]), and spontaneous/induced ratios for malignancy strongly influence views on the choice of radiological risk models (i.e. relative vs. absolute risk) (see, e.g. [S12]). Where there is a paucity of human epidemiological data, as in the case of leukaemogenesis by bone-seeking alpha-emitters, animal studies can provide the preliminary data. For example, the finding of induced acute myeloid leukaemia in low dose ^{224}Ra exposed mice at a higher frequency than that of osteosarcoma may have important implications for human radiation risk estimates [H9, H10]. The inhomogeneity of dose, which is inherent in bone-seeking and other internalized radioisotopes, highlights a major systemic uncertainty in radiation oncogenesis, i.e. the identity and *in vivo* distribution of target cells for oncogenesis. The pattern of isotope distribution and decay in relation to organ specific target cells is probably the major determinant of oncogenesis by these isotopes, yet very little is known about target cell identity and even less about distribution.

139. In conclusion, the highly interactive multi-step nature of oncogenesis demands that systemic factors will greatly influence the probability that a carcinogen-initiated cell in tissue will complete all steps and give rise to an overt malignancy. Positive factors such as dietary and hormonal/growth factor-mediated promotional mechanisms may tend to drive the process forward, while terminal cellular differentiation, programmed cell death, cellular communication, cellular surveillance and dietary/endogenous anti-oncogenic

compounds may restrict or even abrogate tumour development. Any specific judgement on the probability that a single tumour-initiated stem cell will progress to malignancy requires a greater knowledge of the complex interplay between these factors than is currently available. In general, however, it seems certain that the negative factors greatly outweigh the positive and that, although only crudely estimated, perhaps less than one in a million initiated cells complete the full transition to overt malignancy (paragraph 218).

4. Immunodeficiency and cell surveillance mechanisms

140. Some human genetic immunodeficiency diseases, such as the Wiskott-Aldrich syndrome [P3], are characterized by susceptibility to certain neoplasms. However, the role of host immune-response in oncogenesis is a problem that has yet to be satisfactorily resolved (see, e.g. [S43]). In the context of oncogenic mechanisms, some specific comment is necessary.

141. In the case of oncogenic DNA viruses, such as Epstein Barr virus (EBV) that carry transforming genes, there is evidence that immune functions efficiently suppress oncogenesis [P4] and that EBV-carrying lympho-proliferative disorders normally only develop where there is evidence of host immunodeficiency. It has been suggested [K2] that the rather unusual spectrum of human neoplasms that develop in the case of inherited or acquired immuno-deficiency reflects the involvement of oncogenic DNA viruses in tumour aetiology. In such cases the expression of "foreign" viral genes in neoplastic cells could be seen as providing specific targets for host immune functions. Viral oncogenesis often depends on the persistent proliferation of the virus in host tissues (paragraphs 115-118), and this is obviously influenced by the degree to which the host is able to mount an effective immune response against the highly specific "non-self" viral proteins.

142. For oncogenesis mediated by the insertion of a viral sequence close to cellular oncogenes the situation is less clear. The target gene may be activated by the insertion of only a short, non-coding viral sequence (the viral long terminal repeat or enhancer) [J2]. This would not tend to generate immunogenicity in the cell. If, however, the whole viral genome were inserted, the expression of virally encoded proteins could elicit an immune response to eliminate the carrier cell [K2]. The activation of normally silent transposons has been demonstrated in human testicular tumours [B34], and in one case of colon cancer the target *APC* gene had been inactivated by transpositional insertion [M46]. The implication of such activational and insertional events for immune response is however uncertain.

143. In the case of oncogene activation by endogenous processes, i.e. chromosome translocation, gene amplification or point mutation, either normal or minimally modified proteins have been seen to be expressed (paragraphs 28 and 29). Chaemeric fusion proteins (paragraph 71 and Table 1) are a possible exception to this. Consequently, such mechanisms would not, in general, provide strongly antigenic gene products to act as high-affinity "non-self" targets for B- and T-cell mediated immune mechanisms. This conclusion accords with the low immunogenicity seen in most spontaneous neoplasms [K2]. Oncogenic processes associated with gene losses would not obviously have any direct consequences for conventional immune response.

144. T-cell mediated immune recognition depends on the precise presentation of antigens on target cell surfaces through the action of proteins, collectively termed the major histocompatibility complex (MHC), and there is evidence that during the course of their development many tumours develop antigenic determinants that can elicit immune reactions. Tumour antigens have been characterized in a range of human and animal tumours [G14], but the contention that they are capable of stimulating an effective immune reaction may be questioned. Melanoma probably represents the best antigenically characterized human tumour, and around 40 different tumour antigens have been identified using monoclonal antibody techniques. These include antigens of MHC, pigment, growth factor receptor and cell membrane/matrix origin [H36]. A feature of these antigens that illustrates the central problem of tumour immunology is that none are truly tumour-specific; all are expressed, albeit in some cases weakly, by other normal tissues. The lack of specificity of the vast majority of tumour antigens may well underlie the apparent failure of T- and B-cell mediated immune systems to mount an effective response to neoplastic cells arising in tissues. As noted above, the virally-associated human tumours represent a clear and wholly understandable exception to this.

145. Thus, while T- and B-cell mediated immune systems may under some circumstances modify the development of non-viral human tumours, clear evidence that they have the capacity to eliminate early pre-neoplastic cells in tissues is lacking. Indeed, if such efficient systems were to be available, it would be necessary to seek explanations as to why such cells can remain dormant in tissues for long periods prior to promotional stimulation by systemic factors such as hormones (paragraphs 78-97). Also, from an experimental point of view, an explanation is needed for the fact that very large studies with mice, genetically deficient in T-cell immunity, have failed to provide any evidence of elevated tumour susceptibility (see [B25, S42]).

146. Immunodeficiency is a characteristic feature of the ataxia-telangiectasia human genetic disorder [R10]. While the immune defect in the disease may contribute to the increased frequency of lymphoreticular neoplasia in ataxia-telangiectasia, chromosomal rearrangements that are characteristic of the predominant T-cell leukaemias suggest that the underlying defect in DNA metabolism resulting in misrecombination of T-cell receptor genes [R3] may be a more important determinant of neoplasia incidence.

147. There is also evidence that the skin plays a significant role in the body's immune system and that Langerhans' cells in skin originate in bone marrow and are immunocompetent [S28]. With regard to immune effects in carcinogenesis, it has been shown that immunosuppressed patients show an excess of squamous cell carcinomas [K7], and clinical observations have led to suggestions that a depression of the cell-mediated immune function in skin, as a consequence of UV-sensitivity, may contribute towards the incidence of skin neoplasia in XP patients [B14].

148. While there is relatively good understanding of the nature and extent of T- and B-cell mediated immune reactions, the same is not true of the potential defence mechanism provided by natural killer (NK) cells; these appear to recognize abnormal cells without MHC involvement and are far less discriminating in their action than T-cells [B2]. Recognizing certain cell surface receptors that are not necessarily antigenic, NK cells bind and then secrete membrane-perforating proteins that lead to target cell lysis [Y3]. Thus cells misplaced in tissues, cells over-expressing certain membrane proteins and/or cells with conformational membrane changes may be eliminated. The accidental elimination of normal cells by NK cells is known to occur [Y3], and this relatively low specificity of action may provide NK cells with a capacity to eliminate pre-neoplastic cells showing characteristic changes at membrane surfaces. In this general context, NK cells have been shown to exert selective inhibitory effects during post-irradiation haemopoiesis [P8], and a regulatory role for lymphoid cells in selectively preventing the self-renewal and accumulation of early neoplastic cells has also been proposed [G4].

149. The overall extent of NK or NK-like cell function in the elimination of tumour cells and the development of malignancy in man remains uncertain. However, in animal systems it has been shown that the transplantation of cloned NK cells to NK-deficient host mice leads to resistance to radiation-induced thymic lymphoma and the inhibition of lung nodule development following implantation of melanoma tumour cells [W17]. The selective activation of NK cells has also been shown experimentally to inhibit tumour metastasis [H37]. The implications of these observations for radiation carcinogenesis in man remain to be established, but they do provide evidence for the existence of cell-mediated processes that defend against tumour growth and metastasis [H38, Y3]. In spite of this, their apparent lack of specificity poses questions on the overall efficiency of their scavenging capacity.

150. In conclusion, it has been argued that with the exception of a possible viral component, T- and B-cell mediated immune response may not play a major role in moderating human radiation oncogenesis. However, specialized immune functions in certain organs and the existence of non-immunogenic cell surveillance mechanisms imply that a proportion of early pre-neoplastic cells may be eliminated before they become established. Other mechanisms defending against tumour induction or development, including DNA repair, programmed cell death, terminal differentiation and phenotypic suppression, are noted in other Sections of this Annex. Together, these will reduce the probability that a specifically damaged target cell will progress to frank malignancy. An estimate of this probability, while of considerable importance to radiological protection, is extremely difficult to make. Nevertheless, in paragraph 219 a first approximation calculation is illustrated.

III. EXPERIMENTAL INVESTIGATIONS OF CELLULAR AND MOLECULAR MECHANISMS OF RADIATION ONCOGENESIS

151. Given the complexity of the cellular genetic events involved in oncogenesis, how should the principal questions regarding the mechanisms of radiation oncogenesis be framed? With a view to exploring experimental strategies, these questions may be grouped as follows:

(a) what is the nature of radiation-induced initiating events? Is DNA the principal cellular target, and if so, what is the effect of post-irradiation DNA repair on the fate of these potentially initiating lesions?

(b) what is the identity, distribution and radiosensitivity of target cells for the major induced neoplasms?

(c) what are the consequences of an initiating event to a given target cell, and how does this event interact with or determine promotional or progressional events in order to give rise to the overtly neoplastic cellular phenotype?

(d) in what ways do genetic, hormonal and/or environmental factors affect the expression of initial oncogenic damage and the subsequent progression towards malignancy?

(e) how closely can experimentally derived data on oncogenic change be related to other biological/biophysical effects of radiation and, crucially, to *in vivo* human oncogenesis.

152. Unambiguous answers to most of the above questions are not yet possible. The questions serve here only as a framework for discussion. Nevertheless, some specific comment is possible from both *in vitro* and *in vivo* approaches to the problem.

A. EPIDEMIOLOGICAL STUDIES

153. Epidemiological studies of human groups exposed to low-LET radiation show that a range of neoplasms are represented in excess and, broadly, that these do not differ markedly from those arising spontaneously in the population (see, e.g. [U1]). That is not to say that different tissue sensitivities or characteristic mechanisms do not occur for radiation oncogenesis but rather that no unique neoplastic signature of human radiation exposure is, as yet, apparent (paragraphs 223-227). This may be contrasted with the organ-specific neoplasms that characterize exposure to certain chemical agents, e.g. asbestos and mesothelioma, vinyl chloride monomer and hepatic angiosarcoma, benzene and leukaemia and aflatoxin and hepatocellular carcinoma [B22, T16] (paragraphs 91-93). The basis of these observations, although uncertain, may be associated with the evidence that, through energy deposition and chemical radical interaction in DNA, radiation is able to induce a diversity of genomic lesions, ranging from damage to single bases to gross DNA deletions and rearrangements. Again, this may be contrasted with some chemical agents, which have characteristic chemical specificities in their interaction with DNA and also target certain organs (paragraphs 188-203). Thus, the epidemiological characteristics of radiation oncogenesis would be explained, if the spectrum and distribution of induced cellular initiating events was not grossly different from that arising spontaneously and if low-LET radiation simply increased the frequency of the commonly occurring neoplasms, albeit with different levels of excess in different target organs. Although attractive in its simplicity, this hypothesis may need to be modified in the light of molecular information on induced somatic cell mutation. As noted later in Chapter IV, the physiological and biochemical processes governing the uptake, distribution and excretion of radioactive isotopes can lead to dose-inhomogeneity and, subsequently, organ-specific neoplasia. There is limited information on such carcinogenic effects in man [U1, U2]; and Annex F, "Influence of dose and dose rate on stochastic effects of radiation" summarizes some of the relevant animal data.

B. MOLECULAR STUDIES OF MUTAGENESIS AND REPAIR: POSSIBLE IMPLICATIONS FOR NEOPLASTIC INITIATION

154. If, as implied in previous paragraphs, the majority of neoplasms are initiated through gene- and cell-specific somatic mutation, then the molecular characteristics of radiation-induced gene mutation may be informative. Detailed studies of radiation-induced mutation at the *HPRT*, *APRT*, *TK* and *DHFR* loci of mammalian cells show that the principal mechanism of radiation-induced mutation is through gross genetic change, usually DNA deletions [E1, H7, M6, M33, N20, S29, T2, T8, U11]. These data in no way exclude radiation mutagenesis through point mutation, which has been convincingly demonstrated at the *APRT* locus [G5, M33], but rather suggest that ionizing radiation is a relatively weak point mutagen. The molecular analysis of spontaneously arising somatic cell mutants suggests that point mutation may be the predominant spontaneous mutagenic event, although spontaneous deletion mutants have also been characterized [M33, S29, T2].

155. It is, however, important to recognize that most of these data relate to mutation induction in a limited selection of genes and, generally, at relatively high doses and dose rates (see [T8]). In recent studies, it has been shown that *tk* mutations in a murine (L5178Y) cell line are induced in a dose-rate-dependent fashion but, apparently, with an increase in the proportion of multilocus mutations correlating with decreased dose rate [E4]. In this study, mutations at the *hprt* locus, which are thought to be single-locus events, showed no such dose-rate dependence. In contrast, other studies (see [F22, M22]) show that induced *hprt* mutation rates decrease with dose rate or dose fractionation. It has also been demonstrated [M22] that the specific fraction of full *hprt* gene deletion in Chinese hamster ovary cells is not altered by post-irradiation repair processes, suggesting that DNA repair acts with equal fidelity on the majority of potentially mutagenic lesions (see also Annex F, "Influence of dose and dose rate on stochastic effects of radiation"). This latter study also provided preliminary evidence for *hprt* breakpoint hot spots in the 3′ segment of the gene. Since oxygen concentration is known to affect the spectrum of radiation-induced

DNA lesions, it may be an additional and important variable, particularly for DNA base damage that might give rise to point mutations.

156. There is growing evidence that spontaneous and radiation-induced gene deletions in cultured mammalian cells may involve preferential DNA breakage at certain short repeat sequences [M33, M39, M49]. The mechanism for the induction of such deletions remains uncertain but could include the induction of DNA double-strand breaks, followed by recombination and/or replication slippage past secondary DNA structures produced by the pairing of the repeats [M33]. The potential importance of this mechanism for oncogenesis is evidenced by the finding of similar short, direct repeats at the breakpoints of deletions in the *RB* gene in human retinoblastoma, and it also appears that the repeat sequences involved in gene deletions vary according to the locus that is being studied [C25]. The catalytic properties of such repeat sequences, while still to be fully resolved, could therefore be a significant factor in the relative radiosensitivity of different tumour genes and, through this, could be a determinant of the inducibility of the neoplasms with which they are associated. At present the information available is largely restricted to small intragenic deletions, and it is of some importance to determine the relevance of the DNA deletion mechanism noted above for the gross chromosomal losses that characterize some radiogenic neoplasms [B42].

157. A similar picture with respect to gross genetic damage also emerges from molecular studies on the nature of the DNA-repair defect in radiosensitive ataxia-telangiectasia human cells. These data imply that misrepair of DNA double-strand scissions may be the major determinant of ataxia-telangiectasia radiosensitivity and that the misrepair takes the form of DNA deletion and/or rearrangement around the site of the scission [C6, D2] (see also Annex F, "Influence of dose and dose rate on stochastic effects of radiation"). Some of the uncertainties about the relevance of this misrepair mechanism for the ataxia-telangiectasia phenotype have been resolved by the use of a DNA repair assay utilizing cell-free extracts [G16, N15]. Here it has been shown that, whereas nuclear extracts of normal and ataxia-telangiectasia cell lines do not differ markedly in the efficiency with which they rejoin enzyme-induced double-strand breaks in plasmid DNA, they do differ in the fidelity with which certain forms of breaks are repaired; from the data presented it appears likely that the nature of the DNA sequence at the breakpoint may influence repair fidelity. Such *in vitro* approaches may have considerable potential for resolving the molecular mechanisms of oncogenic initiation and could, for example, be used as model systems to explore the importance of double-strand breaks and DNA repeat sequences in the induction of DNA deletions in cloned tumour suppressor genes such as *RB*, *APC* and *p53*. Homologous recombination is thought to be involved in some cases of tumour suppressor gene mutagenesis, and model *in vitro* approaches to this mechanism and its induction by radiation have been described [B31].

158. DNA misrepair may also result in the appearance of DNA translocations as well as deletions, and it is relevant that the predominant, spontaneously arising T-cell neoplasms in ataxia-telangiectasia patients often involve specific chromosomal rearrangement [T6] centred on incorrect recombination of DNA sequences associated with the assembly of mature T-cell receptor genes [R3]. Owing to the apparently small DNA target involved, the efficient induction of such precise translocations by radiation may be questioned (paragraphs 74 and 75). It may be, however, that as a consequence of specific recombination affinity, radiation-induced molecular damage outside the target sequence may catalyse site-specific misrecombination [B42]. Again, this problem could, in principle, be approached using *in vitro* molecular strategies.

159. Overall, the above molecular studies may be used to argue that radiation-induced somatic cell mutations associated with the initiation of oncogenesis are, perhaps, more likely to be specific DNA deletions and/or rearrangements than point mutations. However, there is insufficient evidence to be dogmatic about this important aspect of oncogenic initiation, and it may be that the genomic domain within which a target gene is located is a major determinant of the predominant molecular mechanism of induced genetic change. It may also be oversimplistic to view mutagenic mechanisms as the principal determinant of oncogenesis. A significant factor in the emergence of an established neoplasm will be the degree of proliferative advantage and/or selection associated with early pre-neoplastic events. Thus, while ionizing radiation may be a weak point mutagen for a given gene, the selective advantage conferred to a target cell by a specific point mutation in that gene may in some circumstances outweigh the relatively low overall frequency of such mutations induced within the target cell population. In conclusion, recent attempts to relate specific mutations in radiation-associated human tumours to the mutagenic action of ionizing radiation [V10] highlight the pressing need for more detailed information on the mechanisms of radiation mutagenesis and repair. The induction of cellular repair by low doses of ionizing radiation has been demonstrated in certain experimental systems, but the implications of this for oncogenic processes remain obscure (see Annex F, "Influence of dose and dose rate on stochastic effects of radiation").

C. *IN VITRO* STUDIES WITH CELLULAR SYSTEMS

1. Conventional systems

160. The early work of Reznikoff et al. [R2] provided strategies and techniques for the development of *in vitro* oncogenic cell transformation systems. These clonogenic systems, such as that based on C3H10T½ cells, seek to characterize and quantify radiation-induced changes in quasi-normal cells that mimic or are associated with neoplastic cellular phenotypes, e.g. loss of contact inhibition, growth in semi-solid medium [H6]. The positive and negative arguments on the relevance of these *in vitro* techniques to oncogenesis *in vivo* have been discussed [L2], and it is sufficient here to make only a few general points about their role in the understanding of oncogenic mechanisms.

161. First, irrespective of the detailed cell biology of the systems, *in vitro* studies that relate radiation exposure to the induction of a clonogenic, neoplasia-associated cellular phenotype should be viewed as being potentially informative. Secondly, the characteristics of the established rodent cell systems allow rapid assay of the transformed phenotype and ready manipulation, for the purpose of addressing questions of dose effect, dose rate, radiation quality, post-irradiation repair and tumour promotion. Also of great potential benefit is the possibility that such techniques could be applied to cultured human cells.

162. For the induction of the *in vitro* transformed cellular phenotype there is compelling evidence that the principal target is genomic DNA. The gross morphological cellular changes that signal transformation may be produced by DNA-mediated oncogene transfer, and there is a good correlation between the ability of the given agent to induce cell transformation and its capacity to induce DNA-damage (see also paragraphs 20 and 21). In addition, there is evidence that *in vitro* transformation progresses by at least a two-step process and that many agents and conditions that influence *in vivo* oncogenesis have parallel effects on *in vitro* cell transformation [H6, K10, L3].

163. There remain, however, many uncertainties regarding the true relevance to *in vivo* oncogenesis of quantitative and qualitative studies with many existing *in vitro* systems. The principal *in vitro* cellular systems are based on immortalized rodent cell lines, and quantitative, radiation-induced transformation of normal human diploid cells has yet to be convincingly demonstrated. In the established rodent cell systems there has been considerable controversy on the shape of dose-effect curves [L2], on the influence of radiation quality and, recently, on the existence of a reverse dose-rate effect for high-LET radiations (see [C14]). Overall, the relative simplicity of these systems is appealing, but their direct application to quantitative aspects of human radiological risk is perhaps premature. Some of these aspects are discussed in Annex F, "Influence of dose and dose rate on stochastic effects of radiation".

164. Mechanistic studies of *in vitro* cell transformation indicate that initiating events may, in some instances, be induced at a surprisingly high frequency in an irradiated population of C3H10T½ cells [K3]. Evidence has also been presented that, at low doses, ^{125}I incorporated into DNA is extremely effective at inducing the transformation of BALB/3T3 cells [L18]. Indeed, at ^{125}I levels producing only ~30 decays per cell, the high transformation frequency observed (10^{-4} per surviving cell) implies that only a very small number of unspecified DNA sites need to be damaged to convert the cell to a neoplastic phenotype. Similar conclusions are also emerging from *in vivo*/*in vitro* studies with rat mammary and thyroid clonogens [C5]; such high-frequency induction is, however, difficult to reconcile with the overall picture of specific gene targets for neoplastic initiation that is emerging from studies with human tumours. The molecular mechanisms underlying this process remain obscure, but establishing the generality of such high frequency induced events is of obvious importance. The molecular aspects of the radiation-induced transformed phenotype have been studied using DNA-mediated gene transfer techniques, and although dominantly acting transforming DNA sequences have been shown to be carried by overtly transformed C3H10T½ cells, their identity has yet to be fully established [B3, K22]. The presence of unidentified transforming sequences has been demonstrated in post-irradiation mass cultures of C3H10T½ cells [L2], and recently, DNA transfer techniques have been successfully employed in the molecular cloning of a transforming gene from a radiation-induced C3H10T½ transformant [F20]; it remains to be seen however whether this gene represents the principal target for radiation-induced initiation of C3H10T½ transformation. In addition, *myc* oncogene rearrangement has been characterized in a radiation transformed C3H10T½ clone [S6] and *myc* and *raf* gene expression has been shown to be increased in another such transformed clone [L25].

165. While it is possible that the identification of characteristic gene activation events in *in vitro* transformed cells may allow comment on the broad mechanisms of radiation oncogenesis, it is more likely that such identification will be of greatest value in the understanding the systems themselves. With conventional rodent *in vitro* transformation systems, doubt is likely to remain about the true significance of single cell *in vitro* response to the more complex interactive processes that mediate *in vivo* oncogenesis.

2. Novel systems

166. While quantitative and qualitative data from conventional cell transformation systems will continue to be useful, more attention is now being focused on the potentially more relevant systems that utilize human cells, cells of epithelial origin and cells from haemopoietic tissues (see [C9]). It is already apparent that the conventional criteria for *in vitro* cell transformation, i.e. loss of contact inhibitions/focus formation, growth in semi-solid media, immortalization and relatively rapid progression to an overtly oncogenic phenotype, do not apply generally in cellular systems. Cellular and molecular studies of human neoplasms strongly suggest that different transformational processes may operate in different cell lineages, and this should be reflected in the *in vitro* systems that are employed. The most significant progress that could be anticipated would be the design of *in vitro* cellular systems that were linked, by cytogenetic and molecular studies, to specific *in vivo* neoplastic and pre-neoplastic conditions. It cannot be expected that such systems will be simple or quantitatively precise [H13], but they should reveal more about oncogenic mechanisms than the currently favoured systems based on rodent fibroblast cell lines.

167. New developments in *in vitro* cell transformation have recently been reviewed [C9], and it is sufficient here to highlight a few of the most important findings. Studies with human diploid fibroblasts have been discussed by McCormick et al. [M9], with particular emphasis on the lack of clear evidence for induced malignant transformation in these cells. The immortalization of human fibroblasts, unlike that of cultured rodent cells, appears to be a very rare event and probably represents a rate-limiting step in the pathway towards malignancy. It has been shown, however, that a rare, radiation-induced, immortalized human fibroblast strain may be transformed to a fully malignant phenotype by the introduction of an activated H-*ras* oncogene [N8, N11]. In a series of subsequent experiments [M40] it has been shown that intermittent *in vitro* exposure (total dose 28 Gy) to gamma rays over 50 passages resulted in the immortalization of human fibroblasts but that final malignant conversion could not be demonstrated until the 547th passage (2,800 d in culture). These studies provide a clear demonstration of the multi-step nature of *in vitro* malignant transformation in human fibroblasts and, unfortunately, the difficulties that are faced in obtaining quantitative estimates of induced transformation with these cells.

168. A human hybrid cell system has also been developed in order to quantify radiation effects on a putative tumour suppressor gene encoded on chromosome 11. The quantitative, cellular and molecular aspects of this system are currently under investigation [R4], and good progress may be anticipated. Although based on immortalized strains of human cells and used so far for characterization and chemical carcinogenesis studies, mammary epithelial [S54], kidney epithelial [T18], skin keratinocyte [B7, F6, R18, R19], colonic epithelial [W25] and urinary epithelial cell [R5] systems also show interesting potential for both mechanistic and quantitative studies.

169. Cytogenetic and molecular studies of chemically transformed variants of the SV-HUC human uro-epithelial cell line have been particularly rewarding [K15]. It has been shown that chromosome 3p deletions are characteristic of the high-grade carcinomas produced in transplanted nude mice following *in vitro* chemical transformation. What is particularly noteworthy is that loss of heterozygosity for 3p encoded DNA sequences have been reported in a variety of human carcinomas, thus for the first time providing a putative link between *in vitro* induced cellular damage and carcinogenesis *in vivo*. An extension of this approach to radiation-induced transformation should be encouraged, but it should be recognized that, at present, the assay system as developed does not lend itself to detailed quantitative studies and that the viral immortalization process may influence the transformational response.

170. Novel cell transformation systems that include *in vivo* and *in vitro* phases have been developed for mammary [C5], thyroid [M23] and tracheal [T9] tissues of rodents. In the mammary system, transplantation of dissociated mammary tissue to subcutaneous fat pads has allowed the quantification of differentiating mammary clonogens and, through this, estimates of radiosensitivity. A tissue-dependent post-irradiation repair process has been characterized, as has the induction of dysplastic (pre-neoplastic) lesions resulting from radiation damage to clonogens. The promotional effects of elevated prolactin and glucocorticoid deficiency are evident in these studies, and it is also apparent that neoplastic initiation is a relatively common cellular event [C5].

171. A fat pad transplantation technique also underlies the *in vivo in vitro* studies on thyroid carcinogenesis. The radiation induction of pre-neoplastic lesions was shown to be dependent on hormonal status (thyroid-stimulating hormone), and again, initiating events were observed at a surprisingly high frequency [C5]. Cell-cell interactions have been shown to influence strongly the expression of oncogenesis in both mammary and thyroid systems. Similar findings have been made using an *in vivo in vitro* model of tracheal epithelial transformation in the rat [T10]. Here, direct cell-cell contact in tissues and a diffusible factor from cultured cells have been shown to suppress the expression of early oncogenic changes. In the case of *in vitro*

suppression the factor is believed to be transforming growth factor ß (TGF ß), which may exert its effect through the induction of terminal differentiation [T10]. Thus, the emergence of initiated cells and their subsequent proliferative advantage may depend on their ability to escape from TGF ß mediated terminal differentiation.

172. Despite the increasing knowledge of the complex interactions between growth promoting and inhibitory factors in the regulation of haemopoiesis and associated cell lineage differentiation [D8, M24], transformation systems for cells of haemopoietic origin are at a relatively early stage of development. However, the availability of growth factor-dependent haemopoietic cell lines [D9, G10, S30] and their oncogenic transformation by specific haemopoiesis-related genes [B15, L12] are providing powerful tools with which it may be possible to relate transforming events *in vitro* to those that characterize haemopoietic neoplasms *in vivo*. In the case of osteosarcomagenesis, an *in vitro* system for murine mandibular condyles is being developed to study the cellular and molecular events that mediate skeletoblast differentiation and oncogenic transformation [S15]. In this system it has been shown that *fos* expression precedes the *in vitro* osteogenic differentiation of cartilage cells [C28].

D. *IN VIVO* STUDIES

1. General experimental strategies

173. It has been argued in previous paragraphs that the most plausible molecular form of neoplastic initiation is specific gene mutation that predisposes appropriate target cells to subsequent malignant conversion; studies with familial human neoplasms have also shown that, under some circumstances, it is possible to gain detailed information on the identity of tumour-initiating events in man. However, the central problem for cellular and molecular studies using inducing agents and experimental animal systems is that during the post-irradiation latent period, a number of genetic/epigenetic changes will have accumulated within the evolving neoplastic cell population, and many of them will be represented in the final malignant clone that is available for study. What criteria can be used to determine which of these changes was induced by the carcinogen and is therefore the initiating event?

174. Two main experimental strategies have evolved to approach this crucial question:

(a) to use molecular techniques to search for consistent molecular change in specific genes of the induced neoplasm and attempt to relate any characteristic DNA changes to the known DNA-damaging properties of the inducing agent;

(b) to identify candidate initiating events as consistent molecular and/or chromosomal changes in the overt induced neoplasm and subsequently trace the induction of these events back to the immediate post-treatment proliferation of cells in the target organ.

175. The first strategy has been effectively employed in the putative identification of *ras* proto-oncogenes as principal targets for early events in chemically induced mammary, hepatic and skin carcinomas in rodents (paragraphs 188 and 189). In general, the success of this approach to chemical oncogenesis depends on the induced initiating events being base-pair specific changes in a restricted set of codons of a known gene (see, e.g. [B37]). In this case the chemical specificities of the carcinogen will be immediately apparent and informative. The relative lack of DNA damage specificity following exposure to ionizing radiation may mean that this strategy is less appropriate to radiation oncogenesis. Consistency of molecular genetic change in a given neoplasm infers a major contribution of that change to the success of the malignant clone but need not be informative on the stage in clonal evolution at which the change took place. Point mutation within a limited set of *ras* gene codons has been demonstrated in radiation-induced murine lymphomas [D3, D4, N19], but alone, these data are insufficient to identify *ras* activation as an initiating event for this neoplasm. More recently, however, it was shown that *K-ras* codon mutation spectra in tumours induced by gamma rays are different from those in tumours induced by neutrons [S31]. These data were used to argue that differences in physical properties between the two radiation qualities might influence mutational spectra and hence that *K-ras* activation might represent an initiating event for radiation lymphomagenesis. There is, however, some uncertainty in the biophysical interpretation of these data, and it remains possible that *ras* mutations play a greater role in the development of lymphoma than in its initiation. Even greater problems of interpretation surround other observations of structural and functional changes in oncogenes of radiation-induced animal neoplasms (paragraphs 179-187). In no case is it possible to be confident about the identity of the radiation-induced initiating event (e.g. [F4, S7]). In this area, however, the implementation of polymerase chain reaction techniques (PCR) for rapid gene mutation analysis [E8, R11] during early post-irradiation cell proliferation periods may be expected to have a major impact on future research.

176. The second experimental strategy has been somewhat more successful, particularly in providing comment on the status of characteristic chromosomal changes in radiation-induced haemopoietic neoplasms.

177. Trisomy of chromosome (ch) 15 is a characteristic cytogenetic feature of radiation-induced murine thymic lymphoma. Cytogenetic studies of pre-neoplastic animals strongly suggest that the appearance of the extra ch15 copy is associated with the later stages of neoplastic development. In contrast, the early appearance of a ch 1:5 translocation in a significant proportion of pre-neoplastic animals suggests that this is a better candidate for a lymphoma-initiating event [M7]. There is, as yet, no information regarding the involvement of specific genes in either of these chromosomal changes.

178. The deletion and rearrangement of ch2 is a consistent feature of radiation-induced acute myeloid leukaemia in the mouse [B4, B16, H8]. Using an *in vitro* irradiation and transplantation technique, similar ch2 rearrangements were characterized in rapidly proliferating haemopoietic cell clones within five days of irradiation, and it was concluded that these may represent candidate initiating events for murine acute myeloid leukaemia [B16, S8]. More recently, a strong statistical concordance has been established between radiation-induced ch2 breakpoints in irradiated murine haemopoietic cells and those in acute myeloid leukaemia [B16]. In addition to strengthening the link between ch2 deletion/rearrangement and leukaemic initiation, these data also suggest that induced breakage may occur at specific radiation-sensitive sites on this chromosome. Stable chromosomal changes have also been recorded in irradiated and repopulating haemopoietic cells in the rat [M35].

2. Molecular studies of induced animal neoplasms

179. The molecular aspects of radiation oncogenesis in animal models of thymic lymphoma, myeloid leukaemia and osteosarcoma have recently been reviewed [J2] and are outlined here briefly, together with some observations on rodent skin, mammary and lung carcinogenesis. This whole area has also been explored in a number of recent symposia (see [B28, E7]).

180. ***Thymic lymphoma.*** Studies of thymic lymphomagenesis in mice have provided evidence that an indirect mechanism is involved [K4]. It has been repeatedly shown that thymic lymphomas may develop from immature lymphoid cells present in non-irradiated thymuses that are subcutaneously grafted into split-dose-irradiated, thymectomized recipients [K4, M8]. Since weakly leukaemogenic activity is often present in cell-free extracts of primary lymphomas and its potency increases with serial passage, a viral role in lymphomagenesis was suspected [L4]. Although recombinant retroviral complexes have been reproducibly detected in radiation-induced lymphomas [J2], the specific role of these and their derivation from germ-line ecotropic provirus remains uncertain [J2, N4]. Some evidence for proviral induction by radiation and integration into common genomic domains in lymphomas and derivative cell lines has recently been obtained, but the genes within these domains are not known [J2, S55]. The weight of evidence now tends to favour a role for provirus in lymphoma development rather than initiation, and there are studies that imply that radiation leukaemogenesis in NFS mice does not involve C- and B-type retroviruses [O3]. Indeed, recent evidence suggests that infection by activated viruses is not necessary to explain the indirect induction of radiogenic lymphomas [S56, S57]. It has been proposed that the depletion of T-cell precursors in the bone marrow, together with the depletion of thymic lymphocytes, is sufficient for regenerating thymus cells to undergo pre-neoplastic changes, possibly due to an aberrant expression of genes involved in the growth and differentiation of thymus cells [M50, S56, S57].

181. It has been shown that the injection of syngeneic bone marrow cells into split-dose-irradiated mice can prevent lymphoma development, possibly as a consequence of the rapid repopulation of recipient thymus by donor lymphoid cells [K4, S9]. Overall, it may be concluded that complex cellular processes mediate radiation lymphomagenesis and that direct radiation damage to target cells may not be a prerequisite for the appearance of oncogenic events. In this respect, four interactive factors may be invoked:

(a) activation of potentially leukaemogenic virus from germ-line provirus and subsequent recombination to yield more potent virus;
(b) thymic involution and regeneration, giving a population of virus-susceptible cells;
(c) impairment of cell surveillance mechanisms;
(d) impairment of bone marrow and thymocyte cell function, leading to reduced thymic repopulation and altered gene expression.

In addition, codon mutations in *N-* and *K-ras* oncogenes, T-cell growth factor changes together with specific chromosomal rearrangements have been detected in radiation-induced lymphomas, and some of these have been suggested as early events in lymphomagenesis (paragraph 175, [N19]); in contrast, recent data tend to argue against the involvement of *p53* mutations in radiation-induced and chemically-induced lymphomas [B33]. Attempts to characterize and isolate target cells for radiation lymphomagenesis are also under way [M26].

182. ***Acute myeloid leukaemia.*** There is little evidence to suggest that radiation-induced murine acute myeloid leukaemia proceeds via an indirect (viral) mechanism. In contrast, the specific deletion/

rearrangement of chromosome 2 is a consistent cytogenetic feature of induced murine acute myeloid leukaemia [B4, B16, H8, H44], and evidence has been obtained that ch2 rearrangement is induced directly by x rays in multipotential haemopoietic cells, in some cases generating a cellular phenotype associated with preferential haemopoietic recruitment and/or proliferative advantage [B16, S8]. It has also been shown that ch2 events may be observed in bone marrow cultures established from irradiated mice long before the anticipated appearance of acute myeloid leukaemia [T4] and that the induction of ch2 rearrangement is an early step in leukaemogenesis but is not sufficient for the development of myeloid malignancy [H27, H28]. Preliminary evidence for deletion of the homeobox gene, *hox* 4.1, and activation of the cytokine gene, interleukin-1ß (*Il-1β*), has been obtained in some ch2-rearranged acute myeloid leukaemias [B5, S10, S11]. However, the evidence presented for the involvement of these genes in leukaemic initiation was not compelling, and more recently, detailed molecular analyses of the *Il-1* genomic region on ch2 failed to provide evidence of the structural rearrangements predicted in acute myeloid leukaemia [S32, S33]. In these analyses it was found, however, that some acute myeloid leukaemias show very similar methylation pattern changes in the *Il-1* region, and it was suggested that these may be associated with certain forms of ch2 rearrangement and deletion. Other studies have shown that the ch2-encoded *his-1* locus is involved in virally induced myeloid leukaemia in the mouse and may represent another candidate gene for the initiation of acute myeloid leukaemia [A9].

183. Cytogenetic studies with radiation-induced murine acute myeloid leukaemias and irradiated normal haemopoietic cells have yielded evidence that ch2-encoded fragile sites are involved in leukaemogenic initiation [B16]. These investigations also suggest that the interstitial ch2 sites in question have a strong recombination affinity with the terminal (telomeric) ends of other chromosomes, implying that they may indeed be telomere-like repeat sequences (paragraphs 62 and 63); it was also suggested that the expression of these sites might be influenced by genomic imprinting. More recently, interstitial telomere-like sequences of an inverted repeat form have been cytogenetically mapped close to the relevant ch2 breakpoints, and the use of telomeric sequences as molecular probes has provided some evidence that germ-line variation at certain telomere-like repeat sequences may be associated with genetically determined leukaemogenic radiosensitivity in the mouse [S43]. Following these studies, it has been suggested that the telomere sequences at ch2 fragile sites may promote the formation of recombinogenic secondary DNA structures that are highly radiosensitive [B32]. Finally, while *ras* mutation is not a common feature of murine myeloid leukaemias, the activation of *N-ras* has been reported in radiation-induced myeloid leukaemias in the dog [G17].

184. *Osteosarcoma.* Although weakly oncogenic viruses have been isolated from radiation-induced murine osteosarcomas, there is no evidence for common genomic insertion sites nor is there an obligate requirement for such viruses in osteosarcomagenesis [J2, V8]. A non-essential role for such viruses in oncogenic progression appears, perhaps, to be more likely. Molecular studies have revealed the amplification of a ch15 domain encoding *c-myc* and the *Mlvi-1* proviral integration site in up to 30% of ^{224}Ra-induced osteosarcomas, and evidence for altered expression of *K-ras*, *myc*, *sis*, *abl*, *bas* and *fos* has been reported in some tumours [J2, S59]. Structural and/or expressional changes have also been reported in the *p53* gene of some osteosarcomas, but to date, there is no evidence for consistent structural changes in the retinoblastoma (*rb*) gene [J2, S58]. Although specific comment on the status of these molecular changes in radiation osteosarcomagenesis is not yet possible, the human evidence of *RB* and *p53* gene involvement in the early phases of the human neoplasm [C29, T5] demands further studies with murine osteosarcomas.

185. *Skin carcinomas.* Ionizing radiation induces skin carcinomas in both the mouse and the rat [J3, S7], but little is known of the molecular mechanisms involved. Recently, it has been shown that the activation of *K-ras* and *myc* oncogenes is frequently observed in primary rat skin carcinomas induced by ionizing radiation [S7]; the status of these changes in the oncogenic process remains uncertain, but *myc* seems most likely to function relatively late in skin carcinogenesis [G18]. In murine studies it has been shown that the gene encoding the transin protease is overexpressed in carcinomas but not in benign papillomas. It was inferred from these observations that transin gene expression might be involved in neoplastic progression by enhancing tumour invasiveness [B11].

186. *Mammary carcinomas.* The induction of mammary carcinomas in mice has been studied by isolating mammary epithelial cells at intervals following irradiation *in vivo* and subsequently selecting clonal cell lines *in vitro*. After low *in vitro* passage, isolated cell lines produced normal ductal outgrowth in transplanted mice, but with increasing passage cells became increasingly tumorigenic and invasive. Chromosomal abnormalities and *myc* (but not *ras*) gene expression, increased with passage and tumorigenic potential. On the basis of studies on *rb* and *p53* gene expression it was suggested that alteration of expression of tumour suppressor genes might be an early event in the oncogenic transformation of mammary epithelial cells

[E7]. This *in vitro* system has also been used to investigate the acquisition of angiogenic activity in irradiated mammary cells and its temporal relationship with tumorigenic potential [U12]. Although *ras* proto-oncogene involvement in chemically induced mammary carcinoma in rodents is becoming understood (see [G19]), the situation regarding ionizing radiation has not been resolved.

187. ***Lung carcinomas.*** Lung carcinogenesis has been studied in a number of animal species [M41], and in contrast to the situation in humans it seems at present unlikely that either the *rb* or *p53* gene plays a major role in induced lung neoplasia [G20, M41]. Studies on *ras* gene changes in plutonium-induced rat lung tumours imply that the activation of this gene may be a relatively early event in the generation of proliferative pulmonary lesions [S60], while in the dog, the expression of the epidermal growth factor receptor gene was elevated in a significant proportion of lung tumours and proliferative foci arising after exposure to plutonium [G21].

IV. COMPARATIVE ASPECTS OF ONCOGENESIS BY RADIATION AND CHEMICALS

188. It has been suggested that ionizing radiation may principally, but not exclusively, initiate oncogenesis through mechanisms involving DNA deletion and/or rearrangement. While many chemical agents also induce gross (chromosomal) damage in mammalian cells, the mechanisms of induction are fundamentally different from those of radiation [C3, E3]. In addition, molecular studies of induced somatic mutation show the majority of chemical agents to act principally as point mutagens [S29, T2]. Although the mechanisms of chromosome aberration induction by radiation and by the majority of chemical agents differ in terms of cell cycle dependence, the genomic distribution of damage and the DNA repair/recombination processes involved, there may not be major differences in the final stable forms of many induced chromosomal changes in surviving cells. It should be emphasized, however, that the distribution of these changes within the genome may be expected to be different for radiation and chemical agents. In spite of these uncertainties it appears that the major mechanistic difference at the cellular level between radiation-induced and chemically induced oncogenesis is likely to centre on their relative efficiencies for the induction of neoplasms that are principally initiated through point mutation and activation of proto-oncogenes. Chemical and physical carcinogenesis has been reviewed recently [H46], and the strongest experimental evidence for the existence of such an initiating mechanism for chemical oncogenesis comes from studies of *ras* proto-oncogene activation in some rodent neoplasms. In many chemically induced skin, mammary and hepatic tumours, codon-specific point mutations responsible for *ras* activation correspond to those predicted by the known base-pair-specific mutagenic action of the agent used as the initiator, i.e. *ras* mutation appears to be the initiating event [B6].

189. Recent studies [K8] have extended these observations by showing that following nitrosomethylurea exposure, *ras* activating events may be detected in normal rat mammary glands only two weeks after treatment, i.e. at least two months before the onset of overt neoplasia. It appears, therefore, that these specific chemically induced somatic mutations remain dormant in tissue until promotional, hormone-mediated proliferative responses mobilize *ras* activated cells and allow them to progress towards neoplasia. Broadly, these and other data, e.g. [B37, M42, S61], although currently limited to only a few neoplasms and chemical agents, identify candidate initiating events as point mutations and further strengthen the link between mutagenic and oncogenic mechanisms. However, other studies indicate that *ras* activation is not the only potential initiating event for rat mammary carcinomas and that different initiating mechanisms may have different carcinogen dose and promotional dependencies [Z1, Z2]. Although still at an early stage of development, molecular studies on *in vitro* transformed cells are also consistent with the existence of different molecular mechanisms for radiation and chemical carcinogenesis [C9]. However, for molecular events in a given neoplasm that follow initiating damage, i.e. those contributing towards neoplastic progression, radiation-induced and chemically induced neoplasms may be expected to share some common genetic changes [N7].

190. Two major issues emerge from the suggested mechanistic differences that may distinguish radiation and chemical oncogenesis. First, since different neoplasms may depend for their initiation on different forms of molecular damage to the potentially oncogenic DNA sequence, e.g. point mutations rather than DNA rearrangement or deletion, then differences in

the predominant induced neoplasias following human exposures to radiation and chemical carcinogens may be expected. Secondly, if radiation and chemical agents induce characteristically different spectra of initiating lesions, then different genetically determined post-exposure cellular DNA-repair processes will tend to operate to modify and/or remove that damage. Since the efficiency and fidelity of these repair systems will be a significant determinant of induced oncogenesis, the above differences in repair imply that human genetic susceptibility to induced neoplasia by radiation and chemicals will not necessarily correspond. Although this speculation is broadly supported by the lack of cellular cross-sensitivity between radiation and chemicals in the majority of human genetic diseases showing hypersensitivity to DNA damaging agents [A2, F4, H5], the mutations in these disorders will not be fully representative of those having effects on mutagenesis and oncogenic initiation. This is an important problem in human cancer susceptibility, of which there is insufficient knowledge.

191. Tomatis [T16] has reviewed those chemical agents that are known to have carcinogenic activity in man, and among these are agents for which exposure would occur occupationally (e.g. asbestos, aromatic hydrocarbon derivatives and vinyl chloride monomer), medically (e.g. cyclophosphamide and phenacetin) or environmentally (e.g. aflatoxins, nitrosamines, soots, tars and oils). The majority of these agents do not act directly but require specific endogenous biochemical modification in order to generate the carcinogenic species (see [H46]).

192. Certain workers in the plastics industry are occupationally exposed to vinyl chloride monomer (VCM). The enzyme-mediated activation of VCM (the procarcinogen) to carcinogenic metabolites such as chloroethylene oxide and 2-chloroactelaldehyde occurs principally in the liver. Such activation produces tissue-specific exposure to the direct carcinogen and in the case of VCM produces a very clear excess of the rare hepatic neoplasm, angiosarcoma, in exposed workers [B8].

193. Occupational exposure to aromatic hydrocarbon compounds, in particular benzene, has been associated with the development of haemopoietic neoplasms [T16]. Most polycyclic aromatic hydrocarobons, such as benzo(a)pyrene (BP), are not directly carcinogenic; however, through the action of cytochrome P450-linked mixed function oxidases and epoxide hydrases, BP may be converted to active carcinogens, such as BP 7,8-diol,-9,10 epoxide (see [W18]). Studies with the mouse skin papilloma/carcinoma system suggest that the carcinogenic action of this diol epoxide derivative centres on its capacity to form adducts on the guanine (G) residues of DNA. Misrepair of these adducts results in base-pair substitutions at G residues, and these have been linked with the *ras* proto-oncogene activation events that are believed to initiate mouse skin carcinogenesis (see paragraphs 188-189).

194. As noted earlier, aflatoxin B1 (AFB), present in some fungally contaminated foods, is associated with the prevalence of human liver cancer in parts of southern Africa and eastern Asia [B22]. AFB is metabolized, principally in the liver, by the mixed oxidase enzyme system to produce several products, including a highly reactive 2,3-epoxide derivative. This reacts with the 7 position of guanine residues in DNA and represents a major DNA adduct in the liver of AFB-exposed rats (see [W18]). The importance of this reaction for human liver carcinogenesis has recently been demonstrated by molecular studies on tumour DNA from hepatocellular carcinoma (HCC) patients from regions where the disease is prevalent, probably as a consequence of AFB contamination. These studies revealed that the G→T base substitutions at codon 249 of the *p53* suppressor gene, which might be predicted from AFB epoxide action dominated the *p53* mutational spectrum observed [B23, H34]. As well as highlighting the importance of *p53* suppressor gene mutations for the initiation of HCC, these studies provide the first clear links between environmental carcinogen exposure, procarcinogen activational processes and gene-specific tumour mutations in man. An essentially similar approach with the *p53* gene has been used to study the involvement of specific UV photoproducts in sunlight-mediated human skin carcinogenesis [B36]. In essence, the specific form of *p53* mutation in HCC and skin tumours is providing a signature of human AFB and UV exposure, respectively, [H46]; the potential implications of these data are discussed in paragraphs 221 and 222. However, it should be noted that in the case of the mouse, liver carcinogenesis following chemical exposure may not be associated with consistent *p53* mutation [G20].

195. The *p53* point mutations observed in HCC and other solid tumours [C31, H30, H46, L13] also serve to illustrate the point that the initiation of oncogenesis by chemical agents is in no way restricted to proto-oncogene activation but may also occur via the mutation of tumour suppressor genes. In such cases, the expectation is that those mutations will tend to cluster in the regions of the gene specifying certain active sites in the protein product. Detailed analyses of *p53* gene mutations in human tumours by polymerase chain reaction techniques have provided ample evidence of this [H30, L13] (Figure IV). In the distribution illustrated in the Figure, the horizontal axis represents the 393 codons of the human *p53* gene from N-terminal (NH_2) to C-terminal (COOH) ends. The vertical bars represent the relative proportion of

mutations that occur at each codon of the *p53* gene, as sequenced from 94 different primary tumours, xenografts or cell lines derived from tumours (brain, breast, colon, oesophageal and lung tumours and neurofibrosarcomas, osteosarcomas, rhadomyosarcomas and T-cell lymphomas). The highest percentage is at position 273, which accounted for 13% of all mutations [L13]. Tumour types and *p53* mutations have been tabulated [C31, H30], and further information on tumours of the thyroid and cervix is available [C30, I1, K24]. Some studies show that *p53* mutation can, however, arise at the malignant conversion stage of oncogenic development indicating that *p53* mutational spectra will not always be informative on carcinogenic initiation. Nevertheless, current *p53* mutational analyses have been most informative, and the same approach will doubtless yield important information on the mutational damage sustained by other tumour suppressor genes, such as *APC* [K15, N16], thought to be involved in the initiation of other tumours.

196. Since many environmental chemical carcinogens are subject to specific cellular activation and/or degradative processes, human genetic heterogeneity with respect to these processes may be an important factor in determining the specific dose of the carcinogen to target cells [A7, W19]. These activation/degradative processes will also affect the dose of the carcinogen to different target tissues and thereby influence the spectrum of induced neoplasms.

197. For external radiation, the induction of potentially oncogenic cellular lesions may be viewed as a more direct and genetically less complex process influenced principally by the LET and the penetrative properties of the radiation, by DNA metabolic functions in target cells and, particularly for high-LET radiation, by biophysical factors such as the cross-section of the cellular nucleus of target cells and by the packaging density of the DNA. If, as implied, a significant genetic determinant of the radiation initiation of oncogenesis resides in the activity and fidelity of DNA repair processes, then it may be that there is a greater degree of human genetic variation in cancer susceptibility following exposure to low-LET radiation than there is following high-LET radiation. This speculation derives from observations of the apparent lack of (correct) cellular repair following high-LET irradiation of cultured human cells. If high-LET induced genomic lesions are inherently difficult to repair correctly [C8], then less genetic variation and less influence of repair functions may be anticipated in the human population. The main qualification to this speculation is that it is based on studies of radiation-induced potentially lethal lesions and may not apply in full to potentially mutagenic or oncogenic damage.

198. In contrast, for internal radiation, the chemical and biochemical properties of the isotope will determine *in vivo* metabolic routes for uptake, transport, distribution and excretion (see, e.g. [P5]). All these processes will have genetic determinants, and in this respect, oncogenesis by isotopes taken into the body has some parallels with chemical oncogenesis and may be subject to a greater degree of genetic heterogeneity than predicted for external radiation.

199. For radon, a combination of physical, physicochemical and physiological factors will interact to determine radon inhalation, its concentration in respiratory compartments and the subsequent dose distribution in tissues. The active carcinogenic species following radon exposure is, however, likely to be the daughter nuclides in the decay chain. Hence, the underlying mechanism of radon carcinogenesis will be subject to a series of complex interactive factors involving not only initial radon uptake and distribution but also the biokinetics and half-lives of the radon daughters (see Annex A, "Exposures from natural sources of radiation").

200. More straightforwardly, some alpha-emitting actinides have a high affinity for specific glycoproteins present on bone surfaces and may indeed be bound by metal transport proteins. Consequently, the greatest radionuclide deposition and, thereby, accumulation of alpha-particle dose often occurs at active endosteal bone surfaces. Metabolic factors therefore determine that the principal somatic cells at risk are osteogenic cells at bone surfaces and haemopoietic cells in peripheral marrow close to bone surfaces. Clear evidence for radium-induced osteosarcomas has been obtained in both man and experimental animals. However, alpha particles from some actinides deposited in bone appear to be only weakly leukaemogenic [H9, H10, S16]. It is possible that this latter observation reflects the hypersensitivity of multipotential haemopoietic cells to the lethal effects of track traversals by single alpha particles, in which case there will be a low probability of survival for irradiated target cells; equally, however, the spatial relationship between sites of deposition of radionuclides and target cells and the alpha-particle track LET may also be critical [B26, S16]. In this latter context it is important to recognize that alpha-emitting actinides distribute differently between bone volume and bone surface, and it is, therefore, not appropriate to generalize on the *in vivo* dose to different target cell populations.

201. In the case of radionuclides taken up in particulate form, the action of macrophages in the engulfment, dissolution and nuclide redistribution in tissues is of prime importance. These factors will undoubtedly influence the relationships between dose and target tissues [S46]. In human patients receiving colloidal alpha-emitting thorotrast as a contrast medium, distribution of dose to tissues will have been

subject to cell-mediated effects. In these patients there is evidence of both the accumulation of the isotope in liver and a dramatically increased risk of liver cancer [U1, U2]. Studies have been initiated to relate *p53* mutations in these tumours to potential radiation induced damage [W26].

202. It should, however, be stressed that many of the arguments presented here relate to genetic and physiological effects on the initiation of oncogenesis. Genetic and physiological heterogeneity with respect to promotional and progressive processes in tumour development must be of importance to the overall incidence of induced neoplasia in the population and could indeed be the dominant factors. The relative roles of radiation and chemical agents in these processes are noted in paragraphs 78-114 and discussed in detail elsewhere (see, e.g. [S2, T14]). Here it is sufficient to suggest, that for a highly interactive multi-step disease such as cancer, it is only possible to generalize on the relative roles of radiation and chemical agents in the steps that may currently be defined on the basis of incomplete mechanistic knowledge. Better knowledge should make the task somewhat easier, but it is important to recognize the current extent of ignorance.

203. In conclusion, the mechanisms of oncogenic initiation by radiation and chemicals differ substantially and may be subject to different genetic and physiological factors. Consequently, the determination of relative risk from radiation and chemicals will not be an easy task. A report of the United States National Council on Radiation Protection and Measurements [N10] considers in detail the comparative aspects of the carcinogenicity of ionizing radiation and chemicals, and it is clear from that report and the outline presented here that the determination of relative risk from radiation and chemicals is not at all straightforward. For radiation and those chemical agents with known mechanisms of action on DNA, it may be possible to make some assessments on the basis of molecular dosimetry. In such cases the abundance of initial mutagenic/carcinogenic lesions in the DNA of cells of the target organ following exposure to a carcinogen may provide a crude experimental indicator of potency. However, it should be recognized that for this strategy to have a firm scientific base, it is necessary to know the different spectra of mutagenic lesions and their repair/misrepair characteristics and, perhaps most importantly, to have a much better understanding of the mechanistic differences that characterize the oncogenic processes that drive the induction of different neoplasms. In such a future experimental approach to comparative carcinogenicity it will be essential to be able to relate animal and *in vitro* data to man. In this respect, it should be noted that the current quantitative knowledge of human risk from exposure to ionizing radiation greatly exceeds that for any chemical carcinogen.

V. FUTURE PERSPECTIVES

204. It will have become obvious that although some understanding of the mechanisms of radiation oncogenesis is beginning to emerge, the complexity of the whole process is such that rapid progress on a broad front should not be anticipated. Nevertheless, it should be noted that the main component of understanding has come within the last decade and owes much to the application of modern methods of cell and molecular biology. It may be that the best prospects for the future lie in the strategic implementation of these modern methods, with particular emphasis on the full integration of radiation oncogenesis research into the continually expanding field of cancer biology. A few of the many potential growth points and future needs in research on radiation oncogenesis are briefly discussed in the following Sections.

A. IMPLICATIONS OF ADVANCES IN RELATED RESEARCH

205. During the last few years much progress has been made in elucidating mechanisms of DNA-repair and mutagenesis; some of these advances have been discussed in other Sections. Of particular note is the anticipated availability of molecular probes for genes that determine human sensitivity to radiation and other genotoxic agents (e.g. [F1, G7, H45, K11, K28, T15]). When available, these will find use in the elucidation of human genetic heterogeneity with regard to radiosensitivity, with the final prospect of identifying subpopulations that may carry elevated risks of oncogenesis. In this context, the identification and molecular cloning of tumour genes associated with cancer susceptibility (Table 6) is also of crucial importance. Studies on the latter have largely focused on the dominantly expressing genes of high penetrance, such as *RB*, *WT* and *APC*, but the prospect of identifying less evident genes of low penetrance, which may be more frequent in the population, is probably of greater importance. In addition to increasing the knowledge of oncogenic mechanisms at the human population level, such information may have significant social and economic implications.

206. The characterization of genes involved in mammalian DNA repair and radiosensitivity may also provide the means of identifying (or of generating

through genetic manipulation) radiosensitive, DNA-repair deficient mutants of the mouse. The availability of such mutant strains would provide a very powerful tool for detailed whole animal studies on the relationship between DNA-repair and oncogenesis. Recent studies imply that severe combined immunodeficient (*scid*) mice may have an inherent defect in DNA metabolism that confers cellular radiosensitivity [B27, F12, M10]; mouse mutants of this type could provide valuable models for radiation oncogenesis studies. In a similar way, genetically manipulated mice (transgenics) carrying germ line copies of activated oncogenes (see, e.g. [H15, H24, L26, M11, R20, V9]) may also have an important future role to play in understanding the mechanisms of radiation oncogenesis. In this context, genetically engineered murine models of retinoblastoma and of *p53* deficiency in mice may be particularly valuable [D14, W11]. Other so-called tumour suppressor gene "knock-out" mice will doubtless be available in the near future.

207. Recently, important advances have been made by the successful long-term repopulation of the haemopoietic systems of *scid* immunodeficient mice with engrafted human haemopoietic cells [K28, M12, M13]. These *scid*-human chimaeras may provide the means for studying haemopoietic and leukaemogenic response in an experimental animal system. This general approach, i.e. the use of mouse-human chimaeras, may become an important focus of future studies on human radiation oncogenesis, in that it may allow the study of a range of transplanted human cells in murine host tissues.

208. On a more practical note, two relatively recently developed techniques may have application in the direct assay of radiation-associated somatic cell changes in radiation-exposed human groups. First, a novel technique now allows small samples of human blood to be assayed for the frequency of certain somatic mutations; this technique has been employed to examine residual *HPRT* and glycophorin gene mutations in atomic bomb survivors in Japan [A15, H14, H49, L7]. The technique may have broader application [U13], particularly if it becomes possible to identify gene-specific protein variants associated with haemopoietic neoplasms and to use flow-sorting techniques on blood samples in the same way as recently described for glycophorin A locus variants in bomb survivors [K9]. Secondly, a very powerful molecular technique, polymerase chain reaction (PCR) (see, e.g. [E8, F7, R11]), now allows rapid and specific gene analysis in samples comprising very few cells (conventional methods require much larger samples). If specific genomic changes associated with the initiation of human haemopoietic neoplasms are identified, this technique could, in principle, be employed in conjunction with new automated cytogenetics [P6] and *in situ* chromosome hybridization to detect pre-leukaemic conditions in radiation-exposed individuals.

209. Future molecular approaches to the detection of pre-neoplasia may not however be restricted to the easily accessible haemopoietic and lymphatic systems. In circumstances where a small number of exfoliate cells can be obtained from tissues, polymerase chain reaction techniques have sufficient resolving power to detect specific tumour-associated gene mutations, and this approach has been employed to identify, for example, *p53* gene mutations in cells present in the urine of bladder cancer patients [S44], as well as the *BCR-ABL* gene fusions in pre-leukaemias [M43]. The use of such new molecular and biochemical markers of neoplasia clearly have great potential for the early diagnosis of neoplasia, thereby allowing for early and more effective clinical intervention (see [M34]).

210. However, although the power and speed of polymerase chain reaction techniques may, in principle, be sufficient to contribute to the evaluation of the consequences of human radiation exposure, such as occurred in the immediate vicinity of the Chernobyl accident, it may be argued that there is, as yet, insufficient fundamental knowledge to effectively use the techniques as a screening procedure (see paragraphs 222 and 223).

211. Similar considerations apply in the case of automated cytogenetic screening for stable cytogenetic events, although here there can be no doubt that, if they had been available at the time, they would have greatly facilitated cytogenetic analyses in atomic bomb survivors in Japan (see, e.g. [A5, B17]). Despite these reservations, with increasing technical innovation, the collection and maintenance of archival neoplastic material from radiation-exposed human populations should be given serious consideration. The potential benefit to knowledge that would accrue from such coordinated procedures should not be underestimated.

B. METHODOLOGICAL AND CONCEPTUAL ASPECTS

212. Over many years, a substantial number of experimental animal models of induced neoplasia have been developed. In the long term these models will be most informative if quantitative studies on induced neoplasia are coupled with cellular, cytogenetic and molecular studies of the mechanisms of induction. It may, therefore, be argued that where possible, murine models of neoplasia should be favoured, since for the mouse well-established cytogenetics are available, a detailed genetic map, information on mouse-man genetic homologies, information on the cellular and

molecular aspects of developmental biology and an ever-increasing number of relevant recombinant DNA probes. It is not likely that an equivalent data resource will become available for another mammalian species. This having been said, the rat offers considerable advantages for the study of some model neoplasms, e.g. those of the lung. Where such benefits outweigh technical difficulties, it is obvious that the biological relevance of the animal system should take priority.

213. The degree of commitment that is required to resolve oncogenic mechanisms in whole animal systems is so considerable that animal neoplasms having the greatest relevance to human radiogenic neoplasms should be emphasized. Detailed histopathological comparisons of both neoplastic and pre-neoplastic conditions are crucial to the choice of such animal models. At present mechanistic studies are emphasizing induced leukaemias and osteosarcomas, and it is in these areas that the most rapid progress may be anticipated. However, with a view to representing the whole problem, it will be necessary to approach the broader task of understanding inductive mechanisms for a range of solid tumours, such as those of the breast, liver, kidney, lung and colon. Studies using *in vivo in vitro* transformation systems are already making an important contribution in this area (paragraphs 170-172), and a new dominant mutation predisposing mice to gastro-intestinal tract neoplasms [M25] may be of great value. Since this predisposing gene in the mouse is the homologue of the human *APC* gene (colorectal cancer susceptibility) [S48], there is also the prospect of exploring genetically determined susceptibility to radiation oncogenesis using animal models. Recent findings regarding rodent susceptibility loci for mammary [G23], kidney [W23], liver [B39] and myeloid [S43] neoplasms tend to heighten expectations in this important area of research. The further cytogenetic and molecular study of therapy-related neoplasms in man (see, e.g. [B38, R9, V5, W22]) also holds considerable promise and should be encouraged, particularly since the approach may not only provide direct information on early events in radiation oncogenesis but could also, in principle, contribute towards an understanding of human cancer susceptibility following radiation.

214. Of great importance is the prospect of being able to bridge experimentally between species. One strategy providing for such bridging would be to develop further the organ-specific *in vivo in vitro* approaches to rodent radiation oncogenesis. These experimental systems currently incorporate an *in vitro* phase to reflect the cellular mechanisms and quantitative radiation responses that underlie the *in vivo* induction of relevant radiogenic respiratory, mammary, thyroid and bone neoplasms. If it becomes possible to extend the *in vitro* approach to human tissues, perhaps using transplantation to immune-suppressed mice (paragraph 206), then a direct mechanistic and quantitative comparison between rodent and human *in vitro* phases could be achieved. Such studies, together with quantitative estimates of tumour induction in the whole animal, would then provide for direct extrapolation to mechanisms and risk in man. Existing rodent *in vivo in vitro* transformation systems, as well as providing a potential for the identification of initiating events for the neoplasm in question, have already highlighted the crucial role of hormonal and growth factor effects in the inductive process. The experimental elucidation and quantification of parallel effects in human tissues would be of substantial importance. Thus, while it may not be possible to realize the full theoretical potential of this strategy, it does provide a major goal for future studies and one that unites *in vivo* and *in vitro* approaches to the problem.

215. One important methodological implication of recent advances in cancer research concerns the limitations of current *in vitro* and *in vivo* models of induced neoplastic change for determining the loss of specific DNA sequences in induced tumours. Most of the existing rodent-based animal models of tumorigenesis utilize inbred or closely related hybrid strains of animals; similarly, animal cell culture systems from the mouse, the rat and the hamster are usually of inbred animal strain origin.

216. It has been shown that in outbred human populations, the loss of specific genes from tumours is most easily determined by the molecular analysis of loss of DNA heterozygosity [S19]. Highly inbred animal systems do not allow for this, since for any given autosomal gene the two copies are, by definition, identical, and distinguishing the complete deletion of one of them is not straightforward. Thus, while for the purpose of providing reproducible quantitative estimates of radiation-induced neoplasia it is logical to employ inbred animal strains, this choice can be seen to impose important methodological limitations to the resolution of the molecular mechanisms of oncogenesis. The extension of a selected number of animal and cellular models of radiation tumorigenesis to cross-bred animals, while not a trivial task, now seems to be essential. This will allow the gene deletion mechanism strongly suspected of being involved in radiation oncogenesis to be approached not only in respect to specific candidate genes but also using the more generally applicable new method of determining loss of heterozygosity by analysing highly dispersed and polymorphic DNA repeat sequences, such as polypurine-pyrimidine tracts [C25]. It is notable that this whole approach is already being successfully implemented for animal studies of chemical carcinogenesis (e.g. [B27]). The coupling of these techniques with the rapidly improving techniques of fluorescence *in situ*

hybridization (FISH) for single gene location and "painting" of chromosomes [F18, L19] should further enhance the prospects for resolv-ing mechanisms of radiation oncogenesis at both the molecular and cytogenetic levels.

217. In spite of the optimistic note sounded above, it is most likely that an increased understanding of the molecular mechanisms of oncogenesis will derive from detailed studies of neoplastic phenotypes induced experimentally at relatively high total doses. To what extent will it be possible to provide specific comment on the quantitative aspects of tumour induction at the low doses that are of prime concern in radiological protection?

218. The principal problem in providing any answer to this question concerns the great uncertainties involved in judging the probability with which a single neoplasia-initiated cell in tissue gives rise to a malignancy. As noted elsewhere, the current lack of understanding of the interactive factors that determine this probability is such that even a first approximate calculation is highly dependent on a series of necessary biological assumptions. Nevertheless, it is useful to at least illustrate such an estimation.

219. The assumptions made are as follows:

(a) the human body contains a total of 10^{14} cells;
(b) between one and ten cells per 10,000 have stem-like properties and, as such, are potential targets for induced neoplasia, i.e. 10^{10}-10^{11} target cells per individual;
(c) the typical neoplasia-initiating event centres on single gene inactivation/loss mutations in one of ten possible genes in target cells;
(d) the average acute low-LET induced mutation rate (per cell) for these genes is similar to that observed *in vitro* for the *HPRT* gene i.e. $\sim 10^{-5}$ Gy^{-1};
(e) an acute low-LET exposure of 1 Gy to a population generates a 10% excess risk of malignancy, i.e. one excess tumour for ten exposed individuals;
(f) 1 Gy of low-LET radiation generates 1,000 electron tracks in each cell.

It may then be inferred that:

(a) one excess malignancy occurs within 10^{11}-10^{12} target cells receiving 1 Gy (i.e. 10×10^{10}-10^{11});
(b) the rate of target gene inactivations with ten possible target genes per cell is 10^{-4} Gy^{-1} (i.e. 10×10^{-5});
(c) the number of initiating mutations within these target cells giving rise to a single malignancy is 10^{7}-10^{8} (i.e. $10^{-4} \times 10^{11}$-10^{12});
(d) the probability that a single track intersection of a target cell will give rise to an excess malignancy is 10^{-14}-10^{-15} (i.e. 10^{-11}-$10^{-12} \div 1{,}000$).

In respect to low-LET background radiation of, say, 1 mGy per year, each cell will receive, on average, one track intersection per year. Therefore:

(a) the probability per year of malignancy will be around 10^{-4} [i.e. 10^{10}-10^{11} (target cells) $\times$ 10^{-14}-10^{-15} (probability of malignant conversion)];
(b) for 50 years of exposure this gives a lifetime risk of 5×10^{-3} (50×10^{-4}), i.e. 0.5%;
(c) assuming a natural cumulative frequency of malignancy of 20%, then 1 in 40 (20% ÷ 0.5%) cancers in the population are due to low-LET natural background radiation.

It should be noted that the illustrative calculations above take no account of dose and dose-rate effects for low-LET radiation and that (c) above does not depend on the assumptions made in respect to target cell numbers or on the probability of malignant conversion.

220. The realism of such calculations is, however, highly questionable, depending as it does on a series of biological estimates of frequency, each of which may be incorrect by an order of magnitude or more. However, the exercise points out some questions that need answers from research in cellular and molecular biology if the problems of estimating risk at low doses are to be solved. The most important questions centre on (a) the number of target cells in different tissues; (b) the number of relevant target genes in cells (this may well be dependent on cell type and tissue); (c) the mutagenic mechanism of initiation and the induced mutation rate for different target genes; (d) the mechanisms governing the probability that a given initiated cell will progress to full malignancy.

221. Further to this, epidemiological observations of constant relative cancer risk over time in the atomic bomb survivors in Japan [L20], together with the experimental data outlined in this Annex, imply that radiation acts principally at an early phase in oncogenesis, probably at the initiation stage. Thus, for excess cancer in an irradiated population, the efficiency with which the initiating mutation is induced may be a major factor in the contributions specific neoplasms make to that excess. In this respect, the absence of evidence for any measurable excess of chronic lymphocytic leukaemia (CLL) might be explained by a stringent requirement for CLL initiation by gene-specific chromosome translocation, which has been shown to be involved in the early development of some human T-cell neoplasms [R3]. It has been argued in paragraphs 74 and 75 that such events present very small molecular targets for radiation action, and, on this basis, the T-cell leukaemogenic

potential of radiation might be expected to be low. Experimental evidence for the induction of BCR-ABL gene fusion by high dose x-irradiation has, however, been presented [I3]. Other explanations for this epidemiological observation are also possible. For example, a high sensitivity of T-cell targets to radiation-induced apoptotic death might efficiently remove initiated cells from irradiated target T-cell populations; an explanation of this general form has recently been offered in respect of the differential cancer incidence in the large and small bowel [P15]. It is also important to consider whether cellular and molecular techniques have the potential to distinguish radiation-induced neoplasms from those arising spontaneously or from other forms of carcinogen exposure.

222. As noted in paragraphs 188 and 189, the specificity of many genotoxic chemical agents in their interaction with nucleic acids may provide a characteristic mutational signature in DNA, which infers that cellular exposure to this agent has taken place. In cases where target genes for neoplasia induction have been identified it thus becomes possible to catalogue the DNA base sequence of such mutant genes in human tumours, with a view to identifying characteristic DNA base changes indicative of the action of agents of known mutagenic and carcinogenic potential.

223. Inactivating mutations in the *p53* tumour suppressor gene are strongly suspected of being involved in the early development of a wide range of human solid tumours, and recent analyses of *p53* gene structure in human carcinomas are beginning to provide evidence that tumours of divergent aetiologies arising at various sites do not exhibit the same spectra of mutational change to this gene [C31, H30, H46] (Figure IV). Characteristic *p53* mutations are most evident for hepatocellular carcinoma associated with environmental exposure to aflatoxin B1 [B23, M34, O4] and skin tumours associated with sunlight exposure [B36], but within this rapidly developing field of molecular epidemiology (see also [M34]), parallel advances in relation to other chemical carcinogens and other target genes should be anticipated.

224. Ionizing radiation does not, however, show the same degree of mutagenic specificity as chemical agents and, on current evidence, it may tend to act principally through DNA deletion/ rearrangement rather than base pair change. Nevertheless, in a recent study [V10] rare *p53* gene deletions and base pair changes were shown to characterize radon-associated lung cancer in uranium miners; it may be that this unusual mutational spectrum is associated with alpha-particle-induced damage to the *p53* gene of target respiratory cells. Mutations of the *p53* gene have also been characterized in radiation-associated human sarcomas [B38], and *K-ras* mutation has been shown to be more frequent in radiation-associated follicular carcinomas of the thyroid than in spontaneously arising neoplasms [W22]. In neither case, however, is it possible to be certain that these mutations were specifically induced by the radiation. Even greater uncertainty surrounds the interpretation of the *MOS* gene polymorphisms in normal tissue of radium exposed individuals [H47].

225. The molecular characterization of DNA base pair changes in tumour-associated genes using polymerase chain reaction (PCR) as employed in many of the above studies is a flexible, rapid and reasonably straightforward procedure [E8]. In contrast, the molecular characterization of DNA deletions, particularly those that extend outside the gene of interest, is more difficult, because it demands a detailed knowledge of gene and gene-flanking sequences. While small intragenic DNA deletions will tend to encompass or disturb the reading frame of those sequences encoding functional protein sites, for deletions resulting in loss of the whole gene there is no *a priori* reason why the deletion breakpoints should be characteristic of that gene or of the mutagenic agent in question.

226. There is, however, limited evidence that radiation-induced DNA deletions in mammalian cells may involve specific breakpoints. Whether such deletion breakpoints might be characteristic of radiation-induced damage remains an open question, but the presence of DNA repeat sequence motifs at some DNA sequence breakpoints in somatic cell mutants [M33] and, albeit less certainly, in some neoplasia-associated chromosomal changes [B16, B32] does allow for this possibility. However, on current knowledge, it seems highly unlikely that DNA events of this or other types will be unique to radiation-induced damage (see, e.g. [A14, M33]); if so, this will tend to limit the general utility of molecular analyses for the purposes of discriminating between radiation-induced, chemically induced and spontaneously arising neoplasms in human populations. Nevertheless, the rate of progress in this whole area is such that at present it is prudent to reserve judgement on this crucial issue. Indeed, the unusual *p53* mutation spectrum observed in the lung tumours of uranium miners [V10] hints at the utility of this approach in respect to the *p53* gene.

227. From a predictive viewpoint, the identification of initiating events for radiation oncogenesis is not limited to its potential to discriminate between tumours of inductive and spontaneous origins. Even if it only becomes possible to identify in a more general

fashion the principal categories of induced DNA damage and target genes associated with radiation oncogenesis, there still remain important implications for future research.

228. First, the provision of such data may allow the design of quantitatively reliable cellular systems that mimic or reflect the relevant molecular events. Secondly, it would become possible to specifically explore the post-irradiation repair of the relevant initial DNA lesions (see [W10]), particularly if these were to involve some form of gene or DNA sequence specificity. Thirdly, using Monte Carlo simulations (see, e.g. [N22]) of radiation track structure, it might become possible to link the induction of the initial, potentially oncogenic damage with specific energy loss events in DNA, thus allowing a biologically more realistic microdosimetric extrapolation of radiation effects.

229. However, as noted in paragraph 5, a resolution of the mechanisms of radiation oncogenesis would also provide an essential input into the whole field of cancer research. It is only through such integration that the whole of the complex multi-stage oncogenic process will be better understood, allowing the formulation of realistic cellular and molecular models to replace, or at least complement, the existing empirical approaches to cancer risk projection.

CONCLUSIONS

230. Ionizing radiation induces a broad spectrum of neoplasms in both man and experimental animals. The basic mechanisms of the induction, promotion and progression processes are not yet well understood; however, some points from considerations in this Annex can be summarized.

231. Point mutation, chromosomal translocations and deletions may all play roles in the initiation and progression of neoplasia. Some of these changes are shared by different neoplasms. Others appear to be restricted to certain tumour types.

232. Studies on human susceptibility to neoplasia associated with inherited defects in DNA metabolism or the loss of tumour suppressor genes are making important contributions to the understanding of oncogenic mechanisms and the different modes of inheritance of cancer-proneness in the human population.

233. Neoplastic initiation as a consequence of specific somatic mutation is thought to provide target cells with some degree of proliferative dysregulation. These events may not be phenotypically expressed as preneoplastic conditions until a promotional proliferative signal is received.

234. Point mutations or chromosomal translocations that activate proto-oncogenes or mutations that lead to loss of function of tumour suppressor genes may be considered as potential initiating events for oncogenesis. Relative target sizes for the induction of these events by radiation would tend to favour tumour suppressor genes as the most radiosensitive targets.

235. Strong evidence for tumour suppressor genes as targets for oncogenic initiation has been obtained in studies of germ-line mutations that predispose to cancer. Some of these genes appear to play a central role in the control of the cell cycle.

236. Neoplastic promotion arises mainly as a consequence of induced changes in gene expression in initiated cells. It may occur through the action of specific chemicals, hormones and growth factors on cell surface receptors, and the ensuing proliferative responses may favour the establishment of pre-neoplastic clones in tissues. In some cases the enzyme protein kinase C is thought to mediate promotional processes; changes in intercellular communication may be an important aspect of promotion, but the induction of endogenous DNA damage is also a feature of some strong promoting agents.

237. Neoplastic progression is a complex, multifaceted process that appears to involve a series of subsequent genetic changes within the evolving pre-neoplastic clone of cells; these changes may include changes in growth rate, growth factor response, invasiveness and metastatic potential. The development of intrinsic genomic instability in neoplastic cells may provide the cellular heterogeneity in tumours that drives the progressional process.

238. Both physical and biological factors influence radiation oncogenesis, as shown in experimental animal systems, but few specific details of cellular mechanisms have emerged from quantitative studies. *In vitro* cell transformation studies have highlighted some aspects of cellular oncogenic mechanisms (frequency of potentially initiating events; effects of LET, dose rate and repair; and neoplastic promotional mechanisms). While *in vitro* studies on specific gene involvement in radiation-induced cell transformation

have yet to yield detailed information on the molecular mechanisms of oncogenic initiation by radiation, novel transformation systems, already making an impact in chemical carcinogenesis, show considerable potential.

239. Cell mutagenesis and DNA repair data may be used to argue that oncogenic initiation following ionizing radiation may occur more frequently through DNA rearrangement/deletion than through point mutation, but this may well depend on the gene in question. Chromosomes or cellular oncogenes have been shown to be changed in a number of radiation-induced experimental neoplasms, but the temporal position and role of most of these changes are uncertain. In the case of murine acute myelogenous leukaemia, the induced initiating event is thought to be a specific chromosomal rearrangement/deletion leading to the loss of critical genes. In contrast, other studies suggest that point mutations in *ras* proto-oncogenes may be initiating events for radiation-induced murine thymic lymphomas. Some progress is also being made in the molecular characterization of radiation-induced osteosarcomas and tumours of the skin, breast and lung.

240. There are a number of mechanistic differences between chemical and radiation oncogenesis, including differences in DNA damage induction/repair and the activational/degradative processes that influence the carcinogenicity of many chemicals. An important difference in oncogenic mechanisms may derive from the relative efficiency with which chemical carcinogens and radiation induce point mutations. It is suggested that radiation and chemical oncogenesis are subject to differing degrees of human genetic variation.

241. Molecular studies with certain human tumours have drawn attention to the possibility that specific point mutation in tumour genes may serve as a signature of prior exposure to chemical carcinogens. On current knowledge, the same approach may not be equally informative for ionizing radiation exposures, but the possible preferential involvement of DNA repeat sequences in radiation-induced DNA deletion and of certain DNA bases in point mutations may provide a focus for further study.

242. The development of new methods of investigation promises further advances in understanding. Novel *in vitro* cell transformation systems and cellular/molecular studies with these and with neoplasms induced in outbred animals may be a productive area for the study of oncogenic mechanisms. Recent advances in the construction of transgenic and chimaeric mice, new cellular cytogenic and molecular approaches to the assay of *in vivo* somatic cell changes, and studies on radiation-associated human tumour cells appear to have great potential.

243. In order to take advantage of modern methods of cell and molecular biology and to anticipate further technical advances, tumour material obtained from radiation-exposed human populations should be systematically stored. This material may prove to be a very important resource for future molecular studies of oncogenic mechanisms.

Table 1
The function and chromosomal location of some human oncogenes
[A13, B1, C7, M36, S63]

Classification	*Oncogene*	*Chromosomal location*	*Product/function* [a]
Growth factor	*SIS*	22q 12-13	PDGF β chain
	HST-1	11q 13	FGF family
	INT-2	11q 13	FGF family
Tyrosine kinase	*ERB B1*	7q 12-13	EGF receptor
	ERB B2/NEU	17q 21	EGF receptor-like
	FMS	5q 34	CSF-1 receptor
	KIT	4q 11-12	SCF receptor
	SRC	20q 12-13	Expressed in nerve cells
	YES	18q 21	Expressed in spleen and brain
	FPS/FES	15q 25-26	Expressed in granulocytes/monocytes
	FYN	6q 21	Bound to T-cell receptor
	LCK	1q 32-35	Bound to CD4/CD8 complex
	BCR/ABL	22q 11/9q 34	Chaemeric protein (CML)
Serine/threonine kinase	*MOS*	8q 11	Oocyte maturation
	RAF/MIL	3p 25	Function downstream of *RAS*
GTP binding protein [a]	*H-RAS*	11p 15]	Message transduction, mutated in many tumour types
	K-RAS	12p 12]	
	N-RAS	1p 13-22	Amplified in neuroblastoma
Regulatory factors	*JUN*	1p 31-32	Binds Fos (transcription factor)
	FOS	14q 21-31	Binds Jun (transcription factor)
	MYB	6q 22-24	Expressed in erythroblasts
	MYC	8q 24	Transcription/replication factor
	N-MYC	2p 23-24	Amplified in neuroblastoma
	ERBA	17q 11-21	Thyroid hormone receptor
	PML/RArα	15q 21/17q 11	Chaemeric protein (transcription factor)
	HFL/E2A	17q 22/19p 13	Chaemeric protein (transcription factor)
	PBX/E2A	1q 23/19p 13	Chaemeric protein (transcription factor)
	HOX11	10q 24	Transcription factor
Others	*BCL-2*	18 q 21	Control of apoptosis

[a] GTP: guanosine triphosphate; PDGF: platelet-derived growth factor; FGF: fibroblast growth factor; EGF: epidermal growth factor; CSF: colony stimulating factor; SCF: stem cell factor; CML: chronic myelogenous leukaemia.

Table 2
Suppressor genes in human tumours
[W14]

Chromosomal location	Tumour type
Detected by cell hybridization or chromosome transfer	
1p	Neuroblastoma
3p	Renal carcinoma
6	Endometrial carcinoma
9	Endometrial carcinoma
11	Neuroblastoma; cervical carcinoma; Wilms' tumour

Chromosomal location	Tumour type
Detected through loss of heterozygosity or direct molecular probing	
1p	Melanoma; multiple endocrine neoplasia type 2; neuroblastoma; medullary thyroid carcinoma; pheochromocytoma; ductal cell carcinoma
1q	Breast carcinoma
3p	Small cell lung carcinoma; adeno carcinoma of lung; cervical carcinoma; von Hippel-Lindau disease, renal cell carcinoma
5q	Familial adenomatous polyposis; colorectal carcinoma
9q	Bladder carcinoma
10q	Astrocytoma; multiple endocrine neoplasia type 2
11p	Wilms' tumour; rhabdomyosarcoma; breast carcinoma; hepatoblastoma; transitional cell bladder carcinoma, lung carcinoma
11q	Multiple endocrine neoplasia type 1
13q	Retinoblastoma; osteosarcoma; small cell lung carcinoma; ductal breast carcinoma; stomach carcinoma; bladder carcinoma; colon carcinoma
17p	Small cell lung carcinoma; colorectal carcinoma; breast carcinoma, osteosarcoma; astrocytoma squamous cell lung carcinoma
17q	Neurofibromatosis type 1
18q	Colorectal carcinoma
22q	Neurofibromatosis type 2; meningioma; acoustic neuroma; pheochromocytoma

Table 3
Consistent chromosomal changes in leukaemias and lymphomas
[S45]

Neoplasm	*Chromosome aberration*
Leukaemias	
Chronic myeloid leukaemia	t(9;22)(q34;q11)
Acute myeloid leukaemia	
M1	t(9;22)(q34:q11)
M2	t(8;21)(q22;q22)
M3	t(15;17)(q22;q12)
M4 with abnormal eosinophils	inv(16)(p13q22)
M5a	t(9;11)(p22;q23)
M1, M2, M4 with increased basophils	t(6;9)(p23;q34)
M1, M2, M4, M5, M6	Monosomy 5/del(5q) Monosomy 7/del(7q) Trisomy 8
Chronic lymphocytic leukaemia	t(11;14)(q13;q32) Trisomy 12
Acute lymphocytic leukaemia	t(9;22)(q34;q11) t(4;11)(q21;q23)
Acute B-cell leukaemia	t(8;14)(q24;q32) t(2;8)(p12;q24) t(8;22)(q24;q11)
Acute T-cell leukaemia	inv(14)(q11q32) t(14;14)(q11;q32) t(8;14)(q24;q11) t(10;14)(q24;q11) t(11;14)(p13;q11)
Lymphomas	
Burkitt's lymphoma	t(8;14)(q24;q32) t(2;8)(p12;q24) t(8;22)(q24;q11)
Small non-cleaved cell lymphoma, large cell immunoblastic lymphoma	t(8;14)(q24;q32)
Follicular small cleaved cell lymphoma	t(14;18)(q32;q21)
Small cell lymphocytic lymphoma	Trisomy 12
Small cell lymphocytic transformed to diffuse large cell lymphoma	t(11;14)(q13;q32)
Polycythaemia vera	
Polycythaemia vera	del(20q)

Table 4
Consistent chromosomal changes in solid tumours
[S45]

Neoplasm	*Chromosome aberration*
Alveolar rhabdomyosarcoma	t(2;13)(q37;q14)
Bladder carcinoma	Structural changes of 1 i(5p) Structural changes of 11
Breast carcinoma	Structural changes of 1 t/del(16q)
Ewing's sarcoma, Askin's tumour/neuroepithelioma	t(11;22)(q24:q12)
Kidney carcinoma	t/del(3)(p11-21) t(5;14)(q13;q22)
Large bowel cancer	Structural changes of 1 Trisomy 7 Structural changes of 17
Lipoma	t(12)(q13-14)
Malignant melanoma	t/del(1)(p12-22) t(1;19)(q12;p13) t/del(6q)/i(6p) Trisomy 7
Meningioma	Monosomy 22
Mixed salivary gland adenoma	t(3)(p21) t/del(8)(q12) t/del(12)(q13-15)
Myxoid liposarcoma	t(12;16)(q13-14;p11)
Neuroblastoma	del(1)(p31-32)
Ovarian carcinoma	t(6;14)(q21;q24) Structural changes of 1
Prostatic carcinoma	del(7)(q22) del(10)(q24)
Retinoblastoma	Structural changes of 1 i(6p) del(13)(q14)/-13
Small cell lung carcinoma	del(3)(p14p23)
Synovia sarcoma	t(X;18)(p11;q11)
Testicular teratoma/seminoma	i(12p)
Uterine carcinoma	Structural and numerical changes of 1
Wilms' tumour	Structural changes of 1 t/del(11)(p13)

Table 5
Viral associations in human oncogenesis
[W16]

Virus (type)	*Associated tumours*	*Other risk factors*
T-cell viruses (RNA)	T-cell leukaemia/lymphoma	[a]
Lentiviruses (RNA)	Kaposi's sarcoma, lymphoma	Concurrent viral infections Immune deficiency
Herpes virus (DNA) Epstein-Barr virus	 Burkitt's lymphoma Immunoblastic lymphoma Nasopharyngeal carcinoma	 Malaria Immune deficiency Dietary components HLA genotype
Herpes simplex	Cervical neoplasia (?)	Papilloma viruses, tobacco
Cytomegalovirus	Kaposi's sarcoma (?) Cervical neoplasia (?)	Immune deficiency HLA genotype
Hepatitis B viruses (DNA)	Liver cancer	Aflatoxin, alcohol, tobacco
Papilloma viruses (DNA)	Cervical and anal neoplasia Laryngeal carcinoma Skin carcinoma	Tobacco, herpes virus and immune deficiency X rays, tobacco Sunlight, genetic factors influencing skin pigmentation

[a] Considerable uncertainty.

Table 6
Estimates of the frequency of some cancer-prone human mutations

Mutation	*Principal neoplasms*	*Phenotypic manifestation*	*Chromosomal location*	*Frequency per live births*
Ataxia-telangiectasia (homozygotes)	Leukaemias, lymphomas	Autosomal recessive	11/a/	~ 1 per 100,000
Ataxia-telangiectasia (heterozygotes)	Mammary carcinomas	Autosomal recessive	11/a/	1 per 100 [a]
Retinoblastoma	Retinoblastoma, osteosarcoma	Autosomal dominant	13q	~ 1 per 20,000
Wilms-aniridia	Nephroblastoma	Autosomal dominant	11p	~ 1 per 30,000
Basal cell nevus syndrome	Skin carcinoma, medulloblastoma	Autosomal dominant	9q	< 1 per 50,000
Neurofibromatosis	Neurofibromas, CNS tumours	Autosomal dominant	17q	~ 1 per 5,000
Familial adenomatous polyposis	Colorectal carcinomas	Autosomal dominant	5q	~ 1 per 10,000
Non polyposis colorectal cancer	Colorectal carcinomas	Autosomal dominant	2p	[b]
Familial breast cancer	Mammary and ovarian carcinomas	Autosomal dominant	17q	[c]
Li-Fraumeni syndrome	Wide range of malignancies	Autosomal dominant	17p	< 1 per 50,000

[a] The number and location of ataxia-telangiectasia genes has yet to be conclusively determined; the number of genetic complementaion groups in ataxia-telangiectasia is the major determinant of heterozygote frequency.
[b] Accounts for around 14% of colorectal cancers in the population.
[c] It has been estimated that as many as 1 in 200 women carry one of a number of genes that predispose breast cancer (paragraph 127).

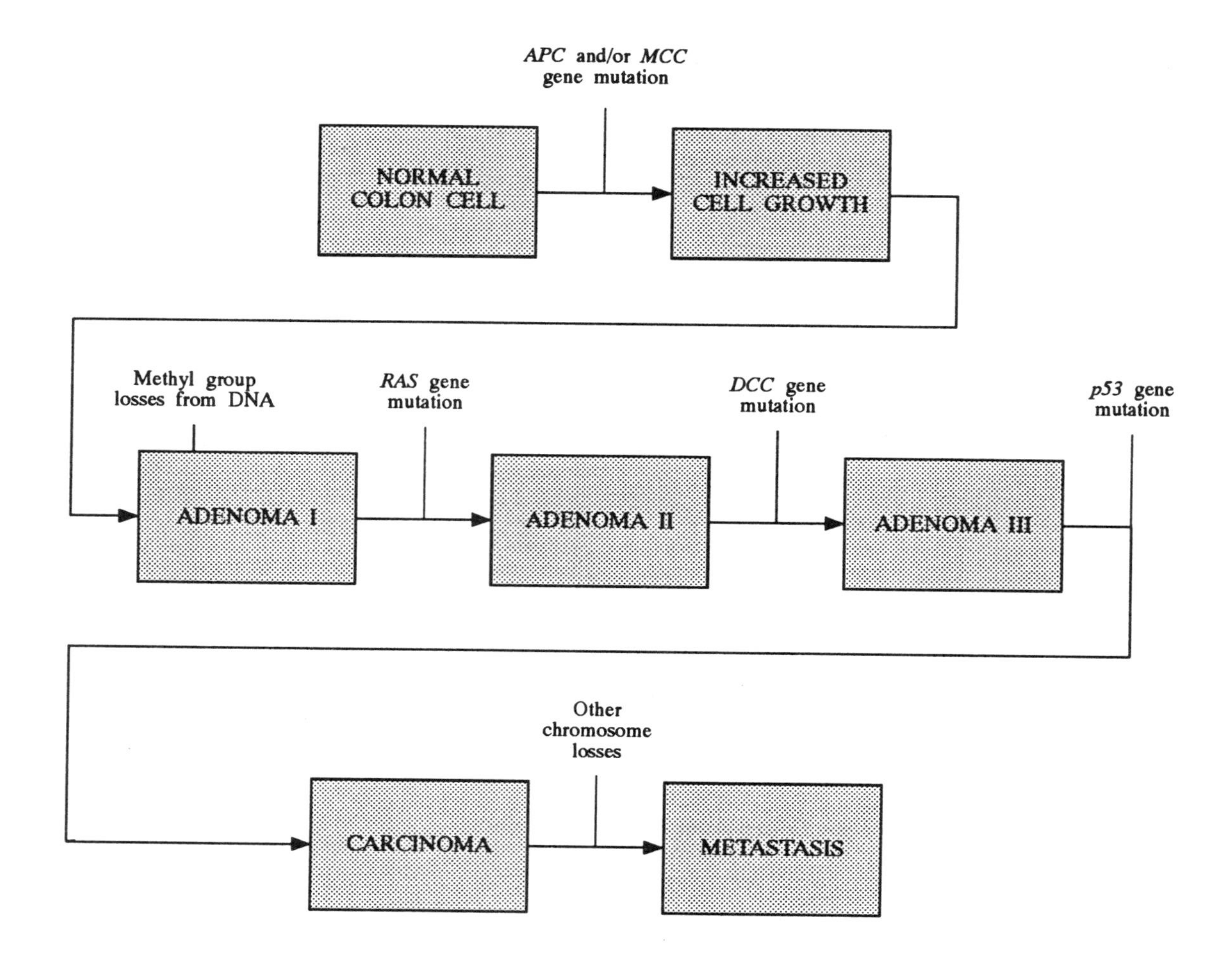

Figure I.
Multi-step colorectal carcinogenesis.
[F8]

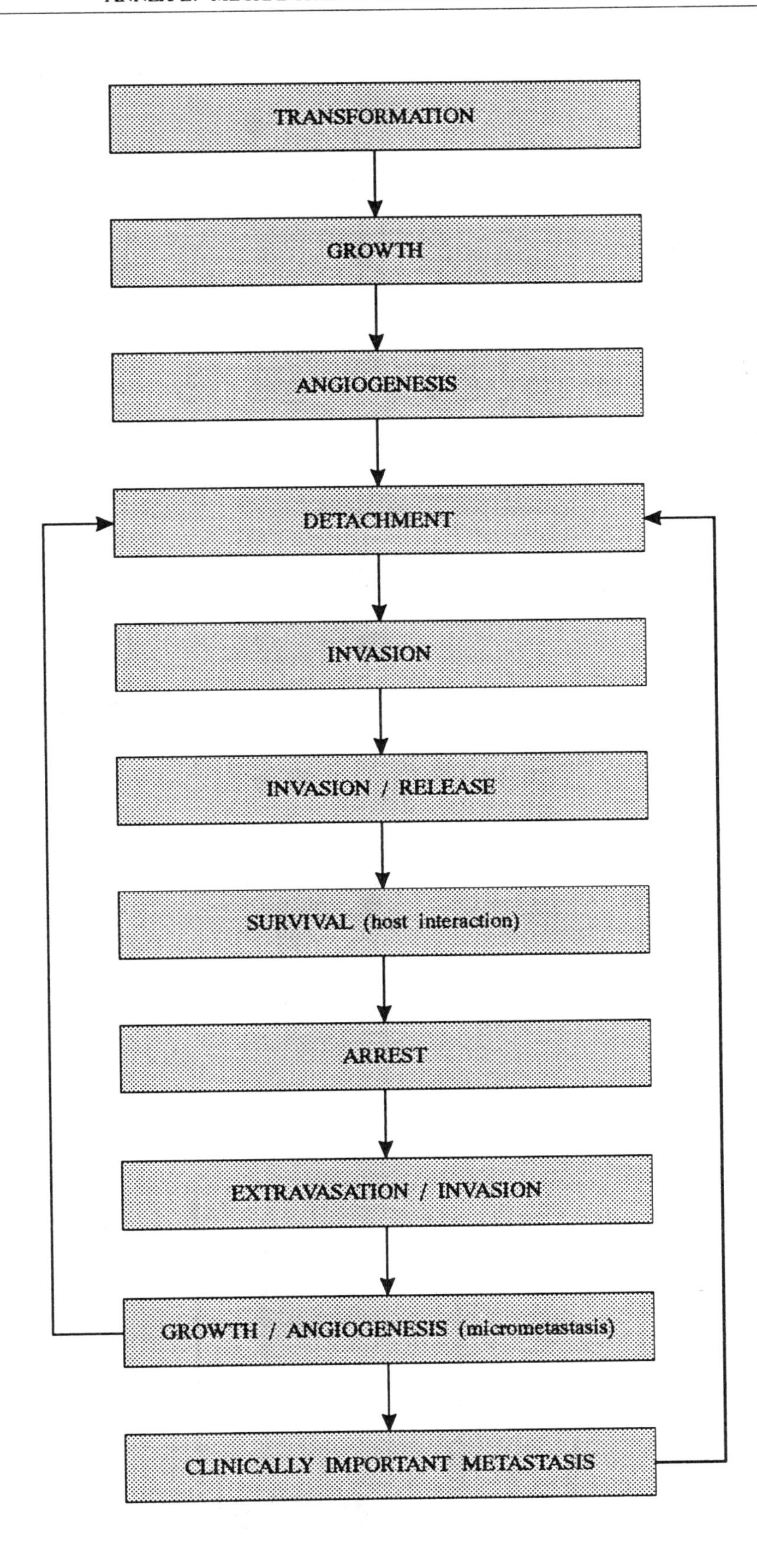

Figure II.
Possible steps involved in the metastatic spread of solid tumours.
[H42]

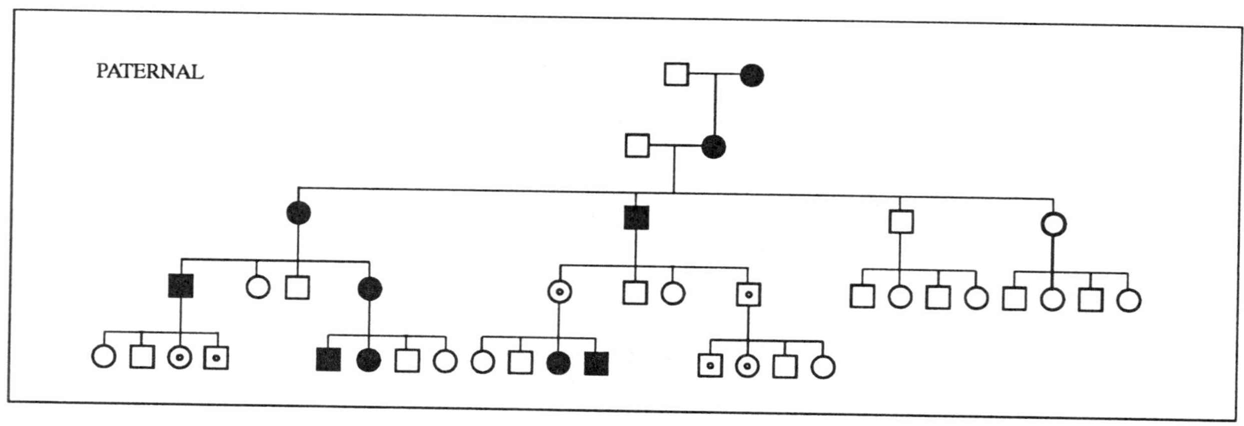

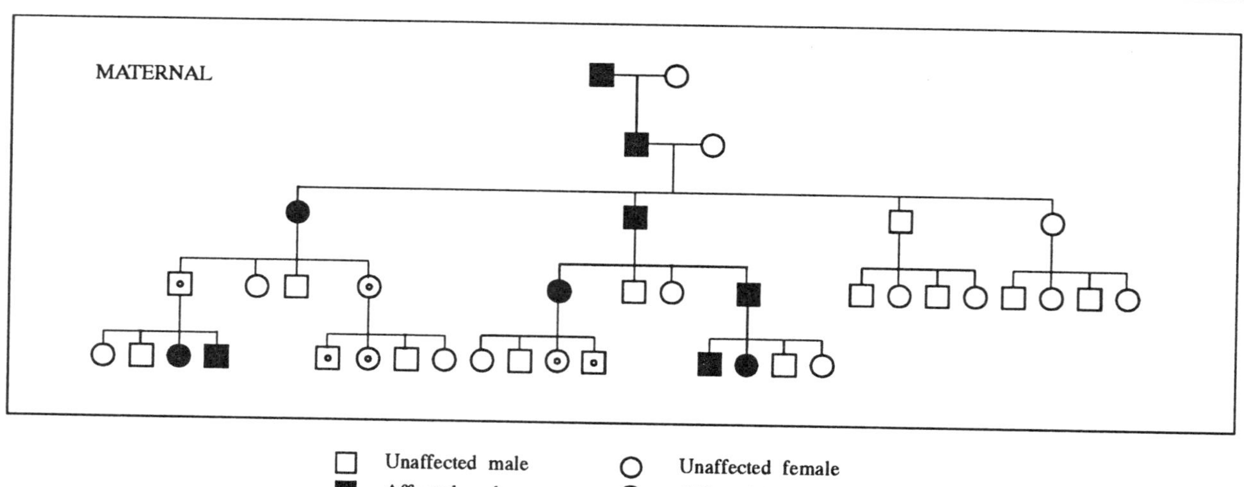

Figure III.
Idealized pedigrees for maternal and paternal genomic imprinting.
[H19]

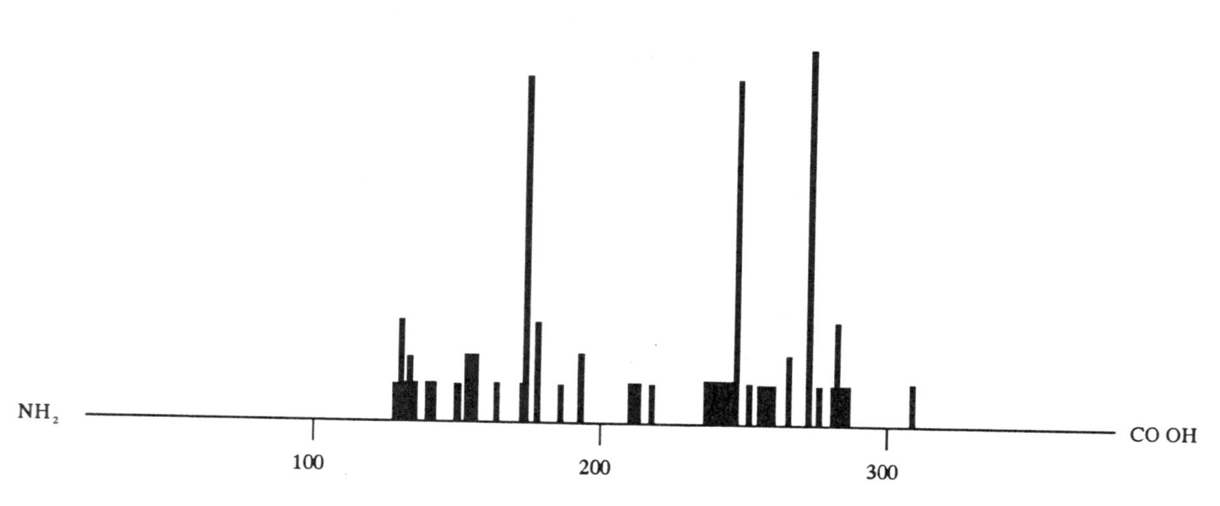

Figure IV.
The distribution of *p53* tumour cell gene mutations in man observed in a wide range of human neoplasms. The horizontal axis represents the 393 condons of the *p53* gene from the NH_2 to the CO OH terminals.
[L13]

References

A1 Alberts, B. (ed.). Molecular Biology of the Cell. Garland, New York, 1988.

A2 Ames, B.N. and J. McCann. Validation of the salmonella test. Cancer Res. 41: 4192-4195 (1981).

A3 Arlett, C.F. The radiosensitivity of cultured human cells. p. 424-430 in: Radiation Research. Volume 2. (E.M. Fielden et al., eds.) Taylor and Francis, London, 1987.

A4 Anisimov, V.N. Carcinogenesis and aging. Adv. Cancer Res. 40: 365-415 (1983).

A5 Awa, A.A. Chromosome aberrations in A-bomb survivors in Hiroshima and Nagasaki. p. 180-190 in: Chromosome Aberrations: Basic and Applied Aspects. (G. Obe and A.T. Natarajan, eds.) Springer Verlag, Berlin, 1990.

A6 Anathaswamy, H.N. and W.E. Pierceall. Molecular mechanisms of ultraviolet radiation carcinogenesis. Photochem. Photobiol. 52: 1119-1136 (1990).

A7 Ayesh, R., J.R. Idle, J.C. Richie et al. Metabolic oxidation phenotypes as markers for susceptibility to lung cancer. Nature 312: 169-170 (1984).

A8 Arch, R., K. Wirth, M. Hofman et al. Participation in normal immune responses of a metastasis-inducing splice variant of CD44. Science 257: 682-685 (1992).

A9 Askew, D.S., C. Bartholomew, A.M. Buchberg et al. His-1 and His-2: Identification and chromosomal mapping of two common sites of integration in a myeloid leukaemia. Oncogene 6: 2041-2047 (1991).

A10 Ames, B.N. Endogenous DNA damage as related to cancer and ageing. Mutat. Res. 214: 41-46 (1989).

A11 Ames, B.N. and L.S. Gold. Too many rodent carcinogens: mitogenesis increases mutagenesis. Science 249: 970-971 (1990).

A12 Arlett, C.F. Human cellular radiosensitivity - the search for the diagnostic holy grail or a poisoned chalice. Adv. Radiat. Biol. 16: 273-292 (1992).

A13 Aaronson, S.A. Growth factors and cancer. Science 254: 1146-1153 (1991).

A14 Akagi, T., K. Morota, H. Iyehara-Ogawa et al. Mutational specificity of the carcinogen 3-amino-1-methyl-5H-pyrido[4,3-b]-indole in mammalian cells. Carcinogenesis 11: 841-846 (1990).

A15 Akiyama, M., K. Nakamura, M. Hakoda et al. Somatic cell mutation in atomic bomb survivors. J. Radiat. Res. (Suppl): 278-282 (1991).

A16 Aaltonen, L.A., P. Peltomaki, F.S. Leach et al. Clues to the pathogenesis of familial colorectal cancer. Science 260: 812-815 (1993).

B1 Bishop, J.M. The molecular genetics of cancer. Science 235: 305-311 (1987).

B2 Bonavida, B. and S.C. Wright. Multistage model of natural killer cell mediated cytotoxicity involving NKCF as a soluble cytotoxic mediators. Adv. Cancer Res. 49: 169-187 (1987).

B3 Borek, C., A. Ong and H. Mason. Distinctive transforming genes in x-ray transformed mammalian cells. Proc. Natl. Acad. Sci. (USA) 84: 794-798 (1987).

B4 Breckon, G., A. Silver and R. Cox. Consistent chromosome changes in radiation-induced murine leukaemias. p. 179-184 in: Kew Chromosome Conference III. (P.E. Brandham and M.D. Bennett, eds.) HMSO, London, 1988.

B5 Blatt, C. and L. Sachs. Deletion of a homeobox gene in myeloid leukaemias with a deletion of chromosome 2. Biochem. Biophys. Res. Commun. 156: 1265-1270 (1988).

B6 Barbacid, M. Ras genes. Annu. Rev. Biochem. 56: 779-878 (1987).

B7 Borek, C. Oncogenes in human cell transformation in vitro. p. 223-230 in: Cell Transformation Systems and Radiation Induced Cancer in Man. (K. Chadwick, B. Barnhart and C. Seymour, eds.) Adam Hilger, Bristol, 1989.

B8 Bartsch, H. and R. Montesano. Mutagenic and carcinogenic effects of vinyl chloride. Mutat. Res. 32: 93-114 (1975).

B9 Bryant, P.E. and A.C. Riches. Chromosome damage and oncogenic transformation in mouse 10T1/2 cells following restriction endonuclease treatment. p. 309-314 in: Cell Transformation Systems and Radiation Induced Cancer in Man. (K. Chadwick, B. Barnhart and C. Seymour, eds.) Adam Hilger, Bristol, 1989.

B10 Boehm, T., L. Mengel-Gaw, U.R. Kees et al. Alternating purine-pyrimidine tracts may promote chromosomal translocations seen in a variety of human lymphoid tumours. EMBO J. 8: 2621-2631 (1989).

B11 Bowden, G.T., D. Jaffe and K. Andrews. Biological and molecular aspects of radiation carcinogenesis in mouse skin. Radiat. Res. 121: 235-241 (1990).

B12 Bremner, R. and A. Balmain. Genetic changes in skin tumour progression: correlation between presence of a mutant ras gene and loss of heterozygosity on mouse chromosome 7. Cell 61: 407-417 (1990).

B13 Boldogh, I., S. AbuBakar and T. Albrecht. Activation of proto-oncogenes: An immediate early event in human cytomegalovirus infection. Science 247: 561-563 (1990).

B14 Bridges, B.A. Some DNA repair-deficient syndromes and their implications for human health. p. 47-57 in: Environmental Mutagens and Carcinogens. (T. Sugimura et al., eds.) A.R. Liss, New York, 1982.

B15 Boettiger, D., S. Anderson and T.M. Dexter. Effect of src infection on long term marrow cultures: increased self-renewal of haemopoietic progenitor cells without leukaemia. Cell 36 (3): 763-773 (1984).

B16 Breckon, G., D. Papworth and R. Cox. Murine radiation myeloid leukaemogenesis: a possible role for radiation sensitive sites on chromosome 2. Genes, Chrom. Cancer 3: 367-375 (1991).

B17 Bender, M.A., A.A. Awa, A.L. Brooks et al. Current status of cytogenetic procedures to detect and quantify previous exposures to radiation. Mutat. Res. 196: 103-159 (1988).

B18 Bos, J.L. The ras gene family and human carcinogenesis. Mutat. Res. 195: 225-271 (1988).

B19 Baker, S.J., S. Mankowitz, E.R. Fearon et al. Suppression of human colorectal carcinoma cell growth by wild type p53. Science 250: 912-915 (1990).
B20 Blackburn, E.H. Structure and function of telomeres. Nature 350: 569-572 (1991).
B21 Basset, P., J.P. Bellocq, C. Wolf et al. A novel metalloproteinase gene specifically expressed in stromal cells of breast carcinomas. Nature 348: 699-704 (1990).
B22 Bannasch, P., D. Keppler and G. Weber (eds.). Liver Cell Carcinoma. Kluwer Academic, Dordrecht, 1989.
B23 Bressac, B., M. Kew, J. Wands et al. Selective G to T mutations of p53 gene in hepatocellular carcinoma in southern Africa. Nature 350: 429-431 (1991).
B24 Bodmer, W.F. Inherited susceptibility to cancer. p. 98-124 in: Introduction to the Cellular and Molecular Biology of Cancer. (L.M. Franks and N.M. Teich, eds.) Oxford University Press, Oxford, 1991.
B25 Beverley, P. Immunology of cancer. p. 406-433 in: Introduction to the Cellular and Molecular Biology of Cancer. (L.M. Franks and N.M. Teich, eds.) Oxford University Press, Oxford, 1991.
B26 Breckon, G. and R. Cox. Alpha particle leukaemogenesis. Lancet 335: 656-657 (1990).
B27 Biedermann, K.A., J.R. Sun, A.J. Giaccia et al. Scid mutation in mice confers hypersensitivity to ionizing radiation and a deficiency in DNA double-strand break repair. Proc. Natl. Acad. Sci. (USA) 88: 1394-1397 (1991).
B28 Broerse, J.J. and D.W. van Bekkum (eds.). The relevance of animal models of radiation carcinogenesis in the light of development in molecular biology. Radiat. Environ. Biophys. 30: 161-257 (1991).
B29 Bianchi, A.B., N.M. Navone, C.M. Aldaz et al. Overlapping loss of heterozygosity by mitotic recombination on mouse chromosome 7F1-ter in skin carcinogenesis. Proc. Natl. Acad. Sci. (USA) 88: 7590-7594 (1991).
B30 Barnes, D.M., A.M. Hanby, C.E. Gillett et al. Abnormal expression of wild type p53 protein in normal cells of a cancer family patient. Lancet 340: 259-263 (1992).
B31 Benjamin, M.B. and J.B. Little. X rays induce inter-allelic homologous recombination at the human thymidine kinase gene. Mol. Cell. Biol. 12: 2730-2738 (1992).
B32 Bouffler, S.B., A. Silver, D. Papworth et al. Murine radiation myeloid leukaemogenesis: the relationship between interstitial telomere-like sequences and chromosome 2 fragile sites. Genes, Chrom. Cancer 6: 98-106 (1993).
B33 Braithwaite, O., W. Bayona and E.W. Newcomb. p53 mutations in C57BL/6J murine thymic lymphomas induced by gamma-irradiation and N-methylnitrosourea. Cancer Res. 52: 3791-3795 (1992).
B34 Bratthauer, G.L. and T.G. Fanning. Active LINE-1 retrotransposons in human testicular cancer. Oncogene 7: 507-510 (1992).
B35 Blattner, W.A. (ed.). Epidemiology of HTLV-I and associated diseases. p. 251-265 in: Human Retrovirology: HTLV. Raven Press, New York, 1990.
B36 Brash, D.E., J.A. Rudolph, J.A. Simon et al. A role for sunlight in skin cancer: UV-induced p53 squamous cell carcinoma. Proc. Natl. Acad. Sci. (USA) 88: 10124-10128 (1991).
B37 Beer, D.G. and H.C. Pitot. Proto-oncogene activation during chemically induced hepatocarcinogenesis in rodents. Mutat. Res. 220: 1-10 (1989).
B38 Brachman, D.G., D.E. Hallahan, M.A. Beckett et al. p53 gene mutations and abnormal retinoblastoma protein in radiation-induced human sarcomas. Cancer Res. 51: 6393-6396 (1991).
B39 Buchman, A., R. Bauer-Hofmann, J. Mahr et al. Mutational activation of the c-Ha-ras gene in liver tumours of different rodent strains: correlation with susceptibility to hepatocarcinogenesis. Proc. Natl. Acad. Sci. (USA) 88: 911-915 (1991).
B40 Bourne, H.R. and H.E. Varmus. Oncogenes and cell proliferation. Curr. Opin. Genet. Dev. 2: 1-3 (1992).
B41 Barlow D.P. Methylation and imprinting: From host defense to gene regulation. Science 260: 309-310 (1993).
B42 Bouffler, S., A. Silver and R. Cox. The role of DNA repeats and associated secondary structures in genomic instability and neoplasia. BioEssays 15: 409-412 (1993).
B43 Billen, D. Response to comments of K.F. Baverstock and J.F. Ward. Radiat. Res. 126: 388-389 (1991).
B44 Billen, D. Spontaneous DNA damage and its significance for the "negligible" dose controversy in radiation protection. Radiat. Res. 124: 242-245 (1990).
B45 Baverstock, K.F. Comments on commentary by D. Billen. Radiat. Res. 126: 383-384 (1991).
C1 Curtis, S.B. The cellular consequences of binary misrepair and linear fixation of initial biophysical damage. p. 312-317 in: Radiation Research. Volume 2. (E.M. Fielden et al., eds.) Taylor and Francis, London, 1987.
C2 Curtis, S.B. Lethal and potentially lethal lesions induced by radiation - a unified repair model. Radiat. Res. 106: 252-270 (1985).
C3 Cox, R. Comparative mutagenesis in cultured mammalian cells. p. 33-46 in: Progress in Environmental Mutagenesis. (M. Alacevic, ed.) Elsevier, Amsterdam, 1980.
C4 Cooper, G.M. Cellular transforming genes. Science 218: 801-806 (1982).
C5 Clifton, K.H., K. Kamiya, K.M. Groch et al. Quantitative studies of rat mammary and thyroid clonogens, the presumptive cancer progenitor cells. p. 135-146 in: Cell Transformation Systems and Radiation Induced Cancer in Man. (K. Chadwick, B. Barnhart and C. Seymour, eds.) Adam Hilger, Bristol, 1989.
C6 Cox, R., P.G. Debenham, W.K. Masson et al. Ataxia-telangiectasia: a human mutation giving high frequency misrepair of DNA double strand scissions. Mol. Biol. Med. 3: 229-244 (1986).
C7 Cooper, G.M. Oncogenes. Jones and Bartlett, 1990.
C8 Cox, R. A cellular description of the repair defect ataxia-telangiectasia. p. 141-153 in: Ataxia-telangiectasia. (B.A. Bridges and D.G. Harnden, eds.) John Wiley & Sons, Chichester, 1982.
C9 Cox, R. and J.B. Little. Oncogenic cell transformation in vitro. Adv. Radiat. Biol. 16: 137-155 (1992).

C10 Cooper, J.A. and P. Whyte. RB and the cell cycle: entrance or exit. Cell 58: 1009-1011 (1989).

C11 Colburn, N.H., E. Farber, B. Weinstein et al. American cancer society workshop conference on tumour promotion and anti-promotion. Cancer Res. 47: 5509-5513 (1987).

C12 Cleaver, J.E. DNA repair in man. p. 61-85 in: Genetic Susceptibility to Environmental Mutagens and Carcinogens. (A.D. Bloom and L. Spatz, eds.) March of Dimes, New York, 1989.

C13 Cox, R. and W.K. Masson. Radiosensitivity in cultured human fibroblasts. Int. J. Radiat. Biol. 38: 575-576 (1980).

C14 Charles, M., R. Cox, D. Goodhead et al. CEIR forum on the effects of high-LET radiation at low doses/dose rates. Int. J. Radiat. Biol. 58: 859-885 (1990).

C15 Cohen, L.A. Diet and cancer. Sci. Am. 257: 42-50 (1987).

C16 Cohen, S.M. and L.B. Ellwein. Cell proliferation in carcinogenesis. Science 249: 1007-1011 (1990).

C17 Christian, B.J., L.J. Loretz, T.D. Oberly et al. Characterization of human uroepithelial cell immortalized in vitro by simian virus 40. Cancer Res. 47: 6066-6073 (1987).

C18 Chen, P.-L., Y. Chen, R. Bookstein et al. Genetic mechanisms of tumour suppression by the human p53 gene. Science 250: 1576-1578 (1991).

C19 Cattanach, B.M. and C.V. Beechey. Chromosome imprinting phenomena in mice and indications in man. Chromosomes Today 10: 135-148 (1990).

C20 Collins, M. Death by a thousand cuts. Curr. Biol. 1: 40-142 (1991).

C21 Cerutti, P.A. Pro-oxidant states and tumour promotion. Science 227: 375-381 (1985).

C22 Cheresh, D.A. and J.R. Harper. Arg-Gly-Asp recognition by a cell adhesion receptor requires its 130 kDa alpha subunit. J. Biol. Chem. 262: 1434-1437 (1987).

C23 Collard, J.G., M. Van de Poll, A. Scheffer et al. Location of genes involved in invasion and metastasis on human chromosome 7. Cancer Res. 47: 6666-6670 (1987).

C24 Cattanach, B.M. Chromosome imprinting and its significance for mammalian development. in: Genome Analysis Series. Volume 2. (K. Davis and S. Tighleman, eds.) Cold Spring Harbour Laboratory Press, Cold Spring Harbour, 1991.

C25 Canning, S. and T.P. Dryja. Short, direct repeats at the breakpoints of deletions of the retinoblastoma gene. Proc. Natl. Acad. Sci. (USA) 86: 5044-5048 (1989).

C26 Cox, R.D. and H. Lehrach. Genome mapping: PCR based meiotic and somatic cell hybrid analysis. BioEssays 13: 193-198 (1991).

C27 Crowell, P.L., R.R. Chang, Z. Ren et al. Selective inhibition of isoprenylation of 21-26-kDa proteins by the anticarcinogen d-limonene and its metabolites. J. Biol. Chem. 266: 17679-17685 (1991).

C28 Closs, E.L., A.B. Murray, J. Schmidt et al. c-fos expression precedes osteogenic differentiation of cartilage cells in vitro. J. Cell Biol. 111: 1313-1323 (1990).

C29 Chandar, N., B. Billig, J. McMaster et al. Inactivation of p53 gene in human and murine osteosarcoma cells. Br. J. Cancer 65: 208-214 (1992).

C30 Crook, T., D. Wrede, J.A. Tidy et al. Clonal p53 mutation in primary cervical cancer: association with human-papillomavirus-negative tumours. Lancet 339: 1070-1073 (1992).

C31 Caron de Fromental, C. and T. Soussi. Tp53 tumour suppressor gene: a model for investigating human mutagenesis. Genes, Chrom. Cancer 4: 1-15 (1992).

C32 Clarke, A.R., C.A. Purdie, D.J. Harrison et al. Thymocyte apoptosis induced by p53-dependent and independent pathways. Nature 362: 849-852 (1993).

D1 de Klein, A., A.G. van Kessel, G. Grosveld et al. A cellular oncogene is translocated to the Philadelphia chromosome in chronic myelocytic leukaemia. Nature 300: 765-767 (1982).

D2 Debenham, P., M. Webb, M. Jones et al. Molecular studies on the nature of the repair defect in ataxia-telangiectasia and their implication for cellular radiobiology. J. Cell Sci. (Suppl.) 6: 1977-1983 (1987).

D3 Diamond, L.E., E.W. Newcomb, L.E. McMorrow et al. In vivo activation of mouse oncogenes by radiation and chemicals. p. 532-537 in: Radiation Research. Volume 2. (E.M. Fielden et al., eds.) Taylor and Francis, London, 1987.

D4 Diamond, L.E., I. Guerrero and A. Pellicer. Concomitant K- and N-ras gene point mutations in clonal murine lymphomas. Mol. Cell. Biol. 8: 2233-2236 (1988).

D5 Doherty, P.C., B.B. Knowles and P.J. Wettstein. Immunological surveillance of tumours in the context of major histocompatibility complex restriction of T-cell function. Adv. Cancer Res. 42: 1-55 (1984).

D6 Defrensne, M.P., A.M. Rongy, R. Greimers et al. Cellular aspects of radiation leukaemogenesis in C57BL/Ka mice. Leuk. Res. 10: 783-789 (1986).

D7 Dubos, C., E.V. Pequignot and B. Dutrillaux. Localization of γ-ray induced chromatid breaks using a three consecutive staining technique. Mutat. Res. 49: 127-131 (1978).

D8 Dexter, T.M. and H. White. Growth without inflation. Nature 344: 380-381 (1990).

D9 Dexter, T.M., J. Garland, D. Scott et al. Growth of factor-dependent haemopoietic precursor cell lines. J. Exp. Med. 152: 1036-1047 (1980).

D10 Duesberg, P.H. Retroviruses as carcinogens and pathogens: expectations and reality. Cancer Res. 47: 1199-1220 (1987).

D11 Dutton, D.R. and G.T. Bowden. Indirect induction of a clastogenic effect in epidermal cells by a tumour promotor. Carcinogenesis 6: 1279-1284 (1985).

D12 Dowdy, S.F., C.L. Fasching, D. Aranjo et al. Suppression of tumorigenicity in Wilms' tumour by the p15.5-p14 region of chromosome 11. Science 254: 293-295 (1991).

D13 Djabali, M., L. Selleri, P. Parry et al. A trithorax-like gene is interrupted by chromosome 11q23 translocations in acute leukaemias. Nat. Genet. 2: 113-118 (1992).

D14 Donehower, L.A., M. Harvey, B.L. Slagle et al. Mice deficient for *p53* are developmentally normal but susceptible to spontaneous tumours. Nature 356: 215-219 (1992).

D15 Dittmer, D., P. Sibani, G. Zambetti et al. Gain of function mutations in p53. Nat. Genet. 4: 42-46 (1993).

E1 Evans, H.H., J. Mencl, M.F. Horng et al. Locus specificity in the mutability of L5178Y mouse lymphoma cells: The role of multilocus lesions. Proc. Natl. Acad. Sci. (USA) 83: 4379-4383 (1986).

E2 Elkind, M.M. Cell killing in radiation tumorigenesis. p. 513-518 in: Radiation Research. Volume 2. (E.M. Fielden et al., eds.) Taylor and Francis, London, 1987.

E3 Evans, H.J. Molecular mechanisms in the induction of chromosomal aberrations. p. 57-74 in: Progress in Genetic Toxicology. (D. Scott et al., eds) Elsevier, Amsterdam, 1977.

E4 Evans, H.H., M. Neilsen, J. Mencl et al. The effect of dose-rate on X-radiation-induced mutant frequencies and the nature of DNA lesions in mouse lymphoma L5178Y cells. Radiat. Res. 122: 316-325 (1990).

E5 Enoki, Y., O. Niwa, K. Yokoro et al. Analysis of clonal evolution in a tumour consisting of psv2neo-transfected mouse fibrosarcoma clones. Jpn. J. Cancer Res. 81: 141-147 (1990).

E6 Egan, S.E., G.A. McClarty, L. Jarolim et al. Expression of H-ras correlates with metastatic potential: evidence for direct regulation of the metastatic phenotype in 10T½ and N1H 3T3 cells. Mol. Cell. Biol. 7: 830-837 (1987).

E7 Elkind, M.H., J.S. Bedford, S.A. Benjamin et al. Oncogenic mechanisms in radiation-induced cancer (meeting report). Cancer Res. 51: 2740-2747 (1991).

E8 Erlich, H.A., D. Gelfand and J.J. Sninsky. Recent advances in the polymerase chain reaction. Science 252: 1643-1651 (1991).

E9 El-Deiry, W.S., S.E. Kern, J.A. Pietenpol et al. Definition of a consensus binding site for p53. Nat. Genet. 1: 45-49 (1992).

E10 Editorial. Keeping track of the translocations. Nat. Genet. 2: 85-86 (1992).

E11 Ellis, R.E. Negative regulators of programmed cell death. Curr. Opin. Genet. Dev. 2: 635-641 (1992).

E12 Eng, C., F.P. Li, D.H. Abramson et al. Mortality from second tumours among long-term survivors of retinoblastoma. J. Natl. Cancer Inst. (in press, 1993).

F1 Friberg, E.C. and P.C. Hanawalt (eds.). Mechanisms and Consequences of DNA Damage Processing. A.R. Liss, New York, 1988.

F2 Fry, R.J.M. and B.A. Carnes. Age, sex and other factors in radiation carcinogenesis. p. 195-206 in: Low Dose Radiation: Biological Bases of Risk Assessment. (K.F. Baverstock and J.W. Stather, eds.) Taylor and Francis, London, 1989.

F3 Foulds, L. Neoplastic Development. Volume 2. Academic Press, New York, 1975.

F4 Frazier, M.E., T.M. Seed, L.L. Scott et al. Radiation-induced carcinogenesis in dogs. p. 488-493 in: Radiation Research. Volume 2. (E.M. Fielden et al., eds.) Taylor and Francis, London, 1987.

F5 Folkman, J. Tumour angiogenesis. Adv. Cancer Res. 43: 175-204 (1985).

F6 Fusenig, N.B., P. Boukamp and D. Breitkreuzt. Transformation of human skin epithelial cells in vitro: concepts and stages of transformation. p. 45-56 in: Cell Transformation Systems and Radiation Induced Cancer in Man. (K. Chadwick, B. Barnhart and C. Seymour, eds.) Adam Hilger, Bristol, 1989.

F7 Farr, C.J., R.K. Saiki, H.A. Erlich et al. Analysis of RAS gene mutations in acute myeloid leukaemia by polymerase chain reaction and oligo-nucleotide probes. Proc. Natl. Acad. Sci. (USA) 85: 1629-1633 (1988).

F8 Fearon, E.R. and B. Vogelstein. A genetic model for colorectal tumourigenesis. Cell 61: 759-767 (1990).

F9 Fearon, E.R., S.R. Hamilton and B. Vogelstein. Clonal analysis of human colorectal tumours. Science 238: 193-197 (1987).

F10 Franke, U. A gene for Wilms' tumour? Nature 343: 692-694 (1990).

F11 Fearon, E.R., K.R. Cho and J.M. Nigro et al. Identification of a chromosome 18q gene that is altered in colorectal cancers. Science 247: 49-56 (1990).

F12 Fulop, G.M. and R.A. Phillips. The scid mutation in mice causes a general defect in DNA repair. Nature 347: 479-482 (1990).

F13 Fuciarelli, A.F., B.J. Wegher, W.F. Blakely et al. Yields of radiation-induced base products in DNA: effects of DNA conformation and gassing conditions. Int. J. Radiat. Biol. 58: 397-415 (1990).

F14 Fialkow, P.J. Clonal origin of human tumours. Ann. Rev. Med. 30: 135-176 (1979).

F15 Furstenburger, G., V. Kinzel, M. Schwartz et al. Partial inversion of the initiation-promotion sequence of multi-stage tumourigenesis in the skin of NMRI mice. Science 230: 76-78 (1985).

F16 Furstenburger, G., B. Schurich, B. Kaina et al. Tumour induction in initiated mouse skin by phorbol esters and methyl methanesulphonate: correlation between chromosomal damage and conversion in vivo. Carcinogenesis 10: 749-752 (1989).

F17 Folkman, J. and M. Klagsbrun. Angiogenic factors. Science 235: 442-447 (1987).

F18 Fuscoe, J., J. Gray, E. Hildebrand et al. Human chromosome-specific DNA libraries: Construction and availability. Biotechnology 4: 537-552 (1986).

F19 Farr, C., J. Fantes, P. Goodfellow et al. Functional reintroduction of human telomeres into mammalian cells. Proc. Natl. Acad. Sci. (USA) 88: 7006-7010 (1991).

F20 Fryer, G.A. and I. Gurvits. Isolation and identification of an oncogene induced by gamma irradiation in C3H 10T½ cells. p. 146 in: Radiation Research: A 20th Century Perspective. Volume 1. (J.D. Chapman et al., eds.) Academic Press, San Diego, 1991.

F21 Farmer, G., J. Bargonetti, H. Zhu et al. Wild-type p53 activates transcription in vitro. Nature 358: 83-86 (1992).

F22 Furuno-Fukushi, I., A.M. Ueno and H. Matsudaira. Mutation induction by very low dose-rate gamma rays in cultured mouse leukaemia cells L5178Y. Radiat. Res. 115: 273-280 (1988).

F23 Feinberg, A.P. Genomic imprinting and gene activation in cancer. Nat. Genet. 4: 110-113 (1993).

G1 Goodhead, D.T. Biophysical models of radiation action. p. 306-311 in: Radiation Research. Volume 2. (E.M. Fielden et al., eds.) Taylor and Francis, London, 1987.

G2 Goodhead, D.T. Saturable repair models of radiation action in mammalian cells. Radiat. Res. 104: 558-567 (1985).

G3 Graham, F.L., A.J. van der Eb and H.L. Heijneker. Size and location of the transforming region in human adenovirus type 5 DNA. Nature 251: 687-691 (1974).

G4 Grossman, Z. and R.B. Herberman. Immune surveillance without immunogenicity. Immunol. Today 7: 128-131 (1986).

G5 Glickman, B.W., E.A. Drobetsky, J. deBoer et al. Ionizing radiation induced point mutations in mammalian cells. p. 562-567 in: Radiation Research. Volume 2. (E.M. Fielden et al., eds.) Taylor and Francis, London, 1987.

G6 Greaves, M.F. Speculations on the cause of childhood acute lymphoblastic leukaemia. Leukaemia 2: 120-125 (1988).

G7 Gatti, R.A., I. Berkal, E. Boder et al. Localization of an ataxia-telangiectasia gene to chromosome 11q 22-23. Nature 336: 577-580 (1988).

G8 Goldstein, S. Replicative senescence: the human fibroblast comes of age. Science 249: 1129-1133 (1990).

G9 Gentner, N.E. and D.P. Morrison. Determination of the proportion of persons in the population-at-large who exhibit abnormal sensitivity to ionizing radiation. p. 253-262 in: Low Dose Radiation: Biological Bases of Risk Assessment. (K.F. Baverstock and J.W. Stather, eds.) Taylor and Francis, London, 1989.

G10 Greenberger, J.S., M.A. Sakakeemy, R.K. Humphries et al. Demonstration of permanent factor-dependent multipotential (erythroid/neutrophil/basophil) haemopoietic progenitor cell lines. Proc. Natl. Acad. Sci. (USA) 80: 2931-2935 (1983).

G11 Gopalakrishna, R. and S.H. Barsky. Tumour promotor-induced membrane-bound protein kinase C regulates haematogenous metastasis. Proc. Natl. Acad. Sci. (USA) 85: 612-616 (1988).

G12 Guirguis, R., E. Schiffman, B. Lin et al. Detection of autocrine mobility factor in urine as a marker of bladder cancer. J. Natl. Cancer Inst. 80: 1203-1211 (1988).

G13 Gatti, R.A. and M. Swift (eds). Ataxia-telangiectasia: Genetics, Neuropathology and Immunology of a Degenerative Disease of Childhood. A.R. Liss, New York, 1985.

G14 Ghosh, B.C. and L. Ghosh. Tumour Markers and Tumour Associated Antigens. McGraw-Hill, New York, 1988.

G15 Green, M.H.L., C.F. Arlett, J. Cole et al. Comparative human cellular radiosensitivity III. γ radiation survival of cultured skin fibroblasts and resting T-lymphocytes from the peripheral blood of the same individual. Int. J. Radiat. Biol. 59: 749-765 (1991).

G16 Ganesh, A., P. North and J. Thacker. Repair and misrepair of site-specific DNA double strand breaks by human cell extracts. Mutat. Res. 299:3-4: 251-259 (1993).

G17 Gumerlock, P.H., F.J. Meyers, B.A. Foster et al. Activated c-N-ras in radiation-induced acute nonlymphocytic leukaemia: twelfth codon aspartic acid. Radiat. Res. 117: 198-206 (1989).

G18 Garte, S.J., F.J. Burns, T. Ashkenazi-Kimmel et al. Amplification of the c-myc oncogene during progression of radiation-induced rat skin tumours. Cancer Res. 50: 3073-3077 (1990).

G19 Gould, M.N., K.H. Clifton, K. Kamiya et al. Quantitative and molecular comparison of initiation frequency of mammary carcinogenesis by radiation and chemical carcinogens. Radiat. Environ. Biophys. 30: 221-223 (1991).

G20 Goodrow, T.L., R.D. Storer, K.R. Leander et al. Murine p53 intron sequences 5-8 and their use in polymerase chain reaction/direct sequencing analysis of p53 mutations in CD-1 mouse liver and lung tumours. Mol. Carcinog. 5: 9-15 (1992).

G21 Gillett, N.A., B.L. Stegelmeier, G. Kelly et al. Expression of epidermal growth factor receptor in plutonium-239-induced lung neoplasms in dogs. Vet. Pathol. 29: 46-52 (1992).

G22 Gazzolo, L. and M. Duc Dodon. Direct activation of resting T lymphocytes by human T-lymphotropic virus type 1. Nature 326: 714-717 (1987).

G23 Gould, M.N. and R. Zhang. Genetic regulation of mammary carcinogenesis in the rat by susceptibility and suppressor genes. Environ. Health Perspect. 93: 161-167 (1991).

G24 Gishizky, M.L. and O.N. Witte. Initiation of deregulated growth of multipotent progenitor cells by bcr-abl in vitro. Science 256: 836-839 (1992).

H1 Hayes, W. The Genetics of Bacteria and their Viruses. Blackwells, Oxford, 1964.

H2 Hofer, K.G., C.R. Harris and J.M. Smith. Radiotoxicity of intracellular Ga-67, I-125 and H-3. Int. J. Radiat. Biol. 28: 225-241 (1975).

H3 Hofer, K.G. and R.L. Warters. Cell lethality after selective irradiation of the DNA replication fork. Radiat. Environ. Biophys. 24: 161-174 (1985).

H4 Haluska, F.G., Y. Tsujimoto and C.M. Croce. Oncogene activation by chromosome translocation in human malignancy. Annu. Rev. Genet. : 321-345 (1987).

H5 Hanawalt, P.C. and A. Sarasin. Cancer prone hereditary diseases with DNA processing abnormalities. Trends Genet. 2: 124-129 (1986).

H6 Hall, E.J. and T.K. Hei. Oncogenic transformation with radiation and chemicals. Int. J. Radiat. Biol. 48: 1-18 (1985).

H7 Hei, T.K., E.J. Hall and C.A. Waldren. Mutation induction and relative biological effectiveness of neutrons in mammalian cells. Radiat. Res. 115: 281-291 (1988).

H8 Hayata, I. Partial deletion of chromosome 2 in radiation induced myeloid leukaemia in mice. p. 277-293 in: Radiation-Induced Chromosome Damage in Man. (I. Ishihara and M.S. Sasaki, eds.) A.R. Liss, New York, 1983.

H9 Humphreys, E.R., J.F. Loutit, I.R. Major et al. The induction by Ra-224 of myeloid leukaemia and osteosarcoma in male CBA mice. Int. J. Radiat. Biol. 47: 239-247 (1985).

H10 Humphreys, E.R., J.F. Loutit and V.A. Stones. The induction by Pu-239 of myeloid leukaemia and osteosarcomas in female CBA mice. Int. J. Radiat. Biol. 51: 331-339 (1987).
H11 Heim, S. and F. Mitelman. Primary chromosome abnormalities in human neoplasia. Adv. Cancer Res. 52: 2-43 (1989).
H12 Herrlich, P. and H. Ponta. Nuclear oncogenes convert extracellular stimuli into changes in the genetic programme. Trends Genet. 52: 112-116 (1989).
H13 Hall, E.J. Finding a smoother pebble: A workshop summary. p. 401-412 in: Cell Transformation Systems and Radiation Induced Cancer in Man. (K. Chadwick, B. Barnhart and C. Seymour, eds.) Adam Hilger, Bristol, 1989.
H14 Hakoda, M., M. Akiyama, S. Kyouizumi et al. Increased somatic cell mutant frequency in atomic bomb survivors. Mutat. Res. 201: 39-48 (1988).
H15 Hanahan, D. Dissecting multistep tumorigenesis in transgenic mice. Annu. Rev. Genet. 22: 479-519 (1988).
H16 Holliday, R. A different kind of inheritance. Sci. Am. 260: 40-48 (1989).
H17 Hinds, P.W., C. Finlay and A.J. Levine. Mutation is required to activate the p53 gene for cooperation with the ras oncogene and transformation. J. Virol. 63: 739-746 (1989).
H18 Herskowitz, I. Functional inactivation of genes by dominant negative mutations. Nature 329: 219-222 (1987).
H19 Hall, J.G. Genomic imprinting: Review and relevance to human diseases. Am. J. Hum. Genet. 46: 857-873 (1990).
H20 Hori, T., E. Takahashi, T. Ishihara et al. Distamycin A-inducible fragile sites and cancer proneness. Cancer Genet. Cytogenet. 34: 177-187 (1988).
H21 Hastie, N.D. and R. Allshire. Human telomeres: fusion and interstitial sites. Trends Genet. 5: 326-330 (1989).
H22 Harley, C.B., A.B. Futcher and C.W. Greidner. Telomeres shorten during ageing of human fibroblasts. Nature 345: 458-460 (1990).
H23 Hockenberry, D., G. Numez, C. Milliman et al. Bcl-2 is an inner mitochondrial membrane protein that blocks programmed cell death. Nature 348: 334-336 (1990).
H24 Hanahan, D. Transgenic mice as probes into complex systems. Science 246: 1265-1275 (1990).
H25 Hecht, F. and B.K. Hecht. Fragile sites and chromosome breakpoints in constitutional rearrangements. I. Amniocentesis. Clin. Genet. 26: 169-173 (1984).
H26 Hecht, F. and B.K. Hecht. Fragile sites and constitutional chromosome rearrangements. II. Spontaneous abortions, stillbirths and newborns. Clin. Genet. 26: 174-177 (1984).
H27 Hayata, I., T. Ichikawa and Y. Ichikawa. Specificity in chromosomal abnormalities in mouse bone marrows induced by the difference of the conditions of irradiation. Proc. Jpn. Acad., Ser. B 63: 289-292 (1987).
H28 Hayata, I. Leukaemogenesis and chromosomal abnormalities: Experimental animals. Acta Haematol. Jpn. 48: 181-187 (1985).
H29 Harris, H. The analysis of malignancy by cell fusion: the position in 1988. Cancer Res. 48: 3302-3306 (1988).
H30 Hollstein, M., D. Sidransky, B. Vogelstein et al. p53 mutations in human cancers. Science 253: 49-53 (1991).
H31 Harrington, L.A. and C.W. Greidner. Telomerase primer specificity and chromosome healing. Nature 353: 451-454 (1991).
H32 Hatano, M., C.W.M. Roberts, M. Minden et al. Deregulation of a homeobox gene, Hox 11, by the t(10;14) in T-cell leukaemia. Science 253: 79-82 (1991).
H33 Hart, I.R., N.T. Goode and R.E. Wilson. Molecular aspects of the metastatic cascade. Biochim. Biophys. Acta 989: 65-84 (1989).
H34 Hsu, I.C., R.A. Metcalf, T. Sun et al. Mutational hotspot in the p53 gene in human hepatocellular carcinomas. Nature 350: 427-428 (1991).
H35 Hall, J.M., M.K. Lee, B. Newman et al. Linkage of early onset familial breast cancer to chromosome 17q21. Science 250: 1684-1689 (1990).
H36 Herlyn, M. and H. Koprowski. Melanoma antigens: immunological and biological characterisation and clinical significance. Annu. Rev. Immunol. 6: 283-308 (1988).
H37 Hanna, N. Inhibition of experimental tumour metastasis by selective activation of natural killer cells. Cancer Res. 42: 1337-1342 (1982).
H38 Herberman, R.B. and J.R. Ortaldo. Natural killer cells: their role in defenses against disease. Science 214: 24-30 (1981).
H39 Harvey, D.M. and A.J. Levine. p53 alteration is a common event in the spontaneous immortalization of primary BALB/c murine embryo fibroblasts. Genes Dev. 5: 2375-2385 (1991).
H40 Haas, O.A., A. Argyriou-Tirita and T. Lion. Parental origin of chromosomes involved in the translocation t(9;22). Nature 359: 414-416 (1992).
H41 Holmberg, M. Is the primary event in radiation-induced chronic myelogenous leukaemia the induction of the t(9;22) translocation? Leuk. Res. 16: 333-336 (1992).
H42 Hart, I.R. and A. Saini. Biology of tumour metastasis. Lancet 339: 1453-1457 (1992).
H43 Hall, J.G. Genomic imprinting and its clinical implications. N. Engl. J. Med. 326: 827-829 (1992).
H44 Hayata, I., M. Seki, K. Yoshida et al. Chromosomal aberrations observed in 52 mouse myeloid leukaemias. Cancer Res. 43: 367-373 (1983).
H45 Hoeijmakers, J.H. and D. Bootsma. DNA repair: two pieces of the puzzle. Nat. Genet. 1: 313-314 (1992).
H46 Harris, C.C. Chemical and physical carcinogenesis: advances and perspectives for the 1990s. Cancer Res. 51 (Suppl.): 5023s-5044s (1991).
H47 Hardwick, J.P., R.A. Schlenker and E. Huberman. Alteration of the c-mos locus in "normal" tissues from humans exposed to radium. Cancer Res. 49: 2668-2673 (1989).
H48 Hossain, M.Z., L.R. Wilkens, P.P. Mehta et al. Enhancement of gap junctional communication by retinoids correlates with their ability to inhibit neoplastic transformation. Carcinogenesis 10: 1743-1748 (1989).

H49 Hakoda, M., M. Akiyama, Y. Hirai et al. In vivo mutant T cell frequency in atomic bomb survivors carrying outlying values of chromosome aberration frequencies. Mutat. Res. 202: 203-208 (1988).

H50 Hartwell, L.H. and T.A. Weinert. Checkpoints: controls that ensure the order of cell cycle events. Science 246: 629-634 (1989).

H51 Helin, K. and E. Harlow. The retinoblastoma protein as a transcriptional repressor. Trend, Cell Biol. 3: 43-46 (1993).

H52 Haig, D. and C. Graham. Genome imprinting and the strange case of the insulin-like growth factor II receptor. Cell 64: 1045-1046 (1991).

I1 Ito, T., T. Seyama, T. Mizuno et al. Unique association of p53 mutations with undifferentiated but not with differentiated carcinomas of the thyroid gland. Cancer Res. 52: 1369-1371 (1992).

I2 Ijdo, J.W., A. Baldini, R.A. Wells et al. FRA 2B is distinct from inverted telomere repeat arrays at 2q13. Genomics 12: 833-835 (1992).

I3 Ho, T., T. Seyama, T. Mizuno et al. Induction of BCR-ABL fusion genes by in vitro X-irradiation. Jpn. J. Cancer Res. 84: 105-109 (1993).

J1 Jacob, F. and E.L. Wollman. Sexuality and the Genetics of Bacteria. Academic Press, New York, 1961.

J2 Janowski, M., R. Cox and G. Strauss. The molecular biology of radiation-induced carcinogenesis: thymic lymphoma, myeloid leukaemia and osteosarcoma. Int. J. Radiat. Biol. 57: 677-691 (1990).

J3 Jaffe, D. and G.T. Bowden. Ionizing radiation as an initiator: effects on proliferation and promotion time on tumor incidence in mice. Cancer Res. 47: 6692-6696 (1987).

J4 Joshi, G.P., W.J. Nelson, S.H. Revell et al. X-ray induced chromosome damage in live mammalian cells and improved measurements of its effects on their colony forming ability. Int. J. Radiat. Biol. 41: 161-181 (1982).

J5 Jones, P.A. and J.D. Buckley. The role of DNA methylation in cancer. Adv. Cancer Res. 54: 1-24 (1990).

J6 Jacobson, S., V. Zaninovic, C. Mora et al. Immunological findings in neurological diseases associated with antibodies to HTLV-1. Ann. Neurol. 23 (Suppl 1): 196-200 (1988).

K1 Knudson, A.G. Genetics of human cancer. Annu. Rev. Genet. 20: 231-251 (1986).

K2 Klein, G. and E. Klein. Evolution of tumours and the impact of molecular oncology. Nature 315: 190-195 (1985).

K3 Kennedy, A.R., J. Cairns and J.B. Little. Timing of the steps in transformation of C3H10T1/2 cells by x-irradiation. Nature 307: 85-86 (1984).

K4 Kaplan, H.S. On the natural history of the murine leukaemias. Cancer Res. 27: 1325-1340 (1967).

K5 Kasid, U., A. Pfeifer, R.R. Weichselbaum et al. The ras oncogene is associated with a radiation resistant human laryngeal cancer. Science 237: 1039-1040 (1987).

K6 Kerbel, R.S., C. Waghorne, C. Korczak et al. Clonal dominance of primary tumours by metastatic cells. Cancer Surveys 7(4): 597-629 (1988).

K7 Kinlen, L. Immunologic factors. p. 494-505 in: Cancer Epidemiology and Prevention. (D. Schotlenfeld and J. Fraumeni, eds.) Saunders, Philadelphia, 1982.

K8 Kumar, R., S. Sukumar and M. Barbacid. Activation of ras oncogenes preceding the onset of neoplasia. Science 248: 1101-1104 (1990).

K9 Kyoizumi, S., N. Nakamura, M. Hakoda et al. Detection of somatic mutations at the glycophorin A locus of erythrocytes of atomic bomb survivors using a single beam flow sorter. Cancer Res. 49: 581-588 (1989).

K10 Kennedy, A.R. Initiation and promotion of radiation-induced transformation in vitro: relevance of in vitro studies to radiation-induced cancer in human populations. p. 263-277 in: Cell Transformation Systems and Radiation Induced Cancer in Man. (K. Chadwick et al., eds.) Adam Hilger, Bristol, 1989.

K11 Komatsu, K.S., S. Kodama, Y. Okumura et al. Restoration of radiation resistance in ataxia-telangiectasia cells by the introduction of normal human chromosome 11. Mutat. Res. 235: 59-63 (1990).

K12 Kern, S.E., K.W. Kinzler, A. Bruskin et al. Identification of p53 as a sequence-specific DNA-binding protein. Science 252: 1708-1710 (1991).

K13 Kanno, Y. Modulation of cell communication and carcinogenesis. Jpn. J. Physiol. 35: 693-707 (1985).

K14 Klingelhutz, A.J., S.-Q. Win, E.A. Bookland et al. Allelic 3p deletions in high grade carcinomas after transformation in vitro of human uroepithelial cells. Genes, Chrom. Cancer 3: 346-357 (1991).

K15 Kinzler, K.W., M.C. Nilbert, L.-K. Su et al. Identification of FAP locus genes from chromosome 5q21. Science 253: 661-665 (1991).

K16 Kastan, M.B., O. Onvekwere, D. Sidransky et al. Participation of p53 protein in the cellular response to DNA damage. Cancer Res. 51: 6304-6311 (1991).

K17 Kern, S.E., J.A. Pietenpol, S. Thiagalingam et al. Oncogenic forms of p53 inhibit p53-regulated gene expression. Science 256: 827-830 (1992).

K18 Katinka, M.D. and F.M. Bourgain. Interstitial telomeres are hotspots for illegitimate recombination with DNA molecules injected into the macronucleus of Paramecium primaurelia. EMBO J. 11: 725-732 (1992).

K19 Kang, C., X. Zhang, R. Ratliff et al. Crystal structure of four stranded *Oxytricha* telomeric DNA. Nature 356: 126-131 (1992).

K20 Krowczyska, A.M., R.A. Rudders and T.G. Kronftiris. The human minisatellite consensus at breakpoints of oncogene translocations. Nucleic Acids Res. 18: 1121-1127 (1990).

K21 King, M.-C. Breast cancer genes: how many, where and who are they? Nat. Genet. 2: 89-90 (1992).

K22 Krolewski, B. and J.B. Little. Molecular analysis of DNA isolated from the different stages of x-ray induced transformation in vitro. Mol. Carcinog. 2: 27-33 (1989).

K23 Kramer, A. and W.H. Blattner. The HTLV-1 model and chronic demyelinating neurological diseases. p. 204-214 in: Concepts in Viral Pathogenesis. (A.L. Notkins and M.B.A. Oldstone, eds.) Springer Verlag, New York, 1989.

K24 Kaelbling, M., R.D. Burk, N.B. Atkin et al. Loss of heterozygosity on chromosome 17p and mutant p53 in HPV-negative cervical carcinomas. Lancet 340: 140-142 (1992).

K25 Kadhim, M.A., D.A. Macdonald, D.T. Goodhead et al. Transmission of chromosomal instability after plutonium α particle irradiation. Nature 355: 738-740 (1992).

K26 Kuerbitz, S.J., B.S. Plunkett, W.V. Walsh et al. Wild type p53 is a cell cycle checkpoint determinant following irradiation. Proc. Natl. Acad. Sci. (USA) 89: 7491-7495 (1992).

K27 Kawakatsu, H., R. Shiurba, M. Obara et al. Human carcinoma cells synthesize and secrete tenascin in vitro. Jpn. J. Cancer Res. 83: 1073-1080 (1992).

K28 Kyoizumi, S., M. Akiyama and Y. Hirai. Spontaneous loss and alteration of antigen receptor expression in mature CD4 T-cells. J. Exp. Med. 171: 1981-1999 (1990).

K29 Kapp, L.N., R.B. Painter, L.C. Yu et al. Cloning of a candidate gene for ataxia-telangiectasia group D. Am. J. Hum. Genet. 51: 45-54 (1992).

L1 Lloyd, D.C., R.J. Purrott, G.W. Dolphin et al. The relationship between chromosome aberrations and low-LET radiation dose to human lymphocytes. Int. J. Radiat. Biol. 28: 75-90 (1975).

L2 Little, J.B. The relevance of cell transformation to carcinogenesis in vivo. p. 396-413 in: Low Dose Radiation: Biological Bases of Risk Assessment. (K.F. Baverstock and J.W. Stather, eds.) Taylor and Francis, London, 1989.

L3 Little, J.B. Influence of noncarcinogenic secondary factors on radiation carcinogenesis. Radiat. Res. 87: 240-250 (1981).

L4 Lieberman, M. and H.S. Kaplan. Leukaemogenic activity of filtrates from radiation-induced lymphoid tumors of mice. Science 130: 387-388 (1959).

L5 Lapis, K., L. Liotta and A. Rabson (eds.). Biochemistry and Molecular Genetics of Cancer Metastasis. Martinus Nijhoff, The Hague, 1986.

L6 Ling, V., A.F. Chambers, J.F. Harris et al. Quantitative genetic analysis of tumour progression. Cancer Metastasis Rev. 4: 173-194 (1985).

L7 Langlois, R.G., W.L. Bigbee, S. Kyouizumi et al. Evidence for increased somatic cell mutations at the glycophorin A locus in atomic bomb survivors. Science 236: 445-448 (1987).

L8 Landsvater, R.M., C.G.P. Mathew, B.A. Smith et al. Development of multiple endocrine neoplasia type 2A does not involve substantial deletions of chromosome 10. Genomics 4: 246-250 (1989).

L9 Le Beau, M.M. Chromosomal fragile sites and cancer specific breakpoints - A moderating viewpoint. Cancer Genet. Cytogenet. 31: 55-61 (1988).

L10 Liotta, L.A. Tumour invasion and metastases: role of the basement membrane. Am. J. Pathol. 117: 339-348 (1984).

L11 Little, J.B. and J. Nove. Sensitivity of human diploid fibroblast cell strains from various genetic disorders to acute and protracted radiation exposure. Radiat. Res. 123: 87-92 (1990).

L12 Lang, R.A., D. Metcalf, N.M. Gough et al. Expression of a haemopoietic growth factor cDNA in a factor dependent cell line resulting in autonomous growth and tumourigenicity. Cell 43(2): 531-542 (1985).

L13 Levine, A.J., J. Momand and C.A. Finlay. The p53 tumour suppressor gene. Nature 351: 453-456 (1991).

L14 Loewenstein, W.R. Junctional intercellular communication: the cell to cell membrane channel. Physiol. Rev. 61: 829-913 (1981).

L15 Leder, A., A. Kuo, R.D. Cardiff et al. v-Ha-ras transgene abrogates the initiation step in mouse skin tumorigenesis: effects of phorbol esters and retinoic acid. Proc. Natl. Acad. Sci. (USA) 87: 9178-9182 (1990).

L16 Little, M., V. Van Heyningen and N. Hastie. Dads and disomy and disease. Nature 351: 609-610 (1991).

L17 Lupulesco, A. Hormones and Carcinogenesis. Praegar Press, New York, 1982.

L18 LeMotte, P.K., S.J. Adelstein and J.B. Little. Malignant transformation induced by incorporated radionuclides in BALB/3T3 mouse embryo fibroblasts. Proc. Natl. Acad. Sci. (USA) 79: 7763-7767 (1982).

L19 Lucas, J., A. Awa, Y. Kodama et al. Rapid translocation frequency analysis in human decades after exposure to ionising radiation. Proc. Natl. Acad. Sci. (USA) 89: 53-63 (1992).

L20 Land, C.E. and W.K. Sinclair. The relative contributions of different organ sites to the total cancer mortality associated with low dose radiation exposure. p. 31-58 in: Annals of the ICRP. ICRP Publication 22. Pergamon Press, Oxford, 1991.

L21 Lee, E.Y., H. To, J.Y. Shew et al. Inactivation of the retinoblastoma susceptibility gene in human breast cancers. Science 241: 218-221 (1988).

L22 Leone, A., U. Flatlow, C.R. King et al. Reduced tumour incidence, metastatic potential and cytokine responsiveness of nm23-transfected melanoma cells. Cell 65: 25-35 (1991).

L23 Liotta, L.A., P.S. Steeg and W.G. Stetler-Stevenson. Cancer metastasis and angiogenesis: an imbalance of positive and negative regulation. Cell 64: 327-336 (1991).

L24 Leib-Mosch, C., R. Brack-Werner, T. Werner et al. Endogenous retroviral elements in human DNA. Cancer Res. 50 (Suppl.): 5636s-5642s (1990).

L25 Leuthauser, S.W.C., J.E. Thomas and D.L. Guernsey. Oncogenes in X-ray-transformed C3H10T½ mouse cells and in X-ray-induced mouse fibrosarcoma (RIF-1) cells. Int. J. Radiat. Biol. 62: 45-51 (1992).

L26 Laviguer, A., V. Maltby, D. Mock et al. High incidence of lung, bone, and lymphoid tumors in transgenic mice overexpressing mutant alleles of the p53 oncogene. Mol. Cell. Biol. 9: 3982-3991 (1989).

L27 Loeb, L.A. Endogenous carcinogenesis. Cancer Res. 49: 5489-5496 (1989).

L28 Lane, D.P. p53, guardian of the genome. Nature 358: 15-16 (1992).

L29 Lowe, S.W., E.M. Schmitt, S.W. Smith et al. p53 is required for radiation-induced apoptosis in mouse thermocytes. Nature 362: 847-849 (1993).

L30 Land, C.E., M. Tokunaga, S. Tokuoka et al. Early onset breast cancer in A-bomb survivors. Lancet 342: 237 (1993).

M1 Mole, R.H. Dose response relationships. p. 403 in: Radiation Carcinogenesis. (J.D. Boice and J.F. Fraumeni, eds.) Raven Press, New York, 1985.

M2 Mole, R.H. Radiation-induced acute myeloid leukaemia in the mouse. Leuk. Res. 10: 859-865 (1986).

M3 Moreau-Gachelin, F., A. Tavitian and P. Tambourin. Spi-1 is a putative oncogene in virally induced murine erythroleukaemias. Nature 331: 277-280 (1988).

M4 Monpezat, J.P., O. Delattre, A. Bernard et al. Loss of alleles on chromosome 18 and on the short arm of chromosome 17 in polyploid colorectal carcinomas. Int. J. Cancer 41: 404-408 (1988).

M5 Mitelman, F. and S. Heim. Consistent involvement of only 71 of the 329 chromosomal bands of the human genome in primary neoplasia-associated rearrangements. Cancer Res. 48: 7115-7119 (1988).

M6 Moore, M.M., A. Amtower, G.H.S. Strauss et al. Genotoxicity of γ-irradiation in L5178Y mouse lymphoma cells. Mutat. Res. 174: 149-154 (1986).

M7 McMorrow, L., E.W. Newcomb and A. Pellicer. Identification of a specific marker chromosome early in tumour development in γ-irradiated C57BL/6J mice. Leukaemia 2: 115-119 (1988).

M8 Muto, M., T. Sato, I. Hayata et al. Reconfirmation of indirect induction of radiogenic lymphomas using thymectomized, irradiated B10 mice grafted with neonatal thymuses from Thyl congenic donors. Cancer Res. 43: 3822-3827 (1983).

M9 McCormick, J.J. and V.M. Maher. Towards an understanding of the malignant transformation of human fibroblasts. Mutat. Res. 199: 273-292 (1988).

M10 Malynn, B.A., T.K. Blackwell, G.M. Fulop et al. The scid defect affects the final step of the immunoglobulin VDJ recombinase mechanism. Cell 54: 453-460 (1988).

M11 Muller, W.J., E. Sinn, P.K. Pattenhale et al. Single step induction of mammary adenocarcinoma in transgenic mice bearing the activated c-neu oncogene. Cell 54: 105-115 (1988).

M12 McCune, J.M., R. Namikawa, H. Kaneshima et al. The SCID-hu mouse: murine model for the analysis of human haematolymphoid differentiation and function. Science 241: 1632-1639 (1988).

M13 Mosier, D.E., R.J. Gulizia, S.M. Baird et al. Transfer of a functional human immune system to mice with severe combined immunodeficiency. Nature 335: 256-259 (1988).

M14 Monk, M. Genomic imprinting. Genes Dev. 2: 921-925 (1988).

M15 Murray, A. Telomeres: all's well that ends well. Nature 346: 797-798 (1990).

M16 Metcalf, J.C., T.R. Hesketh, G.A. Smith et al. Early response pattern analysis of the mitogenic pathway in lymphocytes and fibroblasts. J. Cell Sci. 3 (Suppl.): 199-228 (1985).

M17 Margolis, B., A. Zilberstein and C. Franks et al. Effect of phospholipase C-γ overexpression on PDGF-induced second messengers and mitogenesis. Science 248: 607-610 (1990).

M18 Moore, K.V., P. Vieira, D.F. Fiorentino et al. Homology of cytokine synthesis inhibitory factor (IL-10) to the Epstein-Barr virus gene BCR F1. Science 248: 1230-1234 (1990).

M19 Maraschin, J., B. Dutrillaux and A. Animas. Chromosome aberrations induced by etoposide (VP-16) are not random. Int. J. Cancer 46: 808-812 (1990).

M20 Mittelman, F., Y. Manolova, G. Manolov et al. High resolution analysis of the 5q-marker chromosome in refractory anemia. Hereditas 105: 49-54 (1986).

M21 Moloney, W.C. Radiogenic leukaemia revisited. Blood 70: 905-908 (1987).

M22 Morgan, T.L., E.W. Fleck, B.J.F. Rossiter et al. Molecular characterization of X-ray induced mutations at the HPRT locus in plateau phase Chinese hamster ovary cells: the effect of dose, dose fractionation and delayed plating. p. 207-214 in: Cell Transformation Systems and Radiation Induced Cancer in Man. (K. Chadwick, B. Barnhart and C. Seymour, eds.) Adam Hilger, Bristol, 1989.

M23 Mulcahy, R.T., M.N. Gould and K.H. Clifton. Radiogenic initiation of thyroid cancer: a common cellular event. Int. J. Radiat. Biol. 45: 419-426 (1984).

M24 Metcalf, D. Molecular Control of Blood Cells. Harvard University Press, Boston, 1988.

M25 Moser, A.R., H.C. Pitot and W.F. Dove. A dominant mutation that predisposes to multiple intestinal neoplasia in the mouse. Science 247: 322-324 (1990).

M26 Muto, M., E. Kubo, H. Kamisaku et al. Phenotypic characterization of thymic prelymphoma cells of B10 mice treated with split-dose irradiation. J. Immunol. 144: 849-853 (1990).

M27 Murray, A.W. and H.W. Kirschner. What controls the cell cycle. Sci. Am. 264: 56-63 (1991).

M28 Marx, J. The cell cycle: spinning farther afield. Science 252: 1490-1492 (1991).

M29 Moyzis, R.K. The human telomere. Sci. Am. 265: 34-41 (1991).

M30 Murray, A.W. and D.J. Fitzgerald. Tumour promotors inhibit metabolic co-operation in co-cultures of epidermal and 3T3 cells. Biochem. Biophys. Res. Comm. 91: 395-401 (1979).

M31 Mitchel, R.E.J., N.J. Gragtmans and D.P. Morrison. Beta-radiation-induced resistance to MNNG initiation of papilloma but not carcinoma formation in mouse skin. Radiat. Res. 121: 180-186 (1990).

M32 Moolgavkar, S.M. Hormones and multistage carcinogenesis. Cancer Surveys 5: 635-648 (1986).

M33 Meuth, M. The structure of mutations in mammalian cells. Biochim. Biophys. Acta 1032: 1-17 (1990).

M34 Marx, J. Zeroing in on individual cancer risk. Science 253: 612-616 (1991).

M35 Muxinova, K.N. and G.S. Mushkacheva. Cellular and molecular mechanisms for the changes of the haemopoietic system in case of long-term irradiation. Energoatomizdat, Moscow, 1990.

M36 Muramatsu, M. Introduction to Molecular Medicine. Nankoda, Tokyo, 1992.

M37 Mitchel, R.E.J. and A. Trivedi. Chronic exposure to ionizing radiation as a tumor promoter in mouse skin. Radiat. Res. 129: 192-201 (1992).

M38 Malkin, D., K.W. Jolly, N. Barbier et al. Germline mutations of the p53 tumor-suppressor gene in children and young adults with second malignant neoplasms. N. Engl. J. Med. 326: 1309-1315 (1992).

M39 Monnat, R.J., A.F.M. Hackman and T.A. Chiaverotti. Nucleotide sequence analysis of human hypoxanthine phosphoribosyl transferase (HPRT) gene deletions. Genomics 13: 777-787 (1992).

M40 Mihara, K., L. Bai, Y. Kano et al. Malignant transformation of human fibroblasts previously immortalized with ^{60}Co gamma rays. Int. J. Cancer 50: 639-643 (1992).

M41 Masse, R. Lung cancer in laboratory animals. Radiat. Environ. Biophys. 30: 233-237 (1991).
M42 Miyamoto, S., S. Sukumar, R.C. Guzman et al. Transforming c-Ki-ras mutation is a preneoplastic event in mouse mammary carcinogenesis induced in vitro by N-methyl-N-nitrosourea. Mol. Cell. Biol. 10: 1593-1599 (1990).
M43 Maurer, J., J.W.G. Janssen, E. Thiel et al. Detection of chimeric BCR-ABL genes in acute lymphoblastic leukaemia by the polymerase chain reaction. Lancet 337: 1055-1058 (1991).
M44 Maniatis, T. and H. Weintraub. Gene expression and differentiation. Curr. Opin. Genet. Dev. 2: 197-198 (1992).
M45 Mehta, P.P., J.S. Bertram and W.R. Lowenstein. The actions of retinoids on cellular growth correlate with their actions on gap junctional communication. J. Cell Biol. 108: 1053-1065 (1989).
M46 Miki, Y., I. Nishisho, A. Horii et al. Disruption of the APC gene by a retrotransposal insertion of L1 sequence in a colon cancer. Cancer Res. 52: 643-645 (1992).
M47 Murray, A.W. Creative blocks: cell cycle checkpoints and feedback controls. Nature 359: 599-604 (1992).
M48 Mules, E.H., J.R. Testa, G.H. Thomas et al. Cancer in relatives of leukaemic patients with chromosomal rearrangements at rare (heritable) fragile-site locations in their malignant cells. Am. J. Hum. Genet. 44: 811-819 (1989).
M49 Morris, T. and J. Thacker. Formation of large deletions by illegitimate recombination in the HPRT gene of primary human fibroblasts. Proc. Natl. Acad. Sci. (USA) 90: 1392-1396 (1993).
M50 Muto, M., E. Kubo and T. Sado. Cellular events during radiation induced thymic leukaemogenesis in mice: abnormal T cell differentiation in the thymus and defect of thymocyte precursors in the bone marrow after split dose irradiation. J. Immunol. 134: 2026-2031 (1985).
N1 Natarajan, A.T. and G. Obe. Molecular mechanisms involved in the production of chromosomal aberrations. Chromosoma 90: 120-127 (1984).
N2 Nusse, R. The activation of cellular oncogenes by retroviral insertion. Trends Genet. 2: 244-247 (1986).
N3 Nowell, P.C. Mechanisms of tumour progression. Cancer Res. 46: 2203-2207 (1986).
N4 Newcomb, E.W., R. Binari and E. Fleissner. A comparative analysis of radiation and virus induced leukaemias in BALB/C mice. Virology 140: 102-112 (1985).
N5 Nishizuka, Y. The role of protein kinase C in cell surface signal transduction and tumour promotion. Nature 308: 693-698 (1984).
N6 Nicholson, G. and L. Milas (eds.). Cancer Invasions and Metastasis: Biologic and Therapeutic Aspects. Raven Press, New York, 1984.
N7 Niwa, O., Y. Enoki and K. Yokoro. Overexpression and amplification of the c-myc gene in mouse tumours induced by chemicals and radiations. Jpn. J. Cancer Res. 80: 212-218 (1989).
N8 Namba, M., K. Nishitani, F. Fukushima et al. Multistep neoplastic transformation of normal human fibroblasts by Co-60 gamma rays and Ha-ras oncogenes. Mutat. Res. 199: 415-423 (1988).
N9 Nowell, P.C. Cytogenetics of tumour progression. Cancer 65: 2172-2177 (1990).
N10 National Council on Radiation Protection and Measurements. Comparative carcinogenicity of ionizing radiation and chemicals. NCRP Report No. 96 (1989).
N11 Namba, M., K. Nishitani, T. Kimoto et al. Multistep neoplastic transformation of normal human fibroblasts and its genetic aspects. p. 67-74 in: Cell Transformation Systems and Radiation Induced Cancer in Man. (K. Chadwick, B. Barnhart and C. Seymour, eds.) Adam Hilger, Bristol, 1989.
N12 Nurse, P. Universal control mechanisms regulating onset of M phase. Nature 344: 503-508 (1990).
N13 Nicolson, G.L., K.M. Dulski and J.E. Trosko. Loss of intercellular junctional communication correlates with metastatic potential in mammary adenocarcinoma cells. Proc. Natl. Acad. Sci. (USA) 85: 473-475 (1988).
N14 Newbold, R.F. Metabolic co-operation in tumour promotion and carcinogenesis. p. 301-317 in: Functional Integration of Cells in Animal Tissues. (J.D. Pitts and M.E. Finbow, eds.) Cambridge University Press, Cambridge, 1982.
N15 North, P., A. Ganesh and J. Thacker. The rejoining of double strand breaks in DNA by human cell extracts. Nucleic Acids Res. 18: 6205-6210 (1990).
N16 Nishisho, I., Y. Nakamura, Y. Miyoshi et al. Mutations of chromosome 5q21 genes in FAP and colorectal cancer patients. Science 253: 665-669 (1991).
N17 Neuman, W.L., M.L. Wasylyshyn, R. Jacoby et al. Evidence for a common molecular pathogenesis in colorectal, gastric and pancreatic cancer. Genes, Chrom. Cancer 3: 468-473 (1991).
N18 Nevins, J.R. E2F: A link between the Rb tumor suppressor protein and viral oncoproteins. Science 258: 424-429 (1992).
N19 Newcomb, E.W., M. Corominas, W. Bayona et al. Multistage carcinogenesis in murine thymocytes: involvement of oncogenes, chromosomal imbalances and T cell growth factor receptor. Anticancer Res. 9: 1407-1415 (1989).
N20 Nicklas, J.A., J.P. O'Neill, T.C. Hunter et al. In vivo ionizing irradiations produce deletions in the hprt gene of human T-lymphocytes. Mutat. Res. 250: 383-396 (1991).
N21 Newton, J.A., A.K. Black, C.F. Arlett et al. Radiobiological studies in the naevoid basal cell carcinoma syndrome. Br. J. Dermatol. 123: 573-580 (1990).
N22 Nikjoo, H. and D.T. Goodhead. The relative biological effectiveness (RBE) achievable by high- and low-LET radiations. p. 491-502 in: Low Dose Radiation: Biological Bases of Risk Assessment. (K.F. Baverstock and J.W. Stather, eds.) Taylor and Francis, London, 1989.
N23 Norbury, C. and P. Nurse. Animal cell cycles and their control. Annu. Rev. Biochem. 61:441-470 (1992).
O1 Onions, D.E. and O. Jarrett (eds.). Naturally occurring tumours in animals as a model for human disease. Cancer Surv. 6: 1-181 (1987).
O2 Oberle, I., F. Rousseau, D. Heitz et al. Instability of a 550 base pair DNA segment and abnormal methylation in fragile X syndrome. Science 252: 1097-1102 (1991).

O3 Okumoto, M., R. Nishikawa, M. Iwai et al. Lack of evidence for the involvement of type-C and type-B retroviruses in radiation leukaemogenesis of NFS mice. Radiat. Res. 121: 267-273 (1990).

O4 Ozturk, M., B. Bressac, A. Puisieux et al. p53 mutation in hepatocellular carcinoma after aflatoxin exposure. Lancet 338: 1356-1359 (1991).

O5 Ootsuyama, A. and H. Tanooka. Threshold-like dose of local ß irradiation throughout the life-span of mice for induction of skin and bone tumours. Radiat. Res. 125: 98-101 (1991).

P1 Ponder, B. Gene losses in human tumours. Nature 335: 400-402 (1988).

P2 Pippard, E.C., A.J. Hall, D.J.P. Barker et al. Cancer in homozygotes and heterozygotes of ataxia-telangiectasia and xeroderma pigmentosum in Britain. Cancer Res. 48: 2929-2932 (1988).

P3 Perry, G.S., B.D. Spector, L.M. Schuman et al. The Wiskott Aldrich syndrome in the USA and Canada. J. Pediatr. 97: 72-79 (1980).

P4 Purtillo, D.T. and G. Klein. Introduction to Epstein-Barr virus and lymphoproliferative diseases in immunodeficient individuals. Cancer Res. 41: 4209 (1981).

P5 Priest, N.D. (ed.). Metals in Bone. MTP Press, Lancaster, 1984.

P6 Piper, J. and C. Lundsteen. Human chromosome analysis by machine. Trends Genet. 3: 309-313 (1987).

P7 Ponder, B.A.J. and M.M. Wilkinson. Direct examination of the clonality of carcinogen-induced colonic epithelial dysplasia in chimeric mice. J. Natl. Cancer Inst. 77: 967-976 (1986).

P8 Pantel, K., J. Boertman and A. Nakeff. Inhibition of haemopoietic recovery from radiation-induced myelosuppression by natural killer cells. Radiat. Res. 122: 168-171 (1990).

P9 Paterson, M.C., N.E. Gentner, M.V. Middlestadt et al. Hereditary and familial disorders linking cancer proneness with abnormal carcinogen response and faulty DNA metabolism. p. 235-267 in: Epidemiology and Quantification of Environmental Risk in Humans from Radiation and Other Agents. Volume 96. (A. Castellani, ed.) NATO ASI Series A, 1986.

P10 Pitts, J.D. and M.E. Finbow. The gap junction. J. Cell Sci. 4: 239-266 (1986).

P11 Petrusevska, R.T., G. Furstenburger, F. Marks et al. Cytogenetic effects caused by phorbol ester tumour promotors in primary mouse keratinocyte cultures: correlations with the convertogenic activity of TPA in multistage skin carcinogenesis. Carcinogenesis 9: 1207-1215 (1988).

P12 Ponder, B.A. Inherited predisposition to cancer. Trends Genet. 6: 213-218 (1990).

P13 Peters, G. Oncogenes at viral integration sites. Cell Growth Differ. 1: 503-510 (1990).

P14 Panozzo, J., D. Bertoncini, D. Miller et al. Modulation of expression of virus-like elements following exposure of mice to high- and low-LET radiations. Carcinogenesis 12: 801-804 (1991).

P15 Potten, C.S., Y.Q. Li, P.J. O'Connor et al. A possible explanation for the differential cancer incidence in the intestine based on distribution of the cytotoxic effects of carcinogens in the murine large bowel. Carcinogenesis 13(12): 2305-2312 (1992).

P16 Peltomaki, P., L.A. Aaltonen, P. Sistonen et al. Genetic mapping of a locus predisposing to human colorectal cancer. Science 260: 810-812 (1993).

R1 Radford, I.R., G.S. Hodgson and J.P. Matthews. Critical DNA target size model of ionizing radiation-induced mammalian cell death. Int. J. Radiat. Biol. 54: 63-79 (1988).

R2 Reznikoff, C.A., J.S. Bertram, D.W. Brankow et al. Quantitative and qualitative studies of chemical transformation of cloned C3H mouse embryo cells sensitive to post confluence inhibition of cell division. Cancer Res. 33: 3239-3249 (1973).

R3 Rabbitts, T.H., T. Boehm and L. Mengl-Gaw. Chromosomal abnormalities in lymphoid tumours: mechanisms and role in tumour pathogenesis. Trends Genet. 4: 300-304 (1988).

R4 Redpath, J.L., C. Sun, M. Coleman et al. The application of a human hybrid cell system to studies of radiation-induced neoplastic cell transformation: quantitative cellular and molecular aspects. p. 85-90 in: Cell Transformation Systems and Radiation Induced Cancer in Man. (K. Chadwick, B. Barnhart and C. Seymour, eds.) Adam Hilger, Bristol, 1989.

R5 Reznikoff, C.A., E.A. Bookland, A.J. Klingelhutz et al. SV-HUC-1: a human urinary tract epithelial cell line for multistep in vitro transformation studies. p. 57-66 in: Cell Transformation Systems and Radiation Induced Cancer in Man. (K. Chadwick, B. Barnhart and C. Seymour, eds.) Adam Hilger, Bristol, 1989.

R6 Robbins, P.D., J.M. Horowitz and R.C. Mulligan. Negative regulation of human c-fos expression by the retinoblastoma gene product. Nature 346: 668-671 (1990).

R7 Reik, W. and M.A. Surani. Genomic imprinting and embryonal tumours. Nature 338: 112-113 (1989).

R8 Reik, W. Genomic imprinting and genetic disorders in man. Trends Genet. 5: 331-336 (1989).

R9 Rowley, J.D., H.M. Golumb and J.W. Vardiman. Non-random chromosome abnormalities in acute leukaemia and dysmyelopoietic syndromes in patients with previously treated malignant disease. Blood 58: 759-763 (1981).

R10 Roifman, C.M. and E.W. Gelfand. Heterogeneity of the immunological deficiency in ataxia-telangiectasia. p. 273-285 in: Ataxia-Telangiectasia: Genetics, Neuropathology and Immunology of a Degenerative Disease of Childhood. (R.A. Gatti and M. Swift, eds.) A.R. Liss, New York, 1985.

R11 Rovera, G., B.A. Reichard, S. Hudson et al. Point mutations in both transforming and non-transforming codons of the N-ras proto-oncogenes of Ph+ leukaemias. Oncogene 4: 867-872 (1989).

R12 Robbins, P.D., J.M. Horowitz and R.C. Mulligan. Negative regulation of human c-fos expression by the retinoblastoma gene product. Nature 346: 668-671 (1990).

R13 Radler-Pohl, A., J. Pohl and V. Schirrmacher. Selective enhancement of metastatic capacity in mouse bladder carcinoma cells after transfection with DNA from liver metastases of human colon carcinoma. Int. J. Cancer 41: 840-846 (1988).

R14 Roe, D. (ed.). Diet, Nutrition and Cancer: From Basic Research to Policy Implications. A.R. Liss, New York, 1983.

R15 Rittling, S.R. and D.T. Denhardt. p53 mutations in spontaneously immortalized 3T12 but not 3T3 mouse embryo cells. Oncogene 7: 935-942 (1992).

R16 Reik, W. Imprinting in leukaemia. Nature 359: 362-363 (1992).

R17 Richards, R.I. and G.R. Sutherland. Heritable unstable DNA sequences. Nat. Genet. 1: 7-9 (1992).

R18 Rhim, J.S., J.H. Yoo, J.H. Park et al. Evidence for the multistep nature of in vitro epithelial cell carcinogenesis. Cancer Res. 50 (Suppl): 5653s-5657s (1990).

R19 Rhim, Y.S., J.H. Park and G. Jay. Neoplastic transformation of human keratinocytes by polybrene-induced DNA-mediated transfer of an activated oncogene. Oncogene 4: 1403-1409 (1989).

R20 Ruther, U., D. Komitowski, F.R. Schubert et al. c-fos expression induces bone tumours in transgenic mice. Oncogene 4: 861-865 (1989).

R21 Rotter, V., O. Foord and N. Navot. In search of the functions of normal p53. Trend, Cell Biol. 3: 46-49 (1993).

S1 Stehelin, D., H.E. Varmus, J.M. Bishop et al. DNA related to the transforming gene(s) of avian sarcoma viruses is present in normal avian DNA. Nature 260: 170-173 (1976).

S2 Streffer, C. and W. Muller. Radiation risk from combined exposures to ionizing radiations and chemicals. Adv. Radiat. Biol. 11: 173-210 (1984).

S3 Swift, M. and C. Chase. Cancer and cardiac deaths in obligatory ataxia-telangiectasia heterozygotes. Lancet I: 1049-1050 (1983).

S4 Swift, M., P.J. Reitnauer, D. Morrell et al. Breast and other cancers in families with ataxia-telangiectasia. N. Engl. J. Med. 316: 1289-1294 (1987).

S5 Strong, L. Genetic and environmental interactions. Cancer 40: 1861-1866 (1977).

S6 Sawey, M.J. and A.R. Kennedy. Activation of oncogenes in radiation induced malignant transformation. p. 433-438 in: Low Dose Radiation: Biological Bases of Risk Assessment. (K.F. Baverstock and J.W. Stather, eds.) Taylor and Francis, London, 1989.

S7 Sawey, M.J., A.T. Hood, F.J. Burns et al. Activation of c-myc and c-k ras oncogenes in primary rat tumours induced by ionizing radiation. Mol. Cell. Biol. 7: 932-935 (1987).

S8 Silver, A., G. Breckon, W.K. Masson et al. Studies on radiation myeloid leukaemogenesis in the mouse. p. 494-500 in: Radiation Research. Volume 2. (E.M. Fielden et al., eds.) Taylor and Francis, London, 1987.

S9 Sado, T., H. Kamisaku, H. Kubo et al. Role of T-cell precursors in the bone marrow in thymic lymphomagenesis induced by split dose irradiation in B10 strain mice. p. 190 in: Proceedings of the 8th International Congress of Radiation Research. Volume 1 (1987).

S10 Silver, A., G. Breckon, J. Boultwood et al. Studies on putative initiating events for radiation-oncogenesis. p. 387-395 in: Low Dose Radiation: Biological Bases of Risk Assessment. (K.F. Baverstock and J.W. Stather, eds.) Taylor and Francis, London, 1989.

S11 Silver, A., J. Boultwood, G. Breckon et al. Interleukin-1ß gene deregulation associated with chromosomal rearrangement: a candidate initiating event for murine radiation-myeloid leukaemogenesis? Mol. Carcinog. 2: 226-233 (1989).

S12 Storer, J.B., T.J. Mitchell and R.J.M. Fry. Extrapolation of the relative risk of radiogenic neoplasms across mouse strains and to man. Radiat. Res. 114: 331-353 (1988).

S13 Sager, R. Genetic instability, suppression and human cancer. in: Gene Regulation in the Expression of Malignancy. Cancer Surv. 3: 321-334 (1984).

S14 Schirrmacher, V. Cancer metastasis. Adv. Cancer Res. 43: 1-74 (1985).

S15 Schmidt, J., E.I. Closs, E. Luz et al. Induction of osteogenic maturation and neoplastic transformation of in vitro differentiating skeletoblasts by C-type retroviruses from radiation-induced osteosarcomas. p. 239-250 in: Cell Transformation Systems and Radiation Induced Cancer in Man. (K. Chadwick, B. Barnhart and C. Seymour, eds.) A. Hilger, Bristol, 1989.

S16 Spiers, F.W. and J. Vaughan. The toxicity of the bone-seeking radionuclides. Leuk. Res. 13: 347-350 (1989).

S17 Sugarbaker, J.P., L.L. Gunderson and R.E. Wittes. Colorectal cancer. p. 800-803 in: Cancer: Principles and Practices of Oncology. (V.T. de Vita et al., eds.) Lippencott, Philadelphia, 1985.

S18 Sager, R. Tumour suppressor genes: the puzzle and the promise. Science 246: 1406-1412 (1989).

S19 Scrable, H.J., C. Sapienza and W.K. Cavanee. Genetic and epigenetic losses of heterozygosity in cancer predisposition and progression. Adv. Cancer Res. 54: 25-62 (1990).

S20 Sasaki, M., M. Okamoto, C. Sato et al. Loss of constitutional heterozygosity in colorectal tumours from patients with familial polyposis coli and those with non-polyposis colorectal carcinoma. Cancer Res. 49: 4402-4406 (1989).

S21 Sutherland, G.R. and R.N. Simmers. No statistical association between common fragile sites and non-random chromosome breakpoints in cancer cells. Cancer Genet. Cytogenet. 31: 9-16 (1988).

S22 Shippen-Lentz, D. and E.H. Blackburn. Functional evidence for an RNA template in telomerase. Science 247: 546-552 (1990).

S23 Sieweke, M.H., N.L. Thompson, M.B. Sporn et al. Mediation of wound-related Rouse sarcoma virus tumourigenesis by TGF-ß. Science 251: 1656-1663 (1990).

S24 Sandford, K.K. and R. Parshad. Detection of cancer prone individuals using cytogenetic response to X-rays. p. 113-129 in: Chromosome Aberrations: Basic and Applied Aspects. (G. Obe and A.T. Natarajan, eds.) Springer Verlag, Berlin, 1990.

S25 Seabright, M. High resolution studies on the pattern of induced exchanges in the human karyotype. Chromosoma 40: 333-346 (1973).

S26 Sabatier, L., M. Mulems, M. Prieur et al. Specific sites of chromosomal radiation-induced rearrangements. p. 211-224 in: New Trends in Genetic Risk Assessment. (G. Jolles and A. Cordier, eds.) Academic Press, New York, 1989.

S27 Sapienza, C. Genomic imprinting and dominance modification. Ann. N.Y. Acad. Sci. 564: 24-28 (1989).

S28 Stingl, G., S.I. Katz and I. Clement. Immunologic functions of Ia-bearing epidermal Langerhan cells. J. Immunol. 121: 2005-3013 (1978).

S29 Sankaranarayan, K. Ionizing radiation and genetic risks. III. Nature of spontaneous and radiation-induced mutations in mammalian in vitro systems and mechanisms of induction of mutations by radiation. Mutat. Res. 258: 75-97 (1991).

S30 Schrader, J.W. and R.M. Crapper. Autogenous production of a haemopoietic growth factor, persisting-cell-stimulating factor, as a mechanism for transformation of bone marrow derived cells. Proc. Natl. Acad. Sci. (USA) 80: 6892-6896 (1983).

S31 Sloan, S.R., E.W. Newcomb and A. Pellicer. Neutron radiation can activate k-ras via a point mutation in codon 146 and induces a different spectrum of ras mutations than does gamma radiation. Mol. Cell. Biol. 10: 405-408 (1990).

S32 Silver, A.R.J., W.K. Masson, A.M. George et al. The IL-1a and ß genes are closely linked (<70kb) on mouse chromosome 2. Somat. Cell Mol. Genet. 16: 549-556 (1990).

S33 Silver, A.R.J., A.M. George, W.K. Masson et al. DNA methylation changes in the IL-1(2F) chromosomal region of some radiation-induced acute myeloid leukaemias carrying chromosome 2 rearrangements. Genes, Chrom. Cancer 3: 376-881 (1991).

S34 Stanbridge, E.J. The evidence for human tumour suppressor genes. p. 3-13: in: Genetic Basis for Carcinogenesis. (A.G. Knudson et al, eds.) Taylor and Francis, London, 1990.

S35 Shippey, C.A., M. Layton and L.M. Secker-Walker. Leukaemia characterised by multiple sub-clones with unbalanced translocations involving different telomeric segments. Genes, Chrom. Cancer 2: 14-17 (1990).

S36 Starling, J.A., J. Maule, N.D. Hastie et al. Extensive telomere repeat arrays in mouse are hypervariable. Nucleic Acids Res. 18: 6881-6888 (1990).

S37 Sen, D. and W. Gilbert. Formation of parallel four-stranded complexes by guanine-rich motifs in DNA and its implications for meiosis. Nature 334: 364-366 (1988).

S38 Schultz, R.M., S. Silberman, B. Persky et al. Inhibition by human recombinant tissue inhibitor of metalloproteinases of human amnion invasion and lung colonization by murine B16-F10 melanoma cells. Cancer Res. 48: 5539-5545 (1988).

S39 Steeg, P.S., G.B. Bevilacqua, L. Kopper et al. Evidence of a novel gene associated with low tumour metastatic potential. J. Natl. Cancer Inst. 80: 200-204 (1988).

S40 Sugahara, T., T. Aoyama, M. Ikebuchi et al. (eds). Proceedings of the International Conference on Risk Assessment of Energy Development and Modern Technology. Kyoto Health Research Foundation (1989).

S41 Srivastava, S., Z. Zou, K. Pirollo et al. Germ line transmission of a mutated p53 gene in a cancer-prone family with Li-Fraumeni syndrome. Nature 348: 747-749 (1990).

S42 Sell, S. Basic Immunology: Immune Mechanisms in Health and Disease. Elsevier, New York, 1987.

S43 Silver, A. and R. Cox. Telomere-like DNA polymorphisms associated with genetic predisposition to acute myeloid leukaemia in irradiated CBA mice. Proc. Natl. Acad. Sci. (USA) 90: 1407-1410 (1993).

S44 Sidransky, D., A. von Eschenbach, Y.C. Tsai et al. Identification of p53 gene mutations in bladder cancers and urine samples. Science 252: 706-709 (1991).

S45 Sheer, D. Chromosomes and cancer. p. 269-295 in: Introduction to the Cellular and Molecular Biology of Cancer. (L.M. Franks and N.M. Teich, eds.) Oxford University Press, Oxford, 1990.

S46 Snipes, M.B. Long-term retention and clearance of particles inhaled by mammalian species. Crit. Rev. Toxicol. 20: 175-211 (1991).

S47 Sidransky, D., P. Frost, A. von Eschenbach et al. Clonal origin of bladder cancer. N. Engl. J. Med. 326: 737-740 (1992).

S48 Su, L.-K., K.W. Kinzler, B. Vogelstein et al. Multiple intestinal neoplasia caused by a mutation in the murine homolog of the APC gene. Science 256: 668-670 (1992).

S49 Stallings, R.L., N.A. Doggett, K. Okamura et al. Chromosome 16 - specific DNA sequences that map to chromosomal regions known to undergo breakage/ rearrangement in leukaemia cells. Genomics 13: 332-338 (1992).

S50 Sherman, M.L., R. Datta, D.E. Hallahan et al. Ionizing radiation regulates expression of the c-jun proto-oncogene. Proc. Natl. Acad. Sci. (USA) 87: 5663-5666 (1990).

S51 Shimoyama, Y. and S. Hirohashi. Cadherin intercellular adhesion molecule in hepatocellular carcinomas: loss of E-cadherin expression in an undifferentiated carcinoma. Cancer Lett. 57: 131-135 (1991).

S52 Smith, S.A., D.F. Easton, D.G.R. Evans et al. Allele losses in the region 17q12-21 in familial breast and ovarian cancer involve the wild-type chromosome. Nat. Genet. 2: 128-131 (1992).

S53 Sutherland, G.R., E.A. Haan, E. Kremer et al. Hereditary unstable DNA: a new explanation for some old genetic questions? Lancet 338: 289-292 (1991).

S54 Stamper, M.R. and J.C. Bartley. Induction of transformation and continuous cell lines from normal human mammary epithelial cells after exposure to benzo[α]pyrene. Proc. Natl. Acad. Sci. (USA) 82: 2394-2398 (1985).

S55 Schmidt, J., A. Luz and V. Erfle. Endogenous murine leukaemia viruses: frequency of radiation-activation and novel pathogenic effects of viral isolates. Leuk. Res. 12: 393-403 (1988).

S56 Sado, T. Experimental radiation carcinogenesis studies at NIRS. p. 36-42 in: Proceedings of the International Conference on Radiation Effects and Protection, March 18-29, 1992, Mito, Ibaraki, Japan (1992).

S57 Sado, T., H. Kamisaku and E. Kubo. Bone marrow-thymus interactions during thymic lymphomagenesis induced by fractionated radiation exposure in B10 mice: analysis using bone marrow transplantation between Thy 1 congenic mice. J. Radiat. Res. 32 (Suppl. 2): 168-180 (1991).

S58 Strauss, P.G., K. Mitreiter, H. Zitzelsberger et al. Elevated p53 RNA expression correlates with incomplete osteogenic differentiation of radiation-induced murine osteosarcomas. Int. J. Cancer 50: 252-258 (1992).

S59 Sturm, S.A., P.G. Strauss, S. Adolph et al. Amplification and rearrangement of c-myc in radiation-induced murine osteosarcomas. Cancer Res. 50: 4146-4153 (1990).

S60 Stegelmeier, B.L., N.A. Gillett, A.H. Rebar et al. The molecular progression of plutonium-239-induced rat lung carcinogenesis: Ki-ras expression and activation. Mol. Carcinog. 4: 43-51 (1991).

S61 Sakai, H. and K. Ogawa. Mutational activation of c-Ha-ras genes in intraductal proliferation induced by N-nitroso-N-methylurea in rat mammary glands. Int. J. Cancer 49: 140-144 (1991).

S62 Saint, R. and P.L. Wigley. Developmental regulation of the cell cycle. Curr. Opin. Genet. Dev. 2: 614-620 (1992).

S63 Solomon, E., J. Borrow and A.D. Goddard. Chromosome aberrations and cancer. Science 254: 1153-1160 (1991).

S64 Swift, M., D. Morrell, R.B. Massey et al. Incidence of cancer in 161 families affected by ataxia-telangiectasia. N. Engl. J. Med. 325: 1831-1836 (1991). See also Correspondence, N. Engl. J. Med. 326: 1357-1361 (1991).

S65 Sakamoto, H., M. Oyamada, K. Enomoto et al. Differential changes in expression of gap function proteins connexin 26 and 23 during hepatocarcinogenesis in rats. Jpn. J. Cancer Res. 83: 1210-1215 (1992).

S66 Saul, R.L. and B.N. Ames. Background levels of DNA damage in the population. Basic Life Sci. 38: 529-535 (1986).

T1 Tanooka, H. Monoclonal growth of cancer cells: experimental evidence. GANN 79: 657-665 (1988).

T2 Thacker, J. The nature of mutants induced by ionizing radiation in cultured hamster cells. Mutat. Res. 160: 267-275 (1986).

T3 Trent, J.M., E.J. Stanbridge, H.L. McBride et al. Tumourigenicity in human melanoma cell lines controlled by introduction of human chromosome 6. Science 247: 568-571 (1990).

T4 Trakhtenbrot, L., R. Krauthgamer, P. Resnitzky et al. Deletion of chromosome 2 is an early event in the development of radiation-induced myeloid leukaemia in SLJ/J mice. Leukaemia 2: 545-550 (1988).

T5 Toguchida, J., K. Ishizaki, M.S. Sasaski et al. Preferential mutation of paternally derived RB gene as the initial event in sporadic osteosarcoma. Nature 338: 156-158 (1989).

T6 Taylor, A.M.R. Cytogenetics of ataxia-telangiectasia. p. 53-81 in: Ataxia-Telangiectasia. (B.A. Bridges and D.G. Harnden, eds.) John Wiley and Sons, Chichester, 1982.

T7 Taalman, R.D.F.M., N.E.G. Jaspers, J.M.J. Scheres et al. Hypersensitivity to ionizing radiation in vitro in a new chromosomal breakage disorder, the Nijmegen Breakage Syndrome. Mutat. Res. 112: 23-32 (1983).

T8 Thacker, J. Radiation-induced mutation in mammalian cells at low doses and dose rates. Adv. Radiat. Biol. 16: 77-117 (1992).

T9 Terzaghi-Howe, M. Induction of pre-neoplastic alterations by X-rays and neutrons in exposed rat tracheas and isolated tracheal epithelial cells. Radiat. Res. 120: 352-363 (1989).

T10 Terzaghi-Howe, M. Interactions between cell populations influence expression of the transformed phenotype in irradiated rat tracheal epithelial cells. Radiat. Res. 121: 242-247 (1990).

T11 Trosko, J.E., C.L. Chang and B.V. Madhukar. Modulation of intercellular communication during radiation and chemical carcinogenesis. Radiat. Res. 123: 241-251 (1990).

T12 Trosko, J.E., C.L. Chang, B.V. Madhukar et al. Intercellular communication: a paradigm for the interpretation of the initiation/promotion/progression model of carcinogenesis. in: Chemical Carcinogenesis: Modulation and Combination Effects. (J.C. Arcos, ed.) Academic Press, New York, 1992.

T13 Tanaka, K., I. Satokata, Z. Ogita et al. Molecular cloning of a mouse DNA repair gene that complements the defect of group A xeroderma pigmentosum. Proc. Natl. Acad. Sci. (USA) 86: 5512-5516 (1989).

T14 Trosko, J.E., V.M. Riccardi, C.C. Chang et al. Genetic predisposition to initiation or promotion phases in human carcinogenesis. p. 13 in: Biomarkers, Genetics and Cancer. (H. Anton-Guirgis and H.T. Lynch, eds.) Van Nostrand Reinhold, New York, 1985.

T15 Thompson, L.H., K.W. Brookman, N.J. Jones et al. Molecular cloning of the human XRCCI gene, which corrects defective DNA strand break repair and sister chromatid exchange. Mol. Cell. Biol. 10: 6160-6171 (1990).

T16 Tomatis, L., C. Agthe, H. Bartsch et al. Evaluation of the carcinogenicity of chemicals: a review of the monograph program of the International Agency for Research on Cancer (1971 to 1977). Cancer Res. 38: 877-885 (1978).

T17 Toguchida, J., T. Yamaguchi, S.H. Drayton et al. Prevalence and spectrum of germline mutations of the p53 gene among patients with sarcoma. N. Engl. J. Med. 326: 1301-1308 (1992).

T18 Tveito, G., I.L. Hansteen, H. Dalen et al. Immortalization of normal human kidney epithelial cells by nickel(II). Cancer Res. 49: 1829-1835 (1989).

T19 Takahashi, R., T. Hashimoto, H.J. Xu et al. The retinoblastoma gene functions as a growth and tumor suppressor in human bladder carcinoma cells. Proc. Natl. Acad. Sci. (USA) 88: 5257-5261 (1991).

T20 Tauchi, H. and S. Sawada. Suppression of gamma and neutron induced neoplastic transformation by ascorbic acid in Balb/c3T3 cells. Int. J. Radiat. Biol. 63: 1-6 (1993).

T21 Tatsumi, K., A. Fujimori, A. Tachibana et al. Concurrent analysis of mutagenesis by ionizing radiation at the APRT and HPRT loci in human lymphoblastoid cells. in: Low Dose Irradiation and Biological Defense Mechanisms. (T. Sugahara et al., eds.) Elsevier Science Publishers, Amsterdam, 1992.

U1 United Nations. Sources, Effects and Risks of Ionizing Radiation. United Nations Scientific Committee on the Effects of Atomic Radiation, 1988 Report to the General Assembly, with annexes. United Nations sales publication E.88.IX.7. United Nations, New York, 1988.

U2 United Nations. Genetic and Somatic Effects of Ionizing Radiation. United Nations Scientific Committee on the Effects of Atomic Radiation, 1986

Report to the General Assembly, with annexes. United Nations sales publication E.86.IX.9. United Nations, New York, 1986.

U3 United Nations. Ionizing Radiation: Sources and Biological Effects. United Nations Scientific Committee on the Effects of Atomic Radiation, 1982 Report to the General Assembly, with annexes. United Nations sales publication E.82.IX.8. United Nations, New York, 1982.

U4 United Nations. Sources and Effects of Ionizing Radiation. United Nations Scientific Committee on the Effects of Atomic Radiation, 1977 report to the General Assembly, with annexes. United Nations sales publication E.77.IX.1. United Nations, New York, 1977.

U11 Urlaub, G., P. Mitchell, E. Kas et al. Effects of γ-rays at the dihydroifolate reductase locus: deletions and inversions. Somat. Cell Mol. Genet. 12: 555-566 (1986).

U12 Ullrich, R.L. Cellular and molecular changes in mammary epithelial cells following irradiation. Radiat. Res. 128: 5136-5140 (1991).

U13 Umeki, S., S. Kyoizumi, Y. Kusunoki et al. Flow cytometric measurement of somatic cell mutations in Thorotrast patients. Jpn. J. Cancer Res. 82: 1349-1353 (1991).

V1 Varmus, H. and J.M. Bishop (eds.). Biochemical mechanisms of oncogene activity: proteins encoded by oncogenes. Cancer Surveys 5: (1986).

V2 Vousden, K.H. and C.J. Marshall. Three different activated ras genes in mouse tumours: evidence for oncogene activation during progression of a mouse lymphoma. EMBO J. 4: 913-917 (1984).

V3 Van der Bliek, A.M. and P. Borst. Multidrug resistance. Adv. Cancer Res. 52: 165-204 (1989).

V4 Van der Hoof, A. Stromal involvement in malignant growth. Adv. Cancer Res. 50: 159-196 (1988).

V5 Van den Berghe, H., K. Vermaelen, C. Mecucci et al. The 5q-anomaly. Cancer Genet. Cytogenet. 17: 189-255 (1985).

V6 Van der Mey, A.G.L., P.D. Maaswinkel-Mooy, C.J. Cornellisse et al. Genomic imprinting in hereditary glomus tumours: evidence for new genetic theory. Lancet 2: 1291-1294 (1989).

V7 Van Duin, M., J. deWit, H. Odijk et al. Molecular characterisation of the human excision repair gene ERCC-1: cDNA cloning and amino acid homology with the yeast DNA repair gene RAD 1O. Cell 44: 13-23 (1986).

V8 Van der Rauwelaert, E., J.R. Maisin and J. Merregaert. Provirus integration and myc amplification in ^{90}Sr induced osteosarcomas of CF1 mice. Oncogene 2: 215-222 (1988).

V9 Verbeek, S., M. van Lohuizen, M. van der Valk et al. Mice bearing the E mu-myc and E mu-pim-1 transgenes develop pre-B-cell leukaemia prenatally. Mol. Cell. Biol. 11: 1176-1179 (1991).

V10 Vahakangas, K.H., J.M. Samet, R.A. Metcalf et al. Mutations of p53 and ras genes in radon-associated lung cancer from uranium miners. Lancet 339: 576-580 (1992).

W1 Watson, J.D. (ed.). The Molecular Biology of the Gene. Benjamin Commings, New York, 1988.

W2 Waxman, J. and K. Sikora (eds.). The Molecular Biology of Cancer. Blackwells, Oxford, 1989.

W3 Woodruff, M. Tumour clonality and its biological consequences. Adv. Cancer Res. 50: 197-229 (1988).

W4 Weinstein, I.B. Protein kinase, phospholipid and control of growth. Nature 302: 750-751 (1983).

W5 Weinberg, R.A. Oncogenes and the Molecular Origins of Cancer. Cold Spring Harbour Laboratory, 1989.

W6 Wallace, M.R., D.A. Marchuk, L.B. Andersen et al. Type 1 neurofibromatosis gene: identification of a large transcript disrupted in three NF1 patients. Science 249: 181-186 (1990).

W7 Woloschak, G.E., C.L. Chin-Mei and P. Shearin-Jones. Regulation of protein kinese C by ionizing radiation. Cancer Res. 50: 3963-3967 (1990).

W8 Wheelock, E.F. and M.K. Robinson. Endogenous control of the neoplastic process. Lab. Invest. 48: 120-139 (1983).

W9 Werness, B.A., A.J. Levine and P.M. Howley. Association of human papilloma virus type 16 and 18E6 proteins with p53. Science 248: 76-79 (1990).

W10 Ward, J.F. DNA damage and repair. p. 403-421 in: Physical and Chemical Mechanisms in Molecular Radiation Biology. (W.A. Glass and M.N. Varma, eds.) Plenum Press, New York, 1991.

W11 Windle, J.J., D.M. Albert, J.M. O'Brien et al. Retinoblastoma in transgenic mice. Nature 343: 665-669 (1990).

W12 Ward, J.F. The yield of DNA double stand breaks produced intracellularly by ionizing radiation: a review. Int. J. Radiat. Biol. 57: 1141-1150 (1990).

W13 Wagner, S. and M.R. Green. A transcriptional tryst. Nature 352: 189-190 (1991).

W14 Weinberg, R.A. Tumour suppressor genes. Science 254: 1138-1146 (1991).

W15 Weiss, L. Principles of Metastasis. Academic Press, Orlando, 1985.

W16 Wyke, J.A. Viruses and cancer. p. 203-229 in: Introduction to the Cellular and Molecular Biology of Cancer. (L.M. Franks and N.M. Teich, eds.) Oxford University Press, Oxford, 1990.

W17 Warner, J.F. and G. Dennert. Effects of a cloned cell line with NK activity on bone marrow transplants, tumour development and metastasis in vivo. Nature 300: 31-34 (1982).

W18 Wigley, C. and A. Balmain. Chemical carcinogenesis and precancer. p. 148-174 in: Introduction to the Cellular and Molecular Biology of Cancer. (L.M. Franks and N.M. Teich, eds.) Oxford University Press, Oxford, 1990.

W19 Wolf, C.R. Cytochrome P-450: Polymorphic multigene families involved in carcinogen activation. Trends Genet. 2: 209-214 (1986).

W20 Weinstein, B. Growth factors, oncogenes and multistage carcinogenesis. J. Cell Biochem. 33: 213-224 (1987).

W21 Weichselbaum R.R., D.E. Hallahan, V. Sukhatme et al. Biological consequences of gene regulation after ionizing radiation exposure. J. Natl. Cancer Inst. 83: 480-484 (1991).

W22 Wright, P.A., E.D. Williams, N.R. Lemoine et al. Radiation-associated and "spontaneous" human thyroid carcinomas show a different pattern of ras oncogene mutation. Oncogene 6: 471-473 (1991).

W23 Walker, C., L.T.L. Goldsworthy, D.C. Wolf et al. Predisposition to renal cell carcinoma due to alteration of a cancer susceptibility gene. Science 255: 1693-1695 (1992).

W24 Willman, C.L., C.E. Sever, M.G. Pallavicini et al. Deletion of IRF-1, mapping to chromosome 5q31.1, in human leukaemia and pre-neoplastic myelodysplasia. Science 259: 968-971 (1993).

W25 Williams, A.C., S. Harper and C. Paraskeva. Neoplastic transformation of a human colonic epithelial cell line: experimental evidence for the adenoma to carcinoma sequence. Cancer Res. 50: 4724-4730 (1990).

W26 Wallin, H., H. Andersson, L.L. Nielsen et al. p53 mutations in human liver tumours induced by alpha-radiation. Cancer Detect. Prev. 17: 91 (1993).

W27 Ward, J.F. Response to commentary by D. Billen. Radiat. Res. 126: 385-387 (1991).

Y1 Yunis, J.J., A.L. Soreng and A.E. Bowe. Fragile sites are targets of diverse mutagens and carcinogens. Oncogene 1: 59-70 (1987).

Y2 Yuspa, S.H. and M.C. Poirier. Chemical carcinogenesis: from animal models to molecular models in one decade. Adv. Cancer Res. 50: 25-70 (1988).

Y3 Young, J.D.E. and Z.A. Cohn. How killer cells kill. Sci. Am. 258: 28-36 (1988).

Y4 Young, R.A. and T.J. Elliott. Stress proteins, infection and immune surveillance. Cell 59: 5-8 (1989).

Y5 Yasukawa, M., T. Terasima and M. Seki. Radiation-induced neoplastic transformation of C3H10T1/2 cells is suppressed by ascorbic acid. Radiat. Res. 120: 456-467 (1989).

Y6 Yonish-Rouach, E., D. Resnitzky, J. Lotem et al. Wild type p53 induces apoptosis of myeloid leukaemic cells that is inhibited by interleukin-6. Nature 352: 345-347 (1991).

Y7 Yamasaki, H., M. Hollstein, M. Mesnil et al. Selective lack of intercellular communication between transformed and non-transformed cells as a common property of chemical and oncogene transformation of BALB/c 3T3 cells. Cancer Res. 47: 5658-5662 (1987).

Y8 Yotti, L.P., C.L. Chang and J.E. Trosko. Elimination of metabolic co-operation in Chinese hamster cells by a tumour promotor. Science 208: 1089-1091 (1979).

Y9 Yu, S., M. Pritchard, E. Kremer et al. Fragile X genotype characterised by an unstable region of DNA. Science 252: 1179-1181 (1991).

Y10 Yasukawa, M., T. Terasima and M. Seki. Radiation-induced neoplastic transformation of C3H10T½ cells is suppressed by ascorbic acid. Radiat. Res. 120: 456-467 (1989).

Z1 Zhang, R., J.D. Haag and M.N. Gould. Reduction in the frequency of activated ras oncogenes in rat mammary carcinomas with increasing N-methyl-N-nitrosourea doses or increasing prolactin levels. Cancer Res. 50: 4286-4290 (1990).

Z2 Zhang, R., J.D. Haag and M.N. Gould. Quantitating the frequency of initiation and cH-ras mutation in in situ N-methyl-N-nitrosourea-exposed rat mammary gland. Cell Growth Differ. 2: 1-6 (1991).

Z3 Zur Hausen, H. Viruses in human cancers. Science 254: 1167-1173 (1991).

ANNEX F

Influence of dose and dose rate on stochastic effects of radiation

---

CONTENTS

INTRODUCTION

1. Radiation-induced malignant disease is the main late somatic effect in human populations exposed to ionizing radiation and the only statistically detectable cause of radiation-induced life shortening at intermediate to low doses. In this dose range the incidence of radiation-induced cancer appears to increase with increasing dose, and the probabilistic nature of the relationship between dose and risk of the disease has led to the use of the term "stochastic" for this type of effect. Quantitative information on the risk of cancer in human populations exposed to ionizing radiation at present comes largely from information available from populations that have been exposed at intermediate to high doses and dose rates. In general, however, for assessing the consequences of environmental and occupational exposure to radiation, risks need to be known for exposures to low doses delivered at low dose rates. Some information is now starting to become available from epidemiological studies on occupationally exposed groups, although at present the results of such studies have substantial statistical uncertainties associated with them. It is likely that for the immediate future quantitative risk estimates will continue to be based on the higher dose/dose-rate studies, although increasingly low-dose studies will provide support for these values.

2. It has been recognized by the Committee for some time that information is needed on the extent to which both total dose and dose rate influence cancer induction in exposed individuals. The two features of the dose response that are most important for evaluation of the risk at low doses are the possible presence of a threshold dose, below which the effects could not occur, and the shape of the dose response. Both these factors have been considered in earlier reports of the Committee.

3. Proving or disproving a threshold on the basis of epidemiological studies or studies on tumour induction in experimental animals is, for most tumour types, likely to be impossible due to statistical uncertainties in both the spontaneous and induced incidences of the disease. Therefore, on the assumption that cellular targets can be altered by single ionizing events, that such damage is unlikely to be error-free and that it may ultimately give rise to a tumour, it is normally assumed that there is no threshold for the neoplastic response. This working hypothesis is consistent with many, but not all observations of induced cancer rates found in animal experiments as well as with observations in epidemiological studies and is considered in some detail in Annex E, "Mechanisms of radiation oncogenesis".

4. Tumour induction resulting from exposures to ionizing radiation has been systematically examined in studies with various species and strains of animals and

for specific tumour types. Physical factors such as dose, dose rate, dose fractionation and radiation quality, as well as biological factors such as age, gender and species which can modify the tumour yield, have been considered. In the majority of cases, the dose-effect relationships obtained are complex, showing first a rise with increasing radiation doses, a peak or plateau at intermediate doses and in many cases a final decline in incidence at high doses. In a few cases the spontaneous incidence of tumours changes very little with increasing radiation dose, and in some studies where there is a high spontaneous incidence this has resulted in a negative correlation with increasing dose at high doses.

5. The Committee noted in the UNSCEAR 1977 Report [U4] a considerable variability in the net incidence of various tumour types at intermediate to high doses, both between different species and, within species, between inbred strains. In many cases a particular tumour could be induced by irradiation in only one or two strains of a given species, raising questions as to whether such tumours represented adequate models of the corresponding human diseases. Similar doubts also applied to some observed forms of dose-response relationships that differed from species to species, although in other cases consistent patterns were found. For these reasons it was concluded that the absolute excess of radiation-induced tumours per unit of dose could not, as a general rule, be extrapolated between species.

6. Despite these reservations, a number of general conclusions were drawn by the Committee in 1977 [U4] relating to the preponderance of tumour types that show an increasing incidence with increasing dose up to a maximum, with a subsequent decline at higher doses. A number of common features in the dose-response data obtained from experimental animals appeared to be consistent with radiobiological effects occurring in single cells, such as cell killing, induction of mutations and chromosome aberrations:

(a) a decrease in the dose rate of low-LET radiation leads, in general, to a decrease of tumour yield, following some inverse function of the exposure time;
(b) high-LET radiation is generally more efficient than low-LET radiation for tumour induction, and the tumour yield often shows little dependence on dose protraction and dose fractionation;
(c) the relative biological effectiveness (RBE) of high-LET compared with low-LET radiation changes with the dose, reflecting the patterns of the dose-response curves for low- and high-LET radiation. At high sublethal doses (>1 Gy) RBE values as low as 1 have been found, but for various tumour types the RBE generally increases with decreasing dose, approaching a maximum at low doses.

These patterns of dose response for low- and high-LET radiation are illustrated in Figure I.

7. It was generally concluded in the UNSCEAR 1977 Report ([U4], Annex G, paragraph 311) that the risk per unit dose of low-LET radiation at low doses and/or dose rates was unlikely to be higher but could be substantially lower than the values derived by linear extrapolation to the range of a few tens of milligray from observations made above 1 Gy. Reduction factors from 2 to 20 were reported between the highest and lowest dose rates tested (1 to 10^{-4} Gy min^{-1}) and between single and extremely fractionated and protracted doses for various animal strains and tumour types.

8. It was specifically noted by the Committee that the Life Span Study of the survivors of the atomic bombings in Japan followed to 1972 gave a risk of leukaemia of 3.5 10^{-3} Gy^{-1} at a mean kerma of 3.3 Gy and 1.8 10^{-3} Gy^{-1} at a mean kerma of 1 Gy, suggesting a reduction factor of 2 for the risk coefficient at the lower dose as compared with that at the higher dose ([U4], Annex G, paragraphs 317 and 318). The Committee in its final estimate of risk adopted a reduction factor of 2.5 for estimating risks at low doses and low dose rates when extrapolating from high dose and dose-rate studies. The Committee also emphasized that this reduction factor was derived essentially from mortalities induced at doses of the order of 1 Gy and that larger reduction factors may be appropriate for assessing risks from occupational or environmental exposure.

9. On the basis of these conclusions by the Committee [U4], the International Commission on Radiological Protection in 1977 [I1] adopted a reduction factor of 2 for assessing the risk of fatalities from radiation-induced leukaemia and solid cancers for radiological protection purposes from high dose and high dose rate studies.

10. In the UNSCEAR 1982 Report [U3] the Committee reviewed information on causes of death in exposed human and animal populations. It concluded that the overwhelming body of evidence showed that at intermediate and low doses, above about 1 Gy (low-LET) life shortening was essentially caused by an increased incidence of tumours. When the contribution to life shortening by these excess tumours was subtracted from total life shortening, there was no evidence of other non-specific mechanisms being involved. The Committee also examined the effect of radiation quality, as well as dose and dose rate, on life-span shortening and reported some conflicting results. For a given total dose, the chronic exposure of mice to both x and gamma rays was less effective than

acute exposure in causing life shortening, suggesting a dose-rate effect on tumour induction. In mice given single acute doses of low-LET radiation, however, the dose response found in different studies varied widely. By pooling many series of studies, an apparently linear relationship was obtained, which might imply no dose-rate dependence. In practice, however, the data could also be fitted with a linear-quadratic relationship, which would be consistent with the observation of a dose-rate effect.

11. In the case of neutron exposure, some studies reported that fractionated or protracted exposures of animals resulted in reduced life shortening compared with single exposures; other studies reported the reverse. The Committee concluded that such variations in response could be due to differences in dose-effect relationships for different tumours in various strains and species. Thus, although life shortening following exposure to high-LET radiation appeared to be fully explained by a higher incidence of tumours, the effect of dose rate on tumour induction as a cause of death was not clear. Further investigations into the effects of dose and dose rate on life shortening in animals exposed to high-LET radiation were needed.

12. In the UNSCEAR 1986 Report [U2], the Committee reviewed evidence at the subcellular and cellular levels relevant to assessing the possible nature of the dose-response relationships for cancer initiation by radiation. It also examined how the initiation of cancerous clones and their progression to clinical tumours may affect the shape of the dose-response relationship. Finally, it examined various models of cancer induction and tested them for compatibility with epidemiological and experimental findings. This provided the basis for some general conclusions on the shape of the dose response and on the uncertainties involved in the assessment of risks at low doses.

13. Three basic non-threshold models of the effect of radiation as a function of dose were considered with respect to both cellular effects and to cancer induction: the linear, the linear-quadratic and the pure quadratic models. Notwithstanding some exceptions, these relationships provided a general framework for a variety of end-points at the cellular level as well as for tumour induction in experimental animals and human populations. The Committee concluded that the vast majority of dose-response curves for induction of point mutations and chromosomal aberrations by low-LET radiation could be represented by a linear-quadratic model at low to intermediate doses; for high-LET radiation, after correction for cell killing, a linear model usually applied. Linearity of the dose response for somatic mutations and terminal chromosomal deletions in some cell lines was noted even for low-LET radiation, although such findings were relatively infrequent.

14. Cell transformation *in vitro* can be regarded as a simplified model of certain stages of radiation carcinogenesis. Cells exposed *in vitro* to low-LET radiation the day after seeding in culture are transformed according to complex kinetics that cannot always be fitted to models used for other cellular effects such as cell killing and the induction of chromosome aberrations. Moreover, dose fractionation (at total doses <1.5 Gy) in some cases enhances transformation frequency, which is inconsistent with a linear-quadratic dependence unless the dose-squared coefficient is negative. In reviewing this material for the UNSCEAR 1986 Report [U2], the Committee felt that further research was needed to elucidate such phenomena, but it was generally considered that these *in vitro* systems gave anomalous results owing to atypical conditions of cellular growth during the early periods after establishment of the culture. Irradiation of non-dividing cells, or cells under exponential conditions of growth, which may be more typical of asynchronously dividing cell populations *in vivo*, produces results that are more consistent with those obtained for other cellular effects. For example, high-dose-rate gamma-irradiation had resulted in a greater transformation frequency per unit dose than low dose-rate exposure. The Committee also noted that in some studies transformation following dose fractionation or dose protraction of high-LET neutron exposure was enhanced at low to intermediate doses, compared with high doses and high dose rates [U2]. In view of the limited extent of such data and the uncertainties regarding the mechanisms involved, further work was needed before these studies could be properly interpreted.

15. The Committee considered that experimental findings on radiation-induced tumours in animals, mainly rats and mice, published since the UNSCEAR 1977 Report [U4] generally supported the view that dose-response relationships for low-LET radiation tended to be curvilinear and concave upward at low dose rates, although for mammary tumours in rats a linear dose response with little dose-fractionation and dose-rate dependence had been obtained. For tumour induction in animals following neutron-irradiation, the response often gave a nearly linear response at low doses, with little dependence on dose rate. In some cases enhancement upon dose fractionation (and possibly dose protraction) had been noted, and at doses above about 0.1 Gy or so the dose-response curve for acute exposure tended to become concave downward. Under such conditions a linear extrapolation to risks at low doses from information at intermediate or high doses and dose rates would underestimate the risk of tumour induction to a variable degree.

16. Review of dose-response relationships for radiation-induced tumours in man indicated that for low-LET radiation in some cases (leukaemia and

cancer of the thyroid, lung and breast), the data available were consistent with linear or linear-quadratic models. For breast cancer, linearity was considered more probable as the incidence was little affected by dose fractionation. From this review [U2], the Committee concluded that for low-LET radiation linear extrapolation downwards from effects measured at doses of about 2 Gy would not overestimate the risk of breast cancer and, possibly, thyroid cancer and would slightly overestimate the risk of leukaemia. There were insufficient data on lung cancer to permit any assessment of the effect of dose rate on tumour induction. On the basis of data on the incidence of bone sarcomas in experimental animals after intakes of beta-emitting radionuclides, it was considered that linear extrapolation could overestimate the risk of their occurrence at low doses. Dose-response curves for radionuclides with long effective half-times do, however, present great difficulty in interpretation [N9].

17. For radiation-induced cancers of most other organs, only data from experimental animals were available on dose-response relationships. For low-LET radiation, linear-quadratic dose-response relationships are commonly found, with pronounced dose-rate and dose-fractionation effects at intermediate doses. The Committee concluded in the UNSCEAR 1986 Report [U2] that if similar curves applied to cancers in man, a linear extrapolation of risk coefficients from acute doses in the intermediate dose region to low doses and low dose rates would very likely overestimate the real risk, suggesting that a reduction factor of up to 5 might apply.

18. For high-LET radiation, human information for lung cancer and bone sarcoma induction was reviewed [U2]. Although the data were limited, they suggested that for lung cancer induction in miners exposed to radon and its decay products, the response was linear initially; at high exposures, however, because of flattening of the response, linear extrapolation could underestimate the risk. The incidence of bone sarcomas after internal contamination by radium isotopes was interpreted as being distorted by a pronounced inverse relationship between accumulated dose and latent period.

19. On the basis of epidemiological studies and experimental investigations it was recommended in the UNSCEAR 1988 Report [U1] that a reduction factor was needed to modify the risks of cancer calculated from exposures to low-LET radiation at high doses and high dose rates for application to low doses and low dose rates, suggesting that an appropriate value for most cancers would lie in the range 2-10, although no specific values were recommended ([U1], Annex F, paragraph 607). For exposure to high-LET radiation, no dose or dose-rate reduction factor was considered necessary for assessing risks at low doses and low dose rates. The Committee indicated that this was a topic that it would consider in its future programme of work.

20. A number of other organizations have considered the effect of dose and dose rate on tumour induction. These include the United States National Council on Radiation Protection and Measurements (NCRP), the Committee on Biological Effects of Ionizing Radiation (BEIR) of the National Research Council of the United States, the United States Nuclear Regulatory Commission (NRC), the International Commission on Radiological Protection (ICRP) and the National Radiological Protection Board (NRPB) of the United Kingdom. Their estimates of reduction factors for calculating cancer risks at low doses and low dose rates are given in Table 1.

21. In 1980, the NCRP reviewed the influence of dose and its distribution in time on dose-response relationships for tumour induction resulting from exposure to low-LET radiation. It was concluded, largely on the basis of animal studies, that the number of cancers induced at low doses and low dose rates are likely to be lower than they are at high doses and high dose rates by a reduction factor in the range 2-10 [N1]. The BEIR V Committee reached similar conclusions on values for the reduction factor that could be obtained from animal studies [C1]. The NCRP [N1] used at that time the term "dose-rate effectiveness factor (DREF)" for this reduction factor, which has also been referred to as "linear extrapolation overestimation factor (LEOF)" and a "low dose extrapolation factor (LDEF)" [P2, P3]. The NCRP [N1] also concluded that human data were insufficient to allow the shape of the dose-response curve to be established or to provide a basis for confident judgements about any diminution in health risks at low doses and dose rates. In view of the complexity and wide spectrum of tumorigenic responses to radiation found in experimental animals, as well as the lack of information on the detailed mechanisms of such responses in animals or man, more specific reduction factors for either individual tumour types or total tumour incidence were not given.

22. In its 1990 recommendations [I2], the ICRP drew attention to the fact that theoretical considerations, experimental results in animals and other biological organisms, and even some limited human experience suggested that cancer induction per unit dose at low doses and low dose rates of low-LET radiation should be less than that observed after high doses and high dose rates. In making a determination of the appropriate value of a reduction factor to be used for radiation protection purposes, the ICRP considered the following:

(a) the wide range of reduction factors obtained in animal experiments (2-10), which may have been obtained for a broader range of doses than human data and therefore may include higher values than are relevant;
(b) the results of statistical analyses of the data on survivors of the atomic bombings in Japan, which do not seem to allow for a reduction factor of much more than about 2;
(c) the human evidence that shows little effect of dose fractionation for some tumour types, with others indicating possible effects of up to 3 or 4 at most;
(d) reduction factors adopted by other organizations for risk estimation at low doses and low dose rates.

23. Based on these considerations, the ICRP adopted in its 1990 recommendations a reduction factor of 2, "recognizing that the choice is somewhat arbitrary and may be conservative". It was recognized that this recommendation on the reduction factor "can be expected to change if new, more definitive information becomes available in the future". In these recommendations the ICRP called this reduction factor the dose and dose-rate effectiveness factor (DDREF).

24. The Committee has identified the need to keep under review information relevant to the assessment of risks at low doses and low dose rates. This Annex reviews data on dose and dose-rate effects for both high- and low-LET radiation with the aim of improving the basis for estimating risks at low doses and low dose rates. It considers first the role of biophysical models in understanding the response of cells to radiation of different qualities and their application in assessing the effect of dose and dose rate on cellular responses. Experimental data on the effect of dose rate in both experimental animals and cells in culture are then reviewed, with emphasis on studies of the effects of low-LET radiation. Relevant epidemiological data are also summarized.

25. Previous UNSCEAR reports have proposed both doses and dose rates at which reduction factors would be expected to apply. Thus in the UNSCEAR 1986 Report [U2] low doses were taken to be those up to 0.2 Gy of low-LET radiation, while those above 2 Gy were regarded as high doses, with intermediate doses lying between these values. Low and high dose rates were taken to be <0.05 mGy min^{-1} and >0.05 Gy min^{-1}, respectively, with intermediate rates between these two extremes. These upper limits on low doses and low dose rates are substantially higher than those that might be expected to prevail in most cases of human exposure. Thus, the ICRP in 1990 recommended an average annual dose limit for workers of 20 mGy (low-LET) [I2]. The average annual dose limit recommended for members of the public is 1 mGy (low-LET) in addition to exposures to natural background radiation [I2].

26. In practice, the majority of workers receive doses much lower than the recommended dose limits, and actual exposure rates are low (see Annex D, "Occupational radiation exposures"). There will, however, be some individuals (e.g. radiographers in hospitals) exposed over short periods of the working day to substantially higher dose rates than the average, although total doses are low. Lifetime doses for a few workers may also be high even though dose rates are low. Information is, therefore, needed on both total doses and dose rates for which the application of a reduction factor is appropriate. Chapter IV examines the physical, experimental and epidemiological basis for the choice of doses and dose rates below which reduction factors might be expected to apply. The choice of the appropriate unit of time over which to assess dose rate is not straightforward. The experimental data reviewed in this Annex cover a wide range of doses, dose rates and exposure conditions. Cellular studies typically involve irradiation times of minutes to hours, while animal studies can involve exposures of days or weeks. The Committee considers that for assessing the risks of stochastic effects in human populations exposure rates should, in general, be averaged over about an hour, which is in line with the repair time of DNA (deoxyribonucleic acid). However, for consistency and to facilitate the comparison of experiments carried out under different exposure conditions, dose rates are given in this Annex in terms of Gy min^{-1} or mGy min^{-1} as far as is possible.

I. DOSE RESPONSE FROM RADIATION EXPOSURE

A. THEORETICAL CONSIDERATIONS

27. Damage to DNA (deoxyribonucleic acid), which carries the genetic information in chromosomes in the cell nucleus, is considered to be the main initiating event through which radiation causes cancer as well as hereditary disease. Present knowledge on the stages in tumour development is described in Annex E, "Mechanisms of radiation oncogenesis". Damage to the DNA of cells has been directly observed experimentally at absorbed doses in excess of about 1 Gy. The DNA molecule has a double helix structure, and

damage in many forms is observable, including single- and double-strand breaks and base damage [C5, H26, M4, T20]. Damage may be detected, but with greater difficulty, at lower doses (0.05-0.1 Gy) [B13]. Damage to chromosomes in human cells can be observed, either at metaphase or interphase [C9, C10], and has been observed in human peripheral blood lymphocytes at doses down to about 0.02 Gy [L13, L14].

28. The effects of radiation on cellular components are thought to occur either through the direct interaction of ionizing particles with DNA molecules or through the action of free radicals or other chemical products produced by the interaction of radiation with neighbouring molecules. Other more indirect mechanisms have also been proposed. Cells are able to repair both single- and double-strand breaks in DNA over a period of a few hours [B13, M4, M15], but sometimes misrepair can occur. Such damage is thought to be the cause of chromosomal aberrations and may also be the origin of both mutational and cancerous transformations as well as death of the cell [G1, R1, U2, Y2]. Spontaneous single-strand damage can also occur in the absence of radiation or other identifiable insults [B41, L23, S39, V3, V9], but this is unlikely to extend to the full range of types of double-strand, clustered damage that radiation can produce [G21, W9].

29. It is commonly presumed that mutational events in germ cells are due to single biological changes but that carcinogenesis is a multi-stage process in which radiation can induce one or more of the stages involving DNA damage [U1, U2]. Guidance as to likely dose and dose-rate effects may therefore be sought from radiobiological data on the cellular effects that result from DNA damage. General mechanistic concepts derived from these data have had a considerable influence on attempts to understand and extrapolate available data on carcinogenesis. It should be recognized, however, that the cellular data are mostly for single-stage radiation effects, principally related to initiation, and that they therefore represent only a part of the complex process of carcinogenesis.

30. It is usually assumed that the primary mutagenic and carcinogenic effects of radiation arise as relatively rare stochastic consequences of damage to individuals cells. Insult from ionizing radiation is always delivered in the form of separate charged particles traversing the cells, each leaving behind a "track" of ionized molecules. Each discrete track consists of the stochastic spatial array of initial ionizations and excitations of molecules in the cell along the path of a primary charged particle and all its secondaries as they pass through the cell in $\leq 10^{-12}$ s [P9, P10]. The pattern of ionizations in each track is governed by cross-sections (probabilities) for individual molecular interactions. Each track is therefore different but has statistical features characteristic of the radiation. On the nanometre scale of DNA and radical diffusion distances in cells, many of the individual ionizations are likely to occur alone and far from any others in the same track, especially for low-LET radiations. However, many other ionizations occur in clusters of dimensions comparable to those of DNA. This clustering is particularly marked for high-LET radiations, but it is also common in tracks of low-LET radiations, largely because of the likelihood of low-energy secondary electrons being produced within the cell [B25, G6, G16, M27, N10]. Because the radiation insult is always in the form of discrete tracks, the radiobiological process may be described in terms of damage to particular target material, using concepts of target theory. In its general form, target theory assumes that the observed all-or-nothing effect is caused by one or more radiation tracks passing through the cell and directly or indirectly causing specific damage to critical components within it. Almost all biophysical models of radiation action incorporate at least some essential concepts of target theory. Model descriptions of the possible radiobiological mechanisms are usually constructed on selected assumptions and deductions [E2, G3, G5]. An approach based on the general concepts of target theory can describe essential elements of the mechanism of radiation insult in an approximately model-independent way. It can indicate how biological processes may modify the simplest responses and how there may be a dependence on physical parameters such as dose rate. This description could apply to any single radiation-induced stage of the multi-stage process of carcinogenesis and to some combinations of stages. Within this general description many specific models can and have been constructed, based on their own specific mechanistic or phenomenological assumptions (see [B33, C5, G17, G22, H23, K5, K6, M34, M39, R12, T21]).

1. Single-hit target theory

31. In the simplest form of target theory, a direct "hit" of any type (i.e. one or more ionizations) in a critical component by a radiation track is assumed to lead, with certainty, to the observable effect in that cell. In this case, the frequency of affected cells in an irradiated population of cells should increase with dose according to the probability of a cell receiving one or more critical hits. Assuming that the hits occur randomly according to a Poisson distribution in a homogeneous population, then the frequency, f, of cells with one or more hits is

$$f = 1 - e^{-n} = 1 - e^{-\lambda D} \quad (1)$$

where n is the mean number of critical hits per cell at dose D and λ is the mean number of critical hits per cell per unit dose. For small n (that is, low frequency effects and/or low doses), the dose response is approximately linear, with

$$f \approx \lambda D \quad (2)$$

At higher frequencies the dose response takes the form of equation 1, which saturates at high frequency because, after the first critical hit in a cell, subsequent hits in it cannot lead to additional effect. If a negative effect is being measured, such as frequency of surviving cells (that is, cells without a critical hit), then the dose response is

$$f^1 = 1 - f = e^{-\lambda D} \quad (3)$$

where f^1 is the frequency of cells without a critical hit. This very simple form of target theory, where every elementary hit is biologically effective, may be applicable to the inactivation of many molecules in the dry state and to some viruses, but it is not, in general, appropriate for micro-organisms and mammalian cells, because of their well-established capacity to repair radiation damage and the consequent modification of dose response.

32. More refined forms of single-hit target theory could include variable probability of effect depending on the type ("severity") of a hit and on the cellular reparability of the damage and could also include extension of the size of the target for indirect effects. Provided that the tracks act totally independently of one another in regard to each of these processes, the dose response should still conform to equations 1-3 because the final effective damage should still be randomly distributed among the cells [L3]. The numerical value of λ should now be modified to reflect the combined probability, per cell and per unit dose, of all these single-track processes leading to final effective damage. Indirect effects should increase the value of λ, while biochemical repair should reduce it. Therefore, experimental observation of linear or exponential dose response does not, of itself, indicate that damage cannot be modified and/or repaired by the cell.

2. Multi-track effects

33. Further extension of concepts of target theory can consider additional contributions from two or more tracks, which may modify the probability of effect due to the damage from single tracks alone. Since this modification may be positive or negative, it may introduce corresponding visible curvature to the dose response. Ways in which multiple tracks could increase the probability of effect include the following:

(a) reduction in efficiency of cellular repair of individual points of damage by increasing the overall burden of damage (for example, by partial saturation of the repair process [G17, S40, W10] or induction of damage-fixation processes);

(b) interaction or interference between points of damage to make them less repairable [C5, C28, K6] (for example, formation of exchange events within or between chromosomes [H23]);

(c) production of a series of other independent changes that together increase the overall probability of the final effect (for example, to cause a single-stage effect [K5] or to cause multiple stages in full neoplastic transformation [M39]).

By contrast, decreases in the probability of effect by multiple tracks could occur by the following means:

(d) enhancement of cellular repair (for example, induction of additional repair capabilities [B37, G5, O3, P8]);

(e) elimination of some of the cells from the population by transferring them to a state in which the effect cannot be expressed (for example, by loss of cell viability).

Other processes, such as multi-track perturbation of the cell cycle, have the potential either to increase or to decrease the probability of effect. The reduction of dose rate increases the time intervals between tracks and therefore is likely to alter the contributions from these multiple-track processes.

34. Simple mathematical extension of equations 1-3, now to include multi-track effects, may be made by means of a general polynomial. Those equations are therefore replaced in general by

$$f = 1 - e^{-(\alpha_1 D + \alpha_2 D^2 ...)} \quad (4)$$

For low-frequency effects, the equation is

$$f \approx \alpha_1 D + \alpha_2 D^2 ... \quad (5)$$

and for negative effects it is

$$f^1 = 1 - f = e^{-(\beta_1 D + \beta_2 D^2 ...)} \quad (6)$$

designating the coefficients as β_1 and β_2 to denote that these are negative effects.

35. Attempts to interpret and apply the coefficients α_1, α_2, ... and β_1, β_2, ... must usually rely on particular assumptions of radiobiological mechanisms. Many investigations, including experiments, theory and model formulations, are aimed at identifying the assumptions that may be most reasonable under given circumstances. Without such mechanistic considerations, the coefficients provide no more than fitted values, which may be valid only in the limited range of the experimental data themselves. Quite different mechanistic assumptions can lead to equations such as

equations 4-6, either directly or as the first terms of polynomial expansion approximations. For example, a dose-squared term can arise directly from two tracks damaging separate chromosomes, which then undergo an exchange interaction, or from two tracks creating deletions in complementary chromosomes, causing the loss of both alleles of a gene. By contrast an apparent dose-squared term can arise from multiple tracks increasing the overall burden of damage in a cell and thereby partially saturating a repair system and reducing the probability of repair of particular damage from any one track [G17, S40, W10]. The reliability of extrapolations to low doses, below the range of the fitted data, may depend substantially on the appropriateness of the mechanistic assumptions for these single cellular effects as well as their relevance to carcinogenesis. For example, for exchange aberrations there would be a clear expectation of a substantial linear term to the lowest doses owing to the ability of a single track to damage two separate chromosomes; such a one-track occurrence would be much less probable for a deletion of two identical alleles, but much more probable for a single deletion, which alone may be adequate to enhance carcinogenesis. In the case of saturable repair, extrapolation to low doses would depend largely on the competition between repair and fixation/misrepair processes and whether any types of damage are essentially unrepairable.

36. When the equation is applied to describe a low-frequency effect, such as carcinogenesis or mutagenesis, arising from a given initial population of cells, it may be convenient to separate out the influence of radiation-induced loss of cell viability by replacing equation 5 with

$$f \approx (\alpha_1 D + \alpha_2 D^2 + ...) S(D) \quad (7)$$

where S(D) is the fraction of cells which survive dose D. S(D) itself may be described by the form of equation 6. With high-LET radiation, it may be necessary to consider also correlations between induction of the initial carcinogenic damage and loss of cell viability by the same radiation track [G15]. Additional non-linearity may arise if adjacent cells can be involved in control of the growth of an altered cell.

37. It is frequently found that only the first two terms of the polynomials in equations 4-7 are needed to describe the experimental data. Most effects on cells (e.g. chromosome aberrations) resulting from low to intermediate doses are fitted, therefore, to a linear-quadratic equation without including powers of dose greater than D^2. This simplification may be reasonable for radiobiological mechanisms underlying some of the possible multi-track processes described in paragraph 33, particularly under processes (a) and (b) and especially if only two-track interactions occur. A two-term polynomial is unlikely, however, to be adequate to describe and interpolate over the full dose response, if it includes processes (c) and (d). From reviews of published data it can be deduced that considerable differences are observed between cells of different origins with respect to the values of α_1 and α_2 [B6, B7, T6]. For a dose response that can be fitted with only the first two terms in the polynomials in equations 4-7 the quotient α_1/α_2 equals the dose at which the linear and quadratic components contribute equally to the observed cellular damage.

38. An example of the type of response of equation 7 is provided by observations of myeloid leukaemia frequency in male CBA/H mice after 10 different doses of x rays in the range 0.25-6 Gy inclusive, delivered at 0.5 Gy min^{-1} [M14] (Figure II). Median survival in all groups was similar, and there was essentially no association between induction period and dose. The results were fitted by a four-term polynomial of the form

$$(\alpha_1 D + \alpha_2 D^2)\, e^{-(\beta_1 D + \beta_2 D^2)} \quad (8)$$

and four simplifications of it. The only functions with all parameters significantly greater than zero were:

$$\alpha_2 D^2\, e^{-\beta_1 D} \quad \text{and} \quad \alpha_1 D\, e^{-\beta_2 D^2} \quad (9)$$

The latter function was rejected because no cell survival response depending solely on D^2 is known. The observed data could therefore be well fitted by the function

$$\alpha_2 D^2\, e^{-\beta_1 D} \quad (10)$$

although none of the alternative functions could be rejected on statistical grounds. A similar dose response for myeloid leukaemia induction in CBA mice was reported by Di Majo [D2].

3. Low doses and low dose rates: microdosimetric considerations

39. For a homogeneous cell population, the dose response for an effect arising solely from a single track interacting independently with cellular target(s) should conform with equation 1 and should be simply linear with dose (equation 2) if the frequency of effect is small. It should extend linearly down to zero dose, with no threshold, because reducing the dose simply reduces the number of tracks proportionately and, consequently, the frequency of effect. The dose response should be independent of dose rate, because the time interval between tracks is irrelevant if the tracks are acting totally independently. There may, of course, be many other interactions that are adequately repaired and do not manifest themselves as damage.

40. If the cell population is inhomogeneous, with subpopulations of differing sensitivity, the dose response for single-track effects in each subpopulation should follow the form of equation 1, and the overall response should therefore show a decreasing sensitivity with increasing dose. Any other deviations from the form of equation 1 must be due to the effect of multiple tracks in some way or another. These deviations, however, need not be obviously apparent over all portions of the dose response. Hence, apparent linearity over an experimentally accessible portion of the dose response does not guarantee that only single-track processes are involved in that region or that extrapolation to lower dose is linear. In general, it is expected that multi-track processes may depend on dose rate as the mean time interval between tracks is varied. Referring to the example above, simple expectations are that a reduction of dose rate would reduce the effectiveness of radiation acting via processes (a) and (b) (paragraph 33). Predictions for the other processes are less clear, because they are likely to depend on the timings of the particular processes in relation to the intervals between tracks and the overall irradiation time. For most single-stage processes, it may be expected that at very low dose rates multi-track effects will become negligible, because the tracks become effectively independent in time; in this limit the dose response should conform to equations 1-3.

41. Available experimental and epidemiological data on radiation carcinogenesis can be considered in terms of three regions of the dose response on the basis of fundamental microdosimetric considerations assuming that the cell nucleus is the relevant sensitive volume to define the limit of possible multi-track effects. These are illustrated in Figure III by schematic dose-response curves, consistent with the form of equation 7, for frequency of an effect such as a type of tumour induced by gamma rays, neutrons or alpha particles. The upper part of the Figure shows the response plotted against dose on a linear scale. The lower part shows the identical curves plotted on a logarithmic scale to magnify the lower dose region; on this part a separate dose axis is provided for each radiation type. The logarithmic plot also marks on a common axis the mean number of tracks per cell nucleus (assuming spherical nuclei of 8 μm diameter for these illustrations). In this way, the correspondence between dose and number of tracks can be read off for each radiation. This correspondence has been calculated [C25, G5] by established microdosimetric methods based on experimental and theoretical data [B42, C24, G2, G4, Z2]. In this Figure the dose scale is divided into three approximate dose regions, as described below.

42. ***Dose region I (low-dose region).*** In this dose region there are so few radiation tracks that a single cell (or nucleus) is very unlikely to be traversed by more than one track. In this region of "definite" single-track action (less than ~0.2 mGy for ^{60}Co gamma rays; see Section IV.A), the dose response for single-cell effects is almost bound to be linear and independent of dose rate. This is because varying the dose proportionately varies the number of cells singly traversed, and varying the dose rate varies only the time between these independent events. These simple expectations would be violated only if the rare multi-traversals greatly enhanced the probability of effect, such as may be the case if radiation carcinogenesis requires two radiation-induced stages well separated in time. There are no epidemiological or experimental data in or near this region for low-LET radiation, although a few may approach it for high-LET alpha particles and neutrons [C25, D5]. There is, therefore, little direct information about how a cell or a tissue may respond to the damage from a single radiation track.

43. This is, however, the region of main concern in radiation protection. For example, a worker who has received uniform whole-body gamma-ray exposure spread over a year equal to an annual equivalent dose limit of 50 mSv [I1], corresponding to an absorbed dose of 50 mGy (Q = 1), will have received over the full year an average of about 50 electron tracks through each cell nucleus in his body. Multi-track processes should then be relevant only if they operate over long periods of time comparable at least to the times between tracks (days). If, instead, the irradiation is uniform with only 1 MeV neutrons (and ignoring attenuation, energy degradation or gamma-ray production in the body), then the 50 mSv limit corresponds to 5 mGy of neutrons (Q = 10) and an average of about 0.05 directly ionizing tracks (mostly high-LET recoil protons from the indirectly ionizing neutrons) through each cell nucleus during the year. These tracks must clearly act independently unless multi-track processes persist over very long periods of time, extending to many years. Exposure is seldom uniform in the body or in time, and cell nuclei have a variety of sizes and shapes. Nevertheless, the dose and dose-rate region of main practical relevance in radiation protection (0-50 mSv per year) is characterized by small average numbers of tracks per cell with long intervals of time between them. Effects are, therefore, likely to be dominated by individual track events, acting alone. This dominance will be even greater with the introduction of the ICRP recommendations of 1990 [I2] which propose an average annual limit of equivalent dose of 20 mSv and increased radiation weighting factors for neutrons (>100 keV to 2 MeV, w_R = 20).

44. For the purposes of this microdosimetric criterion for a low dose, the cell nucleus (approximated here as an 8 μm diameter sphere) has been considered to be the sensitive volume in which multiple tracks may be

able to influence the effects of one another. This choice is based on the assumption that radiation carcinogenesis is due to radiation damage to the nuclear DNA of a single cell and that biochemical processes, including repair and misrepair, may operate over the full dimensions of the nucleus. If influence can extend over larger distances, say from tracks in the cell cytoplasm or in adjacent cells, then the microdosimetric criterion for a low dose would need to be decreased. Conversely, if smaller regions can act totally autonomously in respect of initial radiation damage and its repair or misrepair, then the criterion would be increased. In the extreme, if each short (say, 6 base pair) segment of DNA were totally autonomous for damage and repair, then the microdosimetric criterion for a low dose of low-LET radiation would be as large as 10^9 mGy [G6]. This is clearly much too large compared to the doses at which multi-track processes have been observed experimentally by curvature of dose-response or dose-rate dependence in cellular and animal systems (Chapter II). Criteria for designating low doses and low dose rates are discussed further in Chapter IV.

45. *Dose region II (intermediate-dose region).* In this dose region it is commonly assumed that tracks act independently if a linear term (α_1) is obtainable by curve-fitting to equations such as 4-7. However, for most of the epidemiological and experimental animal data used for dose-response curve fitting, the lowest dose at which a significant effect is obtained is usually towards the higher doses of this dose region, when individual cells may, in fact, have been traversed by considerable numbers of tracks.

46. The assumption of one-track action for this region considers that the relevant metabolic processes of the cell are not influenced by the additional tracks in any way that could alter the efficiency of these processes and, therefore, the expression of the ultimate biological damage of each individual track. This region of the dose response, then, should be independent of dose rate. On these assumptions, it is conventional to interpolate linearly from this region to zero dose in order to deduce the effectiveness of low doses and low dose rates of radiation, dose region I. Such interpolation is based on the coefficient α_1 in equations 4-7 and on the assumption that it remains unchanged even to very low doses and very low dose rates in dose region I. There are a number of radiobiological studies, mostly with cells *in vitro*, but also from animals exposed at different dose rates, which suggest that this common assumption is not universally valid (see Sections I.A.4, I.A.5, II.A. and II.B).

47. *Dose region III (high-dose region).* In this dose region, there are often clearly observable multi-track processes causing upward or downward curvature of the dose response, including cooperative effects and also competing processes such as cell killing. Dependence on dose rate is, therefore, usually to be expected because of time dependence in the multi-track process. Mechanisms in this dose region need to be adequately understood and described if such data are to be used for curve-fitting and extrapolation, together with data from dose region II, to the low doses and low dose rates of prime relevance in radiation protection.

4. Radiation quality and relative biological effectiveness

48. A very wide range of radiobiological data on the doses required to produce a given level of effect have shown that high-LET radiation, including neutrons and alpha particles, is more effective than low-LET radiation [S12]. This greater effectiveness is usually particularly marked in the regions of intermediate and low dose, which implies that the individual high-LET tracks have a greater probability of effect than a very much larger number of low-LET tracks. Thus the concentration of energy deposition within the high-LET tracks more than compensates for the reduced number of tracks per unit dose.

49. The relative biological effectiveness (RBE) values of particular relevance in radiation protection are those that apply in the true low-dose region I, in which tracks are most likely to act individually. At these minimally low doses the RBE of a given radiation should be constant and independent of dose and dose rate, because varying the dose for both high- and low-LET radiation varies only the number of cells that are traversed by single tracks. This RBE, at minimal doses, could in principle be calculated by direct comparison of measured effectiveness per unit dose of neutrons and low-LET radiation in the low-dose region I, or from experimental measurements of the effectiveness of single tracks of the radiation. Current experimental methods have not been able to achieve this.

50. Instead, it is conventional to assume that the RBE at minimal doses is also the maximum RBE and that it can be estimated as the ratio of the α_1 values of the two radiations, determined by fitting equations such as 4-7 to the available data at intermediate and high doses. This method assumes that the multiple tracks in the intermediate-dose region do not influence the effectiveness of each other at all and, consequently, that the α_1 values are constant down to zero dose and independent of dose rate. This assumption is best supported for high-LET radiation, for which *in vitro* radiobiological data usually show strongly linear dose responses that vary little with dose rate, with some data approaching the true single-track region. Notable exceptions have been reported, however, in

cellular, animal and human systems (see, e.g. [C22, C25, D5, F9, F10, J2, K8, H9, M28, R13, S13, T7, T8, U16]). The assumption of constant α_1, independent of dose rate, for low-LET reference radiation is also called into question by data from numerous studies on cellular, and some animal, systems (e.g. [B34, C12, C20, F1, F10, F13, F4, I8, K8, M16, M33, O4, S3, S14, S32, T2, W6]). The general approach of estimating risks of high-LET radiations by means of RBE values would not be applicable to effects that were qualitatively different for, or unique to, high-LET radiations. There are indications that such unique effects may arise in some cellular systems, including the induction of sister chromatid exchanges by irradiation of human lymphocytes before stimulation [A11, A4, S42] and the radiation induction of chromosomal instabilities in haemopoietic stem cells [K9]. There are also indications of qualitative differences in early cellular changes during the development of mammary tumours in mice [U25] and in other *in vivo* effects [H33].

5. Deviations from conventional expectations

51. The conventional approach to estimating both absolute biological effectiveness and relative biological effectiveness at minimal doses is based on the assumption of constant α_1 values from dose region II down to zero dose and independence of dose rate. There are, in principle, many ways in which this may not be the case.

52. For single-cell effects, the assumption may not hold if there are significant multi-track processes in the intermediate-dose region. Such processes could include, for example, the induction of multiple independent steps in radiation carcinogenesis, cellular damage-fixation processes and the induction of enhanced repair by small numbers of tracks. There is strong evidence of induction of repair or amplification of gene products in microbes [S41] and some such indications in mammalian cells [L15, W6]. Possibilities that have been suggested to explain observed dose-rate dependence of neutron-induced cell transformation include promotion by multiple tracks or enhancement of misrepair [H10], variations of cell sensitivity with time [B30, R5] and induction or enhancement of repair [G5].

53. The general approach described in this Annex would also need appreciable modification if the biological effect of interest required damage to more than one cell or if it is influenced by damage to additional cells. For example, van Bekkum et al. [V1] and Mole [M14] have hypothesized that radiation tumorigenesis involves the transfer of DNA from one radiation-inactivated cell to an adjacent radiation-damaged cell. In this case the true low-dose region I of action by individual tracks alone would correspond to even lower doses than in Figure III, because the volume containing the target would need to be enlarged to include adjacent cells. This two-cell hypothesis could be experimentally testable with epithermal neutrons, whose individual proton-recoil tracks are too short to hit the nuclei of two adjacent cells [G5].

54. Some of the above processes allow, in principle, for the possibility of a true threshold in the dose-effect curve, especially for low-LET radiation. The most basic, although not sufficient, condition for a true dose threshold is that any single track of the radiation should be totally unable to produce the effect. Thus, no biological effect would be observed in the true low-dose region (region I), where cells are hit only by single tracks. There is little experimental evidence to demonstrate such a situation, although collaborative studies in six laboratories on the induction of unstable chromosomal aberrations in blood lymphocytes given acute doses of x rays of 0, 3, 5, 6, 10, 20, 30, 50 and 300 mGy were able to demonstrate significant increases in aberration yield at doses greater than 20 mGy. Below 20 mGy the observed dicentric yield was generally lower than in controls, but not significantly so. Excess acentric aberrations and centric rings, on the other hand, were higher than in controls, although the increase was generally not significant. It was concluded that even though these studies involved scoring chromosome aberrations in a total of about 300,000 metaphases some variation was observed between the different laboratories involved, and the lack of statistical precision did not allow linear or threshold models at doses below 20 mGy to be distinguished [L14]. Data on the induction of stable chromosome aberrations in blood lymphocytes from individuals of various ages have also been reported [L1] for doses in the range 50 to 500 mGy. In lymphocytes from newborns chromosome aberrations increased roughly in proportion to the dose. In young adults, however, aberrations were not detected at doses of 50 and 100 mGy and for adults not even at 200 mGy. The difference in detection of aberrations was attributed to a high background of aberrations in older ages, compared with the newborn. Of the aberrations examined, one-break terminal deletions were the best indicators of exposure at low doses.

B. MULTI-STAGE MODELS OF CARCINOGENESIS

1. Multi-stage models

55. In order to become fully malignant, a cell needs to undergo a number of phenotypic changes (see Annex E, "Mechanisms of radiation oncogenesis").

Evidence from diverse sources suggests that changes can be considered as occurring in many stages. This Section describes quantitative models that have been previously developed for multi-stage carcinogenesis. The true nature of the individual biological changes is considered in more detail in Annex E.

56. The first stochastic multi-stage model for the development of full malignancy from a normal cell was proposed in 1954 by Armitage and Doll to account for observations that the age-specific incidence rates for many adult carcinomas were proportional to a power of age [A8]. According to this model, which has been widely used in risk assessment, a normal cell can undergo progressive deterioration in a finite number of stages to reach full malignancy. The authors later proposed a two-stage model in which cells multiply exponentially after undergoing the first change and become malignant after the second change [A9]. A similar two-stage model was proposed for carcinogenesis in animals [N8].

57. None of the above models take into account the growth and development of the normal tissue. A model that does include growth and differentiation was proposed by Knudsen et al. for embryonal tumours [H24, K7]. This model has subsequently been developed to a form that is claimed to give a good qualitative description of the age-specific incidence curves of all human tumours [M17, M38] and an excellent quantitative fit to incidence data for several human tumours that were tested [M42]. The working hypothesis underlying this model is based on a genetic regulatory schema postulated by Comings in 1973 [C27]. However, the formalism and parameters of the model are not dependent on the particular biological identities of the critical targets and changes. According to the schema all cells contain genes, termed "oncogenes", capable of coding for transforming factors that can release the cell from normal growth constraints. The oncogenes are expressed during histogenesis and tissue renewal and are normally controlled by diploid pairs of regulatory genes, termed "anti-oncogenes". A cell acquires the malignant phenotype when an oncogene is expressed at an appropriately high level, owing either to inactivation of both of the appropriate pair of anti-oncogenes or by direct activation of the oncogene itself. This latter may occur, for example, if the oncogene becomes positioned adjacent to a promoter as a result of chromosomal rearrangement or viral insertion. This two-stage model presupposes that human tumours most commonly arise by mutations of the anti-oncogenes. Evidence for this process of carcinogenesis comes from, among other things, analyses of familial tumours, such as childhood retinoblastoma and Wilms' tumour and adult familial polyposis carcinoma of the colon. Studies of these tumours indicate that an inactivated anti-oncogene can be inherited, which means that it is present in this stage in all cells of the individual, greatly increasing the potential for malignancy to develop. Nevertheless, in such an individual at least one other event is necessary for malignancy. In a normal individual, whose cells carry only normal pairs of anti-oncogenes, at least two changes should be necessary. It is recognized that this two-stage model may not apply to some tumours that are due to direct oncogene activation and that may be characterized by specific chromosome rearrangements, possibly including lymphoma and leukaemia [M42].

58. In this two-stage model, agents that act as mutagens, to increase the probability of inactivating either one or both of the anti-oncogenes, may be regarded as tumour "initiators". Tumour "promoters" may be assumed to modify cell kinetics and in particular to encourage clonal expansion by greater mitotic activity of cells that have undergone the first-stage change, thereby increasing the chances that at least one of them subsequently undergoes the second change and hence becomes malignant [M41, M42].

59. To apply these multi-stage models to environmental mutagens, one or more of the rates of mutation, or of other changes, may be made a function of dose [M38]. Dose rate or duration of exposure would also need to be considered in relation to the kinetics of the normal and changed cells [M39]. When the two-stage model was fitted to data on lung cancer in mice exposed to a single acute dose of gamma rays, the results were consistent with the hypothesis that brief exposure to radiation acts by enhancing the rate of the first mutation in a proportion of the cells [C21]. It might be expected that subsequent exposure, either by protraction or as a later brief second exposure, would also be capable of inducing by chance the second mutation in those few cells that had undergone the first mutation.

60. A two-stage model of induction of osteosarcoma by alpha particles was formulated by Marshall and Groer [M34] to fit the entire dose-time-response data from radiation in man and dog. The model assumed two alpha-particle-induced initiation events and a subsequent promotion event not related to radiation. Competition by alpha-particle killing of cells was included. The model predicted that the tumour rate should become independent of dose rate at less than 10 mGy d^{-1} and that over the lower dose range of the available data the rate would be proportional to dose squared and at high doses become independent of dose (plateau). On the assumption that the two initiation events arise from damage to two different structures in the cell (rather than to one structure that must be damaged at two separate times), it was concluded that at doses of less than ~400-1,000 mGy the tumour rate

would be predominantly due to a linear component of dose, because both structures are damaged by a single alpha-particle track [M34, M35]. In an earlier two-stage model for radiation carcinogenesis, Burch [B35] assumed that the two changes (regarded as chromosome breaks) needed to be caused by radiation at different times and, as a consequence, the tumour rate at low doses depended purely on the dose squared.

61. The net effect of protracting of radiation exposure would generally be difficult to predict from multi-stage models, because it would depend on a complex combination of the effect of dose rate on each individual mutagenic or other change; the cell kinetics, and therefore cell numbers, between the changes; and whether or not there is a preferred or required temporal relationship between the changes themselves. Even within the relative simplicity of a two-stage model, clear expectations for dose and dose-rate dependence would require determining numerous parameters of the model, including their radiation dependence (dose, dose rate, quality), for the particular cancer [L24]. There is clearly scope, in principle, for expectations of reduced effectiveness at reduced dose rates, owing for example to reduced mutation rates at each stage or to selective disadvantage in growth kinetics for cells that have undergone the first change relative to normal cells. Conversely, there is also scope for expectations of increased effectiveness at reduced dose rates, due for example to increased rates of mutation at each stage (by analogy, perhaps, with the increased transformation and mutation rates reported with high-LET radiation in some *in vitro* systems [H9, J2, M28, R13]) or to selective advantage and clonal expansion of cells that have undergone the first change. The range of possible expectations becomes even wider in the likely event that carcinogenesis depends on more than two stages, particularly if radiation as well as other environmental or spontaneous factors can play a role in a number of these changes.

2. Thresholds in the dose-effect relationships

62. A necessary, but not sufficient, condition for an absolute threshold in the radiation dose-effect relationship is that any single track produced by the radiation is totally incapable of producing the biological effect. This absolute criterion can be considered at three levels of changes in the carcinogenic process: the initial elementary physicochemical changes to biological molecules, the repairability and combinations (if any) of molecular damage required to produce single-stage cellular changes, and the combinations (if any) of separate cellular changes required for a cell to reach full malignancy. Even when the criterion does apply, multi-track effects may be sufficient to preclude a true threshold, although the dose response should then tend to zero slope as the dose tends to zero.

63. Biophysical analyses based on Monte Carlo simulations of radiation track structure show clearly that all types of ionizing radiation should be capable of producing, by single-track action, a variety of damage to DNA, including double-strand breaks alone or in combination with associated damage to the DNA and adjacent proteins [C26, G6, G20]. In essence, this is because all ionizing radiation produces low-energy secondary electrons, and these can cause localized clusters of atomic ionizations and excitations over the dimensions of the DNA helix. Hence, for these types of early molecular damage there can be no real prospect of a threshold in the dose-response relationship for any ionizing radiation. This statement is even more categorical for high-LET radiation, which is capable of producing even greater clusters of ionizations and excitations over the dimensions of DNA and its higher-order structures (see Table 2 [G6, G20]).

64. Expectations of a dose threshold for cellular effects depend on the assumptions that are made regarding cellular repair and the combinations of molecular damage that are required to cause the effect. Very many different mechanistic biophysical models have been proposed to explain radiation-induced cellular effects such as cell inactivation, mutation and chromosome aberrations. Some of these models have been summarized by Goodhead [G3, G19]. There has developed from these models a near-consensus that the biologically critical damage by which single tracks can lead to cellular effect is dominated by local properties of the track structure over dimensions of 0.1-50 nm. The mechanistic models variously assume that the cellular effect is the result of the following: DNA double-strand breaks either singly [C5, C23, R12], both singly and in pairs [P7] or in larger numbers [G22]; pairs of DNA single-strand breaks [R15] or simple damage to pairs of unspecified atoms such that the damage to each is due to single ionizations or excitations only, independent of radiation quality [K6, Z1]; pairs of unspecified chromatin damage [H23, V4]; localized clusters of radiation damage in unspecified molecular targets, either singly or in targets of dimensions similar to DNA [G16, G20] or nucleosomes [G18, G20] depending on radiation quality, or singly and in pairs in targets of unspecified dimensions [C28]; unspecified single or double lesions, probably in DNA, but qualitatively similar independent of radiation quality [T21]; multiple (two or more) ionizations in small structured targets [B36]; or damage to DNA and associated nuclear membrane [A7]. In all these mechanistic models a single radiation track from any radiation is capable of producing the full damage and hence the cellular effect.

65. In agreement with these mechanistic models, track structure analyses, as well as simple linear extrapolations to low dose of measured biochemical damage, indicate that a single track, even from the lowest-LET radiation, has a finite probability of producing one, or more than one, double-strand break in a cell (Table 3). Hence, cellular consequences of a double-strand break or of interactions between them should be possible even at the lowest doses or dose rates. This expectation would be contradicted for low-LET radiation only if cellular repair of small numbers of double-strand breaks, even with associated damage, were totally efficient in all the cells. There is no evidence to demonstrate this, but existing experimental assays are not able to test it extensively due to limited resolution of types and quantities of damage.

66. In addition to mechanistic models of cellular effect, as above, there are current phenomenological models based on correlation of effect with patterns of radiation energy deposition over much larger distances of ~1μm [B33, F12, H25, K5]. Even these approaches, with one exception [H25, K5], agree that a single radiation track can produce the cellular effect. The one exception agrees for high-LET radiation, but it assumes that for low-LET radiation the damage from a number of tracks has to accumulate before any cellular effect is possible. This assumption leads to an initial slope of zero, although not a true threshold. Experimental support for this assumption is lacking.

67. Despite their very different assumptions and almost without exception, these biophysical models lead to the common view that a single track of any ionizing radiation is capable of producing cellular changes, including mutations and chromosome aberrations. On this basis no absolute dose threshold would be expected for the individual cellular changes responsible for individual stages of the carcinogenic process. The difficulty of experimentally proving, or disproving, this expected total lack of a dose threshold for single cellular changes is complicated by the possibilities of adaptation or induced repair after small numbers of tracks [C20, I8, M33, O3, O4, P8, S3, S32, W6]. However, unless such "adaptation" is so fast that it can act with total efficiency on the very first track itself, it would not be able to introduce a true dose threshold, although it might complicate the shape of the dose response at slightly higher doses and also its dose-rate dependence.

68. The final level at which an absolute dose threshold might exist is at the two (or more) stages of two-stage (or multi-stage) carcinogenesis. The simplest such situation would arise if the malignancy required that radiation should bring about both changes and that they should be well separated in time. Then, one track would be totally unable to achieve this, and so even would any single, brief exposure. If the exposure were protracted or repeated, or if the time separation were not required, but if a single track were still incapable, then the slope of the dose response would tend to zero as the dose tended to zero (as, for example, in a pure dose-squared dependence). Although this would not imply a true threshold, the risk would become vanishingly small at the lowest doses. There are, however, many ways in which these requirements could, in principle, be violated and thereby introduce a finite slope without a threshold or vanishing risk. These include:

(a) if malignancy could result from the two essential changes occurring at the same time from a single track, especially if it were a high-LET track;
(b) if one or other of the two changes could occur spontaneously, or as a consequence of other environmental factors, so that only one radiation-induced change was necessary, as suggested, for example, when the two-stage model was fitted to lung tumours in mice after brief exposure to radiation [C21]; the occurrence of spontaneous tumours does also indicate that all the changes can occur without radiation;
(c) if the cells of an individual already had one change due to inheritance so that only one radiation change was sufficient for malignancy;
(d) if the malignancy could result from a single radiation-activated oncogene instead of solely from a pair of inactivated anti-oncogenes;

69. In view of these many possibilities, it would be difficult to conclude on theoretical grounds that a true threshold should be expected even from multi-stage mechanisms of carcinogenesis, unless there were clear evidence that it was necessary for more than one time-separated change to be caused by radiation alone. The multitude of animal and human data showing an increase in tumours after a single brief exposure to radiation and also the occurrence of spontaneous tumours in the absence of radiation, implies that these restrictions do not apply in general. These theoretical considerations cannot preclude the possibility of particular situations where the probability of an effect at low doses may be very small, and even practically negligible, compared with that at higher doses. This topic is considered further in Annex E, "Mechanisms of radiation oncogenesis".

C. MECHANISMS OF DOSE-RATE EFFECTS IN MAMMALIAN CELLS

70. For low-LET radiation, dose rate has been shown to be a major factor in the response of mammalian cells. Since the early days of cellular radiobiology, the sparing effects of dose protraction have been interpreted as reflecting increased repair of induced cellular damage. The magnitude of dose-rate effect for cell

inactivation varies between different cell strains; this is reflected usually, but not always, by the extent of the shoulder on acute dose-response curves [H2].

1. Repair of DNA damage

71. There is strong evidence from a range of *in vitro* cellular studies that the most significant detrimental effects of radiation derive from its ability to damage DNA in mammalian cells (see Annex E, "Mechanisms of radiation oncogenesis"), and if this is the case then it can be assumed that the fidelity of repair of induced DNA damage is a major determinant of the dose-rate effect, although there are many other factors involved in the subsequent development of a tumour following the initial DNA lesion. Direct evidence on this issue has been obtained through studies with radiosensitive mutants of mammalian cells that carry defects in DNA processing.

72. Ataxia-telangiectasia (AT) is an autosomal recessive genetic disease with complex clinical manifestations [M10]. Radiotherapeutic observations provide clear evidence of the *in vivo* sensitivity of ataxia-telangiectasia patients to low-LET radiation. Studies *in vitro* show ataxia-telangiectasia radiosensitivity to have a cellular basis, and for acute doses AT cells show a two- to threefold increase in their sensitivity to the lethal and clastogenic effects of low-LET radiation [L5, T5]. However, most importantly, the ataxia-telangiectasia mutation(s) almost completely abolishes both the capacity of cells to repair x-ray-induced potentially lethal damage and any sparing effect of gamma-ray dose protraction. The effect of the ataxia-telangiectasia mutation(s) on human cellular radiosensitivity was most dramatic after chronic gamma-ray exposure at a dose rate of 2 mGy min^{-1}; where after an accumulated dose of 2 Gy, the number of unrepaired lethal lesions in a normal cell strain was ~0.3 per cell, while the corresponding value for ataxia-telangiectasia strains was ~5.0 [C12]. These data, together with those on potentially lethal damage repair after acute doses, have been used to argue that the rate at which cells sustain radiation damage is a major factor in the efficiency of repair and that ataxia-telangiectasia cells are blocked in a major radiation repair pathway [C12]. Biochemical studies so far appear to have failed to identify a consistent DNA-repair defect in ataxia-telangiectasia cases, including DNA double-strand break rejoining [L5, T4]. However, using a molecular assay based on the cell-mediated rejoining of restriction endonuclease induced DNA double-strand breaks in plasmid DNA substrates, some evidence for reduced fidelity of double-strand break rejoining has been obtained in the Sv40-transformed ataxia-telangiectasia cell line [C13, T4]. However, further studies failed to observe a similar effect with a related plasmid [G11], suggesting that an apparent effect on overall transfection frequency is related not only to repair deficiency but also to sensitivity of potential transfectants to the selective agent. A reduction in repair fidelity has also been reported in a radiosensitive mutant of V79 Chinese hamster cells [D1], but there are still no data on dose-rate effects in this mutant. It might be expected that inaccurate repair of double-strand breaks *in vivo* might lead to increased ionizing radiation mutability. Ataxia-telangiectasia cells, however, show normal spontaneous or ultraviolet mutability, and although they show increased chromosome rearrangements following exposure to ionizing radiation, they show either a reduced mutability or an increased incidence of mutation similar to normal cells [G11, T22]. In Annex E, "Mechanisms of radiation oncogenesis", it is noted that cell mutagenesis and DNA repair data may be used to argue that oncogenic initiation following ionizing radiation may occur more frequently through DNA deletions and/or rearrangements than through point mutations. There is, however, insufficient evidence at present on this important aspect of oncogenic initiation.

73. A correlation between reduced dose-rate effects for cell inactivation and deficiency in DNA double-strand break repair has also been established in radiosensitive mutants of CHO Chinese hamster cells [K1, T3] and L5178Y mouse lymphoma cells [B10, E4, E5, W5], further strengthening the link between dose-rate effects and the repair of a specific radiation-induced DNA lesion. In addition, some of the above data also indicate that the fitted initial slopes, α_1, of dose-effect curves are not constant and may be modified by cellular repair processes.

74. The extent to which radiation-induced DNA damage may be correctly repaired at very low doses and very low dose rates is beyond the resolution of current experimental techniques. If DNA double-strand breaks are critical lesions determining a range of cellular responses, including perhaps neoplastic transformation, then it may be that wholly accurate cellular repair is unlikely even at the very low lesion abundance expected after low dose and low-dose-rate irradiation [T5].

75. Radiation-induced molecular damage to both DNA strands at the same point has a finite probability of generating a scission in the initial DNA substrate, with nucleotide base modifications on both strands. Repair enzyme activity may remove these but, in doing so, it will create a secondary substrate that cannot be returned to its original undamaged form without the presence of the necessary template [F3]. In the absence of such aids to repair, the lesions will tend to be misrepaired, producing intrachromosomal dele-

tions or interchromosomal translocations that are the hallmarks of radiation damage in mammalian cells (see Annex E, "Mechanisms of radiation oncogenesis", and [E1]). The existence of such radiation-induced double-strand DNA lesions, which may be extremely difficult to repair correctly, would imply the absence of threshold for initial damage to DNA, even when there are very few double-strand breaks, and hence absence of thresholds for stable changes to individual cells.

76. This postulate may be contrasted with that for ultraviolet, where there is experimental evidence that biologically critical cellular damage arises as a consequence of the induction of ultraviolet photoproducts that principally affect the nucleotide bases on one strand of the DNA duplex. Ultraviolet-modified bases may be excised from the damaged strand by DNA repair complexes, leaving a gapped strand that may then be accurately filled with the appropriate nucleotides using the coding sequence of the undamaged strand as a template [F3, M2].

77. From a mechanistic standpoint such single-strand damage excision processes, which also act on many chemically induced DNA base adducts, may be regarded as potentially error-free [M2], although even here mistakes in copying may occur. Thus, although in principle the efficient (subsaturation) operation of single-strand excision processes in cells could result in wholly accurate repair and a dose-effect relationship with a threshold at low doses, in practice such thresholds are unlikely to exist for the initial damage to DNA from ionizing radiation. Apparent low-dose thresholds for the ultraviolet-inactivation and mutation of cultured human cells have, however, been demonstrated [M2].

2. Effect of dose rate

78. A number of studies have been reported on the influence of dose rate from low-LET radiation on cell mutagenesis. In cultured rodent cells, radiation mutagenesis may be considerably reduced by dose protraction [T2, T5]. In contrast, in a human lymphoblast system, continuous exposure to radiation from tritiated water [L6] or from daily exposure to x-ray doses <0.1 Gy [G11] failed to produce any reduction in induced mutation frequency. This response may not, however, be characteristic of the response that would be obtained for normal cells *in vivo*. In human TK6 cells, the *hprt* and *tk* mutation frequencies after acute x-irradiation and continuous gamma-irradiation (0.45 and 4.5 mGy min^{-1}) showed linear responses and no dose-rate dependency [K4]. The dose rate of 0.45 mGy min^{-1} is one of the lowest used for mutation studies of cells in culture. While it is possible that these observations highlight a real difference between human and rodent cells in a low-dose radiation response and in the potential for repair, there are complex issues regarding dose-rate effects on cell mutagenesis that need to be considered [T5].

79. For the induction of unstable chromosome aberrations (dicentrics and acentric rings) in human lymphocytes by low-dose and low-dose-rate radiation, there has been considerable interlaboratory variation in aberration yield, so the magnitude of any dose-rate effect at low doses is not clear [L14]. It has been concluded, however, that at low doses, taking all data together, aberration yield is probably linear with dose and independent of dose rate [E1]. Recently, however, observations on the existence of a radiation-induced adaptive response in human lymphocytes have raised questions about the response at low doses. In these experiments it has been shown, for example, that lymphocytes exposed to an x-ray dose of 0.01 Gy (corresponding to an average of 10 tracks per cell) become adapted so that only about half as many chromatid deletions are induced by a subsequent challenge with high doses (e.g. [W7]). The mechanisms and generality of this potentially important post-irradiation response have yet to be established, but it has been shown that cellular protein synthesis is necessary for the development of the adaptive response and that a dose of 0.01 Gy from x rays reproducibly induces the synthesis of a number of cellular proteins (putative repair enzymes) not found in unirradiated lymphocytes [W7]. The effect of radiation on cellular processes has recently been reviewed by Wolff [W4].

80. A number of models have been published that ascribe the repair of radiation damage in the quadratic region of the dose response to a reduction in sublethal or submutagenic damage. Thus, Leenhouts et al. [L20] modelled cellular damage and its repair in terms of induced DNA double-strand breaks; these may be reduced in number in a cell either by the repair of single-strand breaks or by the repair of double-strand breaks, which might not always be perfect. On this basis, three regions of the dose response can be distinguished: an acute dose-rate region (>60 Gy h^{-1}), where exposures are very short compared with the repair rate of sublethal or submutagenic damage and where a linear quadratic dose-effect relationship is measured; a region of protracted dose rate, where the radiation effect decreases with decreasing dose rate; and a region of lower dose rates, where the repair of sublethal damage is essentially complete and the dose-rate effect is essentially negligible. These different regions will not necessarily be the same for all cell types. Similar patterns of response could be obtained, however, if the feature of cellular response giving rise to the quadratic component included a component that could be attributed to the saturation of repair processes.

D. SUMMARY

81. Guidance on expected effects at low doses and low dose rates can be sought from the quantitative models that have been developed to describe the available radiobiological and epidemiological data. Radiobiological data for effects on single cells under a variety of conditions have led to the development of many quantitative models, mechanistic or phenomenological, for single radiation-induced changes in the cells. Multi-stage models of radiation carcinogenesis, based on epidemiological or animal data, assume that a series of two or more changes is required before a cell becomes malignant and that radiation can induce at least some of these changes. The biophysical concepts underlying the different models can be described in terms of general features of target theory, because the insult of ionizing radiation is always in the form of finite numbers of discrete tracks. In this way fundamental expectation can be sought on the nature of overall dose responses, their dependence on dose rate and their features at the low doses that are of greatest practical relevance. Radiation carcinogenesis involves complex changes after the initial cellular damage. The cellular effects and concepts of appropriate models have been emphasized in this Chapter. Other aspects, including organ effects, are considered later in this Annex.

82. Dose responses can be subdivided into regions. In region I, a negligible proportion of cells (or cell nuclei) are intersected by more than one track and hence dose responses for single-stage effects can be confidently expected to be linear and independent of dose rate. In region II, many tracks intersect each cell (or nucleus), but multi-track effects may not be observed in the experimental data, so independent single-track action is commonly assumed, although true linearity and dose-rate independence hinge on the validity of this assumption. In region III, multi-track effects are clearly visible as non-linearity of dose response, and hence dose-rate dependence, is likely. The simpler forms of the dose-response relationship can be expanded as a general polynomial, with only the dose and dose-squared terms being required to fit most experimental data, although sometimes a separate factor is added to account for competing effects of cell killing at higher doses. The induction of an effect can then be represented by an expression of the following form:

$$I(D) = (\alpha_1 D + \alpha_2 D^2)\, e^{-(\beta_1 D + \beta_2 D^2)} \qquad (11)$$

in which α_1 and α_2 are coefficients for the linear and quadratic terms for the radiation response and β_1 and β_2 are linear and quadratic terms for cell killing. It is generally assumed that at sufficiently low doses, α_1 will be constant and independent of dose rate. In this approach it is common to regard the fitted linear coefficient as being constant and fully representative of the response extrapolated down to minimally low dose and dose rate. However, there are in the literature data from numerous studies that violate this simple expectation, for both low-LET and high-LET radiation. Many of these imply that multi-track effects can occur in the intermediate-dose region (II) and that even when the dose response appears linear it may be dose-rate dependent and non-linear at lower doses.

83. Low-dose and low-dose-rate expectations based on multi-stage processes of carcinogenesis depend crucially on the detail of the radiation dependence of the individual stages and on the tissue kinetics. Expectations could, in principle, readily range between two opposite extremes. On the one hand a linear term could be absent entirely, implying vanishing risk as the dose tends to zero, as should be the case if two (or more) time-separated radiation steps were required. On the other hand, there could be, right down to the lowest doses, a clear linear term that even increases with decreasing dose rate, as may occur if either of the stages can occur spontaneously and if there is clonal expansion between them.

84. Consideration has also been given to the possible existence of a true dose threshold in the response to radiation. It is highly unlikely that a dose threshold exists for the initial molecular damage to DNA, because a single track from any ionizing radiation has a finite probability of producing a sizable cluster of atomic damage directly in, or near, the DNA. Only if the resulting molecular damage, plus any additional associated damage from the same track, were always repaired with total efficiency could there be the possibility of a dose threshold for consequent cellular effects. Almost all of the many biophysical models of radiation action assume that there is no such threshold for single-stage changes in cells. Multi-stage models of carcinogenesis could lead to expectations of a dose threshold, or a response with no linear term, under particular, highly restricted sets of assumptions. Available data imply that these restrictions do not apply in general to all tumours, although they may in some particular cases. These fundamental considerations cannot preclude practical situations where the possibility of effects at low doses may be very small or where significant tissue damage is necessary for particular types of tumour to develop.

II. DOSE-RESPONSE RELATIONSHIPS IN EXPERIMENTAL SYSTEMS

85. To provide an experimental basis for assessing the effects of dose rate on cancer induction in man, information is available from a number of sources. Tumour induction in animals provides the main source, but both the transformation of cells in culture and the induction of somatic and germ cell mutations are also valuable for assessing the influence of dose and dose rate on the initiating event(s) resulting from damage to DNA. The following Sections review information from these areas of research that are relevant to considerations of dose-rate effects for cancer induction by both low- and high-LET radiation.

86. In the UNSCEAR 1986 Report [U2] information on dose-response relationships for mutations, chromosomal aberrations in mammalian cells, cell transformation and radiation-induced cancer were reviewed. Three basic non-threshold models were considered for both cellular effects of radiation and for cancer induction: linear, linear-quadratic and pure quadratic models (Figure IV). It was concluded that for most experiments and end-points the prevailing form of the dose-response relationship at intermediate to high doses of low-LET radiation is concave upward and can be represented by an equation of the form

$$I(D) = (\alpha_0 + \alpha_1 D + \alpha_2 D^2) S(D) \qquad (12)$$

in which α_0 is the spontaneous incidence, α_1 and α_2 are coefficients for the linear and quadratic terms for the specific cellular response and S(D) is the probability of survival of transformed cells having received the absorbed dose D. The probability of survival may be expressed as

$$S(D) = e^{-(\beta_1 D + \beta_2 D^2)} \qquad (13)$$

where β_1 and β_2 are coefficients of the linear and quadratic terms of cell killing. For mammalian cells exposed to low-LET radiation, values of the parameter α_1/α_2 for mutations and chromosome aberrations (equivalent to the dose at which the linear and quadratic terms contribute equally to the response) cluster around 1 Gy (geometric mean, 1.27 Gy) while values of the parameter β_1/β_2 for cell sterilization are generally much higher, in the range 2-10 Gy (geometric mean 7.76 Gy) [B27]. The difference appears to be due mainly to higher values of the linear term for cell killing, in accordance with conclusions that, at least at low doses, the loss of proliferative capacity of cells is caused by damage that is not all observable as chromosomal changes at mitosis [B31, B38]. Some may be associated with less severe damage [B13].

87. An example was given in the UNSCEAR 1986 Report [U2] of how the range of survival parameters for cell lines of varying sensitivity for cell killing would affect the shape of the dose-response curve for tumour induction, and hence the reliability of extrapolation from risks obtained at intermediate doses to the low doses that are generally of practical concern. In this analysis [U2], the Committee selected two values of the α_1/α_2 quotient for tumour yield (or mutation/aberration yield) applying to x rays and gamma rays: 0.5 Gy and 2.0 Gy. For survival characteristics, the bone marrow stem cell was selected as the most sensitive. Its survival curve is described by β_1 = 0.4 Gy^{-1} and β_2 = 0.08 Gy^{-2} [B5]. For the least sensitive cell, a hypothetical cell line was assumed with survival parameters β_1 = 0.1 Gy^{-1} and β_2 = 0.08 Gy^{-2} [B5]. To normalize the data, a lifetime cumulative incidence at 3 Gy of 150 cases per 10,000 population (150 10^{-4} Gy^{-1}) was assumed. The results in terms of the cumulative tumour incidence from doses of 1 mGy to 4 Gy for all combinations of α_1/α_2 and β_1/β_2 are plotted in the upper part of Figure V. In the lower plot of Figure V, the data have been redrawn giving relative risks normalized to the same value of the α_1 coefficient.

88. From this analysis, three conclusions can be drawn. First, the sensitivity to cell killing has a more pronounced effect on the shape of the dose-response relationships than the α_1/α_2 quotient. Secondly, for the cells most sensitive to killing (S_{min}, minimal survival), the relationship is concave downward, with maxima at 2-2.5 Gy. Since such curves are not observed for human cancers after exposure to low-LET radiation (i.e. reaching maximum values at doses of about 2 Gy), it seems likely that the assumed sensitivity is too high for *in vivo* irradiation. This would be consistent with the lower sensitivity of single cells irradiated *in situ*. Thirdly, for the cells least susceptible to killing (S_{max}, maximum survival), the overestimate of the tumour yield per unit dose at low doses by linear extrapolation from 1-2 Gy down to 0.001-0.01 Gy ranges from 3.0-2.5 at α_1/α_2 = 0.5 Gy, to 1.2-1.3 at α_1/α_2 = 2 Gy, respectively.

89. The maximum overestimation of the risk results from totally neglecting cell killing. In such a case the overestimate of the risk at low doses from risks observed at high doses, D, can be calculated from equation 12:

$$DDREF = (\alpha_1 D + \alpha_2 D^2)/\alpha_1 D = 1 + (\alpha_2/\alpha_1) D \qquad (14)$$

The extent of overestimation of the risk corresponds to the dose and dose-rate effectiveness factor (DDREF) of ICRP [I2].

90. Linear extrapolation from 3, 2 and 1 Gy down to a low dose of, say, 0.01 Gy for cellular systems with a range of α_1/α_2 quotients between 0.5 Gy and 2 Gy would thus involve the overestimates of radiation effect shown in the Table below. Thus, for a cell response with an α_1/α_2 quotient of 1.0 Gy, if the risk is assessed at 2 Gy then linear extrapolation to assess the risk at low doses will overestimate the risk coefficient by a factor of about 3. If the risk is assessed at 3 Gy, however, the DDREF would be 4. In practice, the available epidemiological and experimental data on tumour incidence generally do not allow reliable estimates to be made of α_1 and α_2, and tumour incidence data up to about 2 Gy are frequently compatible with linear or linear-quadratic models, although a variety of dose-response curves have been obtained (Figures VII-XV). This type of modelling approach does, however, indicate that tumour induction rates at low doses, when based on information obtained at intermediate doses, will, in the absence of significant cell killing, tend to be overestimated by linear extrapolation.

α_1/α_2 (Gy)	DDREF		
	3 Gy	2 Gy	1 Gy
0.5	7	5	3
1.0	4	3	2
2.0	2.5	2	1.5

91. Of concern for radiation protection is how cellular damage by ionizing radiation manifests itself as long-term effects, with cancer induction and hereditary disease being the main effects of concern at low doses and low dose rates. The induction of hereditary disease by ionizing radiation may be readily explained in terms of damage to the genetic material that is manifested in future generations. For cancer induction in both animals and humans the situation is more complex, because tumours in somatic tissue can arise many years after exposure to radiation, following development through a succession of events. Experimentally, cancer caused by exposure to radiation or other agents appears to be the result of a multi-stage process. In the liver, skin, oesophagus, colon and other complex epithelia the cancer induction process can be considered to consist of three stages: initiation, promotion and progression, which are described in Annex E, "Mechanisms of radiation oncogenesis". An initiating event can result from a single exposure to a genotoxic carcinogen that alters a cell or a group of cells, giving a potential for cancer to develop. This damage may be repaired but it may also be irreversible, although the cell and its progeny may never develop to form a tumour. This initial damage may conform to single- or multi-hit models. Subsequent exposure to tumour promoters permits the neoplastic changes to be expressed in initiated cells, with the result that tumours develop. Further stimulation may therefore aid the progression of the tumour. Some chemical agents act as initiators, some as promoters and others as both [A3]. Radiation can act in a dual capacity, as cancers may appear many years after exposure to radiation without any further radiation stimulus, however, at relatively high doses, radiation damage to surrounding tissue may also play a promotional role in cancer development. Many other environmental factors, including hormones, immunological factors or cigarette smoke, may also play a promoting role after an initiating event.

92. The problems in assessing risks of cancer for exposures to low-LET radiation at low doses and low dose rates, when human data are available mainly at high doses and high dose rates, were summarized by the NCRP [N1]. The dose-response relationships are illustrated in Figure I, which gives schematically data points and possible dose-response curves for cancer incidence. Frequently, as in this example, data points are only available at relatively high doses. The approach commonly used in risk assessment is to fit a linear dose-response relationship to the data (curve B), a procedure that is usually considered to give an upper limit to the risk at low doses [C4, I1, U4]. If this linear relationship is due to single tracks acting independently, then the effect per unit dose (the slope of the line, α_H, or risk coefficient at high doses and high dose rates) would be expected to be independent of dose magnitude and dose rate. In practice, however, this is not generally the case, and experimental data suggest that a linear-quadratic relationship (curve A) will frequently provide a better fit to the data, implying that damage is the result not only of single interactions but also of other, more complex interactions. Other explanations for the quadratic function in the response are also possible, such as saturation of repair processes [T16]. With a progressive lowering of the dose and/or the dose rate, allowing more opportunity for repair of damage and less opportunity for interacting events, a point may ultimately be reached at which damage is produced as a result of single events acting alone, giving a linear response (curve D, slope α_L) with the effect proportional to dose. A similar response would be obtained

by lowering the dose rate alone, as even at high total doses, lesions accumulate more slowly. Thus, experimentally, the effect per unit absorbed dose at low dose rates (even at high total doses) would be expected to become progressively less as the dose rate is lowered. Hence, the limiting slope (α_L of Figure I) would be reached either by reducing the dose to very low values where the effect is independent of dose rate or by reducing the dose rate to very low values where the effect is dependent only on the total dose. On this basis, even fractionated exposures will not necessarily give slopes approaching α_L, as the overall dose response will depend on both the total dose and the dose rate per fraction.

93. In practice, because of statistical limitations it is extremely difficult to detect radiation-induced effects in the low dose range (<0.1 Gy) at any dose rate; thus, there are uncertainties in the determination of the limiting slope, α_L, in both animal and human studies. The initial slope of the dose-response curve can be more readily examined by changing the dose rate, as can be done in studies with experimental animals. In many experiments, however, even at low or intermediate dose rates, the limiting slope may not be reached, and a dose response in between the two slopes α_H and α_L is obtained with slope α_{Exp}. Despite this limitation, animal experiments provide the best indication of the extent to which lowering the dose rate of low-LET radiation, even at intermediate or high total doses, can reduce the effectiveness of radiation in inducing cancer. They therefore provide the most useful guidance on the extrapolation of risks observed at high doses and high dose rates to the low doses and low dose rates generally of concern in radiological protection.

94. The ratio of the slope of the no-threshold, "apparently" linear fit to the high-dose and high-dose-rate data (α_H) to the slope of the linear fit to the low-dose-rate data (α_L or α_{Exp}) has been used as a measure of the dose and dose-rate effectiveness factor. The terms dose-rate effectiveness factor (DREF) [N1], linear extrapolation overestimation factor (LEOF) and low dose extrapolation factor (LDEF) [P2, P3] have also been used for this reduction factor. In this Annex, the term dose and dose-rate effectiveness factor (DDREF) (or, more simply, relative effectiveness) will be used for comparing the response at different dose rates.

95. The data on tumour induction in experimental animals that are most directly useful for the derivation of DDREFs for man are, surprisingly, very restricted in their extent. Significant effects have been obtained mainly with intermediate or relatively high doses, although at very different dose rates. Thus, only limited evaluation of the shape of the overall dose-response curve has been achieved, as is also true for epidemiological studies. In general, a significant increase in tumour incidence in experimental animals is found at doses of about 0.2 Gy and above (see Section II.A). Some radiation-induced cancers have been detected in human populations at relatively low doses. Human data on cancer induction relevant to considerations of dose and dose-rate effects from low-LET radiation are reviewed briefly in Chapter III.

A. TUMORIGENESIS IN EXPERIMENTAL ANIMALS

1. Radiation-induced life shortening

96. Extensive studies in experimental animals have reported radiation-induced life shortening as a result of whole-body external irradiation and as the result of intakes of radionuclides. This is a precise biological end-point that reflects the earlier onset of lethal diseases, an increased incidence of early occurring diseases or a combination of the two. To understand the effects of radiation on life-span it is important to know the underlying cause of death, although this is often difficult and in some cases impossible, as death may be the result of a variety of causes acting together. This is particularly the case in older animals, in which multiple lesions are often present. In contrast, in younger animals a specific pathological lesion can frequently be identified.

97. Life shortening is an effect that must be estimated by comparing irradiated and non-irradiated populations. The different ways of describing and expressing the effect quantitatively have been reviewed in the UNSCEAR 1982 Report [U3]. The mean or median life-span, the per cent cumulative mortality or the age-specific mortality rate may all be regarded as compounded expressions of specific and non-specific causes, acting within each individual to decrease fitness and ultimately to cause death.

98. There has been considerable discussion in the published literature about the specificity or non-specificity of life shortening in experimental animals exposed to ionizing radiation. Life shortening must ultimately be due to an underlying cause, and the lack of specific information frequently results from the lack of detailed pathology. A "specific" cause of death has therefore been taken to mean that irradiated animals die earlier than controls and show a different spectrum of diseases or causes of death. Since not all diseases are readily induced by radiation, interest has centred on whether or not radiation may produce life shortening by inducing tumours and how much of the observed shortening can be accounted for by neoplastic diseases. The words "specific" and "non-specific" have generally been taken to indicate neoplastic and non-neoplastic contributions to life shortening.

99. Life shortening by radiation was comprehensively reviewed in the UNSCEAR 1982 Report [U3]. Although life shortening can only be assessed on the basis of death, an end-point that can be defined precisely in time, it is usually more informative to know the cause of death, as most irradiated animals die of diseases that are unrelated to radiation exposure, complicating the identification of the terminal pathological syndromes. Some of the difficulties in interpreting much of the work were summarized in that Report [U3]. These included the lack of careful pathological observations on the animals at death or of a refined multifactorial analysis, particularly in earlier studies. Some studies at low doses have even reported life lengthening, although any increase has generally not been statistically significant. Another problem is that even when good pathology is available, information is usually collected at death, when it is impossible to assess the contribution of each specific cause to life shortening, since there is no reason to presume that all causes are equally accelerated by irradiation. While serial sacrifice experiments might provide this information, they are time-consuming and expensive. The additional effort required to implement this technique is considerable and, as a consequence, such information is uncommon in the literature.

100. Radiation-induced life shortening appears to have been first described in the rat by Russ et al. [R9] and in the mouse by Henshaw [H18]. They reported that irradiated animals had a shorter life-span and appeared to age more rapidly than non-irradiated controls. These and other studies led to the view that the life-shortening action of radiation was due to its enhancement of natural ageing processes. Early reviews of mammalian radiation injury and lethality by Brues et al. [B28] and Sacher [S18] recognized that single acute exposures to radiation tended to displace the Gompertz age mortality function upward and chronic exposure throughout life increased the slope of this function.

101. The concept that radiation-induced life shortening might be equivalent to aging was criticized by Mole [M44], who considered that this view had arisen largely as a result of observations on surviving animals given single large doses in the lethal range. The similarities and differences between natural ageing and radiation-induced life shortening were considered by Comfort [C16]. His review was a significant attempt to differentiate between the various biological effects observed. Neary [N3, N4] regarded theories of ageing as belonging to one of two main groups: those interpreting ageing as due to random events in a population of supposedly uniform individuals and those examining the individual and its component cells. He proposed a theory that ageing proceeds in two successive stages, induction and development, each characterized by appropriate parameters. Experiments reported later from the Soviet Union [V2, V3, V5, V6] tended to show that induction consists of the spontaneous occurrence of lesions in cellular DNA and that development (promotion) results from the activation of endogenous viral genomes by chemical carcinogens or radiation.

102. The first experimental series that allowed analysis of specific causes of death were those of Upton et al. in 1960 [U27] in RF mice. The authors could not, however, establish any clear-cut relationship between life shortening and the incidence of tumours, as the dose-response relationships for different tumour types varied: some increased with dose and some decreased. These data gave some support to the view that radiation could cause non-specific life shortening. A statistical evaluation of these data by Walburg in 1975 [W8], using a method that allowed for competing probabilities of death, indicated that life shortening, which was clearly apparent when all deaths were considered together, disappeared when tumours were excluded from the analysis. Table 4 shows the mean age at death adjusted for competing probabilities of death, for deaths from all causes and from all non-neoplastic diseases, of female RF mice exposed to 1 and 3 Gy of ^{60}Co gamma-radiation (0.067 Gy min^{-1}) at 10 weeks of age compared with data from controls. For these mice, myelogeneous leukaemia, thymic lymphosarcoma and endocrine tumours were induced or accelerated by irradiation. When only non-neoplastic causes of death were considered, there was no significant effect on life shortening, and the mean age at death increased in irradiated animals relative to controls.

103. In a series of studies in mice Storer [S33] noted in the dose range 1-5 Gy from x rays a tendency for neoplastic diseases to occur earlier in irradiated than in control mice. In extensive studies by Upton et al. [U21, U28] in male and female RF mice exposed to either fast neutrons or to gamma rays, detailed pathology was not performed, but the authors considered that the death of irradiated animals was characteristically associated with tumours and degenerative diseases of old age, although the induction of neoplasms could not entirely account for life-span shortening. These data were subsequently analysed in more detail by Walburg [W8], who demonstrated that, in the absence of tumour induction, life shortening was negligible, at least for exposure to gamma rays in the dose range of 1-3 Gy.

104. A number of more recent publications have also addressed the question of life-span shortening in mice. In general, the conclusions have been that for doses of up to a few gray, life-span shortening is due to an increase in tumour incidence. Thus, Grahn et al. [G23] showed that at doses up to 4 Gy life shortening was due to excess tumour mortality, although at higher

doses decreased life expectancy was not accompanied by a parallel increase in tumour incidence. Maisin [M45] attributed life shortening in BALB/c and C57BL mice at intermediate doses essentially to thymic lymphoma and at higher doses to glomerulosclerosis. Similar conclusions have been reached by other authors [L21, L22] in studies with rats; and the same is true for dogs in the series of Andersen et al. [A5], according to an analysis by Walburg [W8].

105. For exposures to high-LET radiation similar conclusions can be drawn. In an analysis of causes of death in B6CF1 mice exposed to single and fractionated doses of fission neutrons Thompson and Grahn [T12] concluded that practically all (>90%) of the excess mortality could be attributed to tumour deaths.

106. From his comprehensive review of published data, Walburg [W8] concluded that at the low to intermediate doses of practical interest in radiation protection, life shortening after irradiation may principally be explained by the induction or acceleration of neoplastic diseases. This conclusion was supported by Storer [S19], although it was recognized that at higher doses other mechanisms were involved in early radiation damage.

107. The majority of comprehensive studies that give quantitative information on the effects of dose, dose fractionation and dose rate on life-span shortening have used the mouse as the experimental animal. Substantial differences in sensitivity have, however, been noted between strains and between the sexes. A review of 10 studies involving about 20 strains of mice given single exposures to x or gamma radiation showed that estimates of life shortening ranged from 15 to 81 days Gy^{-1}, although the majority of values (9 of 14 quoted in the review) were between 25 and 45 days Gy^{-1} with an overall unweighted average of 35 days Gy^{-1} [G8]. In general, in the range from about 0.5 Gy to acutely lethal doses, the dose response was either linear or curvilinear upwards. In male BALB/c mice exposed to acute doses of ^{137}Cs gamma rays (4 Gy min^{-1}), life shortening was a linear function of dose between 0.25 and 6 Gy with a loss of life expectancy of 46.2 ± 4.3 days Gy^{-1} [M5]. The effects of acute single doses on life-span shortening in other species are summarized in the UNSCEAR 1982 Report [U3].

108. The sensitivity to tumour induction has also been shown to depend on age at exposure as well as the gender of the animals. Thus, the lifetime excess of neoplasia in Sprague-Dawley rats following exposure to gamma rays from ^{60}Co decreased by a factor of about 10 in 9-month-old rats as compared to animals irradiated *in utero*, and the spectrum of tumours was different. The higher incidence of tumours observed in the fetal-exposed group appeared to be mainly due to the high sensitivities of the central nervous system and gonads during organogenesis. Differences in tumour incidences were observed between male and female rats and between the incidences of primary cancers and benign tumours in the different groups of animals [M29].

109. Partial-body irradiation is much less effective than whole-body irradiation in causing life shortening. Thus for female ddY/SLC mice following head or lower body exposure to doses of 1.9 Gy from x rays, life shortening was 23 and 26 days Gy^{-1}, respectively, with almost no further life shortening up to 7.6 Gy. After irradiation of the trunk with 1.9 Gy, life shortening was 38 days Gy^{-1}, with a further increase of 6 days Gy^{-1} at doses up to 7.6 Gy. In contrast, for whole-body exposures between 0.95 and 5.7 Gy, the mean survival time decreased linearly with increasing dose, with a loss of life expectancy of 37 days Gy^{-1} [S37]. Extensive studies on the effects of incorporated radionuclides have also shown a reduction in life-span as a result of tumour induction resulting from intakes of radionuclides. Some of these studies are described later in this Chapter in sections which relate to effects on specific organs and tissues. It is noteworthy that in a number of studies, where non-fatal tumours are induced in particular organs and tissues, this does not necessarily lead to a loss of life-span (e.g. [M24]).

110. *Summary*. It may be concluded on the basis of a number of studies that, although irradiated animals do experience, on the average, a shorter life-span than non-irradiated controls, the hypothesis that life shortening at low to intermediate doses up to a few gray of low-LET radiation is due to the same causes of death as is normal in the animals (although appearing earlier in time) is not substantiated by experimental evidence. In general, life shortening as a result of exposure to ionizing radiation arises largely as a result of an acceleration or higher incidence of fatal tumours in irradiated populations. At higher doses that are well into the lethal range, a non-specific component of life shortening becomes apparent from cellular damage to the blood vasculature and other tissues. This does not imply that dose-response relationships for tumour induction and life shortening are directly comparable, because even for the same radiation dose, the mean latent period of some tumours in a given species can be influenced by a number of factors including the dose, dose rate, gender and age at exposure. Furthermore, some tumours that may be induced are non-fatal and do not influence life-span. If the induction of fatal tumours is the main influence on life shortening, however, then a comparison of survival following various patterns of exposure should provide some indication of the effects of dose, dose rate and dose fractionation on tumour induction.

(a) Dose fractionation

111. In the UNSCEAR 1982 Report [U3], the Committee reviewed data on fractionated exposures in which a given dose of whole-body irradiation was split into a series of doses given in two or more fractions. The dose per fraction, fractionation interval and total time of irradiation are all interacting variables that cannot normally be separated. Frequently, therefore, the comparison is between a single exposure given acutely and the same dose given in fractions over a period of time. Fractionation of a given dose into two equal or unequal fractions at an interval of about a day or less has, in general, not altered life shortening significantly, although such a dose-fractionation schedule can decrease acute effects significantly [G8, M21]. Longer dose-fractionation intervals have been more comprehensively studied. In some cases survival has been unaltered or only slightly prolonged by fractionation [G8, K2, L16, U18]; in others it was slightly shortened [A5, C15, M22]. Many of the differences are perhaps due to differences from one animal strain to another in sensitivity to the induction of various tumour types, although a number of studies have also demonstrated how the spectrum of diseases that can result in life shortening may be influenced by the pattern of radiation exposure. Thus, Cole et al. [C15] examined the influence of dose fractionation on the life-span of LAF1 female mice. Animals were exposed either to an acute dose of 6 Gy (250 kVp x rays) or to about 7 Gy given in two, four or eight equal fractions separated by 8 weeks, 19 days or 8 days, respectively. Irradiation shortened survival in all the groups compared with controls, but the greatest effect was seen in the group given eight fractions, for which the mean age at death was about 15 months compared to about 21 months in the group given a single exposure. This was attributed to an increased incidence of leukaemia in the eight-fraction group (39%) compared with the single fraction group (13%) and the controls (29%). It was noteworthy that nephrosclerosis, which was the main cause of death in the group given a single dose (53% incidence) was very much reduced in the group given eight fractions (5%).

112. Dose fractionation at progressively longer periods of time seems to decrease the effects of radiation, but again the variability in results obtained has been considerable [A1, A5, G8, M5, M20, S17]. Ainsworth et al. [A1] reported that exposing both male and female B6CF1 mice to fractionated doses of ^{60}Co gamma rays (8.4 Gy total in 24 equal fractions over 23 weeks) produced an approximately threefold "sparing" effect compared to a similar (7.9 Gy) acute dose (corresponding to life shortening of 45 days Gy^{-1} for acute exposure and 18 days Gy^{-1} for fractionated exposure) in both sexes. In contrast, Grahn et al. [G8] compared the effects of 4.5 and 7 Gy from ^{60}Co gamma rays given as acute exposures or as two fractions separated by time intervals between 3 hours and 28 days. No significant effect of dose fractionation on life shortening was found, and the incidence of leukaemia was not altered in any consistent way. In a preliminary experiment, Silini et al. [S16] compared the effects of a single dose of 5 Gy from 250 kVp x rays on adult male C3H mice with the same dose given as two fractions (1.5 and 3.5 Gy) at different intervals of time (4-48 hours). The results suggested an increase in survival time with increasing fractionation interval, but there was considerable variability in the results obtained. The 50% cumulative mortality for the acutely exposed animals was 450 days; for the animals given fractionated exposures at an interval of 36 hours, it was 520 days.

113. A series of papers have been published by Thomson et al. [T7, T10, T12] that compare survival of male B6CF1 mice following single and fractionated exposures. Mice were exposed to ^{60}Co gamma rays either as single exposures or as 24 or 60 weekly fractions. With single exposures the average loss of life-span was 38.5 ± 2.9 days Gy^{-1}, whereas with 24 weekly fractions it was 22.6 ± 2.2 days Gy^{-1} and with 60 weekly fractions 17.5 ± 3.3 days Gy^{-1}. This study therefore showed that prolonged dose fractionation had a significant effect on life-span, reducing the effectiveness of the radiation by a factor of about 2. Table 5 summarizes some early results on the effect of dose fractionation on survival in rodents and beagle dogs.

114. Maisin and his colleagues have reported a series of studies on the effect of dose fractionation on survival in C57Bl and BALB/c mice. A preliminary study compared the survival of C57Bl mice given either a single exposure to x rays (3.5 or 6.5 Gy) or four equal fractions delivered at weekly intervals, with total doses from 2 to 15 Gy [M19]. Although the results for the two patterns of exposure were not strictly comparable, as the cumulative doses were not the same, the data suggested that life shortening after a fractionated exposure was slightly greater (~20%) than after an acute exposure. The disease spectrum was also different for single exposure and fractionated exposure. Thus the incidence of thymic lymphoma nearly doubled with dose fractionation and that of reticulum cell sarcoma B increased even more, while other diseases decreased in incidence.

115. Maisin et al. [M5, M47] reported a more comprehensive study in male BALB/c mice exposed to ^{137}Cs gamma rays (3 Gy min^{-1}) given either as single or fractionated exposures (10 fractions at 24 hour intervals) in the range 0.25-6 Gy. A significant shortening in life-span ($p < 0.05$) was obtained from a dose of 1 Gy for single exposures and from 2 Gy for fractionated exposures. Both patterns of exposure gave

nearly the same linear dependence of survival on dose with a life shortening of 46.2 ± 4.3 days Gy^{-1} for single exposures and 38.1 ± 3.1 days Gy^{-1} for fractionated exposures (Figure VI). After a single exposure malignant tumours were the principal cause of death in the dose range up to about 2-4 Gy; deterministic effects in the lung and kidney were preponderant at higher doses. In general, the total incidence of malignant tumours increased with dose after fractionated exposures, compared with controls, but decreased after single exposure. The difference between the two groups was significant ($p < 0.05$), although neither differed significantly from the controls. This was partly accounted for by an increase in the proportion of animals with two or more tumours after fractionated exposures in the higher dose groups [M25, M47]. The main exception to this trend was thymic lymphoma, where the incidence remained constant after fractionated exposure. This finding is contrary to observations in other studies, as thymic lymphoma incidence can be substantially increased by dose fractionation [K3, M19] and may be explained by the lower doses per fraction used in this study. Deterministic effects (e.g. lung pneumonitis and kidney damage) appeared, however, to diminish significantly with fractionation, and this may have allowed more tumours to develop. In this strain of mice there is, however, a high spontaneous tumour incidence (>60%) which could have influenced the results obtained and which also limits detailed analysis of the results.

116. In a more recent study [M20, M47], 12-week-old C57BlCnb mice, for which there is a lower spontaneous cancer incidence, particularly with respect to thymic lymphoma and lung cancer, were given either single or fractionated exposures (10 fractions separated by 24 hours or 8 fractions separated by 3 hours) to ^{137}Cs gamma rays (3 Gy min^{-1}), with total doses from 0.25 to 6 Gy. The data on tumour incidence and non-cancerous late degenerative changes in the lungs and kidneys were evaluated by the Kaplan-Meier procedure, using cause of death and probable cause of death as criteria. In general, survival appeared to be a linear function of the dose received in all the experimental groups, although survival was longer with fractionated than with single exposures (Table 6). Survival of the control animals was shorter than in the previous studies with C57Bl mice and may have resulted from the use of specific-pathogen-free animals that are more sensitive to non-cancerous late degenerative changes in the lung. Life shortening, calculated by linear weighted regression on dose of the values obtained by the Kaplan-Meier calculation for survival time, amounted to 31.1 ± 2.6 days Gy^{-1} for a single exposure, 19.6 ± 2.9 days Gy^{-1} for a 10-fraction exposure, and 16.5 ± 3.4 days Gy^{-1} for an 8-fraction gamma exposure. Malignant tumours, particularly leukaemia and including thymoma, as well as non-cancerous late degenerative changes were the principal causes of life shortening after a single high-dose exposure to gamma rays. Fractionated exposures, in particular eight fractions delivered 3 hours apart, appeared to result in an earlier and more frequent appearance of leukaemia and solid tumours in the range 1-2 Gy, a finding similar to that obtained with BALB/c mice [M5]. Since the average life-span is longer after fractionation, earlier death after single exposure may be attributed to the development of non-cancerous late degenerative lesions. It was noteworthy, however, that following single exposures the incidence of all tumours except thymoma was significantly less in the low dose groups (0.25-2 Gy) than in the controls (Table 6). This was a significant factor in the observation of an enhanced tumour incidence for animals given fractionated exposures compared with controls.

117. ***Summary***. Studies on experimental animals, mainly mice, have shown no clear trend in effects of dose fractionation on life-span. The results from a number of studies suggest that, when compared with the effects of acute exposures, the effects of dose fractionation are small and, at least for exposure times of up to about a month, simple additivity of the injury from each increment of dose can be assumed. In general, fractionated doses were given at the same dose rate as acute exposures. For fractionation over a longer time period there is a tendency to a longer life-span with a longer interval between the doses. A reduction in life-span shortening by a factor of ~2, compared with acute exposure, was obtained in one study in which the dose was given as 60 weekly fractions.

(b) Protracted exposures

118. There are far fewer studies of the effect of dose rate on life-span in experimental animals. The majority of studies have been undertaken in mice, although some work has also been reported with rats [R9], rabbits [B26], and beagle dogs [F13]. A number of early studies were described in the UNSCEAR 1982 Report [U3], but they relate mainly to early effects of radiation and do not provide any insight into the effects of dose rate on tumour induction.

119. In a series of studies by Bustad et al. [B29] hybrid male mice (C57BLx101) were exposed for 8 hours daily, between the ages of 6 and 58 weeks, to either 1 mGy h^{-1} or 2 mGy h^{-1} from ^{60}Co gamma-radiation giving total doses of 2.9 and 4.8 Gy. The animals were then maintained for their normal life-span. The average life-span for two subgroups of animals exposed to 1 mGy h^{-1} was about 863 days and for two further subgroups exposed to 2 mGy h^{-1} it was about 875 days. The life-span of the control

animals was about 920 days. Although there were some differences in the survival times between the different subgroups of irradiated animals and the controls, no significant increase in tumour incidence was observed in the irradiated animals.

120. Mole et al. [M23] exposed female CBA mice to gamma rays to give daily doses ranging from 0.03 to 0.5 Gy for progressively longer times (from four weeks to the duration of life). The shape of the cumulative mortality curve depended systematically on the particular level of daily exposure and on the cumulative dose, except possibly at the lowest daily dose. However, the total doses received by the animals were high: 0.6-72 Gy, causing substantial tissue damage, and many of the animals died of acute effects. It was concluded that lower total doses were needed for examining the relationship between dose rate and the late effects of exposure. The experimental results are described in detail in the UNSCEAR 1982 Report [U3].

121. More comprehensive studies that are more directly relevant to the effect of dose rate on life-span and tumour induction were undertaken over many years by Grahn et al. [G8, G9]. This work with mice has been summarized in a series of publications. A number of mouse strains and hybrids were exposed for 8 hours daily to gamma rays in doses ranging from 0.003 to 0.56 Gy per day. Exposures began when the mice were 100 days old and continued throughout life [G8, G9, S1]. The results were analysed in terms of the mean survival time after the initiation of the exposures, designated mean after survival (MAS). Thus, the MAS equalled the mean age at death minus 100 days. There was good consistency in the degree of life shortening for cumulative doses above a few gray when expressed as the MAS, between and among the strains as a function of daily dose. The MAS declined exponentially with increasing daily dose, D (in gray), and could be represented adequately by

$$\text{MAS (treated)} = \text{MAS (controls)}\ e^{-4D} \quad (15)$$

At the lowest daily doses, no consistent life shortening was found, and in some groups there appeared to be life lengthening. This was possibly due to any effect of radiation being lost due to variation between the animals (e.g. see Table 4).

122. This information on life shortening in mice exposed at low dose rates has been compared with that at high dose rates [N1]. Since animals exposed at low dose rates were exposed until death, the total dose accumulated by each animal depended on its survival time. Thus, a wide range of total doses is represented in the population exposed at any given dose regimen. However, by calculating mean loss of life-span (in days), in terms of the mean accumulated dose to death, it was shown that in the low dose range, life shortening amounted to 4 days Gy^{-1}. This may be compared with the results of 10 studies summarized by Grahn et al. [G8], which gave an average of about 35 days Gy^{-1} (range: 15-81 days Gy^{-1}) for acute exposures, and those reported for BALB/c mice [M5], which gave 46.2 ± 4.3 days Gy^{-1} at acute doses down to 0.25 Gy.

123. These data suggest that for radiation-induced life shortening either single brief exposures to low-LET radiation or fractionated exposures at high dose rates are about 8-10 times as effective as the same total dose given in a long protracted exposure at low dose rate. In a review of some of these data and allowing for uncertainties, including the effect of age-dependent decreases in sensitivity with increasing age, it was concluded by NCRP [N1] that protracted exposures may be considered to be one fifth to one tenth as effective in the mouse as single, high-dose-rate exposures (at total doses >0.5 Gy), assuming linearity for life shortening in both cases.

124. The above analyses assumed a linear dose response, with no threshold, for doses above 0.5 Gy at high dose rate. Storer et al. [S13] have, however, reported non-linear dose responses for life shortening in female RFM mice. Groups of mice were exposed to either 0.45 Gy min^{-1} or 0.06 mGy min^{-1} from a ^{137}Cs gamma-ray source to give a range of doses from 0.1 to 4 Gy and 0.5 to 4 Gy, respectively. Life shortening was calculated by subtracting the mean survival time in each experimental group from the mean survival time of the appropriate control. The dose-response curve for female RFM mice exposed to ^{137}Cs gamma rays between 0.1 and 4 Gy at high dose rate (0.45 Gy min^{-1}) showed that significant life shortening occurred at doses of 0.25 Gy and above. There was a rapid rise in life shortening with doses up to 0.5 Gy, followed by what appeared to be a generally linear upward trend with a much shallower slope in the range 0.5-4 Gy (Figure VII). In the region up to 0.5 Gy, the relationship between life-shortening and dose could be described by a dose-squared model ($p > 0.80$) or a linear-quadratic model, with the quadratic component predominating above about 0.04 Gy. These mice appear to be more sensitive than other mouse strains. Storer et al. [S13] have speculated that a contributory factor may have been the barrier environment in which the mice were maintained, as Upton et al. [U20] found less life shortening in conventionally housed RFM female mice. For female mice exposed at the intermediate dose rate (0.06 mGy min^{-1}), there was a significant reduction in life-span compared with controls at all doses examined (0.5-4 Gy), and a linear relationship adequately described the dose response ($p > 0.5$), with the intercept being not significantly different from that for controls (Figure VII). The weighted regression line to the intermediate dose-rate

data at total doses above 0.5 Gy could be described by the equation Y = 37.5D, where Y represents the days of life shortening and D is the dose, in gray. For the high-dose-rate data a weighted linear regression could be fitted, giving an intercept of 57.5 days. The equation of the line was Y = 57.5 + 46.3D. It was concluded that the main difference in response at high and intermediate dose rates was an upward displacement of the regression line at high dose rate, reflecting an increased sensitivity at doses up to about 0.5 Gy. At total doses of 1-2 Gy, protraction of the dose reduced life shortening by about one half and at lower doses by a factor of 2 to 3.

125. Thomson et al. [T8] have published information on the survival of male B6CF1 mice exposed for 22 hours per day, 5 days per week, to ^{60}Co gamma radiation at dose rates of 14-126 μGy min^{-1} for 23 weeks, giving total doses between 2.1 and 19 Gy, or at 14-63 μGy min^{-1} for 59 weeks, giving total doses between 5.3 and 25 Gy. For deaths from all causes, linear dose-response curves were obtained with slopes, corresponding to days of life lost per gray, of 15.8 ± 1.6 and 7.7 ± 0.2 for exposures of 23 and 59 weeks, respectively. These values were not significantly altered if the analysis was restricted to those mice dying with tumours, as about 90% of the radiation-specific mortality was tumour-related.

126. Thomson et al. [T8] compared the data they obtained in their study with data previously published [T7, T10, T12] on mice exposed either to single acute (20-minute) exposures or to 24 or 60 fractions given once weekly (20- or 45-minute exposures). The life shortening coefficients for single, fractionated and continuous gamma exposures, expressed as days of life lost Gy^{-1}, are shown in Table 7. Dividing the total dose into 24 once-weekly fractions (total exposure time: 18 hours) reduced the effectiveness of the radiation by about 40% (22.6 days lost Gy^{-1} compared with 38.5 days lost Gy^{-1} for acute exposure). Giving the same total dose almost continuously (total exposure time: 2,530 hours) over 23 weeks reduced the effectiveness by a further 30%. The effect of dose protraction was more pronounced if fractionated and continuous exposures were carried out over about 60 weeks. Forty-five hours of fractionated exposure had about 45% of the effect of acute exposure, and 6,490 hours of almost continuous exposure had only 20% of the effect of the single exposure. Also shown in Table 7 are the days of life lost per weekly fraction for the different exposures. Thus the maximum reduction in effect is obtained by comparing acute exposure with the effect of continuous exposure over 59 weeks, when the effectiveness is reduced by a factor of about 5. However, this comparison will tend to overestimate the effects of protraction, as a fraction of the radiation exposure will not have contributed to tumour initiation, although it could have influenced tumour development. However, the extent of this effect, if any, is difficult to quantify. For comparing the effectiveness of different patterns of exposure it may, therefore, be more appropriate to compare the effect of continuous and fractionated exposures given over the same period of time. On this basis, a reduction in effect in the range of 1.4-2.3 is obtained.

127. In an extended analysis of the data on life shortening obtained in mice exposed to acute or protracted exposure to low doses (less than a few gray) of low-LET radiation, Scott et al. [S34] have developed a model based on the assumption that life shortening from late effects is caused mainly by radiation-induced tumours. The state-vector model adopted for the analysis was kinetic in nature, with a two-step process leading to partition of the irradiated population into two groups: a group with radiation-induced tumours, in which it was assumed that mean survival is relatively independent of the radiation dose, although the incidence in the population is dose-related and a group without induced tumours, in which the mean survival time is nearly identical to an unirradiated control population. The results based on the model were in reasonable agreement with the available experimental data and were consistent with curvilinear dose-response relationships for acute exposures as well as with a reduced effect after fractionated exposure to ^{60}Co gamma rays.

128. The effect of dose and dose rate on life-span has also been examined in rats [M43]. Male Sprague-Dawley rats (3 months old) were exposed to ^{60}Co gamma rays to give 2.83 Gy (304 rats, 1.34 mGy h^{-1}), 1 Gy (505 rats, 78 mGy h^{-1}) and 3 Gy (120 rats, 78 mGy h^{-1}). The mean survival time of the controls (837 ± 147 days) was greater than that of the two groups of animals given about 3 Gy, but there was no difference between the animals given high dose-rate exposures (life-span: 738 ± 160 days) and those exposed at the lower dose rate (726 ± 160 days).

129. There are few studies that have examined the effect of dose rate on life-span and tumour induction in large animals. Carnes and Fritz [C30] have reported the results of a comprehensive study in young adult beagle dogs exposed to ^{60}Co gamma rays to give total accumulated doses of 4.5, 10.5, 15 and 30 Gy at dose rates of 38, 75, 128 and 263 mGy d^{-1}. Hazard models were used to identify trends in mortality associated with radiation exposure. The probability of an acute death (related to haematopoietic aplasia) was positively associated with the total dose received and the dose rate. For late effects, although there was good evidence of an increase in tumour mortality relative to the controls in all the irradiated groups, no relationship was found between tumour mortality and dose rate. There was, however, a clear relationship between

tumour mortality and cumulative dose. This lack of a dose-rate effect may be a consequence of the relatively small range of dose rates used (38-263 mGy d^{-1}); in the majority of rodent studies in which such an effect was observed, the high and low dose-rate exposures varied by a factor of 100 or more (Section II.A.2).

130. ***Summary***. Experimental studies in mice have demonstrated that with protracted exposures over a period of a few months to a year there is less life shortening by factors of 2 to 5 compared with exposures at high dose rates. In two studies in rats and beagle dogs no evidence was found for an effect of dose rate on tumour mortality. This lack of an effect may be a consequence of the fact that the dose rates used in these studies varied by factors of about 60 (rats) and 7 (dogs), while in the mouse studies they varied by a factor of 100 or more. It is noteworthy that not all tumours are a cause of life shortening.

(c) High-LET radiation

131. Since the 1970s, the Argonne National Laboratory has carried out a series of experiments to examine the effect on life shortening of brief, fractionated and protracted neutron exposures. Early results by Ainsworth et al. [A1] indicated that fractionated fission neutron exposures induced more life shortening in male B6CF1 mice than did single exposures. Thus, with a single dose of 2.4 Gy the mean survival time was 636 ± 13 days, whereas with fractionated exposures (various schedules) survival was 553 ± 6 days (controls: 838 ± 13 days). At a lower dose of 0.8 Gy, life shortening was also reduced, but there was less difference between the two treatment schedules, although the data still suggested that life shortening was greatest with fractionated exposures.

132. Data published before 1981 suggested that regardless of the mode of exposure (single, fractionated or chronic) the RBE could be expressed by the relationship RBE = AD^B, where the value of B was approximately −0.5 and that of A (the RBE value at 10 mGy) ranged from 10 to 80, depending on a number of factors, including the instantaneous dose rate of the reference low-LET radiation [T7, T10]. This observation was compatible with suggestions that the RBE increased over a wide range of doses as the inverse of the square root of the neutron dose, to values in excess of 100 [R10].

133. Later studies at the Argonne National Laboratory showed, however, that when total doses are low and the doses per fraction small, there is no significant difference in life shortening between fractionated and single exposures [C18, T18]. When the effects of single brief exposures of male and female B6CF1 mice to 0.83 MeV fission neutrons giving total doses from 10 to 400 mGy [T15] were compared with the effects of 60 equal, once weekly exposures giving doses of from 20 to 400 mGy [T12], the dose-response curves were linear and of similar slope between 0 and 300 mGy. Based on a linear-quadratic fit to the data for female mice, the days of life lost were 46 Gy^{-1} for single exposures and 44 Gy^{-1} for the 60-week fractionated exposure. Data for male mice gave similar results but were less extensive [T12]. At a dose level of about 400 mGy the dose-response curve for single exposures starts to become less steep and to separate from that for fractionated exposures. Overall, a significant effect of exposure pattern was observed at neutron doses in the range 400-600 mGy. Significant augmentation of radiation damage with dose protraction was observed in both sexes from doses above ~600 mGy. No difference in the dose-response curves for mice given 24 equal once-weekly or 60 equal once-weekly exposures was obtained. Although for exposure to neutrons the dose response at intermediate to low doses was linear and independent of dose pattern, this was not the case for exposures to gamma rays. As a consequence, RBE values from 6 to 43 were obtained, depending on the protraction period (1 day, 24 weeks or 60 weeks) [C18]. At low doses there is likely to be a limiting value for the RBE when the dose-response curves for both the neutron and the reference (gamma) radiation are linear. For single low doses, this has been calculated to be 15.0 ± 5.1 for $B6CF_1$ mice [T15]. In a supplementary analysis it was shown that practically all of the excess mortality resulting from radiation exposure (93% ± 8%) could be attributed to tumour deaths [T12].

134. Results obtained by Storer et al. [S13, S27] at Oak Ridge National Laboratory, using RFM and BALB/c mice were similar to those obtained at Argonne National Laboratory. Thus, female BALB/c mice were given total neutron doses between 25 mGy and 2 Gy in a single brief exposure or in equal fractions at either 1- or 30-day intervals. The neutrons were those of a slightly degraded ^{235}U-fission spectrum. After single or fractionated exposures, the extent of life shortening increased rapidly over the 0-0.5 Gy range and then began to plateau. While no significant increase in effectiveness of dose fractionation on life shortening was observed at total doses below 0.5 Gy, between 0.5 and 2 Gy there was an increase. With protracted neutron exposures using a moderated ^{252}Cf source giving dose rates ranging from 1 to 100 mGy d^{-1}, with total doses between 25 and 400 mGy, again no increase in effectiveness on life shortening was observed at doses below 0.5 Gy. It was also concluded that life shortening resulted primarily from an increased incidence and/or an early onset of malignant neoplasms, particularly in the low to moderate dose range [S27].

135. Maisin et al. [M20] have reported that fractionated exposures to high-energy neutrons (d(50MeV)Be; 8 fractions, 8 hours apart) appeared to have a slightly but not significantly greater effect than single exposures on life shortening in male C57Bl mice at doses up to 1.65 Gy. There appeared to be no significant difference in tumour incidence in the two groups, although in animals exposed to 1.65 Gy malignant tumours appeared earlier with fractionated than with single exposures. Life shortening could be described by a linear function of dose up to 3 Gy.

136. The results of these studies on a number of strains of mice are all reasonably consistent and suggest that the dose response for life shortening following exposure to high-LET radiation is a linear function of dose, at least for total doses up to about 0.5 Gy, and that neither dose fractionation nor dose protraction has much effect.

137. *Summary.* A number of studies in mice have examined the effects of dose fractionation and protraction of neutron doses on life-span shortening. Most recent studies have shown that when total doses are low (<0.5 Gy) and the dose per fraction is small there is no significant difference between acute and fractionated exposures. Data on protraction effects are rather limited but again suggest that protraction of exposure from high-LET radiation does not alter life-span shortening.

(d) Summary

138. At radiation doses up to a few gray (low-LET), life shortening in experimental animals appears to be mainly the result of an increase in tumour incidence, although this could also be influenced by the early appearance of some tumours. There is little suggestion that there is a general increase in other non-specific causes of death. At higher doses, into the lethal range, a non-specific component of life shortening becomes apparent due to cellular damage to the blood vasculature and other tissues. Accordingly, life shortening at low to intermediate doses can be used as a basis for examining the effect of dose fractionation and dose protraction on tumour induction.

139. The majority of comprehensive studies on the effect of dose fractionation of low-LET radiation on life-span have used the mouse as the experimental animal. The effect of dose fractionation appears to be very dependent on the strain of mouse and the spectrum of diseases contributing to the overall death rate. For example, in some strains thymic lymphoma incidence is increased by fractionation [M19]. Where this is a major contributor to the fatality rate, dose fractionation can result in a greater loss of life expectancy than acute exposures. Overall there is no clear trend in the effect of dose fractionation on life-span shortening, and the results from a number of studies suggest that, when compared with acute exposures, the effects of dose fractionation are small and in some studies have given either small increases or decreases in life-span. However, at least for exposure times of about a month, simple additivity of the injury from each dose increment can be assumed. One study in mice has reported that the reduction in survival time with eight fractions given 3 hours apart is half that obtained with an acute exposure, although this was accompanied by an enhanced tumour incidence. For fractionation intervals over a longer time there is a tendency to a longer life-span with an increasing interval between the doses, but the variations observed are generally less than those observed with protracted exposures.

140. When the effects in mice of acute exposures to low-LET radiation are compared with those of protracted irradiation given more or less continuously, it is seen that the effectiveness of the radiation decreases with decreasing dose rate and increasing time of exposure. With lifetime exposures there is some difficulty assessing the total dose contributing to the loss of life-span. The results available suggest, however, that with protracted exposures over a period of a few months to a year the effect on life-span shortening is reduced by factors of between about 2 and 5, compared with exposures at high dose rates. The effects of dose rate on tumour induction and life-span shortening have also been examined in rats and beagle dogs, although no significant differences have been seen. In these studies, however, dose rates varied by a factor of 60 or less, whereas in the studies in mice they varied by a factor of more than 100.

141. A number of early studies suggested that fractionated exposures to high-LET radiation induced more life shortening than single exposures. More recent studies have shown, however, that when total doses are low (<0.5 Gy) and the dose per fraction small, there is no significant difference in life shortening between fractionated and acute exposures. Although the data are less extensive than for low-LET radiation, the available information suggests that protraction of exposure does not affect life-span shortening.

2. Tumour induction

142. Information on radiation-induced tumours in experimental animals was extensively reviewed in the UNSCEAR 1977 Report [U4], in the UNSCEAR 1986 Report [U2], by the NCRP [N1], by Upton [U22] and in a comprehensive monograph on radiation carcinogenesis [U23]. Despite a substantial body of research potentially available for analysis, there are in practice

only a limited number of studies on tumour induction in experimental animals following exposure to low-LET radiation that can help to define the dose-response relationship for cancer induction over a reasonable dose range and to assess the influence of dose rate on tumour response. Important information comes from a series of studies with mice reported by Ullrich and Storer [U11-U16]. Although these investigations covered tumour induction in a number of tissues, it is convenient to discuss the results for different tumour types separately, in the context of other studies. It should be stressed, however, that the experimental animals used in many studies are inbred strains, with patterns of disease that are very different from those found in man. One of the main differences among mouse strains is their varying susceptibilities to both spontaneous and radiation-induced tumours; furthermore, within a given strain, there are frequently sex differences in the incidence and time of onset of specific tumour types. For example, the commonly used BALB/c strain has a very high incidence of spontaneous tumours, and the C57Bl strain has a much lower incidence [M25]. A number of tumour types for which information is available are either not found in man (Harderian gland) or appear to require substantial cell killing for their development (ovarian tumour, thymic lymphoma). For a number of other tumours there may be a human counterpart (myeloid leukaemia and tumours of the lung, the breast, the pituitary and the thyroid), but even here there can be differences in the cell types involved and in the development of the tumour. Furthermore, the development of tumours in both man and animals is subject to the modifying influence of various internal and external environmental factors, all of which can potentially influence dose-response relationships. There are also substantial differences in the rates of turnover of cells and in the life-span of the majority of experimental animals and man. Interpreting the results of animal studies and extrapolating them to man is therefore difficult. Nevertheless, such studies can make an important contribution to understanding the influence on tumour induction of factors such as dose rate and dose fractionation, radiation quality, dose distribution, age, disease and other internal and external agents. The use of animals to provide a basis for understanding factors influencing tumour induction applies not only to radiation but also to other agents such as chemicals and is considered further in Annex E "Mechanisms of radiation oncogenesis".

143. In assessing the influence of dose rate on tumour induction, a particular problem is that the dose-response relationship can vary substantially for different tumour types (Figures VIII-XV) [U22]. As a result, published reports describe the dose response in terms of a wide range of functions. Where data fits are given in the published papers that allow tumour incidences at different dose rates to be compared, the relevant information is given. In other cases, however, it has been necessary to fit the data reported. In general, the approach used has been to fit a linear function to the data obtained up to the highest dose at which there is no apparent influence of cell killing on the tumour yield. Generally this is the case for doses up to 2-3 Gy for acute exposures, but for low dose rates higher doses may be used. In some cases the most appropriate dose ranges for assessing dose and dose-rate effectiveness factors (DDREFs) are not clear from the data. In these cases, data fits have been calculated for a number of dose ranges.

144. The data from experimental animals on the effect of dose rate from low-LET radiation on tumour induction that are described in the following Sections are summarized principally in Tables 8-10. Table 8 gives best estimates of the DDREF for a range of tumour types in different animal species, together with information on the dose rates at which the studies were conducted and the dose ranges used for the calculation of the DDREF. Table 9 gives the results of fitting the data from a number of studies in mice over various dose ranges, and Table 10 examines uncertainties in the calculation of DDREF from studies in male and female mice. Results from a number of individual studies are given in Tables 11-15.

(a) Myeloid leukaemia

145. The effect of dose and dose rate on the induction of myeloid leukaemia has been examined in a number of strains of mice. Upton et al. [U21] compared the effect of a wide range of x- or gamma-ray doses in RF mice in the dose range from 0.25 to ~10 Gy. Male mice were substantially more sensitive than females, with an increased incidence of the disease detectable at 0.25 Gy given at a high dose rate (0.8 Gy min^{-1}, 250 kVp x rays). The incidence passed through a maximum at 3 Gy and declined at higher doses (Figure VIII). At doses up to about 1.5 Gy the incidence of the disease appeared to vary roughly with the square of the dose, although a linear dose response would fit the experimental results up to about 2 Gy. Low-dose-rate irradiation was much less effective than acute exposure. At dose rates of 0.04-0.6 mGy min^{-1}, no significant leukaemogenic effects were evident at a total dose of 1.5 Gy, although a significant increase was found at a dose of about 3 Gy. The induction period, as judged by mean age at death of mice with the disease, varied inversely with the dose and dose rate, suggesting that the disease contributed to the overall reduction in the life-span of the population. The exposures at different dose rates entailed time periods of between a few minutes up to about a month, so age effects are unlikely to have affected

tumour response, and differences between acute and chronic exposures appear to be predominantly due to differences in dose rate.

146. A linear fit to the incidence data up to 1 Gy in male mice [U21] exposed to high dose rates (slope: 14.4% ± 3.2% Gy^{-1}) and to 3.1 Gy following low dose rates (slope: 2.8% ± 0.8% Gy^{-1}) suggests that effectiveness at low dose rates decreased by a factor of 5.1 (Tables 8 and 9). A linear fit to the incidence data up to 3.0 Gy at high dose rate (slope 14.3% ± 1.7% Gy^{-1}) gave a similar result. In an earlier analysis of the high-dose and low-dose incidence data obtained up to 3.0 and 3.3 Gy, respectively, a dose-rate effectiveness factor of 6.7 was reported [N1].

147. In female RF mice the incidence of myeloid leukaemia following acute high dose-rate exposure was highly variable, and no clear dose-response relationship was obtained, although an overall increase in incidence was found at doses of 1 Gy or more at 0.067 Gy min^{-1} (Figure VIII) [U12]. At low dose rates, 0.004-0.7 mGy min^{-1}, the incidence of myeloid leukaemia (~6%) in mice exposed to doses between 1 and 6 Gy was approximately double that in controls (3%), but it showed no trend with increasing dose. The variability in results obtained for mice at high dose rates makes any estimates of dose-rate effect very uncertain. Based on a weighted least-squares fit to the data obtained up to 3 Gy at high dose rates (slope 6.8% ± 2.0% Gy^{-1}) and up to 5.8 Gy at low dose rate (slope 1.04% ± 0.38% Gy^{-1}), a dose-rate effectiveness factor of 6.5 is suggested (Table 9). A somewhat higher dose-rate factor (9.6) is obtained if the high-dose data on myeloid leukaemia incidence are compared with low-dose data over the range 0-6.1 Gy.

148. In contrast to these studies involving variations in dose rate, Upton et al. [U19] also examined the incidence of myeloid leukaemia in male RF mice given fractionated doses (2-3 exposures) of 0.75-1.5 Gy from x rays at high dose rates and found it to be similar to the incidence after single acute exposures. Robinson et al. [R3] re-analysed part of Upton's data on male RF mice [U18, U20, U21], considering those irradiated with 250 kVp x rays up to 4.5 Gy (~2,000 male mice) and correcting for competing risks. They obtained a good fit to the experimental data with a linear-quadratic model having an α_1/α_2 value of 0.5 Gy and a β_1/β_2 value of 2.4 Gy. It appears from these data that the decreased incidence of myeloid leukaemia at low dose rate can be interpreted in terms of an increasing linear component of the response and a diminishing quadratic component. The generalization of these results to other tissues is complicated, however, by the fact that the females are less sensitive than the males; also, it has been shown that the incidence of myeloid leukaemia is influenced by a number of host factors, including genetic background, hormonal status and the environment in which the animals are maintained [U19, U20]. Thus, animals maintained in a germ-free environment are less sensitive to the disease than animals housed in conventional facilities. It is not clear, therefore, whether the data suggesting dose-rate effects can be influenced by environmental factors involved in tumour initiation or expression.

149. Ullrich and Storer [U15] have reported dose-rate effects for myeloid leukaemia induction in 10-week-old specific-pathogen-free RFM/Un female mice exposed at 0.45 Gy min^{-1} or 0.083 Gy d^{-1} to ^{137}Cs gamma rays. Comparative data on dose response were obtained up to 2 Gy. Low-dose-rate exposure was much less effective than high-dose-rate exposure; in fact, no significant increase above control levels was observed at the low dose rate at doses up to 2 Gy. At high dose rate, a significant increase in myeloid leukaemia incidence above control levels was apparent at doses of 0.5 Gy and above, although the difference was only significant at 1.5 Gy or more. Even at 3 Gy the incidence was only 5.2%. Although the data could be fitted with either a linear or linear-quadratic model ($p > 0.5$ and $p > 0.8$, respectively), the dose-squared component was not significant, and linearity predominated over the dose range used in the study [U13]. A linear model fitted to the high-dose-rate data gives an incidence of 1.38% ± 0.12% Gy^{-1}, while that fitted to the low-dose rate data gives −0.050% ± 0.096% Gy^{-1}, reflecting the lack of any significant increase in incidence. The data therefore suggest a dose-rate effectiveness factor of infinity with a lower 95% confidence limit of 9.7.

150. Ullrich and Storer [U13] have also given dose-response data on male RFM mice exposed at 0.45 Gy min^{-1} to total doses between 0.1 and 3 Gy. Myeloid leukaemia incidence was higher than in female mice, and it was notable that the dose response could again be fitted with either a linear or a linear-quadratic model, with the linear component predominating over the dose range used in the study. The ratio of the linear slopes indicates that the sensitivity of male RFM mice to myeloid leukaemia ($I = 0.67 + 6.5D$, where I is the incidence in per cent and D is the dose in gray) is greater than that of female mice ($I = 0.63 + 1.4D$) by a factor of nearly 5.

151. The effect of variation in dose rate on the induction of myeloid leukaemia in male CBA/H mice has been examined by Mole et al. [M13]. This strain of mouse is exceptional in that no case of myeloid leukaemia has been observed in more than 1,400 unirradiated male mice, so that every case occurring in irradiated animals can be regarded as radiation-induced [H17] (see Annex E, "Mechanisms of radiation onco-

genesis"). Groups of mice received exposure to ^{60}Co gamma rays continuously over a four-week period (0.04-0.11 mGy min^{-1}) or single brief exposures five days a week for four successive weeks (0.25 Gy min^{-1}) or a single brief exposure (0.25 Gy min^{-1}). Total doses were 1.5, 3 or 4.5 Gy. The results of the study, summarized in Table 11, demonstrate a dose-dependent increase in incidence of myeloid leukaemia in the acutely exposed animals compared with controls, with a higher incidence than those groups given protracted exposure. However, in the groups in which radiation exposure was spread over a period of four weeks, either continuously or in 20 equal fractions (giving differences in dose rate of several thousand-fold), the incidence was the same, and within the dose range used appeared independent of the total cumulative dose. There is no obvious explanation for this result. Mole et al. [M13] speculated that the critical factor determining leukaemogenic frequency in this experiment was not the instantaneous physical dose rate but some biologically important factor correlated with protraction. Nevertheless, the frequency of leukaemia induction was already reduced by protraction of the dose. As a consequence of the lack of a dose-response relationship for myeloid leukaemia incidence with protracted exposure, in contrast to the results for acute exposure, the factor for reduction in myeloid leukaemia induction at low dose rates varies from 2.2 at 1.5 Gy to 5 at 4.5 Gy (Table 11).

152. ***Summary.*** These studies have shown that radiation-induced myeloid leukaemia can be induced in RFM and CBA mice, although there are differences in sensitivity between the strains and between both sexes. For dose rates varying by factors ranging from 100 to more than 1,000, DDREFs between about 2 and more than 10 have been obtained for doses in the 1-3 Gy range given at high dose rates, but there is no consistent trend (Table 8).

(b) Lung cancer

153. Information on the effect of dose and dose rate on carcinogenesis in the respiratory tract from low-LET radiation has come mostly from whole-body exposure of animals to x rays and gamma rays. However, comparative data are also available on the effects of inhaled radionuclides with different effective half-times in the lung; these data provide further information on dose-rate effects.

154. The induction of lung adenocarcinomas at high dose rates (0.4 Gy min^{-1}) and low dose rates (0.06 mGy min^{-1}) has been compared in female BALB/c mice [U12, U15] in the dose range 0.5-2 Gy. Tumour induction was less at low dose rates than at high dose rates. After high dose-rate exposure, the age-correlated incidence (%) could be represented by a linear function [$I(D) = 13.4 + 12D$; $p > 0.5$]; at low dose rates a linear function also gave a good fit to the data [$I(D) = 12.5 + 4.3D$; $p > 0.8$]. Since the authors indicated there were no changes in sensitivity with age over the period of irradiation and the data were adjusted for differences in the distribution of ages at death among the various treatment groups, the differences in slope can be considered to reflect differences in effectiveness at the two dose rates and suggest a dose-rate effectiveness factor of 2.8 (Table 8). The data on lung tumour induction in mice were extended in a further study [U24] which provided information on the dose response at high dose rates (0.4 Gy min^{-1}) in the dose range from 0.1 to 2 Gy. Although the tumour incidence data could again be fitted by a linear model [$I(D) = 10.9 + 11D$; $p > 0.70$)], they could also be fitted by a linear-quadratic model [$I(D) = 11.9 + 4D + 4.3D^2$, $p > 0.70$]. In this equation the linear term was very similar to that obtained for low-dose-rate exposures, and it was concluded that the result was in general consistent with a linear-quadratic model in which the linear term is independent of dose rate at high and low dose rates.

155. Recently, Ullrich et al. [U26] tested the predictions of the linear-quadratic model in a series of studies with BALB/c mice using fractionated exposures. The model predicts that fractionating an exposure using high-dose-rate fractions but with a small total dose per fraction, which would lie on the predominantly linear portion of the dose-response curve, would have an effect similar to that obtained with low dose rates. Mice were exposed to total doses of 2 Gy from ^{137}Cs gamma rays given in different daily fractions (0.1, 0.5, and 1 Gy) at high dose rate (0.35 Gy min^{-1}). The linear-quadratic dose-response curve for lung tumour induction gave an α_1/α_2 quotient of 0.93, indicating that at doses of about 0.9 Gy, the α_1 and α_2 terms contribute equally to the tumour response. At doses substantially below this, the linear term should predominate, giving a tumour induction rate similar to that at low dose rates (0.06 mGy min^{-1}) (Figure IX).

156. The results of the study are shown in Table 12, which gives both the observed incidences of lung adenocarcinomas and those calculated from the predictions of a linear-quadratic model, on the assumption that the effects of each dose fraction are additive and independent of each other. The lung tumour incidence following daily fractions of 0.1 Gy (group 3), which would be on the linear component of the response curve, was comparable to that obtained following low-dose-rate exposure (group 2). If the dose per fraction was increased the quadratic term would be expected to make an increasing contribution to the response, with an increase in the tumour incidence per unit dose, as was indeed observed (groups 4 and 5), although not to

the level obtained with a single exposure to 2 Gy at high dose rate (group 1). The results are seen to be consistent with the predictions of the linear-quadratic model, which can therefore be used to assess the effect of dose rate on tumour response at various doses and dose rates. Table 13 gives both total tumour incidence and radiation-induced excess tumours for a range of doses (0.1-3 Gy) administered at both high and low dose rates. The incidence of tumours has not been calculated at doses above 3 Gy, because at higher doses cell killing is expected to become significant. At the lowest dose (0.1 Gy), the linear term dominates and the tumour incidence is largely independent of the dose rate (DDREF = 1.1). At higher doses, however, the quadratic term becomes of increasing importance at high dose rates, giving a DDREF of about 3.2 at 2 Gy and 4.2 at 3 Gy (mean: 3.7). These experimental data illustrate very clearly the extent to which lowering the dose rate can reduce the tumour incidence. They also suggest that for lung adenocarcinoma in mice, a low dose, at which there is no significant effect of dose rate, is in the range 0.1-0.2 Gy.

157. Extensive long-term studies on the effects of inhaled beta- and gamma-emitting radionuclides in dogs have been reported by McClellan et al. [M1]. Groups of about 100 beagle dogs about 13 months old were exposed to aerosols of a range of radionuclides bound in fused aluminosilicate particles and having different half-lives (^{90}Y: 64 hours; ^{91}Y: 58.5 days; ^{144}Ce: 285 days; ^{90}Sr: 28 years) to give a range of initial lung contents. In this insoluble form, the radionuclides are poorly transportable in the lung tissue and do not readily translocate to the blood. The different radioactive half-lives of the nuclides gave effective half-times in the lung ranging from 2.5 days for ^{90}Y to 600 days for ^{90}Sr. As a consequence, very different dose rates were obtained for the same cumulative dose (Figure X). For ^{90}Y, more than 90% of the total dose to the lung was received within two weeks of exposure, for ^{91}Y, about 90% of the dose was received by six months; while for ^{144}Ce and ^{90}Sr, only 77% and 34% of the total doses were received by one year. The dogs are being observed for their active lifetime, and the study is not yet complete. Some dogs exposed to high radiation doses died early with radiation pneumonitis and fibrosis; others died later with lung tumours. Tumours occurred with absorbed doses to lung ranging from 11 to 680 Gy. Preliminary data on the incidence rates of radiation-induced lung tumours have been reported [G10, H12]. The estimated risk coefficients for lung tumour induction in dogs exposed to ^{90}Y, ^{91}Y, ^{144}Ce and ^{90}Sr at times up to more than 10 years after exposure were 0.036, 0.032, 0.011 and 0.013 Gy^{-1}. Thus, the relative risk of lung cancer in dogs exposed at the higher dose rate from ^{90}Y is about three times the risk observed in dogs exposed at low dose rates.

158. ***Summary.*** Two studies in mice have found an effect of dose and dose rate on lung tumour induction, with DDREFs in the range of 3-4 for doses in the range 2-3 Gy given at high dose rate. Studies in beagle dogs exposed to inhaled, insoluble radionuclides with different effective half-times have given a range of risk coefficients for induced lung cancer that varied by a factor of about 3 between ^{90}Y, which gave the highest dose rate, and ^{90}Sr, which gave the lowest (Tables 8 and 13).

(c) Mammary tumours

159. Mammary carcinogenesis in inbred strains of mice is highly dependent on hormonal, viral, genetic, immunological, dietary and environmental factors [S7, S8]. As a consequence, irradiation may affect mammary carcinogenesis either directly, by affecting the cells of the breast, or indirectly by causing functional changes in the endocrine glands or by activating mammary tumour virus or other viral agents. In some mouse strains there is evidence that ionizing radiation can induce mammary tumours by "abscopal" effects, i.e. tumours can be induced in the mammary tissue irrespective of the area irradiated [B19, S8]. Similar considerations also apply in the rat. Rat mammary tumours can be classified as fibroadenomas and adenocarcinomas [Y3]. The incidence and proportion of these tumour types is very dependent on the strain of rat irradiated.

160. The most extensive experimental data on the induction of mammary tumours by ionizing radiation come from studies in Sprague-Dawley rats. However, in this strain of rat, which is sensitive to the induction of adenocarcinomas by radiation, there is a high spontaneous tumour incidence beyond about 15 months of age, so that in many experimental studies a cut-off period of approximately 12 months is imposed. Near the end of life of these animals the total tumour incidence in controls approaches that seen in irradiated animals, with the result that the absolute excess incidence is increased minimally, if at all. Thus, it may be that the effect of irradiation is to accelerate the appearance of tumours rather than to increase the overall incidence [C14, S8]. For rats of other strains and for other species the incidence of radiation-induced mammary tumours is less than in Sprague-Dawley rats [U11].

161. In Sprague-Dawley rats given whole-body x-irradiation or ^{60}Co gamma-irradiation at 1-2 months of age (0.25-4 Gy), the incidence of tumours at one year increased as a linear function of the dose [B17]. Similar results were obtained by Shellabarger et al. [S6] in the dose range 0.16-2 Gy with ^{60}Co gamma rays. The incidence of mammary tumours in rats

exposed to ^{60}Co at two different dose rates has been reported by Shellabarger et al. [S15]. Groups of rats were exposed at either 0.0003 Gy min^{-1} or 0.1 Gy min^{-1} to give total doses of 0.9 Gy and 2.7 Gy. In animals exposed to 2.7 Gy, the incidence of mammary adenocarcinomas was higher in the high-dose-rate group (8/20, or 40%) than in the low-dose-rate group (4/35, or 11%). With an incidence in controls of 1%-2%, this suggests a dose-rate effectiveness factor of about 4. However, no effect of dose protraction was found in the low-dose group, and for both dose levels, no protraction effect was observed for mammary fibroadenomas or total mammary tumours. The overall incidence of tumours in the animals exposed at low dose rate was also lower than in the animals exposed at high dose rate, largely because of the effect on adenocarcinomas. Shellabarger et al. [S4, S5] have also compared mammary tumour induction in rats given 4-5 Gy from x rays, either in a single exposure or in up to 32 fractions delivered over a 16-week period. No apparent change in the total tumour incidence was observed with dose fractionation, but this may have been because the total dose exceeded the level at which the response reached a maximum with single-exposure irradiation.

162. The incidence of mammary tumours in Sprague-Dawley rats exposed at different dose rates has been reported by Gragtmans et al. [G7]. Groups of approximately 120 SPF rats were either chronically exposed to 200 kVp x rays over a 10-day period, to give doses between 0.3 and 2 Gy, or given acute exposures of 0.6 or 1.8 Gy over one hour. In all dose groups, total tumour incidence was significantly greater than in controls, and by 450 days the average number of tumours per animal exceeded unity for the highest dose groups following both acute exposure (1.52 tumours per animal) and chronic exposure (1.14 per animal) (controls: 0.17 per animal). The best fit to the data up to 450 days was obtained with a linear function with cumulative tumour incidences of 78.3% ± 10.4% Gy^{-1} for acute exposure and 45.5% ± 5.4% Gy^{-1} for chronic exposure. A linear dose response was also obtained for the proportion of animals with tumours at 450 days with parameter values of 40.5% ± 0.4% Gy^{-1} and 24.8% ± 2.4% Gy^{-1} for acute and chronic exposures, respectively. These results indicate dose-rate effectiveness factors in the range 1.6-1.7, which is the same range in which other data on mammary tumour induction fall.

163. The effect of fractionated or single doses of x rays has been reported for WAG/RIJ rats [B23]. The rats were eight weeks old when irradiated and were kept until death. The frequency of fibroadenomas and carcinomas was based on histological examination. Weibull functions were fitted to the dose-response data, and the probability of survival without evidence of a tumour was calculated according to the Kaplan-Meier life-table analysis. The analysis showed that irradiation accelerated the appearance of fibroadenomas and carcinomas. Fractionation of the dose (10 exposures of 0.2 Gy at one month intervals) was only marginally less effective in respect of the effect on appearance time of mammary carcinomas than a single dose of 2 Gy; this study, therefore, provides no evidence for a reduction factor (i.e. DDREF ≈ 1).

164. The effect of dose rate on mammary tumour induction in mice has been reported by Ullrich and Storer [U12, U15]. In female BALB/c mice exposed to ^{137}Cs gamma rays, groups of mice were exposed at either a low dose rate (0.06 mGy min^{-1}) or a high dose rate (0.45 Gy min^{-1}) to give total cumulative doses of 0.5 Gy or 2 Gy. At both dose levels the incidence of mammary adenocarcinomas could be adequately described by linear relationships and was higher at high dose rates [$I(D) = 7.9 + 6.7D$; $p > 0.5$] than at low dose rates [$I(D) = 7.8 + 3.5D$; $p > 0.25$] (Figure XI). The ratio of the slope constants for mammary tumours suggests a dose-rate effectiveness factor of 1.9.

165. These data on mammary tumour induction were extended in a further study [U24] which provided information on the dose response at high dose rates (0.4 Gy min^{-1}) in the dose range from 0.1 to 2 Gy. The incidence of mammary tumours increased rapidly over the dose range up to 0.25 Gy. At higher doses, although there was some response, it was roughly flat. The high initial sensitivity to tumour induction was surprising in the light of the previous results [U12], which, however, were based on fewer data points and doses no lower than 0.5 Gy. Taken together with the previous data, the data obtained up to a dose of about 0.25 Gy were consistent with a linear-quadratic model of the form $I(D) = 7.7 + 3.5D + 150D^2$. The linear term was similar to that obtained after low-dose-rate exposures.

166. Ullrich et al. [U26] have tested the predictions of this linear-quadratic model in a series of studies with fractionated exposures. The fit to the data gives an α_1/α_2 quotient of 0.023, indicating that doses as low as 0.1 Gy will give a significant contribution from the quadratic component. BALB/c mice were exposed to total doses of 0.25 Gy given as daily fractions of either 0.01 Gy or 0.05 Gy. The incidence of mammary tumours for these two groups and for other groups of mice exposed at high dose rate (0.35 Gy min^{-1}) to give total doses of 0.1-0.25 Gy and at low dose rate (0.07 mGy min^{-1}) to give 0.25 Gy are compared in Table 14 with tumour incidences predicted by the linear-quadratic model. Acute daily fractions of 0.01 Gy gave a tumour incidence similar to that observed following low-dose-rate exposure and in

good agreement with model predictions. In general the results demonstrate that for mammary tumour induction, the effects of dose fractionation can be predicted by the linear-quadratic dose-response model. The response of this strain of mouse appears, however, to be markedly different from that of the rat strains described above, as a substantial dose-rate effect is apparent, with an implied DDREF at 0.25 Gy, the highest dose at which tumour incidence was measured, of about 12 (Table 15). In rats evaluation of the DDREF was made at doses up to about 3 Gy (Table 8).

167. *Summary.* A number of studies have been published on the effect of dose rate on mammary tumour induction in rats. These studies give DDREFs from less than 2 to about 4 for dose rates varying by a factor of 150 or more and for doses at high dose rate in the range from about 2 to 3 Gy (Table 8). One study in mice gives an implied DDREF based on an assumed linear-quadratic response of about 12 at 0.25 Gy for dose rates varying by a factor of about 5,000, although interpretation of the data is limited by the lack of information at higher doses.

(d) Pituitary tumours

168. The effect of dose rate on the induction of pituitary tumours in RFM mice has been reported by Ullrich and Storer [U14, U15] for female mice exposed at high dose rates to ^{137}Cs gamma-radiation (0.45 Gy min^{-1}) giving total doses of 0.1-3 Gy. The incidence of these tumours with radiation dose was found to increase at doses of 0.5 Gy or higher, although the response was somewhat irregular and did not differ significantly from controls, even at 2 Gy. The incidence remained at approximately control levels (6%-7%) over the range 0-0.25 Gy, increased to 9%-10% at 0.5 Gy, remained at that level over the range to 2 Gy, and increased to 20.9% at 3 Gy. Both a linear model [$I(D) = 5.7 + 4.4D$; $p > 0.2$] and a linear-quadratic model [$I(D) = 6.3 + 0.8D + 0.013D^2$] adequately described the data. Lowering the dose rate to 0.06 mGy min^{-1} resulted in a reduced tumour incidence up to a total dose of 2 Gy; this incidence was best described by a linear model [$I(D) = 6.3 + 0.7D$; $p > 0.95$]. When the linear dose responses fitted at low and high dose rates were compared, low-dose-rate exposures were found to be less effective in inducing pituitary tumours, by a factor of about 6 (Table 8). However, if a linear-quadratic response is assumed after high-dose-rate exposure [$I(D) = 6.3 + 0.8D + 0.013D^2$], then the linear term is similar at both dose rates, suggesting that the primary effect of dose rate is to alter the dose-squared component. Male RFM mice were exposed only at the higher dose rate, and the incidence of pituitary tumours was too low to warrant analysis.

169. *Summary.* Only one study has been published that allows an estimate to be made of a DDREF for the induction of pituitary tumours. In female mice, a value of about 6 can be obtained for doses up to about 3 Gy given at high dose rate and for dose rates that differ by a factor of about 8,000.

(e) Thyroid tumours

170. Thyroid cancer in animals can be induced by iodine deficiency, chemical carcinogens, and goitrogens, and exposure to ionizing radiation. Information is available from human populations on the effects of both external radiation and internal radiation from intakes of iodine isotopes; it suggests that ^{131}I is less carcinogenic than external radiation (see Chapter III), although whether this is due solely to dose-rate effects or to other factors as well is not clear. In principle, animal studies should be able to provide information on the relative effects of external radiation and ^{131}I, but in practice the reported results present some difficulties in interpretation, and there are species differences in the way thyroid cancer is expressed.

171. Doniac [D4] reviewed a series of studies in rats that could be used to compare the tumorigenic effects of x rays and ^{131}I. Results from three studies suggested that the carcinogenic effect of 11 Gy from acute x-ray exposure was comparable to that of 1.1 MBq of ^{131}I, which would give a dose to the thyroid of about 100 Gy. The dose rates are substantial, and significant cell killing might be expected, although higher doses of ^{131}I are needed to cause atrophy. With this proviso, the data suggest that protracted irradiation from ^{131}I is less damaging, by a factor of about 10, than an acute dose of x rays.

172. Walinder [W2] compared the carcinogenicity of x rays and ^{131}I in adult CBA mice. His results indicated that ^{131}I was one fourth to one tenth as effective as x rays for the production of thyroid adenomas and carcinomas; doses from x rays were 15 Gy and from ^{131}I, 64-160 Gy. He also found that at somewhat lower doses (10 Gy from x rays and 22-110 Gy from ^{131}I), ^{131}I was one half to one tenth as effective as x rays.

173. Whether this difference in effect is due solely to differences in dose rate is difficult to determine, as a number of factors influence the dosimetry of ^{131}I [C8, D4, J1]. As a consequence of the small mass of the thyroid in the rat or mouse, considerable beta-radiation is lost from the peripheral portions and the isthmus. Thyroid cells near the surface may receive as little as 50% of the dose to the central cells, an effect that becomes more important as the gland size decreases. Unlike the dose from external radiation, the dose from

intakes of ^{131}I may be heterogeneously distributed owing to variation in uptake between follicles, although Walinder et al. [W1] have reported measurements of the dose distribution for ^{131}I and ^{132}I in mouse thyroid and found it to be generally uniform, but with decreases at the thyroid edges, as would be expected for a uniform concentration. Walinder et al. [W1] also observed a similar effectiveness of ^{132}I ($T_{½}$ ~ 2.2 h) and x rays on the thyroid in the inhibition of goitrogen-stimulated growth in the CBA mouse and that ^{131}I was one half to one tenth as effective as x rays. Book et al. [B14] observed in the Sprague-Dawley rat a difference in effectiveness of ^{131}I to ^{132}I of about 1:9, in terms of average thyroid dose, for the suppression of thyroid gland weight increase stimulated by goitrogen. The dose distribution in the thyroid gland is similar for the two radionuclides, and the observed difference in radiation is likely to be due to differences in dose rate. Liu et al. [L2] found that the tumour incidence was lower following exposure to ^{131}I than ^{132}I. Although this difference may have been partly due to higher radiation doses from ^{131}I, the dose rate may have also been a factor in the response. Since ^{131}I uptake by the thyroid in laboratory animals varies with environmental temperature and the dietary content of stable iodide, the administration of similar amounts in separate experiments in different laboratories may give rise to varying doses. The usual assumption, for dosimetric purposes, of a single exponential function for loss of activity from the gland may also result in some uncertainty in the calculated doses, although by a factor of less than 2 [C8]. Despite these uncertainties, it seems likely that the differences in the incidence of cancer resulting from intakes of ^{131}I and from exposure to external radiation cannot be readily explained by differences in dose distribution.

174. In a subsequent study, Lee et al. [L4] compared tumour induction in six-week-old female Long Evans rats given ^{131}I or localized x-irradiation of the thyroid. Three groups of 300 rats were injected intraperitoneally with 18, 70 and 200 kBq of sodium ^{131}I-iodide, giving thyroid doses of 0.8, 3.3 and 8.5 Gy (maximum dose rates: 0.17, 0.69 and 1.6 mGy min^{-1}). Three further groups received localized (collimated) x-ray exposures of the thyroid gland giving doses of 0.94, 4.5 and 10.6 Gy (dose rate: 2.8 Gy min^{-1}). Six hundred animals were kept as controls. All the animals surviving to two years (~62%) were killed, and a six-month minimum latent period for radiogenic thyroid cancer was assumed. The doses from ^{131}I in this study were considerably lower than those in the earlier ones. Exposure to ^{131}I was found to be about 40% as effective as x-irradiation at the highest dose for the production of adenomas, but there was no significant difference from x rays at the lower doses. For the production of thyroid carcinomas the two radiations appear to be of equal effectiveness at all three doses, although the statistics were such that the results do not exclude a two- to threefold difference in the effectiveness of x rays and ^{131}I.

175. These differences in effectiveness observed in the studies by Lee et al. [L4] and the earlier rat studies are not easy to explain. They may reflect differences in the doses used, in the ages of animals or in the strains of rats. Female Long Evans rats are also more sensitive than males, which has been attributed to hormonal fluctuations. The results of Lee et al. [L4] provide probably the largest single body of information on thyroid cancer induction by ^{131}I or x rays in an animal model. Furthermore, the dose range was low and more relevant to the assessment of risks from low-level exposures. That study, however, terminated at two years, rather than allowing the animals to live out their natural life-span. This may have prevented the appearance of some late tumours, an important feature, as about two thirds of the animals remained alive at the end of the two-year study.

176. ***Summary.*** Animal data do not support large differences between ^{131}I and x rays for thyroid cancer induction for doses below about 10 Gy. Early experiments that indicated differences of up to a factor 10 were at doses that would have caused appreciable tissue damage. However, differences in tumour response of a factor of about 3 between ^{131}I and x rays cannot be ruled out.

(f) Liver tumours

177. Di Majo et al. [D3] have reported dose-response relationships for liver tumour induction in $BC3F_1$ male mice. Three-month-old mice were exposed to x rays (0.133 Gy min^{-1}) in graded acute doses from 0.5 Gy to 7 Gy. A significant increase in liver tumours was observed from 2 Gy, and the dose response was best fitted by a pure quadratic response [$I(D) = 11.3 + 1.2D^2$] (Figure XII). Although the animals were not exposed at different dose rates, this pattern of dose response would imply that tumour induction would be reduced at lower dose rates.

(g) Harderian gland tumours

178. The induction of Harderian gland tumours at different dose rates has been examined in RFM mice [U12, U14, U15]. This information is included here for the sake of completeness, although it is noted that there is no human counterpart to this tumour. The data are, however, considered to be relevant to understanding the overall response of tissues to radiation. Low-dose-rate exposures (0.06 mGy min^{-1}) were less effective than high-dose-rate exposures (0.45 Gy

min^{-1}), with incidences at 2 Gy being significantly different for the two treatments (Figure XIII). Dose-response relationships at high dose rates suggested a linear-quadratic model for both males [$I(D) = 1.5 + 0.3D + 0.012D^2$; $p > 0.99$] and females [$I(D) = 1.2 + 1.5D + 0.022D^2$; $p > 0.25$], although linearity could only be excluded with confidence for females ($p < 0.05$). At low dose rates, a linear dose response gave the best fit to the data for female mice [$I(D) = 1.2 + 1.5D$; $p > 0.9$], suggesting, as in the case of pituitary tumours, a similar linear response for low and high dose rates, and that the primary effect of lowering the dose rate was to diminish the dose-squared component. On the basis of a simple linear fit to the high- dose-rate dose-response data [$I(D) = 0.93 + 4.7D$; $p < 0.05$], the results for female mice indicate that tumour incidence at low dose rates is reduced by a factor of about 3 for doses of about 2 Gy (Table 8).

179. ***Summary.*** The dose-response for Harderian gland tumours in female mice resulting from high-dose rate exposures can be fitted by a linear-quadratic relationship. The data suggest a DDREF for high-dose-rate exposures of about 3 for doses of about 2 Gy and for dose rates varying by a factor of about 8,000.

(h) Ovarian tumours

180. The induction of ovarian tumours in gamma-irradiated mice has been shown to depend on the dose rate [U12, U21, Y4]. Interpretation of some of the data is complicated, however, by a decrease with age in the susceptibility of the mouse ovary to tumorigenesis. Furthermore, since the stimulus for tumorigenesis is believed to involve killing of oocytes and associated changes in hormonal status [U21], this is likely to contribute to observed dose-rate effects.

181. The induction of ovarian tumours by x rays was studied by Ullrich and Storer [U15] using SPF/RFM female mice exposed at 0.45 Gy min^{-1} and 0.06 mGy min^{-1}. After high-dose-rate exposures, a significant increase in tumour incidence relative to controls was observed for doses of 0.25-3 Gy. In the group exposed at the lower dose rate, no significant increase in incidence was seen until 1 Gy, when the incidence was similar to that observed in the groups receiving 0.25 Gy at higher dose rate (Figure XIV). The high-dose-rate data could be adequately described by a linear-quadratic model with a negative linear component [$I(D) = 2.3 + (-23) D + 1.8D^2$; $p > 0.25$] or by a threshold plus quadratic model [$I(D) = 2.2 + 2.3 (D-D^*)^2$; $p > 0.75$, where the threshold dose, D*, was estimated to be 0.12 Gy] [U14]. Linear and quadratic models were rejected. For the low-dose-rate response linear, quadratic and threshold plus quadratic models could be rejected ($p < 0.01$). The two models that appeared to describe the relationship adequately were a linear-quadratic model [$I(D) = 2.3 + (-3.7)D + 0.068D^2$; $p > 0.25$] and a threshold plus linear model [$I(D) = 2.07 + 14.9(D-D^*)$; $p > 0.75$, where the threshold dose, D*, was estimated to be 0.115 Gy].

182. In female BALB/c mice similar results have been obtained [U15]. Ovarian tumours were readily induced with high-dose-rate exposures (0.40 Gy min^{-1}) to ^{137}Cs gamma rays, giving a 66% incidence at 0.5 Gy, the lowest dose used, compared with a 9.9% incidence at low dose rate (0.06 mGy min^{-1}) for the same total dose (dose-rate effectiveness factor: 6.7, Table 8). As in the case of RFM mice, linearity could be rejected ($p < 0.05$) at low dose rate, and the dose response up to 2 Gy could be described by a linear-quadratic model [$I(D) = 6.0 + 8.3D + 0.05D^2$]. There were insufficient data at high dose rate to define a dose-response function; doses below 0.5 Gy would have been required.

183. This pattern of response for ovarian tumour induction seen in both RFM and BALB/c mice is explained by the mechanism of induction for ovarian cancers, which is considered to involve substantial cell killing. This mechanism will be less effective at low dose rates and may account for the apparent threshold in the response. Linear functions fitted in this Annex to the dose-response data in RFM mice obtained up to 2 Gy for both high- and low-dose-rate exposures [U15] give a crude overall DDREF of 5.5 (range: 4.1-6.8, Table 9), compared with a value of 6.7 for BALB/c mice (Table 8), but because of the mechanisms involved, the extrapolation of these results to man is uncertain.

184. ***Summary.*** The induction of ovarian tumours has been shown in mice to depend on dose rate. DDREFs of 5.5 and 6.7 have been obtained in RFM and BALB/c mice at doses up to 2 Gy for dose rates varying by a factor of about 8,000. Since the stimulus for tumorigenesis is believed to involve killing of oocytes and associated changes in hormonal status, extrapolation of these results to man is uncertain.

(i) Thymic lymphoma

185. A number of investigators have studied the incidence of thymic lymphoma after radiation exposure. However, many of these studies have been concerned with modifying factors that influence the course of the disease or the sequence of events leading to its development rather than with dose-response relationships. An added complication is that dose-response curves of a threshold type have been reported [M5], indicating that cell killing is important in the induction mechanism.

186. Ullrich and Storer [U12, U15] studied the dose-response relationship and dose-rate effects for exposure to ^{137}Cs gamma rays in 10-week-old female RFM/Un mice. The incidence of thymic lymphoma after high-dose-rate exposure (0.45 Gy min^{-1}) was substantially greater than after low dose rates (0.06 mGy min^{-1}) at all doses for which comparable data were given (0.5, 1 and 2 Gy) (Figure XV). In fact, no significant increase in incidence relative to controls was observed after low-dose-rate irradiation up to a total dose of 1 Gy, whereas at high dose rates a significant increase in incidence was observed at doses of 0.25 Gy. Examination of the relationship between the incidence of thymic lymphoma and the radiation dose at high and low dose rates indicated both quantitative and qualitative differences. The dose response after high-dose-rate exposure appeared to have two components. Up to 0.25 Gy, the incidence of thymic lymphoma increased with the square of the dose, with a second, linear component describing the response over the range 0.5-3 Gy. At the lower dose rate the response was best described by a linear-quadratic model with a shallow (perhaps zero) initial linear slope, and linearity could be rejected. Considering that the mechanism of thymic lymphoma induction is thought to involve cell killing or the possible release of viruses and subsequent target cell viral interactions, it is not surprising that somewhat complex dose and dose-rate response relationships have been obtained.

187. An early analysis by the NCRP [N1] gave a dose-rate effectiveness factor of 6.4 for these data. Alternatively, the high- and low-dose-rate data obtained up to 3 and 2 Gy may be fitted with linear models, giving fits of 16.7% ± 1.8% Gy^{-1} and 2.9% ± 1.9% Gy^{-1}, respectively, corresponding to a dose-rate effectiveness factor of 5.8 (Tables 8 and 9). In males [U13] no dose-response data were obtained at low dose rates, but at high dose rates (0.45 Gy min^{-1}) a significant increase in incidence occurred at doses of 0.25 Gy and above, and the data over the entire dose range up to 3 Gy could be adequately fitted by a linear function (6.7% ± 6.9% Gy^{-1}). Overall, males were less sensitive than females by a factor of about 2.4, reflecting the difference of a factor of about 2 in the incidence in controls.

188. An increased incidence of thymic lymphoma has also been reported by Upton et al. [U21] for male and female RFM mice exposed to x rays. Lymphoid neoplasms occurred in about 4%-10% of controls, and the increase in incidence depended on both the total dose and the dose rate, with a significant increase, relative to controls, at doses of about 2 Gy or more. With decreasing dose rate, the effectiveness of gamma-radiation in inducing tumours declined. A linear dose function fitted to both high-dose-rate (0.8 Gy min^{-1}) and low-dose-rate (0.04-0.6 mGy min^{-1}) incidence data for males suggests a dose-rate effectiveness factor of about 2.6 (Table 8) at doses up to about 4 Gy. For females the data are too variable to infer a dose-rate effectiveness factor.

189. In experiments by Maisin et al. [M5], 12-week-old male mice were exposed to single or fractionated (10 equal doses separated at daily intervals) doses from ^{137}Cs gamma rays (4 Gy min^{-1}) in the dose range 0.25-6 Gy. The dose-response curve for thymic lymphoma was of a threshold type, the incidence in irradiated animals rising above that in controls only at 4 and 6 Gy. Single doses were more effective than fractionated exposures at 4 Gy by a factor of about 2; there was no significant difference in response at 6 Gy.

190. ***Summary***. An effect of dose rate on the induction of thymic lymphoma has been demonstrated in RFM male and female mice with DDREFs of about 2.6 and 5.8 for doses of 2 to 4 Gy and for dose rates varying by factors of more than 1,000 (Table 8). As with ovarian tumours there are difficulties in extrapolating these data to man, however, as cell killing appears to be involved in the development of this tumour.

(j) Skin tumours

191. A number of studies have reported that when the radiation dose is fractionated, the incidence of skin tumours decreases in comparison with acute exposures. Hulse et al. [H30] irradiated the skin of three-month-old CBA/H female mice with a ^{204}Tl source. Four different schedules of exposure were used: four equal doses at weekly intervals, four equal doses at monthly intervals, 12 equal doses at weekly intervals and 20 equal doses five days weekly for four weeks. Total doses given were large, 60 Gy or 120 Gy. The tumours occurring after the different irradiation schedules were similar to those seen after single exposures and were mainly dermal tumours at both dose levels. Dividing the total dose into four fractions did not affect tumour yield, whether the exposures were spread over 22 days or 12 weeks. When 20 fractions were given over 25 days, however, the yield was significantly reduced (p = 0.02) to about half that with a single exposure. With 12 fractions given over 11 weeks, the yield was non-significantly reduced (p = 0.09 for both dose groups; p = 0.06 for 60 Gy). It was concluded that a reduction in tumour yield followed multiple fractionation and protraction over several weeks only if the dose per fraction was 5-6 Gy or less. The reduction factor was about 2. For epidermal tumours, of which there were fewer than half the number of dermal tumours, there was a much greater variation in response between the groups. None of the

groups with fractionated exposure had a significantly different tumour yield from the single exposure group, and there was no clear evidence that protraction or fractionation reduced tumour yield. The yield of epidermal tumours was, however, significantly less in the 20-fraction groups (at 6 and 12 Gy total doses) compared with the groups given 4 and 12 weekly fractions.

192. In a series of studies in male CD rats [B40], skin tumour incidence following acute exposure to attenuated 0.7 MeV electrons (1.6-2.4 Gy min^{-1}) was measured at nine doses (20 rats per group) between 5 Gy and 23 Gy. A peaked dose-response curve was obtained, with a maximum tumour incidence at a dose of about 16 Gy. At 10, 14.5 and 23 Gy, the exposures were also split into two equal fractions spaced at intervals of 1, 3 and 6.3 hours. The effect of split doses on tumour yield depended on the position on the dose-response curve. At the lowest split dose the tumour yield declined with a half-time of about 1.8 hours. At the intermediate dose, an initial increase was followed by a decline, with a half-time of 3-4 hours; at the highest dose (23 Gy) the tumour yield increased, presumably as a result of the spacing effect on cell lethality. The maximum effect of dose fractionation (14.5 Gy, two fractions, 6.3 hours) gave a reduction in tumour yield by a factor of about 2.

193. In a more recent series of papers [O5, O6], skin tumour incidence has been measured in female ICR mice. The backs of the animals were repeatedly irradiated with beta particles from ^{90}Sr-^{90}Y (2.24 Gy min^{-1}, surface dose). For doses of 2.5-11.8 Gy per exposure, three times weekly throughout life, 100% incidence of tumours was observed. At doses of about 1.5 Gy per exposure, however, there was a marked delay in the appearance of tumours. In a further study [O7], groups of 30 or 31 mice were irradiated with ^{90}Sr-^{90}Y three times weekly throughout their life with doses of 0.75, 1.0, 1.5 and 8.0 Gy at each irradiation. The study demonstrated that tumours appeared later in the groups given 1.0 or 1.5 Gy per exposure than in the group given 8.0 Gy per exposure, although tumour incidence was 100% with these two doses. At 0.75 Gy per exposure, no tumours appeared within 790 days, although an osteosarcoma and one squamous cell carcinoma did finally appear. There was no effect on the life-span of the animals. In a further group of 50 mice given 0.5 Gy per exposure no tumours were obtained [O8, T11]. This observation of an "apparent" threshold in response may be accounted for by the small number of animals involved, but it is more likely arises as a result of the characteristics of this particular tumour, in which induction appears to be more dependent on dose per fraction than on total dose; single doses of up to 30 Gy alone do not induce tumours. At the higher doses and dose rates tumour development is likely to be influenced by radiation effects on the tissue surrounding initiated cells.

194. ***Summary.*** A series of studies in rodents has shown that when irradiation of the skin is fractionated the incidence of skin tumours is less than with acute exposure. In the majority of studies, however, the total doses have been large, and dose fractionation has been seen to have an effect only for doses per fraction of less than about 5-6 Gy. In general, the effect of dose fractionation under these conditions has been to reduce tumour yield by a factor of about 2. In one study, in which female ICR mice were repeatedly irradiated with beta particles from ^{90}Sr-^{90}Y, an apparent threshold for tumour induction was obtained at a dose per fraction of about 0.5 Gy. This may have been the result of delayed tumour appearance or the influence of radiation damage to surrounding tissues at the high doses and dose rates used.

(k) Tumour induction in rats

195. In male Sprague-Dawley rats (3 months old) exposed to ^{60}Co gamma rays to give 2.83 Gy (304 rats, 2.2 mGy min^{-1}), 1 Gy (505 rats, 1.3 mGy min^{-1}) and 3 Gy (120 rats, 1.3 mGy min^{-1}), an effect of dose rate on overall tumour induction was observed, although this varied with the tumour type [M43]. At lower dose rates the incidence of radiation-induced carcinomas (excluding thyroid, pituitary and adrenals) was lower than at high dose rates for a total dose of about 3 Gy. The frequencies of carcinoma were 6.8% ± 1.9%, 10.1% ± 3.8% and 25.8% ± 8.2% in controls and animals exposed at 1.34 mGy h^{-1} (total dose: 2.8 Gy) and 78 mGy h^{-1} (3 Gy), respectively, implying a reduction in excess cancers by a factor of about 6 at the lower dose rate. Although the incidence of most carcinomas showed an increase with increasing dose rate, the effect was most significant for the digestive and urinary systems.

196. For a group of sarcomas that are poorly inducible in the rat (nervous system, leukaemia, lymphosarcoma, bone and mesothelioma) but frequent in man, no dependence on dose and dose rate was observed. For a second group of sarcomas (angiosarcomas and fibrosarcomas of internal organs and of soft tissue), which are infrequent in man but common in the rat, the incidence did increase with dose (from 1 to 3 Gy), although again it was independent of dose rate.

197. ***Summary.*** The results of this study in male Sprague-Dawley rats indicate that, as with the studies in mice, the effect of dose rate on tumour induction varies between different tissues. For dose rates varying by a factor of about 60 and for a total dose of about 3 Gy, DDREFs in the range from about 1 to 6 have been obtained for tumours in various tissues. Taken

together, the cancer rate was reduced overall by a factor of about 3.

(l) Uncertainties in the calculation of DDREF

198. A particular problem in estimating dose-rate effectiveness factors from the ratio of cancer yields following exposure to acute (high-dose-rate) and chronic (low-dose-rate) irradiations is that very often the standard errors attached to the linear fits to the data are relatively large (Table 9). Formulae have therefore been developed that allow an estimate to be made of uncertainties in the calculation of the DDREF. If α_H and α_L represent the yield coefficients for high and low dose rates, respectively, then the DDREF may be estimated by:

$$\mathrm{DDREF} = \alpha_H/\alpha_L\,[1 + (\sigma_L^2/\alpha_L^2)] \qquad (16)$$

where σ_L is the standard error on α_L. The correction term exists to represent the skewed distribution of the ratio when α_H and α_L are both normally distributed [E8]. The correction is of little importance unless σ_L/α_L exceeds about 0.3. Examples of calculations of DDREF that allow for this correction are shown in Table 10. These values may be compared with the point estimates of DDREF for the same studies given in Table 9. In all cases the values of DDREF that allow for this correction are larger than the values of those that do not, although by very variable amounts; the effect on the estimate of DDREF increases substantially when the standard error σ_L exceeds α_L. The central estimates of DDREF given in Table 8 for the range of tumour types described in this Chapter do not include this correction.

(m) High-LET radiation

199. The implication of the results described earlier, i.e. that at low doses of high-LET radiation the effects of fractionated or protracted exposures on life shortening are very similar to the effect of acute exposures (Section II.A.1.c), would suggest a similar lack of effect on tumour induction in individual tissues. The effects of neutron and alpha-particle irradiation are described separately.

200. ***Neutron irradiation.*** The effects of protracted and fractionated neutron irradiation on the induction of tumours differ in different tissues and have recently been reviewed by Fry [F10]. Grahn et al. [G12] have examined the main categories of cancers found in B6CF1 mice, namely, those of lymphoid and epithelial tissues. The results obtained so far indicate that mortality from lymphoma and leukaemia is greater after fractionated exposures than single exposures, whereas mortality from epithelial tumours is less after the fractionated than single exposures. Since no dose-fractionation effect is seen on the overall life-span in the dose range up to 0.2 Gy, it must be assumed that the two effects cancel each other out.

201. There is little further information to suggest that dose rate influences leukaemogenesis in experimental animals. Upton et al. [U21] did not report any difference between the effects of protracted neutron exposures at low dose rates on the induction of myeloid leukaemia in RFM mice and the effect after single doses. Huiskamp et al. [H28, H29] reported no effect of dose rate on either the induction of acute myeloid leukaemia (AML) or survival in male CBA/H mice exposed bilaterally to fast fission neutrons (mean energy 1 MeV) at 2, 10 and 100 mGy min^{-1} to give a total dose of 0.4 Gy. No AML was observed in the sham-irradiated controls. The observed AML frequencies in the irradiated groups were 11.4%, 12.3% and 9.8%, respectively, indicating that the incidence of AML was not influenced by a fifty-fold change in dose rate. Besides AML, lymphosarcomas were observed in all experimental groups with a suggestion of a slightly higher frequency in the high-dose-rate group, although numbers were small and with no clear trend with increasing dose rate. Although survival was significantly reduced in the exposed animals, it was independent of dose rate.

202. Ullrich [U16] examined the effect of dose rate or dose fractionation on tumour induction in BALB/c mice exposed to total doses of 0.025-0.5 Gy from ^{252}Cf neutrons. The animals were exposed at high dose rate (0.1 Gy in 20 hours daily), or in two equal fractions separated by 24 hours or 30 days, or at low dose rate (0.01 Gy in 20 hours daily). The effect of dose fractionation and dose rate on the tumorigenic response depended very much on the tissue. For ovarian tumours, the response to fractionated exposures was similar to that obtained for a single acute exposure; however, at the low dose rate the response was reduced. This would be consistent with the need for tissue damage and hormonal imbalance for ovarian tumours to manifest themselves. For lung tumour induction splitting the dose into two equal fractions separated by 24 hours had no effect on the response, although separating the fractions by 30 days gave a higher incidence of lung tumours at a total dose of 0.5 Gy (there was no difference at doses up to 0.2 Gy). These results suggest that the number of cells at risk may have increased in the 30-day interval between fractions, possibly as a response to cell killing by the first fraction. This might also explain why the increased effect occurred only when the initial dose was 0.25 Gy or above. For mammary tumours the response to dose fractionation was similar to that for lung tumours. For both lung and mammary tumours the tumour incidence was greater at low dose rates

than with acute exposures, and the increase was most marked at intermediate doses of about 0.1-0.2 Gy. In another study, the induction of Harderian tumours was little different in single exposures and in fractions of 25 mGy up to a total dose of 0.4 Gy [F9]. It has also been reported that, relative to acute exposures, protraction of neutron irradiation advances the time of appearance of mammary tumours in rats [U3].

203. Di Majo et al. [D3] have reported dose-response relationships for liver tumour induction in $BC3F_1$ male mice exposed to fission neutrons. Three-month-old mice given doses from 0.17 to 2.14 Gy (0.05-0.25 Gy min^{-1}) showed an increased tumour incidence in all the irradiated groups [C29, D3]. A linear model gave a best fit to the dose-response data [I(D) = 11.3 + 34.6D], implying that no dose-rate effect would be expected. Because of the different shapes of the dose-response curves for x rays and neutrons (Figure XII), the RBE depended on the dose at which it was calculated, with a value of 13 estimated at 0.17 Gy.

204. ***Summary***. These results indicate that there are differences between tissues in the tumorigenic response following fractionation and changes in dose rate for neutron irradiation. These differences may relate to the different mechanisms of tumorigenesis involved in the different tissues. Taken together, however, any effects of dose rate and dose fractionation on tumour induction in the various animal experiments that have been reported are small.

205. ***Alpha particle irradiation***. Information is also available on tumour induction in experimental animals following intake of alpha-emitting radionuclides. The interpretation of such data is, however, considerably more difficult than is the case for neutron exposure. The spatial and temporal distribution of dose throughout a tissue depends on the age of the animal and the pattern of intake, as well as on the radionuclide itself and the chemical form in which it enters the body. Thus, even for the same radionuclide given in the same chemical form, the distribution of dose may be very different after acute and protracted exposures, and this is likely to affect the tumour yield. This is particularly the case for alpha emitters deposited in the skeleton, where rates of bone turnover that vary both with age and site in the skeleton result in a very heterogeneous deposition of the radionuclide, which in turn can result in quite different distributions and hence dose with various patterns of intake. Local deposition of radionuclides can also produce hot spots that could lead to local cell killing, thus reducing the tumour yield [P11]. Much of the published data has recently been summarized [S28].

206. Two lifetime studies with adult beagle dogs injected with ^{226}Ra to give a wide range of radiation doses, either as a single injection (0.22-370 kBq kg^{-1}) or fractionated (to give total injected activities of 0.88-370 kBq kg^{-1}) have been reported. The data suggest that for both methods of administration, ^{226}Ra was equally effective in inducing skeletal osteosarcomas. However, ^{226}Ra was more effective at inducing osteosarcoma (per unit dose) at low total doses than at high total doses, where cell killing and wasted radiation may be significant [G13, T19].

207. Fabrikant et al. [F11] have compared osteosarcoma induction by alpha-radiation in young male rats given ^{239}Pu (110 kBq kg^{-1}) by intravenous injection, either as a single dose or fractionated over months (37 kBq kg^{-1}, then 19 kBq kg^{-1} at 2, 4, 6 and 8 weeks). Although the number of animals in each group was small (25), the tumour incidence in the two groups (52% and 56%, respectively) did not differ significantly. There was a tendency for tumours in animals given fractionated injections to occur earlier. It was notable that in animals given single injections of ^{241}Am at a similar dose the incidence of bone tumours was about one fourth that in the animals given ^{239}Pu. This is likely to be due to differences in the distribution of the two radionuclides in the skeleton.

208. The effects of dose protraction on osteosarcoma induction have also been examined in female NMRI mice given either single or repeated injections of ^{224}Ra (half-life: 3.5 days) [M40]. One group received a single injection (18.5 kBq kg^{-1}, corresponding to a mean skeletal dose of 0.15 Gy) and the another group received a similar amount in 72 fractions given twice weekly over 36 weeks. In the group given fractionated administration, lymphomas appeared early (13.5%, 42/299 mice; controls 1%, 1/98 mice); osteosarcomas occurred during the second half of life of the animals (7.1%, 21/299; controls 3%, 3/98). In contrast, the group given a single injection did not develop early lymphomas and showed a later occurrence of osteosarcoma with an incidence of 5.8% (17/295). Although the incidence of osteosarcoma was similar up to 800 days in the two experimental groups, after that, it was different: no additional cases of osteosarcoma were observed in the single-injection group, but one third of all osteosarcomas occurred after 800 days in the fractionated group. Because of the very short half-life of ^{224}Ra administered in the study, much of the dose is delivered while the radium is on bone surfaces shortly after administration, and thus local doses will have been significantly higher than the average bone dose calculated (0.15 Gy). In contrast, the dose received following protracted administration would have been more uniformly spread over the skeletal tissues, and this might well have accounted for the observed differences in tumour response.

209. Information is available on lung tumour induction in rodents exposed to alpha emitters. Sanders et al. [S29] compared lung tumour rates in rats exposed by inhalation to aerosols of $^{239}PuO_2$ and $^{244}CmO_2$. The dose distribution throughout the lung was similar for the two radionuclides, although $^{244}CmO_2$ is more soluble in the lung than $^{239}PuO_2$ and, as a consequence, is cleared more rapidly. Despite this, the dose response for lung tumour induction following inhalation of soluble $^{244}CmO_2$ was similar to that for insoluble $^{239}PuO_2$ up to average radiation doses to the lung of a few gray. At greater radiation doses, rats exposed to $^{244}CmO_2$ died earlier from radiation pneumonitis than those exposed to $^{239}PuO_2$, reflecting the differences in dose rate and distribution of activity throughout the lung tissue. The effect of cell killing on tumour induction became apparent at doses of about 2 Gy for $^{244}CmO_2$ and about 30 Gy for $^{239}PuO_2$. Thus, at high total doses, exposure from ^{239}Pu appeared more effective for tumour induction than exposures from ^{244}Cm. Sanders et al. have also shown [S30] that further protraction of the dose from ^{239}Pu by fractionated exposure does not increase the lung tumour incidence in rats, indicating that lung-tumour promotion is not so much a function of the temporal dose-distribution pattern as of the spatial dose-distribution pattern.

210. In further studies on tumour induction in rats exposed to $^{239}PuO_2$, groups of animals were exposed to various levels of activity giving average lung doses between 0.01 Gy and 62 Gy (based on initial lung deposits measured with a ^{169}Yb marker and knowledge of the retention function for plutonium in the lung). This was a large study involving 1,052 female, SPF, Wistar, sham-exposed rats and 2,105 rats exposed in groups to give different initial lung deposits. The dose from inhaled ^{239}Pu is accumulated over an extended time because of the insolubility of the particles and the long retention time in the lung [S43, S20]. Of the 97 primary lung tumours found in this study (93% malignant and 80% carcinomas) 1 was in controls and 96 in exposed rats. Survival was significantly reduced only in rats with lung doses >30 Gy. Of the malignant lung tumours 49 were squamous carcinoma and 22 adenocarcinoma with the remainder consisting of haemongiosarcoma (9), adenosquamous carcinoma (7), and fibrosarcoma (3). No squamous cell carcinomas were found at average lung doses less than 1.5 Gy, and for adenocarcinoma the threshold dose was 3.1 Gy. The other tumour types were seen only at higher lung doses. In this study the predominant tumour type was therefore squamous carcinoma, which is known to develop in the rat lung following the development of squamous metaplasia [S44], which occurs mainly in regions of high deposition of ^{239}Pu, where the local dose would be substantially in excess of the average lung dose. For this tumour type a threshold for the response would therefore be expected, although this would not necessarily be the case for other tumour types or for tumours occurring in man. It was concluded that, at least in the Wistar rat, average lung doses in excess of 1 Gy (20 Sv assuming a radiation weighting factor, w_R, of 20) are needed to give a significant increase in lung tumours.

211. The induction of lung cancer after single or protracted irradiation with alpha particles was also examined by Lundgren et al. [L19] in mice exposed to $^{239}PuO_2$. After single or repeated inhalation exposures giving average lung doses of 2.8 and 2.7 Gy, respectively, lung tumour incidence was about 2.7 times higher after repeated exposures, although the difference between the groups was not significant ($0.05 < p < 0.10$). In contrast, a significant difference was obtained in mice receiving pulmonary doses of 14 Gy in a single exposure or 19 Gy in repeated exposures, the percentage with pulmonary tumours being about 3.5 times greater among the repeatedly exposed mice ($0.01 > p > 0.025$). It seems possible, however, that, as with the study by Sanders et al. [S29], the differences in effect could be attributed to higher dose rates from the single exposures resulting in more cell killing.

212. Some information on the effect of dose rate on the induction of lung tumours has also been obtained following intratracheal instillation of ^{210}Po in saline [L18]. Protraction of the dose over 120 days was more carcinogenic at lower total doses (0.24 Gy) but less carcinogenic at higher doses (2.4 Gy), in comparison with an exposure limited to a 10-day period. However, the development of tumours was also markedly enhanced by the weekly instillation of saline alone, emphasizing the importance of other factors in the expression of radiation-induced cancer.

213. A number of studies have been reported on the exposure of animals, particularly rodents, to varying concentrations of radon and its decay products. Studies at the Pacific Northwest Laboratory in the United States, which have examined the effects of exposure to radon under a range of exposure conditions in experimental animals, have recently been reviewed [C2, C3]. The predominant effect of the inhalation of radon is tumour induction in the respiratory tract. The main tumours arising are adenocarcinomas, bronchiolar carcinomas, adenocarcinomas, epidermoid carcinomas, adenosquamous carcinomas and sarcomas. Acute effects, although species-dependent, do not appear to have occurred at exposure levels of less than 1,000 WLM (3.5 J h m^{-3}). Excess respiratory tract tumours were, however, produced in rats at exposures well below 100 WLM. The results of a series of studies in rats exposed at 5, 50 and 500 WLM per week to give

a range of cumulative exposures are given in Figure XVI. With a few exceptions, the incidence of adenomas and sarcomas was well below 10%. A decrease in exposure rate, at a given exposure level, increased the overall incidence of lung tumours at all but the lowest exposure level (320 WLM). This increase was specifically the result of an increasing incidence of epidermoid carcinomas, most of which (>70%) are fatal. In rats, most (~80%) of the tumours are considered to originate peripherally and to occur at the bronchiolar-alveolar junction. The remaining 20% are considered to be centrally located in association with the bronchi. It should be noted that these are interim results. The shape of the dose-response curve remains uncertain. Most of the exposures below 100 WLM are not yet complete or analysed. At the lowest exposure rate (5 WLM per week), the data suggest that the exposure-rate effect (but not the risk) tapers off, and the risk might still best be described by a linear model, at least at low doses (Figure XVI) [C3].

214. A series of studies has also been conducted by COGEMA in France on the effects of radon exposure [G24, M24]. In these experiments more than 2,000 rats were exposed to cumulative doses of up to 28,000 WLM of radon gas. There was an excess of lung cancer at exposures down to 25 WLM (80 mJ h m^{-3}). Theses exposures were carried out at relatively high concentrations of radon and its decay products (2 J m^{-3}). Above 6,000 WLM, rats suffered increasingly from life shortening due to radiation-induced non-neoplastic causes, thus limiting tumour development. When the dose-response data were adjusted for these competing causes of death, the hazard function for the excess risk of developing pulmonary tumours was approximately linearly related to dose. This suggests that apparent reductions in tumour induction at high doses may chiefly have been the result of acute damage. Later experiments have, however, found that chronic exposure protracted over 18 months at an alpha energy of 2 WL (0.0042 mJ m^{-3}) resulted in fewer lung tumours in rats (0.6%, 3/500 animals, 95% CI: 0.32-2.33) than similar exposures at a potential alpha energy of 100 WL (2 mJ m^{-3}) protracted over 4 months (2.2%, 11/500 animals, CI: 0.91-3.49) or over 6 months (2.4%, 12/500, CI: 1.06-3.74). The incidence of lung tumours in controls was 0.6% (5/800, CI: 0.20-1.49) [M24]. The confidence intervals are, however, wide, and the longer period of exposure (18 months) would in itself have been expected to result in fewer lung tumours. It is significant, however, that no increase in risk was observed with a decrease in exposure rate.

215. The two-mutation (recessive oncogenesis) model of Moolgavkar and Knudson [M38] has been used to model lung tumour induction in rats exposed to radon. This model postulates transitions from a normal cell to an intermediate cell to a malignant cell with quantifiable transition rates and takes account of the growth characteristics of the normal cell and intermediate cell populations. The model describes well the rat lung cancer data following exposure to radon [M6]. The findings suggest that the first mutation rate is very strongly dependent on the rate of exposure to radon progeny and the second mutation rate much less so, suggesting that the nature of the two mutational events is different. The model predicts that (a) in rats radon doubles the background rate of the first mutation at an exposure rate of approximately 0.005 J h m^{-3} wk^{-1} (1.35 WLM wk^{-1}), an exposure rate in the range of exposures to miners; (b) radon doubles the background rate of the second mutation at an exposure rate of about 1.4 J h m^{-3} (400 WLM wk^{-1}); consequently, the hypothesis that radon has *no* effect on the second mutation rate cannot be rejected; and (c) the net rate of intermediate cell growth is doubled at about 0.12 J h m^{-3} wk^{-1} (35 WLM wk^{-1}). The model also predicts a drop in hazard after radon exposures cease, paralleling the exposure-rate effect noted previously, and that fractionation of exposure is more efficient in producing tumours, although further fractionation leads to a decreased efficiency of tumour production.

216. ***Summary.*** It is clearly difficult to generalize from these results on the effects of neutrons and alpha-emitting radionuclides on tumour induction in experimental animals. Despite this, there is little evidence to suggest that, in the absence of cell killing, there is an appreciable enhancement of tumour induction when the dose from alpha-irradiation is protracted or fractionated rather than administered in a single exposure. For the present, the data seem to be reasonably consistent with the assumption of a linear dose-response relationship, at least at low doses.

(n) Summary

217. A number of studies have been published that permit the effect of dose and dose rate on tumour induction in experimental animals exposed to low-LET radiation to be examined. The majority of the data are for external radiation exposure but some information is also available for incorporated radionuclides. The data that have been reported by various authors cover a wide range of dose-response relationships and in general show an increasing risk with increasing dose and dose rate at low to intermediate doses. Although the results from a number of studies can be fitted by linear-quadratic functions, this is by no means universal, and many other dose-response relationships have been obtained. The assessment of the extent to which changing the dose rate increases the effectiveness of the radiation depends, therefore, on the dose range over which the dose and dose-rate effectiveness

factor (DDREF) is calculated. The majority of studies also show that at high doses and high dose rates, cell killing becomes significant and reduces tumour yield. In these circumstances the risk of tumour induction at low doses may be underestimated by fitting a linear function to the data obtained in this region. Estimates of values of DDREF from the different studies that have been reviewed have therefore been made in the dose range in which no cell killing is apparent. The results of these analyses are given in Table 8.

218. A wide range of DDREFs for tumour induction in a variety of different tissues has been found, with most studies being carried out in the mouse. It must be stressed that some of the tumour types for which information is available are not found in man (Harderian gland) and others (ovarian tumour, thymic lymphoma) appear to involve substantial cell killing and/or changes in hormonal status. For other tumours there is a human counterpart (tumours of the lung, breast, pituitary and thyroid), although the tumours involved may not be strictly comparable to the human disease. In practice, the DDREFs found in these two groups are little different, falling in the range from about 1 to 10 or more for dose rates that vary by a factor of 100 or more, and there was no clear trend with tissue type. The data reported on myeloid leukaemia induction in different species and sexes also give DDREFs in the range from 2.2 to >10. The one reasonably consistent finding is that DDREFs for tumour induction in mammary tissue tend to be lower than for tumours in other tissues, although even here one author [U26] has reported a substantial effect of dose fractionation and, hence, a relatively high value of the DDREF (~10) for mice.

219. The main conclusion to be drawn from the results of both the studies on radiation-induced life shortening (Section II.A.1) and those on the induction of specific tumour types is that the tumour response to low-LET radiation is dependent on the dose rate. While the absolute value of the DDREF varies with the conditions of exposure, the animal strain, tissue/tumour type and the dose range over which it is calculated, there is in general a consistent finding that tumour yield decreases with a substantial reduction in the dose rate. There is also some evidence that if the dose rate is sufficiently protracted initiated tumours are unlikely to be fatal in the life-span of the animal. These results may be expected to apply to human tumours as well as to those in experimental animals.

220. A number of the animal studies also indicate that a dose-rate effect cannot necessarily be inferred from exposures at high dose rates alone, as the dose-response data for tumour induction can be adequately fitted by a linear function. This implies the absence of a visible quadratic (i.e. multi-track) function in the dose response, which, according to conventional interpretations, would appear to be a necessary prerequisite for an effect of dose rate on tumour yield. It is thus clear that where information is available only for exposures at high dose rates, as is normally the case for human exposure on which risk estimates are based [C1, I2, U1], any attempt to assess the effect at low doses and low dose rates, and hence a value of the DDREF, by simply attempting to fit a linear-quadratic or similar function to the dose response is unlikely to succeed fully. The limiting factor is the amount of information available at low doses from which the initial linear term (α_L of Figure I) can be accurately determined. In planning future animal studies it should be noted that most information is likely to come from studies on animals exposed at different dose rates rather than from studies that attempt to obtain information on the risks at very low doses. It is to be hoped that more work will be carried out to supplement the very limited information presently available.

221. From the limited and somewhat disparate data on high-LET radiation it is difficult to generalize. There is, however, little experimental data to suggest that, in the absence of cell killing, there is a need to apply a DDREF to tumour incidence data obtained at high dose and dose-rate exposures to calculate risks at low doses and dose rates. Similarly, there is little evidence to suggest that there is an appreciable enhancement of tumour yield when the dose from high-LET radiation is protracted or fractionated. Some data suggest that if radiation exposure is protracted this results in a delay in the appearance of tumours, and in practice they may not arise in the life-span of the animals.

B. *IN VITRO* CELL TRANSFORMATION

222. As has been indicated, oncogenesis is a complex, multi-stage process that is modified by both environmental and physiological factors. *In vitro* cell transformation systems, which have developed rapidly in recent years, have been used to study part of this process in single cells free from host-mediated influences, such as hormonal and immunological factors, and from environmental agents. Even here, however, cell-cell interaction cannot be discounted. Such systems have the advantage that they allow the relative importance of cell killing and transformation to be measured in the same target population of cells. They can also be carried out in a much shorter period of time than animal studies designed to examine tumour induction, and they can be more readily analysed, not having the problem of competing health risks, which is inherent in animal studies.

223. Transformation describes the cellular changes associated with loss of normal control, particularly of

cell division, which results in the development of a neoplastic phenotype. Although exact definitions depend on the experimental conditions, enhanced growth rate, lack of contact inhibition and indefinite growth potential, anchorage-independent growth and the ability to form malignant tumours when transplanted into a suitable host are the main features of the transformation systems currently in use [O1]. Whereas *in vivo* models involve the whole process of carcinogenesis, *in vitro* cell transformation considers events at the level of the initial target cells. However, cell transformation is in itself a complex, multi-stage process by which a cell acquires progressively the phenotypic characteristics of a tumour cell. In practice progression to complete transformation may not occur [L7, L11].

224. The two most common cell lines used in cell transformation assays are the NIH BALB/c3T3 and the C3H10T½ mouse-embryo-derived fibroblast line. There are inevitably disadvantages associated with the use of such cell transformation systems as a model for carcinogenesis in man. The lack of close intercellular contact and the necessity for an artificial growth medium can alter the reactions of cells. Cell handling techniques, such as the degree of trypinization and changes in culture medium, may substantially alter the results obtained [E6, T13]. In particular, in the cultivation of mammalian cells, the properties of serum, constituting 10% of the growth medium of C3H10T½ cells, can be very variable. Thus Hsiao et al. [H27] found large differences in the ability of serum to support the expression of transformed phenotype of C3H10T½ and rat embryo cells. A particular problem with current work on cell transformation is that it is largely based on fibroblasts of rodent origin, whereas tumours of epithelial origin are the main radiation-induced cancers in man. Reliance on data from experimental models that utilize cultured rodent cells for extrapolation to man, without experimental support can, and has, led to serious errors of interpretation [S21]. Thus, a correlation between anchorage-independent growth and the tumorigenic phenotype has been established in rodent cells [F5, O1, S22], which has allowed for the selection of neoplastically transformed cells by growth in soft agar. This does not apply, however, to cultured human cells, as normal human diploid fibroblasts are capable of anchorage-independent growth when cultured in the presence of high concentrations of bovine serum. More relevant cell lines based ideally on human epithelial cell systems are needed for studying mechanisms of tumorigenesis. There are indications that such models can be developed; a recent paper has described transformation in a human colonic epithelial cell line [W11]. A number of studies have also reported neoplastic transformation of human fibroblasts by ionizing radiation and other carcinogens using anchorage-independent growth as an assay (see, e.g. [M26, S23]).

225. Rodent cells seem to have a much greater ability than human cells to undergo the immortalization stage of transformation *in vitro*, either spontaneously or as a result of treatment with a whole range of carcinogens. This may reflect a fundamental difference in their response and must be taken into account in any interpretation of radiation-induced transformation studies employing the currently available rodent cell lines [L9, L11]. Complete transformation of normal human diploid fibroblasts by physical or chemical agents has rarely been achieved [M3, N5]. Immortalization leading to tumorigenicity is a rare event in human diploid cells, whereas certain characteristics of morphological transformation, such as anchorage-independent growth, may be induced quite easily [L10, L11].

226. Nevertheless, there are several general characteristics of cell transformation *in vitro* that support its relevance as a model system for studying the early stages of radiation-induced carcinogenesis *in vivo* and the effects of dose rate. These have been summarized by Little [L11] as follows:

(a) the commonly used cell transformation systems provide quantitative information on the conversion of non-tumorigenic to tumorigenic cells;
(b) there is a high correlation between the carcinogenicity of many chemicals tested in both animals and cell transformation systems. Similar correlations hold for a number of inhibitors and promoters of carcinogenesis that have been tested both *in vitro* and *in vivo*;
(c) cell transformation responds to initiation and promotion similarly to two-stage carcinogenesis in tissues of experimental animals;
(d) transfection assays have shown that cells transformed *in vitro* have activated oncogenes that can be isolated and will transform recipient cells. The DNA of parental, non-transformed cells is inactive in such transfection assays. These findings are analogous to those with human tumours and normal cells in the same DNA transfection assay.

227. Cell transformation systems currently in use divide into two main categories. The first one is short-term explants of cells derived from rodent or human embryos, e.g. Syrian hamster embryo cells. These have the advantage that they are normal cells with a normal karyotype allowing parallel cytogenetic experiments. As such, they have a limited life-span in culture. Immortal transformants are identified by their altered morphology as survivors against a background of senescing normal cells. Spontaneous transformation of these cells occurs at a low frequency (of about 10^{-6} per cell), and in these assays cell survival and transformation frequency are measured in the same cell

culture after about 10 days, the transformed cells being recognized by their distinctive clonal morphology. Being derived from the whole embryo, however, these cultures contain a mixture of cell types, with the possibility that there could be a subpopulation of sensitive target cells.

228. The second category of cell transformation systems is established cell lines that have undergone a growth "crisis" *in vitro*, resulting in the evolution of a derivative cell population capable of indefinite (immortalized) growth. This category includes the NIH BALB/c3T3 and C3H10T½ mouse-embryo-derived fibroblast lines. These cells are highly abnormal and contain a variety of chromosomal rearrangements. If not treated meticulously, the spontaneous level of transformation may increase dramatically. Cell survival and transformation are measured in separate cultures. Survival is normally measured after two weeks and transformation after six weeks, during which time the cultures have reached confluence, and foci of transformed cells that have lost the property of contact inhibition can be seen as distinct colonies that pile up on top of the layer of untransformed fibroblasts. This delay allows for the expression of lethal mutations in the cell population, and these may have a significant effect on the calculation of induced transformation frequencies [A2, E3, M7, S2]. Extrapolation to effects in human epithelial cells *in vivo* from results in these cell systems must be made with caution.

229. Transformed cells are found by scoring characteristic colonies identified in a culture, thus giving a direct measure of the transformation frequency per surviving cell. Many experiments are reported in this way, but information can also be obtained on cell survival as a function of dose, and on the plating effi-ciency. The transformation yield per initial cell at risk can then be determined by correcting for the surviving fraction in the culture and the plating efficiency. This second measure of transformation frequency commonly cannot be calculated from published values of the frequency per transformation of survivors, which may make it difficult to define accurately dose-response relationships.

230. There are a number of other transformation systems in use or under development that attempt to measure more relevant end-points, e.g. thyroid and mammary cell systems in the rat, in which survival and oncogenicity can be measured by transplantation into a fat pad of the animal [C7] and epithelial tissues grown in culture [M31]. As a general rule, the greater the relevance of the measured end-point, the poorer at present is the degree of quantification. Considerable effort continues to be expended in the search for a reliable, relevant and quantifiable human epithelial cell system that would be more representative of the majority of human tumours [C6] and more relevant to determining dose- and dose-rate-related effects.

231. Despite these limitations, transformation assays can provide practical guidance in understanding a number of areas in radiation carcinogenesis:

(a) the shape of dose-response relationships;
(b) the effect of variations in the dose rates of irradiation;
(c) the relative effectiveness of radiation of different qualities;
(d) the modification of radiation effects by interaction with other agents.

With the transformation systems presently available, the experimental cell system chosen to examine a particular end-point should reflect its suitability for answering the question asked. For example, questions about the relative effectiveness of alpha particles compared to gamma rays or about the effect of dose rate require a more quantitative system, such as the Syrian hamster embryo cell or C3H10T½ cell systems, whereas studies of oncogenic mechanisms and the effect of suppressor genes need a more relevant human epithelial cell system [H3]. (This topic is covered in more detail in Annex E, "Mechanisms of radiation oncogenesis".)

1. Dose-response relationships

232. Dose-response relationships for cell transformation following exposure to low-LET radiation were comprehensively reviewed in the UNSCEAR 1986 Report [U2] and more recently by Barendsen [B9]. A knowledge of the factors influencing the response to radiation is important for understanding the influence of dose fractionation and dose rate on cell transformation, and they are briefly summarized here.

233. The pattern of response is very dependent on cell cycle kinetics. The most reliable experimental evidence shows that when measuring the transformation frequency per cell at risk following exposure to low-LET radiation, a linear or linear-quadratic relationship can be fitted to most available data at lower doses, but above about 4-5 Gy cell reproductive death starts to predominate over the observed frequency of transformation per plated cell [B9, H4]. Figure XVII shows the typical form of the dose-response relationship. Parameters were selected by Barendsen [B9] to illustrate the importance of the linear and quadratic terms in the induction of transformation and of cell reproductive death. When expressed as transformation frequency per surviving cell, a plateau in the yield at high doses may be observed with C3H10T½ cells [H4, T1].

234. It is now recognized that measurements of radiation-induced transformation need to be made with cells that have been allowed to attain asynchronous growth by plating at low density at least 40 hours before treatment [H9, H10]. Before 40 hours, transient parasynchronous growth may cause large fluctuations in observed transformation frequencies for relatively small variations in plating time, because the susceptibility of the cell to transformation varies throughout the cell cycle. This may also be affected by radiation-induced cell cycle delay. The failure to recognize the importance of allowing cells to achieve asynchronous growth may account for some of the more complex dose-response relationships that have been observed. For example, Miller et al. [M8, M9] measured the effect on C3H10T½ cells of x-ray doses down to 0.1 Gy delivered just 24 hours after seeding. They found a plateau in the incidence of transformants per surviving cell between about 0.3 and 1.0 Gy (Figure XVIII). With this unusual dose-response curve there could be substantial underestimation of the effect at low doses if projecting from high doses alone on the basis of a linear model.

235. A similarly shaped curve can be fitted to the results of Borek and Hall [B21], which were obtained by irradiating fresh explants of golden hamster embryos either with single doses or with two fractions of x rays. Because of the greater sensitivity of this system, the apparent plateau in response is at doses below 0.1 Gy. However, a linear relationship cannot be excluded on statistical grounds. Similar dose-response kinetics have been observed for experiments performed with asynchronously growing cells and in some cases with cells irradiated in the plateau phase.

236. C3H10T½ cells irradiated at low density 48 hours or more after initial seeding are determined to be growing asynchronously and increasing exponentially [H9, H10]. The dose-response data reported for low-LET radiation, expressed as transformation frequency per surviving cell, can be fitted to a linear model for doses up to about 2 Gy. However, the quadratic model cannot be excluded on statistical grounds. For single exposures to ^{60}Co gamma rays (1 Gy min^{-1}) Han et al. [H5, H6] reported a linear response up to 1.5 Gy for transformation in C3H10T½ cells described by I(D) = 2.58D 10^{-4} Gy^{-1} (Figure XIX), which agrees remarkably well with the dose response obtained up to 2 Gy for acute x-irradiation (4 Gy min^{-1}) of I(D) = 2.50 ± 0.11D 10^{-4} Gy^{-1} by Balcer-Kubiczek et al. [B1] for 36-hour asynchronous cultures (Figure XX; see also paragraph 245). In both of these experiments the lowest dose used was 0.25 Gy. Little [L8] has compared results for two related mouse cell transformation systems: BALB/3T3 and C3H10T½ cells. Following exposure to up to 3 Gy from x rays, the shapes of the dose-response curves differed significantly: that for C3H10T½ cells appeared to follow a linear-quadratic or quadratic relationship, while that for BALB/3T3 cells was nearly linear (Figure XXI). A linear relationship was also obtained for BALB/3T3 cells exposed to beta particles from tritiated water [L11].

237. A linear dose-response relationship for transformation frequency with no suggestion of a threshold was also observed at doses up to 1.5 Gy for golden hamster embryo cells irradiated 72 hours after culture initiation [W3]. Above this dose a rather more shallow increase in transformation frequency per surviving cell was observed. By contrast, Bettega et al. [B11] irradiated asynchronously growing C3H10T½ cells with 31 MeV protons (~2 keV mm^{-1}), finding a transformation frequency per surviving cell that showed a marked change in slope over the dose range examined but in the opposite direction. Between 0.25 and 2 Gy the frequency was observed to increase slowly with dose, but above 2 Gy and up to 7 Gy it steepened very sharply.

238. X-irradiated contact-inhibited (plateau-phase) C3H10T½ cells have also been used to investigate induced transformation [T1]. A steep increase in transformation frequency up to a dose of about 0.5 Gy was observed with a doubling dose of about 0.2 Gy, followed by a slower increase over 1-4 Gy with a doubling dose of 1 Gy and a plateau above 6 Gy. For plateau cells the D_0 was 1.53 Gy. Contact-inhibited cells are perhaps closer to the state prevailing *in vivo*. However, there are technical problems associated with the cell density of plating that may affect the results from confluent cultures, as well as with the more widely used technique of low-density plating of asynchronously growing cells.

2. Dose rate and fractionation

239. Early results for the exposure of C3H10T½ cells to fractionated doses of x rays [H4] and for exposures to high and low dose rates of ^{60}Co gamma rays [H5, H6] using an experimental system involving irradiation of established asynchronously growing C3H10T½ cells, which had been in culture for at least 40 hours, indicated that transformation frequency per surviving cell was reduced significantly with fractionated or protracted exposure as compared with single acute exposures. Analysis of the experimental data suggested fractionation allowed the error-free repair of subtransformation damage.

240. When considering protracted or fractionated exposures to low-LET radiation, the relative times of cell plating and irradiation are important. Complex dose-response relationships have been shown in the

region of 0.3-1.5 Gy when C3H10T½ cells are irradiated soon after seeding (Figure XVIII). Approximate doubling of the transformation frequency per irradiated cell can be observed when doses in this range are given in two fractions [M8]. Higher numbers of equal fractions, up to three or four, spread over 5 hours lead to an almost proportional increase in the observed transformation frequency [H1]. This enhancement was also observed when freshly plated C3H10T½ cells were irradiated with gamma rays to a dose of 1 Gy delivered over 6 hours rather than 10 minutes [H1]. Above a dose of about 1.5 Gy, no enhancement at reduced dose rate was observed. Thus using this particular experimental approach in the dose range of about 0.3-1.5 Gy, the transformation frequency can be enhanced either by splitting the dose into a number of fractions or by protracting the dose over a similar interval. At 2 Gy, no effect was observed. A similar enhancement in the observed transformation frequency per surviving cell has been observed with freshly seeded Syrian hamster embryo cells irradiated with fractionated doses of 0.5 and 0.75 Gy [B21, B22], for similarly treated BALB/3T3 cells at doses below 2 Gy [L8] and for C3H10T½ cells exposed to ^{244}Cm alpha particles giving doses in the range 2 mGy to 3 Gy [B43].

241. This enhancement in transformation with fractionation of the dose has not been observed for other biological effects of low-LET radiation either *in vitro* or *in vivo*, and the explanation appears to lie in the shape of the dose-response curve for cells irradiated soon after seeding, when parasynchronization effects may apply. In the plateau region between 0.3 and 1.5 Gy, where the effect is roughly independent of dose (Figure XVIII), irradiation with two fractions that are assumed not to interact will approximately double the transformation yield. In addition, from this curve, extrapolation from intermediate and high doses will substantially underestimate the true transformation frequency at low doses, particularly when delivered at low dose rate or in several fractions. These results are in contrast to radiobiological expectations, and in view of the interest surrounding them, further, more extensive experiments have been conducted [B1, B2, H6, H9, H10].

242. Han et al. [H6] have compared the transformation frequency in C3H10T½ cells exposed to either single doses (0.25-1.5 Gy; 1 Gy min^{-1}) of ^{60}Co gamma rays or five equal fractions (0.5-3 Gy; 0.5 Gy min^{-1}) separated by 24 hours. Transiently parasynchronous cells were incubated for at least 40 hours before the beginning of irradiation to ensure asynchronous growth. For both patterns of exposure the dose response could be fitted with a linear function, but for fractionated exposures the transformation frequency for surviving cells (0.8 10^{-4} Gy^{-1}) was about a third of that obtained after acute exposure (2.6 10^{-4} Gy^{-1}), indicating a DDREF of 3.2 (Figure XIX). The reduction in the slope with fractionated exposure indicates that subtransformation damage can be repaired even in the dose region where transformation is apparently linearly dependent on the dose. This is clearly contrary to the autonomous single-hit interpretation of the linear dose-response relationship. However, it is possible that linear and quadratic terms are both present, but that the data are insufficient to allow them to be resolved.

243. Similar results have been obtained by Terasima et al. [T1], who compared the induction of cell transformation and cell killing in plateau-phase C3H10T½ mouse cells by single doses or two fractions separated by intervals between 3 and 15 hours. On the linear component of the dose-response curve (up to ~4 Gy) with total doses of 0.9 and 1.9 Gy, fractionation decreased transformation frequency by about 50%, although very variable results were obtained. At the highest dose used (3.7 Gy) the decrease was by a factor of about 2. Watanabe et al. [W3] have reported that for asynchronously growing golden hamster embryo cells exposed to x rays at various dose rates, lower dose rates (0.5 Gy min^{-1}) were less effective in inducing transformations than high dose rates (6 Gy min^{-1}) by a factor of about 2.

244. The use of C3H10T½ cells in plateau phase also demonstrated the repair of potential transformation damage. Results obtained by Terasima et al. [T1, T13] showed that a rapid reduction of transformation frequency occurred over a period of 6-7 hours after a single dose (3.7 Gy) of 200 kVp x rays, if the irradiated cultures were kept in a confluent state before plating cells at a low density for transformation assay. In two of the three media used, the overall transformation frequency was reduced to about one fourth of that obtained with no post-irradiation period of incubation. The results indicated the repair of potential transformation damage had a half-time of about 3 hours. At times longer than about 7 hours the transformation frequency tended to increase again, although the results were widely variable.

245. Balcer-Kubiczek et al. [B1] studied the dose-rate effect in C3H10T½ cells in some detail, using protracted exposure to x rays of transformed and non-transformed cells. In an initial study on 36-hour asynchronous cultures, similar survival curves for both cell types at doses up to 2 Gy (0.4 Gy min^{-1}) were obtained, indicating similar repair capacity of transformed and non-transformed cells, a result consistent with that of Hill et al. [H8]. In a second series of experiments, cell transformation from acute exposure was compared with that from protracted exposure. For

protracted exposure the dose rate was proportional to the total dose, giving a constant exposure time, so that the repair time was equal at all doses levels. The dose-response curves for oncogenic transformation in the low-dose range between 0.25 and 2 Gy were consistent with a linear response, giving parameters of 2.5 ± 0.11 10^{-4}, 1.5 ± 0.03 10^{-4} and 0.87 ± 0.05 10^{-4} Gy^{-1} for acute (<5 min) and 1-hour and 3-hour protracted exposures, respectively (Figure XX). These results indicate that in the linear dose-response range between 0.25 and 2 Gy, oncogenic transformation is reduced by a factor of up to about 3 with protraction of exposure. A linear-quadratic model could also be fitted to the results, but without a common linear term. The results are consistent with a reduction in slope of the dose response as the exposure time is increased.

246. In an extension of this work, Balcer-Kubiczek et al. [B2] examined the effect of dose protraction in the range 0.25-2 Gy with acute exposure and protracted exposures over 1, 3 and 5 hours. Results similar to those of the previous study were obtained for comparable exposure conditions (2.33 10^{-4}, 1.55 10^{-4} and 1.01 10^{-4} Gy^{-1} for acute, 1-hour and 3-hour exposures, respectively). For protraction of the dose over 5 hours, a transformation frequency of 0.56 10^{-4} Gy^{-1} was obtained. Thus, the overall reduction in oncogenic transformation with protraction was by a factor 4.5. Based on an analysis of the dose-response data using a linear-quadratic function, a repair half-time for cell transformation of 2.4 hours (95% CI: 1.8-3.0) was estimated. Interestingly, this compares well with a typical value for chromosomal aberrations of about 2 hours [P5].

247. The effect of dose rate on transformation frequency has also been examined in golden hamster embryo cells exposed to x rays at different dose rates (0.05 Gy min^{-1}, 0.75 Gy min^{-1} and 6 Gy min^{-1}), giving total doses up to 4 Gy. The transformation frequency increased steeply with increasing dose at all dose rates up to a total dose of 1.5 Gy, with the highest dose rate giving a transformation frequency about 1.5 times that of the lowest dose rate at doses of about 1 Gy. At higher doses the increase in transformation frequency was less steep, and at 4 Gy the transformation frequency at the highest dose rate was about twice that at the lowest dose rate [W3].

3. High-LET radiation

248. An extensive series of studies has examined the effects of high-LET radiation on cell transformation. These studies have been confined largely to neutrons, covering a wide range of energies, although some data on the effects of heavy ions (95 MeV ^{14}N, 22 MeV ^{4}He) have also been published [S24]. For acute exposures, the effectiveness of high-LET radiation on transformation induction follows a pattern similar to that for chromosomal aberration induction, cell killing and other cellular end-points [I6, S12]. In a review of published data, Barendsen [B9] suggested that a maximum RBE value of between about 10 and 20 is typically found for 0.4-1 MeV neutrons. These RBE values tend to be higher than the equivalent values for cell reproductive death by a factor of 2-3 [I7] but similar to those found for dicentric aberration induction [I6, L12, S12] and somatic cell gene mutation by high-LET monoenergetic ions [C11]. Barendsen [B8] interpreted this difference as being due to the relatively large linear component found for cell reproductive death induced by low-LET radiation, in comparison with the corresponding value for cell transformation. In a recent review of data on oncogenic transformation of C3H10T½ cells Miller and Hall [M46] noted that irradiation of cells with monoenergetic neutrons having energies between 0.23 and 13.7 MeV to doses of 0.05-1.5 Gy resulted in a linear response for both transformation and cell killing. When compared with results obtained with 250 kVp x rays, all neutron energies were more effective at both cell killing and induction of transformation. Values of the maximum biological effectiveness, RBE_m, were calculated from the initial linear term (α_1, equation 11) for a linear-quadratic model fit to data on low-LET radiation such that

$$RBE_m = \alpha_n / \alpha_x \quad (17)$$

that is, the ratio of the initial slopes for cell transformation following exposure to neutrons, α_n, and x rays, α_x. Both cell survival and the induction of transformation showed an initial increase in effectiveness with increasing neutron energy, reaching a maximum at 0.35 MeV, followed by a subsequent decline (Figure XXII). This pattern of response is generally consistent with microdosimetric predictions, in that the neutron-induced recoil protons are shifted to lower lineal energies as the neutron energy increases, and the effect of heavy recoils is lessened by saturation effects. The results obtained with heavy ions gave RBE values, relative to ^{60}Co gamma rays, of 3.3 for ^{14}N (530 keV μm^{-1}), 2.4 for ^{4}He ions (36 keV μm^{-1}) and 3.3 for ^{4}He ions with a 100 μm Al absorber (77 keV μm^{-1}) [S24].

249. As previously described, fractionated and low-dose-rate exposures to low-LET radiation generally show a decrease in effectiveness for cell transformation. For high-LET radiation, however, such a dose-rate effect is not usually observed, leading to higher values of RBE for low-dose-rate or fractionated exposure conditions. Thus, for fission spectrum neutrons at high dose rate (0.1-0.3 Gy min^{-1}), the RBE for transformation of C3H10T½ cells was about 2.5 when compared with high dose rate (1 Gy min^{-1}) gamma-ray

exposure from ^{60}Co. With protracted exposure (0.86 mGy min^{-1}) or fractionated exposure (five fractions over 4 days at high dose rate) the RBE was about 20. Higher values of RBE might be expected with fractions given at low dose rate [H11]. Some cell transformation experiments have, however, indicated an inverse dose-rate effect, with certain energies of neutrons giving a greater transformation frequency at low dose rates than at high dose rates [H8, H10, H11, M11], although others have not [B3, B4, B12, H7, H20].

250. Hill et al. [H8, H10] first described an inverse dose-rate effect for oncogenic transformation in C3H10T½ cells exposed to fission spectrum neutrons produced by the Janus reactor and suggested that irradiation times of at least 50 minutes were necessary for enhancement of transformation. At low doses, fission neutrons administered either in dose fractions over 5 days [H11] or continuously for 5 days [H8] induced higher frequencies of transformation than cells exposed to single doses (Figure XXIII). Thus at doses in the range 0.025-0.1 Gy, a linear fit to the data at 0.38 Gy min^{-1} gave a transformation frequency of 5.96 10^{-4} Gy^{-1}, while at lower dose rates (0.86 mGy min^{-1}) the frequency of transformation was 5.3 10^{-3} Gy^{-1}. Thus the incidence of transformation increased at the lower dose rate by a factor of about 9, corresponding to a DDREF of 0.11 [H10]. Later studies intended to clarify this effect have failed to find a factor of this magnitude. A two- to threefold enhancement at low dose rates of fission spectrum neutrons has been observed for transformation of fresh cultures of Syrian hamster embryo cells [J2], and a similar response has been found by Redpath et al. [R2, R16] with a HeLa x skin fibroblast human cell hybrid system exposed to fission neutrons from both the Janus and TRIGA reactors. An enhancement in transformation frequency has been found by Yasukawa et al. [Y5]. For C3H10T½ cells exposed to 2 MeV neutrons from a Van de Graaff generator, fractionation of a dose of 1.5 Gy (two fractions of 0.75 Gy at a 3 hour interval) increased the transformation frequency by about 50%, although with 13 MeV neutrons from a cyclotron the transformation frequency was reduced by about 30% with a similar exposure schedule. Enhancement of transformation was also seen by Yang et al. [Y1], who irradiated confluent cells with accelerated argon ions (400 MeV amu^{-1}; 120 keV μm^{-1}) and iron ions (800 MeV amu^{-1}; 200 keV μm^{-1}) and found an enhancement of transformation at low dose rates. This enhancement was found to be greater at lower doses.

251. Several laboratories have reported no inverse dose-rate effect with C3H10T½ cells for other high-LET radiations, such as ^{244}Cm alpha particles [B12] and ^{241}Am alpha particles [H7]. Balcer-Kubiczek et al. [B3, B4, B39] examined the dose-rate effect in some detail, using fission spectrum neutrons from a TRIGA reactor to irradiate exponentially growing or stationary cultures of C3H10T½ cells. No significant inverse dose-rate effect was obtained following exposure to 0.3 Gy at dose rates from 0.005 to 0.1 Gy min^{-1}. These data argue strongly against the hypothesis that differences in proliferative status of C3H10T½ may play a role in the determination of any dose-rate effect. In a second series, consisting of nine experiments, the induction of transformation in actively growing C3H10T½ cells at neutron doses from 0.05 to 0.9 Gy at dose rates of 0.0044 or 0.11 Gy min^{-1} was examined. Again, no discernible dose-rate effect was obtained [B39]. In a third series, concurrent with the second and with the same exposure parameters, mutagenesis at the *hprt* and a_1 in A_L cells was measured, and again no dose-rate effect was observed [B39].

252. Hill [H20], using both 30- and 46-MeV protons on beryllium failed to observe enhancement of transformation for low-dose-rate exposures. No difference in transformation frequency of rat tracheal epithelial cells was obtained in exposures to neutrons at 0.1-0.15 Gy min^{-1} and $\leq$0.18 mGy min^{-1}. There was also no difference in the induction of metaplasia and tumours in tracheal cells exposed at high and low dose-rates. The exposure times for the low-dose irradiation were between 18 minutes and 3 hours [T14].

253. Saran et al. [S35] examined the effect of fractionation of the dose of fission-spectrum neutrons on exponentially growing C3H10T½ cells. With total doses of 0.11, 0.27, 0.54 and 1.1 Gy given either as single doses or in five equal fractions at 24-hour intervals, no significant difference in either cell survival or neoplastic transformation was obtained. In further studies, C3H10T½ cells were exposed to 1 and 6 MeV neutrons giving doses of 0.25 and 0.5 Gy either as single doses or in five fractions given at 2-hour intervals. Again, no significant difference between acute and fractionated exposures was obtained for survival or neoplastic transformation [S36].

254. Miller et al. [M11], investigated the effects of dose fractionation for monoenergetic neutrons of various energies generated by a Van de Graaff particle accelerator. Comparison of C3H10T½ cells exposed to low doses of neutrons given either in a single acute exposure or in five equal fractions over 8 hours showed that, of the wide range of neutron energies studied (0.23, 0.35, 0.45, 5.9 and 13.7 MeV), significant enhancement of transformation occurred only with 5.9 MeV neutrons. Of the neutron energies examined, 5.9 MeV neutrons had the lowest dose-averaged lineal energy and linear energy transfer.

255. From these studies and a comparison of the available transformation data for C3H10T½ cells irradiated with neutrons, a dose-rate enhancement factor

of about 2-3 at low doses (less than 0.3 Gy) and dose rates below 0.01 Gy min^{-1} was suggested [M12]. It was concluded that the enhancement of transformation by fractionated or low-dose-rate exposures to neutrons appears to depend on radiation quality, with some neutron energies both above and below 5.9 MeV showing no dose-rate effect (Figure XXIV).

256. In a further study, Miller et al. [M28, M46] examined transformation induction in C3H10T½ cells exposed to graded doses of 5.9 MeV neutrons given as a single acute exposure (30 mGy min^{-1}) or in five equal fractions 2 hours apart, or continuously over an 8-hour period at low dose rates (from 0.21 to 1 mGy min^{-1}). Although cell survival studies showed no differences in effect with a change in dose rate, oncogenic transformation was enhanced by a factor of 2-3 when the dose rate was reduced (Figure XXV). When the neutron dose was divided into five fractions given over 8 hours, the effect was intermediate between that for acute and low-dose-rate exposures. Further irradiation was given with deuterons with a LET of 40 keV μm^{-1}, approximating the measured dose-mean lineal energy deposited in the nucleus of C3H10T½ cells by 5.9 MeV monoenergetic neutrons. An inverse dose-rate/dose-fractionation effect for the induction of transformation by these high-LET deuterons was observed when the time between each of three fractions for a 0.3 Gy total dose was at least 45 minutes. Although the transformation frequency increased by a factor of about 2, no further enhancement was seen for longer fractionation periods, suggesting that very protracted exposures of high-LET radiation would produce no additional enhancement.

257. A variety of results have thus been reported on the effects of dose rate on cell transformation *in vitro*. The consistent features that have emerged on the response of C3H10T½ cells to various patterns of neutron exposure have recently been summarized [B30, H31]:

(a) enhancement of transformation with dose protraction is not observed with low-LET radiation;
(b) the greatest enhancement for fission neutrons occurred at dose rates below ~10 mGy min^{-1};
(c) for fission (and all other) neutron irradiation at dose rates above ~10 mGy min^{-1}, little or no enhancement is apparent;
(d) monoenergetic neutrons produce a significantly smaller enhancement than do fission neutrons;
(e) charged particles with LET much above 140 keV μm^{-1} produce little or no enhancement;
(f) the effect appears most prominent at doses around 0.2 Gy, with less evidence of enhancement at doses much above or below this.

258. A number of biophysical models have been proposed to account for this inverse dose-rate effect. The relevance of differential radiation sensitivity through the cell cycle was pointed out by Oftedal [O2], and its application to the inverse dose-rate effect observed in transformation studies was first formalized by Rossi and Kellerer [R5], who postulated that cells in a particular "window" of their cycle may be more sensitive to radiation (for the end-point of interest) than cells in the rest of the cell cycle. If this is the case, an acute exposure of cycling cells to high-LET radiation will result in some fraction of these sensitive cells receiving (on average) very large deposits of energy, much greater than required to produce the damage that may lead to oncogenic transformation. On the other hand, if the exposure is protracted or fractionated, a larger proportion of sensitive cells will be exposed, although to smaller (on average) amounts of energy deposited; the total energy deposition per cell would still be sufficient to produce a potentially oncogenic change in the cell. To the extent that this latter postulate may not apply to low-LET radiation, the inverse dose-rate effect would not be expected to apply. To account for the data first published by Hill et al. [H10], suggesting enhancement by a factor of up to 9 with fractionated exposures, a rather short "window" of only about 5 minutes duration was proposed. With the exception of this early report, the data on enhancement due to dose protraction now all suggest an enhancement factor of up to about 2 or 3, and on this basis the model framework proposed by Rossi and Kellerer [R5] has been revised by Brenner and Hall [B30] and Hall et al. [H31], as summarized below.

259. The probability that a particular cell will be exposed to a given number of tracks is given by the Poisson distribution. Thus the probability, P, that a cell will receive at least one track will be

$$P = 1 - e^{-N} \qquad (18)$$

where N is the average number of tracks, which at a dose D (given in Gy), delivered acutely, will be

$$N_a = 5Dd^2/y_F \qquad (19)$$

where y_F is the (frequency) average lineal energy (the microdosimetric correlate of LET (given in keV μm^{-1}) deposited in the nucleus, which is assumed to be spherical with diameter d (given in μm). It is assumed that the entire nucleus is the target. Not all the cells will be in the sensitive phase during a short acute exposure; the proportion in the sensitive phase, Q_a, will be

$$Q_a = \tau/s \qquad (20)$$

where τ is the duration of the sensitive period of the cell cycle and s is the total length of the cycle. Now, assuming that any number of high-LET tracks is equally likely to produce the damage that can lead to transformation, the overall probability will be

$$P_T = Q_a P_a \quad (21)$$

where P_a is given by equations 18 and 19. Thus, the transformation rate due to this process will be

$$T = KQ_a P_a \quad (22)$$

where K is a constant. It seems unlikely that cells in the rest of the cell cycle will be completely insensitive to the induction of transformation. Based on the low-LET dose response where the effect of the sensitive phase should be less evident, the dose-response relationship for cells damaged in phases other than their sensitive phase can be approximated by a linear-quadratic function. Thus, the total transformation rate is

$$T_a = KQ_a P_a + \alpha_1 D + \alpha_2 D^2 \quad (23)$$

If the dose is not delivered acutely but at a dose rate $\dot{D}$ over a time t (= $D/\dot{D}$), then the average number of tracks through each nucleus in the sensitive phase will decrease from N_a to N_c:

$$N_c = N_a \tau/(t + \tau) \quad (24)$$

However, the proportion of cells exposed in the sensitive phase will be increased from Q_a to Q_c:

$$Q_c = (t + \tau)/s \quad (25)$$

For $t + \tau < s$, the overall transformation rate will be

$$T_c = KQ_c P_c + \alpha_1 D + \alpha_2 D^2 \quad (26)$$

where P_c is given by equations 18 and 19. Finally, for an irradiation that is divided into n equal fractions, where the time between fractions is longer than τ, the expressions become

$$N_f = N_a/n \quad \text{and} \quad Q_f = n\tau/s \quad (27)$$

and

$$T_f = KQ_f P_f + \alpha_1 D + \alpha_2 D^2 \quad (28)$$

where P_f is given by equations 18 and 19.

260. Based on the critical assumption of a target size of 8 μm (corresponding to the average size of the nucleus of a C3H10T½ cell) and a value for α_2 of 0.29 10^{-4}, determined from experimental data [M28], the parameters α_1, K and τ were determined as a best parameter fit for the experimental data shown in Figure XXV for 5.9 MeV neutrons. The model fit to the data was obtained with a period of sensitivity of 61 minutes and values for α_1 of 4.0 ± 2.1 10^{-4} Gy^{-1} and for K of 1.3 ± 0.19. This rather longer period of sensitivity, τ, is more reasonable in terms of the period of the entire cell cycle. A feature of the model is that the time between fractions needs to be longer than τ, the length of the sensitive window, for a dose-fractionation effect to be observed. As the time between fractions decreases, the exposure will become increasingly similar to an acute exposure. The model appears to give a reasonable fit to much of the reported experimental data on the C3H10T½ system and predicts little enhancement of effect for alpha-particle irradiation, as is observed. For intermediate-LET radiation, such as fission neutrons, the effect would be confined to intermediate doses, as the model predicts that both acute and continuous transformation rates will have the same initial slopes.

261. The hypothesis that there is a narrow window (about 1 hour) of sensitivity to oncogenic transformation requires that cells be cycling for the inverse dose-rate effect to be observed and therefore predicts no effect for plateau-phase cells. In a further study, Miller et al. [M17] investigated the LET-dependence of the inverse dose-rate effect using charged particles of defined LET. Parallel studies were conducted with plateau-phase and exponentially-growing C3H10T½ cells exposed to single or fractionated doses of charged particles with LETs between 25 and 250 kV μm^{-1}. Doses were delivered in three dose fractions, with various intervals from 0.3 minutes to 150 minutes between the fractions. Dose fractionation with prolonged time intervals enhanced the yield of transformed cells, compared with a single acute dose for a range of LET values between 40 and 120 kV μm^{-1}. Radiations of lower or higher LET did not show this enhancement. This enhanced effect for cycling cells in log phase was not seen for cells in plateau phase, lending strong support to the model by Brenner et al. [B30]. These data by Miller et al. [M17] have also been analysed by Brenner et al. [B16] in the context of their model, but with the additional modification that the constant K was varied to reflect the specific energy deposition in the nucleus with varying LET. They concluded that the observed LET effects were well explained by the model, assuming a period of sensitivity within the cell cycle of about 1 hour. The inverse dose-rate effect disappears at very high-LET because of a reduction in the number of cells being hit and disappears at LET below about 40 kV μm^{-1} because the majority of the dose is deposited at low values of specific energy insufficient to produce the saturation phenomenon central to the effect. At even lower LET damage repair will produce a characteristic "sparing" associated with protraction of x- or gamma-ray doses.

262. In a further analysis, the predictions of the model were tested by Harrison and Balcer-Kubiczek [H34]. Their analyses, based on unweighted least-squares techniques, suggested that there is no unique solution for τ and that its value is critically dependent on the nuclear diameter. There were also difficulties applying the model to other neutron data on cell transformation. It is clear that the model proposed by Brenner and

Hall [B30], or some future derivative of it, will need to be tested for different doses, dose rates and dose-fractionation schemes to fully examine its general applicability. Ultimately a complete understanding of the inverse dose-rate effect must depend on experimental studies designed to elucidate the mechanistic basis of the observations [B45].

4. Summary

263. Cell transformation studies can yield information of practical use in radiation protection in addition to giving insight into the initial mechanisms of carcinogenesis. At present, the most quantitative data can be derived from cell systems that are not typical of the epithelial cell systems involved in most human cancers. The most commonly used cell lines include cultured embryo cells and the mouse fibroblast cell lines C3H10T½ and BALB/c3T3. Thus, when attempts are made to extrapolate to cancer induction in epithelial tissues in man, the biological limitations of these assay systems must be considered. In addition cell transformation studies have proved to be very difficult to standardize and there are technical uncertainties which must be taken into account in assessing the results of any studies. These include the effects of changes in response during the cell cycle, of plating density and of promoters and suppressors, some of which may be normal components of the growth medium, particularly the serum, and therefore difficult to control.

264. Nevertheless, in carefully controlled experiments where asynchronously dividing cells or, in some cases, non-dividing plateau-phase cells have been irradiated, the resulting observations of dose or dose-rate effects for low-LET radiation are in general agreement with those relating to other cellular effects, such as cell killing and the induction of mutations or chromosomal aberrations. Dose-response curves per cell at risk have a number of features in common with tumour induction *in vivo*, showing an initial rise in transformation frequency with increasing dose to a maximum and then a decline. When plotted as transformants per surviving cell, the dose response for low-LET radiation generally shows the expected linear or linear-quadratic relationship tailing off to a plateau at higher doses. When low doses of x rays or gamma rays are delivered at low dose rate or in fractionated intervals, a dose-rate reduction factor of between 2 and 4 is commonly found. It is noteworthy that some experimental data suggest that the linear term in the dose response may alter with dose rate, but this may be accounted for by the lack of precise data at low doses.

265. Exposures to high-LET radiation results in a higher transformation efficiency with a tendency towards a linear relationship, in line with data for chromosomal aberrations and again tending to a plateau at high doses. As expected from this pattern of response, there is no tendency for the response to decrease at low dose rates or with fractionation, and in practice, a number of studies have shown an enhanced effect. The main evidence for an inverse dose-rate effect with high-LET radiation seems to be limited to 5.9 MeV or fission spectrum neutrons, and over the past few years estimates of the magnitude of the increased effect have been reduced, from factors of about 9 to factors of about 2 or 3. Results reported from a number of laboratories have become reasonably consistent, and it has been possible to develop a model that can satisfactorily predict many experimental results. The model is based on the assumption that the target in the cell, taken to be the nucleus, has a "window" in the cell cycle during which it is more sensitive to radiation.

266. With protracted or fractionated exposures there is a greater opportunity for this particular "window" to be hit by at least one track and thus make possible an enhancement of transformation frequency with a reduction in dose rate. The magnitude of any effect will depend on the lineal energy, and with alpha-particle irradiation little enhancement would be expected, as is in fact observed. Although such a model appears to be consistent with much of the experimental data, it will need to be tested at different doses, dose rates and dose-fractionation schedules to fully examine its general applicability. Ultimately a complete understanding of the inverse dose-rate effect must depend on experimental studies designed to elucidate the mechanistic basis of the observations.

267. Despite this apparent explanation for the inverse dose-rate effect, there remains the problem that it is largely based on the results obtained with the C3H10T½ cell system and may well have only limited application to human carcinogenesis. The development of epithelial cell systems that are of much more direct relevance to human cancer should be a research priority. While some qualitative information is becoming available from such cell systems, no quantitative assays appear to be available at present.

C. MUTAGENESIS

268. It is generally believed (and pointed out in Annex E, "Mechanisms of radiation oncogenesis") that the principal mechanism resulting in a neoplastic initiating event is induced damage to the DNA molecule that predisposes target cells to subsequent malignant development. There is also strong evidence linking a number of tumours to specific gene mutations. After the primary initiating event many genetic, physiological and environmental factors will influence the deve-

lopment and subsequent manifestation of a tumour. There is, however, a clear need to understand the role of both dose and dose rate in this initial genetic change. Studies on somatic and germ cell mutations both *in vivo* and *in vitro* are directly relevant to this question, although the results obtained have been somewhat variable. The effect of dose and dose rate on radiation-induced mutation in mammalian cells has been reviewed by Thacker [T5], and a review of specific locus mutation rates in rodents was also prepared by the NCRP [N1].

1. Somatic mutations

269. A number of mutation systems have been described in the literature, but only a few are sufficiently well defined for quantitative studies. Mutation of a single gene is a relatively rare event; the majority of experimental systems are therefore designed to select out cells carrying mutations. Commonly used systems employ the loss of function of a gene product (enzyme) that is not essential for the survival of cells in culture. Thus, cells may be challenged with a toxic drug that they would normally metabolize with fatal consequences. If mutation renders the gene producing the specific enzyme ineffective, the cell will survive, and thus the mutation frequency can be obtained by measuring the survivors. A frequently used example of such a system is that employing the loss of the enzyme hypoxanthine-canon phosphoribosyl transferase (HPRT), which renders cells resistant to the drug 6-thioguanine (6-TG), and of the enzyme thymidine kinase (TK) which gives resistance to trifluorothymidine (TFT). HPRT activity is specified by an X-linked gene *hprt*, while TK is specified by an autosomal gene *tk*, and therefore has to be used in the heterozygous state.

270. There are a number of difficulties with such somatic cell systems, and these have been reviewed [T5]. In particular, the mutation frequency of a given gene is to some extent modifiable, depending on the exact conditions of the experiment. There may also be a period of time for the mutation to manifest itself. In the unirradiated cell the enzyme would normally be produced and thus will be present for some time in the irradiated cell, even if it is no longer being replenished as a result of a specific mutation. An expression time is therefore normally left after irradiation before a cell is challenged by the specific drug. Ideally the mutation frequency would increase with time after irradiation to reach a constant level. This is not always the case, however, and the mutation frequency may reach a peak and subsequently decline. Thus the true mutation frequency may be difficult to determine, and this can present difficulties in studies of the effect of dose rate when exposures can be spread over varying periods of time.

271. Several established cell lines, derived from mouse, hamster or human tissue, have been used to measure mutant frequencies at different dose rates. The cells lines used experimentally can have sensitivities that depend on the stage of the cell cycle; therefore, to ensure as consistent a response as possible, it is preferable to use a stationary culture in plateau phase in which only a limited number of the cells will be cycling in the confluent monolayer [H21, M30]. The range of published data encompasses both a lack of effect of dose rate and a marked effect on induced mutant frequency [T5]. The data presented here are intended to illustrate the range of results available.

272. The first report on the effect of dose rate on hamster cell lines at low dose rates used hamster V79 cells and the *hprt* locus system [T2]. The cells were irradiated at dose rates of 1.7 Gy min^{-1} and 3.4 mGy min^{-1}, with exposures taking up to five days at the low dose rates. A reduction in mutant frequency was obtained at low dose rates with a reduced effectiveness of between about 2.5 and 4 at total doses between about 2 and 12 Gy. The dose-response relationship for mutation and survival was approximately the same. Further studies [C17] used growing V79 cells and compared dose rates of 4 Gy min^{-1} with 8.3 and 1.3 mGy min^{-1}. The authors reported that 8.3 mGy min^{-1} reduced the mutant frequency compared with the high dose-rate exposure, and that, surprisingly, 1.3 mGy min^{-1} increased it.

273. A series of studies in Japan on a number of mouse cell lines [F6, N6, N7, S25, U29] reported that mutation frequency in growing cells was substantially reduced with decreasing dose rate over a range of dose rates from about 5 Gy min^{-1} down to 0.8 mGy min^{-1}. Thus, for mutation resistance to both 6-TG and methotrexate a reduced effectiveness by a factor of about 2, was obtained at low dose rates for L5178Y cells when the linear term (α_1) of the linear-quadratic model fit to high- and low-dose-rate data were compared [N6]. Similar results were also found with Ehrlich ascites mouse tumour cells used in plateau phase with the *hprt* gene locus system. At a dose rate of about 11 mGy min^{-1} compared with 10 Gy min^{-1}, there was a reduction in effectiveness by a factor of about 2, although the extent of the reduction varied with experimental conditions [I5]. It was noteworthy in all these studies that change in mutant frequency with dose rate was parallelled by changes in cell inactivation, which might reflect mechanisms of DNA damage processing [T17].

274. Further studies were reported by Furuno-Fukushi et al. [F7], who used the *hprt* assay for 6-TG resistance and measured cell killing in growing mouse L5178Y cells exposed to 0.5 Gy min^{-1}, 3.3 mGy min^{-1}

and 0.1 mGy min^{-1}. A marked increase in cell survival was observed with decreasing dose rate. At the low dose rate no reduction in the surviving fraction of cells was found up to a dose of 4 Gy, although only about 10% survival was obtained for the same total dose delivered at high dose rate. The induction frequency for mutations found at 3.3 mGy min^{-1} was less than that obtained at the high dose rate (0.5 Gy min^{-1}) by about a factor of about 2. Surprisingly, there was little decrease in mutation frequency at the low dose rate (0.1 mGy min^{-1}) compared with that at 0.5 Gy min^{-1} up to a total dose of about 3 Gy, and at the highest dose (4 Gy) the reduction was between that found at the high and intermediate dose rates. These results therefore suggest an inverse dose-rate effect for the low dose rate compared with the intermediate dose rate.

275. In a subsequent study, LX830 mouse leukaemia cells, which are more sensitive to cell killing by x rays than L5178Y cells and 2-4 times more sensitive to mutation induction, were also exposed to 0.5 Gy min^{-1}, 3.3 mGy min^{-1} and 0.1 mGy min^{-1} [F8]. A slight, but significant increase was observed in cell survival with decreasing dose rate up to a dose of about 1 Gy. Beyond that, increasing doses at the lowest dose rate (0.1 Gy min^{-1}) did not reduce survival further, although the higher dose rates continued to show an exponential decrease in survival with increasing dose. The mutation frequency increased linearly with dose at all three dose rates, but no significant difference in response was found between the different dose rates. This is consistent with the finding that the LX830 cells are deficient in repair and that this produces a nearly dose-rate-independent response for mutation [E4].

276. A very different sensitivity has been reported by Evans et al. [E5], who assayed for the *hprt* gene mutant frequency in the radio-resistant L5178Y-R cells. At very low dose rates (0.3 mGy min^{-1} from x rays), there was little difference in mutation frequency compared with that at 0.88 Gy min^{-1}. The results also indicated the progressive loss of slow-growing mutants.

277. Evans et al. [E7] also compared the effects of dose rate (0.88 Gy min^{-1} and 0.3 mGy min^{-1}) on mutation frequency in two strains of L5178Y cells with differing radiation sensitivities. The induction of mutants at the heterozygous *tk* locus by x-irradiation was dose-rate-dependent in L5178Y-R16 (LY-R16) cells, but very little dose-rate dependence was observed in the case of L5178Y-S1 (LY-S1) cells. This difference may be attributed to the deficiency in DNA double-strand break repair in strain LY-R16. Induction of mutants by x-irradiation at the hemizygous *hprt* locus was dose-rate-independent for both strains, suggesting that in these strains, the majority of mutations at this locus are caused by single lesions.

278. Suspension cultures of human TK_6 cells assayed for mutations at the *hprt* and *rf* loci after exposure to multiple acute doses of 10-100 mGy min^{-1} for 5-31 days showed no significant cell inactivation but linear dose-response functions for mutation. The induction frequency was very similar to that following acute exposures. Similar results were obtained by Koenig and Kiefer [K4], who found no changes in mutant frequency in human TK_6 cells at low dose rates (0.45 and 0.045 mGy min^{-1}).

279. In recent experiments Furuno-Fukushi et al. [F2] examined the induction of 6-TG resistance in cultured near-diploid mouse cells (m5S) in plateau and log phase following exposure to gamma rays at dose rates of 0.5 Gy min^{-1}, 3 mGy min^{-1} and 0.22 mGy min^{-1}. In plateau-phase culture, lowering the dose rate from 0.5 Gy min^{-1} to 0.22 mGy min^{-1} resulted in an increase of cell survival and a marked decrease in induced mutation frequency. A reduction factor of more than about 3 was obtained at 2 Gy from data obtained for high- and low-dose-rate exposures. The frequency at 0.22 mGy min^{-1} was not higher than that obtained at 3 mGy min^{-1}, contrary to previous findings on growing mouse L5178 cells [F7]. In contrast, in log-phase culture, the magnitude of the dose-rate effect was not marked, and up to about 5 Gy almost no differences in mutation frequency were found at the three dose rates examined. These results, together with those indicating an inverse dose-rate effect in growing mouse L5178 leukaemia cells [F7], show that cell growth during protracted irradiation significantly influences the effects of gamma rays, particularly for mutation induction.

2. Germ cell mutations

280. The measurement of germ cell mutation rates presents additional difficulties, as animal studies are needed to demonstrate the mutational response. The effect of dose rate on the induction of specific locus mutations has been reviewed by Searle [S26], by the NCRP [N1] and by Russell and Kelly [R11]. No repair of radiation damage has been demonstrated in mature sperm [N1, R6], reflecting the lack of cytoplasm and enzymic activity. A series of studies involving *in vitro* fertilization and embryonic culture of mouse oocytes has demonstrated, however, that x-ray-induced damage in mature sperm following exposure to 1-5 Gy can be repaired in the fertilized egg. Assay of chromosome aberrations in fertilized eggs treated with various DNA inhibitors has demonstrated that DNA lesions induced in sperm comprise

mainly double-strand breaks and base damage. It remains to be determined if the specific involvement of repair of a particular type of DNA damage leads to chromosome aberrations and mutations in fertilized eggs, and whether there is a dose-rate effect for such damage. No dose-rate effects appear to have been demonstrated so far [M48, M49, M50, M51]. Unlike mature sperm, spermatogonial cells are metabolically active, and repair processes can modify the yield of mutations or chromosomal aberrations with protracted irradiation. Mouse spermatogonial stem cell studies provided the first demonstration of a dose-rate effect for mutational changes.

281. Russell et al. [R6, R11] first showed that specific locus mutation frequencies after chronic exposures to ^{137}Cs gamma rays (≤8 mGy min^{-1}) were lower than after comparable acute x-ray exposures (0.72-0.9 Gy min^{-1}) at doses up to about 6 Gy (Figure XXVI). Similar results were reported by Phillips [P6]. The data available have been summarized by Searle [S26]. For chronic exposures the dose-response data were fitted with a linear function, but for acute exposures a peaked response was obtained; thus, the relative effectiveness of acute and chronic exposures (i.e. the magnitude of the dose-rate effect) varies with the exposure level considered. By comparing the linear fits of the data from 0, 3 and 6 Gy points following acute x-ray exposures with all the data obtained following chronic exposures (at 0.01 and 0.09 mGy min^{-1}), Russell [R7] obtained a ratio of 3.23 ± 0.62. Alternatively, fitting a linear function to the acute data obtained up to 3 Gy, on the assumption of a cell killing function being present at higher doses, gives a ratio of 4.0 [S26].

282. More information on the dose-rate effect for mutation frequencies in spermatogonia has been obtained with various dose rates and fractionation regimes. Russell et al. [R7, R11, R17] reported that mutation frequency decreased markedly as the dose rate is reduced from 900 mGy min^{-1} to 8 mGy min^{-1}, although there appeared to be no further reduction at dose rates down to 0.007 mGy min^{-1}. Because this independence of dose rate had been shown over a more than one thousand-fold range, it was thought unlikely that mutation frequency would be further reduced at even lower dose rates. The mutation frequency obtained at dose rates from 720 to 900 mGy min^{-1}, with total doses up to about 6 Gy, was compared with that obtained at low dose rates, on the basis of linear fits to the data, to give a DDREF of 3.0 ± 0.41, in close agreement with previous estimates [R11].

283. To examine further this dose-rate effect, Lyon et al. [L17] compared the effects of single doses of about 6 Gy from x rays or gamma rays with those of various fractionation regimes. They found that if the gamma-ray exposure was split into 60 equal fractions of 100 mGy, given daily at 170 mGy min^{-1}, the mutation frequency (4.17 10^{-5} per locus) was less than one third of that from a single gamma-ray exposure at the same dose rate (15.39 10^{-5} per locus) and similar to the frequency obtained after giving a comparable dose at 0.08 mGy min^{-1} over 90 days (3.15 10^{-5} per locus). However, if 12 weekly doses of 0.5 Gy from x rays were given acutely the mutation frequency was similar to that found after a single acute exposure (12.61 10^{-5} per locus). It may be concluded that repeated small doses, even if given at a moderately high dose rate, have less mutagenic effect than the same dose given at one time. With fewer fractions (i.e. larger doses per fraction) the effect is intermediate between the response for an acute exposure and chronic exposure (Table 16).

284. These results are very similar to those obtained for lung tumour induction in mice by Ullrich et al. [U26] (Section II.A.2.b), where the incidence of tumours for a given dose again depended on the dose per fraction. A similar explanation can be invoked, namely that with small doses per fraction, in this case ~100 mGy given at a moderately high dose rate, the effect of each fraction will lie predominantly on the linear portion of the dose-response curve, and thus the overall response is similar to that for low-dose-rate exposure. With larger fractions (0.5 Gy) the quadratic function makes an increasing contribution to the response, and thus an effect between acute and chronic exposure conditions is obtained.

285. Based on the above results of dose-rate effects on mutation rates in spermatogonia, a DDREF of 3 has been applied by the Committee since the UNSCEAR 1972 Report [U5] for assessing the risks of hereditary disease at low dose rates. This value of DDREF was also applied in the UNSCEAR 1988 Report [U1].

286. It is also possible to examine the effects of radiation on translocations induced in spermatogonial cells by subsequent examination of the spermatocyte stage. Clear evidence of dose fractionation effects have been observed in the mouse, and these were reviewed by the NCRP [N1] and more recently by Tobari et al. [T9]. Dose-rate reduction factors from 3 to >10 have been obtained.

287. In a recent study [T9], the induction of reciprocal translocations in the spermatogonia of the adult crab-eating monkey *(Macaca fascicularis)* was examined following chronic gamma-irradiation to total doses of 0.3, 1.0 and 1.5 Gy (0.018 mGy min^{-1}, about 0.024 Gy in 22 h d^{-1}). Two or three monkeys were used for each dose level, and in each testis reciprocal translocations were scored in 1,000-1,250 spermatocytes.

The dose-response relationship for the frequency of translocation per cell could be represented by a linear function I(D) = 0.09 + 0.16D, where I(D) is the frequency of translocations (%) and D is the dose in gray. After acute exposure to x rays at high dose rates (0.25 Gy min^{-1}) the dose response was also found to be linear, at least below 1 Gy, and fitted by the equation I(D) = 1.08 + 1.79D [M18]. Thus, at high dose rates the incidence of translocations was higher than at low dose rates by a factor of about 10.

288. In contrast, van Buul et al. [B24] found that, when the testis of the rhesus monkey was exposed to a gamma-ray dose rate of 0.2 mGy min^{-1} to give a total dose of 1 Gy, the yield of translocations was 0.38%, about one half the yield obtained at the same x-ray dose delivered at 0.3 Gy min^{-1} (0.83%). If a correction is made for the RBE of gamma rays, which is possibly about 0.5-0.7, the translocation yield would become more than one half that at high dose rate. It would appear from these results that the dose-rate effect is less pronounced in the rhesus monkey than in the crab-eating monkey.

289. These results suggest that a wide range of dose-rate effectiveness factors may be obtained, depending on the species and strain used for particular study. Reciprocal translocations are, however, two-hit aberrations, and the yield will be very dependent on recovery processes occurring between successive events. The marked difference in dose-rate effects between species may be accounted for by variable rates of repair in different species.

290. Effects of dose rate have also been studied in some of the germ-cell stages present in female mice. Mature and maturing oocytes have a much larger dose-rate effect than that found in spermatogonia [R18], and unlike the situation described earlier for spermatogonia one study has reported that the size of the dose-rate effect continues to increase when the dose rate is lowered below 8 mGy min^{-1}.

291. Selby et al. [S38], using the specific-locus method, examined the effect of dose rate on mutation induction in mouse oocytes irradiated just before birth. Female mice were exposed to 3 Gy of whole-body x-irradiation at dose rates of 0.73-0.93 Gy min^{-1} and 7.9 mGy min^{-1} at 18.5 days after conception. The frequency of specific-locus mutations was assayed in the offspring of both control and exposed animals. The radiation-induced mutation frequency decreased from 6.1 10^{-5} to 4.2 10^{-6} mutations per gray per locus, i.e. by a factor of about 14, between acute and chronically exposed animals. Although the confidence limits of this estimate of the magnitude of the dose-rate effect are wide with an upper bound of infinity, the results indicate that mutational damage in females irradiated just before birth has a pronounced dose-rate effect. The mutation rate following exposures at low dose rates did not differ significantly from that in controls. Similar calculations, based on results of irradiating mature and maturing oocytes at the same dose rates (0.8-0.9 Gy min^{-1} and 8 mGy min^{-1}) [R18, R19], suggest an approximately fourfold reduction in the induced mutation frequency in the adult. With protracted exposure and lower dose rates (0.09 mGy min^{-1}), a further reduction in mutation frequency was obtained. It was concluded that although the confidence limits on these estimates of the reduction factor at low dose rates were large, the results suggested that females irradiated just before birth had a more pronounced dose-rate effect for mutational damage to oocytes than those irradiated later [S38].

292. Irradiation of mice with high-LET radiation from fission neutrons has shown average values of RBE of about 20 (range: 10-45), relative to chronic irradiation with gamma rays, both with spermatogonial and oogonial irradiation [I6, S12]. Spermatogonia show little or no dose-rate effect with fission neutrons [R8] except at high doses (>2 Gy), where there is a suggestion of a reduced effectiveness, presumably due to selective cell killing of the spermatogonial population [B32, R8].

3. Summary

293. Studies on somatic mutations *in vitro* and germ cell mutations *in vivo* are relevant to assessing the effect of dose and dose rate on the primary lesion in DNA involved in tumour initiation, although subsequent tumour expression will depend on the influence of many other factors. The results obtained in different studies on somatic cell mutations in mice have been somewhat variable, but the overall extent of the dose-rate effect indicates a maximum value of about 2-3. A DDREF of about 3 for specific-locus mutations has also been found in mouse spermatogonia for dose rates that vary by a factor of more than 1,000, and for reciprocal translocations DDREFs up to about 10 have been reported, although there appear to be considerable differences between species. Based on these results, a DDREF of 3 for damage to spermatogonia has been applied by the Committee since the UNSCEAR 1972 Report [U5] for assessing the risks of hereditary disease at low dose rates. The DDREF in mature and maturing mouse oocytes appears to be larger than that in spermatogonia, with the main difference being that the mutation rate continues to decrease when the dose rate decreases below 8.0 mGy min^{-1}. Mouse oocytes present just before birth appear to show a more pronounced dose-rate effect than mature or maturing oocytes, with a DDREF of about 14.

III. DOSE AND DOSE-RATE EFFECTS IN HUMAN CANCER

294. In general, epidemiological studies on the induction of cancer in human populations following exposure to low-LET radiation do not provide information on exposures at different dose rates that allow estimates to be made of dose-rate effectiveness factors. Furthermore, dose-response data are generally not available at the low doses needed to make good estimates of the linear component of the dose response (slope α_L, Figure I). There are, however, some human data that can be used to assess likely dose-rate effects; these have been reviewed by the Committee [U1, U2].

295. In the UNSCEAR 1986 Report [U2] it was concluded from a review of dose-response relationships for radiation-induced tumours in man that for low-LET radiation the data available in some cases (lung, thyroid and breast) were consistent with linear or linear-quadratic models. For breast cancer linearity was considered more probable, as the incidence is little affected by dose fractionation. The Committee considered that for low-LET radiation linear extrapolation downwards from effects measured at doses of about 2 Gy would not overestimate the risk of breast and possibly thyroid cancer, would slightly overestimate the risk of leukaemia and would be likely to overestimate the risk of bone sarcoma (see paragraph 16). For radiation-induced cancers of most other organs only experimental data from animals were available on dose-response relationships, for which upward concave curvilinear dose-response relationships with pronounced dose-rate and fractionation effects are commonly found. The Committee concluded that if similar curves are applied to cancers in humans, a linear extrapolation of risk coefficients from acute doses in the intermediate dose region (0.2-2 Gy) to low doses and low dose rates would very likely overestimate the real risk, possibly by a factor of up to 5. Although some reference was made to the data on the survivors of the atomic bombings in Hiroshima and Nagasaki, the data were not fully utilized because of the uncertainties regarding the revision of the dosimetry. It was also noted that bone sarcoma induction after intake of radium isotopes shows a pronounced inverse relationship of latency to dose, resulting in an apparent threshold at low doses. For assessing the risk of lung cancer from exposure to radon the flattening of the response at higher cumulative exposures could result in an underestimation of the risk by linear extrapolation to low doses.

296. In the UNSCEAR 1988 Report [U1] epidemiological data on the effects of low-LET radiation relevant to assessing risks at low doses and dose rates were also summarized. The Committee considered the then most recent data on the atomic bomb survivors in Japan [P4, S9, S10], which took account of the new (DS86) dosimetry. For leukaemia, a significant difference in the excess relative risk per Gy of organ absorbed dose among survivors exposed to 0.5 Gy or more, as opposed to those exposed to lower doses (5.53 versus 2.44, respectively) was noted, suggesting a curvilinear dose-effect relationship for haemopoietic malignancies. For all cancers except leukaemia the excess relative risk associated with higher doses does not differ significantly from that at lower doses (0.41 versus 0.37, respectively) suggesting a linear response. No significant excess risk was observed at doses below 0.2 Gy, however. The scatter of the data points in the low dose region was such that they could be fitted almost equally well by a quadratic, linear-quadratic or linear dose-response relationship [S9].

297. The Committee also reviewed epidemiological studies of individuals exposed to ^{131}I, which suggested that radiation doses from chronic internal exposures are less carcinogenic than similar doses of acute external radiation by a factor of at least 3 [N2] and possibly even 4 [H15], although non-uniformity of dose distribution within the thyroid gland may be a contributing factor. Breast cancer studies involving fractionated exposures provide some information on low-dose and low-dose-rate effectiveness factors. No fractionation effect was evident in a Massachusetts study of breast cancer following multiple fluoroscopic examination [B15]. However, in a similar but larger Canadian study, a non-linear dose response, especially at high dose, appeared to have been found. This would suggest a low-dose and low-dose-rate effectiveness factor greater than 1.

298. From examination of both experimental and human data the Committee concluded that reduction factors will vary with dose and dose rate and with organ system but will generally fall within the range 2-10. No dose or dose-rate reduction factor was considered necessary for high-LET radiation at low doses.

299. Since the publication of the UNSCEAR 1988 Report [U1], more information has become available from epidemiological studies that relate to considerations of dose-rate effects for low-LET radiation. The relevant studies are reviewed below.

A. LEUKAEMIA AND ALL OTHER CANCERS

1. Survivors of the atomic bombings in Japan

300. The follow-up study on the survivors of the atomic bombings in Hiroshima and Nagasaki continues to provide the main source of information on the effects on a population of exposure to ionizing radia-

tion. Information is available from 1950 to 1985 on mortality in just under 76,000 survivors for whom revised estimates of doses based on the new DS86 dosimetry system [R4] have been calculated [S9, S10].

301. The dose-response relationship for cancer mortality among the survivors of the atomic bombings in Japan has been examined by Pierce and Vaeth [P2, P3]. Their aim was to determine the degree of curvature in a linear-quadratic dose-response model that is consistent with the data. From this, possible values for a linear extrapolation overestimation factor (LEOF), which is equivalent to the dose and dose-rate effectiveness factor (DDREF), were derived.

302. Figure XXVII gives dose-responses for leukaemia and all cancers except leukaemia on the assumption of an RBE for neutrons of 10. For both sets of data any estimates of dose above 6 Gy (shielded kerma) have been reduced to 6 Gy. In both cases the data indicate a levelling off in the relative risk at doses above about 3 Gy. This apparent plateau at high doses may be due, at least in part, to cell killing, as appears to be the case in a number of animal studies (see Chapter II) and other human studies [S45], although it may in part be attributed to errors in exposure estimates.

303. Because of uncertainties as to the reason for this plateau, two approaches were taken by Pierce and Vaeth [P2, P3] in evaluating the dose-response data, namely:

(a) the dose range was limited to 0-4 Gy as well as 0-6 Gy. While this restriction in the range of exposures studied reduces the statistical power in studying the dose response, it should alleviate any bias in this relationship due to errors in estimates of high exposures. The linear-quadratic model assumption is also less critical if made over a restricted range of exposures;
(b) adjustments were made for random errors in the dosimetry of about 35% across the whole range of exposure estimates. Again, such errors could bias the shape of the dose-response curves and would lead to risk estimates higher by about 10%. Results of the unadjusted analysis were given for comparison.

The model fit adopted for all cancers except leukaemia was taken with excess relative risk constant in age-at-risk, but depending on age-at-exposure and sex.

304. Estimates of the LEOF were obtained based on the exposure range 0-4 Gy (DS86), with or without adjustment for random errors in dose estimates [P2]. Data were given for leukaemia, for all cancers other than leukaemia as a group and for combined inferences, assuming common curvature in these two disease categories. Estimates of the LEOF from analyses based on the range 0-6 Gy were lower than those based on the 0-4 Gy range. However, even after allowing for random errors in the exposure estimates, there is an indication that the analyses based on the 0-6 Gy range are unduly affected by the levelling off in the dose response beyond 4 Gy. Hence, the analyses based on the 0-4 Gy range are likely to be more relevant for the extrapolation of risks to low doses.

305. For the grouping of all cancers other than leukaemia, the maximum likelihood estimate of LEOF was 1.2, with a 90% confidence interval (CI) ranging from less than 1 to 2.3. However, after adjusting for random errors in the dose estimates, the best estimate of LEOF was 1.4 (90% CI: <1->3.1). Thus the data for all cancers other than leukaemia are fitted well by a linear dose-response model, although they are also consistent with a linear-quadratic model for which the linear extrapolation overestimation factor is between 1 and 3. For leukaemia, the maximum likelihood estimate of the LEOF from the Japanese data was 1.6 (90% CI: 1.0->3.1) without adjustment for random dosimetry errors and 2.0 (90% CI: 1.1->3.1) with adjustment for these errors. Thus, these data for leukaemia suggest that a linear dose-response model does not provide a good fit and that a linear-quadratic model with an LEOF of the order of 2 is to be preferred. For all cancers together an LEOF of 1.7 (90% CI: 1.1-3.1) was obtained with adjustment for random errors. Pierce and Vaeth [P2, P3] emphasized that the use of LEOFs much above 2 would need to be based upon information from experimental studies and that their inferences depended strongly on the assumption that a linear-quadratic model is appropriate for extrapolation to low doses.

306. It is clear that there are a number of limitations in the analysis of these data. The plateaus in the dose response at intermediate doses (Figure XXVII) imply that analyses of the shapes of the dose-response curves that include groups exposed at doses much above 3 Gy are likely to underestimate the contribution of the quadratic component to the dose-response function. Yet it is these same groups that make a significant contribution to the overall assessment of risk at high doses and high dose rates. A further problem lies in determining the initial slope of the dose-response function when only limited data are available at low doses.

2. Exposures from the nuclear industry

307. Several studies have been conducted of nuclear industry workers. In the United States, Gilbert [G14] performed a joint analysis of data from about 36,000 workers at the Hanford site, Oak Ridge National Laboratory and Rocky Flats weapons plant. Neither for

the grouping of all cancers nor for leukaemia was there an indication of an increasing trend in risk with dose. The upper limit of the 90% confidence interval for the lifetime risk corresponded to a value of 8.2 10^{-2} Sv^{-1} for all cancers and 0.6 10^{-2} Sv^{-1} for leukaemia.

308. A recent study of just over 95,000 individuals in the National Registry for Radiation Workers (NRRW) in the United Kingdom examined cancer mortality in relation to dose [K11]. For all malignant neoplasms, the trend in the relative risk with dose was positive but was not statistically significant ($p = 0.10$). Based on a relative risk projection model, the central estimate of the lifetime risk based on these data was 10 10^{-2} Sv^{-1} (90% CI: <0-26 10^{-2}). For leukaemia (excluding chronic lymphatic leukaemia, which does not appear to be radiation-inducible), the trend in risk with dose was statistically significant ($p = 0.03$). Based on a BEIR-V type projection model [C1], the central estimate of the corresponding lifetime risk was 0.76 10^{-2} Sv^{-1} (90% CI: 0.07-2.4 10^{-2}). The NRRW therefore provides evidence of a raised risk of leukaemia associated with occupational exposure to radiation, but, like the combined study of workers in the Untied States [G14], is consistent with the risk estimates for low-dose, low-dose-rate exposures derived for workers by ICRP [I2] from the Japanese survivor data (4 10^{-2} Sv^{-1} for all cancers and 0.4 10^{-2} Sv^{-1} for leukaemia) which include a DDREF of 2. In particular, combining the results of the NRRW and the United States studies produces central estimates for the lifetime risk of 4.9 10^{-2} Sv^{-1} (90% CI: <0-18 10^{-2} for all cancers and 0.3 10^{-2} Sv^{-1} for leukaemia (excluding chronic lymphatic leukaemia) [K11]. These values are similar to the ICRP [I2] risk estimates, and generally support the use of a low DDREF in assessing risks at low doses and dose rates from high dose and dose-rate studies.

309. Information has recently become available from a number of low-dose-rate studies in the former USSR. Kossenko et al. [K10] have followed up the population of about 28,000 persons exposed as a result of the release of radioactive wastes into the Techa river in the southern Urals. The study shows a statistically significant increase in the risk of leukaemia estimated to be 0.85 (CI: 0.24-1.45) per 10^4 PY Gy. This is substantially smaller than the value of 2.94 per 10^4 PY Gy derived for the atomic bomb survivors [S9]. Some risk estimates are also available for cancers in a number of organs and tissues that are similar to those obtained from the atomic bomb survivors, but the confidence intervals are wide. The risk estimates for leukaemia therefore suggest a reduction in risk at low dose rates by a factor of about 3, although the data must be regarded as preliminary. Further extended analyses are planned. Data are also available on the incidence of leukaemia among the workers at the Chelyabinsk-65 nuclear weapons plant [K12]. Film badge data are available on 5085 men in two facilities. Average cumulative doses varied between 0.49 and 2.45 Sv. When compared with USSR national rates for the period 1970-1986, the relative risk of leukaemia appeared to be increased with a relative risk of 1.45 Gy^{-1}, which is about 2.7 times less than that based on the atomic bomb survivors (≥20 years, excess RR = 3.92 Gy^{-1} [S9]).

B. THYROID CANCER

310. A substantial number of studies have reported excesses of thyroid cancer in populations exposed to external radiation. Many of these studies were summarized in the UNSCEAR 1988 Report [U1] and by the NCRP [N2]. The information summarized in [N2] suggested risks of radiation-induced thyroid cancer are greater in children than in adults, by about a factor 2, and that females appear to be more sensitive than males by a factor of 2 to 3. Radiation-induced thyroid cancer risks in a population were calculated to be 7.5 10^{-4} Gy^{-1} and in adults to be about 5 10^{-4} Gy^{-1}.

311. Information on the dose-response relationship for radiation-induced thyroid cancer is available from studies by Shore et al. [S11] on about 2650 persons who received x-ray treatment for purported enlarged thymuses in infancy. The 30 thyroid cancers detected in the irradiated group (<1 expected), when allocated to 5 dose groups, could be fitted by a linear dose-response relationship (Figure XXVIII) $I(D) = 3.46 \pm 0.82$ per 10^4 PY Gy (±1 SE, $p < 0.0001$), although a linear-quadratic relationship could not be excluded.

312. Shore et al. [S11] also examined the effect of dose fractionation, as the number of dose fractions ranged from 1 to 11, with most subjects having 3 or fewer. Three semi-independent variables were tested: number of fractions, dose per fraction, and average interval between fractions. No evidence was obtained for a significant sparing effect for thyroid cancer associated with any of these three fractionation variables, although numerically the excess cancer risk per Gy was greater in the lowest dose-per-fraction group (0.01-0.49 Gy) than in the higher dose-per-fraction groups (0.5-1.99 Gy and 2-5.99 Gy), namely by a factor of 2-3, again possibly reflecting an effect of cell killing.

313. Data on thyroid cancer induction also comes from patients given ^{131}I for diagnostic reasons [H13, H15, H35]. Holm et al. [H13] reported a retrospective study of 10,133 subjects given ^{131}I for suspected thyroid disease. The population (79% females) had a mean age of 44 years. For the 9,639 adults (>20 years of age) the mean calculated thyroid dose was 0.6 Gy,

whereas in the 494 younger subjects the mean dose was 1.6 Gy. Patients were followed for a mean time of 17 years after exposure to ^{131}I. Only patients diagnosed more than 5 years after ^{131}I exposure were included in the analysis. No excess of thyroid cancer was found, although the number of observed cases was small (8 observed, 8.3 expected).

314. For 35,074 patients in Sweden examined for suspected thyroid disorders between 1951 and 1969 the mean follow-up was 20 years [H15, H22]. The mean age at administration of ^{131}I was 44 years; 5% were under age 20 years and the mean dose to the gland was about 0.5 Gy. Persons with a history of external radiotherapy to the head and neck region, or who had been given internal emitters, were excluded from the study. No overall excess risk of thyroid cancer in this group was observed.

315. Further information on thyroid cancer induction is available from groups given ^{131}I for the treatment of hyperthyroidism. Although a number of studies have been reported, no evidence for radiation-induced cancer in these groups has been obtained. Treatment for hyperthyroidism, however, involves the administration of large quantities of ^{131}I giving substantial doses to the thyroid (>20 Gy), which would be expected to result in substantial cell killing [H32].

316. An increased incidence of thyroid nodules has been seen in the inhabitants of the Marshall Islands who were exposed to weapons fallout [C19]. However, although a large proportion of the dose was contributed by short-lived isotopes of iodine (^{132,133,135}I), there was also a contribution from external radiation with only a small proportion of the dose coming from ^{131}I. It is therefore difficult to use the data to assess any effect of dose rate on tumour induction.

317. There are some uncertainties regarding dosimetry in the studies of Holm et al. [H14, H15, H22]. The main factors influencing the calculated thyroid dose are the mass of the gland and the initial uptake of ^{131}I. Animal studies suggest differences in distribution throughout the gland will be of less importance (see Section II.A.2.e). The mean thyroid weight was estimated on the basis of information in the records and available thyroid scintigrams to be <30 g in 42% of the patients, 30-60 g in 38%, and >60 g in 12%. In 8% of patients the thyroid weight was not assessed. No information is given in the paper on the uptake of ^{131}I by the gland, but the calculated doses suggest 30% has been used, in line with recommendations by the ICRP [I3]. Both these parameters may affect the dose calculations, but taken together are unlikely to alter the average doses calculated by more than a factor of 2. The studies therefore suggest that ^{131}I is less carcinogenic than acute exposure to external radiation, although these studies mostly involved adults who appear to be less sensitive to the induction of thyroid cancer than young persons.

C. BREAST CANCER

318. Since the publication of the UNSCEAR 1986 Report [U2] further information has become available on possible effects of dose rate on breast cancer induction. Miller et al. [M32] have reported data from a number of provinces in Canada on mortality from breast cancer in tuberculosis patients irradiated during fluoroscopic examinations. Mortality data have been obtained for 31,710 women treated at sanatoriums between 1930 and 1952, known to be alive in 1950 and followed to 1980. A substantial proportion (26.4%) had received doses to the breasts of 0.1 Gy or more from repeated fluoroscopic examinations during therapeutic pneumothoraxes. The principal difference among sanatoriums was that in Nova Scotia the patients usually faced the x-ray source, whereas in other provinces they were usually turned away from it. Various dose-response models were fitted to the data. The best fit was obtained with a linear dose-response relationship, and it was notable that a greater effect per unit dose was found in Nova Scotia than in the other provinces. Thus, the increases in relative risk were 1.80 and 0.53 Gy^{-1} for Nova Scotia and the other provinces, respectively. In the BEIR V Report [C1] the difference in relative risk was given as a factor of 6. Even allowing for the differences in orientation during exposure this difference in response is surprising, and the authors considered that it could be due to a dose-rate effect. Although the mean numbers of fluoroscopic exposures were similar in the two groups, the dose rate in Nova Scotia was higher by more than an order of magnitude, although not higher than that in the atomic bomb survivors. These results would therefore be consistent with a dose-rate effectiveness factor greater than 1.

D. SUMMARY

319. The human data that are available for assessing the effects of dose rate on tumour induction from low-LET radiation are limited. In general, the information available is from exposures at high dose rates, and little information is available at doses of less than about 0.2 Gy. Analyses of dose-response relationships for solid tumours in the atomic bomb survivors are generally consistent with linearity but also with a small reduction in the slope of the dose-response at lower doses. For leukaemia among the atomic bomb survivors, however, the data are inconsistent with linearity, and the central estimate of the DDREF at low doses is about 2. Model fit to the dose-response

data for the atomic bomb survivors over the dose range 0-4 Gy kerma for all cancers combined, suggests a DDREF in the range of about 1.7 (when adjusted for random errors). For solid cancers alone, however, linearity provides a good fit, although the data are also consistent with a DDREF of the order of 2. This interpretation of the data depends on the assumption that a linear-quadratic model is appropriate for extrapolation to low doses and that the linear term can be adequately resolved. Information on thyroid cancer induction by acute external irradiation compared with low dose-rate exposure from intakes of ^{131}I are consistent with a DDREF of about 3, although there is some question over the contributions that heterogeneity of dose and uncertainties in the dose estimates as well as the effect of age make to the overall reduction in risk. For female breast cancer the information is conflicting. Dose-response relationships for acute exposures and for fractionated exposures at high dose rates are consistent with a linear dose-response relationship. However, comparative data from Nova Scotia and from other Canadian provinces suggest a DDREF greater than one may be appropriate for assessing cancer risks at low dose rates. Although epidemiological studies of low dose-rate exposure should be more relevant for the purposes of radiological protection than studies at high dose rates, the former type of study at present lacks sufficient statistical power to allow risks to be estimated with tight confidence limits. However, the results of studies such as those of radiation workers are consistent with low values of DDREF.

IV. DESIGNATION OF LOW DOSES AND LOW DOSE RATES

320. The choice of bounds for low and high doses of low-LET radiation that are appropriate for decisions on whether to apply dose and dose-rate effectiveness factors (DDREFs) is not straightforward, as it is essential to understand both the physical and biological factors involved and their possible interactions. The physical factors, unlike the biological factors, are well understood as a result of the advances that have taken place in recent years in microdosimetry at the cellular and subcellular levels [B18, B20, G6, P1, R14]. This Chapter reviews the physical, experimental and epidemiological data that can be used as a basis for assessing either the doses or the dose rates below which it would be appropriate to apply a DDREF.

A. PHYSICAL FACTORS

321. The microdosimetric approach to defining low doses and low dose rates uses fundamental microdosimetric arguments that are based on statistical considerations of the occurrence of independent radiation tracks within cells or cell nuclei (Section I.A.3). Photons deposit energy in cells in the form of tracks, comprising ionizations and excitations from energetic electrons, and the smallest insult each cell can receive is the energy deposited from one electron entering or being set in motion within a cell. For ^{60}Co gamma rays and a spherical cell (or nucleus) assumed to be 8 μm in diameter, there is on average one track per cell (or nucleus) when the absorbed dose is about 1 mGy [B18, B20]. This dose, corresponding to one track per cell, on average, varies inversely with volume and is also dependent on radiation quality, being much larger for high-LET radiation [G4, I4].

322. If the induction of cancer by radiation at low doses depends on energy deposition in single cells, with no interaction between cells, there can be no departure from linearity, unless there have been at least two independent tracks within the cell. The number of independent tracks within cells follows a Poisson distribution, as illustrated in Table 17, with the mean number of tracks being proportional to dose. For average tissue doses of 0.2 mGy from ^{60}Co gamma rays, spherical cells (or nuclei) of diameter 8 μm each receive, on average, about 0.2 tracks (Figure III). Hence, Table 17 shows that, in this case, just 18% of the cells receive a dose and 90% of these cells receive only one track. Thus less than 2% of cells receive more than one track. Halving the dose will simply halve the fraction of the total cells affected, and so at such low doses the dose-effect relationship should be linear. There should be no dose-rate effect, because this only affects the time interval between energy deposition in different cells (Section I.A.3). This argument applies to all biological effects where the energy deposited in a cell produces effects in that cell and in no other cell. It is generally thought to apply to cell killing, chromosome aberrations and mutations. Its applicability to transformation and cancer is less certain. It would need modification, for example, if the probability of effect were so enhanced by a second track at a later time that the small minority of such cells were dominant. This could conceivably be the case for multi-stage carcinogenesis if more than one essential stage was likely to be caused by radiation.

323. To employ the microdosimetric argument for assessing low doses, a knowledge of the autonomous sensitive volume within a cell is required. Biological

effects are believed to arise predominantly from residual DNA changes that originate from radiation damage to chromosomal DNA. It is the repair response of the cell that determines its fate. The majority of damage is repaired, but it is the remaining unrepaired or misrepaired damage that is then considered responsible for cell killing, chromosomal aberrations, mutations, transformations and cancerous changes. The link between DNA damage and cellular effects leads to the notion that the cell nucleus is the critical volume that should be used for these microdosimetric estimations of a low dose. A sphere of 8 μm diameter is representative of some cell nuclei; others may be smaller or larger. On this basis a low dose would be estimated to be less than 0.2 mGy. If part of the nucleus alone responds autonomously to radiation insults and repair, then a smaller volume may be appropriate, and the estimate of a low dose would increase. Conversely, if the entire cell or adjacent cells can be involved in a cooperative response, a larger volume may be appropriate. Figure XXIX shows, for various volumes and radiations, the doses that would correspond to this microdosimetric definition of a low dose. The most fundamental corresponding criterion for a low dose rate is that the dose should not be exceeded in a lifetime (say, 60 years), so that there should be negligible scope for radiation to cause multiple changes in a single cell or its progeny. By this criterion, a low dose rate would be less than about 10^{-8} mGy min^{-1}. A less cautious criterion, applicable to single-stage changes only, is that a low dose should not be exceeded in a time characteristic for DNA repair, say a few hours. In this case, a low dose rate would be less than about 10^{-3} mGy min^{-1}.

B. BIOLOGICAL FACTORS

324. A second approach to estimating a low dose and low dose rate is based on direct observations in animal experiments. The results of animal studies designed to examine the effect of dose and dose rate on tumour induction (see Section II.A and Table 8) suggest that an average dose rate of ~0.06 mGy min^{-1} over a few days or weeks may be regarded as low. The choice by the Committee in the UNSCEAR 1986 Report [U2] of a low dose rate to include values up to 0.05 mGy min^{-1} appears to have come directly from dose rates used in animal studies. If it is assumed that dose-rate effects arise when sufficient damage accumulates in a cell within repair times characteristic for DNA damage (a few hours), then a rounded value of 20 mGy may be regarded as a low dose.

325. It should be noted, however, that experimental studies at "high" dose rates were mainly carried out in the range from about 100 to 800 mGy min^{-1} (Table 8), i.e. dose rates more than a thousand times those at the "low" dose rates for which a DDREF between 2 and 10 has been obtained. It seems likely that a reduction in tumour yield similar to that obtained at about 0.06 mGy min^{-1} would have been obtained at dose rates a few times higher, or lower, than this. There are analogies here with the data on mutation yield in mouse spermatogonia, for which a threefold reduction in yield was obtained at 8 mGy min^{-1} compared with 720-900 mGy min^{-1} (Section II.C.2), with no further reduction at 0.007 mGy min^{-1} [R18]. It may be concluded, therefore, on the basis of animal experiments that a low dose rate can be taken to be 0.1 mGy min^{-1} when averaged over about an hour.

326. A third approach to estimating low doses comes from parametric fits to observed dose-response data for cellular effects. As described in Section I.A.2, the effect can be related to dose by an expression of the form

$$I(D) = \alpha_1 D + \alpha_2 D^2 \qquad (29)$$

in which α_1 and α_2, the coefficients for the linear and quadratic terms fitted to the radiation response, are constants and are different for different end-points. This equation has been shown to fit data on the induction of chromosome aberrations in human lymphocytes, for example, and also data on cell killing and mutation induction. For some types of unstable chromosome aberrations in human lymphocytes, the α_1/α_2 quotient is about 200 mGy for ^{60}Co gamma rays [L12], and thus the response is essentially linear up to 20 mGy, with the dose-squared term contributing only 9% of the total response. At 40 mGy the dose-squared term still only contributes about 17% to the overall response. On this basis it could, therefore, be estimated that 20-40 mGy is a low dose.

327. A fourth approach to estimating a low dose is based on the analysis of data from epidemiological studies, in particular from data on the survivors of the atomic bombings in Japan. Analysis of the dose response for mortality from solid cancers in the range 0-4 Gy (adjusted for random errors) has suggested an α_1/α_2 quotient from a minimum of about 1 Gy with a central estimate of about 5 Gy [P2, P3]. An α_1/α_2 quotient of 1 Gy suggests that at a dose of 100 mGy the dose-squared term contributes less than 10% to the response and at 200 mGy the contribution of the dose-squared term is still less than 20%. This would suggest that for tumour induction in humans a low dose can be taken to be less than 200 mGy. There is, in practice, little evidence of a departure from linearity up to about 3 Gy. In the case of leukaemia in the atomic bomb survivors, where there is significant departure from linearity at doses above about 1.5 Gy, the central estimate of α_1/α_2 has been calculated to be

1.7 Gy, with a minimum value less than 1 Gy [P2, P3]. On the basis of this central estimate the dose-squared term would contribute about 10% to the response at a dose of 200 mGy and about 23% at 500 mGy.

C. SUMMARY

328. A number of approaches based on physical, experimental and epidemiological data have been examined for assessing either doses or dose rates for low-LET radiation below which it would be appropriate to apply a dose and dose-rate effectiveness factor (DDREF). The fundamental microdosimetric argument indicates that a low dose, at which fewer than 2% of cells receive more than one track (assuming a cell diameter of 8 μm), is about 0.2 mGy. Since halving the dose will simply halve the fraction of cells affected, at such low doses the dose-effect relationship should be linear. This fundamental microdosimetric approach would have severe practical limitations in radiological protection, and there do not appear to be any experimental or epidemiological data that suggest that it should be applied.

329. Dose-response studies for cells in culture suggest that doses of less than about 20-40 mGy are low; however, epidemiological studies on the induction of solid tumours in the survivors of the atomic bombings in Japan indicate a linear dose response up to about 3 Gy, which suggests that for tumour induction a low dose would be at least 200 mGy. For leukaemia induction there is a significant departure from linearity at doses above about 1.5 Gy, but again a low dose can be taken to be less than 200 mGy.

330. Information on low dose rates for tumour induction can at present be obtained from animal studies. The results of a series of studies in experimental animals that are summarized in Table 8 suggest that a low dose rate can be taken to be less than about 0.1 mGy min^{-1} given over a few days or weeks.

331. The Committee concludes that for the purposes of assessing the risk of tumour induction in man a dose-rate effectiveness factor (DDREF) should be applied either if the total dose is less than 200 mGy, whatever the dose rate, or if the dose rate is below 0.1 mGy min^{-1} (when averaged over about an hour), whatever the total dose.

CONCLUSIONS

332. Information on dose and dose-rate effects on radiation response has been reviewed in this Annex with the aim of providing a basis for assessing the risks of stochastic effects at low doses and low dose rates from information available at high doses and high dose rates.

333. The conventional approach to estimating both the absolute and the relative biological effectiveness of a given radiation at minimal doses is based on the assumption, derived here in general terms of target theory, that the induction of an effect can be approximated by an expression of the form

$$I(D) = (\alpha_1 D + \alpha_2 D^2) e^{-(\beta_1 D + \beta_2 D^2)} \quad (30)$$

in which α_1 and α_2 are coefficients for the linear and quadratic terms for the induction of stochastic effects and β_1 and β_2 are coefficients for linear and quadratic terms for cell killing. This equation has been shown to give a fit to much of the published data on the effects of radiation on cells and tissues, including cell killing, the induction of chromosome aberrations, mutation in somatic and germ cells, cell transformation and tumour induction. For tumour induction it is generally assumed that at sufficiently low doses α_1 will be constant and independent of dose rate. In practice, however, tumour induction has rarely been observed either in experimental animals or in epidemiological studies at acute doses of much less than 200 mGy.

334. The reduction in effect per unit dose observed at low doses and low dose rates, compared with effects at high doses and high dose rates, is termed a dose and dose-rate effectiveness factor (DDREF), although the terms dose-rate effectiveness factor (DREF), linear extrapolation overestimation factor (LEOF) and low-dose extrapolation factor (LDEF) have also been used. At sufficiently low doses, when cell killing can be disregarded, the DDREF can be defined from the previous equation as

$$DDREF = (\alpha_1 D + \alpha_2 D^2)/\alpha_1 D = 1 + (\alpha_2/\alpha_1)D \quad (31)$$

where D is the dose (in gray) at which the effect is measured.

335. In the absence of clear information on the shape of the dose-response curve for tumour induction at low doses, the initial slope, α_1, of the response at low doses can be determined, in principle, from exposures

at low dose rates. There are, however, limited data on dose-rate effects on tumour induction in human populations and no information on the mechanisms influencing tumour development from which quantitative estimates of dose-rate effects can be inferred. Animal studies and experiments on cell transformation and on somatic and germ cell mutation rates are therefore needed to provide insight into the likely effects of both dose and dose rate on tumour induction. Biophysical models of radiation action also provide an approach for understanding how the fundamental interactions of radiation with cells can play a part in dose-rate effects.

336. ***Models of radiation action.*** Guidance on expected effects at low doses and low dose rates can be sought from radiobiological and epidemiological data in terms of the quantitative models that have been developed to describe them. Radiobiological data for effects on single cells under a variety of conditions have led to the development of many quantitative models, mechanistic or phenomenological, for single radiation-induced changes in cells. Multi-stage models of radiation carcinogenesis, based on epidemiological or animal data, assume that one or more changes are required before a cell becomes malignant and that radiation can induce at least some of these changes (see Annex E, "Mechanisms of radiation oncogenesis"). The biophysical concepts underlying the different models are described in terms of general features of target theory, based on the insult of ionizing radiation always being in the form of finite numbers of discrete tracks. In this way fundamental expectation can be sought on the nature of overall dose responses, their dependence on dose rate and their features at the low doses of practical importance.

337. Dose-response relationships can be subdivided into regions. In *region I* a negligible proportion of cells are intersected by more than one track, and hence dose responses for single-stage effects can be confidently expected to be linear and independent of dose rate. In *region II* many tracks intersect each cell, but multi-track effects may not be observed in the experimental data, and hence independent single-track action is commonly assumed, although true linearity and dose-rate independence hinge on the validity of this assumption. In *region III* multi-track effects are clearly visible as non-linearity of dose response and hence dose-rate dependence is likely. The simpler forms of dose response can be expanded as a general polynomial, with only the dose and dose-squared terms being required to fit most experimental data, although sometimes a separate factor is added to account for competing effects of cell killing at higher doses. In this approach it is common to regard the fitted linear coefficient as being constant and fully representative of the response extrapolated down to minimally low dose and dose rate. However, the literature contains data from numerous studies that violate this simple expectation, for both low-LET and high-LET radiation. Many of these imply that multi-track effects can occur in the intermediate-dose region (II) and that even when the dose response appears linear it may exhibit dose-rate dependence and non-linearity at lower doses.

338. Low-dose and low-dose-rate expectations based on multi-stage processes of carcinogenesis depend crucially on the radiation dependence of the individual stages and on the tissue kinetics. Expectations could, in principle, readily range between two opposite extremes. On the one hand there could be the total absence of a linear term, implying vanishing risk as the dose tends to zero, as should be the case if two (or more) time-separated radiation steps were required. On the other hand, there could be a finite slope of the dose response down to zero dose, and this could even increase with decreasing dose rate, as may occur if either of the stages can occur spontaneously and if there is clonal expansion between them (see Annex E, "Mechanisms of radiation oncogenesis").

339. ***Life shortening in experimental animals.*** Radiation-induced life shortening in experimental animals following exposure to both low- and high-LET radiation at low to intermediate doses is mainly the result of an increase in tumour incidence. There is little suggestion that there is a general increase in other causes of death into the lethal range, although degenerative diseases in some tissues may be increased at higher doses. On this basis, life shortening can be used to assess the effect of dose fractionation and protraction on tumour induction.

340. The majority of comprehensive studies on the influence of fractionation of low-LET radiation on life-span have used the mouse as the experimental animal. The effect of fractionation appears to be very dependent on the strain of mouse and the spectrum of diseases contributing to the overall death rate. For example, in some strains thymic lymphoma incidence is increased by fractionation. Where this is a major contributor to the fatality rate, fractionation can lead to a greater loss of life expectancy than acute exposures. Overall there is no clear trend, and the results from a number of studies suggest that, when compared with acute exposures, the effects of fractionation on life-span shortening are small and, at least for exposure times of about a month, simple additivity of the injury from each dose increment can be assumed. For fractionation intervals over a longer time there is a tendency to a longer life-span with an increasing interval between the doses, but the increases in life-span observed are generally less than those found with protracted exposures.

341. When the effects in mice of acute exposures to low-LET radiation are compared with those of protracted irradiation given more or less continuously, the effectiveness of the radiation clearly decreases with decreasing dose rate and increasing time of exposure. With lifetime exposures there is some difficulty assessing the total dose contributing to the loss of life-span. However, the results available suggest that with protracted exposures over a few months to a year the effect on life-span shortening is reduced by factors between about 2 and 5 compared with acute exposures. The effect of dose rate on tumour induction and life-span shortening has also been examined in rats and beagle dogs, although no significant differences have been found. In these two studies dose rates varied by factors of 60 or less, whereas in the studies with mice they varied by factors of 100 or more.

342. A number of early studies suggested that fractionated exposures to high-LET radiation induced more life shortening than single exposures. More recent studies have shown, however, that when total doses are low and the dose per fraction is small, there is no significant difference in life shortening between fractionated and acute exposures. Although the data are limited, the available information suggests that protraction of exposure does not affect life shortening.

343. ***Tumour induction in experimental animals.*** A number of studies have been published that permit the effect of dose rate from low-LET radiation on tumour induction in experimental animals to be examined. The data that have been reported by various authors cover a wide range of dose-response patterns, and with different dose ranges, differing values of DDREF may be calculated. A wide range of DDREFs for tumour induction in different tissues has been found for dose rates generally varying by factors between about a hundred and a thousand or more. Some of the tumour types for which information is available have a human counterpart (myeloid leukaemia and tumours of the lung, the breast, the pituitary and the thyroid), although the tumours involved may not be strictly comparable to the human disease. Other types either have no human counterpart (Harderian gland) or require for their development substantial cell killing and/or changes in hormonal status (ovarian tumour, thymic lymphoma). In practice, the DDREFs found in these two groups are little different, falling in the range from about 1 to 10 or more, and there is no clear trend with tissue type.

344. Myeloid leukaemia has been induced in RFM and CBA mice, although there are differences in sensitivity between the strains and between the sexes. DDREFs between about 2 and more than 10 have been obtained, but with no consistent trend with changing dose rate. A reasonably consistent finding is that DDREFs for tumour induction in mammary tissue in rodents tend to be low, although even here one author has reported a substantial effect of dose fractionation on the tumour response in mice. DDREFs for lung tumour induction also tend to be low, with values falling in the range of about 2-4 following exposure to both external radiation at different dose rates and to inhaled insoluble radionuclides with different effective half-times in the lung. The results of the principal studies that have been reviewed are given in Table 8, together with the dose ranges over which the DDREFs have been estimated.

345. It has also been demonstrated that the effect of fractionation on tumour response depends on the dose per fraction. With small doses per fraction, which lie predominantly on the linear portion of the dose-response curve, the tumour response is similar to that obtained at low dose rates. At higher doses per fraction, the response approaches that obtained for single acute doses.

346. The main conclusion to be drawn from the results of the studies on radiation-induced life shortening and those on the induction of specific tumour types following exposure to low-LET radiation is that tumour induction is dependent on the dose rate, with a reduction in incidence at low dose rates. While the absolute value of the DDREF varies with the conditions of exposure, the animal strain and gender, tissue/tumour type and the dose range over which it is calculated, there is a consistent finding of a difference in tumour yield per unit dose for dose rates varying by factors of between about 100 and in excess of 1,000.

347. The animal studies also indicate that the presence of a dose-rate effect could not necessarily be inferred from dose-response relationships obtained at high dose rates alone, since for a number of studies the dose-response data for tumour induction up to a few gray could be adequately fitted by a linear function. This would imply the absence of a visible quadratic (i.e. multi-track) function in the dose response, which according to conventional interpretation would appear to be a prerequisite for an effect of dose rate on tumour yield. Clearly, when information is available only for exposures at high dose rates, any attempt to assess the effect at low doses and low dose rates, and hence a value of the DDREF, by simply fitting a linear-quadratic or similar function to the dose response is unlikely to be fully successful. The limiting factor is the amount of information available at low doses from which the linear term (α_1 of equation 30) can be accurately defined. For planning future animal studies it is clear that most information is likely to come from studies on animals exposed at different dose rates, rather than from attempting to obtain information on the risks at very low doses. It is

to be hoped that more studies will be carried out to supplement the information presently available.

348. From the limited and somewhat disparate data on high-LET radiation it is difficult to generalize. There is, however, little experimental support for applying a DDREF to high-dose or high-dose-rate exposures to calculate risks at low doses and dose rates. Similarly, there is little evidence to suggest that, in the absence of cell killing, there is an appreciable enhancement of tumour yield when the dose from high-LET radiation is protracted or fractionated.

349. *Cell transformation.* Cell transformation studies can yield information of practical use in radiation protection in addition to giving insight into the mechanisms of carcinogenesis. At present, however, the most quantitative data is derived from the least physiologically relevant cell systems, such as cultured embryo cells or the mouse fibroblast cell lines C3H10T½ and BALB/c3T3. Thus, when attempts are made to extrapolate to cancer induction in man, which occurs mainly in epithelial tissues (lung, gastrointestinal tract), the biological limitations of these assay systems must be considered. In addition there are a number of technical uncertainties that must be taken into account. These include the effects of cell cycle time, of plating density and of promoters and suppressors, some of which may be normal components of the growth medium, particularly the serum, and therefore difficult to control.

350. Nevertheless, in carefully controlled experiments where asynchronously dividing cells or, in some cases, non-dividing plateau-phase cells have been irradiated, the resulting observations on dose or dose-rate effects for low-LET radiation are in general agreement with those relating to other cellular effects, such as cell killing and the induction of mutations or chromosomal aberrations and to tumour induction in animals. Dose-response curves per cell at risk have a number of features in common with tumour induction *in vivo*, showing an initial rise in transformation frequency with increasing dose to a maximum and then a decline. When plotted as transformants per surviving cell, the dose response for low-LET radiation generally shows the expected linear or linear-quadratic relationship tailing off to a plateau at higher doses. When low doses of x rays or gamma rays are delivered at low dose rate or in fractionated intervals, a DDREF of between about 2 and 4 is obtained. Because of the limitations of the experimental system, the range of dose rates applied in experimental animals has not been used, with the maximum range being a factor of about 40. It is noteworthy that some experimental data suggest that the linear term may alter with dose rate, but this may be accounted for by the lack of precise data at low doses.

351. Exposures to high-LET radiation result in a higher transformation efficiency with a tendency towards a linear relationship, in line with data for chromosomal aberrations and again tending to a plateau at high doses. As expected from this pattern of response, there is no tendency for the response to decrease at low dose rates or with fractionation, and in practice, a number of studies have shown an enhanced effect. The main evidence for an "inverse" dose-rate effect with high-LET radiation seems to be limited to 5.9 MeV or fission spectrum neutrons, and over the past few years estimates of the magnitude of the increased effect have been reduced from factors of around 9 to about 2 or 3. Results reported from a number of laboratories have become reasonably consistent, and it has been possible to develop a model that can predict many experimental results.

352. The model is based on the assumption that the target in the cell, taken to be the nucleus, has a "window" in the cell cycle lasting about 1 hour during which it is more sensitive to radiation. With protracted or fractionated exposures there is a greater opportunity for this particular window to be hit by at least one track, and thus the possibility for an enhancement of transformation frequency with a reduction in dose rate. The magnitude of any effect will depend on the lineal energy, and with alpha-particle irradiation little enhancement would be expected, as is in fact observed. Although such a model appears to be consistent with much of the experimental data and has been tested in one series of studies, it is critically dependent on the target size and will need to be examined at different doses, dose rates and dose-fractionation schedules to fully examine its general applicability. Ultimately a full understanding of the inverse dose-rate effect must depend on experimental studies designed to understand the mechanistic basis of the observations.

353. Despite this possible explanation of the inverse dose-rate effect, there remains the problem that it is largely based on the results obtained with the C3H10T½ mouse-embryo-derived fibroblast cell line and may well have only limited application to human carcinogenesis. The development of epithelial cell systems that are of much more direct relevance to human cancer should be a research priority.

354. *Mutagenesis in somatic and germ cells.* Studies on somatic mutations *in vitro* and germ cell mutations *in vivo* are relevant to assessing the effect of dose and dose rate on the primary lesion in DNA involved in tumour initiation, although subsequent tumour expression will depend on the influence of many other factors. The results obtained in different studies on somatic cell mutations in mice have been somewhat variable, but the overall extent of the dose-rate effect

indicates a maximum value of about 2-3. A DDREF of about 3 for specific-locus mutations has been found in mouse spermatogonia for a dose rate of 8 mGy min^{-1} compared with a dose rate of about 900 mGy min^{-1}, although no further reduction in effect was obtained at lower dose rates down to 0.007 mGy min^{-1}, i.e. an overall range in dose rates in excess of a factor of 10^5. Based on these results, a DDREF of 3 for damage to spermatogonia has been applied by the Committee since the UNSCEAR 1972 Report [U5] when assessing risks of hereditary disease at low dose rates. For reciprocal translocations, DDREFs up to about 10 have been reported, although there appear to be considerable differences between species. Reciprocal translocations are, however, two-hit aberrations, and the yield will be very dependent on recovery processes between successive events. The marked differences in dose-rate effects between species may be the result of variable rates of repair. The DDREF in mature and maturing mouse oocytes is larger than that in spermatogonia, with the main difference being that the mutation rate continues to fall when the dose rate decreases below 8 mGy min^{-1}. Mouse oocytes present just before birth show a more pronounced dose-rate effect than mature or maturing oocytes, with a DDREF of about 14.

355. ***Epidemiology***. The human data that are available for assessing the effects of dose rate on tumour induction from low-LET radiation are limited. In general, the information available is from exposures at high dose rates, and little information is available at doses of less than about 0.2 Gy. Analyses of dose-response relationships for solid tumours in the atomic bomb survivors are generally consistent with linearity but also with a small reduction in the slope of the dose-response at lower doses. For leukaemia among the atomic bomb survivors, however, the data are inconsistent with linearity, and the central estimate of the DDREF at low doses is about 2. Model fits to the dose-response data for the atomic bomb survivors over the dose range 0-4 Gy kerma for all cancers combined, suggests a DDREF in the range of about 1.7 (when adjusted for random errors). For solid cancers alone, however, linearity provides a good fit, although the data are also consistent with a DDREF of the order of 2. This interpretation of the data depends on the assumption that a linear-quadratic model is appropriate for extrapolation to low doses and that the linear term can be adequately resolved. Information on thyroid cancer induction by acute external irradiation compared with low dose-rate exposure from intakes of ^{131}I are consistent with a DDREF of about 3, although there is some question over the contributions that heterogeneity of dose and uncertainties in the dose estimates as well as the effect of age make to the overall reduction in risk. For female breast cancer the information is conflicting. Dose-response relationships for acute exposures and for fractionated exposures at high dose rates are consistent with a linear dose-response relationship. However, comparative data from Nova Scotia and from other Canadian provinces suggest a DDREF greater than one may be appropriate for assessing cancer risks at low dose rates. Although epidemiological studies of low dose-rate exposure should be more relevant for the purposes of radiological protection than studies at high dose rates, the former type of study at present lacks sufficient statistical power to allow risks to be estimated with tight confidence limits. However, the results of studies such as those of radiation workers are consistent with low values of DDREF.

356. ***Dose criteria***. The designation of low doses and low dose rates below which it is appropriate to apply dose and dose-rate effectiveness factors (DDREFs) in assessing risks of human cancer resulting from radiation exposure have been considered by the Committee. A number of approaches based on physical, experimental and epidemiological data have been reviewed. It was concluded that for assessing the risks of cancer induction in man a DDREF should be applied either if the total dose is less than 200 mGy, whatever the dose rate, or if the dose rate is below 0.1 mGy min^{-1} (when averaged over about an hour), whatever the total dose.

357. ***Summary***. The dose-response information on cancer induction in the survivors of the atomic bombings in Japan provides no clear evidence for solid tumours for a DDREF much in excess of 1 for risk estimation at low doses and low dose rates of low-LET radiation. For leukaemia, the dose response fits a linear-quadratic relationship with a best estimate of the DDREF of about 2. There is only limited support for the use of a DDREF from other epidemiological studies of groups exposed at high dose rates, although for both thyroid cancer and female breast cancer some data suggest a DDREF of possibly 3 may be appropriate.

358. The results of studies in experimental animals conducted over a dose range that was similar, although generally somewhat higher, than the dose range to which the survivors of the atomic bombings in Japan were exposed, and at dose rates that varied by factors between about 100 and 1,000 or more, give DDREFs from about 1 to 10 or more with a central value of about 4. Some of the animal tumours have no counterpart in human cancer. Similar results to those obtained with animal tumour models have been obtained for transformation of cells in culture, although the DDREFs obtained have not been as large. In a number of these experimental studies linear functions would give a good fit to both the high- and low-dose-rate data in the range from low to intermediate doses. This indicates that if the cellular response can, in principle,

be fitted by a linear-quadratic dose response, in practice it is not always possible to resolve the common linear term for exposures at different dose rates.

359. If the human response is similar to that in experimental animals, then it can be envisaged that at lower dose rates than were experienced in Hiroshima and Nagasaki, a DDREF greater than that suggested by analysis of the dose-response data could be obtained. However, information from human populations exposed at low dose rates suggests risk coefficients that are not very different from those obtained for the atomic bomb survivors, although the risk estimates have wide confidence intervals. Taken together, the available data suggest that for tumour induction the DDREF adopted should, on cautious grounds, have a low value, probably no more than 3. Insufficient data are available to make recommendations for specific tissues.

360. For the purposes of applying DDREFs for assessing cancer risks in man, the Committee concluded either that dose rates less than 0.1 mGy min^{-1} (averaged over about an hour) or acute doses less than 200 mGy may be regarded as low.

361. For high-LET radiation, a DDREF of 1 is at present indicated on the basis that experimental data suggest little effect of dose rate or dose fractionation on tumour response at low to intermediate doses. It is noted that a DDREF of somewhat less than 1 is suggested by some studies, but the results are equivocal and cell killing may be a factor in the tissue response.

362. In the case of hereditary disease, the adoption of a DDREF of 3 is supported by experimental data in male mice, although a somewhat higher value has been found with one study in female mice.

Table 1
Summary of reduction factors for estimating cancer risk at low dose and low dose rates for low-LET radiation

Source		*Year*	*Reduction factor*	*Alternative conditions for applying a reduction factor*		*Ref.*
				Dose (Gy)	*Dose rate*	
Committee on the Biological Effects of Ionizing Radiation	BEIR III	1980	2.25	[a]	[a]	[C4]
	BEIR V	1990				[C1]
	Leukaemia		2	<0.1	[a]	
	Solid cancers		2-10	<0.1	[a]	
International Commission on Radiological Protection	ICRP	1977	2	[b]	[b]	[I1]
		1991	2	<0.2	<0.1 Gy h^{-1}	[I2]
National Council on Radiation Protection and Measurements (United States)	NCRP	1980	2-10	<0.2	<0.05 Gy y^{-1}	[N1]
National Radiological Protection Board (United Kingdom)	NRPB	1988	3	<0.1	<0.1 Gy d^{-1}	[S31]
		1993	2	<0.1	<0.1 mGy min^{-1}	[M36]
United Nations Scientific Committee on the Effects of Atomic Radiation	UNSCEAR	1977	2.5 [c]	[a]	[a]	[U4]
		1986	up to 5	<0.2	<0.05 mGy min^{-1}	[U2]
		1988	2-10	<0.2	<0.05 mGy min^{-1}	[U1]
United States Nuclear Regulatory Commission	NRC	1989	3.3	[a]	<0.05 Gy d^{-1}	[A6]
		1991	2	<0.2	<0.1 Gy h^{-1}	[A10]

[a] Not specified.
[b] For radiological protection purposes.
[c] Could be higher, as discussed in Annex G of the UNSCEAR 1977 Report [U4] (paragraphs 314 and 318).

Table 2
Ionization clusters produced directly in a DNA-related target by a single radiation track [a]
[G6, G21]

Radiation type	*Average number of ionizations [b] in*		
	DNA segment of length 2 nm	*Nucleosome*	*Chromatin segment of length 25 nm*
Gamma rays	1 (0 to >8)	2 (0 to >20)	2 (0 to >45)
Alpha particles	2 (0 to >15)	10 (0 to >90)	50 (0 to >200)

a A similar, or slightly larger, number of excitations are produced, in addition.
b Estimated range in parentheses.

Table 3
Damage products in a single-cell nucleus traversed by a single radiation track [a]
[G6, G21]

Radiation type	*Average number of ionizations*	*Average number of induced breaks [b]*		
		DNA single-strand breaks	*DNA double-strand breaks*	*Chromatin*
Gamma rays	70 (1-1500)	1 (0-20)	0.04 (0-few)	0.01 (0-few)
Alpha particles	23000 (1-100,000)	200 (0-400)	35 (0-100)	6 (0-20)

a Number of the breaks, based on linear extrapolation to low dose of a selection of experimental data, and the range estimated from the microdosimetric variation of single tracks.
b Estimated range in parentheses.

Table 4
Age at death of RF female mice exposed at 10 weeks of age to whole-body gamma-radiation
[W8]

Cause of death	*Dose (Gy)*	*Number of animals*	*Adjusted mean age at death (days) ± SE [a]*	*Difference from controls [b]*
All causes	0	232	577 ± 8	
	1	95	552 ± 13	$p < 0.02$
	3	92	473 ± 17	$p < 0.001$
All causes other than neoplastic	0	104	611 ± 10	
	1	29	650 ± 18	$p > 0.20$
	3	20	657 ± 30	$p > 0.30$

a Study terminated at 799 days of age.
b Data for controls from [U21].

Table 5
Effects of whole-body irradiation and dose fractionation on longevity in rodents and beagle dogs exposed to x rays or gamma rays [a]

Species	*Strain*	*Sex*	*Age (months)*	*Number of animals*	*Total dose (Gy)*	*Fractions*		*Dose rate*	*Longevity*	*Ref.*
						Number	*Spacing (days)*	*(Gy min⁻¹)*	*(months)*	
Rat	Wistar	Male	7.5	45	6	1	-	0.185	17.0	[H19]
				48	6	10	1	0.185	19.7	
				50	6	30	1	0.185	21.4	
				50	0	-	-	-	21.0	
		Female	3	14-16	4.8	6	3.5-14	0.55	21.3	[L16]
						3	3.5-14	0.55	19.3	
						1	-	0.55	19.2	
					2-4	6	3.5-14	0.55	24.8	
						3	3.5-14	0.55	21.9	
						1	-	0.55	21.4	
					1.2	6	3.5-14	0.55	25.9	
						3	3.5-14	0.55	23.9	
						1	-	0.55	25.1	
					0	-	-	-	28.6	
Mouse	RF	Male	1.3	104	1.5	1	-	0.9	15.6	[U28]
				82	1.5	2	2	0.9	16.3	
				77	1.5	2	6	039	16.5	
				314	0	-	-	-	19.1	
	RF	Male	1.3	105	4.5	1	-	0.9	10.3	[U28]
				71	4.5	3	2	0.9	10.8	
				99	4.5	3	5	0.9	11.1	
	LAF_1	Male	3.5	40	6.9	1	-	0.27	21.0 [b]	[C15]
				40	6.8	8	8	0.27	15.0 [b]	
				40	0	-	-		26.5 [b]	
Dog	Beagle	Female	10-12	129	1.0	2, 4	7, 14, 28	0.08	126	[A5]
				23		1	-	0.08	130	
				140	3.0	2, 4	7, 14, 28	0.08	110	
				11		1	-	0.08	125	
				57	0	-	-	-	139	

[a] Summary of early published results.
[b] Median value.

Table 6
Mean life-span and incidence of malignancies in C57Bl mice exposed at 3 months of age to single and fractionated doses of gamma radiation
[M20]

Parameter	*Dose (Gy)*	*Exposure pattern*		
		Single	*8 fractions at 3-hour intervals*	*10 fractions at 24-hour intervals*
Mean life-span (d ± SE)				
Survival	0	606 ± 29		
	0.25	578 ± 38		600 ± 60
	1	540 ± 36	611 ± 62	610 ± 59
	2	532 ± 38	561 ± 22	609 ± 59
	4	478 ± 43	545 ± 55	518 ± 51
Disease incidence (%)				
Thymoma	0	1.27		
	0.25	1.65		4.63
	1	0	1.89	0.86
	2	2.3	5.38	0
	4	13.29	7.83	23.7
All leukaemia	0	20.93		
	0.25	18.18		24.07
	1	15.04	20.75	24.14
	2	13.82	30.11	22.61
	4	26.57	32.17	35.59
Carcinomas and sarcomas	0	16.3		
	0.25	14.04		19.44
	1	8.94	26.42	18.1
	2	14.29	27.96	19.13
	4	16.08	24.39	20.34
All malignancies	0	33.19		
	0.25	28.51		39.81
	1	21.95	45.28	36.2
	2	26.37	51.61	36.52
	4	39.16	51.3	54.24

Table 7
Life shortening from single, fractionated and continuous gamma-ray exposure of mice
[T8]

Type of exposure	*Time pattern*	*Coefficient of life shortening (days lost per Gy)*	*Ref.*
Single		38.5 ± 2.9	[T10]
Fractionated	24 once per week	22.6 ± 2.2	[T10]
	60 once per week	17.5 ± 3.3	[T12]
Continuous	For 23 weeks	15.8 ± 2.2	[T8]
	For 59 weeks	7.7 ± 0.2	[T8]

Table 8
Dose and dose-rate effectiveness factors (DDREFs) for tumour induction by low-LET radiation in experimental animals

Effect	*Animal studied*	*Dose rate (mGy min^{-1})*		*DDREF*			*Ref.*
				Upper range of dose for evaluation (Gy)		*Value*	
		High	*Low*	*High dose rate*	*Low dose rate*		
Harderian gland tumours	RFM female mice	450	0.06	2	2	~3	[U12, U14, U15]
Lung adenocarcinomas	BALB/c female mice	400	0.06	2	2	2.8	[U12, U15]
	BALB/c female mice	350	0.06	2-3	2-3	3.2-4.2	[U6]
Lung cancer [a]	Beagle dogs					~3	[G10]
Mammary tumours	BALB/c mice	350	0.07	0.25	0.25	11.4	[U6]
	Sprague-Dawley rats	100	0.3	0.9	2.7	~1	[S15]
	Sprague-Dawley rats	10-30	0.02-0.14	1.8	2	1.6-1.7	[G7]
	BALB/c mice	450	0.06	2	0.5	1.9	[U12]
	WAG/RIJ rats	(2 Gy)	(2 Gy) [b]	2	2	~1	[B23]
Mammary adenocarcinomas	Sprague-Dawley rats	100	0.3	0.9	2.7	4	[S15]
Myeloid leukaemia	RFM male mice	800	0.04-0.6	1	3	5.1	[U21]
	CBA/H male mice	250	0.04-0.11	1.5-4.5	1.5-4.5	2.2-5	[M13]
	RFM/Un female mice	450	0.06	3	2	9.7-∞	[U15]
	RF female mice	67	0.004-0.7	3	6	~8	[U21]
Ovarian tumours	RFM female mice	450	0.06	2	2	~5.5	[U15]
	BALB/c female mice	400	0.06	2	2	6.7	[U15]
Pituitary tumours	BALB/c mice	450	0.06	3	2	~6	[U14, U15]
Skin tumours	LBA/H female mice	[c]	[c]	6	6	~2	[H30]
Thymic lymphoma	RFM female mice	450	0.06	2	2	5.8	[U12, U15]
	RFM male mice	800	0.04-0.6	4	4	2.6	[U21]
Thyroid tumours [d]	CBA mice	(15 Gy)	(64-160 Gy)	15	64-160	2-10	[W2]
	Long Evans rats	2800	(0.8-8.5 Gy)	0.94-10.6	0.8-8.5	~1	[L4]
	Rats	(11 Gy)	(100 Gy)	11	100	~10	[D4]
Total tumours	Sprague-Dawley male rats	1.3	0.022	2.8	3	~3	[M43]

[a] High dose rate from ^{91}Y; low dose rate from ^{144}Ce or ^{90}Sr.
[b] Ten fractions of 0.2 Gy each.
[c] ^{204}Tl source (fractionated exposure).
[d] High dose rate from x rays; low dose rate from ^{131}I.

Table 9
Tumour incidence in mice and evaluation of dose and dose-rate effectiveness factors (DDREF) for exposure to gamma-radiation
[E8]

High dose rate		*Low dose rate*		*DDREF*			
Dose range (Gy)	*Incidence, α_H (% per Gy) ±1 SE*	*Dose range (Gy)*	*Incidence, α_L (% per Gy) ±1 SE*	*Upper range of dose for evaluation (Gy)*		*Value* [a]	*±1 SE* [b]
				High dose rate	*Low dose rate*		
Myeloid leukaemia (RF male mice) [U21]							
0-1	14.4 ± 3.2	0-3.08	2.8 ± 0.8				
0-1.5	17.4 ± 2.1	0-3.29	2.6 ± 0.7	1	3.08	5.1	3.8-7.0
0-3	14.3 ± 1.7	0-6.21	0.87 ± 0.53				
Myeloid leukaemia (RF female mice) [U21]							
0-3	6.8 ± 2.0	0-3.1	0.99 ± 0.47				
0-5	3.7 ± 1.2	0-5.8	1.04 ± 0.38	3	5.8	6.5	4.5-9.6
		0-6.14	0.71 ± 0.31	3	6.14	9.6	6.3-15
Pituitary tumours (RFM female mice) [U15]							
0-2	2.2 ± 0.8	0-2	0.48 ± 0.70	2	2	4.6	1.8-11.5
0-3	3.9 ± 0.7			3	2	8.1	3.3-20
Harderian gland tumours (RFM female mice) [U15]							
0-1	3.8 ± 1.2	0-1	1.5 ± 0.9				
0-1.5	3.3 ± 0.9	0-2	1.5 ± 0.5	1.5	2	2.2	1.5-3.1
0-2	5.7 ± 1.2						
0-3	5.4 ± 0.7			2	2	3.8	2.7-5.3
Ovarian tumours (RFM female mice) [U15]							
0-0.5	42 ± 22	0-1	1.7 ± 3.5	0.5	2	6.8	3.7-12
0-1	36 ± 9	0-2	6.2 ± 3.9	1	2	5.8	3.5-9.7
0-2	25.6 ± 5.4			2	2	4.1	2.5-6.9
Thymic lymphoma (RFM female mice) [U15]							
0-2	16.7 ± 1.8	0-2	2.9 ± 1.9	2	2	5.8	3.5-9.6

[a] Based on linear fit over dose range specified for evaluation (i.e. α_H/α_L).
[b] Estimated from the fractional standard errors in the acute and chronic incidences.

Table 10
Calculations of DDREF allowing for uncertainties in the dose-response for gamma-radiation at high and low dose rates
[E8]

Effect	*Animal*	*Upper range of dose for evaluation (Gy)*		*DDREF* [a]	*±1 SE*	*Ref.*
		High dose rate	*Low dose rate*			
Myeloid leukaemia	Male mice	1	3.08	5.6	3.8-8.1	[U21]
Myeloid leukaemia	Female mice	3	6.14	11.4	6.3-20	[U21]
Pituitary tumours	Female mice	3	2	25	3-∞	[U15]
Harderian gland tumours	Female mice	2	2	4.2	2.7-6.3	[U15]
Ovarian tumours	Female mice	1	2	8	3.5-18	[U15]

[a] Based on $\alpha_H/\alpha_L\ (1 + \sigma^2L/\alpha^2L)$ of Table 9.

Table 11
Acute myeloid leukaemia in male CBA/H mice exposed to gamma radiation
[M13]

Total dose (Gy)	*Acute exposure* [a]		*Chronic exposure* [b]		*DDREF*
	Number of mice	*Leukaemia (%)*	*Number of mice* [c]	*Leukaemia (%)*	
1.5	99	11	143 (72/71)	5	2.2
3.0	83	17	131 (65/66)	6	2.8
4.5	105	25	131 (65/66)	5	5

[a] Dose rate 0.25 Gy min^{-1}.
[b] Dose rate 0.25 Gy min^{-1} in 20 fractions, 5 days weekly for 4 weeks; or 0.04-0.11 mGy min^{-1} for 28 days continuously.
[c] Two groups of mice used with numbers in parentheses.

Table 12
Lung adenocarcinoma incidence in BALB/c mice exposed to single, fractionated and protracted gamma radiation
[U26]

Group	*Total dose (Gy)*	*Exposure regimen*	*Dose rate (Gy min^{-1})*	*Observed incidence (%)* [a]	*Expected incidence (%)* [b]
1	2	High dose rate	0.35	38.6 ± 5.4	37.3
2	2	Low dose rate	0.083[d]	21.4 ± 2.6	21
3	2	0.1 Gy per fraction	0.35	21.3 ± 3.3	21
4	2	0.5 Gy per fraction	0.35	27.9 ± 4.5	25
5	2	1 Gy per fraction [c]	0.35	30.3 ± 6.4	29
6	2	1 Gy per fraction [c]	0.35	32.9 ± 6.8	29

[a] Incidence ± SE.
[b] Expected incidence based on $I = 11.9 + 4D + 4.3D^2$ (D in Gy).
[c] Two fractions separated by one day (Group 5) and 30 days (Group 6).
[d] 0.083 Gy d^{-1} (0.06 mGy min^{-1}).

Table 13
Lung adenocarcinoma incidence in BALB/c mice estimated from model fits to experimental data for gamma-radiation exposure
[U26]

Dose (Gy)	*Tumour incidence (%)*				*DDREF*
	High dose rate (0.35 Gy min^{-1})		*Low dose rate (0.1 Gy per fraction)*		
	Total	*Excess* [a]	*Total*	*Excess* [a]	
0.1	12.34	0.44	12.30	0.40	1.1
0.2	12.87	0.97	12.70	0.80	1.2
0.3	13.49	1.59	13.10	1.20	1.3
0.5	14.98	3.07	13.90	2.00	1.5
0.93	19.34	7.44	15.60	3.72	2.0
1	20.20	8.30	15.90	4.00	2.1
2	37.1	25.20	19.90	8.00	3.2
3	62.6	50.70	23.90	12.00	4.2

[a] Expected incidence based on $I = 11.9 + 4D + 4.3D^2$ (D in Gy).

Table 14
Mammary adenocarcinoma incidence in BALB/c mice exposed to single, fractionated and protracted gamma radiation
[U26]

Group	*Total dose (Gy)*	*Exposure regimen*	*Dose rate (Gy min^{-1})*	*Observed incidence* [a] *(%)*	*Expected incidence* [b] *(%)*
1	0.1	High dose rate	0.35	9 ± 3.2 [c]	9.6
2	0.2	High dose rate	0.35	15 ± 4.8	14.4
3	0.25	High dose rate	0.35	20 ± 4.6	18.0
4	0.25	Low dose rate	0.1 [c]	7.9 ± 2.1	8.5
5	0.25	0.01 Gy daily fractions	0.05	7.5 ± 2.3	8.5
6	0.25	0.05 Gy daily fractions	0.05	17 ± 4.1	18.3

[a] Incidence ± SE.
[b] Expected incidence based on $I = 7.7 + 3.5D + 150D^2$ (D in Gy).
[c] 0.1 Gy d^{-1} (0.07 mGy min^{-1}).

Table 15
Mammary adenocarcinoma incidence in BALB/c mice estimated from model fits to experimental data for gamma-radiation exposure
[U26]

Dose (Gy)	*Tumour incidence (%)*				*DDREF*
	High dose rate (0.35 Gy min^{-1})		*Low dose rate (0.1 Gy per fraction)*		
	Total	*Excess* [a]	*Total*	*Excess* [a]	
0.05	8.27	0.57	7.89	0.19	3
0.1	9.55	0.85	8.05	0.35	5.3
0.15	11.60	3.9	8.23	0.53	7.4
0.2	14.40	6.7	8.40	0.70	9.6
0.25	17.96	10.26	8.58	0.88	11.7

[a] Expected incidence based on $I = 7.7 + 3.5D + 150D^2$ (D in Gy).

Table 16
Specific-locus mutations in adult spermatogonia of mice exposed to x- or gamma-radiation [L17]

Exposure conditions	*Total dose (Gy)*	*Dose rate ($mGy\ min^{-1}$)*	*Frequency per locus*
^{60}Co gamma rays, 12 fractions weekly	6.15	0.6	$6.26\ 10^{-5}$
^{60}Co gamma rays, 60 fractions daily	6.26	170	$4.17\ 10^{-5}$
X rays, 12 fractions weekly	6.15	600-700	$12.61\ 10^{-5}$
^{60}Co gamma rays, acute	6.36	170	$13.07\ 10^{-5}$
^{60}Co gamma rays, acute	6.70	720	$15.39\ 10^{-5}$
^{60}Co gamma rays, chronic (90 days)	6.18	0.08	$3.15\ 10^{-5}$

Table 17
Proportions of a cell population traversed by tracks at various levels of track density

Mean tracks per cell	*Percentage of cells in population suffering*						*Percentage of hit cells with only 1 track*
	0 tracks	*1 track*	*2 tracks*	*3 tracks*	*4 tracks*	*>5 tracks*	
0.1	90.5	9	0.5	0.015	-	-	95.1
0.2	81.9	16.4	1.6	0.10	-	-	90.3
0.5	60.7	30.3	7.6	1.3	0.2	-	77.1
1	36.8	36.8	18.4	6.1	1.5	0.4	58.2
2	13.5	27.1	27.1	18.0	9.0	5.3	31.3
5 [a]	0.7	3.4	8.4	14.0	17.5	56.0	3.4
10 [a]	0.005	0.05	0.2	0.8	1.9	97.1	0.05

[a] At these values appreciable proportions of the cell population will incur more than 5 tracks.

Table 18
Alternative criteria for upper limits of low dose and low dose rate for assessing risks of cancer induction in man (for low-LET radiation)

Method of estimation	*Low dose (mGy)*	*Low dose rate ($mGy\ min^{-1}$)*
UNSCEAR 1986 Report [U2]	200	0.05
This Annex	200	0.1 [a]
Linear term dominant in parametric fits to single-cell dose responses	20 - 40	
Microdosimetric evaluation of minimal multi-track coincidences in cell nucleus	0.2	10^{-8} (lifetime) 10^{-3} (DNA repair)
Observed dose-rate effects in animal carcinogenesis		0.06
Epidemiological studies of survivors of the atomic bombings in Japan	200	

[a] Averaged over about an hour.

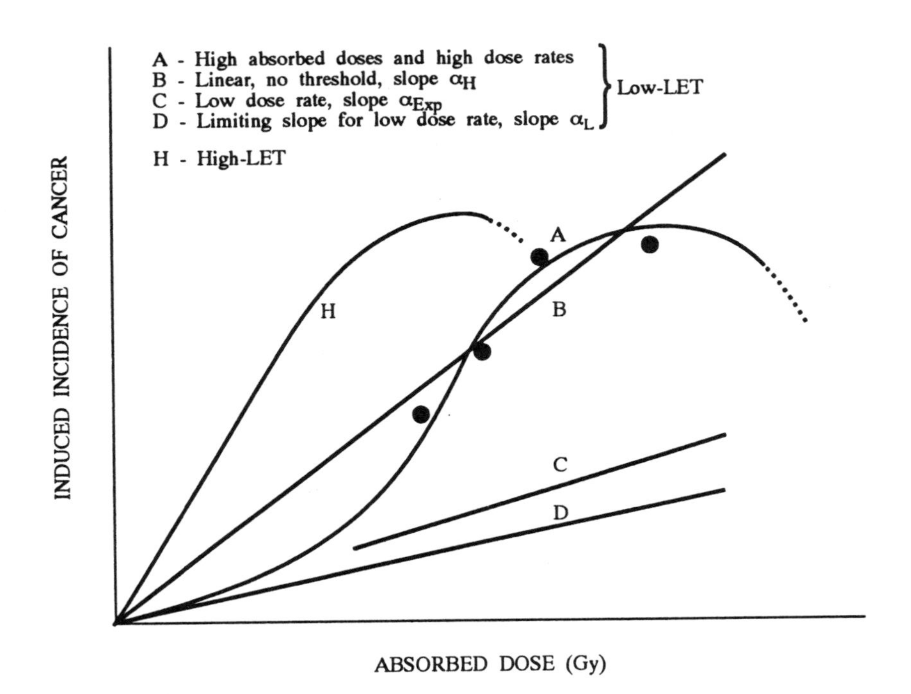

Figure I.
Dose-response relationship for radiation-induced cancer.
Possible inferences are illustrated in extrapolating data available at high doses and high dose rates to response at low doses and dose rates for low-LET radiation.
[N1]

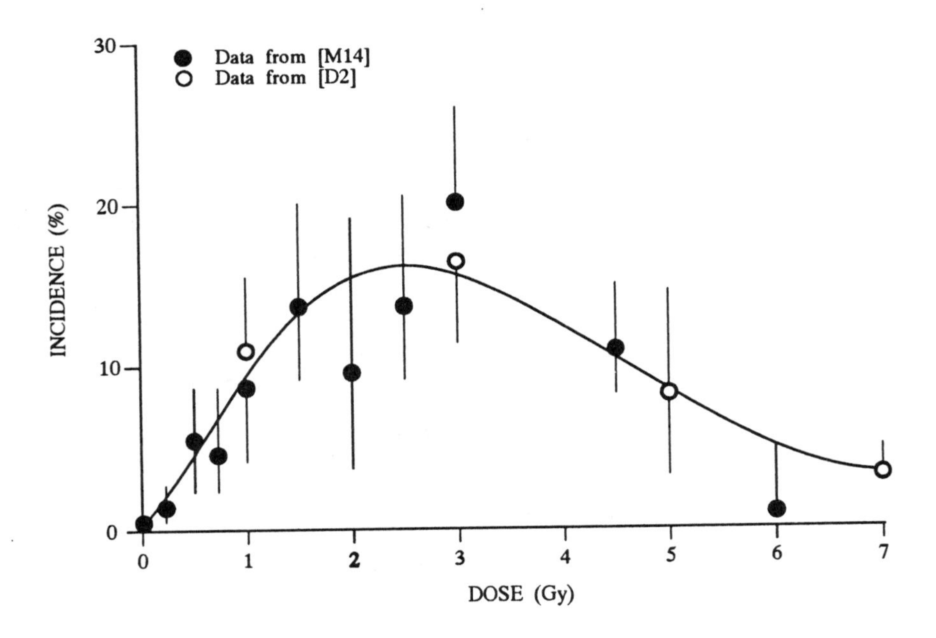

Figure II.
Incidence of myeloid leukaemia in male CBA/H mice following brief exposures to x rays.
[D2, M14]

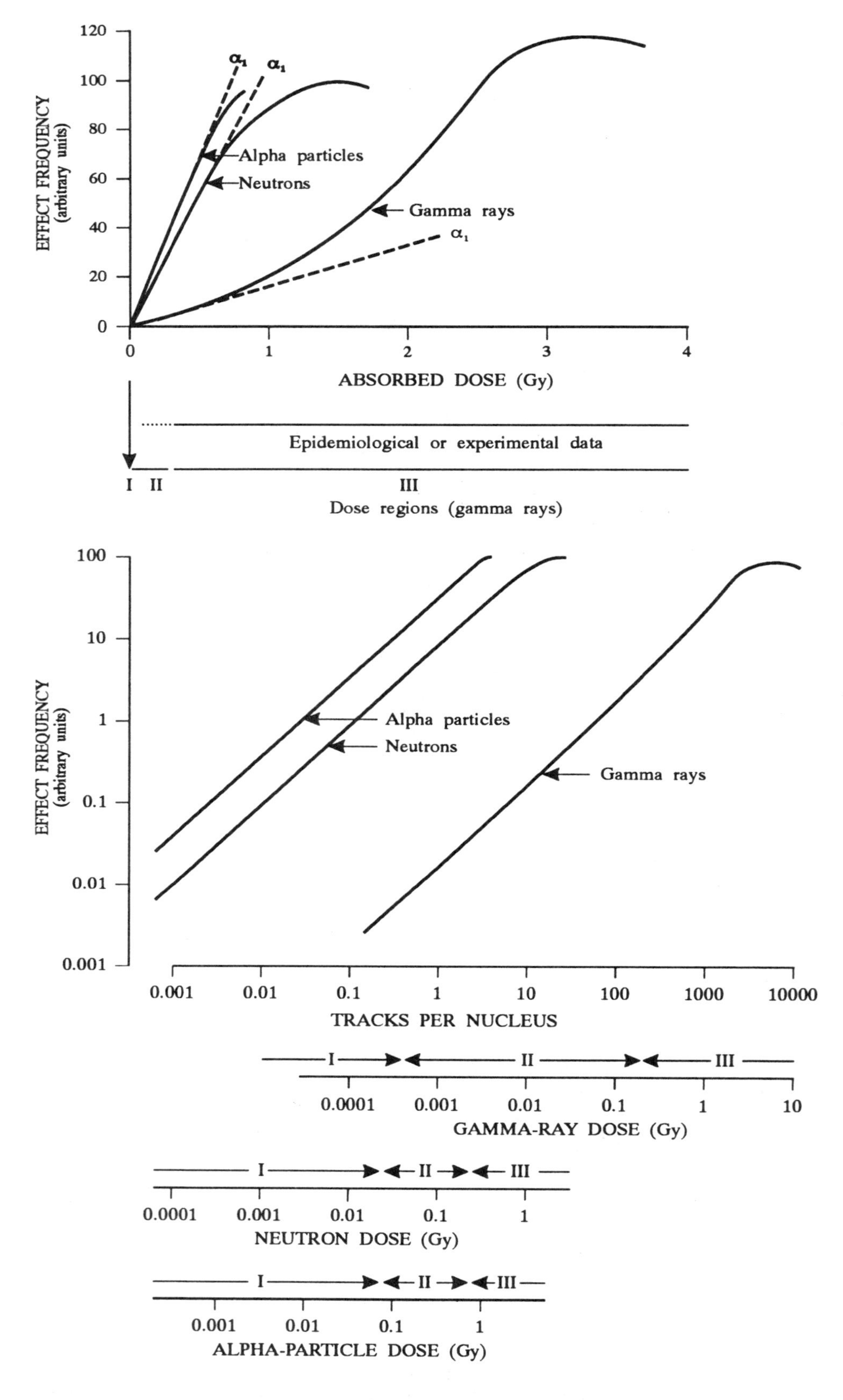

Figure III.
Schematic dose-response relationships for induction of stochastic biological effects by high-LET (slow neutrons and alpha particles) and low-LET (gamma rays) radiation on linear (upper plot) and logarithmic (lower plot) scales.
These example curves do not reflect all types of observed response, and in some *in vivo* systems alpha particles may be less effective than neutrons.
[C25, G5]

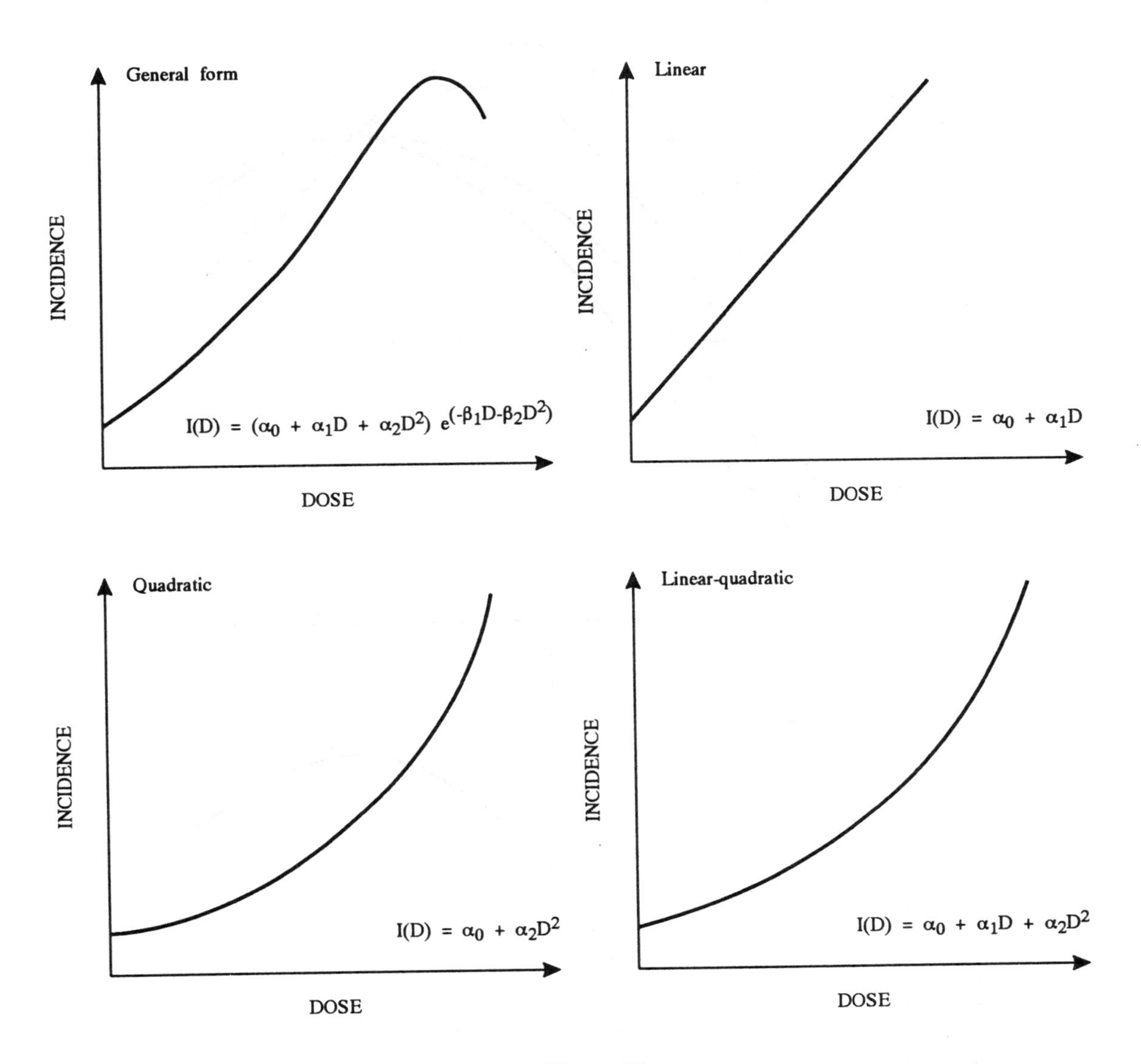

Figure IV.
Various shapes of dose-response curves for tumour induction.
[U2]

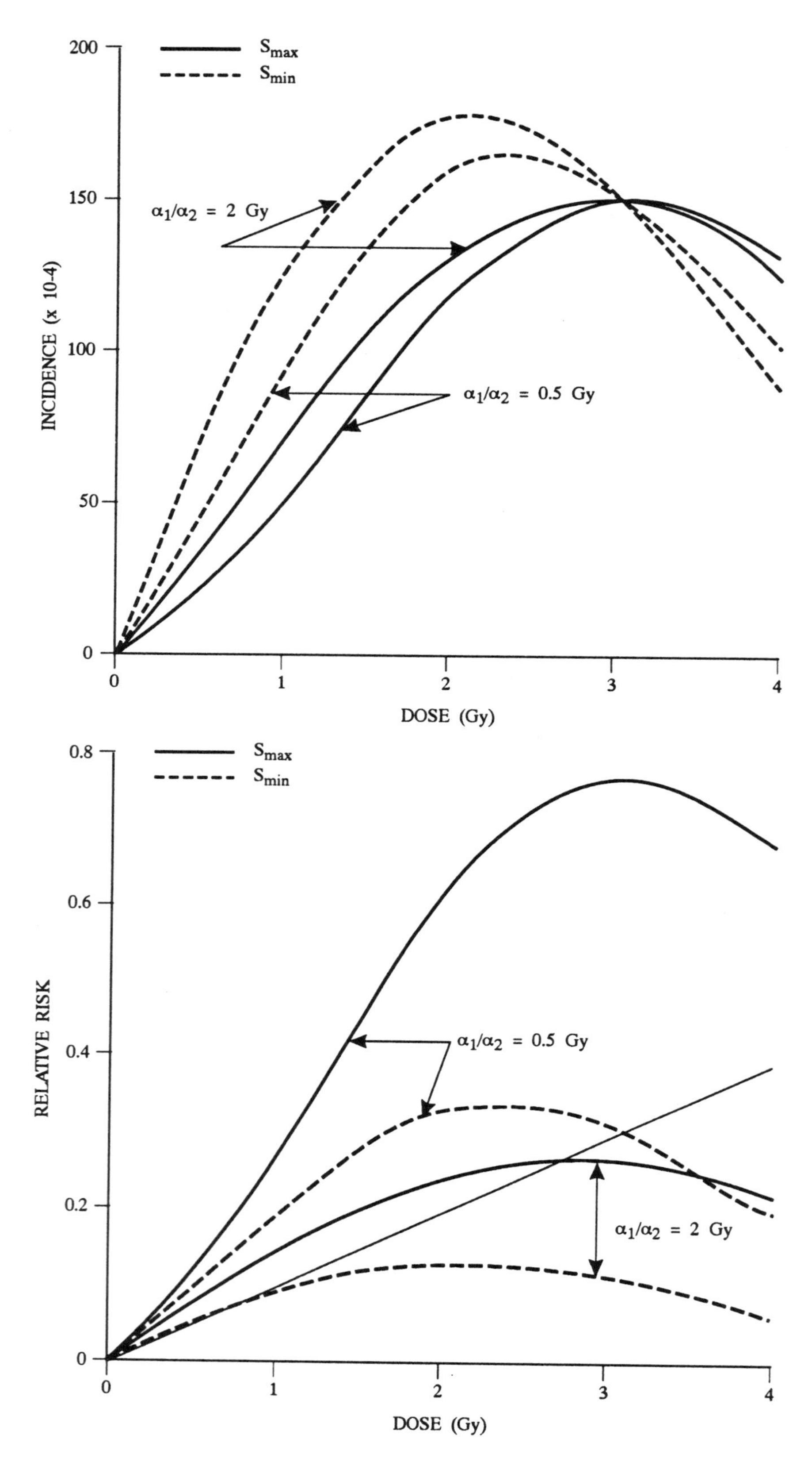

Figure V.
Expected cumulative incidence of radiation-induced cancer according to a linear-quadratic model with cell killing. Cell survival functions S_{max} defined by β_1 = 0.1 Gy^{-1} and β_2 = 0.08 Gy^{-2}, S_{min} defined by β_1 = 0.4 Gy^{-1} and β_2 = 0.08 Gy^{-2}. Incidence (upper plot) normalized to 150 10^{-4} at 3 Gy. Relative risk (lower plot) with normalization to the same value of α_1. [U2]

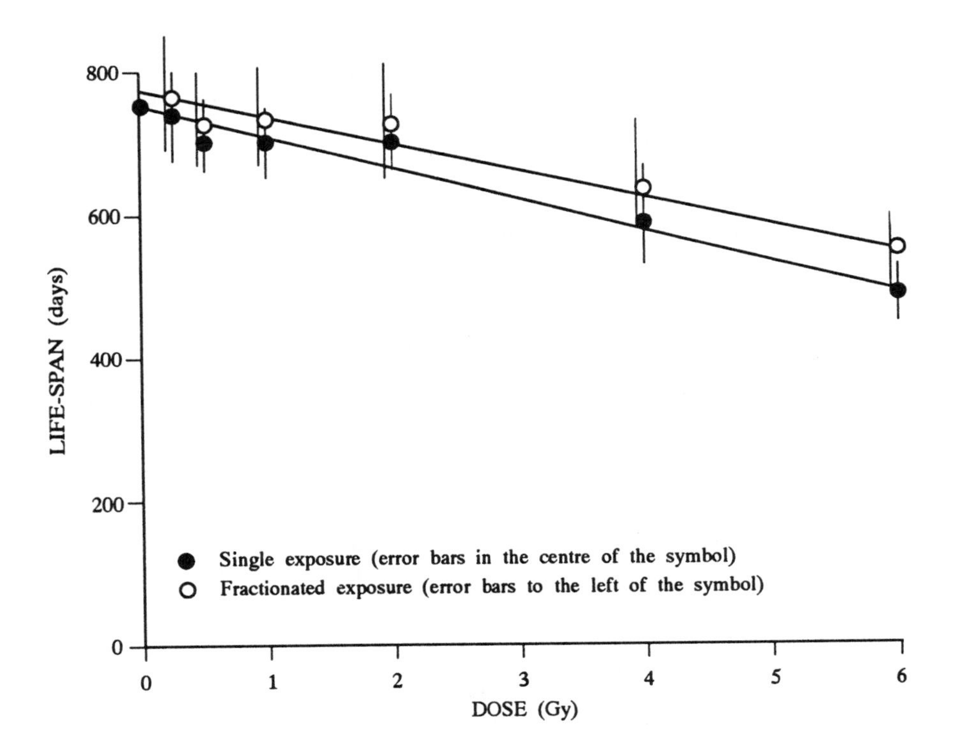

Figure VI.
Life-span reduction in male BALB/c mice following exposure to single or fractionated doses of ^{137}Cs gamma rays.
[M5]

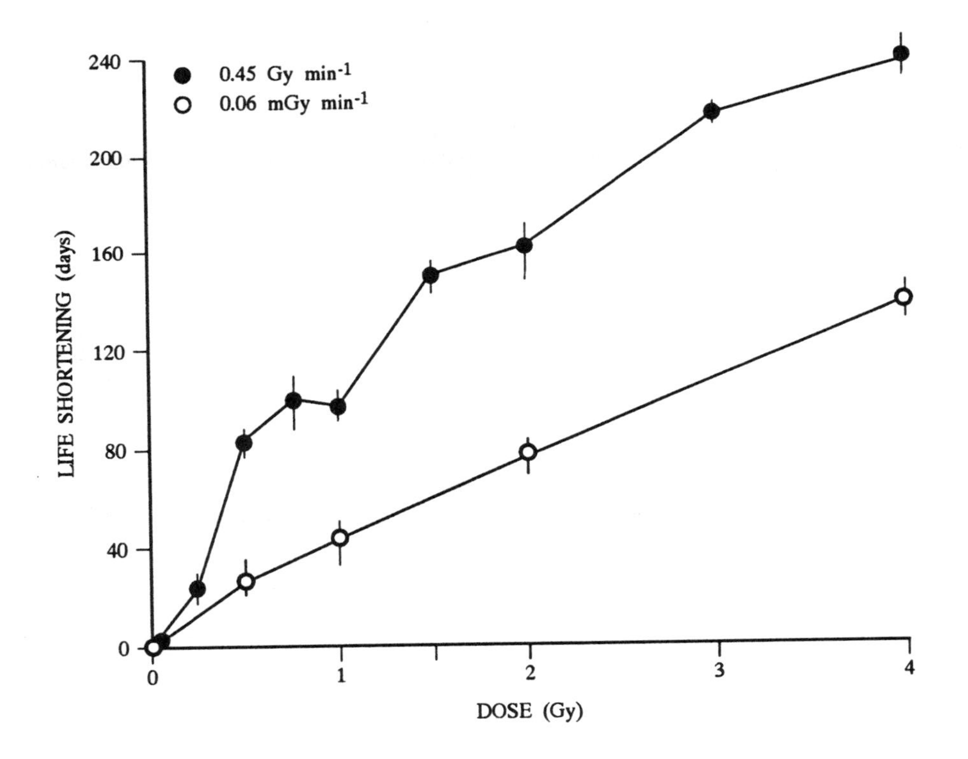

Figure VII.
Life shortening in female RFM mice following exposure to ^{137}Cs gamma rays at high and intermediate dose rates.
[S13]

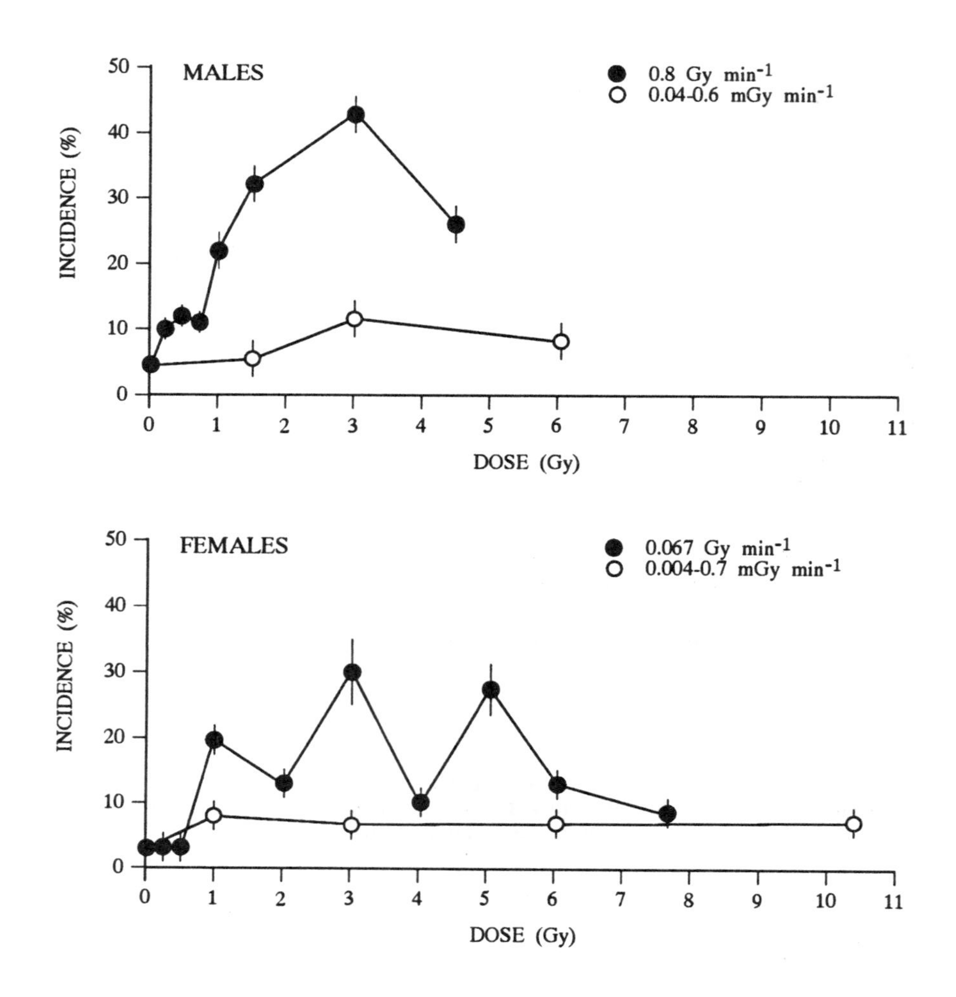

Figure VIII.
Myeloid leukaemia incidence in RF mice following exposure to x rays at high and intermediate dose rates. [U12]

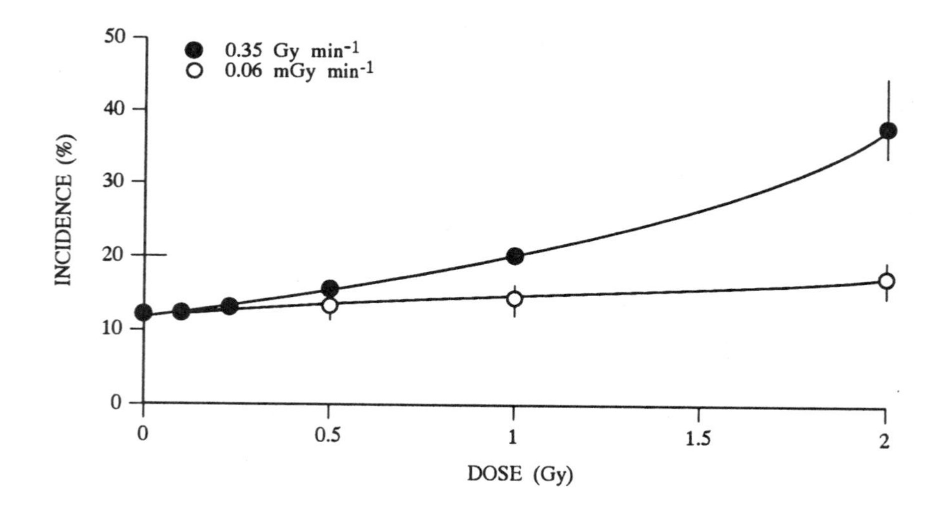

Figure IX.
Lung adenocarcinoma incidence in female BALB/c mice (age-adjusted) following exposure to ^{137}Cs gamma rays at high and intermediate dose rates. [U15, U26]

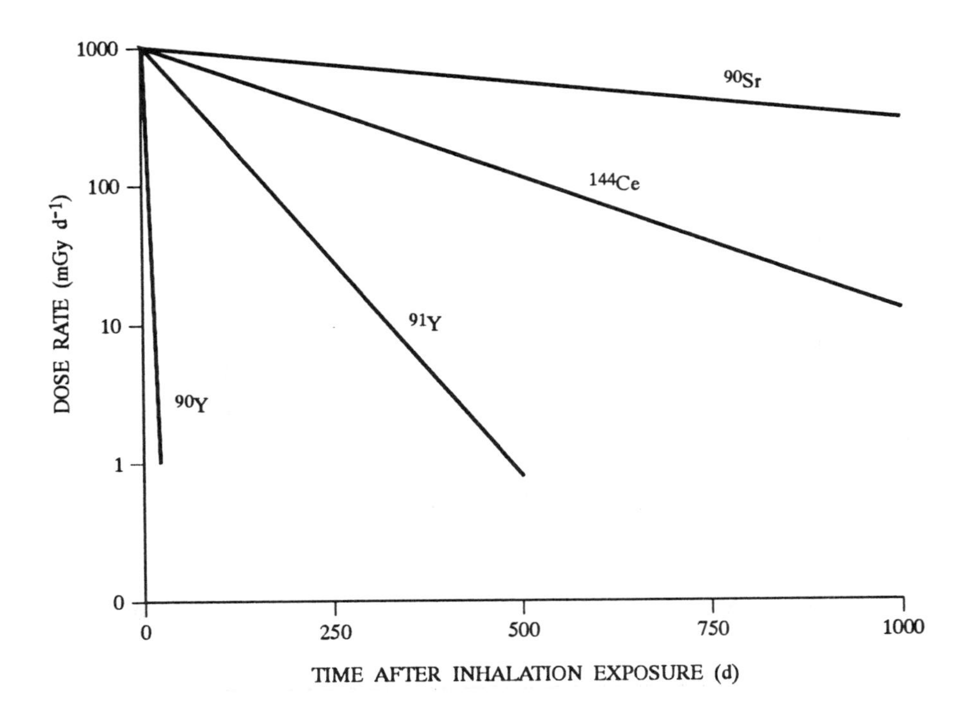

Figure X.
Theoretical beta-radiation dose rates to lungs of beagle dogs for various inhaled radionuclides incorporated in fused aluminosilicate particles. The dose rates have been normalized to an initial dose rate of 1 Gy d^{-1}. [M1]

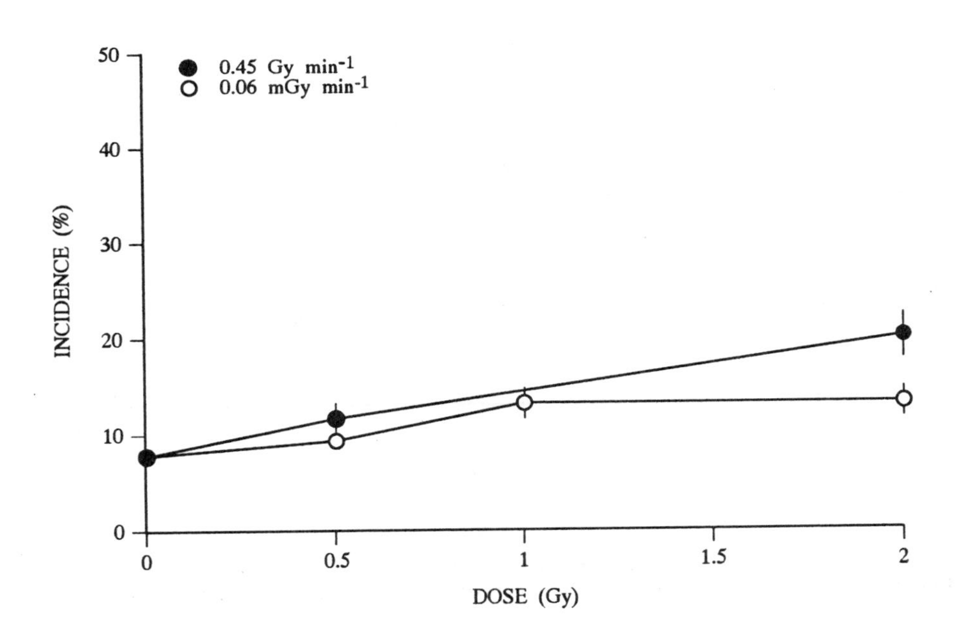

Figure XI.
Mammary tumour incidence in female BALB/c mice (age-adjusted) following exposure to ^{137}Cs gamma rays at high and intermediate dose rates. [U15]

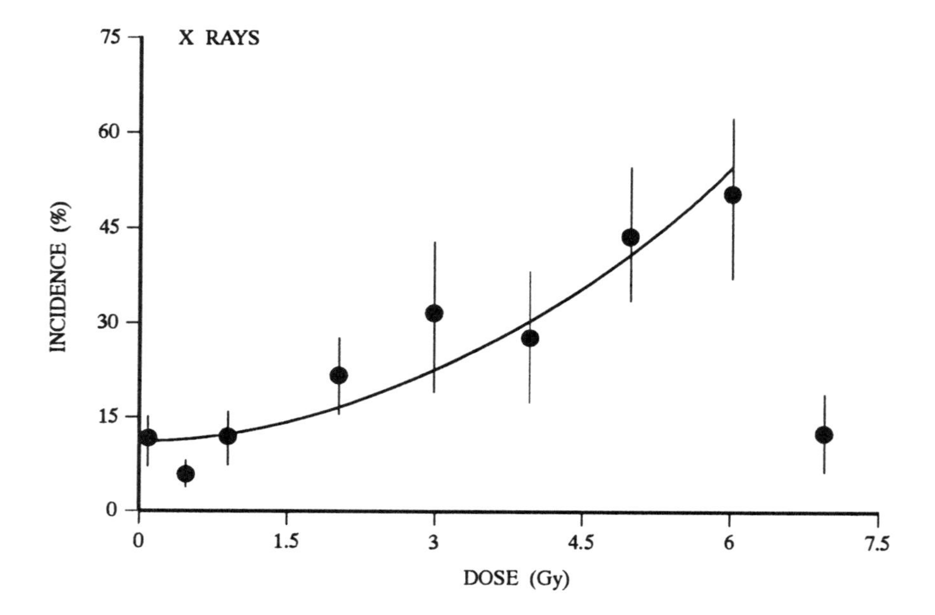

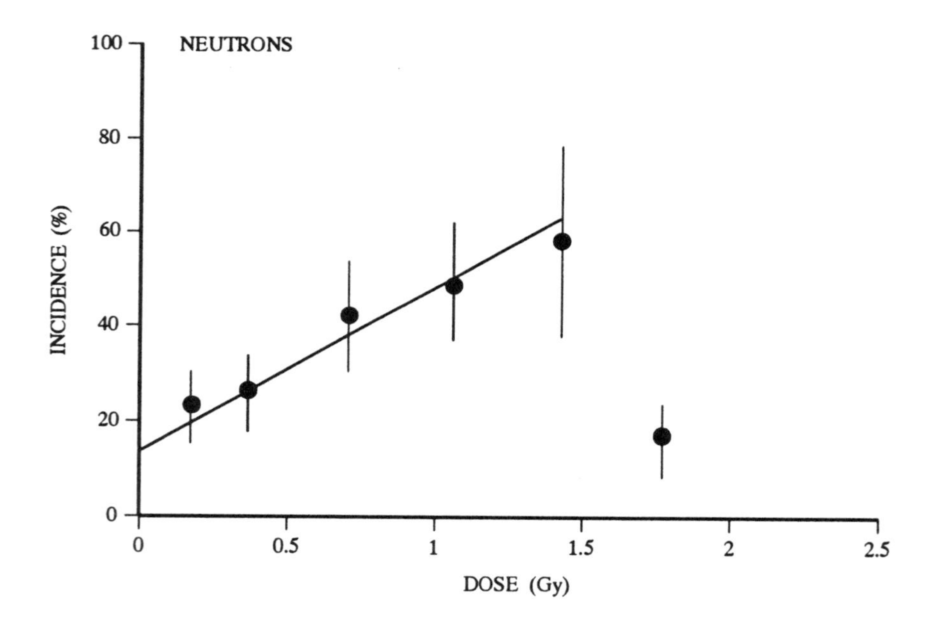

Figure XII.
Incidence of liver tumours in 3-month-old $BC3F_1$ male mice (age-adjusted) following exposure to 250 kVp x rays (upper plot) and fission neutrons (lower plot). **[D3]**

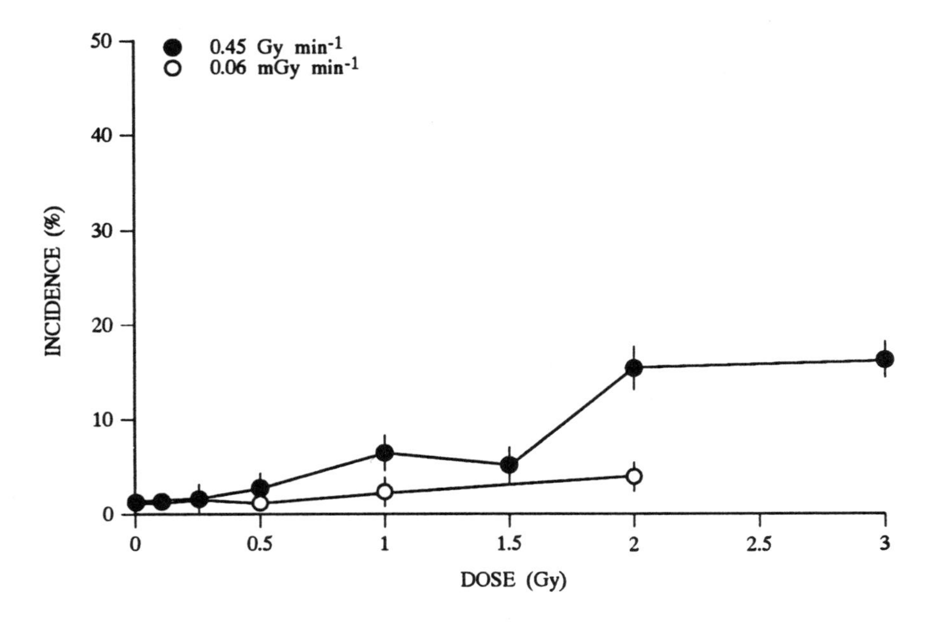

Figure XIII.
Harderian gland tumour incidence in female RFM mice (age-adjusted) following exposure to ^{137}Cs gamma rays at high and intermediate dose rates.
[U12]

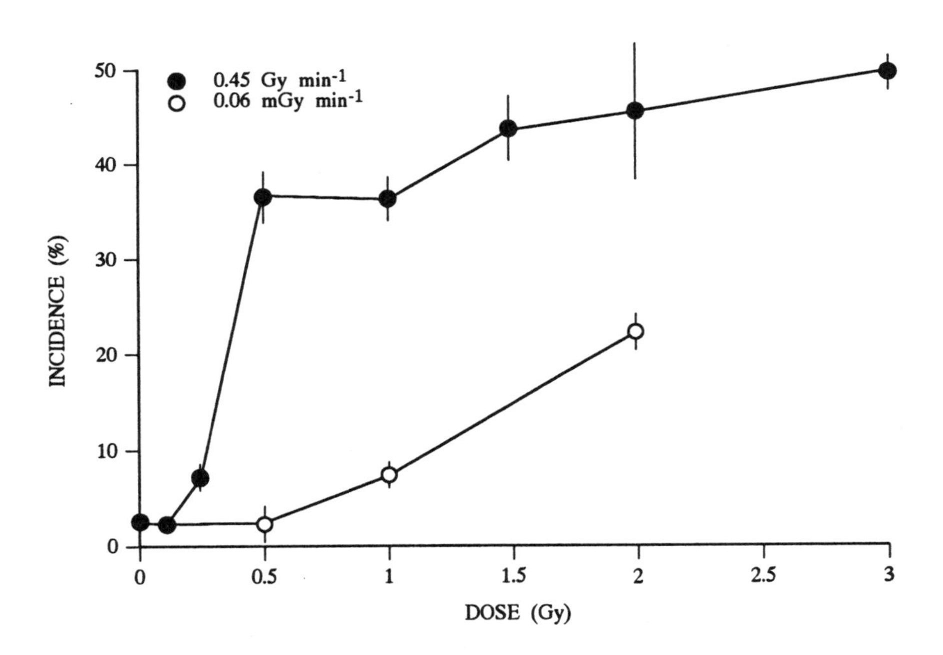

Figure XIV.
Ovarian tumour incidence in female RFM mice (age-adjusted) following exposure to ^{137}Cs gamma rays at high and intermediate dose rates.
[U12]

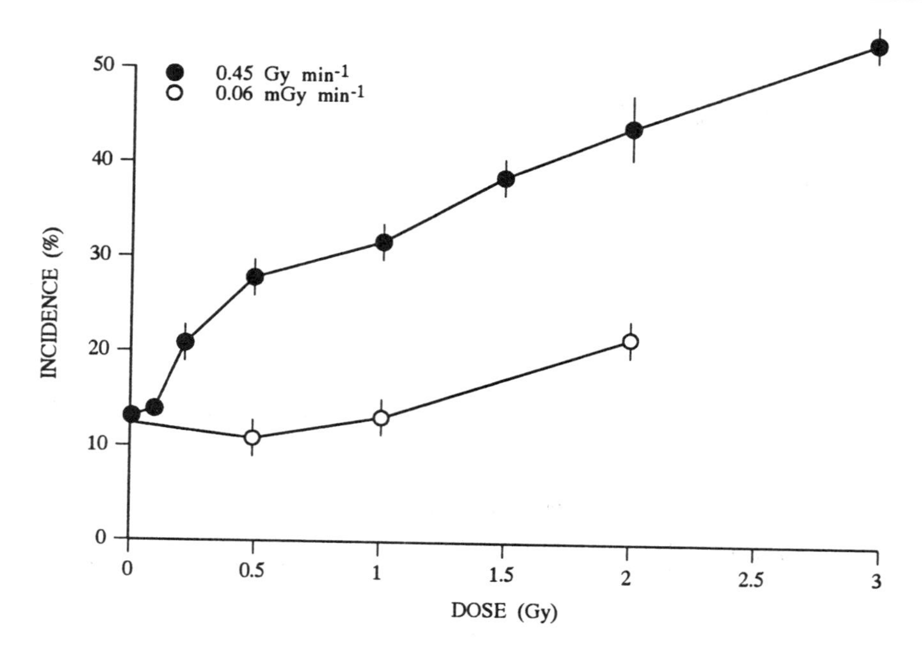

Figure XV.
Thymic lymphoma incidence in female RFM mice (age-adjusted) following exposure to ^{137}Cs gamma rays at high and intermediate dose rates. [U12]

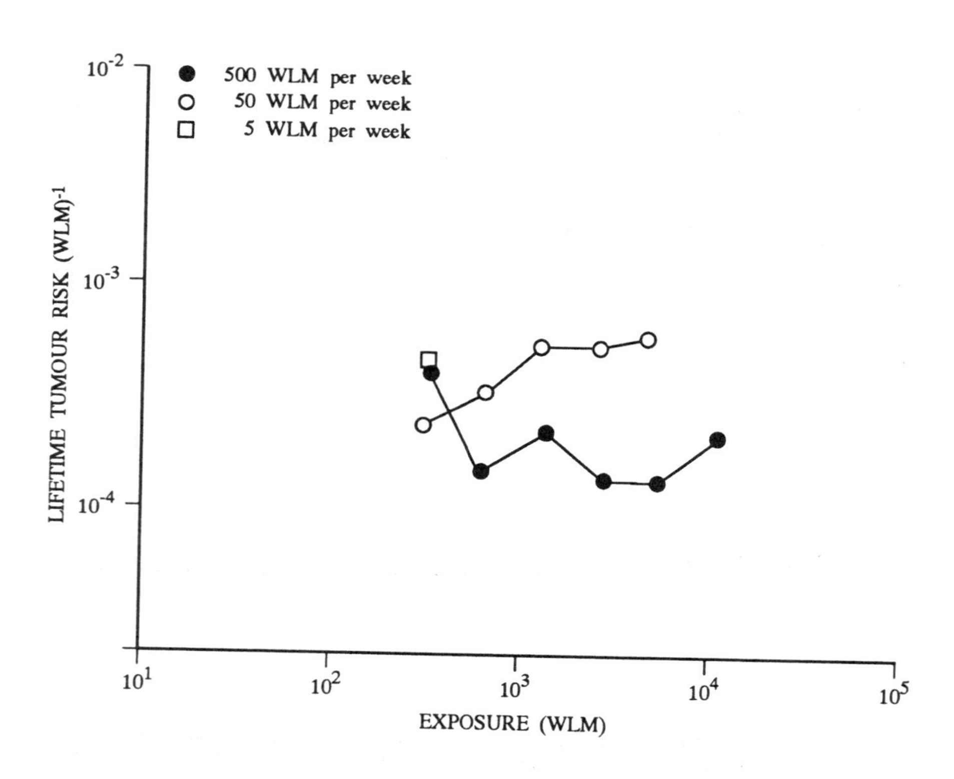

Figure XVI.
Lifetime risk coefficients for tumour induction in rats exposed to radon at various exposure rates. [C3]

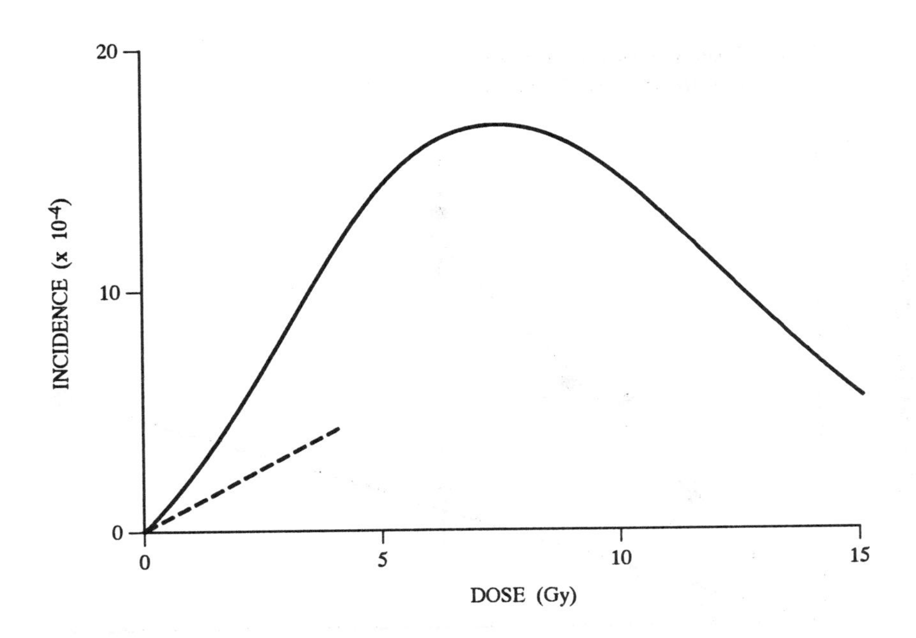

Figure XVII.
General characteristics of incidence of cell transformation per plated cell induced by low-LET radiation. Parameters α_1 = 10^{-4} Gy^{-1}, α_2 = 10^{-4} Gy^{-2}, β_1 = 10^{-1} Gy^{-1} and β_2 = 10^{-2} Gy^{-2} have been selected to illustrate the importance of linear and quadratic terms in the induction of transformations and of cell reproductive death. The broken line represents the initial slope, determined by α_1.
[B9]

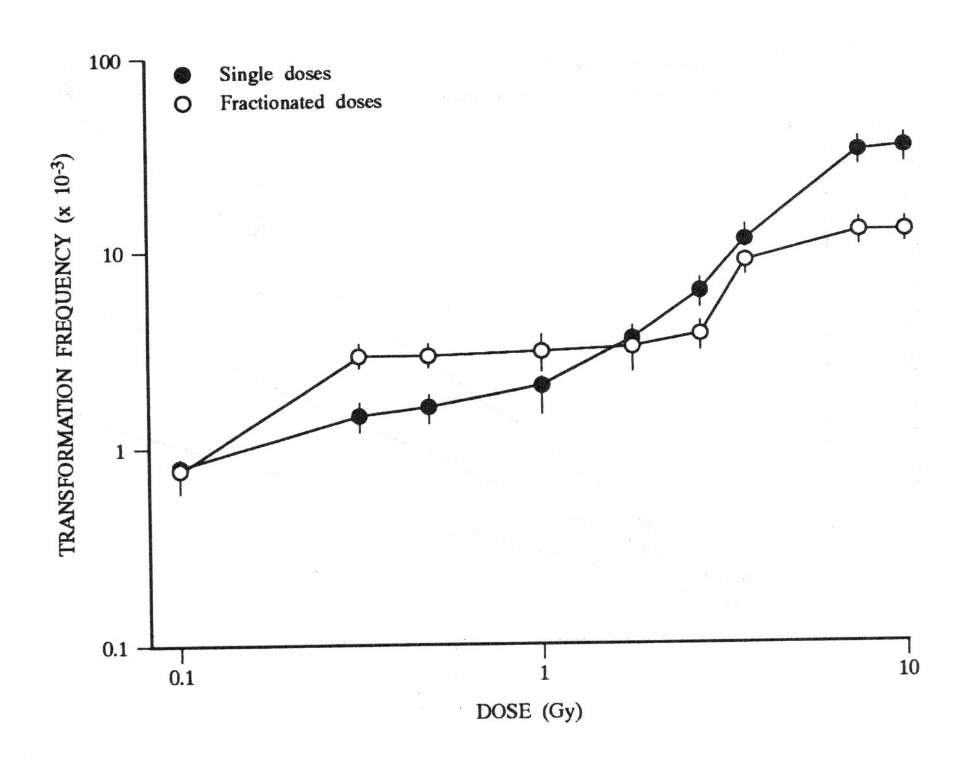

Figure XVIII.
Transformation frequency in C3H10T½ cells following exposure to single or fractionated doses of x rays before the establishment of asynchronous growth of cells.
In the case of fractionated doses, the radiation was delivered in two equal exposures separated by five hours.
[M8]

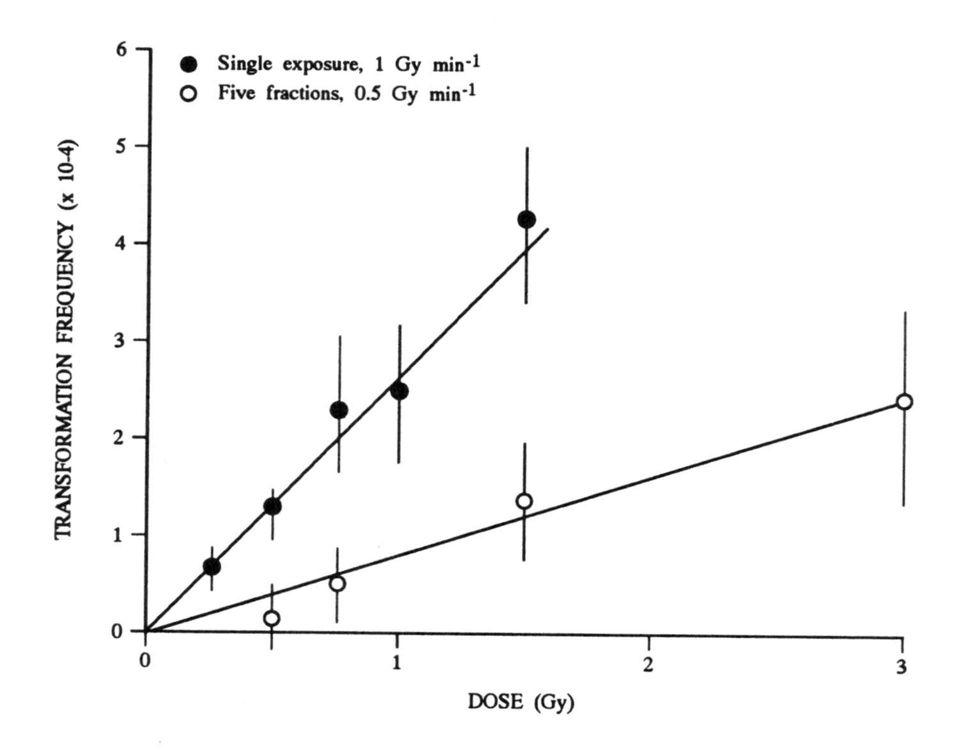

Figure XIX.
Transformation frequency in C3H10T½ cells following exposure to single or fractionated doses of ^{60}Co gamma rays. [H5, H6]

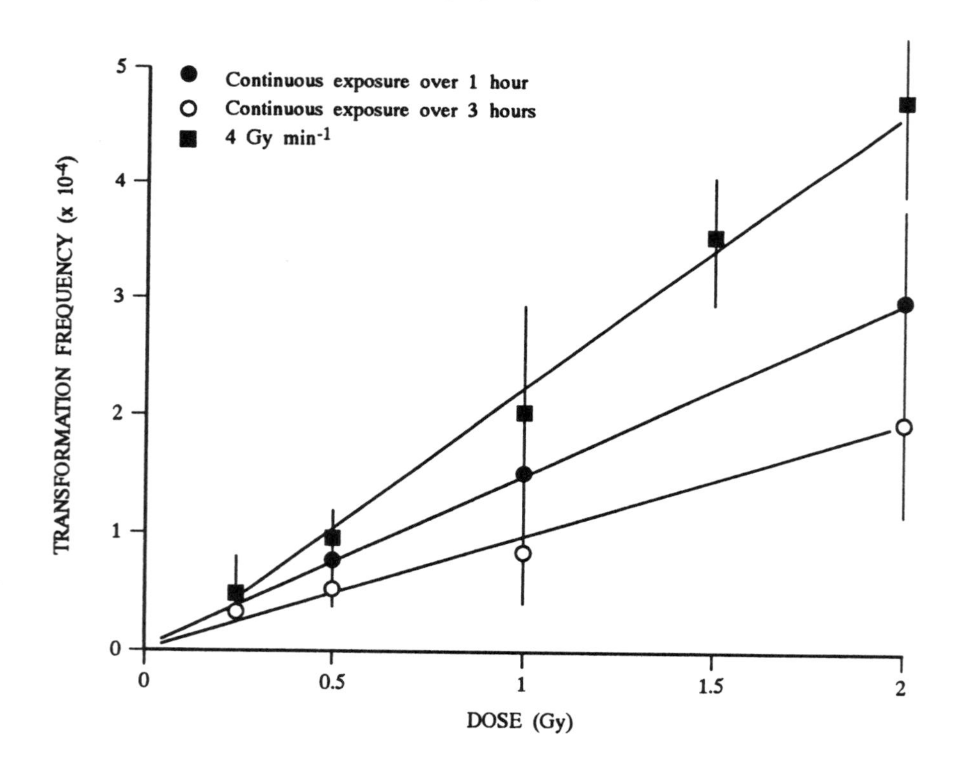

Figure XX.
Transformation frequency in C3H10T½ cells following exposure to single or protracted doses of x rays. Lines are fits to the data with a linear dose-response function. [B1]

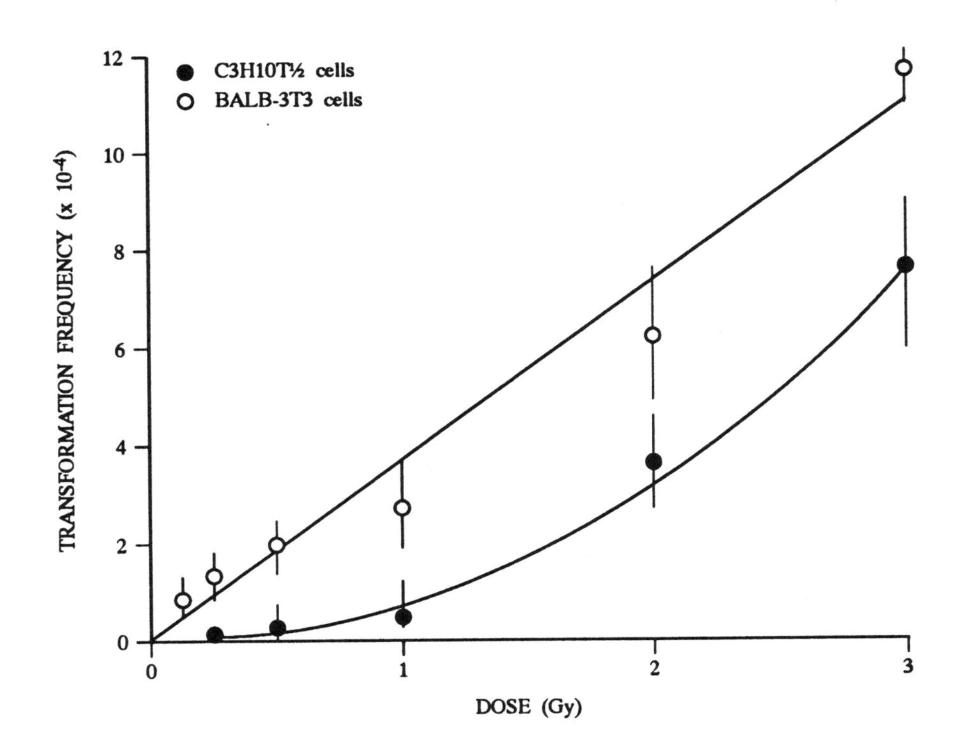

Figure XXI.
Transformation frequency in C3H10T½ and BALB-3T3 cells following exposure to single doses of x rays.
[L11]

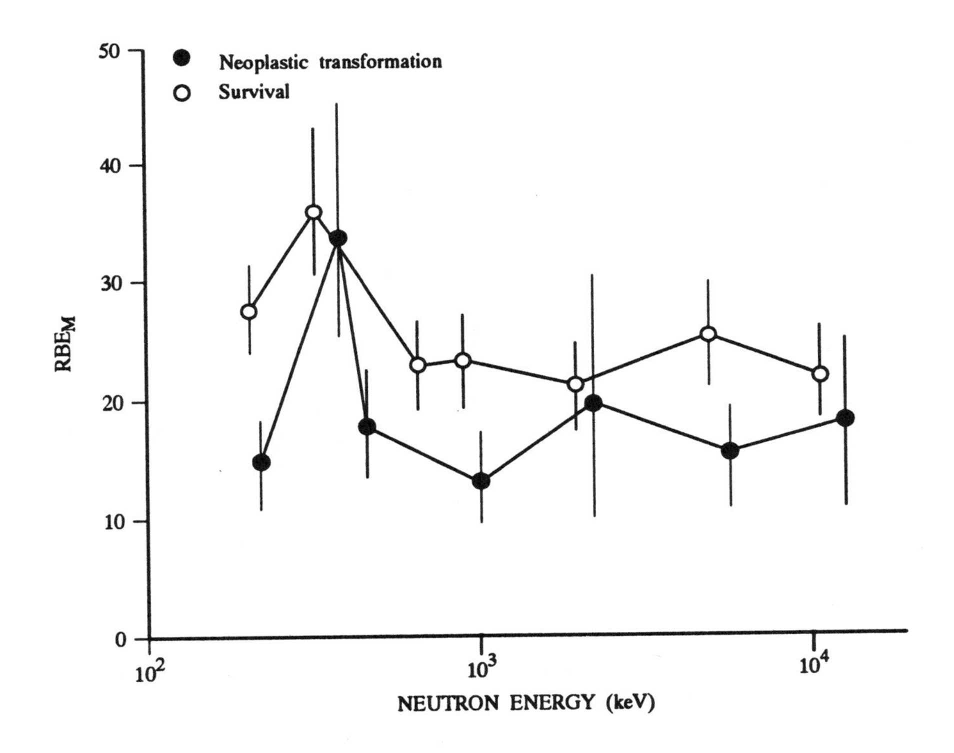

Figure XXII.
Maximal relative biological effectiveness (RBE_M) for survival and neoplastic transformation as a function of monoenergetic neutron energy. RBE_M represents the ratio of the initial slopes of the dose-response curves (α_n/α_x) for each energy.
[M46]

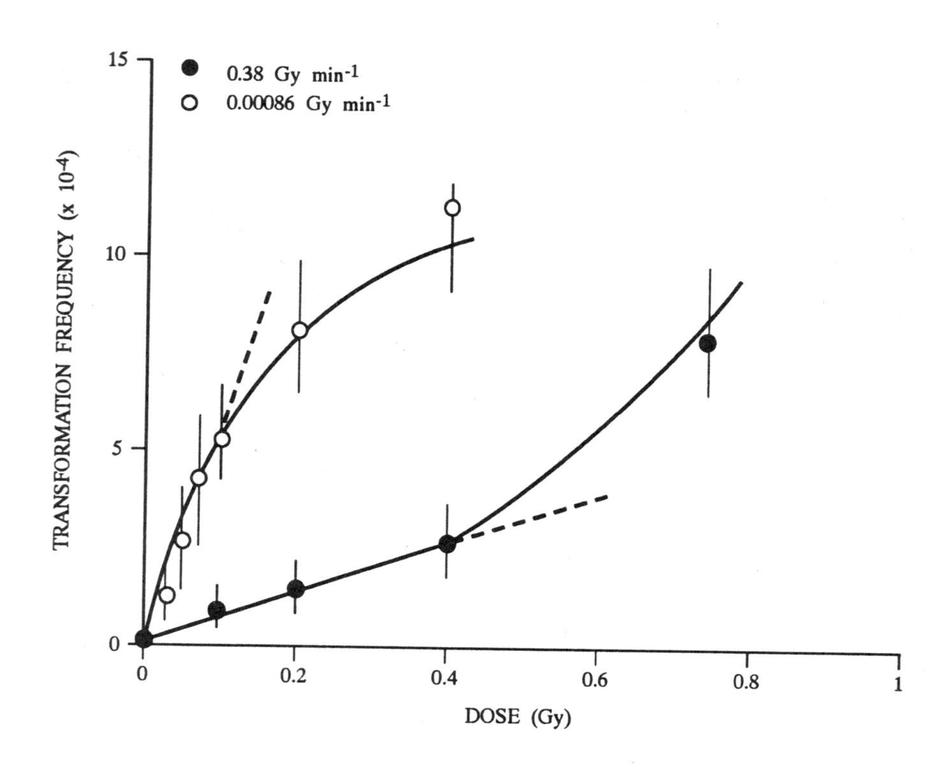

Figure XXIII.
Transformation frequency in C3H10T½ cells exposed to fission spectrum neutrons at high and low dose rates. Broken lines indicate the linear regressions fitted to the initial portions of the curves.
[H11]

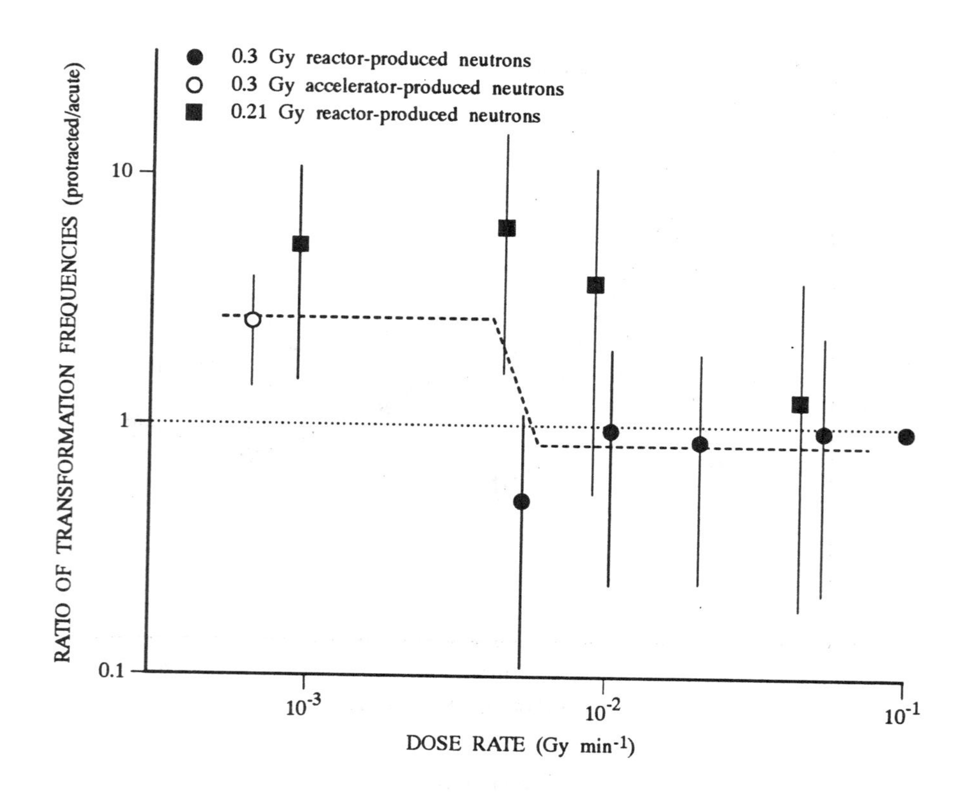

Figure XXIV.
Inverse dose-rate effect in C3H10T½ cells irradiated with fission spectrum and 5.9 MeV neutrons.
[M12]

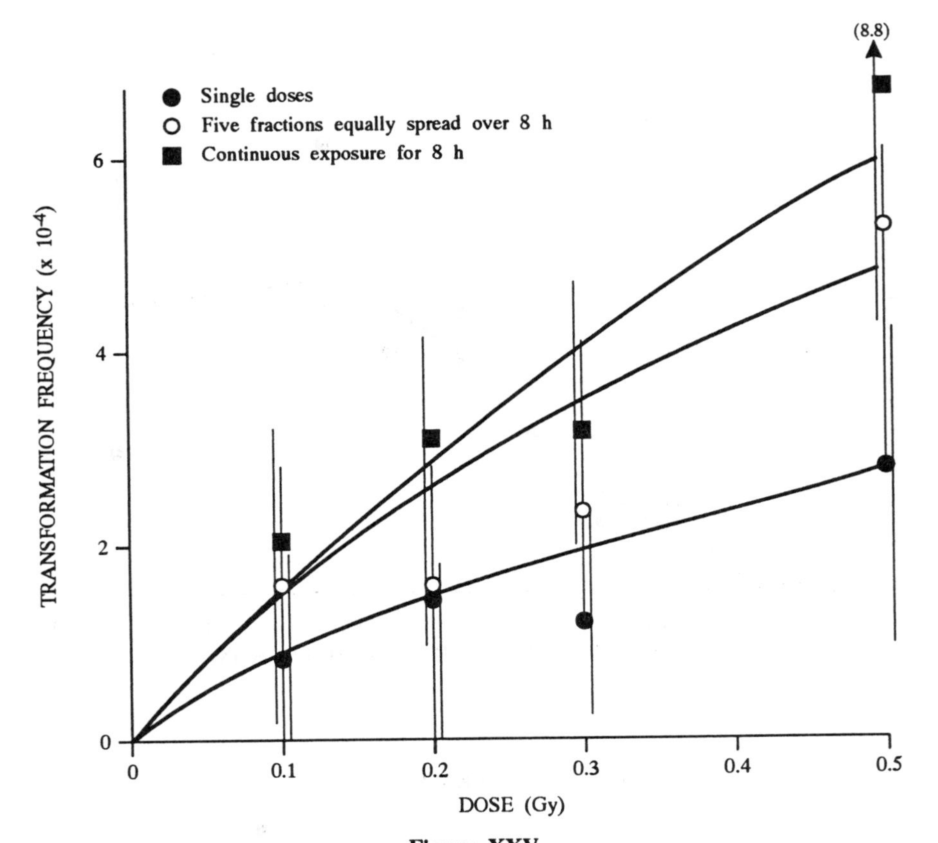

Figure XXV.
Transformation frequency in C3H10T½ cells following exposure to single, fractionated or continued dosesof 5.9 MeV neutrons. The equations and parameters of the fitted curves are given in paragraphs 259 and 260. [B30, M28]

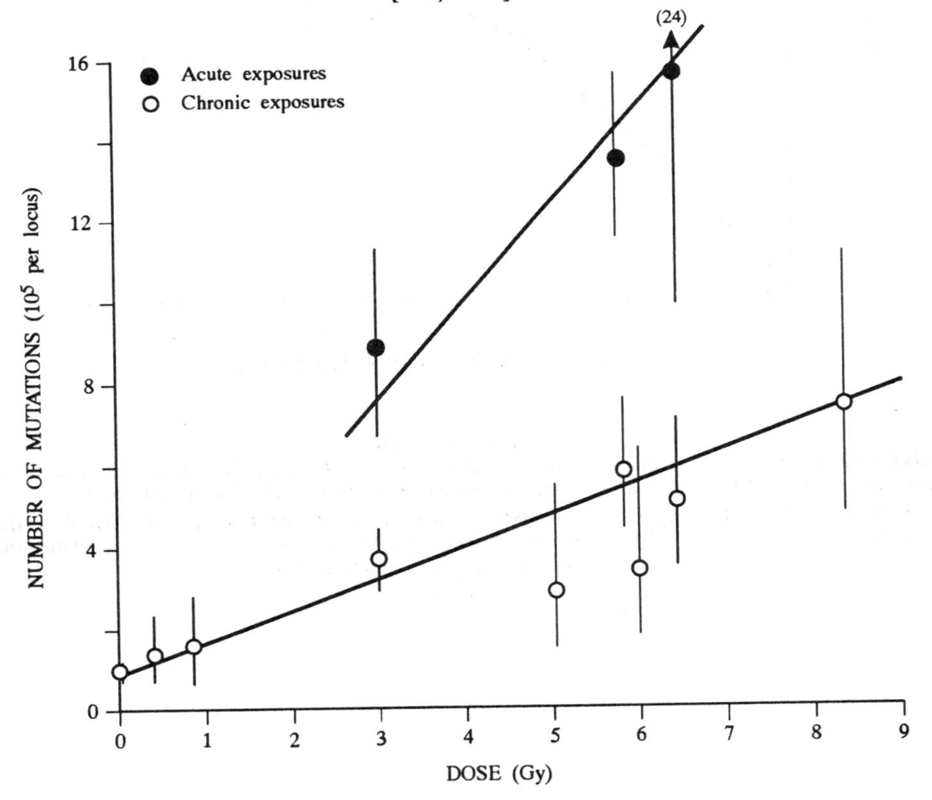

Figure XXVI.
Mutation rate in mouse spermatogonia following acute and chronic exposures. Straight lines of best fit by the method of maximum likelihood for specific-locus data. [R11]

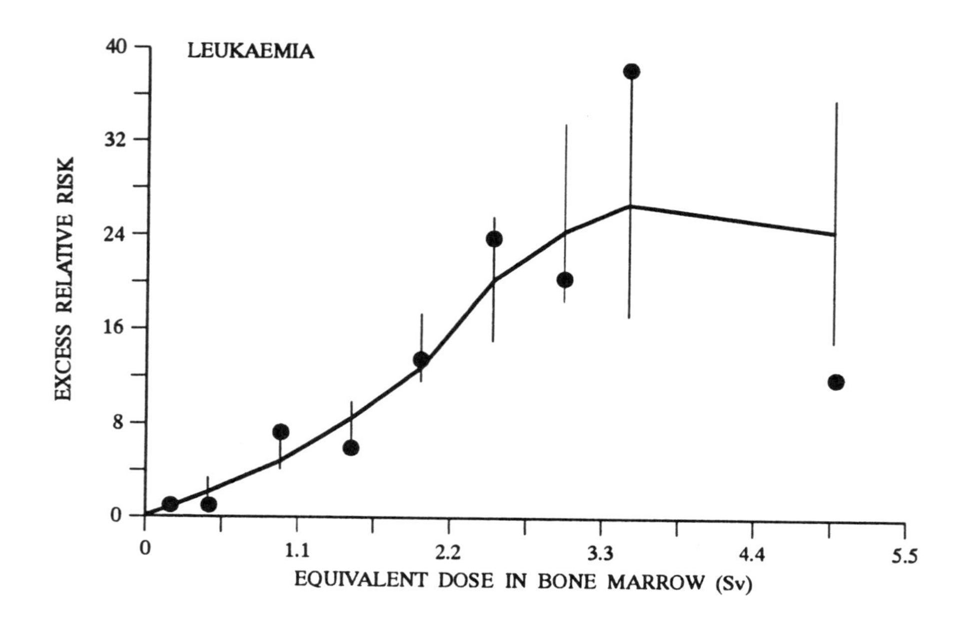

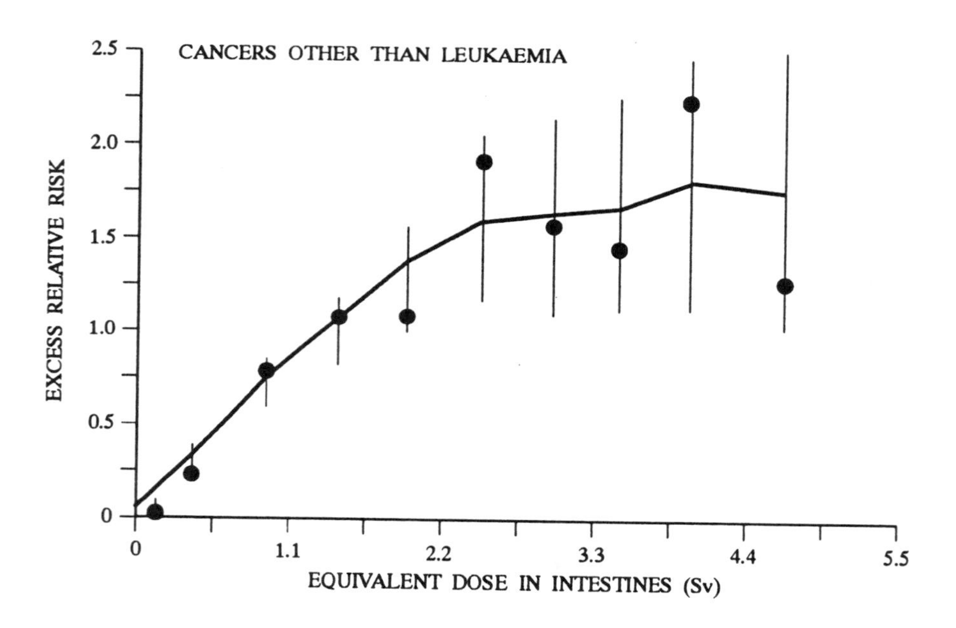

Figure XXVII.
Excess relative risk of mortality from leukaemia and cancers other than leukaemia in the Life Span Study. (DS86 dosimetry, both cities, both sexes, age at exposure groups 0-19, 20-34 and >35 years, 1950-1985). Points are estimated relative risk in each equivalent dose interval, averaging with equal weights over six age-at-exposure and sex groups. RBE is assumed equal to 10. Lines are smoothed average of the points. Error bars refer to the smoothed values.
[P3]

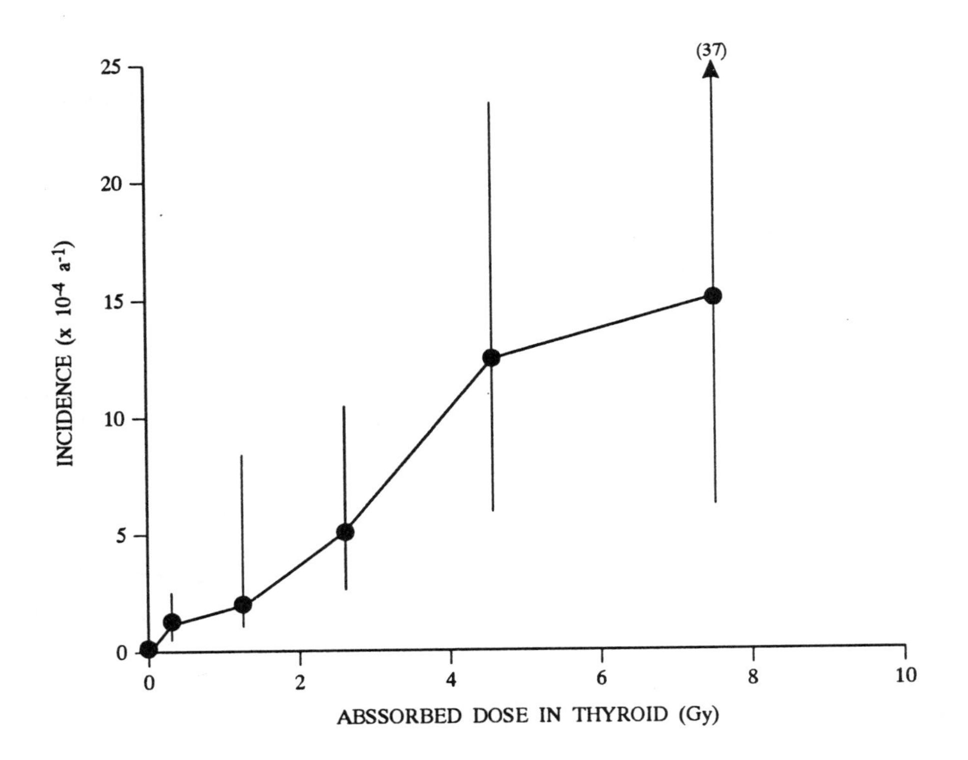

Figure XXVIII.
Adjusted thyroid cancer incidence in relation to radiation dose in the thyroid gland. [S11]

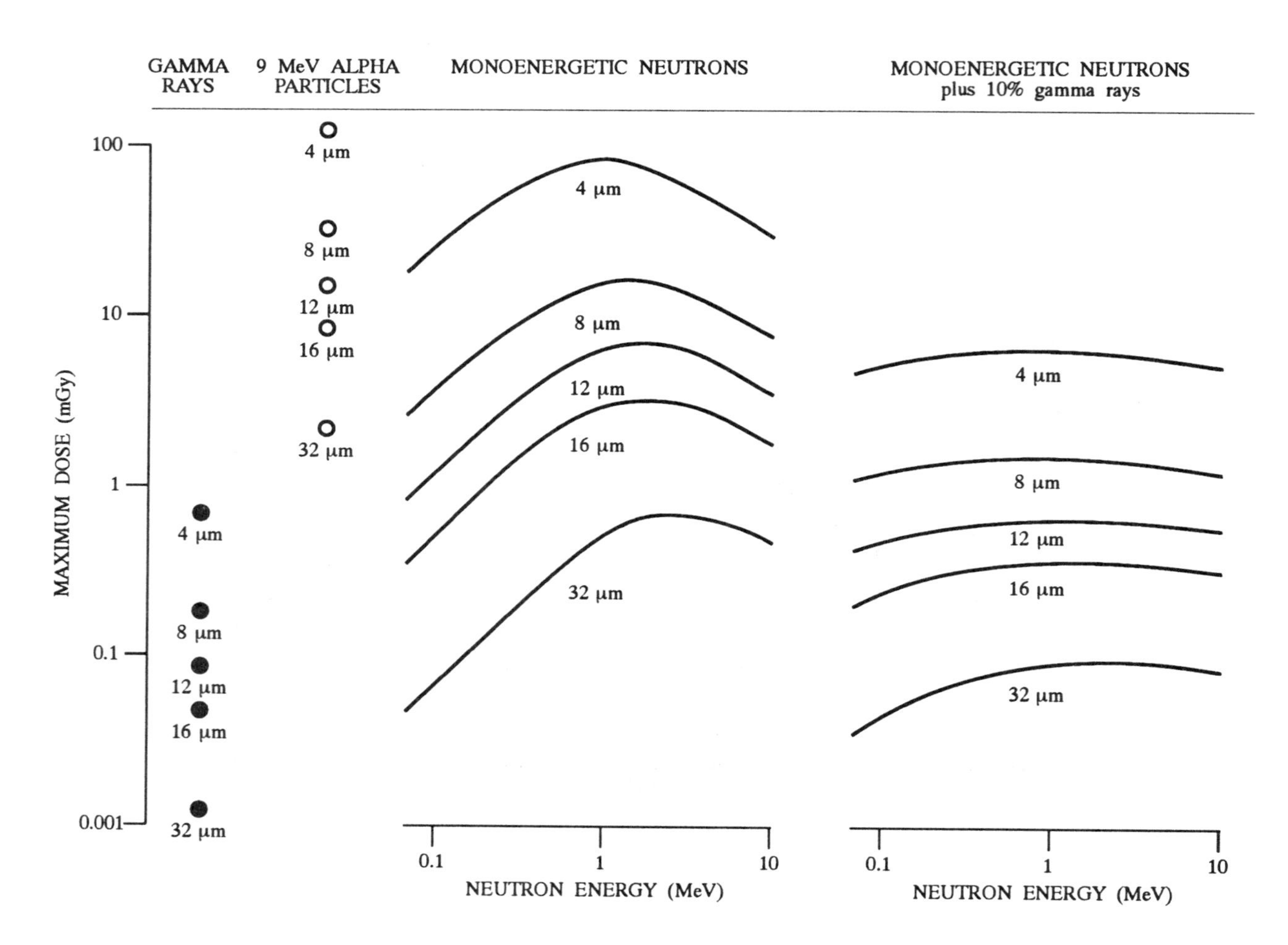

Figure XXIX.
Upper limit of a low dose for various assumed sensitive volumes within a cell.
[G4]

References

A1 Ainsworth, E.J., R.J.M. Fry, P.C. Brennan et al. Life shortening, neoplasia and systematic injuries in mice after single or fractionated doses of neutron or gamma radiation. p. 77-92 in: Biological and Environmental Effects of Low-Level Radiation, Volume 1. STI/PUB/409. IAEA, Vienna, 1976.

A2 Alper, T., C. Marshall and C.B. Seymour. Reply to letter by Elkind et al. Int. J. Radiat. Biol. 53: 961-963 (1988).

A3 Archer, M.C. Chemical carcinogenesis. p. 89 in: The Basic Science of Oncology. (I.F. Tannock and R.P. Hall, eds.) Pergamon Press, Oxford, 1987.

A4 Aghamohammadi, S.Z., D.T. Goodhead and J.R.K. Savage. Production of chromosome aberrations, micronuclei and sister chromatid exchanges by 24-keV epithermal neutrons in human Go lymphocytes. Mutat. Res. 211: 225-230 (1989).

A5 Andersen, A.C. and L.S. Rosenblatt. The effect of whole-body X-irradiation on the median lifespan of female dogs (beagles). Radiat. Res. 39: 177-200 (1969).

A6 Abrahamson, S., M. Bender, C. Book et al. Health effects models for nuclear power plant accident consequence analysis. Low LET radiation. Part II: Scientific bases for health effects models. NUREG/CR-4214 SAND85-7185, Rev. 1, Part II (1989).

A7 Alper, T. Cellular Radiobiology. Cambridge University Press, Cambridge, 1979.

A8 Armitage, P. and R. Doll. The age distribution of cancer and a multistage theory of carcinogenesis. Br. J. Cancer 8: 1-12 (1954).

A9 Armitage, P. and R. Doll. A two-stage theory of carcinogenesis in relation to the age distribution of human cancer. Br. J. Cancer 11: 161-169 (1957).

A10 Abrahamson, S., M. Bender, B.B. Boecker et al. Health effects models for nuclear power plant accident consequence analysis. Modifications of models resulting from recent reports on health effects of ionizing radiation. Low LET radiation. Part II: Scientific bases for health effects models. NUREG/CR-4214, Rev. 1, Add. 1 and LMF-132 (1991).

A11 Aghamohammadi, S.Z., D.T. Goodhead and J.R.K. Savage. Induction of sister chromatid exchanges (SCE) in Go lymphocytes by plutonium-238 α-particles. Int. J. Radiat. Biol. 53: 909-915 (1988).

B1 Balcer-Kubiczek, E.K. and G.H. Harrison. Survival and oncogenic transformation of C3H10T½ cells after extended x irradiation. Radiat. Res. 104: 214-223 (1985).

B2 Balcer-Kubiczek, E.K., G.H. Harrison and B.W. Thompson. Repair time for oncogenic transformation in C3H10T½ cells subjected to protracted x-irradiation. Int. J. Radiat. Biol. 51: 219-226 (1987).

B3 Balcer-Kubiczek, E.K., G.H. Harrison, G.H. Zeman et al. Lack of inverse dose rate effect on fission neutron induced transformation of C3H10T½ cells. Int. J. Radiat. Biol. 54: 531-536 (1988).

B4 Balcer-Kubiczek, E.K., G.H. Harrison and G.H. Zeman. The relationship between dose rate and transformation induction in C3H10T½ cells by TRIGA reactor fission neutrons at 0.3 Gy. p. 529-538 in: Low Dose Radiation: Biological Bases of Risk Assessment. (K.F. Baverstock and J.W. Stather, eds.) Taylor and Francis, London, 1989.

B5 Barendsen, G.W. Radiosensitivity of tumours and related cells in culture. Biomedicine 26: 259-260 (1977).

B6 Barendsen, G.W. Dose fractionation, dose rate and iso-effect relationships for normal tissue responses. Int. J. Radiat. Oncol. Biol. Phys. 8: 181-197 (1982).

B7 Barendsen, G.W. Dose-effect relationships for various responses of mammalian cells to radiations of different linear energy transfer. J. Soc. Radiol. Prot. 4: 143-152 (1984).

B8 Barendsen, G.W. Do fast neutrons at low dose rate enhance cell transformation in vitro? A basic problem of microdosimetry and interpretation. Int. J. Radiat. Biol. 47: 731-734 (1985).

B9 Barendsen, G.W. Physical factors influencing the frequency of radiation induced transformation of mammalian cells. p. 315-324 in: Cell Transformation and Radiation Induced Cancer. (K.H. Chadwick et al., eds.) Adam Hilger, Bristol, 1989.

B10 Beer, J.Z., E. Budzicka, E. Niepokojczycka et al. Loss of tumourigenecity with simultaneous changes in radiosensitivity and photosensitivity during the in vitro growth of L5178Y murine lymphoma cells. Cancer Res. 43: 4736-4742 (1983).

B11 Bettega, D., P. Calzolari, P. Pollara et al. In vivo cell transformations induced by 31 MeV protons. Radiat. Res. 104: 178-181 (1985).

B12 Bettega, D., P. Calzolari, A. Ottolenghi et al. Transformation of C3H10T½ with Cm-244 alpha particles at low and high dose rates. p. 333-340 in: Cell Transformation and Radiation Induced Cancer. (K.H. Chadwick et al., eds.) Adam Hilger, Bristol, 1989.

B13 Birnboim, H.C. and J.J. Jevcak. Fluorometric method for rapid detection of DNA strand breaks in human white blood cells produced by low doses of radiation. Cancer Res. 41: 1889-1892 (1981).

B14 Book, S.A., D.A. McNeill, N.J. Parks et al. Comparative effects of iodine-132 and iodine-131 in rat thyroid glands. Radiat. Res. 81: 246-253 (1980).

B15 Boice, J.D. and R.R. Monson. Breast cancer in women after repeated fluoroscopic examinations of the chest. J. Natl. Cancer Inst. 59: 823-832 (1977).

B16 Brenner, D.J., E.J. Hall, G. Randers-Pehrson et al. Mechanistic considerations on the dose-rate/LET dependence of oncogenic transformation by ionizing radiations. Radiat. Res. 133: 365-369 (1993).

B17 Bond, V.P., E.P. Cronkite, S.W. Lippincott et al. Studies on radiation-induced mammary gland neoplasia in the rat. III. Relation of the neoplastic response to dose of total body radiation. Radiat. Res. 12: 276-285 (1960).

B18 Bond, V.P., L.E. Feinendegen and J. Booz. What is a "low dose" of radiation? Int. J. Radiat. Biol. 53 (1): 1-12 (1988).

B19 Boot, L.M., P. Bentvelzen, J. Calafat et al. Interaction of x-ray treatment, a chemical carcinogen, hormones and viruses in mammary gland carcinogenesis. p. 434-440 in: Oncology. Volume 1. (R.L. Clark et al., eds.) Yearbook Medical Publishers, Chicago, 1970.
B20 Booz, J. and L.E. Feinendegen. A microdosimetric understanding of low-dose radiation effects. Int. J. Radiat. Biol. 53 (1): 13-21 (1988).
B21 Borek, C. and E.J. Hall. Effect of split doses of x-rays on neoplastic transformation of single cells. Nature 252: 499-501 (1974).
B22 Borek, C. Neoplastic transformation following split doses of x-rays. Br. J. Radiol. 52: 845-846 (1979).
B23 Broerse, J.J., L.A. Hennen, M.J. van Zwieten et al. Dose-effect relations for mammary carcinogenesis in different rat strains after irradiation with x-rays and monoenergetic neutrons. p. 507-519 in: Biological Effects of Low-Level Radiation. STI/PUB/646. IAEA, Vienna, 1983.
B24 Buul, P.P.W. van, J.F. Richardson and J.H. Goudzwaard. The induction of reciprocal translocation in Rhesus monkey stem-cell spermatogonia: effects of low doses and low dose rates. Radiat. Res. 105: 1-7 (1986).
B25 Burch, P.R.J. Calculations of energy dissipation characteristics in water for various radiations. Radiat. Res. 6: 289-301 (1957).
B26 Boche, R.D. Effects of chronic exposure to x-radiation on growth and survival. p. 222-252 in: Biological Effects of External Radiation. (N.A. Blair, ed.) McGraw-Hill, New York, 1954.
B27 Brown, J.M. The shape of the dose-response curve for radiation carcinogenesis. Extrapolation to low doses. Radiat. Res. 71: 34-50 (1977).
B28 Brues, A.M. and G.A. Sacher. Analysis of mammalian radiation injury and lethality. p. 441-465 in: Symposium on Radiobiology. (J.J. Nickson, ed.) John Wiley and Sons, New York, 1952.
B29 Bustad, L.K., N.M. Gates, A. Ross et al. Effects of prolonged low-level irradiation of mice. Radiat. Res. 25: 318-330 (1965).
B30 Brenner, D.J. and E.J. Hall. The inverse dose-rate effect for oncogenic transformation by neutrons and charged particles: a plausible interpretation consistent with published data. Int. J. Radiat. Biol. 58: 745-758 (1990).
B31 Barendsen, G.W. Influence of radiation quality on the effectiveness of small doses for induction of reproductive death and chromosome aberrations in mammalian cells. Int. J. Radiat. Biol. 36: 46-63 (1979).
B32 Batchelor, A.L., R.J.S. Phillips and A.G. Searle. A comparison of the mutagenic effectiveness of chronic neutron- and gamma-irradiation of mouse spermatogonia. Mutat. Res. 3: 218-229 (1966).
B33 Bond, V.P. and M.N. Varma. A stochastic, weighted hit size theory of cellular radiobiological action. p. 423-437 in: Radiation Protection. Proceedings of the Eighth Symposium on Microdosimetry. (J. Booz and H.G. Ebert, eds.) EUR-8395 (1983).
B34 Brewen, J.G., R.J. Preston and H.E. Luippold. Radiation-induced translocations in spermatogonia. III. Effect of long-term chronic exposures to gamma-rays. Mutat. Res. 61: 405-409 (1979).
B35 Burch, P.R.J. Radiation carcinogenesis: a new hypothesis. Nature 185: 135-142 (1960).
B36 Burch, P.R.J. and M.S. Chesters. Mammalian cell survival and radiation quality: analysis with allowance for delta tracks. Phys. Med. Biol. 26: 997-1018 (1981).
B37 Burch, P.R.J. and M.S. Chesters. Neoplastic transformation of cells in vitro at low and high dose rates of fission neutrons: an interpretation. Int. J. Radiat. Biol. 49: 495-500 (1986).
B38 Barendsen, G.W. RBE-LET relations for induction of reproductive death and chromosome aberrations in mammalian cells. p. 55-68 in: Proceedings of the Sixth Symposium on Microdosimetry, Brussels, May 1978. (J. Booz and H.G. Ebert, eds.) Harwood Academic Publication, London, 1978.
B39 Balcer-Kubiczek, E.K., G.H. Harrison and T.K. Hei. Neutron dose-rate experiments at the AFRRI nuclear reactor. Radiat. Res. 128: S65-S70 (1991).
B40 Burns, F.J. and M. Vanderlaan. Split-dose recovery for radiation-induced tumours in rat skin. Int. J. Radiat. Biol. 32: 135-144 (1977).
B41 Billen, D. Spontaneous DNA damage and its significance for the "negligible dose" controversy in radiation protection. Radiat. Res. 124: 242-245 (1990).
B42 Booz, J. Microdosimetric spectra and parameters of low-LET radiations. p. 311-344 in: Proceedings of the Fifth Symposium on Microdosimetry. (J. Booz, H.G. Ebert and B.G.R. Smith, eds.) EUR-5452 (1976).
B43 Bettege, D., P. Calzolari, G. Noris Chiorda et al. Transformation of C3H10T½ cells with 4.3 MeV α particles at low doses: effects of single and fractionated doses. Radiat. Res. 131: 66-71 (1992).
B44 Boice, J.D. Jr., D. Preston, G. Faith et al. Frequent chest X-ray fluoroscopy and breast cancer incidence among tuberculosis patients in Massachusetts. Radiat. Res. 125: 214-222 (1990).
B45 Brenner, D.J. and E.J. Hall. Reply to letter by Harrison and Balcer-Kubizek. Int. J. Radiat. Biol. 61: 142 (1992).
C1 Committee on Biological Effects of Ionizing Radiation (BEIR V). Health Effects of Exposure to Low Levels of Ionizing Radiation. United States National Academy of Sciences, National Research Council. National Academy Press, Washington, 1990.
C2 Cross, F.T. A review of experimental animal radon health effects data. p. 476-481 in: Radiation Research: A Twentieth Century Perspective. (J.D. Chapman et al., eds.) Academic Press, San Diego, 1991.
C3 Cross, F.T. Experimental studies on lung carcinogenesis and their relationship to future research on radiation-induced lung cancer in humans. p. 27-35 in: The Future of Radiation Research. BIR Report 22. (G.B. Gerber et al., eds.) British Institute of Radiology, London, 1991.
C4 Committee on Biological Effects of Ionizing Radiation (BEIR III). The Effects on Populations of Exposure to Low Levels of Ionizing Radiation: 1980. United States National Academy of Sciences, National Research Council. National Academy Press, Washington, 1980.
C5 Chadwick, K.H. and H.P. Leenhouts. The Molecular Theory of Radiation Biology. Springer-Verlag, Berlin, 1981.

C6 Chadwick, K.H., C. Seymour and B. Barnhart (eds.). Cell Transformation and Radiation Induced Cancer. Adam Hilger, Bristol, 1989.

C7 Clifton, K.H. Radiation biology in cancer research. p. 501-513 in: 32nd M.D. Anderson Symposium on Fundamental Cancer Research. (R.E. Meyn and H.R. Withers, eds.) Raven Press, New York, 1980.

C8 Clifton, K.H. Thyroid cancer: re-evaluation of an experimental model for radiogenic endocrine carcinogenesis. p. 181-198 in: Radiation Carcinogenesis. (A.C. Upton et al., eds.) Elsevier Press, New York, 1986.

C9 Cornforth, M.N. and J.S. Bedford. A quantitative comparison of potentially lethal damage repair and the rejoining of interphase chromosome breaks in low passage normal human fibroblasts. Radiat. Res. 111: 385-405 (1987).

C10 Cornforth, M.N. and J.S. Bedford. X-ray-induced breakage and rejoining of human interphase chromosomes. Science 222: 1141-1143 (1983).

C11 Cox, R., J. Thacker, D.T. Goodhead et al. Mutation and inactivation of mammalian cells by various ionizing radiations. Nature 267: 425-427 (1977).

C12 Cox, R. A cellular description of the repair defect in ataxia-telangiectasia. p. 141-153 in: Ataxia-Telangiectasia: A Cellular and Molecular Link Between Cancer, Neuropathology and Immune Deficiency. (B.A. Bridges and D.G. Harnden, eds.) Wiley and Sons, Chichester, 1982.

C13 Cox, R., P.G. Debenham, W.K. Masson et al. Ataxia-telangiectasia: a human mutation giving high frequency misrepair of DNA double strand scissions. Mol. Biol. Med. 3: 229-244 (1986).

C14 Cronkite, E.P., C.J. Shellabarger, V.P. Bond et al. Studies on radiation-induced mammary gland neoplasia in the rat. I. The role of the ovary in the neoplastic response of the breast tissue to total- or partial-body x-irradiation. Radiat. Res. 12: 81-93 (1960).

C15 Cole, L.J., P.C. Nowell and J.S. Arnold. Late effects of X-radiation. The influence of dose fractionation on life span, leukaemia and nephrosclerosis incidence in mice. Radiat. Res. 12: 173-185 (1960).

C16 Comfort, A. Natural aging and the effects of radiation. Radiat. Res. (Suppl.) 1: 216-234 (1959).

C17 Crompton, N.E.A., F. Zoelser, E. Schneider et al. Increased mutant induction by very low dose-rate gamma irradiation. Naturwissenschaften 72: S439 (1985).

C18 Carnes, B.A., D. Grahn and J.F. Thomson. Dose-response modelling of life shortening in a retrospective analysis of the combined data for the JANUS programme at Argonne National Laboratory. Radiat. Res. 119: 39-56 (1989).

C19 Conard, R.A. Late effects in Marshall Islanders exposed to fallout 28 years ago. p. 57-71 in: Radiation Carcinogenesis: Epidemiology and Biological Significance. (J.D. Boice Jr. and J.F. Fraumeni Jr., eds.) Raven Press, New York, 1984.

C20 Cai, L. and S.-Z. Liu. Induction of cytogenetic adaptive response of somatic and germ cells *in vivo* and *in vitro* by low-dose X-irradiation. Int. J. Radiat. Biol. 58: 187-194 (1990).

C21 Cardis, E.M. Modelling the Effect of Exposure to Environmental Carcinogens on Incidence of Cancers in Populations. Ph.D. Dissertation, University of Washington, 1985.

C22 Carnes, B.A. and D. Grahn. Neutron issues in the JANUS mouse program. International Colloquium on Neutron Radiation Biology, Maryland, 1990.

C23 Chadwick, K.H. and H.P. Leenhouts. A molecular theory of cell survival. Phys. Med. Biol. 18: 78-87 (1973).

C24 Caswell, R.S. and J.J. Coyne. Microdosimetric spectra and parameters of fast neutrons. p. 97-123 in: Proceedings of the Fifth Symposium on Microdosimetry. (J. Booz, H.G. Ebert and B.G.R. Smith, eds.) EUR-5452 (1976).

C25 Charles, M., R. Cox, D. Goodhead et al. CEIR forum on the effects of high-LET radiation at low doses/dose rates. Int. J. Radiat. Biol. 58: 859-885 (1990).

C26 Charlton, D.E., H. Nikjoo and J.L. Humm. Calculation of initial yields of single and double strand breaks in cell nuclei from electrons, protons and alpha particles. Int. J. Radiat. Biol. 56: 1-19 (1989).

C27 Comings, D.E. A general theory of carcinogenesis. Proc. Natl. Acad. Sci. (USA) 70: 3324-3328 (1973).

C28 Curtis, S.B. Lethal and potentially-lethal lesions induced by radiation - a unified repair model. Radiat. Res. 106: 252-270 (1986).

C29 Covelli, U., V. Di Majo, M. Coppola et al. Neutron carcinogenesis in mice: a study of the dose-response curves. Radiat. Res. 128: S114-S116 (1991).

C30 Carnes, R.A. and T.E. Fritz. Responses of the Beagle to protracted irradiation. I. Effects of total dose and dose rate. Radiat. Res. 128: 125-132 (1991).

D1 Debenham, P.G., N.J. Jones and M.B.T. Webb. Vector-mediated DNA double strand break repair analysis in normal and radiation-sensitive Chinese hamster V79 cells. Mutat. Res. 199: 1-9 (1988).

D2 Di Majo, V., M. Coppola, S. Rebessi et al. Dose-response relationships of radiation-induced Harderian gland tumours and myeloid leukaemia of the CBA/Cne mouse. J. Natl. Cancer Inst. 76: 955-963 (1986).

D3 Di Majo, V., M. Coppola, S. Rebessi et al. Age-related susceptibility of mouse liver to induction of tumours by neutrons. Radiat. Res. 124: 227-234 (1990).

D4 Doniach, I. Effects including carcinogenesis of I-131 and X-rays on the thyroid of experimental animals: a review. Health Phys. 9: 1357-1362 (1963).

D5 Darby, S.C. and R. Doll. Radiation and exposure rate. Nature 344: 824 (1990).

E1 Edwards, A.A., D.C. Lloyd and J.S. Prosser. Chromosome aberrations in human lymphocytes - a radiobiological review. p. 423-432 in: Low Dose Radiation: Biological Bases of Risk Assessment. (K.F. Baverstock and J.W. Stather, eds.) Taylor and Francis, London, 1989.

E2 Elkind, M.M. Kaplan lecture: target theory, linearity and repair/misrepair in radiobiology. p. 296-305 in: Proceedings of the 8th International Congress of Radiation Research, Edinburgh, 1987 (Volume 2). (E.M. Fielden et al., eds.) Taylor and Francis, London, 1987.

E3 Elkind, M.M., F.Q.H. Ngo, C.K. Hill et al. Letter to the editor: Do lethal mutations influence radiation transformation frequencies? Int. J. Radiat. Biol. 53: 849-859 (1988).

E4 Eguchi-Kasai, K., T. Kosaka, K. Sato et al. Reparability of DNA double-strand breaks and radiation sensitivity in five mammalian cell lines. Int. J. Radiat. Biol. 59: 97-104 (1991).

E5 Evans, H.H., M.-F. Horng, J. Mencl et al. The influence of dose rate on the lethal and mutagenic effects of x-rays on proliferating L5178Y cells differing in radiation sensitivity. Int. J. Radiat. Biol. 47: 553-562 (1985).

E6 Elkind, M.M. Physical, biophysical and cell-biological factors that can contribute to neoplastic transformation by fission-spectrum neutrons. Radiat. Res. 128: S47-S52 (1991).

E7 Evans, H.E., M. Nielsen, M. Jaroslav et al. The effect of dose rate on x-radiation-induced mutant frequency and the nature of DNA lesions in mouse lymphoma L5178Y cells. Radiat. Res. 122: 316-325 (1990).

E8 Edwards, A.A. Low dose and low dose rate effects in laboratory animals. NRPB-TM/1-92 (1992).

F1 Fertil, B., P.J. Gueulette, J. Wambersie et al. Dependence of the quadratic model parameters on dose rate (γ rays) and 50 MeV neutrons: an analysis based on the in vitro survival curves of 6 human cell lines. Radiat. Environ. Biophys. 17: 315 (1980).

F2 Furuno-Fukushi, I., K. Aoki and H. Matsudaira. Mutation induction by different dose rates of γ rays in near-diploid mouse cells in plateau and log phase culture. Radiat. Res. (in press, 1993).

F3 Friedberg, E.C. and P.C. Hanawalt (eds.). Mechanisms and Consequences of DNA Damage Processing. A.R. Liss, New York, 1988.

F4 Fry, R.J.M. Radiation protection guidelines for the skin. Int. J. Radiat. Biol. 57: 829-839 (1990).

F5 Freedman, V.H. and S. Shin. Cellular tumorigenicity in male mice: correlation with cell growth in semi solid medium. Cell 3: 355-359 (1974).

F6 Furuno-Fukushi, I. and H. Matsudaira. Mutation induction by tritiated water and effects of deuterium oxide in cultured mouse leukaemia cells. Radiat. Res. 103: 466-470 (1985).

F7 Furuno-Fukushi, I., A.M. Ueno and H. Matsudaira. Mutation induction by very low dose rate gamma-rays in cultured mouse leukaemia cells L5178Y. Radiat. Res. 15: 273-280 (1988).

F8 Furuno-Fukushi, I. and H. Matsudaira. Mutation induction by different dose rates of x-rays in radiation-sensitive mutants of mouse leukaemia. Radiat. Res. 120: 370-374 (1989).

F9 Fry, R.J.M. The role of animal species in low dose extrapolation. p. 109-118 in: Proceedings of the 10th Annual Meeting of the National Council on Radiation Protection and Measurement on Critical Issues in Setting Radiation Dose Limits. NCRP (1982).

F10 Fry, R.J.M. Time-dose relationship and high-LET irradiation. Int. J. Radiat. Biol. 58: 866-870 (1990).

F11 Fabrikant, J.I., T.H. Hsu, D.H. Knudson et al. Effect of LET on radiation carcinogenesis: comparison of single and fractionated doses of ^{239}Pu, ^{241}Am, ^{32}P and X-rays on the production of osteosarcomas in rats. p. 322-346 in: Radionuclide Carcinogenesis. (C.L. Saunders et al., eds.) CONF-720505 (1973).

F12 Feinendegen, L.E., J. Booz, V.P. Bond et al. Microdosimetric approach to the analysis of cell responses at low dose and low dose rate. Radiat. Prot. Dosim. 13: 299-306 (1985).

F13 Fritz, T.E., T.M. Seed, D.V. Tolle et al. Late effects of protracted whole-body irradiation of beagles by cobalt-60 gamma rays. in: Lifespan Radiation Effects Studies in Animals: What Can They Tell Us? (R.C. Thompson and J.A. Mahaffey, eds.) CONF-830951. NTIS, Springfield VA, 1986.

G1 Glickman, B.W., E.A. Drobetsky, J. Boer et al. Ionizing radiation induced point mutations in mammalian cells. p. 562 in: Proceedings of the 8th International Congress of Radiation Research, Edinburgh, 1987. Volume 2. (E.M. Fielden et al., eds.) Taylor and Francis, London, 1987.

G2 Goodhead, D.T. Deductions from cellular studies of inactivation, mutagenesis and transformation. p. 369-385 in: Radiation Carcinogenesis: Epidemiology and Biological Significance. (J.D. Boice Jr. and J.F. Fraumeni Jr., eds.) Raven Press, New York, 1984.

G3 Goodhead, D.T. Biophysical models of radiation-action - introductory review. p. 306-311 in: Proceedings of the 8th International Congress of Radiation Research (Abstract), Edinburgh, 1987. Volume 2. (E.M. Fielden et al., eds.) Taylor and Francis, London, 1987.

G4 Goodhead, D.T. Relationship of microdosimetric techniques to applications in biological systems. p. 1-89 in: The Dosimetry of Ionizing Radiations. Volume 2. (K.R. Kase et al., eds.) Academic Press, Orlando, 1987.

G5 Goodhead, D.T. Spatial and temporal distribution of energy. Health Phys. 55: 231-240 (1988).

G6 Goodhead, D.T. and H. Nikjoo. Track structure analysis of ultrasoft x-rays compared to high- and low-LET radiations. Int. J. Radiat. Biol. 55(4): 513-529 (1989).

G7 Gragtmans, N.J., D.K. Myers, J.R. Johnson et al. Occurrence of mammary tumours in rats after exposure to tritium beta rays and 200-kVp x rays. Radiat. Res. 99: 636-650 (1984).

G8 Grahn, D. and G.A. Sacher. Fractionation and protraction factors and the late effects of radiation in small mammals. p. 2.1-2.27 in: Proceedings of a Symposium on Dose Rate in Mammalian Radiation Biology. (D.G. Brown et al., eds.) CONF-680410. USAEC, Oak Ridge, 1968.

G9 Grahn, D. Biological effects of protracted low dose radiation exposure of man and animals. p. 101 in: Late Effects of Radiation. (R.J.M. Fry et al., eds.) Van Nostrand Reinhold Co., New York, 1970.

G10 Griffith, W.C., B.B. Boecker, R.G. Cuddihy et al. Preliminary radiation risk estimates of carcinoma incidence in the lung as a function of cumulative radiation dose using proportional tumour incidence rates. p. 196-204 in: Inhalation Toxicology Research Institute Annual Report 1986-1987. LMF-120. ITRI, Albuquerque (1987).

G11 Grosovsky, A.J. and J.B. Little. Evidence for linear response for the induction of mutations in human cells by x-ray exposures below 10 rad. Proc. Natl. Acad. Sci. (USA) 82: 2092-2095 (1985).
G12 Grahn, D. and B.A. Carnes. Quoted in [F10].
G13 Goldman, M. Experimental carcinogenesis in the skeleton. p. 214-231 in: Radiation Carcinogenesis. (A.C. Upton et al., eds.) Elsevier, New York, 1986.
G14 Gilbert, E.S., S.A. Fry, L.D. Wiggs et al. Analyses of combined mortality data on workers at the Hanford site, Oak Ridge National Laboratory, and Rocky Flats nuclear weapons plant. Radiat. Res. 120: 19-35 (1989).
G15 Goodhead, D.T., R.J. Munson, J. Thacker et al. Mutation and inactivation of cultured mammalian cells exposed to beams of accelerated heavy ions. IV. Biophysical interpretation. Int. J. Radiat. Biol. 37: 135-167 (1980).
G16 Goodhead, D.T. and D.J. Brenner. Estimation of a single property of low LET radiations which correlates with biological effectiveness. Phys. Med. Biol. 28: 485-492 (1983).
G17 Goodhead, D.T. Saturable repair models of radiation action in mammalian cells. Radiat. Res. 104: S58-S67 (1985).
G18 Goodhead, D.T., D.E. Charlton, W.E. Wilson et al. Current biophysical approaches to understanding of biological effects in terms of local energy deposition. p. 57-68 in: Radiation Protection. Proceedings of the Fifth Symposium on Neutron Dosimetry. (H. Schraube et al., eds.) EUR 9762 (1985).
G19 Goodhead, D.T. Physical basis for biological effect. p. 37-53 in: Nuclear and Atomic Data for Radiotherapy and Related Radiobiology. STI/PUB/741. IAEA, Vienna, 1987.
G20 Goodhead, D.T. The initial physical damage produced by ionizing radiations. Int. J. Radiat. Biol. 56: 623-634 (1989).
G21 Goodhead, D.T. Biophysical features of radiations at low doses and low dose rates. p. 4-11 in: New Developments in Fundamental and Applied Radiobiology. (C. Seymour and C. Mothersill, eds.) Taylor and Francis, London, 1991.
G22 Gunther, K. and W. Schulz. Biophysical Theory of Radiation Action - A Treatise on Relative Biological Effectiveness. Akademie Verlag, Berlin, 1983.
G23 Grahn, D., R.J.M. Fry and R.A. Lea. Analysis of survival and cause of death statistics for mice under single and duration-of-life gamma irradiation. p. 175-186 in: Life Sciences and Space Research. Akadamie Verlag, Berlin, 1972.
G24 Gray, R.G., J. Lafuma and S.E. Paris. Lung tumors and radon inhalation in over 2000 rats: approximate lineariety across a wide range of doses and potentiation by tobacco smoke. p. 592-607 in: Lifespan Radiation Effects Studies in Animals: What Can They Tell Us? (R.C. Thompson and J.A. Mahaffey, eds.) CONF-830951. NTIS, Springfield VA, 1986.
H1 Hall, E.J. and R.C. Miller. The how and why of in vitro oncogenic transformation. Radiat. Res. 87: 208-223 (1981).
H2 Hall, E.J. Radiobiology for the Radiologist. Lippincott, Philadelphia, 1988.
H3 Hall, E.J. Finding a smoother pebble: a workshop summary. p. 401-412 in: Cell Transformation and Radiation Induced Cancer. (K.H. Chadwick et al., eds.) Adam Hilger, Bristol, 1989.
H4 Han, A. and M.M. Elkind. Transformation of mouse C3H10T½ cells by single and fractionated doses of x-rays and fission-spectrum neutrons. Cancer Res. 39: 123-130 (1979).
H5 Han, A., C.K. Hill and M.M. Elkind. Repair of cell killing and neoplastic transformation at reduced dose rates of Co-60 γ-rays. Cancer Res. 40: 3328-3332 (1980).
H6 Han, A., C.K. Hill and M.M. Elkind. Repair processes and radiation quality in neoplastic transformation of mammalian cells. Radiat. Res. 99: 249-261 (1984).
H7 Hieber, L., G. Ponsel, H. Roos et al. Absence of a dose rate effect in the transformation of C3H10T½ cells by α particles. Int. J. Radiat. Biol. 52: 859-869 (1987).
H8 Hill, C.K., F.M. Buonaguro, C.P. Myers et al. Fission spectrum neutrons at reduced dose rates enhance neoplastic transformation. Nature 298: 67-69 (1982).
H9 Hill, C.K., A. Han, F.M. Buonaguro et al. Multifraction of Co-60 gamma rays reduces neoplastic transformation in vitro. Carcinogenesis 5: 193-197 (1984).
H10 Hill, C.K., A. Han and M.M. Elkind. Fission spectrum neutrons at low dose rate enhance neoplastic transformation in the linear low dose region (0-10 cGy). Int. J. Radiat. Biol. 46: 11-15 (1984).
H11 Hill, C.K., B.A. Carnes, A. Han et al. Neoplastic transformation is enhanced by multiple low doses of fission spectrum neutrons. Radiat. Res. 102: 404-410 (1985).
H12 Hahn, F.F., B.A. Muggenburg, B.B. Boecker et al. Insights into radionuclide-induced lung cancer in people from life-span studies in Beagle dogs. p. 521-534 in: Lifespan Radiation Effects Studies in Animals: What Can They Tell Us? (R.C. Thompson and J.A. Mahaffey, eds.) CONF-830951. NTIS, Springfield VA, 1986.
H13 Holm, L.-E., G. Lundell and G. Walinder. Incidence of malignant thyroid tumours in humans after exposure to diagnostic doses of iodine-131. I. Retrospective cohort study. J. Natl. Cancer Inst. 64: 1055-1059 (1980).
H14 Holm, L.-E., G. Eklund and G. Lundell. Incidence of malignant thyroid tumours in humans after exposure to diagnostic doses of iodine-131. II. Estimation of actual thyroid size, thyroidal radiation dose and predicted versus observed number of malignant thyroid tumours. J. Natl. Cancer Inst. 65: 121 (1981).
H15 Holm, L.-E., K.E. Wiklund, G.E. Lundell et al. Thyroid cancer after diagnostic doses of iodine-131: a retrospective cohort study. J. Natl. Cancer Inst. 80: 1132-1138 (1988).
H16 Howe, G.R. Epidemiology of radiogenic breast cancer. p. 119-130 in: Radiation Carcinogenesis: Epidemiology and Biological Significance. (J.D. Boice Jr. and J.F. Fraumeni Jr., eds.) Raven Press, New York, 1984.
H17 Humphreys, E.R. Medical Research Council Radiobiology Unit, United Kingdom. Communication to the UNSCEAR Secretariat (1989).

H18 Henshaw, P.S. Experimental roentgen injury. IV. Effects of repeated small doses of x-rays on the blood picture, tissue morphology and life span in mice. J. Natl. Cancer Inst. 4: 513-522 (1944).

H19 Hursh, J.B., T.R. Noonan, G. Casarett et al. Reduction of lifespan of rats by roentgen irradiation. Am. J. Roentgenol., Radium Ther. Nucl. 74: 130-134 (1955).

H20 Hill, C.K. Is the induction of neoplastic transformation by radiation dependent upon the quality and dose rate? Inst. Phys. Chem. Res. 83: 31-35 (1989).

H21 Hahn, G.M. and J.B. Little. Plateau-phase culture of mammalian cells in an in vitro model for human cancer. Can. Topics Radiat. Res. Quost. 8: 39-83 (1972).

H22 Holm, L.-E., K.E. Wiklund, G.E. Lundell et al. Cancer risk in population examined with diagnostic doses of ^{131}I. J. Natl. Cancer Inst. 81: 302-306 (1989).

H23 Harder, D. The pairwise lesion interaction model. p. 159-170 in: Quantitative Mathematical Models in Radiation Biology. (J. Kiefer, ed.) Springer Verlag, Heidelberg, 1988.

H24 Hethcote, H.W. and A.M. Knudsen. Model for the incidence of embryonal cancers: application to retinoblastoma. Proc. Natl. Acad. Sci. (USA) 75: 2453-2457 (1978).

H25 Hofman, W. and F. Daschil. Biological effects of alpha particles in lung tissue. Radiat. Prot. Dosim. 13: 229-232 (1985).

H26 Hutchinson, F. Chemical changes induced in DNA by ionizing radiation. Prog. Nucleic Acid Res. Mol. Biol. 32: 115-154 (1985).

H27 Hsiao, W.L., C.A. Lopez, T. Wu et al. A factor present in fetal calf serum enhances oncogene-induced transformation of rodent fibroblasts. Mol. Cell. Biol. 7: 3380-3385 (1987).

H28 Huiskamp, R. Acute myeloid leukaemia induction in CBA/H mice by irradiation with fission neutrons as a function of exposure rate. Radiat. Environ. Biophys. 30: 213-215 (1991).

H29 Huiskamp, R., J.A.G. Davids and R.H. Mole. Acute myeloid leukaemia induction in CBA/H mice by irradiation with fission neutrons as a function of exposure rate. p. 258 in: Radiation Research: A Twentieth Century Perspective. Volume 1. (J.D. Chapman, W.C. Dewey and G.F. Whitmore, eds.) Academic Press, San Diego, 1991.

H30 Hulse, F.V. and R.H. Mole. Skin tumour incidence in CBA mice given fractionated exposures to low energy beta particles. Br. J. Cancer 23: 452-463 (1969).

H31 Hall, E.J., R.C. Miller and D.J. Brenner. Neoplastic transformation and the inverse dose rate effect for neutrons. Radiat. Res. 128: S75-S80 (1991).

H32 Holm, L.-E. Malignant disease following iodine-131 therapy in Sweden. p. 263-271 in: Radiation Carcinogenesis: Epidemiology and Biological Significance. (J.D. Boice Jr. and J.F. Fraumeni Jr., eds.) Raven Press, New York, 1984.

H33 Hendry, J.H. The slower cellular recovery after high-LET irradiations, including neutrons, focuses on the quality of DNA breaks. Radiat. Res. 128: S111-S113 (1991).

H34 Harrison, G.H. and E.K. Balcer-Kubiczek. Ambiguity of the Brenner-Hall model. Int. J. Radiat. Biol. 61: 139-142 (1992).

H35 Holm, L.-E., K.E. Wiklund, G.E. Lundell et al. Cancer risk in population examined with diagnostic doses of ^{131}I. J. Natl. Cancer Inst. 81: 302-306 (1989).

I1 International Commission on Radiological Protection. Recommendations of the International Commission on Radiological Protection. ICRP Publication 26. Annals of the ICRP 1(3). Pergamon Press, Oxford, 1977.

I2 International Commission on Radiological Protection. Recommendations of the International Commission on Radiological Protection. ICRP Publication 60. Pergamon Press, Oxford, 1991.

I3 International Commission on Radiological Protection. Limits for Intakes of Radionuclides by Workers. ICRP Publication 30. Annals of the ICRP 2(3/4). Pergamon Press, Oxford, 1979.

I4 International Commission on Radiation Units and Measurements. "Microdosimetry". ICRU Report 36 (1983).

I5 Iliakis, G. The influence of conditions affecting repair and fixation of potentially lethal damage on the induction of 6-thioguanine resistance after exposure of mammalian cells to x-rays. Mutat. Res. 126: 215-225 (1984).

I6 International Commission on Radiation Units and Measurements. The Quality Factor in Radiation Protection. ICRU Report 40 (1986).

I7 International Commission on Radiological Protection. RBE for Deterministic Effects. ICRP Publication 58. Annals of the ICRP 20(4). Pergamon Press, Oxford, 1989.

I8 Ikushima, T. Chromosomal responses to ionizing radiation reminiscent of an adaptive response in cultured Chinese hamster cells. Mutat. Res. 180: 215-221 (1987).

J1 Johnson, J.R. and D.K. Myers. Is ^{131}I less efficient than external irradiation at producing thyroid cancers? p. 289-301 in: Biological Effects of Low-Level Radiation. STI/PUB/646. IAEA, Vienna, 1983.

J2 Jones, C.A., B.A. Sedita, C.K. Hill et al. Influence of dose rate on the transformation of Syrian hamster embryo cells by fission spectrum neutrons. p. 539-546 in: Low Dose Radiation: Biological Bases of Risk Assessment. (K.F. Baverstock and J.W. Stather, eds.) Taylor and Francis, London, 1989.

K1 Kemp, L.M., S.G. Sedgwick and P.A. Jeggo. X-ray sensitive mutants of CHO cells defective in double strand break rejoining. Mutat. Res. 132: 189-196 (1984).

K2 Kohn, H.I. and P. Guttman. Age at exposure and the late effects of X-rays. Survival and tumor incidence in CAF_1 mice irradiated at 1 to 2 years of age. Radiat. Res. 18: 348-373 (1963).

K3 Kaplan, H.S. and M.B. Brown. A quantitative dose-response study of lymphoid-tumour development in irradiated C57 black mice. J. Natl. Cancer Inst. 13: 185-208 (1952).

K4 Koenig, F. and J. Kiefer. Level of dose-rate effect for mutation induction by gamma-rays in human TK6 cells. Int. J. Radiat. Biol. 54: 891-897 (1988).

K5 Katz, R., B. Ackerson, M. Homayoonfar et al. Inactivation of cells by heavy ion bombardment. Radiat. Res. 47: 402-425 (1971).

K6 Kellerer, A.M. and H.H. Rossi. A generalized formulation of dual radiation action. Radiat. Res. 75: 471-488 (1978).

K7 Knudsen, A.G., H.W. Hethcote and B.W. Brown. Mutation and childhood cancer: a probabilistic model for the incidence of retinoblastoma. Proc. Natl. Acad. Sci. (USA) 72: 5116-5120 (1975).

K8 Kronenberg, A. and J.B. Little. Mutagenic properties of low doses of X-rays, fast neutrons and selected heavy ions in human cells. p. 554-559 in: Low Dose Radiation: Biological Bases of Risk Assessment. (K.F. Baverstock and J.W. Stather, eds.) Taylor and Francis, London, 1989.

K9 Kadhim, M.A., D.A. Macdonald, D.T. Goodhead et al. Transmission of chromosome instability after plutonium α-particle irradiation. Nature 355: 738-740 (1992).

K10 Kossenko, M.A. and M.O. Degteva. The follow-up of the population exposed as a result of the release of radioactive wastes into the Techa river. Part 3. Cancer mortality and risk evaluation. Sci. Total Environ. (1993, accepted for publication).

K11 Kendall, G.M., C.R. Muirhead, B.H. MacGibbon et al. Mortality and occupational exposure to radiation: first analysis of the National Registry for Radiation Workers. Br. Med. J. 304: 220-225 (1992).

K12 Koshurnikova, N.A., L.A. Buldakov, G.D. Bysogolov et al. Mortality from malignancies of the hematopoietic and lymphatic tissues among personnel of the first nuclear plant in the USSR. Sci. Total Environ. (1993, accepted for publication).

L1 Lefrancois, D., W. Al Achkar, A. Aurias et al. Chromosome aberrations induced by low-dose gamma-irradiation. Study of R-banded chromosomes of human lymphocytes. Mutat. Res. 212: 167-172 (1989).

L2 Liu, Z.H., C.S. Fu, C.M. Li et al. 131-I and 132-I carcinogenic effects in rat thyroid glands. Chin. Med. J. 95: 641-648 (1982).

L3 Lea, D.E. Actions of Radiations on Living Cells. Second edition. Cambridge University Press, London, 1955.

L4 Lee, W., R.P. Chiacchierini, B. Shleien et al. Thyroid tumours following I-131 or localized x-irradiation to the thyroid and pituitary glands in rats. Radiat. Res. 92: 307-319 (1982).

L5 Lehmann, A.R. The cellular and molecular responses of ataxia-telangiectasia cells to DNA damage. p. 83-101 in: Ataxia-Telangiectasia: A Cellular and Molecular Link Between Cancer, Neuropathology and Immune Deficiency. (B.A. Bridges and D.G. Harnden, eds.) Wiley and Sons, Chichester, 1982.

L6 Liber, H.L., V.H. Ozaki and J.B. Little. Toxicity and mutagenecity of low dose rates of ionizing radiation from tritiated water in human lymphoblastoid cells. Mutat. Res. 157: 77-86 (1985).

L7 Little, J.B. Origins of human cancer. p. 923-939 in: Cold Spring Harbour Conferences on Cell Proliferation. Volume IV. (H.H. Hiatt et al., eds.) Cold Spring Harbour, New York, 1977.

L8 Little, J.B. Quantitative studies of radiation transformation with the A31-11 mouse BALB/3T3 cell line. Cancer Res. 39: 1474-1480 (1979).

L9 Little, J.B. Characteristics of radiation induced neoplastic transformation in vitro. Leuk. Res. 10: 719-725 (1986).

L10 Little, J.B. Induction of neoplastic transformation by low dose-rate exposure to tritiated water. Radiat. Res. 107: 225-233 (1986).

L11 Little, J.B. The relevance of cell transformation to carcinogenesis in vivo. p. 396-413 in: Low Dose Radiation: Biological Bases of Risk Assessment. (K.F. Baverstock and J.W. Stather, eds.) Taylor and Francis, London, 1989.

L12 Lloyd, D.C. and A.A. Edwards. Chromosome aberrations in human lymphocytes: effect of radiation quality, dose and dose rate. p. 23-49 in: Radiation-induced Chromosome Damage in Man. (T. Ishihara and M.S. Sasaki, eds.) A.R. Liss, New York, 1983.

L13 Lloyd, D.C., A.A. Edwards, A. Leonard et al. Frequencies of chromosomal aberrations induced in human blood lymphocytes by low doses of x-rays. Int. J. Radiat. Biol. 53: 49-55 (1988).

L14 Lloyd, D.C., A.A. Edwards, A. Leonard et al. Chromosomal aberrations in human lymphocytes induced *in vitro* by very low doses of X-rays. Int. J. Rad. Biol. 61: 335-343 (1992).

L15 Lücke-Huhle, C., M. Pech and P. Herrlich. Selective gene amplification in mammalian cells after exposure to Co-60 γ rays, Am-241 α particles, or UV light. Radiat. Res. 106: 345-355 (1986).

L16 Lamson, B.G., M.S. Billings, J.J. Gambino et al. Effect of single and divided doses of X-irradiation on longevity in rats. Radiat. Res. 18: 255-264 (1963).

L17 Lyon, M.F., R.J.S. Phillips and H.J. Bailey. Mutagenic effect of repeated small radiation doses to mouse spermatogonia. I. Specific locus mutation rates. Mutat. Res. 15: 185-190 (1972).

L18 Little, J.B., A.R. Kennedy and R.B. McGandy. Effect of dose rate on the induction of experimental lung cancer in hamsters by α radiation. Health Phys. 103: 293-299 (1985).

L19 Lundgren, D.L., A. Gillett and F.F. Hahn. Effects of protraction of the α dose to the lungs of mice by repeated inhalation exposure to aerosols of $^{239}PuO_2$. Radiat. Res. 111: 201-224 (1987).

L20 Leenhouts, H.P. and K.H. Chadwick. The influence of dose rate on the dose-effect relationship. J. Radiol. Prot. 10: 95-102 (1990).

L21 Lamson, B.G., M.S. Billings, R.A. Meek et al. Late effects of total-body roentgen irradiation. III. Early appearance of neoplasms and life-shortening in female Wistar rats surviving 1000R hypoxic total-body irradiation. Arch. Pathol. 66: 311-321 (1958).

L22 Lamson, B.G., M.S. Billings, L.M. Ewell et al. Late effects of total-body irradiation. IV. Hypertension and nephrosclerosis in female Wistar rats surviving 1000R hypoxic total-body irradiation. Arch. Pathol. 66: 322-329 (1958).

L23 Lindahl, T. and B. Nyberg. Rate of depurination of native deoxyribonucleic acid. Biochem. 11: 3610-3621 (1972).

L24 Leenhouts, H.P. and K.H. Chadwick. Analysis of radiation-induced carcinogenesis using a two-stage carcinogenesis model: implications for dose-effect relationships. Radiat. Prot. Dosim. (1993, in press).

M1 McClellan, R.O., B.B. Boecker, F.F. Hahn et al. Lovelace ITRI. Studies on the toxicity of inhaled radionuclides in beagle dogs. p. 74-96 in: Lifespan Radiation Effects Studies in Animals: What Can They Tell Us? (R.C. Thompson and J.A. Mahaffey, eds.) CONF-830951. NTIS, Springfield VA, 1986.

M2 McCormick, J.J. and V.M. Maher. Mammalian cell mutagenesis as a biological consequence of DNA damage. p. 739-749 in: DNA Repair Mechanisms. (P.C. Hanawalt et al., eds.) Academic Press, New York, 1978.

M3 McCormick, J.J. and V.M. Maher. Towards an understanding of the malignant transformation of diploid human fibroblasts. Mutat. Res. 199: 273-291 (1988).

M4 McWilliams, R.S., W.G. Cross, J.G. Kaplan et al. Rapid rejoining of DNA strand breaks in resting human lymphocytes after irradiation by low doses of Co-60 γ rays or 14.6-MeV neutrons. Radiat. Res. 94: 499-507 (1983).

M5 Maisin, J.R., A. Wambersie, G.B. Gerber et al. The effects of a fractionated gamma irradiation on life shortening and disease incidence in BALB/c mice. Radiat. Res. 94: 359-373 (1983).

M6 Moolgavkar, S.H., F.T. Cross, G. Luebeck et al. A Two-mutation model for radon-induced lung tumours in rats. Radiat. Res. 121: 28-37 (1990).

M7 Mendonca, M.S., W. Kurohara, R. Antoniono et al. Plating efficiency as a function of time post-irradiation: evidence for the delayed expression of lethal mutations. Radiat. Res. 119: 387-393 (1989).

M8 Miller, R.C. and E.J. Hall. X-ray dose fractionation and oncogenic transformations in cultured mouse embryo cells. Nature 272: 58-60 (1978).

M9 Miller, R.C., E.J. Hall and H.H. Rossi. Oncogenic transformation of mammalian cells in vitro with split doses of x-rays. Proc. Natl. Acad. Sci. (USA) 76: 5755-5758 (1979).

M10 Miller, R.W. Highlights in clinical discoveries relating to ataxia-telangiectasia. p. 13-21 in: Ataxia-Telangiectasia: A Cellular and Molecular Link Between Cancer, Neuropathology and Immune Deficiency. (B.A. Bridges and D.G. Harnden, eds.) Wiley and Sons, Chichester, 1982.

M11 Miller, R.C., D.J. Brenner, C.R. Geard et al. Oncogenic transformation by fractionated doses of neutrons. Radiat. Res. 114: 589-598 (1988).

M12 Miller, R.C., C.R. Geard, D.J. Brenner et al. The effects of temporal distribution of dose on neutron-induced transformation. p. 357-362 in: Cell Transformation and Radiation Induced Cancer. (K.H. Chadwick et al., eds.) Adam Hilger, Bristol, 1989.

M13 Mole, R.H. and I.R. Major. Myeloid leukaemia frequency after protracted exposure to ionizing radiation: experimental confirmation of the flat dose-response found in ankylosing spondylitis after a single treatment course with X rays. Leuk. Res. 7: 295 (1983).

M14 Mole, R.H. Dose-response relationships. p. 403-420 in: Radiation Carcinogenesis: Epidemiology and Biological Significance. (J.D. Boice Jr. and J.F. Fraumeni Jr., eds.) Raven Press, New York, 1984.

M15 Morgan, W.F., M.C. Djordjevic, R.F. Jostes et al. Delayed repair of DNA single strand breaks does not increase cytogenetic damage. Int. J. Radiat. Biol. 48: 711-721 (1985).

M16 Morgan, G.R., C.J. Roberts and P.D. Holt. The influence of dose-rate on the biological effect of low doses of radiation. p. 129 in: Proceedings of the 8th International Congress of Radiation Research (Abstract), Edinburgh, 1987. Volume 1. (E.M. Fielden et al., eds.) Taylor and Francis, London, 1987.

M17 Miller, R.C., G. Randers-Pehrson, L. Hieber et al. The inverse dose-rate effect for oncogenic transformation by charged particles is dependent on linear energy transfer. Radiat. Res. 133: 360-364 (1993).

M18 Matsuda, Y., I. Tobari, J. Yamagiwa et al. Dose-response relationship of γ-ray induced reciprocal translocations at low doses in spermatogonia of the crab-eating monkey (Macaca fascicularis). Mutat. Res. 151: 121-127 (1985).

M19 Maisin, J.R., G.B. Gerber, M. Lambeit-Collier et al. Chemical protection against long-term effects of whole-body exposure of mice to ionizing radiation. III. The effects of fractionated exposure to C57B1 mice. Radiat. Res. 82: 487-497 (1980).

M20 Maisin, J.R., A. Wambersie, G.B. Gerber et al. Life-shortening and disease incidence in C57B1 mice after single and fractionated γ and high-energy neutron exposure. Radiat. Res. 113: 300-317 (1988).

M21 Metalli, P., G. Silini, S. Casillo et al. Induction of tumours and leukaemia by split doses of X-rays. p. 277-288 in: Radiation-Induced Cancer. STI/PUB/228. IAEA, Vienna, 1969.

M22 Mole, R.H. Patterns of response to whole body irradiation: the effects of dose intensity and exposure time on duration of life and tumour production. Br. J. Radiol. 32: 497-501 (1959).

M23 Mole, R.H. and A.M. Thomas. Life-shortening in female CBA mice exposed to daily irradiation for limited periods of time. Int. J. Radiat. Biol. 3: 493-508 (1961).

M24 Morlier, J.P., M. Morin, J. Chameaud et al. Importance du rôle du débit de dose sur l'apparition des cancers chez le rat après inhalation de radon. C.R. Acad. Sci., Ser. 3 (315): 436-466 (1992)

M25 Maisin, J.R., G.B. Gerber, A. Wambersie et al. Life-span shortening and disease incidence in male BALB/c and C57Bl mice after single, fractionated d(50)-Be neutron or gamma exposure. p. 172-183 in: Lifespan Radiation Effects Studies in Animals: What Can They Tell Us? (R.C. Thompson and J.A. Mahaffey, eds.) CONF-830951. NTIS, Springfield VA, 1986.

M26 Milo, G.E. and J.A. Di Paolo. Neoplastic transformation of human diploid cells in vitro after chemical carcinogen treatment. Nature 275: 130-132 (1978).

M27 Michalik, V. Particle track structure and its correlation with radiobiological endpoint. Phys. Med. Biol. 36: 1001-1012 (1991).

M28 Miller, R.C., D.J. Brenner, G. Randers-Pehrson et al. The effects of the temporal distribution of dose on oncogenic transformation by neutrons and charged particles of intermediate LET. Radiat. Res. 124: S62-S68 (1990).

M29 Morin, M., R. Masse and J. Lafuma. Rôle de l'âge au moment de l'irradiation sur l'induction des tumeurs. C.R. Acad. Sci., Ser. 3 (312): 629-634 (1991).

M30 Mitchell, J.B., J.S. Bedford and S.K. Bailey. Dose rate effects in mammalian cells in culture. III. Comparison of cell killing and cell proliferation during continuous irradiation for six different cell lines. Radiat. Res. 79: 537-551 (1979).

M31 Mothersill, C., C.B. Seymour and M. Moriarty. Development of radiation transformation systems for epithelial cells - problems and perspectives. p. 414-422 in: Low Dose Radiation: Biological Bases of Risk Assessment. (K.F. Baverstock and J.W. Stather, eds.) Taylor and Francis, London, 1989.

M32 Miller, A.B., G.R. Howe, G.J. Sherman et al. Mortality from breast cancer after irradiation during fluoroscopic examinations in patients being treated for tuberculosis. N. Engl. J. Med. 321: 1285-1289 (1989).

M33 Marples, B. and M. Joiner. Cell survival at very low radiation doses. p. 53-55 in: Gray Laboratory Annual Report. Cancer Research Campaign, London, 1989.

M34 Marshall, J.H. and P.G. Groer. A theory of the induction of bone cancer by alpha radiation. Radiat. Res. 71: 149-192 (1977).

M35 Marshall, J.H. and P.G. Groer. Theory of the induction of bone cancer by radiation. II. A possible low-lying linear component in the induction of (bone) cancer by alpha radiation. p. 110-144 in: Radiological and Environmental Research Division, Annual Report. ANL-77-65 (1977).

M36 Muirhead, C.R., R. Cox, J.W. Stather et al. Estimates of late radiation risks to the UK population. Documents of the NRPB, Volume 4(4) (1993).

M37 Moolgavkar, S.H. and D.J. Venson. Two event models for carcinogenesis: incidence curves for childhood and adult tumours. Math. Biosci. 47: 55-77 (1979).

M38 Moolgavkar, S.H. and A.G. Knudsen. Mutation and cancer: a model for human carcinogenesis. J. Natl. Cancer Inst. 66: 1037-1052 (1981).

M39 Moolgavkar, S.H. Model for human carcinogenesis: action of environmental agents. Environ. Health Perspect. 50: 285-291 (1983).

M40 Müller, W.A., A. Luz, B. Murray et al. The effect of dose protraction with a very low radium-224 activity in mice. p. 32-36 in: Risks From Radium and Thorotrast. BIR Report 21. (D.M. Taylor, C.W. Mays, G.B. Gerber et al., eds.) British Institute of Radiology, London, 1989.

M41 Moolgavkar, S.H. Hormones and multistage carcinogenesis. Cancer Surveys 5: 635-648 (1986).

M42 Moolgavkar, S.H. A two-stage carcinogenesis model for risk assessment. Cell Biol. Toxicol. 5: 445-460 (1989).

M43 Morin, M., R. Masse and J. Lafuma. Effects de cancérogènes de l'irradiation gamma à faible débit de dose. C.R. Acad. Sci., Ser. 3 (311): 459-466 (1990).

M44 Mole, R.M. Some aspects of mammalian radiobiology. Radiat. Res. (Suppl.) 1: 124-148 (1959).

M45 Maisin, J.R., A. Decleve, G.B. Gerber et al. Chemical protection against the long-term effects of a single whole-body exposure of mice to ionizing radiation. II. Causes of death. Radiat. Res. 74: 415-435 (1978).

M46 Miller, C.E. and E.J. Hall. Oncogenic transformation of C3H10T½ cells by acute and protracted exposures to monoenergetic neutrons. Radiat. Res. 128: S60-S64 (1991).

M47 Maisin, J.R., A. Wambersie, G.B. Gerber et al. Life-shortening and disease incidence in mice after exposure to gamma rays of high-energy neutrons. Radiat. Res. 128: S117-S123 (1991).

M48 Matsuda, Y. and I. Tobari. Repair capacity of fertilized mouse eggs for X-ray damage induced in sperm and mature oocytes. Mutat. Res. 210: 35-47 (1989).

M49 Matsuda, Y., N. Seki, T. Utsugi-Takeuchi et al. X-ray- and mitomycin C (MMC)-induced chromosome aberrations in spermiogenic germ cells and the repair capacity of mouse eggs for the X-ray and MMC damage. Mutat. Res. 211: 65-75 (1989).

M50 Matsuda, Y., N. Seki, T. Utsugi-Takeuchi et al. Changes in X-ray sensitivity of mouse eggs from fertilization to the early pronuclear stage and their repair capacity. Int. J. Radiat. Biol. 55: 233-256 (1989).

M51 Matsuda, Y., M. Maemori and I. Tobari. Relationship between cell cycle stage in the fertilized egg of mice and repair capacity for X-ray-induced damage in the sperm. Int. J. Radiat. Biol. 56: 301-314 (1989).

N1 National Council on Radiation Protection and Measurements. Influence of dose and its distribution in time on dose-response relationships for low-LET radiation. NCRP Report No. 64 (1980).

N2 National Council on Radiation Protection and Measurements. Induction of thyroid cancer by ionizing radiation. NCRP Report No. 80 (1985).

N3 Neary, G.J. Aging and radiation. Nature 187: 10-18 (1960).

N4 Neary, G.J. Aging and radiation. Am. Heart J. 62: 433-435 (1961).

N5 Namba, M., K. Nishitani, T. Kimoto et al. Multistep neoplastic transformation of normal human fibroblasts and its genetic aspects. p. 67-74 in: Cell Transformation and Radiation Induced Cancer. (K.H. Chadwick, et al., eds.) Adam Hilger, Bristol, 1989.

N6 Nakamura, N. and S. Okada. Dose-rate effects of gamma-ray-induced mutations in cultured mammalian cells. Radiat. Res. 83: 127-135 (1983).

N7 Nakamura, N. and S. Okada. Mutations induced by low doses of gamma-rays with different dose rates in cultured mouse lymphoma cells. paper B-248 in: Proceedings of the 7th International Congress of Radiation Research, Amsterdam, 1983. Martinus Nijhoff, Amsterdam, 1983.

N8 Neyman, J. and E. Scott. Statistical aspects of the problem of carcinogenesis. p. 745-776 in: Fifth Berkeley Symposium on Mathematical Statistics and Probability. University of California Press, Berkeley, 1967.

N9 National Council on Radiation Protection and Measurements. The relative biological effectiveness of radiations of different quality. NCRP Report No. 104 (1990).

N10 Nikjoo, H. Track structure analysis illustrating the prominent role of low-energy electrons in radiobiological effects of low-LET radiations. Phys. Med. Biol. 36: 229-238 (1991).

O1 Otsu, H., M. Yasukawa and T. Terasima. In vitro properties and tumorigenicity of radiation-transformed clones of mouse 10T½ cells. J. Radiat. Res. 24: 118-130 (1983).

O2 Oftedal, P. A theoretical study of mutant yield and cell killing after treatment of heterogeneous cell populations. Hereditas 60: 177-210 (1968).

O3 Oftedal, P. A holistic view of low-level radiation effects in biological systems. Can. J. Phys. 68: 974-978 (1990).

O4 Olivieri, G.J. and S. Wolff. Adaptive response of human lymphocytes to low concentrations of radioactive thymidine. Science 223: 594-597 (1984).

O5 Ootsuyama, A. and H. Tanooka. One hundred percent tumor induction in mouse skin after repeated β irradiation in a limited dose range. Radiat. Res. 115: 488-494 (1988).

O6 Ootsuyama, A. and H. Tanooka. Induction of osteosarcomas in mouse lumbar vertebrae by repeated β irradiation. Cancer Res. 49: 1562-1564 (1989).

O7 Ootsuyama, A. and H. Tanooka. Threshold-like dose of local β irradiation repeated throughout the life span of mice for induction of skin and bone tumours. Radiat. Res. 125: 98-101 (1991).

P1 Paretzke, H.G. Physical aspects of radiation quality. p. 514-522 in: Low Dose Radiation: Biological Bases of Risk Assessment. (K.F. Baverstock and J.W. Stather, eds.) Taylor and Francis, London, 1989.

P2 Pierce, D.A. and M. Vaeth. The shape of the cancer mortality dose-response curve for atomic bomb survivors. RERF TR/7-89 (1989).

P3 Pierce, D.A. and M. Vaeth. Cancer risk estimation from the A-bomb survivors: extrapolation to low doses, use of relative risk models and other uncertainties. p. 54-69 in: Low Dose Radiation: Biological Bases of Risk Assessment. (K.F. Baverstock and J.W. Stather, eds.) Taylor and Francis, London, 1989.

P4 Preston, D.L. and D.A. Pierce. The effect of changes in dosimetry on cancer mortality risk estimates in the atomic bomb survivors. RERF TR/9-87 (1987).

P5 Purrott, R.J. and E. Reeder. Chromosome aberration yields in human lymphocytes induced by fractionated doses of x radiation. Mutat. Res. 34: 437-446 (1976).

P6 Phillips, R.J.S. A comparison of mutation induced by acute x and chronic gamma irradiation in mice. Br. J. Radiol. 34: 261-264 (1961).

P7 Pohlit, W. Interaction of energy depositions and primary radiation lesions along a particle track and between different tracks. Radiat. Prot. Dosim. 13: 271-273 (1985).

P8 Pohl-Ruling, J. Chromosome aberrations in man in areas with elevated natural radioactivity. p. 103-111 in: Berzelius Symposium XV. Umea, Sweden, 1989.

P9 Paretzke, H.G. Radiation track structure theory. p. 89-170 in: Kinetics of Nonhomogeneous Processes. (G.R. Freeman, ed.) Wiley and Sons, New York, 1987.

P10 Paretzke, H.G. Biophysical models of radiation action-development of simulation codes. p. 17-32 in: The Early Effects of Radiation on DNA. (E.M. Fielden and P. O'Neill, eds.) Springer-Verlag, Heidelberg, 1991.

P11 Polig, E., W.S.S. Jee, R.B. Setterberg et al. Local dosimetry of ^{226}Ra in the trabecular skeleton of the Beagle. Radiat. Res. 131: 24-34 (1992).

R1 Rauth, A.M. Radiation carcinogenesis. p. 106 in: The Basic Science of Oncology. (I.F. Tannock and R.P. Hall, eds.) Pergamon Press, Oxford, 1987.

R2 Redpath, J.C., C. Sun, M. Mendonca et al. The application of a human hybrid cell system to studies of radiation-induced cell transformation: quantitative cellular and molecular aspects. p. 85-90 in: Cell Transformation and Radiation Induced Cancer. (K.H. Chadwick et al., eds.) Adam Hilger, Bristol 1989.

R3 Robinson, V.C. and A.C. Upton. Computing-risk analysis of leukaemia and non-leukaemia mortality in x-irradiated male RF mice. J. Natl. Cancer Inst. 60: 995-1007 (1978).

R4 Roesch, W.C. (ed.). US-Japan Joint Reassessment of Atomic Bomb Radiation Dosimetry in Hiroshima and Nagasaki, Final Report. RERF (1987).

R5 Rossi, H.H. and A.M. Kellerer. The dose rate dependence of oncogenic transformation by neutrons may be due to variation of response during the cell cycle. Int. J. Radiat. Biol. 50: 353-361 (1986).

R6 Russell, W.L., L.B. Russell and E.M. Kelly. Radiation dose rate and mutation frequency. Science 128: 1546-1550 (1958).

R7 Russell, W.L. The effect of radiation dose rate and fractionation on mutation in mice. p. 205-217 in: Repair from Genetic Radiation Damage. (F.H. Sobels, ed.) Pergamon Press, New York, 1963.

R8 Russell, W.L. Studies in mammalian radiation genetics. Nucleonics 23: 53 (1965).

R9 Russ, S. and G.M. Scott. Biological effects of gamma-radiation (II). Br. J. Radiol. 12: 440-441 (1939).

R10 Rossi, H.H. The effects of small doses of ionizing radiation: fundamental biophysical characteristics. Radiat. Res. 71: 1-8 (1977).

R11 Russell, W.L. and E.M. Kelly. Mutation frequencies in male mice and the estimation of genetic hazards of radiation in man. Proc. Natl. Acad. Sci. (USA) 79: 542-544 (1982).

R12 Radford, I.R., G.S. Hodgson and J.P. Matthews. Critical DNA target size model of radiation-induced mammalian cell death. Int. J. Radiat. Biol. 54: 63-79 (1988).

R13 Redpath, J.L., C.K. Hill, C.A. Jones et al. Fission-neutron-induced expression of a tumour-associated antigen in human cell hybrids (HeLa x skin fibroblasts): evidence for increased expression at low dose rate. Int. J. Radiat. Biol. 58: 673-680 (1990).

R14 Rossi, H.H. Microscopic energy distribution in irradiated matter. p. 43 in: Radiation Dosimetry. Volume 1. (F.H. Atix and W.C. Roesch, eds.) Academic Press, New York, 1968.

R15 Rossi, H.H. Microdosimetry and radiobiology. Radiat. Prot. Dosim. 13: 259-265 (1985).

R16 Redpath, J.L., C. Sun and W.F. Blakey. Effect of fission-neutron dose rate on the induction of a tumour-associated antigen in human cell hybrids. Radiat. Res. 128: S71-S74 (1991).

R17 Russell, W.L. and E.M. Kelly. Specific-locus mutation frequencies in mouse stem-cell spermatogonia at very low radiation dose rates. Proc. Natl. Acad. Sci. (USA) 79: 539-541 (1982).

R18 Russell, W.L. and E.M. Kelly. Mutation frequencies in female mice and the estimation of genetic hazards or radiation in women. Proc. Natl. Acad. Sci. (USA) 74: 3523-3527 (1977).

R19 Russell, W.L. The genetic effects of radiation. p. 487-500 in: Peaceful Uses of Atomic Energy. STI/PUB/300, Volume 13. IAEA, Vienna, 1972.

S1 Sacher, G.A. and D. Grahn. Survival of mice under duration-of-life exposure to gamma rays. I. The dosage - survival relation and the lethality function. J. Natl. Cancer Inst. 32: 277 (1964).

S2 Seymour, C.B., C. Mothersill and T. Alper. High yields of lethal mutations in somatic mammalian cells that survive ionizing radiation. Int. J. Radiat. Biol. 50: 167-179 (1986).

S3 Shadley, J. and S. Wolff. Very low doses of x-rays can cause human lymphocytes to become less susceptible to ionizing radiation. Mutagenesis 2:95-96 (1987).

S4 Shellabarger, C.J., V.P. Bond and E.P. Cronkite. Studies on radiation-induced mammary gland neoplasia in the rat. VIII. The effect of fractionation and protraction of sublethal total-body irradiation. Radiat. Res. 17: 101-109 (1962).

S5 Shellabarger, C.J., V.P. Bond, G.E. Aponte et al. Results of fractionation and protraction of total-body radiation on rat mammary neoplasia. Cancer Res. 26: 509-513 (1966).

S6 Shellabarger, C.J., V.P. Bond, E.P. Cronkite et al. Relationship of dose of total-body ^{60}Co radiation to incidence of mammary neoplasia in female rats. p. 161-172 in: Radiation-Induced Cancer. STI/PUB/228. IAEA, Vienna, 1969.

S7 Shellabarger, C.J. Modifying factors in rat mammary gland carcinogenesis. p. 31 in: Biology of Radiation Carcinogenesis. (J.M. Yuhas et al., eds.) Raven Press, New York, 1976.

S8 Shellabarger, C.J., J.P. Stone and S. Holtzman. Experimental carcinogenesis in the breast. p. 169-180 in: Radiation Carcinogenesis. (A.C. Upton et al., eds.) Elsevier, New York, 1986.

S9 Shimizu, Y., H. Kato, W.J. Schull et al. Life Span Study Report II, Part I: Comparison of risk coefficients for site-specific cancer mortality based on the DS86 and T65DR shielded kerma and organ doses. RERF TR/12-87 (1987).

S10 Shimizu, Y., H. Kato and W.J. Schull. Life Span Study Report II, Part II: Cancer mortality in the years 1950-1985 based on the recently revised doses (DS86). RERF TR/5-88 (1988).

S11 Shore, R.E., E. Woodard, N. Hildreth et al. Thyroid tumours following thymus irradiation. J. Natl. Cancer Inst. 74: 1177-1184 (1985).

S12 Sinclair, W.K. Experimental RBE's of high-LET radiations at low doses and the implications for quality factor assignment. Radiat. Prot. Dosim. 13: 319-326 (1985).

S13 Storer, J.B., L.J. Serrano, E.B. Darden et al. Life shortening in RFM and BALB/c mice as a function of radiation quality, dose and dose rate. Radiat. Res. 78: 122-161 (1979).

S14 Strniste, G.F. and D.J. Chen. Genotoxicity of chronic, low doses of low- or high-LET radiation in human cells. p. 39 in: Abstracts of Papers for Thirty-third Annual Meeting of the Radiation Research Society. Radiation Research Society, Philadelphia, 1985.

S15 Shellabarger, C.J. and R.D. Brown. Rat mammary neoplasia following Co-60 irradiation at 0.3R or 10R per minute. Radiat. Res. 51: 493-494 (1972).

S16 Silini, G. and P. Metalli. Preliminary results from a split dose experiment on late effects of ionizing radiation in the mouse. Data on life span shortening. p. 207-215 in: Radiation and Aging. (P.J. Lindop and G.A. Sacher, eds.) Taylor and Francis, London, 1966.

S17 Spalding, J.F., J.R. Prine and G.L. Tietjen. Late biological effects of ionizing radiation as influenced by dose, dose rate, age at exposure and genetic sensitivity to neoplastic transformation. p. 3-11 in: Late Biological Effects of Ionizing Radiation. Volume II. STI/PUB/489. IAEA, Vienna, 1978.

S18 Sacher, G.A. A comparative analysis of radiation lethality in mammals exposed at constant average intensity for the duration of life. J. Natl. Cancer Inst. 15: 1125-1144 (1955).

S19 Storer, J.B. Radiation carcinogenesis. p. 453-483 in: Cancer. Volume I. (F.F. Becker, ed.) Plenum Publishing Co., New York, 1975.

S20 Sanders, C.L., K.E. Lauhala and K.E. McDonald. Life-span studies in rats exposed to $^{239}PuO_2$ aerosol. III. Survival and lung tumors. Int. J. Radiat. Biol. (1993, in press).

S21 Stanbridge, E.J. An argument for using human cells in the study of the molecular genetic basis of cancer. p. 1-9 in: Cell Transformation and Radiation Induced Cancer. (K.H. Chadwick et al., eds.) Adam Hilger, Bristol, 1989.

S22 Shin, C., L.C. Padhy and R.A. Weinberg. Transforming genes of carcinomas and neuroblastomas introduced into mouse fibroblasts. Nature 290: 261-264 (1981).

S23 Stevens, C., W.H. Brondyk, A. Burgess et al. Partially transformed anchorage-independent human diploid fibroblasts resulting from over-expression of the c-sis oncogene: mitogenic activity of an apparent mononeric platelet - derived growth factor 2 species. Mol. Cell. Biol. 8: 2089-2096 (1988).

S24 Suzuki, M., M. Watanabe, K. Suzuki et al. Neoplastic cell transformation by heavy ions. Radiat. Res. 120: 468-476 (1989).

S25 Suzaki, N. and S. Okada. Gamma-ray mutagenesis of cultured mammalian cells in vitro and in vivo. Mutat. Res. 43: 81-90 (1977).

S26 Searle, A.G. Mutation induction in mice. Adv. Radiat. Biol. 4: 131-207 (1974).

S27 Storer, J.B. and R.L. Ullrich. Life shortening in BALB/c mice following brief, protracted or fractionated exposures to neutrons. Radiat. Res. 96: 335-347 (1983).

S28 Stather, J.W. Effects of α-particle irradiation on carcinogenesis. Int. J. Radiat. Biol. 58: 871-874 (1990).

S29 Sanders, C.L. and J.A. Mahaffey. Inhalation carcinogenesis of high-fired $^{244}CmO_2$ in rats. Radiat. Res. 76: 384-401 (1978).

S30 Sanders, C.L. and J.A. Mahaffey. Inhalation carcinogenesis of repeated exposures to high-fired $^{239}PuO_2$. Health Phys. 41: 629-644 (1981).

S31 Stather, J.W., C.R. Muirhead, A.A. Edwards et al. Health effects models developed from the UNSCEAR 1988 Report. NRPB-R226 (1988).

S32 Sanderson, B.J.S. and A.A. Morley. Exposure of human lymphocytes to ionizing radiation reduces mutagenesis by subsequent ionizing radiation. Mutat. Res. 164: 347-351 (1986).

S33 Storer, J.B. Radiation resistance with age in normal and irradiated populations of mice. Radiat. Res. 25: 435-459 (1965).

S34 Scott, B.R. and E.J. Ainsworth. State-vector model for life shortening in mice after brief exposure to low doses of ionizing radiation. Math. Biosci. 49: 185-205 (1980).

S35 Saran, A., S. Pazzaglia, M. Coppola et al. Absence of a dose-fractionation effect on neoplastic transformation induced by fission-spectrum neutrons in C3H10T½ cells. Radiat. Res. 126: 343-348 (1991).

S36 Sarahan, A., S. Pazzaglia, M. Coppola et al. Neoplastic transformation of C3H10T½ cells by fractionated doses of monoenergetic neutrons. p. 437 in: Radiation Research: A Twentieth Century Perspective. Volume 1. (J.D. Chapman et al., eds.) Academic Press, San Diego, 1991.

S37 Sato, F., S. Sasaki, N. Kawashima et al. Late effects of whole or partial body X-irradiation on mice: life shortening. Int. J. Radiat. Biol. 39: 607-615 (1981).

S38 Selby, P.B., S.S. Lee, E.M. Kelly et al. Specific-locus experiments show that female mice exposed near the time of birth to low-LET ionizing radiation exhibit both a low mutational response and a dose rate effect. Mutat. Res. 249: 351-367 (1991).

S39 Shapiro, R. Damage to DNA caused by hydrolysis. p. 3-18 in: Chromosome Damage and Repair. (E. Seeberg and K. Kleepe, eds.) Plenum Press, New York, 1981.

S40 Sànchez-Reyes, A. A simple model of repair action based on repair saturation mechanism. Radiat. Res. 130: 139-147 (1992).

S41 Sedgewick, S.G. Inducible DNA repair in microbes. Microbiol. Sci. 3: 76-83 (1986).

S42 Savage, J.R.K. and M. Holloway. Induction of sister chromatid exchanges in d(42 MeV)-Be neutrons in unstimulated human blood lymphocytes. Br. J. Radiol. 61: 231-234 (1988).

S43 Sanders, C.L., K.E. McDonald and J.A. Mahaffey. Lung tumour response to inhaled Pu and its implications for radiation protection. Health Phys. 55: 455-462 (1988).

S44 Sanders, C.L., G.E. Dagle, W.C. Cannon et al. Inhalation carcinogenesis of high-fired $^{239}PuO_2$ in rats. Radiat. Res. 68: 349-360 (1976).

S45 Shore, R.E., N. Hildreth, E. Woodard et al. Breast cancer among women given X-ray therapy for acute postpartum mastitis. J. Natl. Cancer Inst. 77: 689-696 (1986).

T1 Terasima, T., M. Yasukawa and M. Kimura. Neoplastic transformation of plateau-phase mouse 10T½ cells following single and fractionated doses of x rays. Radiat. Res. 102: 367-377 (1985).

T2 Thacker, J. and A. Stretch. Recovery from lethal and mutagenic damage during post-irradiation holding and low-dose-rate irradiation of cultured hamster cells. Radiat. Res. 96: 380-392 (1983).

T3 Thacker, J. and A. Stretch. Responses of 4 x-ray sensitive CHO cell mutants to different radiations and to irradiation conditions promoting cellular recovery. Mutat. Res. 146: 99-108 (1985).

T4 Thacker, J. Inherited sensitivity to x-rays in man. Bio. Essays 11: 58-62 (1989).

T5 Thacker, J. The measurement of radiation-induced mutation in mammalian cells at low doses and dose rates. Adv. Radiat. Biol. 16: 77-124 (1992).

T6 Thames, H.D. and J.H. Hendry. Fractionation in Radiotherapy. Taylor and Francis, London, 1987.

T7 Thomson, J.F., F.S. Williamson, D. Grahn et al. Life shortening in mice exposed to fission neutrons and γ-rays. II. Duration-of-life and long-term fractionated exposures. Radiat. Res. 86: 573-579 (1981).

T8 Thomson, J.F. and D. Grahn. Life shortening in mice exposed to fission neutrons and γ rays. Radiat. Res. 118: 151-160 (1989).

T9 Tobari, I., Y. Matsuda, G. Xiaohung et al. Dose-response relationship for translocation induction in spermatogonia of the crab-eating monkey (Macaca fascicularis) by chronic γ ray irradiation. Mutat. Res. 201: 81-87 (1988).

T10 Thomson, J.F., F.S. Williamson, D. Grahn et al. Life shortening in mice exposed to fission neutrons and γ rays. I. Single and short-term fractionated exposures. Radiat. Res. 86: 559-572 (1981).

T11 Tanooka, H. and A. Ootsuyama. Threshold-like dose response of mouse skin cancer induction for repeated beta irradiation and its relevance to radiation-induced human skin cancer. Recent Results Cancer Res. 128: 231-241 (1993).

T12 Thomson, J.F. and D. Grahn. Life shortening in mice exposed to fission neutrons and γ rays. VII. Effects of 60 once-weekly exposures. Radiat. Res. 115: 347-360 (1988).

T13 Terasima, T., M. Yasukawa and M. Kimura. Radiation-induced transformation of 10T½ mouse cells in the plateau phase: post-irradiation changes and serum dependence. GANN Monogr. Cancer Res. 72: 762-768 (1981).

T14 Terzaghi-Howe, M. Induction of preneoplastic alternations by x-rays and neutrons in exposed rat tracheas and isolated tracheal epithelial cells. Radiat. Res. 120: 352-363 (1989).

T15 Thomson, J.F., F.S. Williamson and D. Grahn. Life shortening in mice exposed to fission neutrons and γ rays. V. Further studies with single low doses. Radiat. Res. 104: 420-428 (1985).

T16 Thacker, J., R.E. Wilkinson and D.T. Goodhead. The induction of chromosome exchange aberrations by carbon ultrasoft x-rays in V79 hamster cells. Int. J. Radiat. Biol. 49: 645-656 (1986).

T17 Thacker, J. The involvement of repair processes in radiation-induced mutation of cultured mammalian cells. p. 612-620 in: Proceedings of the 6th International Congress of Radiation Research, Tokyo, 1979. (M. Okado et al., eds.) Toppan, Tokyo, 1979.

T18 Thomson, J.F., F.S. Williamson and D. Grahn. Life shortening in mice exposed to fission neutrons and x-rays. III. Neutron exposures of 5 and 10 rad. Radiat. Res. 93: 205-209 (1983).

T19 Thompson, R.C. Life-span effects of ionizing radiation in the beagle dog. PNL-6822 (1989).

T20 Teoule, R. Radiation-induced DNA damage and its repair. Int. J. Radiat. Biol. 51: 573-589 (1987).

T21 Tobias, C.A., E.A. Blakely, F.Q.H. Ngo et al. The repair-misrepair model of cell survival. p. 195-230 in: Radiation Biology in Cancer Research. (R.E. Meyn and H.R. Withers, eds.) Raven Press, New York, 1980.

T22 Tatsumi, K. and H. Takebe. γ-irradiation induces mutation in ataxia-telangiectasia lymphoblastoid cells. GANN Monogr. Cancer Res. 75: 1040-1043 (1984).

U1 United Nations. Sources, Effects and Risks of Ionizing Radiation. United Nations Scientific Committee on the Effects of Atomic Radiation, 1988 Report to the General Assembly, with annexes. United Nations sales publication E.88.IX.7. United Nations, New York, 1988.

U2 United Nations. Genetic and Somatic Effects of Ionizing Radiation. United Nations Scientific Committee on the Effects of Atomic Radiation, 1986 Report to the General Assembly, with annexes. United Nations sales publication E.86.IX.9. United Nations, New York, 1986.

U3 United Nations. Ionizing Radiation: Sources and Biological Effects. United Nations Scientific Committee on the Effects of Atomic Radiation, 1982 Report to the General Assembly, with annexes. United Nations sales publication E.82.IX.8. United Nations, New York, 1982.

U4 United Nations. Sources and Effects of Ionizing Radiation. United Nations Scientific Committee on the Effects of Atomic Radiation, 1977 report to the General Assembly, with annexes. United Nations sales publication E.77.IX.1. United Nations, New York, 1977.

U5 United Nations. Ionizing Radiation: Levels and Effects. Report of the United Nations Scientific Committee on the Effects of Atomic Radiation, with annexes. United Nations sales publication E.72.IX.17 and 18. United Nations, New York, 1972.

U11 Ullrich, R.L., M.C. Jernigan, G.E. Cosgrove et al. The influence of dose and dose rate on the incidence of neoplastic disease in RFM mice after neutron irradiation. Radiat. Res. 68: 115-131 (1976).

U12 Ullrich, R.L. and J.B. Storer. Influence of dose, dose rate and radiation quality on radiation carcinogenesis and life shortening in RFM and BALB/c mice. p. 95-113 in: Late Biological Effects of Ionizing Radiation. Volume II. STI/PUB/489. IAEA, Vienna, 1978.

U13 Ullrich, R.C. and J.B. Storer. Influence of γ irradiation on the development of neoplastic disease in mice. I. Reticular tissue tumours. Radiat. Res. 80: 303-316 (1979).

U14 Ullrich, R.L. and J.B. Storer. Influence of γ irradiation on the development of neoplastic disease in mice. II. Solid tumours. Radiat. Res. 80: 317-324 (1979).

U15 Ullrich, R.C. and J.B. Storer. Influence of γ irradiation on the development of neoplastic disease in mice. III. Dose-rate effects. Radiat. Res. 80: 325-342 (1979).

U16 Ullrich, R.L. Tumour induction in BALB/c mice after fractionated or protracted exposures to fission spectrum neutrons. Radiat. Res. 97: 587-597 (1984).

U17 Ullrich, R.L. The rate of progression of radiation transformed mammary epithelial cells as enhanced after low dose rate neutron irradiation. Radiat. Res. 105: 68-75 (1986).

U18 Upton, A.C., F.F. Wolff, J. Furth et al. A comparison of the induction of myeloid leukaemias in x-irradiated RF mice. Cancer Res. 18: 842-848 (1958).

U19 Upton, A.C., V.K. Jenkins and J.W. Conklin. Myeloid leukaemia in the mouse. Ann. N.Y. Acad. Sci. 114: 189 (1964).

U20 Upton, A.C., V.K. Jenkins, H.E. Walburg et al. Observation on viral, chemical and radiation-induced myeloid and lymphoid leukaemia in RF mice. Natl. Cancer Inst. Monogr. 22: 229-347 (1966).

U21 Upton, A.C., M.L. Randolph and J.W. Conklin. Late effects of fast neutrons and gamma-rays in mice as influenced by the dose rate of irradiation: induction of neoplasia. Radiat. Res. 41: 467-491 (1970).

U22 Upton, A.C. Radiobiological effects of low doses. Implications for radiological protection. Radiat. Res. 71: 51-74 (1977).

U23 Upton, A.C., R.E. Albert, F.J. Burns et al. (eds.). Radiation Carcinogenesis. Elsevier, New York, 1986.

U24 Ullrich, R.L. Tumor induction in BALB/c female mice after fission neutron or γ irradiation. Radiat. Res. 93: 506-515 (1983).

U25 Ullrich, R.L. Cellular and molecular changes in mammary epithelial cells following irradiation. Radiat. Res. 128: S136-S140 (1991).

U26 Ullrich, R.L., M.C. Jernigan, L.C. Satterfield et al. Radiation carcinogenesis: time-dose relationships. Radiat. Res. 111: 179-184 (1987).

U27 Upton, A.C., A.W. Kimball, J. Furth et al. Some delayed effects of atomic-bomb radiations in mice. Cancer Res. 20: 1-62 (1960).

U28 Upton, A.C., M.L. Randolph and J.W. Conklin. Late effects of fast neutrons and gamma rays in mice as influenced by the dose rate of irradiation: life-shortening. Radiat. Res. 32: 493-509 (1967).

U29 Ueno, A.M., I. Furuno-Fukushi and H. Matsudaira. Induction of cell killing, micronuclei and mutation to 6-thioguanine resistance after exposure to low-dose-rate gamma-rays and tritiated water in cultured mammalian cells (L5178Y). Radiat. Res. 91: 447-456 (1982).

V1 van Bekkum, D.W. and P. Bentvelzen. The concept of gene transfer-misrepair mechanism of radiation carcinogenesis may challenge the linear extrapolation model of risk estimation for low radiation dose. Health Phys. 43: 231-237 (1982).

V2 Vilenchik, M.M. DNA damage and repair in aging and programmed death of cells. Int. Congr. Gerontol. Kiev 2: 40 (1972).

V3 Vilenchik, M.M. Spontaneous DNA damage and repair. p. 266-267 in: Mechanisms of DNA Damage and Repair. Biological Centre of the Academy of Sciences, Puschino, 1971.

V4 Virsik, R.P., R. Blohm, K.P. Herman et al. Fast, short-ranged and slow, distant-ranged processes involved in chromosome aberration formation. p. 943-955 in: Proceedings of the Seventh Symposium on

Microdosimetry. (J. Booz, H.G. Ebert and H.D. Hartfiel, eds.) EUR-7147 (1981).

V5 Vilenchik, M.M. Molecular Mechanisms of Aging. Nuaka, Moscow, 1970. (in Russian)

V6 Vilenchik, M.M. Initial mechanisms of "natural" and radiation-induced aging. p. 87-97 in: Uspekhi Radiobiologii. Volume 7. (A.M. Kuzin and S.N. Alexandrov, eds.) Atomizdat, Moscow, 1978.

V7 Vilenchik, M.M. Study of spontaneous DNA lesions and DNA repair in human diploid fibroblasts aged in vitro and in vivo. Stud. Biophys. 85: 53-54 (1981).

V8 Vilenchik, M.M. DNA Instability and Late Radiation Effect. Energoatomizdat, Moscow, 1987.

W1 Walinder, G., C.J. Jonsson and A.M. Sjödén. Dose-rate dependence in the goitrogen stimulated mouse thyroid: a comparative investigation of the effects of roentgen 131-I and 132-I irradiation. Acta Radiol., Ther., Phys., Biol. 11: 24-36 (1972).

W2 Walinder, G. Late effects of irradiation on the thyroid gland in mice. I. Irradiation of adult mice. Acta Radiol. Ther. Phys. Biol. 2: 433-451 (1972).

W3 Watanabe, M., M. Horikawa and O. Nikaido. Induction of oncogenic transformation by low doses of x-rays and dose rate effect. Radiat. Res. 98: 274-283 (1984).

W4 Wolff, S. Is radiation all bad? The search for adaptation. Radiat. Res. 131: 117-123 (1992).

W5 Wlodek, D. and W.N. Hittelman. The repair of double strand breaks correlates with radiosensitivity of L5178Y-S and L5178Y-R cells. Radiat. Res. 112: 146-155 (1987).

W6 Wolff, S., U. Afzal, J.K. Wiencke et al. Human lymphocytes exposed to low doses of ionizing radiations become refractory to high doses of radiation as well as chemical mutagens that induce double-strand breaks in DNA. Int. J. Radiat. Biol. 53: 39-48 (1988).

W7 Wolff, S., J.K. Wiencke, U. Afzal et al. The adaptive response of human lymphocytes to very low doses of ionizing radiation: a case of induced chromosomal repair with the induction of specific proteins. p. 446-454 in: Low Dose Radiation: Biological Bases of Risk Assessment. (K.F. Baverstock and J.W. Stather, eds.) Taylor and Francis, London, 1989.

W8 Walburg, H.E. Radiation-induced life-shortening and premature aging. Adv. Radiat. Biol. 7: 145-179 (1975).

W9 Ward, J.F. Response to commentary by D. Billen. Radiat. Res. 126: 385-387 (1991).

W10 Wheeler, K.T. and G.B. Nelson. Saturation of a DNA repair process in dividing and non-dividing mammalian cells. Radiat. Res. 109: 109-117 (1987).

W11 Williams, A.C., S. Harper and C. Paraskeva. Neoplastic transformation of a human colonic epithelial cell line; experimental evidence for the adenoma to carcinoma sequence. Cancer Res. 50: 4724-4730 (1990).

Y1 Yang, T.C., L.M. Craise, M.T. Mei et al. Dose protraction studies with low- and high-LET radiations on neoplastic cell transformation in vitro. Adv. Space Res. 6: 137-147 (1986).

Y2 Yates, J.M., R.W. Tennant and J.D. Regan. Biology of Radiation Carcinogenesis, Proceedings of a Symposium. Raven Press, New York, 1975.

Y3 Young, S. and R.C. Hallowes. Tumours of the mammary gland. p. 31-74 in: Pathology of Tumours in Laboratory Animals. Volume I. (V.S. Turosov, ed.) IARC, Lyon, 1973.

Y4 Yuhas, J.M. Recovery from radiation-carcinogenesis injury to the mouse ovary. Radiat. Res. 60: 321-332 (1974).

Y5 Yasukawa, M., T. Terasima, T. Furuse et al. In vitro neoplastic transformation by neutron beams - relative biological effectiveness and dose fractionation. J. Radiat. Res. 28: 268-273 (1987).

Z1 Zaider, M. and H.H. Rossi. Dual radiation action and the initial slope of survival curves. Radiat. Res. 104: S68-S76 (1985).

Z2 Ziegler, J.F. Helium: stopping powers and ranges in all elemental matter. The Stopping and Ranges of Ions in Matter. Volume 4. Pergamon Press, New York, 1977.

ANNEX G

Hereditary effects of radiation

CONTENTS

INTRODUCTION

1. Evaluation of the hereditary hazard associated with the exposure of human populations to ionizing radiation has been a major concern of the Committee since its inception. Many approaches have been used to formulate optimal predictions of the extent to which a given dose of ionizing radiation will increase the naturally occurring mutation rate of germ cells and of how such an increase will affect the health of future human populations. However, an extremely complex set of problems remains, and there are many questions that cannot be answered given the present state of knowledge.

2. Attempts at risk estimation entail uncertainties, in part because it has not been possible to directly confirm radiation-induced mutations in human populations. Genetic risk estimates have relied on a general knowledge of human genetics and on the extrapolation of results from animal experiments. Limited data from long-term studies on the children of radiation-

exposed parents, particularly those exposed to the atomic bombings of Hiroshima and Nagasaki, may be used to set outside limits on genetic risk estimates. These data indicate that the hereditary effects of moderate irradiation of a large human population are minimal, at least for acute exposure.

3. Progress is being made in several areas of human genetics. There have been major advances in the knowledge of non-traditional inheritance and so-called multifactorial disease in humans. Previous UNSCEAR Reports raised the question of whether, and how, to include estimates of genetic risk for multifactorial diseases. This category of disease represents a heterogeneous group for which the underlying mechanisms are poorly understood, although they clearly have a genetic component. Multifactorial diseases are related in a complex way to other risk factors and to population structure and living conditions. Radiation damage may affect the regulation of genes involved in multifactorial inheritance by many different mechanisms and may also affect the structure and function of single genes. These multifactorial diseases and non-traditional mechanisms of inheritance are discussed in this Annex in order to emphasize the complexity of human genetics and biology, as well as the difficulty of obtaining accurate risk estimates from studies of only a few well-defined disorders in animal models.

4. The understanding of human genetics on a molecular level is increasing extremely rapidly. As discussed in this Annex, new laboratory techniques allow a more precise analysis of the type of genetic damage caused by various agents, including radiation. Eventually, the sequencing and identification of every gene on every chromosome will provide a method of direct access to the effects of radiation on human genes at the molecular level. Knowledge of population genetics, gained from registries of birth defects, is improving estimates of the current incidence of serious birth defects, with which any estimate of risk from radiation may be compared.

5. The knowledge gained from the Japanese experience, from advances in human genetics, and from animal studies should allow uncertainties of risk estimates to be gradually reduced. However, as the difficulties inherent in the estimation procedures become even more apparent, there is increased uncertainty and/or inability to specify appropriate and realistic values. Practical solutions are needed. In this Annex, the complexities involved in making human risk estimates using animal models are pointed out, the best estimates of genetic risk that can be made at this time are discussed, and ways of obtaining information that could lead to more reliable genetic risk estimates are suggested.

I. GENETIC DISEASES IN HUMANS

6. Genetic diseases occur because of alterations to the structure or regulation of DNA in the cells of an organism. Genes are units of heredity, comprised of specific sequences of DNA and carried on the chromosomes and in mitochondria. Mutations (changes in DNA structure, arrangement or amount) occur spontaneously or are caused by physical or chemical agents.

7. Genetic disorders have traditionally been classified into three categories: (a) single-gene disorders, (b) chromosomal aberrations, (c) multifactorial disorders. Although many recent developments in molecular biology and new concepts relating to mechanisms of disease processes have made these distinctions less clear, the classification will be retained for the discussion that follows.

A. SINGLE-GENE DISORDERS

8. Single-gene disorders are usually recognized by their clinical manifestations, but research is now identifying many disorders on the molecular level. Disease traits occur because of mutations to the normal gene. Alleles are alternative forms of a gene at a particular locus, or position on the chromosome. There are two levels on which the genetic constitution of an individual may be considered: the genotype, or particular alleles of a given gene carried by an individual, and the phenotype, or the physical, bio-chemical or physiological characteristics determined by these alleles. These single gene defects are often called Mendelian, after Mendel, who first described these units of heredity.

9. Simple Mendelian traits are inherited by autosomal transmission (i.e. the genes for them are carried on one of the 22 pairs of autosomes, or non-sex chromosomes) or by X-linked transmission (i.e. the genes are carried on the X-chromosome). With autosomal genes, one copy of the gene is normally contributed by the mother and one by the father. X-linked genes will always come from the mother in a male (as he has received a Y-chromosome from his father), or from both parents in a female (since she has received an X-chromosome from each parent).

1. Dominant traits

10. Dominant disorders are those in which there is a clinically recognizable abnormality produced, even if only a single copy (allele) of the gene is abnormal, i.e. in the heterozygous state. On average, the autosomal dominant gene (i.e. the abnormal allele for the trait) will be transmitted to 50% of the offspring of an affected individual. Unaffected individuals will not usually carry or transmit the abnormal gene. Affected individuals will have an affected parent, except in the event of a new mutation of the gene.

11. Autosomal dominant traits are not always expressed to the same degree in all individuals who carry them. In complex genetic and environmental interactions, some members of a family may be severely affected and others only mildly so. There may even be transmitters of a dominant allele who appear phenotypically normal. To describe this phenomenon, the terms penetrance and expressivity have been developed [T9].

12. Heterogeneity is the term used to describe situations in which the same or nearly the same phenotype is produced by different mechanisms. There are many situations in which heterogeneity appears to exist. For instance, homocystinuria can produce a symptom complex that strongly resembles Marfan syndrome [B7].

13. Conversely, it is possible that two different mutations in the same gene will produce different phenotypes. This may occur when the mutations lie in different domains, or regions, of the protein product and thus affect different functions of the same protein. For example, osteogenesis imperfecta types I and II and some occurrences of Ehlers Danlos syndrome may be caused by mutations in the alpha 1 chain of type I collagen, but depending on which portion of the collagen molecule is altered, markedly different diseases occur [B7].

2. Recessive traits

14. Recessive disorders are those that are usually clinically expressed only when both copies of the gene are abnormal (homozygosity). If two different abnormal alleles of the gene are present, the individual is said to be a compound heterozygote. A recessive disorder will also be clinically expressed when there is one abnormal copy and no normal copy of the gene is present (hemizygosity). Hemizygosity occurs normally in males for the X-chromosome; this leads to disease when the single normal copy of a gene carried on the X-chromosome is lost or damaged. This is known as an X-linked disorder. Hemizygosity can also occur in autosomal genes if there is a deletion of part of the chromosome or if one of a pair of chromosomes is lost. When an autosomal recessive condition is present in a family, cases usually occur among siblings. The abnormal copy of the gene (the abnormal allele) may also be carried by other relatives, offspring and parents, but the trait or disease will appear only in the offspring of two individuals who carry the abnormal gene. This type of pairing is rare in the general population.

15. Frequently, homozygotes for autosomal recessive disorders do not reproduce, because the homozygous state of the deleterious gene reduces their biological fitness. For this reason, some autosomal recessive traits must have conferred a selective advantage on the individual during the course of evolution, otherwise the mutation would not be as prevalent in the general population as it is. A mutation may be maintained at relatively high frequency in a population by this kind of selective advantage or because of a founder effect, or because of genetic drift (see glossary) [V10].

16. Consanguineous marriages may also play a role in producing a homozygous individual for a rare autosomal recessive condition. In a consanguineous marriage, the parents of an affected individual are related (e.g. first cousins), which makes them more likely to have inherited the same abnormal allele [L5]. Some human populations have higher rates of consanguineous marriage than others.

17. Occasionally, each parent may carry two different alleles of a particular gene; in this event the offspring could inherit two differently abnormal copies of the gene. This might result in a disease characterized by a combination of the symptoms of two somewhat different diseases. Alternatively, each of the two defective alleles could compensate for the other, resulting in a normal phenotype. This is called complementation.

18. Mutations occur on a regular but unpredictable basis. They are most frequently observed as dominant mutations, since the dominant nature of the gene allows expression and immediate recognition. However, new mutations must be occurring in genes for recessively inherited traits as well. It is estimated that the mutation frequency for some genes is in the range of 1 in 30,000 to 1 in 50,000 live-born individuals, but most mutation rates are probably lower. Some human disorders, such as neurofibromatosis I, have far higher mutation frequencies (1 in 6,000). This difference in mutation frequencies may be influenced by the size of the gene, its vulnerability, its exact position on a chromosome (e.g. at a mutational hot spot) [V3, W3], or by other as yet undefined factors [V5].

3. X-linked traits

19. X-linked traits, as mentioned above, are those in which the gene producing the abnormal phenotype is located on the X-chromosome. Because males do not pass their X-chromosome on to their sons (i.e. the sons are male because they have inherited their father's Y-chromosome), there will be no male-to-male transmission of an X-linked trait in a pedigree. Females, with two X-chromosomes, may or may not manifest an abnormal phenotype for an X-linked trait, depending on whether the trait is dominant or recessive. In addition, the manner in which normal X-inactivation (lyonization) occurs may affect expression. Thus, if by chance the normal allele is on an X-chromosome that is inactivated in more than 50% of the cells, a carrier female may express some features of even a recessive disorder.

B. CHROMOSOMAL ABERRATIONS

20. Each species has a characteristic chromosomal constitution with respect to number and morphology. This is called the karyotype and can be visualized under the microscope at the stage of the cell cycle where condensation occurs. Normally, a human being carries 46 chromosomes in each somatic cell. These comprise 22 homologous pairs of autosomes and one pair of sex chromosomes. The members of a homologous pair are matched with respect to the genetic information that each carries, although they may contain different alleles of the same genes.

21. There are two types of cell division. Mitosis is the usual type that occurs as the body grows and replaces cells. Mitosis involves the precise duplication of each chromosome so that the daughter cells will be identical to the original cell in terms of genetic information. The second type of cell division is meiosis, the specialized process of producing gametes (ova and sperm). During meiosis, the diploid number of 46 chromosomes is reduced to the haploid number, in which only one copy of each chromosome pair will be present.

22. The union of the egg and the sperm at fertilization reestablishes the normal diploid number of chromosomes. Abnormal numbers of chromosomes, breaks, or rearrangements of chromosomes or of segments of them can produce major abnormalities in the affected individual. The presence of abnormal numbers of chromosomes is called aneuploidy (i.e. not euploid). Certain chromosomal rearrangements are not compatible with viability or are selected against by the growth of more vigorous normal cells during development. However, a wide variety of rearrangements (translocations, inversions etc.), breaks and extra or missing chromosome segments may be tolerated.

C. MULTIFACTORIAL AND POLYGENIC INHERITANCE

1. Determining factors

23. The terms polygenic and multifactorial refer to those traits, diseases or congenital anomalies whose development has a genetic component but whose inheritance does not follow standard Mendelian patterns for autosomal dominant, autosomal recessive, or sex-linked transmission, suggesting that more than one gene is involved. Rather, many genes acting in concert are thought to be responsible. If environmental factors appear to play a role in the development of the trait or disease, it is described as multifactorial. These so-called multifactorial disorders are a very heterogeneous group, including about 95% of conditions having a genetic predisposition. They are observed at all ages and in all human populations. Their aetiology is complex, heterogeneous and poorly understood. It is important that this term be used only when referring to a single condition or trait (e.g. clubfeet, not multiple contractures) and that all disorders due entirely to a defect in a single gene be excluded.

24. Observations suggest that there is a gradation of factors contributing to the development of a multifactorial trait and that a certain number of such factors are necessary to produce the trait. If an individual has a susceptible genotype and is exposed to a predisposing environment, the likelihood that he or she will manifest the trait depends upon the accumulation of both genetic and environmental factors beyond a certain threshold. The threshold is the point on a liability scale below which individuals are not affected and above which they are affected [F7].

25. Numerous environmental factors may affect the development of multifactorial traits. Environmental factors include the milieu in which the embryo and fetus develop, including both intrinsic and extrinsic factors such as drugs, airborne toxins, viral or bacterial agents and radiation; abnormalities of maternal metabolism, such as diabetes mellitus, malnutrition, or maternal hyperthermia, may also be a factor [F7, F8].

26. In calculating the recurrence risk for such multifactorial disorders, it is first essential to determine, along with the family pedigree and the preconceptional and prenatal history, whether there are other cases of such disorders in unrelated families who live in the same geographic area. A case cluster of this type would suggest that environmental factors may be particularly important in the aetiology of the defect [B8].

27. Human susceptibility to teratogenic or mutagenic agents, including radiation, may differ between individuals and between humans and mice. Likewise, there

are ethnic or strain differences within a single species. Cleft lip with or without cleft palate can be induced in 100% of offspring of A/J strain mice when pregnant females are treated with corticosteroids on days 11-14 of gestation. By contrast, only 20% of the offspring of C53B1/6 mice given the same treatment will have clefts [F7]. Direct comparisons between humans and mice are not possible; however, ethnic differences are known to exist for multifactorial conditions in humans.

28. Both genetic and environmental factors can influence the development of a given embryo relative to a particular threshold by acting at any point during development. When different strains of mice are crossed and interbred, the picture is further complicated by new combinations of genetic backgrounds. The same is most likely true for humans with different ethnic and genetic backgrounds.

29. Thus, in applying the mouse model to human studies, it must be borne in mind that the embryo's teratogenic (or mutagenic) susceptibility can be influenced by its normal developmental patterns and interactions. Thus an ethnic (strain) or regional group difference in the frequency of an induced malformation could occur even if the primary effect of the teratogen or mutagen was the same in the two strains. This is a very important aspect of the threshold model of multifactorial inheritance.

30. It should also be kept in mind that two or more mutations (or external mutagens) can act together either additively or synergistically on any developmental process. Furthermore, multifactorial systems are heterogeneous, i.e. two individuals who are similarly liabile to develop a particular disorder may be so as a result of completely different genes and/or mechanisms.

31. In humans, there are numerous examples of differences in incidence between different ethnic groups and different geographic regions, as can be observed in studies of neural tube defects. Neural tube defects are a heterogeneous group of anomalies that involve the developing brain and spinal cord. The epidemiologic characteristics of neural tube defects include a higher incidence in females, in lower socioeconomic groups, and in people of Celtic or East Indian ancestry, and prevalence rates that vary substantially in different geographic regions [H4]. While neural tube defects are generally registered as a single category of defect, their causes are heterogeneous and can be influenced by teratogenic exposure or maternal nutritional deficiency or illness. In some families recurrence is frequent, in others only sporadic. Each of these components of the overall category "neural tube defect" is likely to be differentially affected by exposure to various mutagenic agents [V12], and, as with other multifactorial disorders, nutrition and lifestyle, i.e. environment, can have a protective effect as well as a damaging effect. For example, folic acid supplementation has been shown to reduce the recurrence of neural tube defects [W4].

32. It is also important to remember that multifactorial disorders often manifest with different gradations of severity. Thus if a new mutation simply increased the severity of a disorder, it would probably not be noted as a change in the incidence of the disorder in the population.

33. In exploring the relationship between environmental factors and the occurrence of congenital anomalies, one is confronted with an extremely complex situation. In multifactorial disorders, an environmental factor or factors interacts with a susceptible genotype to produce the defect. The uniqueness of this interaction in a given family may preclude generalization to the population as a whole. As a result, it is perhaps not surprising that it is so difficult to define specific environmental factors that correlate significantly and consistently with particular congenital anomalies in humans. This difficulty is particularly relevant to any attempt to predict the effects of radiation exposure on multifactorial disorders.

2. Risk of recurrence within families

34. When determining the risk of recurrence for common multifactorial disorders, empirical data are used, as no single model explains the observed variables. But even empirical data from a large random sample will not take into account the uniqueness of each family, its environment, or the particular events of a given pregnancy that might affect the outcome. Thus, only generalizations can be used for dealing with questions of risk and recurrence. The models developed to describe multifactorial inheritance are just that, models. In no case have all of the specific genes involved and their interactions been defined. Thus it becomes very difficult to predict the effects of a particular type of mutation (e.g. radiation-induced), much less the multiple environmental agents involved [F8, F10].

35. In general, the risk of recurrence for multifactorial disorders is directly related to the severity of the disorder in the proband or index case. This is, in a sense, a dose-response phenomenon, i.e. the more genes that are involved in causing the defect and the more environmental factors that contribute, the more likely the defect is to occur with a severity proportional to both genetic and environmental contributions. Assuming that the potential gene pool of a couple

remains constant and that they continue to live in the same environment, the risk of a congenital anomaly recurring will be greater if the index case child is severely affected than if it is mildly affected [F8, F10].

36. Because in most cases many unknown factors are involved in recurrence, figures for recurrence risk represent average probabilities rather than certainties. Thus, if only one child in a family is affected, the average risk of recurrence is 3%-5% for most multifactorially inherited birth defects. If two siblings are affected, the average risk of recurrence is usually 5%-10%. After three siblings are affected, the risk for a fourth child is 10%-25%. As the number of affected children in a family increases towards a 25% recurrence rate, it becomes essential to ask whether one is perhaps dealing with a specific autosomal recessive trait having variable penetrance rather than with a multifactorial continuum [F10].

37. Mathematical models are available for the distribution and risk of recurrence of many multifactorial disorders [B8]. But it must be made clear that each disorder requires a separate model, and there is no guarantee that recurrence risks will remain the same from one family to another. The basic principles of recurrence risk assessment for a multifactorial disorder are as follows:

(a) the correlation of phenotype between relatives is proportional to the number of alleles in common;
(b) the correlation for offspring is halfway between the risk for parents and that for the general population;
(c) if a disorder is more frequent in one sex, the recurrence risk depends on the sex of subsequent offspring;
(d) if the population frequency is p, the risk among first degree relatives is the square root of p (when heritability is high);
(e) the recurrence risk is higher when more than one member of the family is affected;
(f) the more severe a malformation, the higher the recurrence risk;
(g) the risk to relatives drops off rapidly with increasing remoteness of relation;
(h) monozygous twins are several times more likely to be concordant than dizygous twins, but concordance is never complete (it is usually less than 40%) [S34];
(i) consanguinity increases the risk of polygenic and multifactorial conditions.

38. To estimate recurrence risks with the multifactorial model, two pieces of information are required: the frequency of the condition in the population and the empirical frequency in first-degree relatives of affected individuals. The correlation in liability between first-degree relatives can be estimated by the method of Bonaitie-Pellie et al. [B8]. This method takes into account differences in frequency between sexes and different severity-age classes. Computer programmes are available to derive the risk estimates (e.g. [B8]).

39. It must be reemphasized that it is at present difficult, if not impossible, to discriminate between a multifactorial model and a unifactorial model with incomplete penetrance for most multifactorial conditions in humans, since the different modes of inheritance lead to similar frequencies in relatives [F10]. Understanding of such disorders in humans is primarily empirical at this stage; cases are observed and recorded, but the underlying molecular mechanisms remain obscure. Gradually, more and more human genetic disorders are yielding to new molecular techniques.

D. NON-TRADITIONAL INHERITANCE

40. Many newly recognized mechanisms of gene regulation and genetic disease in humans were not known to classical geneticists and thus have not been considered in previous estimates of either background incidence or risk of heritable disorders following irradiation. Since they could, however, be significantly affected by radiation, they are discussed in this Section in some detail, with the caveat that any estimation of risk must include an understanding and consideration of these additional potential sources of hereditary disease.

1. Mosaicism

41. Mosaicism refers to the presence of both normal cells and cells carrying a mutation within a single individual. Somatic mosaicism results from a gene mutation or chromosomal anomaly arising in a somatic cell. Since the number of cells in the human body (approximately 10^{14}) exceeds the magnitude of the mutation rate for almost all genetic disorders thus far recognized, it seems likely that during the course of embryonic, fetal and postnatal life, virtually the entire repertoire of known mutations might occur within all normal human beings [H3].

42. Mosaicism may result from chromosomal abnormalities (missing or extra chromosomes or parts of chromosomes), from single gene mutations or from changes in gene control, such as X-inactivation, genomic imprinting or loss of imprinting (see below). It may also result from uniparental disomy (see below), gene amplification (see below) or from the incorporation of extrachromosomal DNA.

43. The expected effects of somatic mosaicism would depend on a number of factors, including (a) the type of mutation (deletion, point mutation etc.), (b) the type of gene in which the mutation occurs (housekeeping, structural, regulatory etc.), (c) the locus (or loci) at which the mutation occurs, (d) the domain involved (intron, exon, regulatory region), (e) whether the mutation has led to heterozygosity or homozygosity of the mutant or wild-type allele, (f) the specific cell type(s) involved and the tissues and organs affected, (g) the stage of development in which the mutational event occurs, and (h) the fate of the particular cell lineage in which it arose (migration, mingling, selection etc.). Very different effects would be expected if the mutation occurred in a growing and developing organism rather than in an end-stage differentiated cell.

(a) Chromosomal mosaicism

44. With the advent of chorionic villus sampling in prenatal diagnosis, some interesting and unexpected types of chromosomal mosaicism have been reported, such as confined placental mosaic aneuploidy in fetuses who have intrauterine growth retardation and a normal karyotype [K1]. In some cases, when the fetus is aneuploid, the presence of a normal cell line in the placenta may even explain why a small minority of fetuses afflicted with lethal chromosome anomalies are able to survive to term. This has also been shown in fetuses with altered chromosomes 18 and 13 that survive to term [K2].

45. It seems quite possible that there are genetic reasons why mosaicism is tolerated in some individuals and in some tissues. The mechanisms involved are unknown at this time but could be affected by radiation, making an individual more tolerant to mosaicism and thereby more likely to develop abnormal tissues.

(b) Germ-line mosaicism

46. There have been a number of reports suggesting that mosaic mutations of the germ line may be present in phenotypically normal individuals. Families with Duchenne muscular dystrophy [H3], pseudoachondroplasia [H5], Apert syndrome [A3], osteogenesis imperfecta type II [B11], tuberous sclerosis [H5] and many other disorders [H3] whose transmission is normally either dominant or X-linked have been reported in which parents are phenotypically normal by all known tests but more than one of their children are affected by the disorder.

47. Germ-line mosaicism is a mechanism of mutation that may produce transgenerational effects, as the germ cells of the carrier parent are formed in embryogenesis during the grandmother's pregnancy. Alternatively, if a parent carried mosaicism for a mutation that involved a multifactorial trait, it could be passed through the children and not manifest with visible phenotype until the grandchildren's generation or later [H3].

48. With regard to recurrence risk, the data available on single-gene "new" mutations from the disorders so far characterized on a biochemical or DNA level suggest that many (at least 5%) of what appear to be new mutations may actually represent a substantial parental germ-line mosaicism [H3]. One implication of this is that there may be a real risk for the recurrence of a new dominant mutation in subsequent offspring in what had previously been thought to represent a risk-free situation.

49. Depending on the particular tissue and mutation, some chromosomal anomalies and single-gene mutations may be lethal to the cells, others may be tolerated if they do not have a severe effect on that tissue, while still other mutations may actually have a selective advantage, as in the case of malignancies [F5]. For example, observations on patients with mosaicism for trisomy 8 and tetrasomy 12p support this concept, since mosaicism for these aneuploidies appears to be much better tolerated in fibroblasts that in lymphocytes [P2].

50. Normal cells may occasionally arise in dominant lethal disorders via back-mutation, gene conversion, mitotic crossover, suppressor mutation or double mitotic nondisjunction. They then outgrow the mutant cells, interspersing themselves throughout the body and allowing survival of what would otherwise be a lethal condition. Such may be the explanation for the occasional survival of males with X-linked incontinentia pigmenti [H10] and Melnick Needle syndrome [D6].

51. Mosaicism is a pervasive phenomenon that almost certainly affects all multicellular organisms. When expressed in somatic cells, it can be an important cause of neoplasia and possibly other aspects of the aging process [H3]. Somatic mosaicism can also be an important and sometimes dramatic cause of phenotypic variation in the expression of genetic traits [H3].

52. It should be kept in mind that if a mutation occurs in a DNA repair function, then somatic mutations, and therefore mosaicism, will occur far more frequently (as seen in DNA repair disorders such as Fanconi's anaemia etc. which predispose to cancer). Thus, a radiation-induced mutation would have a very different effect in families with a DNA repair defect than in other people. Likewise, a radiation-induced mutation in a DNA repair gene would affect many other genes as well.

53. In the past, only in the case of chromosomal abnormalities has it been possible to confirm the existence and significance of mosaicism, but the development and application of molecular genetic techniques should provide several approaches for identifying and analyzing a wider range of mosaic states in humans.

2. Genomic imprinting

54. Genomic imprinting is a newly recognized genetic phenomenon in humans. It appears to be a regulatory mechanism by which certain genes are differentially expressed, and thus convey different phenotypic effects, depending on whether they are inherited from the mother or the father. An "imprinted" gene is inactivated. Thus, a paternally imprinted gene would be expressed in a child only when it has been inherited from the mother; the paternal copy would be inactivated [H4].

55. A mechanism such as imprinting might further complicate efforts to estimate hereditary risk from radiation, as paternal vs maternal irradiation could have different influences on the phenotypes of F_1 offspring, even if damage to the genetic material was identical [V6]. In addition, imprinting effects may remain hidden for several generations. This is due to the fact that a mutation in an imprinted gene may remain silent (i.e. inactivated) through many generations before it is actually expressed in offspring.

56. As with the DNA repair genes discussed above, a mutation in a gene that regulates the imprinting process could have pleiotropic effects at multiple gene loci, causing them to be improperly expressed or improperly silenced. Imprinting appears particularly to affect early embryonic development and growth and to play a role in cancer. In other words, if a particular gene inherited from one parent is damaged, it may result in overgrowth or tumour development, while loss of the same gene from the other parent may have no effect.

57. Another line of evidence to support the existence of parent-of-origin differences in gene expression has developed from the study of human chromosome deletion syndromes. There are indications that the parental origin of the chromosome that carries the deletion or translocation may be associated with or modify the clinical manifestations of a number of observed syndromes [H6].

58. Two striking examples are the Prader-Willi and Angelman syndromes. Both are associated with deletions of the same region of the proximal long arm of chromosome 15. The clinical features of the two syndromes are remarkably different. On a cytogenetic level, it has been determined that in Prader-Willi patients with visible chromosomal deletions, the deletion is always of the paternally derived 15q11-13 region, whereas in Angelman patients with visible deletions, the deletion is always of the maternally derived 15q11-13 region [H6]. The deletions in the two syndromes thus apparently involve the critical region(s) of chromosome 15 but result in different phenotypes, depending on the parental origin of the chromosome.

59. These observations strongly suggest that this region of chromosome 15 is imprinted. Presumably there is a gene or group of genes in this region that is expressed only from the maternal chromosome, resulting in Angelman syndrome when deleted, while a second gene or group of genes in this region is expressed only from the paternal chromosome, resulting in Prader-Willi when deleted. A deletion or translocation in this region of chromosome 15 will have quite different effects in different generations, depending on the parent of origin [H6].

60. The concept of checks and balances between the parental contributions is further supported by recent studies on endogenous mouse genes. It has been found that in mice, only the paternally inherited gene for insulin-like growth factor II (Igf-2) is expressed [D1] and only the maternally derived gene for the Igf-II receptor (Igf-2r) is expressed [B6].

61. A second group of chromosomal deletions whose phenotypic effects are now recognized to have a non-random pattern of parental origin are those involved in oncogenesis [H2]. Familial cancer syndromes usually behave as dominantly inherited traits. Loss of the wild-type allele in individual cells is thought to result in loss of a suppressor gene function, which in turn allows oncogenic transformation and the development of tumours. It has recently been recognized that in a large number of sporadic Wilms' tumours there is loss of all or part of chromosome 11. Now that DNA markers allow identification of parental origin, it has been determined that those deletions or losses of chromosome 11 almost always involve the chromosome of maternal origin [S9]. The Philadelphia chromosome translocation associated with leukaemia and other haemopoietic neoplasms has recently been shown to demonstrate parent-of-origin effects, with chromosome 9 always being paternal in origin and chromosome 22 always maternal [H16].

62. Work on the retinoblastoma *(rb)* gene also suggests that there are tissue-specific, parent-of-origin differences in the expression of maternally and paternally derived genes [H2]. For instance, new mutations resulting in retinoblastoma are almost always paternal in origin, whereas sporadic sarcomas or rhabdomyo-

sarcomas with deletions of the *rb* gene almost always involve loss from the maternally derived chromosome 13.

63. Imprinting probably involves modifications of the nuclear DNA in somatic cells in order to produce these parent-of-origin differences in the phenotype. Thus the same nucleotide sequence may confer different phenotypic effects in different generations, depending upon whether it has been inherited from a male or from a female. It is not yet clear at which stage in development genomic imprinting occurs.

64. It should be noted that if the imprinting process or part of it occurs during meiosis, this may be another mechanism for which mutation would have such transgenerational effects. These effects would begin with the radiation exposure of the grandmother, because the formation of an oocyte, which when fertilized will eventually become a new individual, occurs during the *in utero* life of the mother (i.e. during the mother's own embryonic development within the grandmother). The effects of radiation thus might not become apparent for two or more generations following irradiation. Imprintable genes would be expected to be transmitted in a Mendelian manner, but their expression would be determined by the sex of the parent transmitting the gene, by way of this epigenetic form of regulation. Thus, studies of irradiation in females may produce results that are markedly different from those in males, depending on how much of the human genome is imprinted.

65. Now that molecular markers are available, the parental origin of various chromosomes and chromosome segments can easily be traced, and phenotypes dependent upon this phenomenon are being recognized in many areas of biology and medicine. Many human disorders are now being identified as imprinted [H6]. Disorders whose transmission and inheritance have been poorly understood and described as variably penetrant, multifactorial or variably expressed should now be examined for parent-of-origin differences and possible imprinting effects.

66. Imprinting has obvious implications for understanding the hereditary effects of radiation, since parent-of-origin effects would be expected and might be masked in animal experiments, where parents of only one sex are irradiated. Also, the effects of mutations involving imprinted genes may be masked for several generations.

3. Uniparental disomy

67. Uniparental disomy occurs when, in a cell with a normal number of chromosomes, both members of a chromosome pair have been inherited from a single parent. Normally, one chromosome of each pair is maternal in origin and the other paternal. Experiments using translocation chromosomes in mice have shown that at least seven segments of the mouse genome produce marked phenotypic differences in growth, behaviour and survival when uniparental disomy is present; in other segments, no difference is observed [C5, S14]. In other words, for some regions of the genome, a totally different phenotype is observed depending on whether both segments come from the mother or both from the father. Because of extensive homologies between the mouse and human genomes, it is reasonable to expect that the imprinted regions of human chromosomes will follow a similar distribution.

68. Not all cases of the Prader-Willi and Angelman syndromes carry visible cytogenetic deletions. Using molecular markers, many of these cases can be shown to have resulted from uniparental disomy [H6, H15, M2]. In these instances of Angelman syndrome, both members of the chromosome 15 pair have been inherited from the father; in the cases of Prader Willi syndrome with uniparental disomy, both have been inherited from the mother. Uniparental disomy occurs far more frequently than originally assumed [E9]. It may occur through the loss of a chromosome, in the case of a trisomy, or through the duplication or complementation of the remaining chromosome, in the case of a monosomy (i.e. salvage, since monosomy is lethal) [H6]. Irradiation is known to lead to chromosome deletion and loss and could therefore be expected to uncover imprinting and uniparental disomy effects [C17].

69. An interesting corollary of uniparental disomy is that it can, for the following reason, result in a child being affected by an autosomal recessive disorder when only one parent is a carrier for that disorder: if a parent carries a chromosome that contains an abnormal recessive gene and a son or daughter inherits two identical copies of this chromosome (uniparental isodisomy), the son or daughter will now carry two copies of the abnormal gene, i.e. will be homozygous for the mutant gene. Thus, he or she will express an autosomal recessive disorder that has been inherited from only one carrier parent. Precisely this situation has been shown to have occurred in two cases of cystic fibrosis [V11] and a collagen defect [S41]. The percentage of cases where an autosomal recessive disorder is uniparental rather than familial is unknown at this time, but clearly the question deserves further study.

70. The effects of uniparental disomy for chromosome 7 (intrauterine growth retardation) and chromosome 15 (Angelman and Prader-Willi syndromes) have been described above. In addition, a rare,

dominantly inherited human overgrowth syndrome, the Wiedeman-Beckwith syndrome, has been shown to occur in cases with paternal disomy for chromosome 11 [W2]. When familial, this syndrome has been known for some time to be nearly always transmitted through the mother. As discussed above, this again suggests a role for imprinting in growth disorders, as well as in human cancer, since patients with this condition frequently develop several types of cancer.

71. Other chromosomes for which uniparental disomy has been documented are chromosome 4 [C3], chromosome 6 [W6], chromosome 14 [T2], chromosome 16 [K17] and chromosome 21 [W1]. More information will be needed before it can be known if these chromosomes contain imprinted regions. Whether uniparental disomy occurs for other chromosomes remains to be determined. The implications for the hereditary effects of radiation are that damage to a chromosome may lead to loss of part or all of a chromosome, with complementation by the remaining chromosome producing uniparental disomy with increased frequency.

4. Cytoplasmic inheritance

72. Cytoplasmic components are present in the ova but not the sperm. Thus, the elements of the cytoplasm, such as the mitochondria (and possibly the mitotic spindles, endoplasmic reticulum etc.), are initially derived from the mother by cytoplasmic inheritance. One specific type of cytoplasmic inheritance is mitochondrial inheritance. The nucleus is not the only cellular organelle to carry genetic information. The mitochondria contain a separate genome, comprised of over 16,000 base pairs. This genome is circular in structure; both strands of mitochondrial DNA (mtDNA) are transcribed and translated, in contrast to the single coding strand of the nuclear chromosomes, which is usually transcribed in only one direction [M3].

73. Each mitochondrion contains many copies of these circular genomes, and thus each cell (with its many mitochondria) contains thousands of copies of the mitochondrial genome, as opposed to only two copies of each nuclear chromosome. In addition, the mitochondria contain essential enzyme and other protein molecules that are transcribed in the nucleus, translated in the cytoplasm and then transported to the mitochondria.

74. The mitochondrial genome is transcribed as a single messenger RNA (mRNA) that is cleaved into various genetic units. The products of the mitochondrial genes participate in a number of functions, the most important being the energy-generating synthesis of ATP via oxidative phosphorylation. (Of the 69 separate polypeptides known to be required for oxidative phosphorylation, 13 are coded for by the mitochondrial DNA [T3].)

75. As discussed above, the inheritance of mitochondrial DNA follows a strictly maternal line of transmission. Thus a clue to this cytoplasmic mode of inheritance is that a trait is passed only through females, but all (or almost all) offspring are affected or are at risk of being affected (as opposed to X-linked recessive traits, where only males are affected or X-linked dominant traits, where only 50% of the offspring are affected because there are two X-chromosomes).

76. Disorders such as Leber optic atrophy, myoclonic epilepsy with ragged red fibres and progressive external ophthalmoplegia (alone or as part of Kearns-Sayre syndrome) have been shown to be due to mutations in mitochondrial DNA. Mitochondrial disorders tend to have a more severe effect on tissues that require high levels of metabolic energy, such as muscle and brain. The mothers of these cases, and the cases themselves, are often heteroplasmic, meaning that each of their cells carries some normal and some abnormal mitochondria and thus may appear unaffected. Each offspring (and each tissue of offspring) may thus also carry varying proportions of abnormal mitochondria.

77. While the mitochondria have few genes compared to the approximately 100,000 genes in the nuclear genome, mitochondrial genes have a significantly higher rate of spontaneous mutation than nuclear genes [R2]. Thus the daughter of a heteroplasmic mother may develop additional mutations in her mitochondrial genome, and so on down the generations, increasing the likelihood that a child will carry a sufficient number of abnormal mitochondria to become symptomatic and to manifest one of the mitochondrial disorders. It is also likely that the effects of radiation may be more severe for the mitochondrial genome than for the nuclear DNA, but because of heteroplasmy, the effect may not become apparent for one or more generations [W12].

5. Anticipation and allelic expansion

78. Genetic anticipation is a phenomenon in which the phenotype of a disorder becomes progressively more severe in each subsequent generation inheriting the gene. Although until recently this phenomenon was thought not to occur, a number of studies have identified molecular mechanisms by which it can, and does, occur [H8].

79. One mechanism that can cause anticipation is found in the autosomal dominant disorder myotonic muscular dystrophy (MMD). This disorder is highly variable in its expression and is often more severe in the children than in the mildly affected parents. Part of the gene for MMD has recently been isolated and appears to be highly unstable, becoming larger in subsequent generations [H8]. The mutation responsible for fragile-X syndrome, the most common single-gene mental retardation syndrome in humans, has also been identified: it shows a similar instability in both phenotype and gene size in subsequent generations inheriting the mutation [Y3].

80. This type of increase in the size of a particular gene is called allelic expansion and can occur either somatically or during meiosis. In traditional Mendelian genetics, it has always been assumed that genes are essentially stable units of genetic information, and that either a normal allele or a mutant allele carried by the parent will be passed to offspring unchanged. When allelic expansion occurs, however, it has been found that patients with the most severe symptoms have the greatest enlargement of the defective gene, owing to an increase in the number of units of a repetitive sequence in the DNA. The number of repetitive sequence units continues to increase from generation to generation and is associated with a worsening of symptoms, i.e. anticipation [F9].

81. A similar increase in gene size has also been found in the fragile-X syndrome, with expansion of a CGG repeat [Y3], Huntington disease, with expansion of a CAG repeat [H17], and in X-linked spinal bulbar atrophy, also with an expansion of a (CAG)n repeat which occurs in the coding region of the gene for the androgen receptor [L1]. When amplification occurs at the fragile-X site, it is always when the mutation is passed by a female to her children [Y3]; when the Huntington expansion is passed from a male, it can expand rapidly. Thus it seems likely that parent-of-origin effects could play a role in the transmission and expression of the fragile-X phenotype [L2]. Other disorders are likely to involve allelic expansion, or a similar mechanism. For example, unstable sequences called microsatellite DNA have been shown to be associated with familial colorectal cancer [A8, P4, T7].

82. The implications of allelic expansion for radiation are as follows: if certain regions of the genome are more sensitive than others to allelic expansion, radiation damage might cause this sort of mutation to increase at a different rate than classical mutations. There may also be differences between the effects of irradiation of the mother and those of irradiation of the father. Many familial cancers have been demonstrated to have widespread alterations in short repeat DNA sequences, which may predispose to oncogenic events [A8, W11]. In addition, the spontaneous mutation rate in these regions may be unusually high; thus estimates of background incidence of mutations may be different than for other genetic disorders.

6. Gene amplification

83. In gene amplification, an entire gene or portions of it are duplicated. This may lead to an increased expression of gene product, either normal or defective, or to disruption and loss of gene function. Amplification can produce a selective advantage, as in cancer cells that are able to survive chemotherapy by virtue of having amplified the multi-drug resistance (MDR) gene to gain many active copies [S30]. Alternatively, it can produce a disease phenotype, such as Lesch-Nyhan syndrome, in which an internal amplification has been found to disrupt a normal allele for the enzyme hypoxanthine-phosphoribosyl transferase (HPRT), causing loss of gene function and thus leading to the disease [S32].

84. Amplification differs from allelic expansion in that the latter term refers to an increase in the length of a fragment consisting of multiple copies of a short repetitive sequence (for example, [CGG]n) [H8]. Such short repetitive sequences are found throughout the genome, usually flanking structural genes. They are also referred to as a variable length polymorphisms, as the sequences alter the restriction fragment size for a particular gene. Amplification refers to an increase in the number of copies of a longer nucleotide sequence unique to a particular gene. The molecular mechanisms for each may or may not be similar and may or may not be affected by radiation [M3].

7. Transposable elements

85. Transposable elements are sequences of DNA that integrate unstably into the genome at random (or possibly by homologous recombination at specific sequences). These include the Alu and LINE elements [L3, S33]. This integration, if it occurs in the middle of a structural gene or regulatory sequence, can disrupt gene function and produce a mutant phenotype. Transposable elements have long been observed in a number of lower organisms, including yeast, maize and drosophila [L3]. They were suspected in the human genome but until recently had not been proven.

86. However, Dombroski et al. [D5] have identified a LINE-1 transposable element disrupting the factor VIII gene in two haemophilia patients. This element also contains a full-length copy of a gene for reverse transcriptase, making it possible, after the element is

copied to RNA, for the transposable sequence to be copied back into DNA, which can then integrate back into the genome at a new site, often disrupting functional genes [M6]. It is thought that this type of element may have originated with retroviral integration into the human genome. Similar LINE-1 transposable elements have caused mutations in the neurofibromatosis type 1 gene [W10] and the cholinesterase gene [M12]. It seems likely that radiation should be able to mobilize or destabilize such elements, which lead to increased mutation or gene disruption in later generations.

E. SUMMARY

87. Genetic diseases occur because of alterations (mutations) to the structure or regulation of genes in the cell. Traditionally, genetic disorders have been classified into one of three categories: single-gene disorders, chromosomal aberrations and multifactorial disorders. Single-gene traits and disorders are either recessive (i.e. a normal copy of the gene will prevent the disease phenotype) or dominant (i.e. one abnormal copy of the gene will result in expression of the disease phenotype). A single gene can have multiple and apparently unrelated effects on many different tissues; this is called pleiotropism.

88. Phenotypic diversity within a single heritable disorder can be caused by (a) environmental factors, (b) allelic series (an individual with two alleles of a single gene with two different mutations), (c) genetic compounds (mutations in two different genes), (d) mutations in different domain coding regions of the same gene and (e) interaction with the products of other genes in that individual. Similar phenotypes can be caused by the action of any one of several different genes. This is called heterogeneity of disease. Multifactorial traits and disorders are those where a single condition (i.e. not complex disorders or multiple anomalies) is thought to have a genetic component but whose inheritance cannot be explained by single-gene inheritance.

89. Modes of non-traditional inheritance include cytoplasmic inheritance, mosaicism, imprinting and uniparental disomy. These mechanisms may prove to be increasingly important as causal factors in diseases whose inheritance does not follow standard Mendelian patterns of inheritance, and they may well be affected by radiation. Genetic disorders, particularly severe ones that interfere with reproduction, may be the result of new, as opposed to inherited, mutations. Human gene mapping using family pedigrees and restriction fragment length polymorphisms is being used to localize and isolate genes related to specific disorders.

II. MONITORING THE BACKGROUND INCIDENCE OF GENETIC DISEASE

90. The term genetic disease has been used to refer to any disorder (anatomical or metabolic) that is severe enough to interfere with a normal life and that has a genetic component, regardless of the age at which it occurs. The term congenital means present at birth. Congenital anomaly is a more precise term than birth defect and refers to structural anomalies present at birth. There are three major types of structural anomaly that may be apparent at birth [S35]:

(a) malformation, a defective or abnormal formation of a structure from its origin;
(b) deformation, an improper formation of a structure because of some physical impediment (e.g. too little amniotic fluid causes restricted fetal movement, which in turn results in joint contractures);
(c) disruption, an injury to a formed structure caused by an extrinsic or intrinsic force (e.g. amniotic bands disrupting circulation to a limb or digit).

A. REGISTRIES OF CONGENITAL ANOMALIES

1. Types and incidence of congenital anomalies

91. Congenital anomalies are not usually the consequence of Mendelian or chromosomal disorders, which they greatly outnumber. They have the advantage of being easy to document, as birth, surgery and death involve recorded events; moreover, in earlier days, when their nature was less clear, they were considered useful genetic markers. It is now possible to assess fairly accurately whether a congenital anomaly represents a significant problem and whether treatment is available. The anomalies can be classified as major (e.g. hydrocephalus, achondroplasia, amelia) or minor (e.g. skin tags, pigmented nevi, supernumerary nipples, minimal polydactyly).

92. Access to multiple registries allows the development of fairly accurate background rates for congenital anomalies. Some registries reflect concentrations of specific ethnic groups or high rates of consanguinity. Different registries have different incidences of anomalies, reflecting regional, ethnic and temporal variations. However, taken all together, they allow establishing fairly accurate background incidence of various congenital anomalies. Anomalies that are subject to environmental influences, such as neural tube defects, can be identified as varying with social class and region.

93. There is a consistent finding in all populations that 2%-3% of the serious congenital anomalies that will alter the length of life or ability to function normally without medical intervention are ascertained in newoms and that another 2%-3% of serious congenital anomalies are ascertained by 5 years of age [B2]. An additional 5%-13% of minor anomalies are found in all populations [B2, N11]. Efficacious treatment is available for at least one half of the defects, allowing an affected individual to become functional, independent and a contributing member of society. However. the remaining one half of congenital anomalies presently leave the affected individual with considerable disability in spite of therapy.

94. A study by Baird et al. [B3], conducted since publication of the UNSCEAR 1988 Report [U1], used a database of more than 1 million consecutive live births, followed from birth through the age of 25 years, obtained from the British Columbia Health Surveillance Registry through 1983. A hierarchical approach ensured that individuals were not counted more than once. Although the authors generally followed the approach of Trimble and Doughty [T6], they chose to proceed from single-gene disorders (autosomal dominant, autosomal recessive, X-linked) to chromosome disorders and then to multifactorial disorders. Congenital anomalies were considered last. Their analysis was restricted to those relatively common conditions that are generally accepted as having a major genetic component. The aetiological category "genetic unknown" was used when it was evident that the condition had a genetic basis but the inheritance pattern was not known.

95. It is recognized that this approach yields minimal estimates of incidence rates, since cases with relatively mild manifestations may not be diagnosed or may not come to the attention of the ascertainment sources. In addition, the count of multifactorial cases was assumed to be falsely low, because of an inherent bias in the counting process that could be present whenever a case had more than one diagnosis. Only those cases with a single diagnosis were counted as multifactorial. This means that the chance occurrence of a second non-multifactorial diagnosis or a second, unrelated multifactorial diagnosis in the same individual would cause that case to be omitted from the multifactorial category, occurring in the same individual. Baird et al. discussed an adjusted value for this rate that would correct this problem in the methodology.

96. The study found that before they reached the age of 25 years, more than 53 of 1,000 live-born individuals can be expected to have diseases with an important genetic component (see Table 1). The breakdown was as follows: 3.6 per 1,000 for single-gene disorders, consisting of autosomal dominant (1.4 per 1,000), autosomal recessive (1.7 per 1,000) and X-linked recessive disorders (0.5 per 1,000); 1.8 per 1,000 for chromosomal anomalies and 46 per 1,000 for multifactorial disorders, including those present at birth and those whose onset was before the age of 25 years. If all congenital anomalies are considered as part of the genetic load, the total rises to 79 per 1,000 live-born individuals.

97. It was found that if all cases of congenital anomaly (non-genetic as well as genetic) were considered, including those to which no genetic aetiology was attributed, the combined rate of all congenital anomalies was approximately twice that for genetic anomalies alone (i.e. 52,808 per 1 million live births, or 5.3%). If inguinal hernia was added, approximately 6.1% of the live-born in this population had a congenital anomaly (recent Hungarian data found 7.2% [B2]). However, inguinal hernias are easily corrected and are not considered a serious congenital anomaly. The study by Nelson et al. [N11] in Massachusetts found the same level of incidence and genetic distribution as the study by Baird et al. [B2, B3].

98. The point was made that *in utero* diagnosis of genetic abnormality has become increasingly common in recent years, and that this could bias the estimates of genetic defect in live-born children, since a positive test may lead to termination of the pregnancy. The potential impact was calculated from the records of the British Columbia Provincial Prenatal Diagnosis Programme [B2], and it was concluded that the impact of pregnancy termination on the rates in the study was extremely small, with an incidence of approximately 0.027% in the mid-1980s.

99. Baird et al. noted that the present records of the British Columbia Health Surveillance Registry make it possible to identify those cases within the congenital anomaly group that were judged to have a genetic aetiology. This is a considerable advance, because many earlier studies did not attempt to quantify the relative importance of the genetic versus the non-genetic categories within the broader "congenital anomalies" grouping. The other advantage of this study is that it provides follow-up data to age 25 years for at least a portion of the study population; the

follow-up data reveal that many congenital anomalies are not ascertained during the first few months of life.

2. Scope of monitoring

100. There are two approaches to monitoring congenital anomalies: epidemiological, i.e. the detection of outbreaks or clusters of predefined conditions by statistical methods, and teratological, which stresses the importance of clinical details in the search for unusual events, either rare malformations or unusual combinations of malformations, that may indicate the introduction of a new teratogen [W8].

101. In attempting to calculate the genetic consequences of any agent, be it a drug, a chemical or radiation, it is essential to begin with an accurate estimate of the background incidence rate for a given genetic disease or congenital anomaly. Previous reports on the genetic effects of radiation [C1, C2, U1, U2, U3, U4] raised the issue of background incidence. These reports relied heavily on data that are now almost 20 years old, and that were derived primarily from two sources [C13, C14]. A number of developments in recent years should make it possible to improve the accuracy of background estimates and to address the question of which genetic disorders and congenital malformations are most informative and worthy of inclusion in the study. There are now numerous registries of birth defects worldwide, each with unique features and each with advantages and disadvantages; these should all be taken into account when attempting to assess background incidence for human populations in general. Likewise, the accuracy of specific diagnosis has been greatly improved and refined in recent years, providing more precise definitions of significant defects.

102. There are bound to be regional, ethnic and temporal variations in the incidence of congenital malformations. For example, a study comparing congenital malformations in Aboriginal and non-Aboriginal newborns using the Western Australia Congenital Malformations Registry found that although the birth prevalence of all malformations was 3.5% for both groups, nervous system and cardiovascular defects and cleft lip and palate were significantly more prevalent in Aborigines and pyloric stenosis and urogenital defects were significantly less prevalent [B9]. In another example, Sikhs in British Columbia were found to have a significantly higher rate of neural tube defects than the general population, which is largely of northern European extraction [H4]. Many alarms generated by the International Clearinghouse for Birth Defects Monitoring Systems [W8] have, upon further investigation, yielded negative results.

103. Stochastic temporal variations in incidence may result in apparent clusters of a particular congenital anomaly or group of anomalies. While it is important to investigate such increases, it is probably not appropriate to rely on registries containing substantial deviations from the majority of registries in estimating background incidences of congenital malformations. However, if the concern is for a specific region, e.g. the Ukraine, where the reactor accident occurred, the background incidence of genetic disease for that particular population should be used, if it is available, to provide the baseline from which to calculate any increase in risk. Japan has regional monitoring programmes [K18]. It should be kept in mind, however, that any effect from a specific mutagen is likely to be obscured by the effects of social disruption, as some of the commoner malformations, e.g. neural tube defects [H4], are known to be greatly influenced by diet and standard of living [S16].

104. One other point to bear in mind is that, within a category of congenital malformation, there are often multiple subcategories with divergent causes and incidences, i.e. heterogeneity. For example, neural tube defects are generally classified as a single category, yet the cause of this defect can be single-gene mutation, chromosomal anomaly, teratogenic exposure, nutritional deficiency or ethnic predisposition. In some families recurrences are frequent, while in others the cases are sporadic; some cases can be caused by physical disruption such as amniotic bands. High lesions (anencephaly and thoracic spina bifida) differ from low lesions (lumbosacral spina bifida), and cases that occur in the presence of other birth defects differ from those that occur alone [H4]. Each of these components of the overall category "neural tube defect" could be differently affected by exposure to various mutagenic agents, and yet they are usually grouped together.

105. Registries may also differ in other aspects. It is important to consider the following sources of variation when comparing them: (a) exclusion or inclusion of stillbirths, (b) effects of prenatal diagnosis (rates of incidence may be lower owing to increased prenatal diagnosis and selective abortion for particular anomalies), (c) number of people contained in the registry (too small a sample may not yield statistically significant results), (d) ascertainment, as mentioned below and (e) duplication of reporting (multiple congenital anomalies may be reported singly as well as collectively).

106. According to Cordero [C9], if registries are to be useful in surveillance, epidemiological and other kinds of studies, they must contain four critical elements of information: who, what, when and where. Once these elements are specified, i.e. number of cases (what), divided by the population (who), in a specified area (where) and for a specific time period (when), incidence rates can be calculated [C9].

107. The collection of data can be either active or passive. With an active system, the registry has trained staff who follow a particular methodology to ascertain infants with birth defects and to collect data. With a passive system, the registry relies on reports from sources such as physicians, hospitals or vital records departments [C9].

108. Active systems have several strengths: (a) they have fairly complete ascertainment, (b) they can obtain data in a timely fashion, (c) they can include quality control measures for the data gathering process, (d) they define the type of data to be collected and (e) they usually allow for the follow-up of cases. A disadvantage of active systems is their cost, which tends to limit the sample size of the population to be studied. This, in turn, limits the registry's ability to collect sufficient data for some types of epidemiological studies [C9].

109. Passive systems have one major strength, low cost, which allows them to cover larger populations with a minimum of resources. Their disadvantages include a lack of diagnostic specificity, little control over time delays in obtaining data and measurable underreporting of data. In some passive systems, the quality of the data cannot be evaluated. Moreover, few systems provide a means to track cases, making follow-up studies impossible.

110. The process of finding persons with the disease under study is referred to as ascertainment. It is important to bear in mind that methods of ascertainment are bound to differ between registries, often resulting in the under- or overreporting of a particular birth defect in a particular population. For example, physicians in Hungary were paid for every instance of congenital hip dysplasia they reported; this malformation subsequently comprised an artificially high percentage of overall birth defects in Hungary. It is also important to bear in mind that many birth defects do not become apparent until after the first few months of life. Thus, a registry that reports only birth prevalence may be underreporting.

111. An alternative approach for complete ascertainment is to review medical records. In the United States, every baby born in a hospital has a medical record that generally indicates if birth defects are present. The strengths of this approach include nearly complete ascertainment, the ability to achieve population-based ascertainment and a lower cost than if every baby were examined independently,i.e. not by its own physician. Its disadvantages include labour intensiveness, inefficiency and cost [C9].

112. Some programmes, e.g. those in Sweden, Australia and Atlanta, Georgia in the United States, do not routinely record possible exposures during pregnancy. Such programmes are usually found in areas where it is relatively easy to go back to medical records and to contact the parents of the damaged infant if exposure information is thought to be of interest. In other programmes, such as the Central-East France programme and the large hospital-based programme in Italy, information on possible exposures during pregnancy is collected at the same time the malformed infant is reported, but no similar data are collected for normal infants. A third group of programmes, including one in Mexico, Spain and South America, has ongoing case-control data collection, in which information on possible exposure is obtained for each malformed infant and for a control (normal) infant born at the same hospital. Each technique has its advantages and disadvantages, but in areas of the world where it may not be possible to follow up an observation by interview at some time after birth, collecting exposure data on a case-control basis seems the most effective technique [C9].

B. CONSIDERATIONS ON BACKGROUND INCIDENCE

1. Sentinel Mendelian diseases

113. The concept that certain phenotypes were so obvious that they could not be missed led to the idea that their frequencies could be easily monitored for sudden increases. It is not difficult to establish the background incidence of autosomal-dominant disorders, especially those that have a strong selective disadvantage, the prevalence of which is maintained in the population by an equilibrium between constant mutation pressure and selection (see [V8, V10]).

114. Theoretically, in situations where illegitimacy can be ruled out and genetic heterogeneity can be recognized, this method should lead to reliable estimates of the spontaneous mutation rate and its increase because of a mutagenic agent. Such mutations are called sentinel mutations, because they are expected to indicate mutation rate increases caused by a new agent in the environment. Czeizel [C13, C14] enumerated 15 sentinel anomalies that are thought to be caused by dominant new mutations and that can be diagnosed at birth or shortly thereafter. However, the molecular aetiologies of these disorders, which are beginning to be defined, appear to be very heterogeneous. Thus, it may not be valid to apply one estimate to the group as a whole, as each subgroup might be expected to have a different rate of mutation. Moreover, as suggested by Strobel et al. [S39], such sentinel mutations are too rare to easily provide realistic mutation rate increases. Furthermore, continuous screening of very large populations would be required.

115. From the experience accumulated so far, it is extremely unlikely that human populations will ever be exposed to mutagenic agents that will cause an observable statistically significant increase in this type of disorder above the natural rate of mutation (see paragraph 213). The Hungarian data were used to test whether the Chernobyl accident in April 1986 had led to any increase of new mutations [C15]. No evidence was found that it had. This is, however, not surprising, because according to Strobel [S39], for a mutation incidence of 3 per 10,000, it would have been necessary to screen of a population of almost 2 million newborns distributed in two samples of equal size (before and after irradiation) to recognize an increase of 30% in 95% of instances. A smaller increase would require an even greater sample size. Down's syndrome alone (7.02 per 10,000) is more common than all the sentinel mutations taken together. But even for it, a population of approximately 1 million newborns would be necessary to recognize a statistically significant change, and Hungary has only about 150,000 live births per year [C14, C15] (see paragraphs 213 and 338).

116. Many autosomal-dominant disorders, especially many rarer ones, are thought to be maintained in the population by an equilibrium between mutation and selection. This may be true for such disorders as neurofibromatosis, Marfan syndrome and autosomal-dominant types of osteogenesis imperfecta. Other disorders, such as bilateral retinoblastoma or haemophilia, were probably maintained by such an equilibrium in the past, but successful therapy is very likely to have upset this equilibrium in recent decades. Assuming constant mutation rates, the incidence of such disorders is bound to increase until a new equilibrium has been reached unless there are counteracting circumstances, for example, artificial selection.

117. It is, however, very unlikely that the more common disorders are maintained by an equilibrium between mutation and selection. The mechanisms that have caused the present-day incidence of many dominant diseases are unknown. It follows that dominant and X-linked diseases cannot be subdivided easily into those whose incidence is maintained by an equilibrium between mutation and negative selection and those in which a selective advantage under certain living conditions has been the decisive factor. More complicated situations may occur and the equilibrium conditions may change over time, depending on living conditions.

118. There are, of course, a great number of fairly rare and, in most cases, very rare disorders that may indeed be maintained by an equilibrium between mutation and selection, but for an overall estimate of the mutational component, it is not the number of these disorders but their combined incidence that is important in calculating risk. Since they are mostly lethal at an early age, fertility is 0 and there is a 100% mutational component, i.e. all cases are caused by a new mutation, rather than inherited from the parents. These disorders comprise only about 1/30 of the entire group of dominant and X-linked disorders. In other disorders, the mutational component is smaller, and for some of the most common ones, it may not exist at all. In some earlier UNSCEAR Reports, the Committee estimated the mutational component of the entire group as 15%. In this, the medical geneticists may have been persuasive, having in mind the more severe and debilitating forms of genetic disease (this would be understandable, since these diseases are the ones most frequently seen in daily practice), but in the general case, the estimate is high.

119. To place an increase in morbidity due to autosomal dominant and X-linked radiation-induced mutations in proper perspective, it should be remembered that the natural spontaneous mutation rate, the causes of which are unknown, is not a constant. The best known factor that influences the mutation rate is paternal age. For some autosomal-dominant anomalies, such as achondroplasia, acrocephalosyndactyly (Apert syndrome), Marfan syndrome, myositis ossificans and probably many others, the mutation rate at a paternal age of 40-45 is four to six times higher than at a paternal age of 20-25 [V8]. Modell and Kulieve [M10] have calculated how much a given shift in the distribution of paternal ages in a population would change mutation rates. They compared the mutation rates expected with the present paternal age distributions with those expected if all fathers were less than 30 years old at the time of birth of their child. They found that even a relatively small shift in the distribution of paternal ages, and especially a reduction in the fraction of older fathers, could influence the mutation rate for such paternal-age-dependent mutations appreciably.

120. Not all known dominant mutations show such a strong increase with paternal age (for details see [V8]). In recent decades, and with a decrease in the average number of children per marriage, a decrease in the fraction of older fathers has been observed in many populations, and a corresponding reduction in the number of such paternal-age-dependent new mutants has to be assumed in the developed countries. Hence, even a relatively small shift in paternal age distribution, especially an increase or a reduction of older fathers, could influence the mutation rate for such paternal-age-dependent mutations appreciably, probably much more than could a change in exposure to mutagenic agents, e.g. radiation.

2. Autosomal recessive diseases

121. Searle and Edwards [S16] stressed that the degree of inbreeding influences only the immediacy of

the effects and that in the absence of a strong heterozygote disadvantage it will affect only slightly the total number of casualties. That is, in a population with a high rate of inbreeding (i.e. consanguinity), damage due to homozygosity of mutations becomes visible sooner. The authors assumed for their calculations a rate of 1% first-cousin matings.

122. Estimates of the manifestation of homozygotes in future generations depend critically on consanguinity rates. In industrialized countries, the rate of first-cousin matings has dropped to one or a few per thousand in recent decades. Since this reduction is caused on the one hand by greater mobility and on the other hand by smaller numbers of children (and, hence, a reduction in the number of available cousins), the decrease will probably continue and also occur in the populations of countries only now becoming industrialized. However, even if consanguinity can be neglected in the future, it is open to question whether effects distributed to thousands of generations should be considered at all in genetic risk estimates. It may be most reasonable to assume that civilization will develop in about the same direction as it has in recent centuries and that gene therapy and/or prenatal diagnosis at the zygote level will eventually become routine, especially for autosomal recessive diseases that involve mostly simple enzyme defects.

123. In humans, few data on phenotypic deviations in heterozygotes of autosomal-recessive diseases are available [V5], and those that are related primarily to enzyme studies. As a rule, heterozygotes have about half the activity of normal homozygotes for the product of the gene affected by the mutation, which in many cases is an enzyme. This reduced activity is, however, in most cases sufficient for normal function.

124. Finally, it should not be forgotten that the background incidence of recessive mutations, and especially of recessive diseases, in human populations is not constant from one disease or population to another. The human species is a patchwork of extremely different frequencies of recessive genes. The breaking up of isolated subpopulations and having strong intermixture between them will not lead to a reduction of frequencies of all recessive genes in a similar fashion, but it will lead to an assimilation of gene frequencies and especially to an appreciable reduction of frequencies of genes that had become common in one or a few populations owing to random drift. This, in turn, will lead to a general decrease of homozygotes of autosomal-recessive diseases, as a consequence of the Hardy-Weinberg Law [V10]. This decrease will then be followed by a very slow increase in gene frequencies, because fewer alleles will be eliminated in homozygotes. This is the complex background against which any possible effect of additional radiation should be viewed, since any attempt to derive an estimate of increased risk will depend on population structure.

3. Chromosomal diseases

125. There is general agreement that estimates of chromosomal disease incidence at birth disregard the great majority of (numerical and unbalanced, structural) chromosomal aberrations in human germ cells and early zygotes. Most embryos and fetuses with chromosomal aberrations die some time during embryonic life. It seems very unlikely that more than 1% of all conceptions with recognizable, chromosomally aberrant phenotypes survive to birth [V10]. This is a reasonable but cautious estimate, i.e. the true fraction of survivors might well be lower. The number of zygotes dying in the first days after fertilization, before implantation, cannot be estimated, but it may be appreciable. In studies of chromosomes of human sperm, the fraction of those showing chromosome aberrations is high [B12, K13, K14, K15, K16, M4, M5, S42]. It is, of course, unknown which of these chromosomally abnormal cells are still able to fertilize; but the use of this method of sperm karyotyping for mutagenicity testing, especially in men exposed to high doses of mutagenic agents, such as radiation, should be encouraged. Studies of ova used during *in vitro* fertilization suggest that human ova also have a high fraction of spontaneous chromosomal aberrations.

126. Calculations similar to those for paternal age effects in autosomal-dominant and X-linked recessive diseases have been performed for numerical chromosomal aberrations, such as Down's syndrome, to determine maternal age effects. The baseline is especially variable for trisomies, because the spontaneous mutation rate increases with the age of the mother: the risk for mothers above 40 is 10-20 times higher than that for 20-year-old mothers [H12]. The conclusion reached is therefore the same as for paternal age and dominant mutations: even a small shift in the distribution of maternal ages in a human population, and especially in the fraction of mothers above 35, will alter the incidence of trisomy syndromes at birth much more than any probable increase caused by radiation.

4. Congenital anomalies and multifactorial diseases

127. The background incidences of congenital anomalies and multifactorial diseases are not easy to establish. The UNSCEAR 1986 Report [U2] gave a figure of 60,000 per million for congenital anomalies and 600,000 per million for other multifactorial dis-

eases [U2]. BEIR V [C1] estimated congenital abnormalities as 20,000-30,000 per million and subdivided "other disorders of complex aetiology" into three categories: heart disease (600,000), cancer (300,000) and selected others (300,000). These three figures add up to more than 1 million, so they cannot be meant to be mutually exclusive. These discrepancies reflect the difficulties in attempting to establish reliable background incidence mentioned earlier in this Annex.

128. The seemingly simple task of determining the incidence of congenital malformations at birth continues to pose problems; results from one study to the next may show considerable differences, occasionally because of real differences between populations but much more often because of differences in ascertainment and classification. To predict a possible increase attributable to a specified radiation dose experienced by the germ cells of parents, the mutational component of this incidence needs to be estimated. This involves estimating the frequency and degree of genetic determination of single anomalies and their modes of inheritance, which, as discussed earlier, is very difficult to achieve and must be individualized. Furthermore, any possible selective disadvantages of such anomalies under present and earlier living conditions (and, if possible, in populations of industrialized countries and of developing countries with poor medical systems) should be known. This information is needed to estimate which part of the genetic component of a certain anomaly is lost in every generation and which is therefore replaced by new mutants. Even then, the estimate would be of the right order of magnitude only if there were an equilibrium between mutation and selection [H1].

129. In the British Columbia registry data, 4.6% of individuals were noted to have a multifactorial condition by age 25 years (Table 1) [B3]. Many congenital anomalies are consistent with the concept of multifactorial inheritance. A few are caused by environmental factors such as teratogenic drugs or, very rarely, irradiation during pregnancy. For many congenital anomalies, no cause can be identified; they are attributable to an accumulation of random processes during early embryonic development. However, data from radiation experiments in mice suggest that some may also be caused by irregularly manifesting dominant mutations. Their frequency may increase after the irradiation of fathers. For example, Ehling [E1, E8] and Selby et al. [S21, S24, S25, S28] have shown that the irradiation of mouse spermatogonia may lead to occurrence of a wide array of skeletal malformations. The genetic variation that influences some malformations may, indeed, have a strong mutational component. It is remarkable, on the other hand, that studies on the association of malformations with known genetic polymorphisms, such as the ABO blood groups (see [V4, V10]) and the major histocompatibility system [T4], have failed to point to any such association.

130. Some aspects of mammalian embryology should be mentioned here, since they are relevant to estimation of risk. Mammalian development is not entirely pre-programmed; rather it is influenced to a significant degree by the environment of the developing embryo. In the event of physical or chemical insult, the embryo has an remarkable ability to catch up and correct the damage. Many buffering effects are built into biologic systems, such that if one element is disrupted, others may be able to compensate. In addition, the evolution of gene duplication has led to a biological system of buffering, such that if one gene is knocked out, others may be able to take over its function. There appear to be thresholds during the course of development and aging, such that timing is extremely important. Mutations that upset the timing of events (heterochronic mutations) may produce unpredictable results [W7].

131. The incidence of all types of multifactorial diseases given in the UNSCEAR 1986 Report [U2], 660,000 per million, was based on the study of Czeizel et al. in Hungary [C12], which considered morbidity up to the age of 70, and some individuals had more than one disease. The Hungarian study comprised incidence estimates for 26 such multifactorial diseases, which were classified according to ICD and subdivided into three groups:

(a) very severe (schizophrenia, multiple sclerosis, epilepsy, myocardial infarction);
(b) moderately severe and/or episodic or seasonal (Graves' disease, diabetes, gout, affective psychoses, duodenal ulceration, asthma);
(c) less severe (varicose veins, atopic dermatitis etc.).

With the exception of epilepsy, none of these diseases causes death in the age group 0-19 years, but they are among the leading causes of death in advanced age. Such incidence estimates are extremely useful for many purposes, but in the context of radiation risk estimation, these prevalence estimates need to be carefully analysed to further identify subsets of conditions that may potentially respond to an increase in mutation rate. Such analysis is necessary because of the following:

(a) a major part of morbidity for many of these diseases is not the result of genetic predisposition or inescapable environmental exposure or both but is the result of voluntary and avoidable behaviour. Type 2 diabetes is one example; coronary heart disease and gout are other examples;
(b) in some of these diseases, the quality of life is not impaired decisively, providing that the individual finds a way of adapting his or her lifestyle to the disease;

(c) parameters such as the attitude of the society, the number of doctors and the quality of the health care system influence whether a disease is diagnosed and how much detriment it causes.

The relative importance of these factors may vary in different populations and may vary over time within the same population.

C. MOLECULAR AND BIOCHEMICAL STUDIES OF SPONTANEOUS AND RADIATION-INDUCED MUTATIONS

132. In addition to numerous types of DNA damage leading to stable, heritable mutations (i.e. single base deletions, base-pair modifications, strand breaks, base-pair substitutions, nondisjunction etc., that lead to nonsense, missense, frameshift, chromosomal mutations etc.), the site of a particular mutation must also be taken into account when attempting to analyse its impact on genetic risk. The relevance of various sites of mutation and their effect on cell function is of crucial importance in understanding the effect of molecular damage on phenotypic abnormality. Thus, a knowledge of molecular damage can be important in predicting genetic risk.

1. Location and effects of mutations

133. Structural mutations occur in the coding region of a gene, altering the protein product of a single gene. If the change occurs in a sequence that codes for a non-critical region of the protein, it will have little or no effect and will be well tolerated (e.g. amino acid substitution into the non-active site of an enzyme). If, however, it occurs in a critical region, it may impair the function of the protein (e.g. the disruption of the disulfide bridge in the oxygen-carrying haemoglobin molecule, which results in sickle-cell anaemia).

134. While the structure, and thus the function, of the gene product will not be affected by mutations in regulatory regions, the amount of gene product synthesized may be. Loss of promoter function will render a gene inactive even though its structural integrity remains intact, making the mutation difficult to identify, the loss of other regulatory elements, such as repressors, enhancers etc. may result in the loss of responsiveness to environmental conditions (e.g. liver cytochromes, which are upregulated in response to toxic insult).

135. If the protein serves a single, limited function, its loss or overproduction may have only a minor effect on the survival of the organism (e.g. the loss of tyrosine hydroxylase, which results in albinism). However, if the gene product is a regulatory protein involved in a pathway that amplifies its effect, the effects of the mutation may be far-reaching or even devastating to the organism (e.g. protein kinase proto-oncogenes, in which activating mutations lead to cancer). Other examples include molecules like the chaperonins, which regulate the secondary structural folding of many different proteins; *p53*, which has a dominant negative effect; the ubiquitins, which regulate the degradation of all messenger RNA molecules such that they are not transcribed into protein indefinitely; transport proteins, which carry the gene products to their proper location in the cell; genes involved in gene inactivation, such as dosage compensation resulting from X-chromosome inactivation in females [T3].

136. Likewise, if the gene product is a structural molecule essential to the development and maintenance of normal anatomy, such as connective tissue constituents, the loss of this type of gene function will have far-reaching effects for the organism as a whole (e.g. defective keratin which leads to epidermis bullosa, and defective collagen, which leads to osteogenesis imperfecta). Moreover, any gene involved in the synthetic pathway of such structural elements will have major effects (e.g. defective hydroxylase enzyme, which leads to mucopolysaccharidoses and concomitant skeletal changes).

137. In molecules where there is a repeating structure, any type of mutation in these repeating segments of the gene will destroy the structure of the whole molecule. For example, collagen contains multiple repetitive elements, such that any mutation in the third amino acid of the repeat disrupts the entire secondary structure of the glycoprotein.

138. Recent developments in cancer research suggest that somatic mutations are responsible for most, if not all, leukaemias, lymphomas and solid tumours [C6, M11, S11]. This is generally due to the loss or mutation of an oncogene suppressor gene function (as, for example, retinoblastoma or Wilms' tumour) or to an "activating" mutation in an oncogene that renders it immune to normal regulation (e.g. *RAS* in colon cancer). There are also many hot spots for mutation throughout the genome; since these regions show a higher frequency of mutation than other regions of the genome, they may be far more sensitive to mutagenic agents [V3].

139. The failure of crossover during meiosis can lead to non-disjunction, resulting in the loss or gain of large regions of chromosomal material. Thus, this single event can adversely affect many genes (e.g. trisomy 21 causes Down's syndrome, while most other trisomies and monosomies are not compatible with life.) Mutations that disrupt this genetically regulated process will have major ramifications.

140. Mutations in one region of a gene may produce a phenotype that is completely different from mutations in another region. This is particularly true for genes coding for products with multiple domains, such as connective tissue molecules (for example, dislocated lens of the eye and rupture of the aorta are both caused by mutations in the fibrillin gene) [V10].

141. It has also become apparent that alternative splicing of messenger RNA molecules occurs (e.g. the messenger RNA for several different hormones can be produced from one gene); that there are "genes within genes" (e.g. the neurofibromatosis locus); and that some genes code for precursors that are then cleaved enzymatically to yield the active product (e.g. prothrombin to active thrombin, encephalon to endorphin). Thus, one gene can, in effect, code for several products.

142. It is now clear that damage to mitochondria (including those in ova) must also be considered in genetic risk estimates. In the past it was assumed that damage to DNA was the only concern, but changes to other components of the cell structure, such as mitochondria, may affect subsequent generations [W12].

(a) Nature and origin of spontaneous mutations in human Mendelian disease

143. A large number of spontaneously arising mutations that cause disease states in humans have been described. Only a few are known at the molecular level. As of 1990, molecular data were available for some 76 Mendelian diseases in humans [S3]. For 33 of these, the predominant event is a point mutation (base-pair change), and for 39 it is a length mutation (mostly DNA deletions, but sometimes duplications or other gross changes). In the 4 remaining diseases, both point mutations and length mutations occur. These relative frequencies may be revised as more data become available, but for now, it can be assumed that point mutations and length mutations each account for about half of the Mendelian diseases [S7].

144. In spontaneously occurring mutations, point mutations (i.e. mutations in which a single base pair is altered or deleted) do not appear to be distributed at random throughout the genome. This is thought to be related to the sequence organization of the gene and its genomic context [S7]. CpG dinucleotide sequences, when present in a gene, provide hot spots for transition-type mutations (i.e. A to G or G to A and C to T and T to C). Vertebrate DNA is highly methylated at the cytosine residue, and about 90% of 5-methyl-cytosine occurs within CpG sequences. At the level of the gene, C to T transitions and the corresponding G to A transitions in the complementary DNA strand occur at a high frequency within these methylated regions; this is thought to be due to the propensity of 5-methylcytosine to undergo spontaneous deamination to form thymine [C10]. It can be anticipated that each gene will have its own susceptibility pattern, and it is not known whether these patterns will be similar in humans and in mice. Other endogenous damage to DNA is thought to come from replication errors and from oxidative attack mediated by chemical radicals [A9].

145. Examples of non-random point mutations that have been identified in human cancer biology studies include the point mutations in codons 12, 59 and 61 of the *RAS* genes involved in myeloid leukaemia, lung cancer etc. and those in codons 110-307 of the *P53* tumour suppressor gene in diverse types of cancers. Such site preferences have long been known to occur in visible chromosomal changes in neoplasias, particularly leukaemias and lymphomas, and molecular studies are now shedding light on these specificities.

146. There is good evidence that the breakpoints of length mutations are also non-randomly distributed. Of 60 small (<20 bp) deletions at the 23 loci studied, 59 had direct repeats of 2-8 bp. For large deletions, sequence homologies and repetitive sequences such as Alu located within or between genes appear to play important roles. The mechanisms involved in the generation of deletions and duplications are listed in Table 2.

147. Data from a number of well-analysed spontaneous gene deletions are consistent with mechanisms that assume base mispairing between repeat sequences and slippage during replication; homologous unequal recombination between evolutionarily related genes; homologous unequal recombination between repetitive sequences such as Alu; and non-homologous recombination. There is circumstantial evidence supporting the hypothesis that repetitive sequences may play an important role in chromosome pairing [S3]; if true, the deletions and duplications that have been found to be associated with spontaneously arising mutations in many diseases may represent the inevitable by-products of occasional mispairing.

148. Examples of deletions arising as a result of non-homologous recombination are provided by some alpha-thalassemias [N12, O1], some beta-thalassemias [A5, H11] and some complex thalassemias [J1]. In all these deletions, the 5' breakpoints were mapped either in or close to Alu sequences. The interpretation is that these deletions presumably arose during DNA replication (when sequences widely separated in the linear DNA molecule might be physically close to one another as a result of anchorage to the nuclear matrix and chromatin loop formation) as a consequence of non-homologous intrachromosomal breakage and reunion events [A5, V2]. The models proposed differ in some details.

149. Intragenic partial deletions (well over 300 are now known) appear to be the most common defect leading to Duchenne and Becker muscular dystrophies [D2, F6, G5, K8]. Less common are intragenic duplications that appear to duplicate one or a few exons by the tandem duplication of a portion of the gene, presumably by unequal crossing-over between repeat elements [H13, K8]. Data have also been published suggesting that duplications can arise as an intrachromosomal event through unequal sister-chromatid exchange [H14].

150. Thus, in spontaneously occurring mutations there occur both point mutations (base-pair changes) and length mutations, which include DNA deletions (small and large), insertions, rearrangements and duplications. The length mutations are occasionally microscopically detectable as chromosomal aberrations. Several other mechanisms of mutation are involved in spontaneously occurring mutations in humans, including gene conversion and mutation due to the insertion of mobile, or transposable, genetic elements. (Transposable elements are also discussed in Section I.D.) The term gene conversion describes the local transfer of DNA sequences from one gene to a related gene elsewhere in the genome in an event that resembles a double crossover [M1]. Gene conversion events leading to disease phenotypes are now well documented in humans. One example is congenital adrenal hyperplasia due to 21-hydroxylase deficiency [D7, H7, U12]. There are two 21-hydroxylase genes in humans, one of which is a non-functional pseudogene; if any of the inactivating sequences in the pseudogene are introduced into the functional gene by gene conversion, there will be a deficiency of the enzyme. Other examples include spontaneous mutations at the HLA-A and thymidine kinase (TK) loci in human somatic cells *in vitro*, in which gene conversion has been shown to play a significant role (see [S5]).

(b) Radiation-induced mutations in mammalian experimental systems

151. Data from mouse mutation studies (with x- or gamma- and neutron irradiation) have provided most of the information on the genetic effects of radiation. They have been reviewed from time to time [E4, F3, F4, R8, R9, R10, S1, S3, S4, S5, S6, S7, S13, S19]. Points of interest include the following:

(a) spermatogonia, post-meiotic male germ cells and mature and immature oocytes differ in their sensitivity to the induction of mutations by radiation;
(b) the yield of mutations varies between gene loci;
(c) a majority of radiation-induced mutations are lethal in the homozygous condition (i.e. two copies of the same mutant gene);
(d) the relative frequency of various molecular changes seen in the mutational event differs between spontaneous mutation and radiation-induced mutation; and
(e) in mice, the frequencies of radiation-induced recessive and dominant mutations differ.

152. Russell et al. [R3], in a detailed genetic and molecular characterization of large numbers of specific-locus mutations collected at the d, se and c loci, have shown that the simple phenotypic classification of specific-locus mutations can effectively separate mutations into the following three categories: multi-locus deletions, presumed intragenic mutations and viable null mutations. Comparisons between mutations induced in different germ-cell stages, spontaneous mutations and mutations induced by low-LET radiation, neutrons and ethylnitrosourea (ENU) have shown that there are marked qualitative differences between spontaneous and induced mutations and between mutations induced by low-LET radiation, neutrons or ENU in different germ-cell types. A total of 264 radiation-induced mutations and 45 spontaneous mutations were classified in this way. Most of radiation-induced mutations studied in the mouse and in mammalian *in vitro* systems, however, are either presumed to be or actually demonstrated to be DNA deletions; however, the relative proportions of point mutations versus deletions vary with the locus and the test system under study [S7]. In one study [R13], 31 mutations were analysed by Southern blot analysis with a tyrosinase cDNA clone and with other probes, which identified 13 radiation-induced and one spontaneous mutation to be deletions or rearrangements ranging from 36 to 2,000 kb. The fact that such large viable deletions can be recovered suggests that 1 or 2 Mb of DNA including and surrounding the c-locus harbour no genes essential for viability or fertility.

153. There are also hot spots for radiation-induced breaks, as observed in the chromosomes of blood lymphocytes in human radiotherapy patients. These hot spots are in T bands, which are very rich in both GC and Alu sequences, suggesting that at least some radiation-induced deletions may arise by mechanisms similar to those inferred for naturally occurring deletions mediated to Alu sequences [R13]. (T bands, which are a subset of R bands, represent only 15% of all bands, but contain 65% of mapped genes and 42% of x-ray-induced breaks [S7]).

154. The findings in mouse studies are consistent with the view that in mouse germ cells, most radiation-induced mutations are DNA deletions. This has now been shown to be the case by molecular methods for a number of mutations [S4]. However, most work done on the effects of germ-cell irradiation have been done in males; female germ cells may have very

different susceptibility to different types of induced mutation at different stages. Surprisingly large deletions can be tolerated in viable mice [C18].

155. Data on the induction of mutations that lead to observable congenital structural abnormalities in the progeny of irradiated mice suggest that these abnormalities are not very sensitive end-points. In addition, it should be mentioned that different strains of mice may have different sensitivities to radiation [N15, N16], although the work of Favor et al. [F17, F18] suggests no strain differences when using radiation and ethylnitrosourea.

156. From available studies that have analysed the molecular nature of mutations, the following conclusions may be drawn:

(a) ionizing radiation induces very few point mutations;
(b) when ionizing radiation induces mutations in enzymatic proteins, the changes lead to altered enzyme activity or lack of enzyme activity; the molecular changes may include a mixture of events at the DNA level, ranging from point mutations to intragenic DNA deletions, multilocus deletions, or rearrangements;
(c) the limited data on radiation-induced mutations at the haemoglobin loci in mice suggest that radiation induces deletions, duplications and translocations, but not point mutations.

The fact that radiation-induced mutations are likely to differ from spontaneous mutations in the type of mutation produced, the frequency and the sites affected must also be considered, and indeed expected. The above examples offer a convincing argument that a simple, direct correlation between the number of mutations and the degree of mutation damage would be exceedingly difficult, if not impossible, to demonstrate in either animal or human studies.

2. Protein studies

157. Quantitative and qualitative protein variations in the children of atomic bomb survivors were examined, using a variety of methods. Presumed new mutations were verified by carefully excluding false paternity. No increase in comparison with the controls was observed. The number of loci screened was 6.67 10^5 in the exposed group (parents within 2 km of the centre of the atomic bombings) and 4.67 10^5 in the non-exposed group. Three new mutants were identified in each group. The mutation rates per locus per generation were estimated to be 6 10^{-6} (95% CI: 2-15 10^{-6}; exposed group) and 6.4 10^{-6} (95% CI: 1-19 10^{-6}; non-exposed group) [N7, N9].

158. For the monitoring of large population groups, another approach has been suggested that avoids the logistically most difficult part of protein studies, namely contacting the families and collecting the blood samples [V9]. In most countries, practically all newborns are screened for inherited metabolic diseases such as phenylketonuria (PKU). A few drops of blood are put on a special test card that is sent to a screening centre. A method has been developed by which haemoglobin (Hb) and other proteins can be extracted from this card and studied by electrophoretic methods [A4]. In a pilot project in Japan, blood samples from 40,003 newborns (for Hb variants) and 30,659 individuals (for other protein variants), were screened, representing altogether 722,719 gene loci. In three instances, the transmission test was negative but there was no evidence for non-paternity. These three individuals can be regarded as new mutants. From these data, the following mutation rates were estimated: 5.2 10^{-6} per locus per generation, 2.0 10^{-8} per codon and 6.0 10^{-9} per base. These data are in good agreement with other spontaneous mutation rates (see [V10]).

159. Given the number of offspring included in the study by Neel et al. [N9] and the relatively low gonadal exposure of parents in the exposed group, it would be premature to use these data to speculate on the biological mechanisms of radiation-induced mutations. But one likely conclusion can be drawn: medium- to low-dose irradiation in humans does not induce an unexpectedly large number of mutations detectable at the protein level. As discussed later, radiation does not cause significant visible genetic damage in humans in the next generation, and the result for proteins just noted seems to decrease the likelihood that radiation could enhance the long-term genetic load in the human population by producing many recessive mutations. Many radiation-induced recessive mutations in the mouse are deletions, as evidenced by studies with the seven recessive test loci [R3]. From widespread experience in medical genetics it would be expected that such deletions, if induced in human gene loci coding for known enzyme proteins, would reduce enzyme activity by about one half. Such effects have not been observed at a higher rate in children of irradiated parents in Japan.

160. The methods for assessing protein variants in children of parents exposed to the atomic bombings tend to be very time-consuming and personnel-intensive. They might be applicable to the monitoring of a limited population group that has been exposed to relatively high doses of radiation (or any other mutagenic agent), but they are not suited for the long-term screening and monitoring of large population groups.

D. SUMMARY

161. The estimation of additional genetic risk is meaningful only in relation to the spontaneous mutation rate. Thus, in attempting to calculate the genetic consequences of any agent including radiation, it is essential to begin with an accurate estimate of the background incidence rate for a given genetic disease or congenital anomaly.

162. There are now numerous registries of birth defects worldwide, each with unique features and each with advantages and disadvantages; these should all be taken into account when attempting to assess the background incidence for human populations in general. Access to multiple registries allows the development of fairly accurate background rates for congenital anomalies. Registries have different incidences of different anomalies with regional, ethnic and temporal variations in specific birth defects. However, when they are taken all together, fairly accurate background incidences for various congenital anomalies can now be established. Anomalies that are subject to environmental influences, such as neural tube defects, can be identified as varying with social class and region.

163. There is a consistent finding in all populations of 2%-3% incidence of serious congenital anomalies that will alter the length of life or ability to function normally without medical intervention that are ascertained in newborns. Another 2%-3% of serious congenital anomalies are ascertained by 5 years of age. An additional 5%-13% of minor anomalies are found in all populations.

164. Dominant mutations, together with X-linked mutations, are usually considered to provide the most important contribution to an increase in genetic disease that results from exposure to environmental mutagens. Contributions from autosomal recessive mutations would have less impact initially and would not be expected to be evident for many generations.

165. There is general agreement on the background incidence of autosomal dominant disorders. There is even less difficulty in establishing a baseline for autosomal-dominant diseases that have a strong selective disadvantage, the prevalence of which is maintained in the population by an equilibrium between constant mutation pressure and selection. These sentinel mutations are expected to indicate increases in the mutation rate caused by a new mutagenic agent in the environment. However, sentinel mutations are too rare to provide a basis for estimating realistic mutation rate increases. Continuous screening of very large populations would be required, but from the experience accumulated so far, it is extremely unlikely that human populations will ever be exposed to mutagenic agents that will cause an observable increase above the natural rate of mutation.

166. Other factors, such as paternal age, may greatly influence the rate of occurrence of certain autosomal dominant congenital anomalies; thus a shift in paternal age distribution within a population may have a greater effect on incidence than a change in exposure to radiation or other mutagenic agents. Maternal age may influence the rate of chromosomal anomalies such as Down's syndrome in a similar fashion.

167. Both heterozygote advantage and heterozygote disadvantage have been observed in autosomal recessive diseases in humans [V10]. Induced recessive mutations may cause harm in four ways:

(a) partnership with a defective allele already established in the population;
(b) partnership with another recessive mutation induced at the same locus;
(c) the formation of homozygous descendants of the induced mutation; that is, identity by descent;
(d) heterozygous effects (i.e. a carrier of the gene may have adverse effects).

Estimates of the manifestation of homozygotes in future generations depend critically on the assumptions made about consanguinity rates.

168. The incidence of visible structural anomalies or unbalanced translocations in chromosomal disease has been based on population studies on newborns; they do not include data from studies on spontaneous abortions. Most fetuses with numerical chromosomal anomalies (e.g. monosomy or trisomy) do not survive to birth. Thus, any radiation-induced increase of non-disjunction and/or early chromosome loss is likely to lead to an increase in the rate of spontaneous abortion rather than to an increase in chromosomally abnormal newborns. Thus, any increase in structural and numerical chromosomal aberration among newborns attributable to additional radiation of the parents would very probably be small and would depend on the age structure of the population.

169. It is important to estimate the mutational component of the incidence of congenital malformations. This involves estimating the frequency and degree of genetic determination of single anomalies and their modes of inheritance, which is very difficult to do, and indeed must be individualized. The complex genetic basis of most malformations makes it almost impossible to be sure of the effects of specific chemical or physical agents such as radiation.

170. In addition to multiple types of DNA damage leading to heritable mutations (i.e. single base dele-

tions, base-pair modifications, strand breaks, base-pair substitutions, nondisjunction etc., leading to nonsense, missense, frameshift, chromosomal mutations etc.), the site of a particular mutation must be taken into account when attempting to analyse its impact on genetic risk. Structural mutations occur in the coding region of a gene, altering the protein product of a single gene. Mutations in regulatory regions may affect the amount of gene product expressed or the time at which it is expressed. The type of gene in which a mutation occurs, e.g. a gene with limited function or a gene coding for a regulatory factor, will influence the extent of the mutation's harm to the organism. Failure of crossover during meiosis can lead to nondisjunction and may have a serious detrimental effect on the organism (chromosomal effects). Mutations in one region of a gene may produce a phenotype that is completely different from that caused by a mutation within another region. Mutations that upset the timing of events may produce unpredictable results (heterochronic effects).

171. It had been assumed that DNA damage was the only concern in radiation damage, but it now appears that changes in other components of the cell structure, such as the mitochondria, may have effects that are transmitted to subsequent generations. Mutations that affect the non-traditional mechanisms of inheritance (e.g. the methylation that might be involved in genomic imprinting) could affect numerous genes and have consequences that might not become visible for several generations.

III. GENETIC RISK ESTIMATION

172. Radiation exposure of the germ cells of animals, and therefore presumably also of humans, causes mutations and chromosomal aberrations that in turn may lead to genetic defects or diseases in the offspring and in later generations. Studies of atomic bomb survivors, industrial accidents and occupational and medical exposures have allowed some rough estimates to be made of genetic effects following human exposure to radiation. However, the paucity of direct observations regarding the genetic effects of radiation in humans has led to considerable uncertainty in the estimates of overall genetic risk and of the relative proportions of the various types of mutations that may occur from radiation. Animal experiments, most of them in mice, have been undertaken in an attempt to further quantify these effects. Although mice or other animals and humans differ in many ways that are biologically important, it has been necessary to assume similar responses in extrapolating the results of mouse and other animal studies to human populations.

173. In previous UNSCEAR Reports, the Committee described the various methods used to make genetic risk estimates and applied them to the available data. The history of these and other attempts to estimate the genetic risk of radiation has been described by Sankaranarayanan [S2, S3, S4, S5, S8]. Much has been learned about the limitations of these methods and about the molecular nature of the mutations that must be taken into account in estimating risk.

174. In the early 1970s, the following conclusions were derived from studies of animals, predominantly mice, and they were thought also to apply to human beings [S13, V6]:

(a) even at a relatively low dose, radiation leads to a sterile phase in males because it kills most of the spermatogonia; the testicular tissue is later repopulated by repeated division of a few especially resistant A spermatogonia;

(b) in the male mouse, a majority of visible chromosomal aberrations that are present in the F_1 offspring are induced in the pre-sterile phase, i.e. in postmeiotically irradiated male germ cells. Thus, if a human male is irradiated, chromosomal aberrations are not likely in the next generation unless conception occurs less than about 6-8 weeks after irradiation;

(c) in the female mouse, chromosomal anomalies may be induced, most of which lead to the death of the zygote at a very early stage of development (equivalent to early abortions in humans). The same is true for chromosomal aberrations that are induced in male germ cells and that are present in the zygote;

(d) in the hours around fertilization there is increased susceptibility to the induction of aneuploidies, especially the loss of single chromosomes, e.g. the X-chromosome;

(e) acute irradiation at relatively high dose leads to a considerable increase in recessive mutations in both sexes;

(f) a strong dose-rate effect has been observed in spermatogonia and in oocytes: chronic irradiation induces only about one third of the recessive mutations that are induced by acute irradiation. A dose-rate effect is also present for predisposition to dominant mutations;

(g) many radiation-induced mutations, especially those induced in postspermatogonial cell stages, have been identified as deletions. Many induced recessive mutations were found to be lethal in the homozygous state;

(h) dominant mutations with clear-cut phenotypic effects and full penetrance are induced relatively rarely; dominant effects within multifactorial genetic systems, e.g. mutations affecting the skeleton, appear to be more common. However, before extrapolating this result to humans, the much easier and more detailed assessment of human anomalies should be considered;

(i) most translocations induced in spermatogonia are unable to pass through meiosis; they do not lead to abortions or to malformed offspring.

These conclusions have since been supplemented on the basis of data from further studies in animals and humans. The results of these studies will be discussed in the following Sections.

A. HUMAN STUDIES

1. Genetic follow-up studies on the survivors of the atomic bombings

175. While people who were exposed to radiation have been shown to suffer direct effects from that exposure, such as increased cancer rates, the data on the survivors of the atomic bombings of Hiroshima and Nagasaki indicate that acute irradiation at moderate doses has a negligible adverse effect on the health of the subsequent generation. Any minor effects that may be produced are so small that they are submerged in the background noise of naturally occurring mutational effects; they have not been demonstrated even by the refined epidemiological methods that have been employed over the last five decades [N7, N8, N9].

176. The first steps towards organizing a genetic follow-up study at Hiroshima and Nagasaki were taken in 1946, and the full programme was initiated in 1948. Now, after 45 years, that programme, conducted by the Radiation Effects Research Foundation (formerly the Atomic Bomb Casualty Commission), has become the largest and longest-running exercise in genetic epidemiology ever carried out. In recent years, the significance of the study has been greatly enhanced by the revised radiation dose estimates for survivors that became available in 1986. All of the accumulated data have now been analysed on the basis of the revised dose system.

177. The study has had two phases. In the early years (1947-1954), because of the Japanese ration system, it was possible to register virtually all pregnant women in the two cities at the end of the fifth month of their pregnancy and to arrange that once the child was born, it would be examined by a Japanese physician especially instructed in the diagnosis of congenital malformations. The first phase of the study collected the following data on each child: presence of congenital defect, viability at birth, survival through the first two weeks of life, birth weight and sex. What made it unusual was that because of the pre-birth registration, it was a prospective study embracing a total newborn population; studies of this type are less prone to bias than retrospective studies, in which at some fixed date one attempts to reconstruct pregnancy outcomes over a preceding period. About one third of the infants who were examined under this study were reexamined at the age of 9 months. All children born before May 1946 were excluded from the study of heritable genetic effects, since they may have been conceived prior to the bombings and received *in utero* exposures [N3].

178. In the second phase of the study (1954 to the present), the births continued to be registered until 1985, but the clinical programme was terminated. The data now collected are on the survival of liveborn infants, the occurrence of cancer in the children and, for selected subsets of the registered children, physical development, the presence of chromosome abnormalities and the occurrence of mutations that alter certain characteristics of the proteins of blood serum and red blood cells. The birth registry was also extended backwards in time, to include all infants born between 1 May 1946 (i.e. conceived after the bombings) and December 1947 (after the latter date infants would have been registered in the earlier programme). By now, the cohort of all children born to survivors of the atomic bombings who received significant exposures to radiation at the time of the bombings and who still live in Hiroshima and Nagasaki is thought to be complete. Significant exposure to radiation is defined as having been within 2,000 meters of the hypocentre of either bomb; individuals in this category are spoken of as proximally exposed, while those more distant from the hypocentre are referred to as distally exposed. The cohort of children born to a parent or parents who were proximally exposed consists of 31,150 individuals. An age- and sex-matched control group of 41,066 children was established by selection from the much larger group of children in the two cities born to parents in the distally exposed category. The number of children drawn from these cohorts for the second phase of the study varied according to the indicator. The average gonadal dose (parents combined) for the proximally exposed category was about 0.4 Sv, the actual dose varying somewhat from study to study depending on which children were included. The dose curve is quite asymmetrical, skewed to the right, with some parents having received combined gonadal doses as high as 2.5 Sv [N7, N8, N9]. The results of the various end-points studied are summarized in the paragraphs below.

179. ***Untoward pregnancy outcome.*** Because major congenital defect, stillbirth and neonatal death are inter-related, these end-points have been treated as a single entity, termed "untoward pregnancy outcome" and defined as an outcome resulting in a child with major congenital defect and/or a stillbirth and/or death within the first two weeks of life. Between 1948 and 1954, data were collected on these outcomes for a total of 76,617 births in Hiroshima and Nagasaki; data on 69,706 of them were sufficiently complete in all respects to permit inclusion in the analysis [N3, O2]. In later analysis the category of untoward pregnancy outcome is separated into stillbirths and congenital anomalies, giving eight end-points in all for analysis.

180. ***Pre-reproductive deaths among liveborn children (exclusive of those resulting from a malignant tumour).*** The frequency of death of live-born children has been analysed through 1985, when the mean age of the members of the study groups, if still surviving, would have been 26.2 years. In the two cohorts assembled for the second phase of the study, there are 67,202 individuals, among whom there had been 2,584 deaths by 1985 [K3, N3, Y2].

181. ***Cancer incidence.*** Data on malignancies occurring before age 20 have been collected on all children born at Hiroshima and Nagasaki after May 1946, i.e. on all children conceived following the exposure of their parents and on a suitable set of control children in the two cities. There were 43 malignant tumours in the 31,150 children of proximally exposed parents and 49 such tumours in 41,066 children of distally exposed or unexposed parents. The incidence of leukaemia (a malignancy of particular interest because of the study of Gardner et al. [G2], see Section III.A.2) is essentially the same in the children of parents one or both of whom were proximally exposed as it is in the children of parents who were not significantly exposed [Y1].

182. ***Frequency of certain types of chromosomal abnormalities (balanced structural rearrangements of chromosomes and abnormalities in sex chromosome number).*** Among the 8,322 children of the proximally exposed who were studied, 19 showed sex-chromosome abnormalities and 23, chromosomal rearrangements; among the control group of 7,976 children, 24 showed sex-chromosome abnormalities and 27, chromosomal rearrangements. Since there is no known instance of a parent with a sex-chromosome abnormality transmitting it to a child, all children with sex-chromosome aneuploidy were assumed to result from a mutation in the germ cells of the preceding generation. With respect to the chromosomal rearrangements, only one child in each group was shown to result from a mutation in the preceding generation [A6]. It must be noted, however, that the youngest children in the chromosome study were 13 years of age at the start of the study, and the study thus could not be expected to yield adequate data on the frequency of cytogenetic anomalies associated with increased mortality rates, such as unbalanced autosomal structural rearrangements and autosomal trisomies. Most patients with these aberrations will already have died by the age of 13. A possible exception is Down's syndrome (i.e. trisomy 21), but even in these cases, a high percentage of the patients may have died during childhood and early youth, mostly from recurrent infections but also from congenital malformations of the heart and other organs, given the living conditions prevalent in post-war Japan. The data on sex chromosomal abnormalities and balanced autosomal structural rearrangements should, however, be relatively unbiased.

183. ***Frequency of mutations affecting certain characteristics of proteins.*** A total of 667,404 tests were performed for protein mutations that alter electrophoretic mobility or enzyme activity in the children of the proximally exposed parents, and 466,881 tests were performed in the children of parents who did not receive significant exposures. The appropriate family studies on the 747 rare protein variants detected revealed that there were four mutations in the children of the proximally exposed and three in the control children [N4].

184. ***Sex ratio.*** The most pertinent data on the effect of parental radiation on sex of the child derives from the situation where the mother was exposed and the father unexposed. In this case, the sons would be expected to manifest the deleterious effects of radiation-induced X-linked dominant and X-linked recessive mutations as well as loss of the Y-chromosome, whereas the daughters would experience the effect of only the dominant mutations. A radiation effect should manifest itself as a relative decrease in male offspring, i.e. the sex ratio (male births/female births) should decrease. In fact, at the time the data were last analysed, there was an insignificant increase in the sex ratio, i.e. the data were counter-hypothesis [S10].

185. ***Physical development of child.*** The physical development of a subset of the children of exposed and control parents was studied at birth and at age 8-10 months [N3] and during the school years [F11, F12, F13, F14, F15]. The data for the most part pertain to height, weight, and chest circumference.

186. A variety of analyses of these seven data sets (and in later publications presented as eight data sets) has failed to reveal a statistically significant effect of parental radiation on the indicator. The average combined gonadal dose of acute ionizing radiation received by the proximally exposed parents (0.4 Sv) approximates that which in the past had been estimated to be a genetic doubling dose for mice. The

statistical power of these studies is such that the absence of an effect of parental exposure to the bombings on any of the indicators suggests that humans may not be as sensitive to the genetic effects of radiation as had for some years been projected on the basis of the murine doubling dose data.

187. The argument can be, and was, carried a step further. The investigators of the genetic effects of the atomic bombings accepted the proposition that some mutations did indeed result from the exposures to the atomic bombings and that this corpus of data should reflect the first-generation impact of these mutations on the population. The proposition was bolstered by the increase in chromosomal damage and somatic cell mutations observed in lymphocytes and red blood cells of the atomic bomb survivors [A7, N1], as well as by the increase in leukaemia and other malignant neoplasms in survivors [P3]. Accordingly, an effort has been made to estimate from these data the doubling dose of radiation for humans [N7, N9]. The doubling dose (relative) approach was felt to be imperative in this setting, as it would confer a perspective on the relative risks of radiation that would be lacking with the direct (absolute) approach. But although simple in principle, the doubling dose concept has been difficult to implement: for the estimate to have maximum accuracy, it requires the widest possible spectrum of genetic end-points, each weighted as to its importance in the total phenotypic burden imposed on a population by spontaneous mutation.

188. The doubling dose approach requires estimating the contribution of spontaneous mutation in the parental generation to each indicator anomaly or mutation. For technical reasons, this is not feasible for the sex ratio and the physical measurements. The approach also requires deriving a simple linear regression of each indicator on dose. This was judged to be not justified for balanced chromosomal rearrangements, where only a single mutation was observed in the children of both exposed and of unexposed parents. There remained five indicators from which to derive the regressions. (Since the data for the three indicators that were eliminated from the calculation did not suggest a radiation effect, their elimination should not bias the calculation.)

189. To derive a doubling dose, the impact of spontaneous mutation on the indicator in the parental generation must be estimated for each indicator. The value for sex-chromosome aneuploids and for loci encoding for proteins may be directly determined from the appropriate family studies. The value for the other three indicators has been estimated from the genetic literature. These three estimates are relatively uncertain and should improve with time. The background incidence for these indicators and the parental mutational component in the indicator, expressed in absolute terms and as a per cent, are given in Table 4 [N5]. The range given for three of the indicators reflects uncertainty as to the exact magnitude of the mutational component.

190. The data can be used for two different types of calculations. In Table 4, the doubling dose of radiation in relation to the contribution of spontaneous mutation to the indicator has been calculated for lower confidence limits of 99%, 95% and 90%. In principle, such estimates may be combined if it is assumed that the true doubling dose is the same for all the phenomena under study. Such an assumption is not warranted in this situation, the radiation literature suggesting that the doubling dose for the genetic phenomena resulting in untoward pregnancy outcomes, F_1 (first generation) mortality and F_1 cancer may be lower than the doubling dose for sex chromosome aneuploids and the nucleotide substitutions, which were the predominant end-points of the protein studies. The minimal doubling dose at the 95% probability level for the first three indicators combined was estimated to be between 0.63 and 1.04 Sv; for the last two, it was estimated to be 2.71 Sv.

191. Since these five end-points are essentially independent of one another, the most probable doubling dose for the totality of phenomena measured by these end-points can be obtained by summing these five regressions, summing the estimated contribution of spontaneous mutation to the various indicators and dividing the latter by the former [N9].

192. The resulting estimate was between 1.7 and 2.2 Sv, with the range again reflecting some of the uncertainty in estimating the contribution of the parental mutation to the end-point. The investigators considered this estimate conservative, for two reasons: (a) as noted, certain indicators for which there is no evidence for a radiation effect could not, for technical reasons, be included in the estimate, and (b) the data on socio-economic status, which were routinely collected on a subset of the population, suggested a slightly lower status for the proximally exposed survivors [K3]. This fact might increase the frequency of untoward pregnancy outcomes and death among live-born infants in this group and so give an upward bias to the estimate of the genetic effect of radiation.

193. As the investigators pointed out, the extrapolation of these results to the effects of chronic (or small and intermittent) exposures to ionizing radiation requires the selection of an appropriate dose-rate reduction factor. For the murine data, which was for the most part collected at doses of 3 and 6 Gy, a dose rate reduction factor of 3 has been employed. In the light of the much lower gonadal exposures experienced by proximally exposed survivors at Hiroshima and Nagasaki, the investigators elected to employ a

dose rate reduction factor of 2 [N6]. This resulted in a minimal estimate of the doubling dose for humans for chronic exposure to ionizing radiation, approximately 4.0 Sv.

194. The error in this estimate is indeterminate but must be considerable. First, there is the statistical error inherent in the estimation procedures, which is relatively large in relation to the regressions. Next, there is the error inherent in the present uncertainty concerning the contribution of parental mutation to such indicators as untoward pregnancy outcomes and early death. In addition, there is a potential error in the use of a dose-rate reduction factor of 2 in extrapolating from the effects of acute to chronic radiation. The fact that three additional indicators could not, for technical reasons, be incorporated into the estimate renders it conservative, as was already mentioned, but does not reduce its error. Finally, the human controls are not as accurately defined as would be the controls in a similar mouse study. Although the control parents were taken from the distally exposed group (they had been 2.5 km or more from the hypocentre of the bomb), it is not possible to ascertain that they were not exposed to radiation from other sources.

195. Some further guidance as to the lower limit of this estimate may be derived from the fact that although the average conjoint parental dose of acute radiation experienced by the proximal survivors was 0.4 Sv (a dose which in past UNSCEAR Reports was thought on the basis of murine experiments to approximate a doubling dose for acute exposures), it was not observed to have a significant effect on any of the eight indicators (see paragraph 186). This would be very unlikely if the true doubling dose for acute radiation is as low as 0.4 Sv. From the lower 95% confidence limits cited earlier, it seems unlikely that the human doubling dose for acute ionizing radiation under these circumstances is less than 1.0 Sv, and for chronic ionizing radiation, less than 2.0 Sv. The estimation of the doubling dose for humans must be regarded as a dynamic and continuing process, subject to revision as further data become available. Furthermore, it must be recalled that any estimate of the doubling dose is time- and place-specific, reflecting the genotype-environment interaction at a particular time. This is certainly true of the estimate based on the Hiroshima-Nagasaki experience.

196. In evaluating the importance to be accorded to the results of this study vis-a-vis the results of the more controlled murine experiment (see following Sections), four considerations stand out: (a) it is based directly on human data, (b) the indicators (congenital malformation, early death, cancer and syndromes attributable to sex-chromosome aneuploidy) are highly relevant to human affairs, (c) since the study includes virtually all the children ever to be born to exposed parents at Hiroshima and Nagasaki, it provides a total appraisal of the genetic effects of exposures to the atomic bombings rather than a snapshot in time, (d) the findings are of necessity obtained at doses compatible with human survival and hence do not require the degree of extrapolation from the much higher (for humans, unrealistically higher) doses employed in the murine experiments.

2. Epidemiological study of leukaemia cases at Sellafield

197. Many epidemiological studies have been carried out on populations exposed to radiation [A2, B5, C7, C11, C15, D3, K7, L4, S8]. One in particular raised concern about the harmful hereditary effects of chronic exposure. In 1990, Gardner et al. [G1, G2] reported the results of a case-control study of leukaemia and lymphoma among young people near the Sellafield nuclear plant in the United Kingdom. The study involved 52 cases of leukaemia and 22 cases of non-Hodgkin's lymphoma. The increased incidence of leukaemia among children near Sellafield was associated with recorded whole-body penetrating radiation to the fathers who worked at the Sellafield plant before conception. The authors suggested that the radiation exposures of the fathers caused mutations in their germ cells that, when transmitted to their children, caused those children to develop leukaemia. The authors pointed out that since low doses were involved, there were important potential implications for radiobiology and for the protection of radiation workers and their children. Those fathers who were employed at the Sellafield nuclear plant and whose children developed leukaemia had received total doses of ≥100 mSv before conception and doses of ≥10 mSv in the 6 months before conception.

198. The implications of Gardner's conclusions, if correct, would be far-reaching, since they suggest that as small a dose as 10 mSv, delivered at a low dose rate to the fathers, is sufficient to cause a large increase in the incidence of leukaemia among their children. The authors point out that their results on leukaemia conflict with the results available for children of parents exposed to radiation at Hiroshima and Nagasaki; they suggested that the difference might be explained by the fact that the exposures in Japan were acute, with a high dose rate, and those in Sellafield were chronic, with a low dose rate.

199. From extensive studies in mice it has been known for some time that chronic exposure over a prolonged period has an important effect on mutational response to radiation. However, that effect is in the opposite direction from that hypothesized by Gardner, since protracted radiation induces only one third as many mutations in spermatogonia as high-dose-rate

radiation [R6, R12]. Recent results on other populations provide no support for the conclusions of Gardner et al. [G1, G2]. Indeed, when Yoshimoto et al. [Y1] calculated the slope of the dose-response curve for the incidence of cancer below the age of 20 years versus conjoint parental dose, using linear multiple regression, they found negative slopes both for leukaemia and for all cancers combined. (The standard error of the slope, in each case, was larger than the absolute value of the slope.) The average radiation exposures of the survivors of the atomic bombings were much higher than those of the fathers employed at the Sellafield nuclear plant.

200. In addition, the statistically significant increase in relative risk of leukaemia found for fathers employed at the Sellafield nuclear plant was due almost entirely to only four affected children. Most of the other affected children had fathers employed in other industries. The conclusions of Gardner et al. are inconsistent with expectations from the risk estimates presented in this Annex, both from the doubling dose method and the direct method. Although the Gardner study used accepted procedures and appears to have been carefully done, it should be kept in mind that its conclusion is based on a correlation and is not consistent with other observations of exposed parents, and it may be a chance observation. A correlation alone cannot show causation. Furthermore, this particular correlation is heavily dependent on a very small number of cases and is contradicted by all of the studies that have been done in other populations with similar exposures (see paragraph 208).

201. The chromosomal translocations resulting in proto-oncogene activation that characterize the early phases of many leukaemias and lymphomas would tend to produce phenotypic effects incompatible with embryogenesis [E7]. For this reason such events are unlikely to be genetic determinants of leukaemia that could account for the Gardner et al. [G1, G2] findings. However, specific gene losses are also believed to characterize the early phases of some leukaemias [W11]. Since predisposition to some solid tumours of childhood (retinoblastoma and Wilms' tumour) is known to involve suppressor gene loss, a germ-line origin for some fraction of human leukaemias related to loss of specific genes or loss of suppressor gene function cannot be excluded as having a possible causal relationship in childhood cancer. Even in the case of leukaemia associated with proto-oncogene translocation, recent observations imply that germ-line-mediated epigenetic events (imprinting) can affect the subsequent formation of the translocation in somatic cells of the offspring [H16]. In the mouse there is more direct molecular evidence of germ-line mutations resulting in a predisposition to leukaemia/lymphoma. In one case this predisposition centres on the loss of the *p53* tumour suppressor gene [D8]; in the other it centres on changes to the structure of an anonymous telomere-like repeat sequence that may represent a heritable chromosomal fragile site [S43]. None of these observations serve, however, to account for the extraordinarily high induced mutation frequency that is necessary to explain the epidemiological findings at Sellafield. Modern molecular genetic techniques allow the identification of the parent from whom a particular chromosome has been inherited. If it could be demonstrated that in every case of leukaemia, the defective chromosome(s) was(were) inherited from the father, this would at least lend support to Gardner's hypothesis. However, no such cytogenetic or molecular studies have been done on the Sellafield cases [E7]. Had there been such a biological follow-up, it is likely that some of the children with leukaemia would have been found to have chromosome rearrangements in only a fraction of their somatic cells. Such a finding would have been more consistent with a mutation of somatic origin rather than with the hypothesis that the mutation came from the father.

202. A large number of individually rare genetic diseases are known to increase the risk of cancer in both the homozygous and heterozygous states. Some of these predispose to leukaemia and lymphoma and others to other types of cancer. Leukaemias would be expected to make up only a small fraction of the induced genetic disorders predicted by the risk estimates developed in this Annex. Thus, if a dose of radiation as low as 10 mSv induced a cluster of leukaemias, as suggested by Gardner, that same dose would be expected to induce an increase in other diseases in the same population. Since no such epidemic of genetic diseases has been reported at Sellafield [E7] or in long-term follow-up in the Russian Federation [K12, P5] or around other nuclear plants [A2], it seems highly unlikely that the conclusions of Gardner et al. are correct.

203. There are some data from mice that could support Gardner's conclusion. Studies by Nomura [N13, N14] found that there were significant increases in tumour incidence in the progeny of x-irradiated male and female mice in some strains, suggesting that the different genetic backgrounds of different human ethnic groups could influence radiation susceptibility. The dose-effect relationship was clear-cut for male post-meiotic stages and less clear-cut for spermatogonial stages. Oocytes at late follicular stages were resistant to x rays in the range 0.36-1.08 Gy but highly sensitive to higher doses. At the highest dose, 5.04 Gy, the tumour incidence in the offspring was around 30% following irradiation of spermatids in the male or oocytes in the female. This incidence was six times higher than the tumour incidence observed in untreated controls. Matings to the F_3 generation

demonstrated that the tumours were heritable and dominant, with about 40% penetrance on average. Some strains of mice had different sensitivities to these heritable effects of radiation. Other strains, however, showed no increase in heritable tumours with equivalent doses of radiation. While the dose used in Nomura's studies, 5.04 Gy was far higher than that calculated for the Sellafield workers and well above the doubling dose used in estimating genetic risks, the studies do indicate that heritable tumours can be induced by radiation.

204. Nomura [N17] has proposed three possible reasons for the differences between the Sellafield studies and other studies on human populations:

(a) different germ-cell susceptibility to leukaemia-causing mutations in Japanese and English people (similar to different susceptibility in different strains of mice);
(b) different germ-cell stages exposed in the two populations;
(c) different postnatal tumour-promoting environments.

Nomura noted that lung cancer, for example, had a seven times higher incidence in white uranium miners than in non-white miners who had received equal doses, although this was not a hereditary effect. He cited mouse studies demonstrating that the offspring of mice irradiated before conception show persistent hypersensitivity to tumorigenesis when exposed postnatally to tumour-promoting agents, developing clusters of tumours.

205. However, there are difficulties with Nomura's conclusions as well. The UNSCEAR 1986 Report [U2] reviewed the results of Nomura on the induction of dominant mutations causing tumours, and Selby [S21] and Sankaranarayanan [S4] also reviewed those results in detail. Most of Nomura's results are on pulmonary adenomas. A major difficulty in applying Nomura's results to risk estimation is the high control frequency found for each end-point studied. Attempts to extrapolate from mice to humans become especially uncertain if only a few different abnormalities are studied and if each of them occurs at much higher frequencies in mice than in humans. In addition, the high control frequencies make it much more difficult to evaluate the strength of the evidence on transmission and penetrance.

206. While Nomura treated his data as if each offspring with a tumour represented a dominant mutation, it seems much more likely that the tumours were threshold traits and that most of the affected offspring were non-mutational variants [S21]. Although it is probable that radiation can induce mutations that predispose individuals to develop tumours, the extent to which it does so is unclear from Nomura's work. There is no indication that parents were randomized or that offspring were coded in Nomura's experiments, and without such precautions it becomes especially difficult to interpret experiments for end-points having such high control frequencies (for example, 4.7% for pulmonary adenomas). According to a report of the International Agency for Research on Cancer [I2], positive results in lung tumour bioassay in susceptible strains of mice "may be strongly suggestive of carcinogenicity but are not conclusive by themselves". The report advises that when positive results are found in this assay, replicating them in another laboratory would greatly increase confidence in them, and a long-term, full-fledged bioassay might be necessary to remove all doubt.

207. Nomura's results on pulmonary adenomas and leukaemia suggest that the offspring of heavily irradiated male mice should have a high frequency of induced tumours. A recent small experiment by Takahashi et al. [T8] on liver tumours supports this view. Although it would seem, from this work, that it should be easy to find increased numbers of tumours in progeny carefully autopsied at time of natural death, no effect was found by Kohn et al. [K9] or by Cosgrove et al. [C19] in mice exposed to 5.3-7.2 Gy or 6.0 Gy of acute x rays, respectively. In both studies the offspring of both experimental and control groups developed many tumours. The Cosgrove et al. study also found no difference in longevity between experimental and control groups.

3. Epidemiological studies on other human populations

208. The Sellafield report stimulated other studies on radiation exposure in human populations as well as a reevaluation of previous studies. In addition to studies on the Japanese atomic bomb survivors, studies have been conducted on patients receiving radiation treatment for diseases such as rheumatoid spondylitis [L4, S8]; on populations living in areas with elevated background radiation in India [K7], Brazil [B5], Canada [A2], the Russian Federation [B4, K12, P5, T5] and China [C7, C11, D3]; on the population in Hungary exposed to fallout from the Chernobyl accident [C15, C16]; and on x-ray technicians [T1].

209. The only effect found in children of therapeutically irradiated patients and in x-ray technicians was a sex ratio shift in the direction expected if additional X-linked recessive lethal mutations are induced in the X-chromosomes of irradiated females and X-linked dominant mutations in the X-chromosomes of irradiated males. However, results from sex ratio studies are not easily interpreted and have not yet been found suitable for the estimation of genetic risk.

210. Two areas in southern China (near Yangjiang) with especially high levels of natural background radiation were studied. The radiation arises from radionuclides in fine particles of monazite that are washed down year after year from nearby mountains. These areas have been inhabited for about 800 years; the families of about 80,000 present-day inhabitants have been living there for more than two generations. The annual gamma-ray exposure is about three times that of the control population, which is similar to that of average population groups in other parts of the world. In this population, parameters such as cancer mortality, incidence of congenital malformations and other health impairments were studied, generally with negative results [C7, C11, D3]. One result, however, is of special interest: Down's syndrome (trisomy 21) was found to be far more common in the exposed than in the control group. To put this result into proper perspective, a number of factors must be considered. Incidence in the control group is much lower than in all other populations for which fairly reliable incidence figures are available. An incidence of only 1.8 cases per 10,000 births is without parallel in the international literature. Even the incidence of 8.7 cases per 10,000 births found in the exposed group is lower than the incidences reported in most population groups outside of China, which have been found to be 13-14 per 10,000. The most obvious explanation is that the diagnosis and/or reporting of Down's syndrome cases has been incomplete in both series and less complete in the control than in the exposed sample. The incidence of Down's syndrome in six other Chinese populations was compared with that of these two population groups. It ranged between 2.7 per 10,000 and 6.2 per 10,000, i.e. between the figures for the irradiated and the control groups. Again comparison with international figures suggests underreporting of varying degrees.

211. It is common knowledge that the incidence of meiotic non-disjunction, and therefore of Down's syndrome, increases sharply with advancing maternal age. Thus, first hypothesis of the Chinese scientists was that the difference between the two groups was caused by a difference in the age distribution of the mothers. And indeed, 12.02% of mothers in the exposed group, as compared with only 4.44% in the control group, were older than 35 years at the birth of the children included in the study. But even in the younger age group (below 35 years), the difference between irradiated and control populations remains significant (3.6 per 10,000 versus 0.5 per 10,000).

212. The observed differences between exposed and unexposed population groups is very probably caused by a combination of two factors: different age distribution of mothers and underreporting, especially in the control population. In the light of these two biases, the study results cannot demonstrate an additional radiation effect; indeed they cannot even be regarded as hinting at such an effect. This outcome highlights some of the problems encountered in assessing large populations for induced effects. As is described in detail in Section II.A, the accurate ascertainment of index cases is both difficult and crucial.

213. No change in the incidence of genetic disease in Hungary was detected by Czeizel after the Chernobyl accident [C15]. The lack of effects in studies of populations in areas of varying background is only to be expected, given the low statistical power of the investigations. Although some studies have included large population groups, the dose differences have been too small to observe statistically low risk effects (see paragraph 115). The most useful human data are still those collected at Hiroshima and Nagasaki.

B. METHODS OF RISK ESTIMATION: ANIMAL STUDIES

214. Animal data, especially those collected in mouse studies, still provide a basis for genetic risk estimation in humans. Extensive work has been done to try to develop accurate animal models for estimating human genetic risk following radiation exposure. The data on survivors of the atomic bombings that are becoming available suggest many additional animal studies that would be useful. Thus, despite the criticisms and limitations of each of the methods outlined below, animal studies are still invaluable and should be continued and refined as greater understanding of the complexity of the problem is gained.

215. It has been assumed, based on general principles of radiation genetics, that mutations induced by radiation are more likely to be neutral or harmful than beneficial and that the frequency of mutations will increase linearly with increasing dose. Two main methods are used in animal experiments (primarily mouse) that attempt to quantify genetic risk: the doubling dose (or indirect) method and the direct method. Since they have been described and used with varying emphasis in previous UNSCEAR Reports [U1, U2, U3, U4], as well as in other reports on radiation effects, such as those of the Committee on the Biological Effects of Radiation (BEIR) of the United States National Research Council [C1], they are discussed only briefly here, with a mention of their respective advantages and disadvantages.

216. Both methods extrapolate from animal data on induced mutations to risk of genetic disease in humans, although in different ways, as discussed below. The terms direct and indirect refer to whether the estimate of damage in the first generation is based directly on phenotypic damage found in mice in first-

generation progeny (direct method) or whether it is based on extrapolation back to the first generation from a prediction at genetic equilibrium (indirect method). Although the frequency of harmful effects from induced mutations (from the exposure of a single generation) would be expected to decrease beyond the first generation, owing to negative selection, it should be kept in mind that some of the genetic effects of radiation, e.g. aneuploid segregants from certain translocations or mutations leading to abnormal imprinting in the gametes of first-generation offspring, might not manifest until the second or subsequent generations.

1. The doubling dose (indirect) method

(a) Concept

217. The doubling dose method is used to estimate expected risk to a population under conditions of continuous irradiation, expressed in terms of the natural prevalence of genetic diseases. It is based on the concept that with stable population structure and living conditions, there is a balance between mutations that arise spontaneously and those that are eliminated by selection every generation. When an additional mutation source (such as radiation exposure) is introduced, the population will eventually (over a number of generations, depending again on mutation rate and selection) reach a new equilibrium between mutation and selection. It is the additional risk at this new equilibrium that is estimated with this method. Estimates of risk for the first or subsequent generations are then obtained from that at equilibrium using assumptions on the persistence of mutations in the population.

218. The method involves the estimation of the doubling dose, which thus is used to designate the method. The doubling dose is the dose of radiation required to produce as many mutations in a generation as those arising spontaneously. It is obtained by dividing the spontaneous rate at a set of gene loci by the rate of induction by radiation at the same set of loci. The doubling dose currently used in risk estimation is 1 Gy for low-LET, low-dose-rate irradiation conditions and is based on mouse data. The choice of this value has been discussed in previous UNSCEAR Reports.

219. The risk is estimated from three quantities used in the following equation:

$$\text{Risk per unit dose} = P\,F_m / D_d \qquad (1)$$

where P denotes the natural prevalence of the disease class under consideration, F_m, the mutational component and D_d is the doubling dose.

220. The doubling dose in experimental animals, especially mice, is defined as the radiation dose that doubles the spontaneous mutation rate (not the incidence or prevalence of a certain condition). Lüning and Searle [L6] have reviewed doubling doses for various genetic parameters. From their report, two aspects are obvious:

(a) there is an appreciable difference between estimates of doubling doses for various end-points. In mice, these end-points are defined as dominant and recessive mutations leading to defined phenotypes; dominant mutations affecting the skeleton; recessive lethals; and chromosomal translocations leading to semi-sterility. It should be noted that in humans, there may be other more meaningful end-points, and they may not be so well defined or consistent;

(b) the confidence intervals of these estimates are very large. Earlier UNSCEAR Reports [U1, U2, U3, U4] used a doubling dose of 1 Sv for irradiation at low dose rates. This estimate, based mainly on data from studies of seven recessive mutations in mice, is probably at least of the correct order of magnitude. The doubling dose might, however, be quite different for other end-points (i.e. other types of genetic effects), such as predisposition to cancer. This limitation or possibility should be kept in mind.

221. Regarding attempts to estimate doubling doses for some of the end-points examined in the offspring of atomic bomb survivors, Ehling [E8] concluded that the doubling doses based on data available from the atomic bomb survivors were not significantly different from estimates of doubling doses based on data from mice (see direct method, below). The absolute effects in humans are much too small to permit such a conclusion, and the end-points are too different to allow direct comparison. This does not, however, mean that no attempt should be made to estimate the doubling dose from human data or to compare it with that from the mouse data. In view of the overwhelming difficulties in arriving at rationally founded risk estimates, all reasonable approaches should be tried and optimized as far as possible, and the results compared. The application by Neel et al. [N8, N9] of the doubling dose method to studies of human populations was discussed earlier in this Chapter.

222. Since the doubling dose method uses the concept of mutation-selection equilibrium, the method can be applied to conditions whose prevalence can be attributed to this mechanism. All autosomal dominant and X-linked conditions (combined prevalence of 10,000 per million) have been traditionally considered to belong to this group; they are also the conditions for which the relationship between mutation and disease can be considered straightforward.

223. Autosomal recessive diseases require the combination of two mutant alleles to manifest the condition and are strongly dependent on population structure, in addition to selective factors. For these the relationship between mutation and disease is less direct. For multifactorial conditions, as mentioned earlier, the complexities of interactions between genes and with the environment preclude any direct relationship between mutation and disease, and this makes the application of the doubling dose method for these diseases very uncertain.

224. In order to circumvent at least some of the difficulties in risk estimation for the rather large group of multifactorial diseases, the concept of the mutational component was first introduced in the BEIR 1972 report and was subsequently elaborated upon by Crow et al. [C20]. Estimates of the mutational component are based on equilibrium theory. Although this approach was used in the BEIR V report to estimate the mutational components for congenital abnormalities and with these to obtain tentative risk estimates for this class of disorders, the Committee [U1, U2] refrained from doing so.

225. There has been no new empirical data that would warrant revision of the risk estimates presented in the UNSCEAR 1988 Report [U1]. However, arguments questioning the validity of some of the assumptions used and suggesting that these risk estimates for Mendelian diseases may be conservative have been advanced [S6, S7]. Nonetheless, for the present, the Committee favours the view that it is prudent to retain the 1988 estimates, if only because it is better to err on the side of caution. These estimates are presented in Table 5.

(b) Strengths and weaknesses

226. The major strength of the doubling dose method is that the risks are expressed in terms of the background load of genetic diseases, so that some tangible perspective can be derived to indicate whether the projected increases are trivial, small or large. Furthermore, it has the apparent advantage that whole classes of genetic diseases can be handled as units. However, many of the assumptions used seem open to doubt and have recently been discussed [S6, S7, V6].

227. The existence of a balance between mutation and selection (and its corollary, the mutational component) are among the central assumptions of the method. As discussed in Chapter II.B, even for Mendelian conditions, the assumption of mutation-selection equilibrium may be applicable to only a small fraction of these. This means that the prevalence value (for these and X-linked conditions) of 10,000 per million used in the risk equation may be high. For multifactorial conditions, the estimation of mutational components is still fraught with considerable uncertainties.

228. Another significant difficulty in application of the doubling dose method for genetic risk estimation lies in establishing the baseline of spontaneous mutations. (It should be mentioned that use of the term spontaneous does not mean that these mutations occur without cause. It simply means that in this context they are not caused by the agent of interest, namely additional radiation.) The disorders caused by spontaneous mutations may be very different and may occur in proportions very different from those caused by radiation. The doubling dose method assumes that spontaneous mutations have the same rate relative to mechanisms as do radiation-induced mutations. As pointed out above, however, there is evidence that this is not the case.

229. The use of the doubling dose method to analyse human populations assumes a stable population and environment. However, human populations are constantly shifting, and there are times, particularly during war, when there are shortages of food and health care, with increased infection and illness. Such conditions may well have an adverse effect on the radiation sensitivity of humans and their susceptibility to the mutagenic effects of radiation. Furthermore, human populations (including isolated, inbred groups) are genetically heterogeneous in comparison with mouse laboratory strains, which have been bred through multiple generations to be highly homogeneous.

230. Further discussions on the doubling dose method centre on the data on the molecular nature, specificities and mechanisms of origin of mutations underlying human Mendelian diseases and on the nature of radiation-induced mutations in mammalian experimental systems [S4, S5, S6, S7]. These suggest that (a) the doubling dose method may be applicable only to a small proportion of Mendelian diseases, (b) the doubling dose for autosomal dominant diseases may be higher than 1 Gy (i.e. lower relative risk) and (c) risk estimates for these presented in the 1988 Report are conservative, but provide a margin of safety in radiological protection.

2. The direct method

(a) Concept

231. The so-called direct method for genetic risk estimation was suggested by Ehling in 1974 [E8], with the intention of circumventing many of the difficulties encountered in the practical application of the doubling dose method. This has allowed the Committee to make

alternative estimates of genetic risks [U1, U2, U3]. The direct method of genetic risk estimation has as its basis a measure of the extent of induced phenotypic damage found in the offspring of mice exposed to radiation. Damage in the first generation would be expected to result almost entirely from induced dominant mutations, including deletions, that can have a range of penetrance from complete to low. The procedure for estimating genetic risk by this method is shown mathematically below:

$$\text{Risk per unit dose} = F_d M N \qquad (2)$$

where the risk per unit dose applies to the expected number of significant, radiation-induced dominant diseases in humans per million live-born in the first-generation progeny of irradiated parents; F_d is the frequency of radiation-induced dominant mutations per unit dose; M is the multiplication factor, i.e. the reciprocal of the fraction of total mutations thought to affect the body system(s) under study; and N is the number of children born in the population for which risk is being estimated, which is usually 1 million.

232. The multiplication factor has been assumed by the Committee in the past to be 10 for skeletal damage [U4] and 36.8 for cataracts [U3] (see Table 7). (The derivation factor and some qualifications concerning its use are discussed below.) The direct method has been used to estimate risk in only the first generation, although assumptions about the persistence of mutations in the population could permit the extrapolation of first-generation estimates to later generations. Dominant mutations are those that show clear-cut phenotypic effects in heterozygotes of the F_1 generation. Experiments for inducing and registering such mutations in the mouse have been performed almost since the beginning of radiation genetic studies in the 1930s and have often been reviewed (see, for example, [R10, S21]). End-points studied include mutations affecting the skeleton, the eye lens (leading to cataracts); dominant visible mutations, i.e. those in the living mouse recognizable with the naked eye; litter size reduction; congenital malformations; tumours; and effects on behaviour (see [S22]).

233. The UNSCEAR 1986 Report [U2] included, in consideration of the direct method, an estimate of the frequency of induction of sublethal effects that kill between birth and early life. Infant mortality is undoubtedly much higher in mice than in humans, because human mothers make great efforts to keep their young alive. Thus, it is important to realize that a large fraction of the sublethal effects in mice probably correspond to serious disorders in humans that may not be lethal early in life. An estimate of the amount of induced damage expected from unbalanced products of induced balanced reciprocal translocations has also been presented in evaluating genetic risk according to the direct method [U1, U2]. This estimate is based on the frequencies of induction of translocations in several species, including primates, and it uses various assumptions to determine the risk that a live-born child will be genetically abnormal. Details of such calculations were presented in the UNSCEAR 1986 and 1988 Reports [U1, U2].

234. A fundamental assumption of the direct method is that the genetic damage observed in mice can be related to genetic damage observed in humans. Critics of the method doubt that this can be done. Mutations can range from those with minimal effect to those with devastating effects on a particular organism, and the opportunity to observe the phenotypic consequences of induced dominant mutations in mice provides a sense of the seriousness of the induced mutations. For example, the largest data set used in the direct method was a sample of 37 dominant skeletal mutations [S23, S24, S25]. The two clinical geneticists involved in the first application of the direct method, McKusick and Carter, both concluded that approximately half of the 37 mutations would represent a serious health problem in humans [U4]. The many structural similarities between the skeletons and lenses of mice and humans make it much simpler to address the question of whether effects seen in mice relate to serious genetic diseases in humans. For example, almost all of the bones in the feet are similar in the two species. As a result, it is much easier to compare foot malformations between humans and mice than, for example, between humans and mammals with hooves. Molecular studies of mice and humans have shown marked similarities at the DNA level and have even proved to be useful in predicting the location of genes in chromosomes in humans based on their location in mice [S17]. Such similarities increase the chances that extrapolations of induced dominant damage from mice to humans may be reasonably valid.

235. Some induced dominant skeletal and cataract mutations in mice appear to be homologous to mutations known in humans. Other mutations seem to have different effects in the two species. These differences between the effects of mutations in mice and humans would be an especially serious complication if the direct method depended on recognizing the same disorders in mice and humans. It does not, however. Instead, the basis for comparison between the species comes from thinking of the malformations caused by many dominant mutations as threshold traits, according to the threshold concept advanced by Wright [W9]. Some dominant mutations shift the distribution entirely over the threshold, in which case they are simple dominants with full penetrance. Other dominant mutations shift the distribution only partially over the threshold, in which case they have incomplete pene-

trance. Many dominant mutations affect several developmental pathways and can thus influence several distributions of underlying factors relative to thresholds. Many mutations that cause genetic diseases, including those of complex aetiology, can be thought of as acting in this way in all mammals.

236. In the direct method, an attempt is made to determine the effects of induced mutations on the entire range of underlying factors and distributions that must exist in normal development. The genetic background of the mouse provides a very large number of different threshold traits on which the effects of induced mutations can be tested. Mutations can be detected that occur anywhere in the genome and that involve any type of molecular damage, providing that the mutation is capable of shifting a distribution over a threshold, such that a phenotypic effect is revealed in a first-generation offspring. The mouse, or other experimental mammal, used in the direct method thus becomes a tool for revealing the effects of induced mutations on the vast array of threshold traits present. It is hoped that by carefully looking for effects on threshold traits in first-generation offspring of mice, and by evaluating them for severity, some idea may be obtained of the likely effects of radiation in inducing serious genetic diseases in humans.

(b) Application and qualifications

237. The most recent application by the Committee [U1] of the direct method is summarized as follows. The expected approximate frequencies of induction of genetically abnormal children per million live-born, following 0.01 Gy of exposure of males, are 10-20 for mutations having dominant effects, 0 for recessive mutations and 1-15 for unbalanced products of reciprocal translocations. A footnote indicated that risk from dominant sublethal mutations is estimated to be 5-10. For exposure of the female, the same categories, reported in the same order, have risks of 0-9, 0 and 0-5. No estimate is available for dominant sublethal mutations in the female.

238. A difficulty with the direct method is that risk is estimated for only a small part of the total damage of concern to humans. Skeletal malformations and cataracts have been used because they can be examined in detail in the mouse. A few other end-points, for example adenomas in the lungs [N13], have been investigated, but it is not yet clear how to apply such end-points in the direct method. Much discussion and several lines of argument went into the choice of the multiplier of 10 to extrapolate from induced serious skeletal damage to induced serious total damage.

239. Several of the geneticists most familiar with genetic diseases in mice and humans felt that the number 10 was a reasonable figure to use in making such an extrapolation. Russell had suggested using 10, and Selby [S23] had suggested a range of 5 to 20. The Committee examined McKusick's catalogue of Mendelian inheritance in man [M7] and concluded that about one fifth of the diseases listed involved the skeleton [U4]. Although McKusick's catalogue gives no indication of the relative incidences of the diseases listed, in a rough way this analysis suggested that it might be appropriate to multiply the skeletal effects by 5 to derive total serious damage. However, the Committee noted that because there is a bias of ascertainment for skeletal effects, the true multiplier must be larger than 5. Since pleiotropy is common for genetic diseases in both species, it seemed that the multiplier should not be too much larger than 5, and 10 seemed to be a useful round number that would suggest little precision. McKusick [M8] agreed that the factor of 10 was reasonable, recognizing that the catalogue does not reflect the human genome in reality.

240. In view of these and other considerations, the Committee adopted 10 as the multiplication factor, and the estimate of risk, calculated as it was from data on mice, was assumed to be approximately correct for humans. Another limitation in using the direct method is that both skeletal and cataract mutations are connective tissue disorders, and it is anticipated that the genes involved in other tissues may respond differently to DNA damage. As more is learned about the relationships between DNA damage and phenotypic changes, it is expected that the multiplication factor will require adjustment, perhaps for each tissue type.

241. The Committee estimated that paternal exposure to 0.01 Gy per generation would lead to 20 serious dominant disorders per million live-born. According to the BEIR V report [C1], this figure was estimated to be between 5 and 15. Risk from exposure of the mother was estimated to be 0%-44% of that from paternal exposure (see Table 3).

242. Starting with the UNSCEAR 1982 Report [U3], the Committee included, in addition to skeletal malformation, dominant eye cataracts in its direct estimates. The radiation-induced mutation rate for such cataracts was established by mouse experiments mainly by Ehling et al. [E5, E6]. Dominant cataracts of various types are known to occur in humans and can be diagnosed in mice relatively easily. Again, the problem arises of finding a way of extrapolating from a very limited selection of mutations observed in mice to all loci expressing dominant mutations of clinical relevance in humans.

243. The multiplication factor suggested by Ehling to convert the dominant cataract rate to an overall mutation rate was again based on McKusick's catalogue of autosomal phenotypes [M7]. The number of well-established dominant mutations, 42, was assumed to be the same in man and mouse. This ratio is then used to convert the induced mutation rate of dominant cataracts to the estimate of the overall dominant mutation rate. As new knowledge of the human situation is gained, it should be possible to readjust the multiplication factor.

244. Ehling et al. [E8] have recovered more than 85 independent dominant cataracts in the mouse. About one third were observed in radiation genetic experiments. Combined experiments with the well-known specific-locus test (the seven specific recessive mutations) [E3] showed that the yield of dominant cataract mutations was one fourth that of specific-locus mutations.

245. Using an argument similar to that mentioned above for skeletal mutations, the dominant cataract mutation frequency was estimated to be 0.45-0.55 10^{-6} mutations per 0.01 Gy per gamete for high-dose-rate exposure. For low-dose-rate exposure, this estimate was divided by 3, yielding an estimate of 0.15- 0.18 10^{-6} mutations per gamete. Again using the McKusick catalogue listings [M7] and a multiplier of 36.8, a risk estimate of 6-7 10^{-6} serious dominant disorders per 0.01 Gy of paternal exposure was derived. Both estimates, that based on skeletal mutations and that based on cataract mutations, are similar, considering the multiple assumptions they require. The Committee decided in favor of a rough estimate of 10-20 serious dominant disorders per million live-born [U3].

246. Several correction factors are needed to estimate risk by the direct method. All estimates of phenotypic damage are based on high-dose-rate exposures, even though risk is estimated for low-dose-rate exposures. It is necessary to assume that the dose-rate effect for serious dominant damage is the same as that seen for specific-locus mutations, which are recessive mutations at one of seven genes in the mouse. (The predictive value of the specific-locus data seems stronger in this regard because many of the mutations at the *s* locus, which is one of the seven genes studied in the specific-locus test, are associated with reduced size, suggesting an associated dominant effect [R5].) Most data used in the direct method also come from experiments using fractionated exposures, which were administered with the expectation of increasing the mutation frequency. These experiments require correction factors, again based on specific-locus data, for the fractionation effect.

247. The estimate of genetic risk to the female depends on the assumption that the relationship for induced dominant damage and specific-locus mutations will be the same as that for the male. No experiments have been conducted studying the induction of skeletal anomalies or cataracts following the irradiation of female mice, and qualitative differences in the mutations in the two sexes could affect the level of induced damage to an important extent.

248. Even though many large experiments have been conducted to learn about the induction of mutations in mammals, the direct method still rests upon relatively few experiments including few mutations. The total includes only 42 dominant skeletal mutations and 12 dominant cataract mutations [S8, U3, U4], a small number on which to base such an important application, particularly when the mouse and human disorders may be quite different. It would be reassuring to have much more data collected on different strains or species; this would provide some indication of whether the frequency of induced dominant damage is highly dependent on the genetic background of the animals being examined. It would also be helpful to confirm the conceptual model on a molecular level. The direct method has only been used to estimate the genetic risk of serious genetic diseases, but since this is the information about genetic risk that is most needed, this is not a serious limitation of the method.

249. Although the direct method requires no information on the incidence of genetic diseases in a particular human population, it is important to have such an estimate to help put the mouse estimates into perspective. The incidences presently used in the doubling dose method (see above) are probably not valid for this purpose, however, for two reasons: (a) they include many conditions that are probably far less serious than those used in the direct method and (b) they are based on the incidences of disorders instead of the incidences of individuals with disorders. Concerning the latter point, it is relevant to note that many of the dominant skeletal mutations cause numerous effects, sometimes on other body systems as well [S24]. In spite of this, when estimating risk by the direct method, the number of affected individuals (which corresponds to the number of induced mutations) is used instead of the total number of malformations. This would seem to be a reasonable approach, since only one individual is disabled as the result of each mutation.

(c) Strengths and weaknesses

250. The principal advantage of the direct method of risk estimation is that it makes no assumptions regarding spontaneous mutations with similar genetic mechanisms or phenotypic effects, and no assumptions are necessary regarding the mutational component in complex diseases or malformations. The method relies,

however, on extrapolations from mice to humans and from a small fraction of dominant mutations, for example those affecting the skeleton or the lens, to all dominant mutations. In these repects, the so-called doubling dose (or indirect) method is much more direct: doubling doses have been estimated not only in mice, with subsequent extrapolation to humans, but also in humans, from the results of studies on atomic bomb survivors. In addition, estimates of the spontaneous incidence of dominant mutations and their increase in relation to a certain radiation dose were based not only on certain categories but on all such mutations.

251. The indirect method requires two main steps. In the first, the absolute number of mutations in relation to a certain dose and quality of radiation is estimated. This estimate is compared in the second step with the spontaneous mutation rate (or the assumed mutational component of complex conditions). The direct method requires only the first of these steps. The logical relationship between the two approaches should be kept in mind when the so-called direct approach is discussed in the following paragraphs. Selby [S22] correctly distinguishes between the indirect method as a method of relative risk estimation and the direct method as a method of absolute risk estimation. Moreover, an absolute risk estimate should always be put into perspective by relating it to spontaneous mutations, i.e. by transforming it into a relative estimate.

252. Many of the criticisms of the doubling dose method also apply to the direct method. In addition, there are a few points of criticism from the viewpoint of medical genetics. It is certainly too simplistic to calculate the multiplication factor from the number of different dominant skeletal malformations and cataracts in humans in comparison with the total number of known, dominantly inherited human phenotypes. The phenotypes enumerated in McKusick's catalogue of 1975 [M7] are a mixture of moderately common, relatively rare and extremely rare phenotypes. There have been many changes and additions to the catalogue since 1975. Many new entries in the category of confirmed human skeletal and cataract disorders, as well as many additional multiple anomaly disorders involving skeleton and cataracts should be included in such a calculation. One purpose of McKusick's catalogue is to permit the medical geneticist a quick orientation in the vast area of genetically determined human phenotypes. It has never been McKusick's intention to say anything about the incidence or prevalence of such phenotypes or their mutational origin.

253. The life expectancy of a mouse (approximately two to three years) is very much shorter than that of a human being. Certain genetic defects that lead to hereditary cataract in humans later in life simply have no time to manifest themselves in mice. Thus, only cataracts manifesting at birth or a short time afterwards can be assumed to be genetically homologous to the mouse cataracts recorded for use with the direct method. It must also be kept in mind that all experiments considered in the direct method have been done on male mice. The genetic risk for the offspring of irradiated female mice could be considerably different.

254. The estimate from skeletal anomalies may be criticized on similar grounds. For example, it is well known to anatomists that minor, and sometimes not so minor, variations of the human skeleton are widespread. Many, if not most of these variants have no clinical significance at all. In this context it should be remembered that human populations are mixed genetically, whereas the mouse populations used in experiments are often inbred strains. The best way to arrive at reasonable extrapolations to relevant mutation rates in humans would be to compare the patterns of manifestation of skeletal mutants and cataracts in the mouse with homologous dominantly inherited diseases in the human skeleton and eye, as documented and described in the medical genetic literature. For example, as Selby suggests [S22], it would be particularly reassuring if mouse mutant [S31] involving cleidocranial dysplasia could be identified for which there is a homologous human syndrome .

255. Selby [S22] suggested that clinical geneticists could help to classify animals as to clinical severity. In his opinion, the biggest advantage of the direct method is that it includes within its scope the irregularly inherited disorders, which constitute 85% of the serious genetic disorders in humans. The direct method requires no assumption that spontaneous and induced mutations have approximately the same likelihood of causing harm, no knowledge of the current incidence of serious genetic disorders in the human population, no estimate of how many of the irregularly inherited disorders are multifactorial or dominant disorders with low penetrance and no knowledge of the persistence of mutations in the population. However, these advantages are offset by the fact that it does not allow correlating a possible increase in mutations of known incidence with the spontaneous occurrence rates of relevant traits in human populations.

256. Another difficulty with the direct method is that risk is measured for only a small portion of the total damage of concern to humans. Skeletal malformations and cataracts are used because they can be examined in detail in the mouse. Much discussion, and several lines of argument, went into the choice of the multiplier of 10 to extrapolate from induced serious skeletal damage to induced serious total damage. However, both skeletal and cataract mutations are disorders of connective tissue, and it is likely that the DNA

damage in these tissues will be somewhat different from that in other tissues. As more is learned about the relationships between DNA damage and phenotypic damage, it would not be surprising for the multiplication factor to require some adjustment because of tissue differences. Multifactorial disorders and disorders of complex aetiology are probably far more common than is accounted for by a multiplier of 10.

257. A major shortcoming of the direct method has been the uncertainty about the inclusion of risk from serious disorders of multifactorial (complex) aetiology, which make up the great majority of the human genetic load. Because radiation-induced mutations often have incomplete penetrance [S23, S24], it would not be surprising if many disorders of complex aetiology involve mutations with incomplete penetrance. Other important classes of induced damage for which the aetiology is not presently understood might be overlooked if only those mutations are included that have proven transmissibility or meet particular presumed mutation criteria, as has been done thus far in applying the direct method. In addition, generations beyond the F_1 could express visible effects of induced mutations that involve non-traditional mechanisms of inheritance, such as genomic imprinting, not all of which will be visible in the F_1 generation.

258. In conclusion, the direct method, at least in its present form, does not allow estimating the expected increase of dominant phenotypes overall in humans. However, it has provided an enormous amount of information in carefully controlled conditions. In addition, it does not contradict the doubling dose estimates from data on the atomic bomb survivors and seems to be a useful alternative approach to the problem of estimating genetic damage in humans. If molecular analyses are used, the method could probably be developed to provide additional interesting information on the genetic basis of some irregularly inherited anomalies and on genetic effects in humans.

C. EXPERIMENTAL STUDIES

1. New experimental data relevant to risk estimation

259. Basic data on the genetic effects of radiation continue to be derived from earlier animal experiments. A major study in progress, assessing dominant damage in mice, is intended to have direct relevance to the estimation of genetic risk in humans. This study and others on the genetic effects of radiation are reviewed in this Section.

260. The results of studies of dominant skeletal and cataract mutations in mice remain the foundation of the direct method of genetic risk estimation. Ehling [E2] reported that three of his presumed dominant mutations were indeed shown to transmit their effects in a dominant manner. Selby and Selby [S23, S24, S25] conducted a large breeding-test experiment whose main purpose was to determine conclusively that the dominant skeletal mutations induced by exposure of stem-cell spermatogonia to low-LET radiation were indeed dominant mutations. It is noteworthy that many of the dominant mutations were shown to have incomplete penetrance and variable expressivity (and thus might or might not be truly autosomal dominant). Selby [S20] later demonstrated the statistically significant induction of dominant skeletal mutations in stem-cell spermatogonia following acute x-irradiation with 6 Gy or 1 Gy + 5 Gy (24-hour interval) or exposure to ethylnitrosourea [S26].

261. Ehling et al. [E3, K10] demonstrated that acute gamma radiation induces dominant cataract mutations in mouse stem-cell spermatogonia and in post-spermatogonial stages. This fractionated experiment and two later ones that yielded induced mutation frequencies that were not significantly higher than in controls were used in the UNSCEAR 1982 Report [U3] to apply the direct method to cataracts. The resulting risk estimate, based on cataract data, was 10 genetically abnormal children per 0.01 Gy of paternal exposure to low-dose-rate, low-LET radiation. It was used in the UNSCEAR 1982 Report [U3] and in the UNSCEAR 1986 and 1988 Reports [U1, U2] as the lower bound of the risk estimate made by the direct method. Ethylnitrosourea has also been shown to induce dominant cataract mutations [F1]. Many dominant cataract mutations exhibit incomplete penetrance and variable expressivity [F2, G6].

262. Selby et al. [S20] are using the assessment of dominant damage approach [S22] to investigate the induction of dominant mutations in stem-cell spermatogonia, with emphasis on skeletal and cataract mutations. Results to date [S29] are presented for 6 Gy of low-LET ionizing radiation, delivered either as 0.04 mGy min^{-1} ^{137}Cs gamma radiation (chronic) or 0.89 Gy min^{-1} x radiation (acute), and for a matched control. The frequencies of mice with possibly serious cataracts in the different groups were as follows: chronic irradiation, 5/1,502 (0.33%); acute irradiation, 4/1,290 (0.31%); and matched control, 5/1,693 (0.30%). The frequencies of mice with severe skeletal malformations were as follows: chronic irradiation, 11/1,291 (0.85%); acute irradiation, 20/1,193 (1.68%); and matched control, 23/1,457 (1.58%). When less severe skeletal malformations were included, the frequencies were chronic irradiation, 25/1,291 (1.94%); acute irradiation, 37/1,193 (3.10%); and matched control, 41/1,457 (2.81%). No significant differences were observed.

263. Graw et al. [G6] conducted experiments on the induction of dominant cataract mutations in stem-cell spermatogonia in mice, as detected in first-generation offspring produced in matings with untreated females, and found no significant effect of radiation up to 5.1 Gy + 5.1 Gy (24-hour interval). The reason for this lack of effect is not known, but at least the results are consistent with a low frequency of induction of cataract mutations. Specific-locus data collected in the same experiments showed that both treatments were clearly effective in inducing other types of mutations.

264. Selby [S21] reanalysed the published data of Graw et al. to assess whether there had been a significant increase over control in the frequency of cataracts. The findings led Selby to suggest that many of the cataracts found in such experiments may result from induced mutations with such low penetrance that proof of transmission is unlikely.

2. Studies of mutations in mouse oocytes

265. For many years estimates of the genetic risk to offspring of exposed women have been more uncertain than those of the risk to offspring of exposed men. Large-scale experiments using neutrons or x rays do not show that specific-locus mutations are induced in the immature arrested primary oocytes in the mouse (i.e. oocytes ovulated more than six weeks after irradiation). Russell [R11] presented a series of arguments suggesting that it might be reasonable to apply the apparently negligible risk for this germ-cell stage in the mouse to immature arrested primary oocytes in women, even though the arrested oocytes of mice are in diffuse diplotene (dictyate stage) and those in women are in a more condensed state (typical diplotene). Russell [R11] also argued, however, that for the sake of caution one might want to consider the possibility that the human arrested oocyte could be as mutationally sensitive as the most sensitive oocyte stages in the mouse, namely, the maturing and mature oocytes. To provide a basis for such extrapolation, he provided four different fits for the low-level radiation, specific-locus experiments in female mice. Only the highest frequency (0.44 times that in spermatogonia) was significantly above the control value. Russell concluded that genetic risk in the female is probably less than that in the male, and the Committee has applied the value of 0.44 in the direct method when calculating the upper limit for risk following maternal exposures [U1, U2].

266. Dobson and Straume [D4] suggested that it is inappropriate to base risk estimates for human arrested primary oocytes on the specific-locus data collected for arrested primary oocytes in the mouse. They demonstrated [S37] that the target for cell death in arrested primary oocytes of mice is not the DNA but rather the plasma membrane or something similar to it in terms of geometry and location in the cells. They have suggested that in Russell's large 0.5 Gy specific-locus experiment using x rays [R11], which provided most of the basis for concluding that risk for this stage might be negligible, the oocytes that survived the membrane damage would have received doses substantially lower than 0.5 Gy. They suggested that the estimate of risk based on a 0.5 Gy exposure might be much lower than it should be. In the UNSCEAR 1986 Report [U2] it was noted that current concepts of microdosimetry agreed with Russell's view that the distribution of ionizations from x rays would be so diffuse that the dose to the large nucleus of an oocyte could not differ appreciably from the exposure of 0.5 Gy administered.

267. Many more details of the Monte Carlo calculations by Straume et al. have now been published [S38], however, and those calculations suggest that there is a very small fraction of oocytes in the 0.5 Gy x-ray experiment that received as little as about 0.2 Gy to their DNA and there is a very small fraction of the oocytes that received as little as about 0.1 Gy to their plasma membrane. Furthermore, their calculations indicated significant coupling between the plasma membrane and nuclear doses, such that when the dose to the membrane was lower than average, the dose to the nucleus tended also to be low, and vice versa. In the view of Straume et al. [S38], only oocytes with the lowest dose to DNA (presumably about 0.2 Gy) survived, so Russell's finding of no mutations in 92,059 offspring [R11] was for a dose of only about 0.2 Gy instead of the 0.5 Gy administered. In their view, Russell's data do not suggest as low a mutation frequency as he estimated. Even if the interpretation of Straume et al. is accepted, however, it should be noted that the data from Russell's large 0.5 Gy experiment provide no basis for concluding that arrested primary oocytes are highly mutable, or even mutable, because no specific-locus mutations were found.

268. Besides providing evidence that the arrested primary oocytes in Russell's 0.5 Gy experiment may have received a lower dose than had been thought, Straume et al. [S38] demonstrated the induction of genetic damage in those oocytes by exposure to monoenergetic 0.43 MeV neutrons. They selected this form of radiation because of its short track lengths, which they say permits the recoil protons to deposit energy in the nucleus without traversing the plasma membrane. As a result, there would presumably be little or no correlation between energy deposition in the plasma membrane and the DNA, and oocytes receiving higher doses could survive. The two types of induced genetic damage detected in mice that had been superovulated using hormonal injections 8-12

weeks after irradiation were (a) chromosome aberrations, detected in oocytes arrested at metaphase I, and (b) dominant lethals, detected by the success with which cultured two-cell embryos survived to the morula or the blastocyst stage or hatched from the zona pellucida and formed a sheet of trophectoderm with a proliferated inner cell mass. The induction of both types of genetic damage was reported to be significant, with 6.0% chromosome aberrations and 16.9% dominant lethality at 0.25 Gy.

269. Although the authors demonstrated the induction of genetic damage in arrested primary mouse oocytes, it is not clear whether these types of genetic damage, detected following superovulation, are relevant to the genetic damage that would be seen in the offspring of irradiated females. They referred to the work of Griffin and Tease (next paragraph) and to much earlier work by Brewen et al. [B10] on the induction of chromosome aberrations in maturing mouse oocytes, and they state that the intrinsic mutational sensitivity of mouse immature oocytes is not very different from that of maturing oocytes. They claimed that their results make it possible to estimate genetic risk for women more confidently using the substantial amount of genetic data previously available for maturing oocytes in the mouse. The risk estimates presented in the UNSCEAR 1986 Report [U2] ranged from the lower limit of zero, based on the assumption that the mutational sensitivity of immature human oocytes is similar to that of immature mouse oocytes, to the upper limit of about 9, based on the assumption that the sensitivity of the human oocytes is similar to that of mature and maturing mouse oocytes. The latter is 0.44 times that for spermatogonia. Thus, the Committee took the position that risk in the female could be as high as Straume et al. now suggest that it should be.

270. Griffin and Tease [G7] provided the first clear evidence of the induction of genetic damage in arrested primary mouse oocytes by radiation (or by any agent, for that matter). Young (4-5 weeks-old) female mice were exposed to whole-body gamma radiation at a mean dose rate of 0.1 mGy min^{-1} until they received a total of 1, 2 or 3 Gy. Eight weeks after the end of the treatment, they were induced to superovulate by hormonal injections, and metaphase II oocytes were screened for numerical and structural chromosome anomalies. Hyperhaploidy (i.e. the presence of an extra chromosome) was used to assess the effect of the radiation on chromosome segregation. Several kinds of structural anomalies could also be detected in these cells. Again, the extent to which this genetic damage seen in superovulated oocytes would affect the health of the progeny of such females is unknown. The chromosome aberrations reported are probably not compatible with survival, but they may indicate a low level of induction of smaller types of rearrangements that might be viable.

271. Returning to studies on immature oocytes, Selby et al. [S28] found that females acutely irradiated near birth later produced as many as four or five litters, in sharp contrast to adult females, which became sterile after one or two litters following such an acute exposure [R7]. Based on the known radiosensitivities to cell killing of the different oocyte stages present near the time of birth, it seems likely that this experiment provided the mutation frequencies for pachytene and perhaps diplotene oocytes. Unlike in the adult female, the mutations found following an acute exposure were not restricted to the first six weeks after treatment; in fact, all mutations were found later or much later than this. No evidence was found for induction of mutations when females were exposed to 3.0 Gy at a moderately low dose rate near the time of birth.

272. As discussed above, it is uncertain whether the finding of no induction of specific-locus mutations in arrested primary oocytes of adult female mice can be extrapolated to women. If the degree of condensation of the chromosomes has an important bearing on the mutational response, those immature oocytes with condensed chromosomes that are present near the time of birth, which were studied by Selby et al. [S28], may be more comparable to the vast majority of oocytes in women than any other oocyte stage studied in the mouse. The finding of no mutation induction in those oocytes at moderately low dose rates suggests there may be no reason to abandon the view that mutation induction in female mice could be negligible compared to that in male mice.

3. Induction of translocations in primates

273. Van Buul [V1] and Adler and Erbelding [A1] conducted studies on the induction of reciprocal translocations in various strains of monkeys. Based on these results, there appear to be significant strain differences in monkeys. The frequency for stump-tailed macaques represents the lowest induction rate per gray ever recorded for an experimental mammal [V1]. This may raise questions about differences between primates and mice and about the validity of using mice to study radiation risk for humans. Generoso et al. [G3, G4] also found strain differences in mice for the induction of reciprocal translocations.

4. Induction of dominant mutations causing congenital malformations

274. Mutation studies aimed at detecting anomalies present at birth in mice and rats often examine fetuses

late in pregnancy instead of soon after birth, to avoid the problem of mothers eating grossly abnormal offspring. Earlier work was discussed in previous UNSCEAR Reports [U1, U2, U3], and recently there has been a detailed review of these studies [S21]. While some experiments have shown clear-cut effects of mutagens, others have shown weak effects or no effect at all for strong mutagens. Because of this inconsistency and the high levels sometimes found in controls, Lyon and Renshaw [L10] concluded that, in humans, the incidence of malformations is likely to be a relatively insensitive indicator of an increased mutation rate. Many of the congenital malformations are probably threshold traits (see Section I.C), and some of them are fairly common in the strains used. There is also reason to believe that some of the anomalies might result from spontaneous mutations with low penetrance that are segregating in the stocks [S21]. Selby pointed out that the randomization of parents in such studies, which does not appear to be standard practice, would help to guard against misinterpretations and improve the usefulness of the results [S21].

275. Nomura [N16] has almost doubled the sizes of his samples for studies of the induction of congenital malformations in mice by x-rays. The statistically significant induction of congenital malformations was shown for acute irradiation of post-spermatogonial stages, stem-cell spermatogonia, oocytes in adult females that were ovulated within 6 weeks after irradiation and oocytes present in 21-day-old mice. Nomura reported that frequencies of congenital malformations increased with dose for spermatozoa, stem-cell spermatogonia and mature and maturing oocytes of the adult. However, the slope of the simple regression line of dose versus frequency was statistically significantly above zero only in the mature and maturing oocytes. While much importance was given to the clear linear relationship between dose and mutation frequency found in spermatogonia between 0 and 2.2 Gy, the much lower mutation frequency reported for 5.0 Gy was ignored. In the total data reported, 42% of the anomalies found by Nomura were open eyelid, 25% were dwarfism and the rest were tail anomalies or cleft palate. Most of the mice with open eyelid showed only a small unilateral gap, and it was felt that had they been born, most would have been indistinguishable from normal mice by a few days after birth.

5. Results of the direct method to estimate risk

276. The experiments of Ehling [E1] and of Selby et al. [S23] both yielded estimates of an induced frequency of about 4 10^{-6} dominant skeletal mutations per gamete per 0.01 Gy for low-dose-rate irradiation, after applying correction factors derived from specific-locus experiments. As explained in describing the concept of the direct method, this frequency was multiplied by 0.5 (for severity), by 10 (multiplication factor for total damage) and by 1 million, to yield the estimate that 0.01 Gy of paternal exposure would result in 20 genetically abnormal children per million live births. In the UNSCEAR 1982 Report [U3], risk in the female was considered possibly negligible or, at most, 44% of that in the male, yielding the range 0-9 for 0.01 Gy of maternal exposure. The correction factors used to estimate maternal risk came from the suggestion of Russell [R11], based on specific-locus data in mice. Data on the induction of dominant cataract mutations were used in that same report to derive an estimate of 10 genetically abnormal children per 0.01 Gy of paternal exposure to low-dose-rate, low-LET radiation as the lower bound of the risk estimate made by the direct method.

277. Selby et al. [S29] point out that the preliminary results of assessment of dominant damage experiments in progress show no large error of underestimation in the direct estimate of genetic risk following paternal irradiation, even if that estimate is applied to all genetic disorders causing serious handicaps. They suggest that the data from an assessment of dominant damage experiment using protracted exposure [S29] could be used to derive an estimate of genetic risk as follows: subtraction of control results from experimental results will yield the frequency of induced serious genetic disorders. The estimate of genetic risk per 0.01 Gy could be calculated by dividing the induced frequency by 600 and then by multiplying it both by 10 (to expand to all body systems) and by 1 million to obtain an estimate of genetic risk expressed per million live births. Many of the correction factors and assumptions used before in applying the direct method would thus no longer be needed. Multiplication by the correction factors of 0 and 0.44, derived from specific-locus results, would yield an estimate of maternal risk, as was done previously.

278. If a mouse dies during the first few weeks of life, most of the types of phenotypic damage discussed above would not be detected. The omission of early deaths from induced dominant mutations would be a serious deficiency in a risk estimate. The assessment of dominant damage experiments [S29] are specifically designed to circumvent this problem by including extraordinary efforts to examine the skeleton of every mouse living beyond three weeks of age. This eliminates overlooking serious mutations because of early deaths. In the UNSCEAR 1986 Report [U2] the Committee made an estimate for protracted gamma radiation of the frequency of induction of dominant mutations causing death between birth and early life.

That estimate was based in part on an analysis by Selby and Russell [S27] of first-generation litter-size reduction in 14 radiation experiments involving 158,490 litters. That experiment yielded the estimate that for 0.01 Gy of low-LET, low-dose-rate paternal irradiation, there would be 19 deaths caused by dominant mutations between conception and three weeks of age for every million F_1 mice that would have lived to that age in the absence of irradiation.

279. The data of Lüning [L7], from one large experiment, yielded a similar estimate, 24 induced deaths per million. While the data of Selby and Russell could not be used to partition the total mortality rate into that occurring before and after birth, the data of Lüning [L7] and of Searle and Papworth [S15] could be used for this purpose. Based on these three data sets, the Committee estimated that the induction rate of dominant genetic changes causing death between birth and weaning would be 5-10 cases per million births per 0.01 Gy [U2]. This estimate has since been referred to as the "frequency of dominant sublethal effects". Although no such estimate has yet been made for maternal risk, it would seem reasonable to make a rough estimate by assuming that risk in the female is possibly negligible and, at most, 44% of that in the male, as has been done for other end-points. Risk in the female would thus be about 0-5 for dominant sublethal effects.

280. It should be noted that the chances that children with any one of many different serious birth defects will survive is heavily dependent on the sophistication of the medical technology available. The risk estimate for dominant sublethal effects based on the mouse is thus probably especially relevant when considering genetic risk from radiation in countries where advanced medical technology is less readily available. Baseline risk estimates are very difficult to obtain in such countries.

281. Table 3 shows the estimate of genetic risk based on the mouse model. It is noteworthy that there is no longer a separate listing for unbalanced products of reciprocal translocations. Those effects are presumably already included in the new risk estimate. It is important to note that research specifically aimed at understanding the induction of translocations in mice or other species, especially primates, must be carefully followed to see whether the mouse model, as applied in Table 3, could lead to a large underestimation of risk. Appropriate additions could be made to the Table if needed.

282. All modes of inheritance that could lead to first-generation effects are presumably included in the estimates given in Table 3, regardless of whether the aetiology is understood. Earlier work [S23] showed that an important part of the total consists of dominant mutations with full or incomplete penetrance.

283. Studies on skeletal and cataract mutations have shown that many of these mutations are recessive lethal mutations that have effects in heterozygotes [K11, S18]. Roughly 10% of the earlier direct estimate of risk based on the skeleton was thought to result from balanced translocations that acted like dominant mutations [S18].

284. The equilibrium estimate is the frequency of induced damage expected in each generation if the hypothetically increased mutation frequency stays constant until an equilibrium is reached. The estimate of genetic risk for the first generation could be extrapolated to an estimate at equilibrium if the persistence of mutations were well enough known. This is the reverse of the procedure that is necessary to estimate first-generation risk from equilibrium risk by the indirect method. Persistence, however, is rather well known only for the better understood diseases, such as those caused by simple dominants. For these, it is thought to be about 5 generations, although this is very dependent on the specific disorder. In the past, the Committee assumed that mutations responsible for disorders of complex aetiology persist for about 10 generations [U3], but this is an especially uncertain estimate. The discussion of multifactorial disease and non-traditional inheritance in this Annex underlines the difficulty of understanding the persistence of mutations that cause serious genetic diseases in humans.

285. In view of these uncertainties, no attempt is made to estimate risk at genetic equilibrium using the direct method. An equilibrium estimate is probably much less necessary for reaching decisions than a first-generation estimate, since as knowledge of genetics and medicine advances, ways may be found to reduce future impacts. As noted elsewhere, it would be useful to extend the direct method to at least a few later generations by measuring induced dominant damage following radiation exposure of successive generations.

6. Mouse versus human genes

286. Comparisons between humans and mice have been extremely useful in understanding development and genetic disease. The homology and sequence conservation between mouse and human genes is extensive. However, there are also notable differences in the expression of disease phenotypes. Several of the most frequent human disease mutations (e.g. neurofibromatosis) are not observed in mice. The most frequent mouse mutations (e.g. W locus) are rarely seen in humans. Furthermore, a number of human disease genes have been isolated, the abnormal mouse homologues of which do not produce any alteration in phenotype (e.g. Duchenne muscular dystrophy and Lesch Nyhan disease). Thus, the same mutation may

lead to disease in one species but not in another. There also appear to be marked strain differences in mice with regard to the severity of the phenotypic defect produced by a particular gene mutation. This type of strain variation in mice is probably comparable to the ethnic differences observed in humans [L11].

287. In addition to differences in disease phenotypes, there are also significant differences between mice and humans in early developmental processes, placentation and types of congenital anomalies. For instance, monozygous twinning is rare in most strains of mice but occurs quite frequently in humans [N2].

D. GENETIC RISK ESTIMATES

288. Some new information relevant to estimating the genetic effects of radiation has been presented in this Annex. There has, however, been no reason to revise the risk estimates, although the uncertainties could well be widened in view of the many complexities that are emerging. The genetic risk estimates of the Committee are summarized here and compared with those of other groups, national and international.

1. Estimates of UNSCEAR

(a) Dominant and X-linked diseases

289. The Committee has not changed its estimate of the incidence of dominant and X-linked diseases in the population since the UNSCEAR 1972 Report [U5]. This value of 10,000 cases per million live births divided by the doubling dose of 1 Gy, multiplied by a mutational component of 100% for these diseases and by a continuing dose of 0.01 Gy per generation gives an equilibrium estimate of 100 cases per million live births. The first generation increment (15 cases per million live births) is assumed to be 15% of that at equilibrium and the second generation increment (13 cases per million live births) is 15% of the equilibrium less the first generation cases (100-15 cases per million live births). These results are listed in Table 5.

(b) Recessive diseases

290. The Committee has estimated that autosomal recessive diseases occur at a rate of 2,500 per million live births. Calculations based on a combination of data from observations on human populations and from mouse experiments suggested that an extra dose of 0.01 Gy of low-LET radiation to each parent in a stable population with a million live-born offspring would induce up to 1,200 extra recessive mutations [S16]. From these data it was calculated that partnership with an established or newly induced recessive allele in the population would produce about one extra child with a recessive disorder in the following 10 generations (per million born in each generation). About 10 extra cases of recessive diseases would be expected from this dose by the tenth generation, assuming about 1% of first-cousin matings.

(c) Chromosomal diseases

291. Based on extensive cytogenic data from human populations, the Committee estimated that visible structural anomalies or unbalanced translocations occur at the rate of 400 per million live births [U1, U2, U3]. The indirect method of estimation (doubling dose of 1 Gy) thus gives an incidence rate at equilibrium of 4 cases per million live births from a continuing dose rate of 0.01 Gy per generation. The first-generation increment has been assumed to be three fifths of the equilibrium value [U3], giving 2.4 cases per million live births. The second-generation increment is three fifths of the remainder: $3/5 \times (4 - 2.4) = 1$ case per million live births.

292. The estimate of genetic risk was based on evidence that about 9% of individuals with unbalanced chromosome rearrangements survive to birth. The question of how many such rearrangements can be induced by radiation is not easily answered. Comparative studies in mice, rhesus monkeys, marmoset monkeys, crab-eating monkeys and human males have revealed striking differences (see the UNSCEAR 1986 Report [U2], Table 21, page 128). One interesting point should be noted: many spontaneously occurring translocations in humans are Robertsonian in type, but it has been concluded from mouse data that radiation does not induce such Robertsonian translocations [F16].

293. For numerical chromosomal diseases (mainly trisomies), the Committee has used a figure for the current incidence of 3,400 per million live births [U2]. The increase following radiation exposure could not be calculated but was assumed to be very small, based on mouse data. The human data from the Japanese studies also support a small risk.

294. Studies in the mouse have shown that the rates of aneuploidy induction in male and female germ cells by radiation were of the same order of magnitude ($2\text{-}7\ 10^{-2}$ per Gy) and were not very different from those reported by various authors for translocation induction in spermatogonia [P1]. The oocyte, when irradiated at the time of fertilization, is especially susceptible to chromosome loss, especially loss of the X-chromosome. However, most monosomic human zygotes do not survive early pregnancy; even the great majority of surviving 45 X-zygotes are thought to be attributable not to nondisjunction or chromosome loss during meiosis but to mitotic events during early

pregnancy. Moreover, most trisomies do not survive to birth [H9]. Hence, in view of the well-known high incidence of chromosomal anomalies among spontaneous abortions, any radiation-induced increase in nondisjunction and/or early chromosome loss is likely to lead to an increase in the rate of spontaneous abortion rather than to more chromosomally abnormal newborns, as explained in greater detail in earlier UNSCEAR Reports. This conclusion is corroborated by a study in the mouse [R1], in which the frequency of chromosomal radiation effects was followed from zygotes to early and late embryos. The fraction of chromosomally disturbed germ cells, which was very high at the beginning, was found to be practically zero in embryos surviving to birth.

295. In the UNSCEAR 1982 Report [U3] (Table 8, page 525), 12 studies were listed that addressed the question of whether pre-conceptual irradiation of mothers increases the incidence of Down's syndrome. Four studies described a significant increase in this syndrome; eight studies failed to show such an effect. The studies included women who had been exposed at some time in their lives to small doses of radiation for medical reasons. Obviously, they were not an unbiased population sample; there is ample opportunity for the action of confounding variables. On the other hand, the data do not allow dismissing the possibility that low radiation doses enhance the risk for autosomal nondisjunction in female human meiosis, at least under certain conditions (see also the studies of populations living in areas of high natural background radiation in India and China, discussed in Section III.A.2). The Japanese data do not support an increased risk for live-borns with trisomies.

(d) Congenital anomalies and multifactorial diseases

296. In the UNSCEAR 1988 Report [U1], the Committee estimated the incidence of congenital anomalies and multifactorial diseases to be 60,000 and 600,000 per million live births, respectively, but did not estimate the increase caused by radiation [U1]. In the UNSCEAR 1977 and 1982 Reports [U4, U3] the Committee had used a doubling dose of 1 Gy and a mutational component of 5%, but the uncertainties did not justify continuing this procedure, given the higher estimated incidence of these conditions of varying seriousness that can arise throughout a lifetime. The study of the survivors of the atomic bombings in Japan indicates no increase in congenital anomalies or multifactorial disorders subsequent to parental irradiation [N8, N9]. In theory, a system of continuous registration of these conditions that is complemented by ad hoc studies on special problems, such as genetic data (for example empirical risks in families) or environmental factors (radiation, drugs and environmental chemicals), is the best system for answering questions of incidence and causation. However, in view of the complex genetic basis of most malformations and of multifactorial diseases, it is impossible to estimate increases caused by radiation, and no such estimate was attempted in the UNSCEAR 1988 Report [U1].

2. Estimates of BEIR, ICRP AND NUREG

297. While the BEIR III Committee [C2] relied mostly on the direct method to estimate first-generation risk for genetic disorders and traits that cause a serious handicap at some time during a lifetime, the BEIR V Committee [C1] described the direct method but stated that the "Committee had little confidence in the reliability of the individual assumptions required by the direct method let alone the product of a long chain of uncertain estimates that follow from these assumptions. Therefore, they did not place heavy reliance on the direct method in making their risk estimates, but used it only as a test of consistency". The BEIR V Committee discussed relatively few of the many assumptions used in the indirect method, which it did apply. In contrast, the United States Nuclear Regulatory Commission report [N10], in discussing the BEIR V report, noted that the direct method involved fewer uncertainties than the indirect and was thus preferable.

298. The BEIR V report presented a much higher current incidence for genetic disorders than the UNSCEAR 1988 Report [U1] (Table 5). It concluded that the current incidence is 1,247,300 genetic effects per million live-born offspring. Risk was not estimated for the 1,200,000 of these effects that consisted of heart disease, cancer and selected other diseases. Regarding these three categories, they concluded as follows: "The magnitude of the genetic component in susceptibility to heart disease and other disorders with complex aetiologies is unknown. Because of great uncertainties in the mutational component of these traits and other complexities, the committee has not made quantitative risk estimates for them. The risks may be negligibly small, or they may be as large or larger than the risks for all other traits combined". For the remaining genetic disorders (current incidence of 47,300 per million), the estimate of first-generation risk of radiation-induced genetic effects per 0.01 Sv of exposure was between 16 to 53 per million live births (Table 5). Of that total, between 1 and 15 were estimated to be clinically mild.

299. The risk of congenital anomalies was given in the BEIR V report [C1] as about 10 in the first generation and 10-100 at equilibrium for 0.01 Sv of additional radiation. These estimates assumed that the

relevant malformations consist of those caused in part by multifactorial inheritance in combination with a threshold and in part by irregularly manifesting dominant mutations. The overall mutational component was estimated to be between 5% and 35%. The upper limit (35%) was then used to estimate the increase (Table 5). The result is quite uncertain. Moreover, the argument is based in part on results of twin studies, which are misleading for congenital malformations since the background incidence of most congenital abnormalities is increased in monozygous twinning, apparently because of the special conditions that produce monozygotic twin pregnancies [V10].

300. The ICRP estimated the component of risk for multifactorial diseases from radiation exposure to be 0.5 10^{-2} Sv^{-1} and the total for severe hereditary effects for all generations to be 1 10^{-2} Sv^{-1} (see Annex B in [I1]). The ICRP risk coefficients [I1, S44] relied heavily on the UNSCEAR 1988 risk estimates [U1], with some important additions. The effect of 0.01 Gy per generation per million live births on the incidence of Mendelian and chromosomal diseases was taken to be 120 at equilibrium [S44], as in Table 5. The natural prevalence of congenital abnormalities was taken to be 6%, as in Table 5, and of other multifactorial disorders 65%. Assuming a doubling dose of 1 Gy of low-dose-rate, low-LET radiation, an average mutational component of 5% and a weighting factor of one third for severity of effects, the risk coefficient for all multifactorial diseases, including congenital anomalies, becomes 120 per million live births at equilibrium for exposure to 0.01 Gy per generation [I1, S44], or 1.2 10^{-2} Sv^{-1}. The total risk coefficient for all Mendelian, chromosomal and multifactorial diseases is thus 2.4 10^{-2} Sv^{-1} at equilibrium. However, when the total population is considered, the genetically significant dose will be markedly lower than the total dose received over a lifetime. If it is assumed that the mean age at reproduction is 30 years and the average life expectancy at birth is 70-75 years, the dose received by 30 years is about 40% of the total dose. The risk coefficient for the total population is thus 0.4 × 2.4 10^{-2} Sv^{-1}, or 1 10^{-2} Sv^{-1} at equilibrium, i.e. when the effects are summed over all generations [I1, S44]. The corresponding risk coefficient summed over the first two generations only would be 0.2 10^{-2} Sv^{-1}.

301. The NUREG Committee [N10] expressed genetic risk per 480,000 live births instead of per million live births. This figure is an estimate of first generation offspring in the United States, predicted from the 1978 demographic data of 1 million persons of all ages (i.e. 16,000 live births per year for 30 years). Its combined first-generation risk estimate for single-gene disorders, chromosome aberrations (including aneuploidy) and congenital abnormalities was 30 radiation-induced genetic disorders, and its first-generation estimate for selected irregularly inherited diseases (having a normal incidence of 576,000 per 480,000 live births, which is equivalent to the current incidences used by the BEIR V Committee), was 35 radiation-induced genetic disorders. The Committee stressed the "extremely tenuous nature of these numerical estimates for diseases of complex aetiology in light of the very large uncertainties involved" [N10].

302. The NUREG Committee pointed out that its estimate of risk from unbalanced translocations, as well as the estimate in the UNSCEAR 1988 Report [U1], was based on an estimate of the frequency of balanced translocations at least an order of magnitude higher than that actually observed cytologically in the offspring of the atomic bomb survivors [A7]. It thus may be that the risk estimates in the UNSCEAR 1988 Report [U1] for this category of genetic disease are too high.

3. Re-evaluation of doubling dose estimates in mice and humans

303. It has been suggested that, for humans, the doubling dose of acute low-LET ionizing radiation of the gonads is 0.3-0.4 Sv, with limits of 0.1-1 Sv [C1, U2]. That estimate appears to be based primarily on the data summarized by Lüning and Searle [L6], namely, data on semi-sterility (i.e. reciprocal translocations), the seven-locus (or specific locus) system of Russell [R4], dominant visible mutations recovered in the course of specific-locus studies, dominant skeletal mutations and recessive lethals. The average of these values was 0.31 Sv. When a dose-rate reduction factor of 3 was employed for conversion to the effect of chronic radiation, the doubling dose for chronic and/or intermittent radiation was about 1 Sv, with lower and upper limits of 0.3 and 3 Sv. It has been suggested that for chronic radiation the doubling dose is not less than 1 Sv [C1]. This estimate was based on a wider variety of end-points of genetic damage than those used by Lüning and Searle, and the confidence limits for some of the additional end-points were very wide.

304. In view of the apparent discrepancy between these estimates and those resulting from the follow-up studies on the children of atomic bomb survivors, Neel and Lewis [N7] compared the findings on mice and humans point-by-point. They concluded that because of biological differences between the two species, a precise comparison was impossible for many end-points. For instance, the newborn mouse corresponds roughly, in terms of development, to a human fetus at 100 days of gestation [N7]. The data on congenital malformations in mouse fetuses following paternal irradiation were obtained by sacrificing pregnant mice at day 18 or 19 of gestation, equivalent to less than

100 days of human fetal development [K5, K6]. Because in humans some fraction of the corresponding defects would be lost through early miscarriage and in most studies go unrecorded, and because the very immature mouse fetus cannot be subjected to the same type of physical examination as a newborn infant, the mouse and human data are not comparable. Furthermore, the polytocous nature of mouse reproduction results in pre- and postnatal competition between litter mates, which does not exist in humans. This competition renders a comparison of the two species with respect to postnatal mortality following radiation uncertain and complicates any extrapolation. Finally, since several of the mouse strains employed in radiation research were originally developed for research on cancer, it may not be entirely valid to compare the results of Nomura [N14, N15] on mice with the results obtained in Hiroshima and Nagasaki, particularly since the tumour types that dominate Nomura's data are not those associated with germ-line mutations in humans.

305. Given the manner in which the recent estimate of the human genetic doubling dose resulting from acute radiation (the Japanese studies) was derived, the mouse estimate that would seem to be most comparable to the human would be that based on locus-specific phenotype studies. In Table 6, the findings for eight different types of locus-specific phenotype studies in the mouse are compared. These studies are of rather uneven informational content, and some not quite congruous studies are combined, particularly those in which the results had not previously been incorporated into doubling dose estimates. The simple, unweighted average of the results of these eight types of tests is 1.35 Gy. Applying the dose rate factor of 3 customarily applied to such data in the light of the results of Russell et al. [R6], the estimate of the murine genetic doubling dose of chronic ionizing radiation becomes about 4 Gy. As for the human data, it is difficult to develop a precise error term for these data.

306. The potential difference between acute and chronic exposure and between different types of radiation needs further study. Searle and Edwards [S16] in particular have shown an increase in translocations with protracted exposure to low levels of high-LET radiation (i.e. alpha particles and fission neutrons).

307. It will be noted that the results obtained with different test systems appear to vary widely. Since for several of these estimates (e.g. electrophoretic variants and recessive visible mutations), only a single mutation has been encountered in the controls, the error of the estimate is large. There may also be real differences between systems. The data of Russell et al. [R5] indicate significant differences among the seven loci in their system with reference to radiation-induced rates. Similar data on locus differences in spontaneous locus mutability are beginning to emerge for humans [N7]. Thus, it should not be regarded as surprising if different systems yield different estimates, and there is no objective basis for preferring the results from one system over those derived from another.

308. This summary of the mouse data indicates the need to consider the results from many systems in arriving at a balanced view of the genetic effects of radiation. It should be noted that the studies in Japan (Section III.A.1) involve end-points that reflect the input of many loci. There may, however, be an additional reason for differences between the results of the different mouse systems: inadvertent selection in some of the murine systems of the more mutable loci for study. For example, the valuable and much used seven-locus test system developed by Russell [R5] was developed on the basis of known, contrasting phenotypes associated with each of the loci in question. This was the key to developing the test crosses, which permitted rapid locus scoring for mutation. It now seems possible that this derivation of the system may have introduced inadvertent selection for loci with relatively high spontaneous and induced mutation rates. This and the possible strain differences in mice again raises the question of ethnic differences in humans: could different genetic backgrounds result in loci with differing susceptibility to mutation?

309. Although the error in both the mouse and human estimates is, for various reasons, indeterminate but presumably large, these considerations, in the view of Neel and Lewis, may bring the mouse and human results into much better congruence than appeared to be the case in the past. There is, of course, no reason why two species differing in as many respects as mice and humans should have identical doubling doses, but there is also no reason to think they should be unequal. Given the difference in the end-points used for the two species, this congruence is somewhat surprising and should be regarded with caution.

4. Molecular biological developments

310. Sankaranarayanan [S3, S4, S5, S6, S7] considered at length the impact of molecular biology on the estimation of genetic risk from ionizing radiation and made a number of points. In genetic risk estimation, adverse genetic consequences have generally been viewed through the prism of naturally occurring genetic diseases. The concept of radiation-induced genetic disease relies on the premise that the types of events induced are similar to those arising spontaneously; this was supported by the recovery in experimental systems of induced mutations at selected gene loci, the phenotypes of which were similar to those of spontaneous mutations. This idea continues to catalyse

the search for increases in the frequencies of known dominant or X-linked genetic diseases in human populations exposed to radiation (e.g. as a result of the Chernobyl accident [C15] and the atomic bombings of Hiroshima and Nagasaki).

311. However, as discussed in Section II.C, molecular data for Mendelian diseases and for radiation-induced mutations in experimental systems now demonstrate that (a) while the types of events are indeed similar, those that lead to naturally occurring Mendelian diseases show specificities both in their distribution and their mechanisms of origin and (b) the overlap in mechanisms between spontaneous and induced mutations may be small. Thus, the probability that ionizing radiation will induce the specific mutations that result in known Mendelian diseases is likely to be small. It is not to be implied that gonadal radiation exposures have no adverse genetic effects. Rather, the message is that the frame of reference used, namely naturally occurring Mendelian diseases, may not be entirely adequate [S7].

312. With regard to the two standard methods of risk estimation using animal models the following may be noted. The size of the multiplication factor used in the direct method is partly based on an understanding of the relative damage to different body systems from spontaneous mutations. As noted earlier, the estimate of this is uncertain. It would be subject to additional uncertainty if the very large numbers of genes that can mutate to cause damage to different body systems respond to radiation damage to very different extents.

313. With the doubling dose method, the risk is estimated by multiplying the natural prevalence of autosomal dominant and X-linked diseases by the relative mutation risk. A number of arguments suggest that the value of the natural prevalence may need to be revised downwards and that of the doubling dose upwards; as a consequence, the estimate of risk will be lower than at present. These arguments are as follows:

(a) since radiation generally induces deletions, and assuming that only about 50% of naturally occurring Mendelian diseases are due to deletions, clearly the value of the natural prevalence used in the risk estimation should be lower, pertaining only to the subset of genes that are responsive to induced deletions;

(b) the estimate for a doubling dose of 1 Sv is based primarily on mouse data for recessive visible mutations at seven loci, which may be more mutable than most genes. Genes that mutate to recessives have been observed to do so at a higher rate than those that mutate to dominants. This suggests that if a doubling dose based on recessives is used for estimating the risk of dominant genetic disease, the risk will be overestimated;

(c) the risk estimation used in the doubling dose method assumes that genes that mutate at high rates spontaneously will also mutate at high frequencies after irradiation. This assumption is open to doubt. A high spontaneous rate depends, among other factors, on the size and sequence of the gene and on the types of mutational mechanisms involved. A high induction rate is more dependent on whether a random change in the gene can give rise to the phenotype being measured [S7].

314. Again, as emphasized above, the growing understanding of non-traditional mechanisms by which genetic diseases may arise (see Section I.D) has introduced another dimension of complexity and may influence estimations of genetic risk, depending on how these mechanisms respond to radiation.

E. SUMMARY

315. Two main methods have been used in animal experiments (primarily mouse) that attempt to quantify genetic risk from exposure to radiation: the doubling dose (also referred to as the indirect) method and the so-called direct method. Both methods involve collecting similar or identical data on radiation exposures and abnormalities in offspring. However, they use different approaches in extrapolating animal data to humans. The terms direct and indirect refer to whether the estimate of damage in the first generation is based directly on phenotypic damage found in mice in first-generation progeny (direct method) or whether it is based on extrapolation back to the first generation from a prediction at genetic equilibrium (indirect method). Although the frequency of harmful effects from induced mutations (from the exposure of a single generation) would be expected to decrease beyond the first generation, owing to negative selection, it should be kept in mind that some of the genetic effects of radiation, e.g. aneuploid segregants from certain translocations, or mutations leading to abnormal imprinting in gametes of first generation offspring, might not manifest until the second or subsequent generations.

316. The doubling dose (or indirect) method of genetic risk estimation expresses risk in relation to the natural incidence of mutations and genetic diseases that are evident at birth in the general population. The doubling dose is the amount of radiation necessary to produce twice as many mutations as would occur spontaneously in the population in a generation. It is obtained by dividing the average rate of spontaneous

mutations at a given set of gene loci by the rate of induction of mutations at the same set of loci. The reciprocal of the doubling dose is the relative mutation risk. A low doubling dose means a high relative mutation risk, and vice versa. This method is generally used to estimate risks under equilibrium conditions. The currently used doubling dose estimate, 1 Sv, for low-dose-rate or chronic exposures to sparsely ionizing radiation such as x rays or gamma rays is based primarily on mouse data on autosomal recessive mutations at seven specific loci and is expected to be at least of the correct order of magnitude. One difficulty of the doubling dose method in estimating the risk of autosomal dominant and X-linked diseases in man is to specify correctly the mutational component, or the component of a given disorder that is due to genetic mutation.

317. In the direct method, the estimated rates of induction of dominant mutations affecting the skeleton or causing cataracts in the eye of the mouse are used to derive estimates of the total risk of dominant genetic disease to the first-generation (F_1) progeny of an exposed human population. Assumptions about the persistence of mutations in the population, however, could permit extrapolating first-generation estimates to later generations. The direct method and the doubling dose method each has its inherent advantages and disadvantages in using the results of animal experiments to calculate the risks in humans of induction of hereditary disorders caused by radiation. It is thus recommended that both methods continue to be used and compared. Caution should be exercised, however, when extrapolating mouse studies to humans: there are notable differences between mice and humans in disease expression, early development, placentation and types of congenital anomalies that are most frequent. There are also strain differences in mice, which are probably comparable to ethnic differences in humans.

318. While people who have been exposed to radiation have been shown to suffer direct effects from exposure, such as increased cancer rates, the data on survivors of the atomic bombings indicate that acute irradiation with moderate doses of ionizing radiation has a negligible adverse effect on the health of the subsequent generation. A number of different indicators, such as untoward pregnancy outcome, cancer in the children of exposed parents and mutations affecting certain protein characteristics, have been used to infer doubling doses. Several types of analyses of seven data sets failed to reveal a statistically significant effect of parental radiation for various indicators. The average combined gonadal dose of acute ionizing radiation received by the proximally exposed parents (0.4 Sv) approximates that which in the past had been estimated to be a genetic doubling dose for mice. The statistical power of these studies is such that the absence of an effect of parental exposure to the atomic bombings on any of the indicators suggests humans may not be as sensitive to the genetic effects of radiation as has for some years been projected on the basis of murine doubling-dose data.

319. The estimate obtained from the studies on the atomic bomb survivors suggests that a doubling dose estimate for humans of between 1.7 and 2.2 Sv for acute irradiation and 4.0 Sv for chronic exposure, should be used. It also suggests that the genes used in the specific locus studies in mice may be more radiosensitive than most genes in humans. Studies of populations living in areas of high background radiation, or exposed to radiation through accidents, support the conclusions from the Japanese studies, i.e. that humans have little risk of hereditary damage from moderately low exposures to ionizing radiation. The potential differences between acute and chronic exposures and between different types of radiation require further study.

IV. FUTURE PERSPECTIVES

A. MOLECULAR INVESTIGATIONS

320. So far, the hereditary effects of radiation have been discussed and assessed mainly at the level of phenotypes. Indeed, changes in phenotypes are of primary interest to society. There are, however, complex problems of methodology in estimating such effects, as discussed in the previous Chapters. Many uncertainties have to be bridged by assumptions and extrapolations. On the other hand, basic research in genetics, and especially in human genetics, is concentrating more and more on the structure of genes themselves and their products. To allow using these new technologies in testing for radiation effects, new approaches have been, or are being, developed at the levels of gene DNA and proteins.

321. In view of the difficulties in assessing mutational effects at the phenotypic and gene-product levels, on the one hand, and recent progress in studying DNA sequences directly, on the other, it is not surprising that the possibility of studying possible radiation effects directly in the DNA has been explored. A number of approaches have been suggested, including the following:

(a) sequence analysis;
(b) analysis of restriction fragment length polymorphisms;
(c) RNase A and gradient denaturation electrophoresis analysis of mutational change;
(d) detection of deletions, insertions and rearrangements by single restriction enzyme digest;
(e) determination of mini-satellites to allow unique identification of particular segments of DNA;
(f) amplification of small amounts of DNA by the polymerase chain reaction;
(g) refined cytogenetic analysis by chromosome *in situ* hybridization (chromosome painting).

322. At first glance, a comparison of the DNA sequences in parents and children would be the most promising approach. Assuming a spontaneous base-pair mutation rate of 10^{-8} and about 6-7 10^9 base pairs in the diploid human genome, there would be 60-70 spontaneous new mutants in a child's genome [T3]. Any statistically significant increase should be attributed to induced mutations. At present, however, sequencing would not be sufficiently precise and would be too time-consuming and expensive to allow carrying out the large number of tests needed to obtain statistically significant results. Further progress in techniques is awaited. The analysis of restriction fragment length polymorphisms is still too time-consuming and expensive to be used for tracing mutations in population studies, although it can be applied to individual cases. Many, if not most, radiation-induced changes of the genetic material are structural chromosomal aberrations, such as deletions, insertions and reciprocal translocations. Larger changes of these kinds can be ascertained by conventional cytogenetic techniques. More recently, however, techniques have been developed in which cytogenetics has been combined with hybridization. The resolution power of such methods, while not approaching that of sequencing DNA base pair by base pair, is much better than that of conventional cytogenetics [N8]. Such methods could also be used for studying human and animal germ cells.

323. Methods of DNA analysis are not yet contributing to risk assessment. Nevertheless, some of the approaches mentioned above, or others, may help one day to improve appreciably the understanding of genetic radiation risks. Even now, however, it may be asked whether and to what degree such studies will further knowledge of possible health hazards. Some of these hazards could adversely affect the health of the current generation, or that of their children and grandchildren. In conjunction with studies of the children of atomic bomb survivors, work is proceeding on such methods of hazard assessment, and lymphoblastoid cell lines are being established for further study.

B. THE HUMAN GENOME PROJECT

324. The human genome (the gene complement of all of the chromosomes) is estimated to comprise approximately 3 10^9 base pairs of DNA and to contain 50,000-100,000 functionally expressed genes [M9]. The Human Genome Project, now in progress, is an international cooperative effort to map and eventually sequence the entire DNA content of the human genome. It is expected that the results will offer clues to the molecular causes and possible treatment of more than 4,000 known genetic diseases, as well as many others with a suspected genetic link [C4]. The project may well revolutionize the approach to human disease and mutation, bringing a shift from estimates based on indirect methods to estimates based on molecular analysis.

325. Both short- and long-term goals have been established for the Human Genome Project. Short-term (five-year) goals include mapping (as opposed to immediately sequencing) the human genome, and mapping and sequencing the genomes of non-human model organisms, including those of bacteria (Escherichia coli), yeast (Saccharomyces cerevisiae), nematode (Caenorhabditis elegans), fruit fly (Drosophila melanogaster) and laboratory mouse (Mus musculus) [U11]. It is felt that mapping will allow scientists to search for specific genes of medical and biological importance, as nearly 95% of the human genome comprises what are presumed to be non-functional sequences [C4]. In the meantime, new sequencing technologies will be developed that will facilitate the eventual sequencing of the entire human genome.

326. For the physical mapping (cytogenetically or molecularly based), one of the initial goals is to assemble a map of sequence tagged sites. These are short sequences of DNA that occur only once in the genome and thus uniquely identify a mapped gene or other marker. The order and spacing of these sequences will allow them to be used as signposts for assigning positions to subsequently mapped genes and will provide a uniform system for reporting data, regardless of the mapping strategy or technique used. Sequence tagged sites will be reported as pairs of oligonucleotide primers that have been tested and shown to produce a polymerase chain reaction product that identifies a single band in a Southern blot with total DNA from a human male [C4].

327. The short-term goal for genetic linkage mapping is to enhance the resolution of present maps that are based on DNA polymorphisms. Over 2,000 of these polymorphisms are already known, and eventually the map should provide an average interval size between adjacent loci of about 2 centimorgans [S36]. The mapping will allow maps of overlapping clones and

panels of genetic markers, along with sequence tagged sites, to be used in positioning a genetic defect, greatly facilitating the identification of genes for specific diseases and malformations.

328. The mapping and sequencing of non-human genomes will allow scientists to work with simpler systems (i.e. smaller genomes) and to manipulate and study the structure and function of mapped genes in the intact organism, which is extremely difficult to do in humans. Because many essential genes are largely conserved over species boundaries, insights gained from animal models can often be applied to the study of human genes [C4]. According to researchers who support the project, the traditional manner of searching for an abnormal gene is unnecessarily costly and wasteful of the scientist's time; it is, moreover, practically untenable for genetically complex defects such as Alzheimer's disease, cancer or schizophrenia [C8]. A positional approach (as opposed to a functional approach) makes it possible to isolate the abnormal genes when the structure and function of the gene product are unknown. It was the positional method that led to the cloning of the genes for cystic fibrosis and neurofibromatosis. It has an even greater advantage for polygenic and multifactorial disorders [C8].

329. The long-term goal of the project is to sequence the entire human genome. The undertaking should be completed in 15 years [W5]. Because the information gained from the mapping and sequencing of genes for human disease, as well as for traits such as sex and intelligence, will have profound social implications, 3%-7% of the budgets for most genome projects have been allocated for studying the ethical, legal and social implications of the information. The purpose of these studies is to anticipate and address implications for individuals and society in areas such as health insurance and prenatal testing and will develop policy options, e.g. in areas where there might be conflict of interest, to ensure that the information is used for the benefit of individuals and society [U11].

330. The Human Genome Project is expected to have at least four corollary benefits [W5]:

(a) it will provide a direct method for analyzing mutation rates, as well as the effects of particular mutagens (including radiation), using human DNA. Thus, risk estimates will be far more accurate than at present, and the various complicating factors will be able to be defined and analysed individually;
(b) new laboratory technologies will be developed to achieve the goals of the project;
(c) new computer technology will be applied to molecular biology, with a concomitant development of new hardware, software and database designs to support and facilitate the massive scale of the undertaking;
(d) the identification and cloning of medically and biologically important genes will, in turn, furnish scientists with material for research on their identity, structure and function for many years to come. From the standpoint of the hereditary effects of radiation, it is expected that once the human genome has been sequenced, a much better understanding of radiation biology, susceptible areas of the human genome and the tracing of suspected damage will be possible.

CONCLUSIONS

331. The present situation in radiation genetic risk estimation can be summarized as follows: (a) current risk estimates for Mendelian diseases appear to be conservative and to provide an adequate margin of safety in radiation protection; and (b) while none of the methods used for risk estimation is free of uncertainties, in the absence of more reliable methods it would not be prudent to abandon any of the approaches or to alter the risk estimates presented in the UNSCEAR 1986 and 1988 Reports [U2, U1]. New data and understanding have served primarily to increase the complexity of the task of risk estimation.

332. Some relatively reliable data are available on the incidence of chromosomal aberrations and on a few rare dominant or X-linked conditions (sentinel mutations) in humans. It is, in principle, possible to determine the background spontaneous incidence of congenital anomalies at birth in a human population. However, to do so requires a sophisticated logistical network that includes, among other things, a precise definition of end-points. To allow comparing data from various countries and different time periods within the same country, international coordination is necessary. The Hungarian registry is a good example of a national screening system.

333. Even with data from such a system at hand, it is not yet possible to predict an increase in the incidence of congenital anomalies attributable to a specific exposure of the gonads to radiation, since such a prediction would require estimating the mutational component of such an increase. An estimation of this com-

ponent would in turn require much more thorough knowledge of the genetic basis of these anomalies and the involvement of environmental factors.

334. Observations on human populations and experiments with animals are improving risk estimation; however, both of these methods require considerable extrapolation: from a very few sentinel mutations to all genetic disease, and from animal to human. It must, therefore, be kept firmly in mind that both the direct and the doubling dose method still provide only rough estimates of risk. Because both methods require extrapolation and estimation, the terms direct and indirect (or doubling dose) are not entirely accurate. It might be more appropriate to refer to the two methods as the absolute method and the relative method, or perhaps as the first-generation method and the equilibrium method.

335. The direct and doubling dose methods have yielded risk estimates that are of a similar order of magnitude; because each method has its advantages and drawbacks, it would seem prudent to continue using both to derive information that is as complete as possible. The estimates obtained should be regarded as lower limits, with the caveat that radiation effects on multifactorial disease, gene regulation and non-traditional forms of inheritance are not well understood and may require different methods of estimation.

336. One purpose of this Annex has been to point out the difficulties that are inherent in any attempt to quantitatively predict the health hazards to future generations caused by exposures to ionizing radiation. Such predictions, based on extrapolations from animal experiments and on the direct observation of exposed population groups, are possible in genetically simple and straightforward situations, such as for cytogenetically visible chromosomal aberrations or rare dominant and X-linked diseases. For all other groups of diseases, such an estimate is not yet possible and will probably remain impossible for some time to come. The studies on the children of atomic bomb survivors at Hiroshima and Nagasaki suggest that the adverse effects on the first generation of progeny from a single moderate radiation dose will probably be only minor. A more specific statement cannot be made at this time.

337. When considering mutations on the molecular level, several points should be kept in mind. The relative frequency of the various molecular changes seen in spontaneous mutation differs from that seen in radiation-induced mutation. It has been noted that most spontaneous mutations tend to be small point mutations, while a majority of radiation-induced mutations are larger DNA deletions. The fact that radiation-induced mutations are likely to differ from spontaneous mutations in the type of mutation produced, frequency and sites affected, and in the disease phenotypes produced, must also be considered and, in fact, expected in any attempt at risk estimation. It should also be kept in mind that almost all work done on the effects of germ-cell irradiation on phenotypic damage in progeny has been done in males; female germ cells may have very different susceptibility to different types of induced mutation at different stages, particularly during *in utero* development of the female. These points offer convincing arguments that a simple, direct correlation between the number of mutations and the degree of mutation damage would be exceedingly difficult, if not impossible, in both animal and human studies.

338. Many newly recognized mechanisms of gene regulation and genetic disease in humans were not known by classical geneticists and thus have not been considered in previous estimates of genetic risk. They could, however, be significantly affected by radiation. Any estimation of risk must understand and consider these additional potential sources of hereditary disease; however the current state of knowledge of non-traditional mechanisms such as genomic imprinting and allelic expansion (see Section I.D) is limited. It may be assumed that these mechanisms could have trans-generational effects and would not necessarily manifest in the F_1 or even the F_2 generation, but there are few data with which to quantify risk.

339. From a purely scientific point of view, then, the problem cannot be defined more precisely at this time, and numerous questions require further examination. Thus, risk estimates can be made only with great uncertainty. It remains impossible to make any responsible statement on the morbidity of genetic effects in middle and advanced age in humans, but a preliminary statement regarding morbidity and mortality in young age might be attempted. Almost the only empirical data available for such an estimate are the data on children of survivors of the atomic bombings at Hiroshima and Nagasaki, since the extensive experimental animal work can only approximate effects in humans.

340. The study of children of the atomic bomb survivors has shown that the long-term monitoring of certain risk groups is possible. However, despite a relatively large sample size and exposure to relatively high radiation doses, the outcome of this study has been largely negative so far; i.e. it has found little or no convincing evidence that radiation influences the incidence of congenital malformations (or other multifactorial conditions). In view of this result, it can hardly be imagined that an even larger risk group would lead to positive findings. Studies on populations living in areas of high natural background radiation in various parts of the world, such as China, Brazil and southern India, have also demonstrated no clear evidence of any genetic risk from exposure to radiation.

341. The situation for multifactorial diseases, which include not only congenital disorders but also disorders with onset at all ages, is still more difficult. Complex systems of intertwined genetic polymorphisms in combination with a great variety of mutations leading to disease in human populations are becoming evident to medical genetic researchers. Estimates of incidence and even prevalence in a population critically depend on parameters such as the definition of disease in general and the delineation of diseases from the range of normal variability of conditions. Moreover, epidemiological research has shown that the incidence and prevalence of many such diseases differ from one population to another, and even within the same population from one time period to another, mainly owing to environmental factors.

342. A series of recommendations can be formulated to assist future attempts at risk estimation. It is first of all recommended that studies in both mice and humans of genetic damage due to radiation should be carried to the molecular level. Information from the Human Genome Project will be especially helpful in this regard. Since it is now possible to determine which chromosomes were inherited from which parent, it can be determined on a molecular level whether a mutation in a child was inherited from the parent with higher exposure to radiation.

343. However, it is likely to be a long time before the findings of the Human Genome Project provide definitive ways of estimating genetic risk from radiation. In the meantime, information is needed on the possibility that radiation induces mutations that cause specific genetic disorders with non-traditional inheritance. If it can be shown that some mechanisms leading to abnormal development differ considerably between mice and humans, experiments must be designed to indicate whether such differences are likely to lead to substantially different radiation risks in the two species. Taking mouse studies to a molecular level would help to make this comparison.

344. In addition, a formal protocol should be established for follow-up studies on heritable effects in the event of accidents involving ionizing radiation; such investigations may yield a great deal of information on human genetic risk that could not be obtained in any other way.

345. Additional information is needed on the induction of phenotypic damage observed in the progeny of irradiated experimental mammals. It would be useful to have data on body systems other than those involving skeletal and cataract mutations. It would be especially valuable if data could be developed that would, in some straightforward way, permit estimates of the risk of inducing dominant mutations that affect predispositions to cancer. More animal experiments are also needed to determine the risk of nondisjunction, Robertsonian translocations, autosomal recessive mutations manifesting in subsequent generations and the role of radiation in upsetting nontraditional mechanisms of disease inheritance, such as genomic imprinting and transposable elements.

346. Several obvious gaps in knowledge exist regarding the induction of dominant phenotypic damage. Until such damage is measured in offspring following the irradiation of oocytes (probably mature and maturing oocytes in mice), the direct method can be applied to women only by assuming that the relationship between the sexes is the same as predicted from specific-locus results. Estimates are needed for the phenotypic damage that results when both males and females are exposed to high-LET radiation.

347. Additional experiments using different strains of mice or other small experimental mammals could indicate the extent to which genetic background determines the overall level of induced dominant genetic damage. It would also be useful to determine the extent of induced phenotypic damage following several successive generations of radiation exposure. Such results could validate the assumptions used in extrapolating from the first-generation direct estimate to later generations.

348. It is known that Mendelian diseases in mammals can be induced by radiation. It seems likely that risk estimation can become more precise as more human genes are sequenced, mutation spectra analysed and mechanisms unravelled. It is therefore essential that scientists making genetic risk estimates keep abreast of progress in molecular biology.

349. New mouse *in vivo* test systems should be designed, including tests for dominant mutations, which take into account the homologies between the human and mouse genomes. Molecular studies with somatic cell mutations, both spontaneous and induced, will extend the knowledge of mutation spectra and mechanisms.

350. In well-studied experimental systems, most radiation-induced mutations are recessive and are due to DNA deletions. If human germ cell responses are similar, such mutations will accumulate in the gene pool. Given the very low levels of inbreeding in present-day human populations, homozygosity for induced recessives may occur only rarely. Thus it would be useful to have assessments, instead, of the overall adverse health effects in heterozygote carriers of induced recessive mutations. In humans, a useful starting point would be to compare the health of normal individuals with that of obligate heterozygotes for known recessive mutations.

Table 1
Incidence of genetic or partially genetic diseases having serious health consequences before the age of 25 years [a] [B3]

Category	*Rate per million live births*	*Percentage of total births*
Part A: Serious diseases with known genetic aetiology		
Dominant	1,395	0.14
Recessive	1,655	0.17
X-linked	532	0.05
Chromosomal	1,845	0.18
Multifactorial	46,583	4.64
Genetic unknown	1,164	0.12
Total	53,175	5.32
Part B: Serious congenital anomalies		
All congenital anomalies (ICDA codes 740-759)	52,808	5.28
Congenital anomalies with genetic aetiology (included in Part A above)	26,584	2.66
Part C: Serious genetic diseases and congenital anomalies		
Disorders in Part A (above) and congenital anomalies not included	79,392	7.94

[a] Based on the British Columbia Health Surveillance Registry in a study of 1,169,873 births from 1952 to 1983.

Table 2
Examples of molecular mechanisms that cause spontaneous deletions and duplications [S7]

Mechanism	*Example*
Replication slippage in tandem repeats	Some beta-globin structural variants Some mutations in factor VII and factor IX genes
Unequal homologous recombination-related genes	Most alpha-thalassemias, anomalous trichromacy
Unequal homologous recombination between Alu repeats	Some alpha-globin gene deletions Low-density lipoprotein receptor gene deletions and duplications Fabry disease, steroid sulphatase deficiency
Nonhomologous recombination with one breakpoint in or near Alu repeats	Some deletions in alpha, beta and complex thalassemias Lipoprotein lipase deficiency
Unequal sister chromatid exchange	Some dystrophin gene duplications
Gene conversion involving a functional gene and a pseudogene	21-hydroxylase deficiency (adrenal hyperplasia)

Table 3
Genetic risk estimates for serious effects in humans from 0.01 Gy of low-LET radiation from application of the direct method to mouse data

Basis of estimate	*Expected frequency in the first generation (Number per million live births)*	
	From exposure of males	*From exposure of females*
Phenotypic changes in mice living 3 weeks or longer dying between birth and 3 weeks of age	 10-20 [a] 5-10 [b]	 0-9 [c] 0-5 [c]
Total, each sex	15-30	0-14
Total, both sexes	15-44 [d]	

[a] Lower estimate based on induced cataracts; multiplication factor 36.8. The data, collected at high dose rates, have been corrected based on specific locus results.
[b] Based on many experiments on the amount of induced death and on two experiments that indicate that part of total occurring after birth.
[c] Data unavailable. Estimate assumed to be 44% of result with irradiated males, an upper bound suggested by specific-locus experiments. Because of qualitative differences in mutations between males and females, there is additional uncertainty in this risk estimate.
[d] Includes risks for all types of inheritance, including translocations, unbalanced products of reciprocal translocations and reciprocal translocations that act like dominant mutations.

Table 4
Estimates of minimal gametic doubling doses from analysis of end-points of genetic effects in survivors of the atomic bombings
[N5]

Genetic effect	*Observed total background incidence*	*Estimated mutational contribution to background incidence* [a]	*Mutational component* [b] *(%)*	*Regression parameters*	*Doubling dose (Sv)* [c] *at lower confidence limit of*		
					99%	*95%*	*90%*
Untoward pregnancy outcome	0.0502	0.0017-0.0027	3.4-5.4	β: 0.0026±0.0028 α: 0.039±0.0058	0.14-0.23	0.18-0.29	0.21-0.33
F_1 mortality	0.0458	0.0016-0.0026	3.5-5.7	β: 0.00076±0.0015 α: 0.063±0.0018	0.51-0.83	0.68-1.10	0.81-1.32
F_1 cancer	0.0012	0.00002-0.00005	2.0-4.0	β:-0.00008±0.00028 α: 0.0010±0.00033	0.04-0.07	0.05-0.11	0.07-0.15
Sex-chromosome aneuploids	0.0030 [d]	0.0030	100	β: 0.00044±0.00069 α: 0.0025±0.00043	1.23	1.60	1.91
Loci encoding for proteins	0.000013 [d]	0.000013	100	β:-0.00001±0.00001 α: 0.00001±0.00001	0.99	2.27	7.41

[a] Per diploid locus.
[b] Equal to mutational contribution divided by observed total background incidence (× 100 for %).
[c] The doubling dose is equal to α/β (equivalent to the reciprocal of the excess relative risk per sievert). The minimal doubling dose is the reciprocal of : β/α + the normal derivate at the desired probability level times the square root of the variance of β/α.
[d] Observed zygotic mutation rates.

Table 5
Incidence of genetic disease and risk estimates in humans from 0.01 Gy of low-LET radiation from application of the indirect method

Genetic disease	*Incidence per million live births*		*Effect of 0.01 Gy per generation per million live births*				
			UNSCEAR [U1]			*BEIR V [C1]*	
	UNSCEAR [U1]	*BEIR V [C1]*	*First generation*	*Second generation*	*Equilibrium*	*First generation*	*Equilibrium*
Autosomal dominant	10,000		15	13	100		
Clinically severe		2,500				5-20	25
Clinically mild		7,500				1-15	75
X-linked		400				<1	<5
Autosomal recessive	2,500	2,500	0.05	0.05	15	<1	Very slow increase
Chromosomal							
Structural anomalies	400	600	2.4	1	4	<5	Very little increase
Numerical anomalies	3,400	3,800	[a]	[a]	[a]	<1	<1
Congenital anomalies	60,000	20,000-30,000	Not estimated			10	10-100
Multifactorial diseases	600,000		Not estimated				
Heart disease		600,000				Not estimated	
Cancer		300,000				Not estimated	
Selected other		300,000				Not estimated	
Total			17	14	120		

[a] Probably very small.

Table 6
Estimates of gametic doubling doses for acute, high-dose irradiation of spermatogonia derived from specific-locus, specific-phenotype systems in the mouse
[N7]

System	*Origin of treated males*	*Doubling dose (Gy)*	*Reference*	
			Data summarized in	*Calculated by*
Russell seven-locus	101 × C3H	0.44	[E5, S12]	[N7]
Dominant visibles	Various	0.16	[L6]	[L6]
Dominant cataract	101/E1 × C3H/E1	1.57	[F3]	[F3]
Skeletal malformations	101	0.26	[E1]	[L6]
Histocompatibility loci	C57B1/6JN	>2.60	[B1]	[B1]
Recessive lethals	DBA	0.51	[S40]	[L6]
	C3H/HeH × 101/H	0.80, 1.77	[L8]	[B1]
	DBA, C3H	4.00	[L9]	[B1]
Loci encoding for proteins	Various	0.11	[N7]	[N7]
Recessive visibles	C3H/HeH × 101/H	3.89	[L8]	[N7]

Table 7
Correction factors used with the direct method to obtain estimates of risk of dominant genetic disease in humans [S6]

Step	*Quantity or correction factor*	*Correction procedure*	*Result*
	Skeletal mutations		
1A	Mutation frequency (1 + 5 Gy; 24-h fractionation, γ rays)	37 ÷ 2646	1.4 10^{-2}
1B	Mutation rate (per 0.01 Gy)	Divide (1A) by 600	2.3 10^{-5}
1C	Correction for dose fractionation and dose-rate effects [a]	Multiply (1B) by 1/1.9 and 1/3	4.0 10^{-6}
1D	Extrapolation from skeletal effects to all dominants (proportionality correction factor) [b]	Multiply (1C) by 10	40 10^{-6}
1E	Correction for severity	Divide (1D) by 2	20 10^{-6}
	Risk of dominant genetic disease to the first-generation progeny per 0.01 Gy of paternal exposure		20 10^{-6}
	Cataract mutations		
2A	Mutation frequency (4.55 + 4.55 Gy; 24-h fractionation; γ rays)	6 ÷ 5,231	1.15 10^{-3}
2B	Mutation rate (per 0.01 Gy)	Divide (2A) by 910	1.26 10^{-6}
2C	Correction for dose fractionation and dose-rate effects [c]	Multiply (2B) by 1/1.2 and 1/3	3.5 10^{-7}
3A	Mutation frequency (5.34 Gy acute γ rays)	3 ÷ 10,212	0.29 10^{-3}
3B	Mutation rate (per 0.01 Gy)	Divide (3A) by 534	5.5 10^{-7}
3C	Correction for dose-rate effect	Multiply (3B) by 1/3	1.8 10^{-7}
4A	Mutation frequency (6 Gy, acute γ rays)	3 ÷ 11,095	0.27 10^{-3}
4B	Mutation rate (per 0.01 Gy)	Divide (4A) by 600	4.5 10^{-7}
4C	Correction for dose-rate effect	Multiply (4B) by 1/3	1.5 10^{-7}
5	Average of (2C), (3C) and (4C) weighted by the number of mutants		2.6 10^{-7}
6	Extrapolation from dominant cataracts to all dominants [d]	Multiply (5) by 36.8	~10 10^{-6}
	Risk of dominant genetic disease to the first-generation progeny per 0.01 Gy of paternal exposure		~10 10^{-6}

[a] The correction factors are based on specific-locus experiments carried out at Oak Ridge.
[b] Based on the McKusick catalogue of autosomal phenotypes, 1975 edition [M7]; at that time, it was estimated that about 74 out of 328 clinically important autosomal dominant conditions in man involved one or more parts of the skeleton (about 20%); however, since skeletal defects are more easily diagnosed than those of other organ systems, the true figure was assumed to be about 10%.
[c] The correction for dose-fractionation effects (1/1.2) is based on concurrent specific-locus studies in Neuherberg.
[d] Based on the McKusick catalogue of autosomal phenotypes, 1978 edition [M7]; at that time, it was estimated that 20 out of 736 of all known and proven dominant mutations (2.7%) were associated with one or another form of cataract in man; recent analysis by Favor [F3], based on the McKusick catalogue of autosomal phenotypes, 1986 edition [M7], shows that these numbers are, respectively, 28 and 1,172, i.e. 2.4% of known dominant mutations are associated with cataracts. The multiplication factor is therefore 41.

Glossary

allele	an alternative form of a gene at a given locus. Being diploid organisms, humans may have two alleles at a given locus, i.e. a normal and a mutant allele. Abbreviation of allelomorph
allelic association	the association of two alleles at distinct loci beyond chance expectation. Normally a consequence of close linkage: loci within a megabase usually show some allelic association
allelic disorders	disorders, which may be phenotypically different, that are due to mutations in the same gene
alu repetitive sequence	repetitive sequence found about 500,000 times in human genome. The sequence contains a recognition site for the restriction enzyme AluI and is around 300 base pairs in length.
amplification	an increase in the number of copies of a particular DNA fragment. Can occur under natural circumstances, e.g. amplification of a repeat sequence, as in fragile-X syndrome, or during laboratory procedures such as cloning or polymerase chain reaction
aneuploid	a chromosome number that is not an exact multiple of the haploid number; an individual with an aneuploid chromosome number. Usually refers to an absence (monosomy) or an extra copy (trisomy) of a single chromosome
annealing	see hybridization
anticipation	phenomenon in which the severity of a genetic condition appears to become more severe and/or arise at an earlier age with subsequent generations
antisense strand (of DNA)	the non-coding strand of the DNA double helix that serves as the template for mRNA synthesis
association	the occurrence of an allele with a disease more often than chance should allow
autosome	any chromosome other than a sex chromosome. Men have 22 pairs of autosomes and an X- and a Y-chromosome; women have the same autosome pairs and two X-chromosomes. In the Paris convention, written 46XY and 46XX
bacteriophage	see phage. Bacterial virus used as a vector for cloning segments of DNA
band	a chromosomal segment defined by distinct staining. Both lighter and darker segments are called bands and are numbered from the centromere outwards, with smaller bands classified by a second number. Bands 11, 12, 13, 21, 22, 31 could be a continuous series.
base pair (bp)	in the DNA double helix, a purine and pyrimidine base on each strand that interact with each other through hydrogen bonding. The number of base pairs is often used as a measure of the length of a DNA segment, e.g. 500 bp.
base sequence	the order of nucleotide bases in a DNA molecule. Length is usually defined in base pairs.
blastomere	one of the cells produced by cleavage of a fertilized ovum, forming the blastoderm
breakpoint	refers to sites of breakage when chromosomes break (and recombine)
carrier	an unaffected individual who is heterozygous at a particular locus for a normal gene and an abnormal gene which, although it may be detectable by laboratory tests, is not expressed phenotypically. Variously used to cover both permanent non-expression in recessives and X-linked recessives and temporary non-expression in dominants (e.g. Huntington's chorea). More recently used to describe unaffected individuals who carry unstable or dynamic mutations that can expand and cause a genetic condition in offspring
cDNA	complementary DNA. The synthetic DNA equivalent of messenger RNA (mRNA) with a sequence complementary to the DNA strand from which it is derived
cDNA library	a collection of clones containing inserts of overlapping cDNA fragments representing expressed sequences (mRNA). cDNA libraries differ from one tissue or cell type to another.

centimorgan (cM) — the unit of genetic distance defined as the length of a segment of chromosome which has a 1% chance of recombining at meiosis. See also recombination percentage. Equivalent segments of chromosomes usually recombine more frequently at oogenesis than at spermatogenesis. Because even numbers of recombinant events between two strands cancel out, the recombination percentage is always less than the genetic distance and can never exceed 50%. The percentage recombination and the genetic distance in centimorgans are very similar when linkage is close (i.e. less than 10%).

centromere — the part of the chromosome by which it is moved at cell division and which separates it into two arms, appearing as a distinct "waist" on microscopy. Point of spindle attachment to the chromosome during meiosis and mitosis

chimaera — an organism compounded from two or more zygotes. A mosaic is formed from variant cells derived from the same zygote.

chiasma — the crossing of chromatid strands of homologous chromosomes during meiosis

chorionic villus sampling — procedure used to obtain fetal cells for prenatal diagnosis; involves biopsy of the placental membranes. Now usually done transabdominally from 8 weeks of pregnancy

chromatid — during mitosis each chromosome replicates into two DNA strands called chromatids. At meiosis recombination is due to chiasmata between non-identical pairs of chromatids.

chromatin — the composite of DNA and proteins that comprises chromosomes

chromosome — thread-like, deep-staining bodies situated in the nucleus. They are composed of DNA and protein and carry the genetic information.

cis — on the same chromosome, usually quite close. The opposite of trans, which relates to the other homologue. Cis effects are due to physical action between segments of the same DNA strand; trans effects are due to diffusion. Historically implies on the same chromosome. In molecular biology refers to an effect on a gene directed by the sequence of that gene or very close to it on the same chromosome (in contrast to trans effects, which are produced by other factors, such as the transcription factors encoded by other genes). The terms are commonly used to describe factors that influence gene expression.

cleavage — mitotic segmentation of the fertilized ovum, the size of the zygote remaining unchanged and the cleavage cells, or blastomeres, becoming smaller and smaller with each division

clone — a group of individual organisms or cells derived from a single individual by asexual reproduction

cloning — production of genetically identical cells (clones) from a single ancestral cell; cloning is utilized in molecular biology to propagate single or discrete DNA fragments of interest.

coding sequence — those parts of the gene from which the genetic code is "translated" into amino acid sequences of a protein

co-dominant — when both alleles are expressed in the heterozygote

codon — a group of three adjacent nucleotides that codes for particular amino acids or for the initiation or termination of the amino acid chain

codon usage — given the degeneracy of the genetic code, refers to the preference of codons used to specify particular amino acids. Often differs among species and among different genes and proteins

complementary — two nucleotide sequences are complementary when they can form a perfect double helix because they have a mirror-image relationship

compound heterozygote — an individual who has different mutant alleles at a given locus

congenital — existing at, and usually before, birth; referring to conditions present at birth, regardless of their causation

consanguinity — relationship by descent from a common ancestor; a consanguineous mating is between individuals who have one or more common ancestors. As all individuals have common ancestors it is usually restricted to couples with a common pair of grandparents, e.g. first cousins.

consensus sequence	a minimum nucleotide sequence found to be common (although not necessarily identical) in different genes and in genes from different organisms that is associated with a specific function. Examples include binding sites for transcription factors and splicing machinery.
conserved sequence	base sequence in a DNA molecule (or an amino acid sequence in a protein) that has remained essentially unchanged throughout evolution
contiguous gene syndrome	syndrome due to abnormalities of two or more genes that map next to each other on a chromosome; most often caused by a deletion that involves several contiguous genes
contig map	genetic map showing the order of (contiguous) DNA fragments in the genome
cosmid	a cloning vector derived from a natural bacterial parasite capable of accommodating up to 40 Kb of DNA (see plasmid)
coupling	when alleles from two loci are known to be on the same chromosome; the opposite of repulsion. Also, all alleles derived from one parent
crossing-over	the exchange of segment of a chromosome in meiosis. Small chromosomes usually have a single chiasma, so that of the four chromosomes entering gametes two are hybrid and two unchanged, e.g. if the parental chromosomes are ABCDE and abcde, the gametes could be ABCDE, ABcde, abCDE and abcde. The middle two are recombinant chromosomes with a crossover between loci B and C.
DNA	deoxyribonucleic acid. The long double-stranded molecule whose sequence of the four possible nucleotide bases provides the genetic information. The strands are held together by hydrogen bonds between nitrogenous bases that constitute the code: adenine (A) and thymine (T) which pair with each other, and guanine (G) and cytosine (C), which pair with each other.
DNA marker	a DNA sequence variation that is easily detectable; examples include restriction fragment length polymorphisms and dinucleotide and trinucleotide repeat polymorphisms.
DNA methylation	attachment of methyl groups to DNA, most commonly at cytosine residues. May be involved in regulation of gene expression
DNA polymerase	enzyme responsible for replication of DNA
DNA sequence	the relative order of base pairs
degeneracy	(of the genetic code) different codons code for the same amino acid
deletion	loss of a portion of a gene or chromosome; a type of mutation; a synonym of deficiency
diploid	containing two chromosome sets. The normal condition of most human cells except gametes; megakaryocytes, Purkinje cells and a few others have multiple sets.
dizygotic	twins derived from two distinct zygotes
domain	a discrete portion of a protein (and corresponding segment of gene) with its own function. A protein may have several different domains and the same domain may be found in different proteins.
dominant	a trait that is expressed in the heterozygote, sometimes only late in life
dominant mutations	mutations that produce an abnormal clinical phenotype (disorder or trait) when present in the heterozygous state
dominant negative mutations	heterozygous mutations in which the product of the mutant allele interferes with the function of the product normal allele
doubling dose	the dose of radiation that, under a given set of conditions, will lead to an overall mutation frequency that is double the spontaneous frequency
downstream	a DNA sequence is written from the left, or 5', direction or to the right, or 3' direction. Downstream refers to the 3' direction, i.e. the stop codon for a gene is downstream (3') of the coding sequences of that gene.
dysmorphology	study of abnormalities of morphologic development
electrophoresis	an analytical method used to separate nucleic acid, peptide or protein fragments based on size and charge of the molecule; typically smaller fragments travel further through the media (gel) in which separation is carried out.

enchromatin — darkly stained chromatin

enhancers — DNA sequences that increase transcription of a nearby gene; they can act in either orientation, may be either 5' or 3' to the gene or within an intron.

euchromatin — the chromatin that is thought to contain active or potentially active genes. Light (vs. dark) bands on G-banding

exon — a region of a gene containing a coding sequence. Most genes have several exons separated by introns, which are usually longer.

expressivity — the extent to which a genetic defect is expressed

F_1, F_2 etc. — the first (F_1) or second (F_2) generation of progeny of a mating

founder effect — a genetic effect due to the establishment of a new population by a few original founders who carry only a small fraction of the total genetic variation of the original population, with the consequence that some mutant alleles may reach unusually high frequencies in the new population. [Examples: the 2,000 Dutch settlers in South Africa in the 17th and 18th centuries, who did not marry outside the small ethnic group, eventually giving rise to a population of about 3 million. Frequency of familial hypercholesterolemia (FH) heterozygotes: 1/85 to 1/100 and 95% of mutations accounted for by only three alleles. Likewise, the current population of French Canadians of 5.8 million descended from 7,000 French settlers between 1608 and 1763. One familial hypercholesterolemia mutation accounts for about 60% of the heterozygotes in this group.]

frameshift mutation — a mutation that alters the normal triplet reading frame so that codons downstream from the mutation are out of register and not read properly

fragile site — gap or defect noted in the continuity of a chromosome when stained, e.g. fragile-X site. Many are apparent only when cells are cultured under special conditions.

gamete — mature reproductive cell (sperm or ovum); contains a haploid set of chromosomes (23 for humans)

gene — the unit responsible for transmitting an inherited character; the region of DNA that specifies the synthesis of a protein

gene targeting — artificial modification of a gene in a specific and directed fashion. Typically refers to substituting one DNA sequence for another to inactivate a gene or introduce or correct a mutation in a gene

genetic locus — a specific position or location in the genome

genetic fingerprint — a pattern of restriction fragments detected by probes that recognizes alleles at highly polymorphic loci; this is effectively unique to all individuals except identical twins.

genetic marker — an allele used in following the inheritance pattern of loci in cell lines, pedigrees or populations

genetic distance — the functional distance between two loci defined through recombination; it is measured in centimorgans; for small values (<10%) it is approximately equal to the recombination percentage.

genetic drift — the tendency for variations to occur in the genetic composition of small isolated inbreeding populations by chance. Such populations become genetically different from the original population from which they were derived.

genome — the complete genetic composition of an individual's chromosome; the complete set of genes characteristic of a species

genome DNA — DNA from a genome containing all coding (exon) and non-coding (intron and other) sequences, in contrast to cDNA, which contains only coding sequences

genomic library — a collection of clones containing DNA inserts of overlapping DNA fragments representing the entire genome of an organism

genotype — the alleles present in an individual at a locus or loci under consideration

germ cell — see gamete

germ-line mosaicism — presence of two or more cell lines in the gonadal cells. Implies risk of transmission of mutations present in the gonads to offspring

gonadal mosaicism	see germ-line mosaicism
haploid	containing one chromosome set as found in gametes after meiosis. The normal condition for gametes. The human haploid number is 23, half the diploid number of 46.
hemizygous	the condition of cells with respect to genes when only one set is present, as for genes on the X-chromosome in the male
heterochromatin	chromatin composed of repetitive DNA; stains as dark (versus light) bands in G-banding
heterozygote	an individual with two different alleles at a particular locus (adj. heterozygous)
histones	proteins associated with DNA in chromosomes
homeobox domain	a short DNA sequence common to a group of DNA binding proteins involved in pattern formation in early embryogenesis
homologies	similarities found in DNA or protein sequences when individuals of the same or different species are compared
homologous	matched. The other of a pair of chromosomes
homologous chromosomes	chromosomes containing the same linear gene sequences. In a normal mating, 1 of a pair of homologous chromosomes is derived from each parent. Humans normally have 22 pairs of homologous chromosomes and 2 X-chromosomes or 1 X- and 1 Y-chromosome.
homologous recombination	substitution of a segment of DNA by another that is identical (homologous) or nearly so. Occurs naturally during meiotic recombination; also used in the laboratory for gene targeting to modify the sequence of a gene
housekeeping genes	genes that encode proteins necessary for basic cellular functions. They are expressed in virtually all cells.
human gene therapy	insertion of normal DNA directly into cells to correct a genetic defect
hybridization (annealing)	the artificial conjunction of two complementary DNA strands, one of which usually carries a radioactive marker. Also used for the production of cells containing chromosomes from more than one species
imprinting	phenomenon in which an allele at a given locus is altered or inactivated depending on whether it is inherited from the mother or the father. Implies a functional difference in genetic information depending on whether it is inherited from the father or the mother
in situ hybridization	use of a nucleic acid probe to detect the presence of a DNA sequence in chromosome spreads or in interphase nuclei or of an RNA sequence in cells. It is used to map gene sequences to chromosomal sites and to detect gene expression.
insert	in molecular genetics, refers to DNA sequence of interest that has been inserted into a cloning vector such as a plasmid or bacteriophage
insertion	type of mutation in which a DNA sequence of variable length is inserted into a gene disrupting the normal structure of that gene
intron (intervening sequences)	the DNA sequences that interrupt the protein-coding sequences of a gene. The region of a gene that separates exons or coding sequences. They are removed during processing of mRNA. Introns may contain sequences involved in regulating expression of a gene.
karyotype	the chromosome set; the number, size and shape of the chromosomes of a somatic cell may be displayed diagrammatically as an idiogram.
kilobase (kb)	a thousand bases. A common unit for specifying the size of genes and physical distances along a DNA region
library	collection of clones in which overlapping genomic or cDNA fragments have been inserted into a particular cloning vector
linkage	the non-independent meiotic segregation of alleles at different loci, which is usually because the loci concerned are all on the same chromosome, and only separable by recombination. Linked loci are within measurable genetic distance of one another on the same chromosome, or are members of the same linkage group, e.g. on the same chromosome. Distant loci on the same chromosome may show independent segregation and now show linkage. They are then described as syntonic.

linkage disequilibrium	see allelic association
locus	the position on a chromosome. Usually that of a gene, but may refer to a DNA marker
lod score	a statistical method used to determine if a set of linkage data indicates two loci are linked or unlinked. A lod (log of odds ratio) score of +3 (1,000:1 odds) is commonly accepted to indicate that linkage exists, and a score of -2 (100:1 odds against) excludes linkage.
mapping	the process of determining the location of a gene by either direct observation or family study
marker	a detectable physical location on a chromosome. It can be a restriction enzyme cutting site, a gene, or a di- or trinucleotide repeat polymorphism whose presence and inheritance can be monitored.
maternal inheritance	inheritance pattern displayed by mitochondrial genes that are propagated from one generation to the next through the mothers; the mitochondria of the zygote comes almost entirely from the ovum.
megabase (Mb)	one million base pairs of DNA sequence roughly equal to 1 cM of genetic distance
Mendelian	a trait obeying Mendel's first law of independent segregation of the alleles at the same locus conveyed by each parent
meiosis	the type of cell division that occurs during gamete formation and results in the halving of the diploid somatic number of chromosomes so that each gamete is haploid and contains one of each chromosome pair. These post-meiotic chromosomes are usually partly paternal and partly maternal in origin.
messenger RNA (mRNA)	processed RNA that serves as a template for protein synthesis or for synthesis of cDNA
microsatellite	highly polymorphic DNA marker comprised of mononucleotides, dinucleotides, trinucleotides or tetranucleotides that are repeated in tandem arrays and distributed throughout the genomes. The best studies are the CA (alternatively GT) dinucleotide repeats. They are used for genetic mapping.
minisatellites	highly polymorphic DNA markers comprised of a variable number of tandem repeats that tend to cluster near the telomeric ends of chromosomes. The repeats often contain a repeat of 10 nucleotides. They are used for genetic mapping.
missense mutation	mutation that causes one amino acid to be substituted for another
mitochondrial (mt) DNA	DNA distinct from nuclear DNA in that it is mostly unique sequence DNA and codes for proteins that reside in mitochondria
mitosis	the type of cell division that occurs in somatic cells
monogenic	a synonym of Mendelian, i.e. governed by only one gene
monozygotic	twins derived from a single zygote
morphogenesis	evolution and development of form, as the development of the shape of a particular organ or part of the body
mosaicism	an individual with substantial proportions of two or more cell lines derived from a single zygote
motif	three-dimensional structure of gene product (protein) with known or implied function, i.e. DNA binding, traverse membrane etc. Often inferred from cDNA sequence
multifactorial	refers to the type of inheritance determined by many factors including both genes and the environment. If these are assumed additive, estimates of heritability may be made. In Mendelian and infective disorders a single factor will have a deciding role in manifestation, although not necessarily in severity or the potential for prevention or treatment. See also polygenic
mutation	a permanent and heritable change in genetic material (includes point mutations, deletions and changes in number or structure of chromosomes)
mutation frequency	number of mutations observed divided by number of progeny or cells examined
non-disjunction	failure of two members of a chromosome pair to disjoin (separate) during cell division
nonsense mutation	mutation that changes a codon for an amino acid to a termination or stop codon and leads to premature termination of translation

nucleosome — the basic structural unit of chromatin, in which DNA is wrapped around a core of histone molecules

nucleotide — a purine or pyrimidine base to which a sugar (ribose or deoxyribose) and 1, 2 or 3 phosphate groups are attached

nucleus — the organelle in eukaryotic cells that contains the genetic material

oligonucleotide — a short piece of DNA, typically 5-50 nucleotides

oncogene — a gene, one or more forms of which is associated with cancer. Many oncogenes are involved, directly or indirectly, in controlling the rate of cell growth.

open reading frame — a stretch of DNA following an initiation codon that does not contain a stop codon. Open reading frames in a nucleotide sequence suggest an exon and therefore a gene.

Paris convention — the notation system in which the karyotype is defined by the number of chromosomes followed by the sex chromosomes and information, if any, on an abnormality, e.g. 46XY, 47XHY (+21); 45XO; 47XXY. The position on a chromosome is defined by p and q (petit and queue) for the short and long arm and then by numbers defining bands and sub-bands, which are numbered outwards from the centromere. Usually there are 2-4 major bands and 2-5 minor bands, the term band covering both deeply and lightly staining segments.

pedigree — a diagrammatic representation of a family history

penetrance — the frequency of expression of a trait or genotype. The proportion of individuals observed to show a particular phenotypic effect of a mutant gene compared with the number expected on the basis of Mendelian inheritance

phage — a virus that infects bacteria and is a useful cloning vector for medium size pieces of DNA between 5 and 25 kb

phenocopy — an environmentally induced mimic of a genetic disorder

phenotype — the appearance (physical, biochemical and physiological) of an individual that results from the interaction of environment and genotype. Often used to define the consequences of a particular mutation

physical map — a map of physical landmarks on a DNA fragment or chromosome measured in base pairs. Landmarks include restriction endocnucleose recognition sites, DNA sequence and chromosomal bands.

plasmid — extrachromosomal small circular DNA molecule capable of autonomous replication within a bacterium. Commonly used as a cloning vector for small pieces of DNA, typically 50-5,000 bases

poly A RNA — RNA transcript that contains a tail of poly A residues at its 3' end; implies that an RNA sequence is mRNA. The poly A residues serve as stop signals to terminate transcription.

polyamines — compounds with many amino groups that are associated in the cell with nucleic acids

polygenic — inheritance determined by many genes at different loci, each with small additive effects. A simple example is height within either sex. See also multifactorial

polymerase — see DNA polymerase, RNA polymerase

polymerase chain reaction (PCR) — a method to amplify a DNA sequence using a heat-stable polymerase and two sets of primers that define the sequence to be amplified. Several variations have been developed for specific needs. May be combined with reverse transcription of mRNA to cDNA to amplify an mRNA, so-called RT-PCR

polymorphism — the occurrence in a population of two or more genetically determined forms in such frequencies that the rarest of them could not be maintained by mutation alone. Used in various distinct senses, especially in RFLPs where it is used to imply alternative forms. Usually implies commonest allele is less than 99% so that over 2% of individuals are heterozygous.

polyploid — an abnormal chromosomal complement that exceeds the diploid number and is an exact multiple of the haploid number

positional cloning	strategy for identifying and cloning a gene based on its location in the genome rather than on the biologic function of its product. Usually involves linking the gene locus of interest to one that has already been mapped
pre-mutation	a permanent and heritable change in a gene that does not have phenotypic consequences (does not cause disease) but predisposes to a "full" mutation that may
primary transcript	the initial RNA transcript of a gene, before processing to mRNA; it contains introns as well as exons.
primer	short polynucleotide chain that anneals to a nucleic acid template and promotes copying of the template from the primer site
proband	a synonym of propositus or proposita. The affected individual who brings the family to medical attention
probe	single-stranded DNA or RNA molecule of specific base sequence, labelled either radioactively or by other means, that is used to detect a complementary base sequence by hybridization. A labelled fragment of DNA (usually labelled with a radioactive isotope) used to identify a complementary sequence
promoter	a sequence on a gene that is upstream (5') to coding sequences to which RNA polymerase binds and initiates transcription of a gene
protein	a large molecule composed of one or more chains of amino acids in a specific sequence; the sequence is determined by the sequences of nucleotides in the gene coding for the protein. Proteins are required for the structure, function and regulation of the body's cells, tissues and organs, and each protein has unique functions. Examples are hormones, enzymes and antibodies.
pseudogene	sequence of DNA that is very similar to a normal gene but has been altered slightly so that it is not expressed
RNA	ribonucleic acid, the nucleic acid found mainly in cytoplasm. Messenger RNA (mRNA) transfers genetic information from the nucleus to the ribosomes in the cytoplasm and acts as a template for the synthesis of polypeptides; transfer RNA (tRNA) transfers activated amino acids from the cytoplasm to messenger RNA; ribosomal RNA (rRNA) is a component of the ribosomes that function as the site of polypeptide synthesis.
reading frame	register in which translation machinery reads the genetic triplicate code
recessive	a trait that is expressed in individuals who are homozygous for a particular allele
recessive mutations	mutations that produce an abnormal clinical phenotype when present in the homozygous or hemizygous state. Heterozygosity for the mutation, i.e. carrier state, may often be detected in persons whose clinical phenotype is normal.
recombinant DNA	DNA that is artificially transferred from the genome of one organism to that of another
recombinant DNA molecules	DNA molecules of different origins that are combined and manipulated in the laboratory
recombinant DNA technologies	laboratory procedures used to manipulate DNA fragments, e.g. cut, modify and ligate, and introduce them into an organism so that their number can be amplified as the organism replicates, i.e. cloning
recombination	the formation of a new combinations of linked genes by crossing-over between their loci during meiosis
recombination percentage	equivalent segments usually recombine more frequently at oogenesis than at spermatogenesis. Because even numbers of cut-and-join events between two strands cancel out, the recombination percentage, often termed theta, is always less than the genetic distance and can never exceed 50%. They are almost the same at less than 10%, which is just over 10 cM.
repulsion	when specific alleles at two different loci are derived from different parents. The opposite of coupling
restriction enzyme	bacterial-derived enzyme that recognizes a specific, short nucleotide sequence and cuts DNA at that site
restriction fragments	DNA fragments that result from digestion of DNA with restriction enzymes

restriction endonuclease	a group of enzymes each of which cleaves DNA at specific base sequences (recognition site)
restriction map	a map of a DNA sequence with restriction enzyme recognition sites serving as landmarks
restriction site	shortened term for restriction endonuclease recognition sequence
retrovirus	RNA viruses that encode the enzyme reverse transcriptase so that their RNA can be transcribed into DNA in the host cell; modified retroviruses are used as vectors to introduce genes (or portions thereof) of interest into eukaryotic cells.
reverse transcriptase	an enzyme that catalyses the synthesis of DNA from an RNA template (and thus can also make cDNA from mRNA)
RFLP	restriction fragment length polymorphism. The occurrence of two or more alleles in a population differing in the lengths of fragments produced by a restriction endonuclease
RNA polymerase	enzyme that synthesizes (transcribes) RNA from a DNA template
RNA splicing	process by which introns are removed from primary RNA transcripts, leaving only exons that encode the amino acid sequence of a protein
segregation	separation of alleles at meiosis
sequencing	determination of the order of nucleotides in a DNA or RNA fragment, or the order of amino acids in a protein
sequencing gel analysis	electrophoretic technique by which nucleotide size differences as little as a single base pair can be discerned
sequence-tagged sites (STSs)	short sequences of genomic DNA for which the base sequence is known. Polymerase chain reaction can be used to amplify the known sequences, which can serve as physical landmarks for mapping.
sex chromosome	the chromosomes that primarily govern sex determination (XX in women and XY in men). The other chromosomes are autosomes.
somatic cells	all cells in the body except gametes and their precursors
somatic cell hybrid	a hybrid cell line derived from fusion of cells from different sources. Human/rodent hybrids containing a small amount of human genetic material, such as a single chromosome, are used in human gene mapping.
somatic mosaicism	the presence of two or more cell lines in somatic (non-germinal) cells
Southern blotting	a technique, developed by E.M. Southern in 1975, for transferring DNA to a backing sheet prior to hybridization. Northern and Western blots are non-eponymous variations relating to RNA and protein analyses. DNA is fractionated by electrophoresis, transferred to a membrane (blotted) and detected by a complementary labelled probe that hybridizes to the DNA, revealing information about its identity, size and abundance.
splicing	removal of introns during the processing of mRNA
stop codon	one of the three codons (UAG, UAA or UGA) that cause termination of protein synthesis
synteny	loci on the same chromosome which may or may not be within range of detection through cosegregation
tandem repeat sequences	multiple copies of the same base sequence on a chromosome. When the number of repeats varies in the population, they are useful as DNA markers.
telomeres	refers to the ends of chromosomes that contain characteristic repetitive DNA sequences
termination codon	see stop codon
transfection	transfer of a DNA fragment into prokaryotic or eukaryotic cells
trans	(a) historically implies on a different chromosome; (b) in molecular biology, refers to an effect on a gene caused by a factor distinct from the sequence of that gene, in contrast to cis effects, which are encoded in the sequence of the gene. Cis and trans are commonly used to describe factors that influence gene expression. On different chromosomes, usually quite close. The opposite of cis
transcript	refers to an mRNA molecule that encodes a protein
transcription	the synthesis of an RNA molecule (transcript) from a DNA template in the cell nucleus catalyzed by RNA polymerase

transcription start site	site within a gene where transcription of RNA begins
transgenic	containing foreign DNA. For example, transgenic mice contain foreign DNA sequences in addition to the complete mouse genome
translation	assembly of amino acids into peptides based on information encoded in mRNA, i.e. mRNA sequence of bases is translated into sequence of amino acids in a peptide or protein. Occurs on ribosomes
translocation	the transfer of genetic material from one chromosome to another non-homologous chromosome, usually through a reciprocal event at meiosis
trisomy	the state of having three homologous chromosomes instead of the usual pair, as in trisomy 21 (Down's syndrome)
triploid	a cell with three times the haploid number of chromosomes, i.e. three copies of all chromosome types
uniparental disomy	situation in which an individual has two homologous chromosomes (or chromosomal segments) from one parent and none from the other. May be heterodisomy if both chromosomes from the single parent are present orisodisomy if two copies of the same parental chromosome are present
unique sequence DNA	non-repetitive DNA that potentially codes for mRNA and protein
upstream	a DNA sequence is written from the left, or 5', direction to the right, or 3' direction. Upstream refers to the 5' direction, i.e. regulatory elements of a gene are typically located upstream (5') of the coding sequences of that gene.
vector	the vehicle into which DNA is inserted prior to cloning in bacteria. Includes plasmids, phage and cosmids
X-inactivation	the random turning off of all the genes on one of the X-chromosomes in somatic cells during early embryonic development
X-linked	genes carried on the X-chromosome. The term sex-linked should only be used on the very rare occasions both X- and Y-chromosomes are involved.
zygote	the diploid cell resulting from the union of the haploid male (sperm) and female (ovum) gametes

References

A1 Adler, I.D. and C. Erbelding. Radiation-induced translocations in spermatogonial stem cells of Macaca fascicularis and Macaca mulatta. Mutat. Res. 198: 337-342 (1988).

A2 Atomic Energy Control Board, Canada. Symposium on Leukemia Clustering. (V. Elaguppillai, J.P. Goyette, G. Hill et al., eds.) Ottawa, Canada, 1992.

A3 Allanson, J. Germinal mosaicism in Apert syndrome. Clin. Genet. 29: 429-433 (1986).

A4 Altland, K., M. Kaempfer and M. Forssbohm. Mass screening technique for detecting globin variants from newborn dried blood samples. p. 143-157 in: Proceedings of an International Symposium on Chemical Mutagenesis, Human Population Monitoring and Genetic Risk Assessment. Progress in Mutation Research. Volume 3. (K.C. Bora, ed.) Elsevier, Amsterdam, 1982.

A5 Anand, R., C.D. Boehm, H.H. Kazazian et al. Molecular characterization of a beta-thalassemia resulting from a 1.4 kb deletion. Blood 72: 636-641 (1988).

A6 Awa, A.A., T. Honda, S. Neriishi et al. Cytogenetic studies of the offspring of atomic bomb survivors. p. 166-183 in: Cytogenetics: Basic and Applied Aspects. (G. Obe and A. Basler, eds.) Springer Verlag, Berlin, 1987.

A7 Awa, A.A., K. Ohtaki, M. Ito et al. Chromosome aberration data for A-bomb dosimetry reassessment. p. 185-202 in: New Dosimetry at Hiroshima and Nagasaki and Its Implications for Risk Estimates. NCRP Proceedings No. 9 (1988).

A8 Aaltonen, L.A., P. Peltomäki, F.S. Leach et al. Clues to the pathogenesis of familial colorectal cancer. Science 260: 812-816 (1993).

A9 Ames, B.N. Endogenous DNA damage as related to cancer and aging. Mutat. Res. 214: 41-46 (1989).

B1 Bailey, D.W. and H.I. Kohn. Inherited histocompatibility changes in progeny of irradiated and unirradiated inbred mice. Genet. Res. 6: 482-484 (1965).

B2 Baird, P.A. Measuring birth defects and handicapping disorders in the population: The British Columbia Health Surveillance Registry. Can. Med. Assoc. J. 136: 109-111 (1987).

B3 Baird, P.A., T.W. Anderson, H.B. Newcombe et al. Genetic disorders in children and young adults: a population study. Am. J. Hum. Genet. 42: 677-693 (1988).

B4 Baisogolov, G.D. and I.P. Shishkin. The course of pregnancy and the condition of infants born to the patients treated for Hodgkin's disease. Med. Radiologiya 5: 35-37 (1985).

B5 Barcinski, M.A., M.C. Abreu, J.C.C. de Almeida et al. Cytogenetic investigation in a Brazilian population living in an area of high natural radioactivity. Am. J. Hum. Genet. 27: 802-806 (1975).

B6 Barlow, D.P., R. Stoger, B.G. Herrmann et al. The mouse insulin-like growth factor type-2 receptor is imprinted and closely linked to the Tme locus. Nature 349: 84-87 (1991).

B7 Beighton, P. (ed.). McKusick's Heritable Disorders of Connective Tissue. Fifth edition. Mosby, St. Louis, 1993.

B8 Bonaiti-Pellie, C. and C. Smith. Risk tables for genetic counselling in some common congenital malformations. J. Med. Genet. 11: 374-377 (1974).

B9 Bower, C., R. Forbers and M. Seward. Congenital malformations in aborigines and non-aborigines in western Australia, 1980-1987. Med. J. Aust. 151: 245-248 (1989).

B10 Brewen, J.G., H.S. Payne and I.-D. Adler. X-ray-induced chromosome aberrations in mouse dictyate oocytes. II. Fractionation and dose rate effects. Genetics 87: 699-708 (1977).

B11 Byers, P.H., P. Tsipouras, J.F. Bonadio et al. Perinatal lethal osteogenesis imperfecta (OI type II): a biochemically heterogeneous disorder usually due to new mutations in the genes for type I collagen. Am. J. Hum. Genet. 42: 237-248 (1988).

B12 Brandriff, B.F. and L.A. Gordon. Human sperm cytogenetics and the one-cell zygote. p. 183-194 in: Biology of Mammalian Germ Cell Mutagenesis. Banbury Report 34. (J.W. Allen et al., eds.) Cold Spring Harbor Laboratory Press, New York, 1990.

C1 Committee on the Biological Effects of Ionizing Radiations (BEIR V). Health Effects of Exposure to Low Levels of Ionizing Radiation. United States National Academy of Sciences, National Research Council. National Academy Press, Washington, 1990.

C2 Committee on the Biological Effects of Ionizing Radiations (BEIR III). The Effects on Populations of Exposure to Low Levels of Ionizing Radiation: 1980. United States National Academy of Sciences, National Research Council. National Academy Press, Washington, 1980.

C3 Carpenter, N.J., B. Say and N.D. Barber. A homozygote for pericentric inversion of chromosome 4. J. Med. Genet. 19: 469-471 (1982).

C4 Caskey, C.T. and R.G. Worton. ASHG Human Genome Committee Report: The human genome project: Implications for human genetics. Am. J. Hum. Genet. 49: 687-691 (1991).

C5 Cattanach, B.M. Mammalian chromosome imprinting. Genome 31: 161-162 (1989).

C6 Cavenee, W.K. The genetic basis of neoplasia: the retinoblastoma paradigm. Trends Genet (Dec.): 299-300 (1986).

C7 Chen, Deqing et al. Cytogenetic investigation in a population living in the high background radiation area in China. Chin. J. Radiol. Med. Prot. 2: 61-63 (1982).

C8 Collins, F. Genome project can benefit search for disease genes. Hum. Genome News 2(3): 1-2 (1990).

C9 Cordero, J.F. Registries of birth defects and genetic diseases. p. 65-77 in: The Pediatric Clinics of North America: Medical Genetics I. (J.G. Hall, ed.) W.B. Saunders, Philadelphia, 1992.

C10 Coulondre, C., J.H. Miller, P.J. Farabaugh et al. Molecular basis of base substitution hotspots in Escherichia coli. Nature 274: 775-780 (1978).

C11 Cui, Yanwei et al. Hereditary diseases and congenital malformation survey in high background area. Chin. J. Radiol. Med. Prot. 2: 55-57 (1982).

C12 Czeizel, A.E., K. Sankaranarayanan, A. Losonci et al. The load of genetic and partially genetic diseases in man. II. Some selected common multifactorial diseases: estimates of population prevalence and of detriment in terms of years of lost and impaired life. Mutat. Res. 196:259-292 (1988).

C13 Czeizel, A.E. Hungarian surveillance of germinal mutations. Hum. Genet. 82: 359-366 (1989).

C14 Czeizel, A.E. Population surveillance of sentinel anomalies. Mutat. Res. 212: 3-9 (1989).

C15 Czeizel, A.E., C. Elek and E. Susánszky. The evaluation of the germinal mutagenic impact of Chernobyl radiological contamination in Hungary. Mutagenesis 6: 285-288 (1991).

C16 Czeizel, A.E. Incidence of legal abortions and congenital abnormalities in Hungary. Biomed. Pharmacother. 45: 249-254 (1991).

C17 Cattanach, B.M. Chromosome imprinting and its significance for mammalian development. in: Genome Analysis Series. Volume 2. (K. Davies and S. Tighlman, eds.) Cold Spring Harbor Laboratory Press, New York, 1991.

C18 Cattanach, B.M., M.D. Burtenshaw, C. Rasberry et al. Large deletions and other gross forms of chromosome imbalance compatible with viability and fertility in the mouse. Nat. Genet. 3: 56-61 (1993).

C19 Cosgrove, G.E., P.B. Selby, A.C. Upton et al. Life-span and autopsy findings in the first-generation offspring of x-irradiated male mice. Mutat. Res. (1993, in press).

C20 Crow, J.F. and C. Denniston. The mutation component of genetic damage. Science 212: 888-893 (1981).

D1 DeChiara, T.M., E.J. Robertson and A. Efstradiadis. Parental imprinting of the mouse insulin-like growth factor II gene. Cell 64: 849-859 (1991).

D2 den Dunnen, J.T., P.M. Grootscholten, E. Bakker et al. Topography of the Duchenne muscular dystrophy gene: FIGE and cDNA analysis of 194 cases reveals 115 deletions and 13 duplications. Am. J. Hum. Genet. 45: 835-847 (1989).

D3 Deng, Shaozhuang et al. Birth survey in high background radiation area. Chin. J. Radiol. Med. Prot. 2: 60 (1982).

D4 Dobson, R.L. and T. Straume. Mutagenesis in primordial mouse oocytes could be masked by cell-killing: Monte-Carlo analysis. Abstract of the 15th Annual Meeting of Environmental Mutagen Society, Montreal, Canada, 1984.

D5 Dombroski, B.A., S.L. Mathias, E. Nanthakumar et al. Isolation of an active human transposable element. Science 254: 1805-1808 (1991).

D6 Donnenfeld, A.E., K.A. Conard, N.S. Roberts et al. Melnick-Needles syndromes in males: a lethal multiple congenital anomalies syndrome. Am. J. Med. Genet. 27: 159-173 (1987).

D7 Donohue, P.A., C. Van Doip, R.H. McLean et al. Gene conversion in salt-losing congenital adrenal hyperplasia with absent complement C4B protein. J. Clin. Endocrinol. Metab. 62: 995-1002 (1986).

D8 Donehower, L.A., M. Harvey, B.L. Slagle et al. Mice deficient for *p53* are developmentally normal but susceptible to spontaneous tumours. Nature 356: 215-219 (1992).

E1 Ehling, U.H. Dominant mutations affecting the skeleton in offspring of x-irradiated male mice. Genetics 54: 1381-1389 (1966).

E2 Ehling, U.H. Evaluation of presumed dominant skeletal mutations. p. 162-166 in: Chemical Mutagenesis in Mammals and Man. (F. Vogel et al., eds.) Springer Verlag, Berlin, 1970.

E3 Ehling, U.H., J. Favor, J. Kratochvilova et al. Dominant cataract mutations and specific-locus mutations in mice induced by radiation or ethyl-nitrosourea. Mutat. Res. 92: 181-192 (1982).

E4 Ehling, U.H. and J. Favor. Recessive and dominant mutations in mice. p. 389-428 in: Mutation, Cancer and Malformation. (E.H.Y. Chu and W.M. Generoso, eds.) Plenum Press, New York, 1984.

E5 Ehling, U.H., D.J. Charles, J. Favor et al. Induction of gene mutations in mice: the multiple end-point approach. Mutat. Res. 150: 393-401 (1985).

E7 Evans, H.J. Ionizing radiations from nuclear establishments and childhood leukaemias - an enigma. BioEssays 12: 541-549 (1990).

E6 Ehling, U.H. Induction and manifestation of hereditary cataracts. p. 354-367 in: Assessment of Risk from Low Level Exposure to Radiation and Chemicals: A Critical Overview. (A.D. Woodhead et al., eds.) Plenum Press, New York, 1985.

E8 Ehling, U.H. Genetic risk assessment. Annu. Rev. Genet. 25: 255-280 (1991).

E9 Engel, E. and C.D. DeLozier-Blanchet. Uniparental disomy, isodisomy, and imprinting: probable effects in man and strategies for their detection. Am. J. Med. Genet. 40: 432-439 (1991).

F1 Favor, J. A comparison of the dominant cataract and recessive specific-locus mutation rates induced by treatment of male mice with ethylnitrosurea. Mutat. Res. 110: 367-382 (1983).

F2 Favor, J. Characterization of dominant cataract mutations in mice: penetrance, fertility and homozygous viability of mutations recovered after 250 mg/kg ethylnitrosourea paternal treatment. Genet. Res. 44: 183-197 (1984).

F3 Favor, J. Risk estimation based on germ-cell mutations in animals. Genome 31: 844-852 (1989).

F4 Favor, J., A. Neuhäuser-Klaus, J. Kratochvilova et al. Towards an understanding of the nature and fitness of induced mutations in germ cells of mice: homozygous viability and heterozygous fitness effects of induced specific-locus, dominant cataract and enzyme-activity mutations. Mutat. Res. 212: 67-75 (1989).

F5 Fialkow, P.J., J.W. Singer, W.H. Raskind et al. Clonal development, stem-cell differentiation, and clinical remissions in acute nonlymphocytic leukemia. N. Engl. J. Med. 317: 468-473 (1987).

F6 Forrest, S.M., G.S. Cross, A. Speer et al. Preferential deletion of exons in Duchenne and Becker muscular dystrophies. Nature 329: 638-640 (1987).

F7 Fraser, F.C. The multifactorial/threshold concept - uses and misuses. Teratology 14: 267-280 (1976).

F8 Fraser, F.C. The genetics of common familial disorders - major genes or multifactorial? Can. J. Genet. Cytol. 23: 1-8 (1981).

F9 Fu, Y.H., D.P.A. Kuhl, A. Pizzuti et al. Variation of the CGG repeat at the fragile X site results in genetic instability: resolution of the sherman paradox. Cell 67: 1047-1058 (1991).

F10 Fuhrmann, W. and F. Vogel. Genetic Counseling, 3. Springer Verlag, New York, 1983.

F11 Furusho, T. and M. Otake. A search for genetic effects of atomic bomb radiation on the growth and development of the F_1 generation. 1. Stature of 15- to 17-year-old senior high school students in Hiroshima. RERF TR/4-78 (1978).

F12 Furusho, T. and M. Otake. A search for genetic effects of atomic bomb radiation on the growth and development of the F_1 generation. 2. Body weight, sitting height, and chest circumference of 15- to 17-year-old senior high school students in Hiroshima. RERF TR/5-78 (1978).

F13 Furusho, T. and M. Otake. A search for genetic effects of atomic bomb radiation on the growth and development of the F_1 generation. 3. Stature of 12- to 14-year-old junior high school students in Hiroshima. RERF TR/14-79 (1979).

F14 Furusho, T. and M. Otake. A search for effects of atomic bomb radiation on the growth and development of the F_1 generation. 4. Body weight, sitting height, and chest circumference of 12- to 14-year-old junior high school students in Hiroshima. RERF TR/1-80 (1980).

F15 Furusho, T. and M. Otake. A search for genetic effects of atomic bomb radiation on the growth and development of the F_1 generation. 5. Stature of 6- to 11-year-old elementary school pupils in Hiroshima. RERF TR/9-85 (1985).

F16 Ford, C.E., E.P. Evans and A.G. Searle. Failure of irradiation to induce Robertsonian translocations in germ cells of male mice. p. 102-108 in: Conference on Mutations: Their Origin, Nature and Potential Relevance to Genetic Risk in Man, Jahrkonferenz 1977. Zentraallaboratorium für Mutagenitätprufung, Harald Boldt Verlag, Boppard, 1978.

F17 Favor, J., A. Neuhäuser-Klaus and U.H. Ehling. Radiation-induced forward and reverse specific locus mutations and dominant cataract mutations in treated strain BALB/c and DBA/2 male mice. Mutat. Res. 177: 161-169 (1987).

F18 Favor, J., A. Neuhäuser-Klaus and U.H. Ehling. The induction of forward and reverse specific-locus mutations and dominant cataract mutations in spermatogonia of treated strain DBA/2 mice by ethylnitrosourea. Mutat. Res. 249: 293-300 (1991).

G1 Gardner, M.J., A.J. Hall, M.P. Snee et al. Methods and basic data of case-control study of leukaemia and lymphoma among young people near Sellafield nuclear plant in West Cumbria. Br. Med. J. 300: 429-434 (1990).

G2 Gardner, M.J., M.P. Snee, A.J. Hall et al. Results of case-control study of leukaemia and lymphoma among young people near Sellafield nuclear plant in West Cumbria. Br. Med. J. 300: 423-428 (1990).

G3 Generoso, W.M., K.T. Cain, C.V. Cornett et al. Comparison of two stocks of mice in spermatogonial response to different conditions of radiation exposure. Mutat. Res. 249: 301-310 (1991).

G4 Generoso, W.M., K.T. Cain, C.V. Cornett et al. Difference in the response of two hybrid stocks of mice to x-ray induction of chromosome aberrations in spermatogonial stem cells. Mutat. Res. 152: 217-223 (1985).

G5 Gillard, E.F., J.S. Chamberlin, E.G. Murphy et al. Molecular and phenotypic analysis of patients with the deletion-rich region of the Duchenne muscular dystrophy (DMD) gene. Am. J. Hum. Genet. 45: 507-520 (1989).

G6 Graw, J., J. Favor, A. Neuhäuser-Klaus et al. Dominant cataract and recessive specific-locus mutations in offspring of X-irradiated male mice. Mutat. Res. 159: 47-54 (1986).

G7 Griffin, C.S. and C. Tease. Gamma-ray-induced numerical and structural chromosome anomalies in mouse immature oocytes. Mutat. Res. 202: 209-213 (1988).

H1 Haldane, J.B.S. The rate of spontaneous mutation of a human gene. J. Genet. 31: 317-326 (1935).

H2 Hall, J.G. Genomic imprinting. Curr. Opin. Genet. Develop. 1: 34-39 (1991).

H3 Hall, J.G. Review and Hypotheses. Somatic mosaicism: observations related to clinical genetics. Am. J. Hum. Genet. 43: 355-363 (1988).

H4 Hall, J.G., J.M. Friedman, B.A. Keena et al. Clinical, genetic and epidemiological factors in neural tube defects. Am. J. Hum. Genet. 43: 827-837 (1988).

H5 Hall, J.G., J.P. Dorst, R. Rotta et al. Gonadal mosaicism in pseudoachondroplasia. Am. J. Med. Genet. 28: 143-151 (1987).

H6 Hall, J.G. Genomic imprinting: review and relevance to human disease. Am. J. Hum. Genet. 46: 857-873 (1990).

H7 Harada, F., A. Kimura, T. Iwanaga et al. Gene-conversion-like events cause steroid 21-hydroxylase deficiency in congenital adrenal hyperplasia. Proc. Natl. Acad. Sci. (USA) 84: 8091-8094 (1987).

H8 Harley, H.G., J.D. Boork, S.A. Rundle et al. Expansion of an unstable DNA region and phenotypic variation in myotonic dystrophy. Nature 355: 545-551 (1992).

H9 Hassold, T.J. and P. Jacob. Trisomy in man. Annu. Rev. Genet. 18: 69-77 (1984).

H10 Hecht, F. and B.K. Hecht. The half chromatid mutation model and bidirectional mutation in incontinentia pigmenti. Clin. Genet. 24: 177-179 (1983).

H11 Henthorn, P.S., D.L. Mager, T.J. Hutsman et al. A gene deletion ending with a complex array of repeated sequences 3' to the human beta-globin gene cluster. Proc. Natl. Acad. Sci. (USA) 83: 5194-5198 (1986).

H12 Hook, E.B. Surveillance of germinal human mutations for effections of putative environmental mutagens and utilization of a chromosome registry in following rates of cytogenetic disorders. p. 141-165 in: Cytogenetics: Basic and Applied Aspects. (G. Obe and A. Basler, eds.) Springer Verlag, Berlin, 1987.

H13 Hu, X., A.H.M. Burghes, P.N. Ray et al. Partial gene duplication in Duchenne and Becker muscular dystrophies. J. Med. Genet. 25: 369-376 (1988).

H14 Hu, X., A.H.M. Burghes, D.E. Bulman et al. Evidence for mutation by unequal sister chromatid exchange in the Duchenne muscular dystrophy gene. Am. J. Hum. Genet. 44: 855-863 (1989).

H15 Hulten, M., S. Armstrong, P. Challinor et al. Genomic imprinting in an Angelman and Prader-Willi translocation family. Lancet 338: 638-639 (1991).

H16 Haas, O.A., A. Argyriou-Tirita and T. Lion. Parental origin of chromosomes involved in the translocation t(9:22). Nature 359: 414-416 (1992).

H17 Huntington Disease Collaborative Group. A novel gene containing a trinucleotide repeat that is expanded and unstable on Huntington disease chromosomes. Cell 72: 971-983 (1993).

I1 International Commission on Radiological Protection. 1990 Recommendations of the International Commission on Radiological Protection. ICRP Publication 60. Pergamon Press, Oxford, 1991.

I2 International Agency for Research on Cancer (IARC). Long-term and short-term assays for carcinogens: a critical appraisal. (R. Montesano et al., eds.) IARC Publication 83 (1986).

J1 Jagadeeswaran, P., D. Tuan, B.G. Forget et al. A gene deletion ending at the midpoint of a repetitive DNA sequence in one form of hereditary persistence of fetal hemoglobin. Nature 296: 469-470 (1982).

K1 Kalousek, D.K. and J.F. Dill. Chromosomal mosaicism confined to the placenta in human conceptions. Science 221: 665-667 (1983).

K2 Kalousek, D.K. and B. McGillivray. Confined placenta mosaicism and intrauterine survival of trisomies 13 and 18. Am. J. Hum. Genet. 41: A278 (1987).

K3 Kato, H., W.J. Schull and J.V. Neel. A cohort-type study of survival in the children of parents exposed to atomic bombings. Am. J. Hum. Genet. 18: 339-373 (1966).

K4 Kazakov, V.S., E.P. Demidchik and L.N. Astakhova. Thyroid cancer after Chernobyl. Nature 359: 21-22 (1992).

K5 Kirk, M. and M.F. Lyon. Induction of congenital anomalies in offspring of female mice exposed to varying doses of X-rays. Mutat. Res. 106: 73-83 (1982).

K6 Kirk, M. and M.F. Lyon. Induction of congenital malformations in the offspring of male mice treated with X-rays at the pre-meiotic and post-meiotic stages. Mutat. Res. 125: 75-85 (1984).

K7 Kochupillai, N., I.C. Verma, M.S. Grewal et al. Down's syndrome and related abnormalities in an area of high background radiation in coastal Kerala. Nature 262: 60-61 (1976).

K8 Koenig, M., A.H. Beggs, M. Moyer et al. The molecular basis for Duchenne versus Becker muscular dystrophy: correlation of severity with type of deletion. Am. J. Hum. Genet. 45: 498-506 (1989).

K9 Kohn, H.I., M.L. Epling, P.H. Guttman et al. Effect of paternal (spermatogonial) X-ray exposure in the mouse: life span, X-ray tolerance and tumour incidence of the progeny. Radiat. Res. 25: 423-434 (1965).

K10 Kratochvilova, J. and U.H. Ehling. Dominant cataract mutations induced by gamma-irradiation of male mice. Mutat. Res. 63: 221-223 (1979).

K11 Kratochvilova, J. Dominant cataract mutations detected in offspring of gamma-irradiated male mice. J. Hered. 72: 301-307 (1981).

K12 Krestinina L.Yu., M.M. Kosenko and V.A. Kostyuchenko. Lethal developmental defects in descendants of a population residing in the area of a radioactive trace. Med. Radiol. 6: 30-32 (1991). (in Russian)

K13 Kamiguchi, Y. and K. Mikamo. An improved, efficient method for analyzing human sperm chromosomes using zona-free hamster ova. Am. J. Hum. Genet. 38: 724-740 (1986).

K14 Kamiguchi, Y., H. Tateno and K. Mikamo. Dose-response relationship for the induction of structural chromosome aberrations in human spermatozoa after in vitro exposure to tritium beta-rays. Mutat. Res. 228: 125-131 (1990).

K15 Kamiguchi, Y., H. Tateno and K. Mikamo. Types of structural chromosome aberrations and their incidence in human spermatozoa x-irradiation in vitro. Mutat. Res. 228: 133-140 (1990).

K16 Kamiguchi, Y., H. Tateno and K. Mikamo. Micronucleus test in 2-cell embryos as a simple assay system for human sperm chromosome aberrations. Mutat. Res. 252: 297-303 (1991).

K17 Kalousek, D.K., S. Langlois, I. Barrett et al. Unparental disomy for chromosome 16 in humans. Am. J. Hum. Genet. 52: 8-16 (1993).

K18 Kuroki, Y. and H. Konishi. Monitoring of congenital anomalies in Japan. p. 59-64 in: Proceedings of International Conference on Radiation Effects and Protection, Mito, Ibaraki, Japan, March 18-20, 1992.

L1 La Spada, A.R., E.M. Wilson, D.B. Lubahn et al. Androgen receptor gene mutations in X-linked spinal and bulbar muscular atrophy. Nature 352: 77-79 (1991).

L2 Laird, C.D. Possible erasure of the imprint on a fragile X chromosome when transmitted by a male. Am. J. Med. Genet. 38: 391-395 (1991).

L3 Lambert, M.E., J.F. McDonald and I.B. Bernstein (eds.). Eukaryotic Transposable Elements as Mutagenic Agents. Cold Spring Harbour, New York, 1988.

L4 Lejeune, J., R. Turpin and M.O. Rethore. Les enfants nes de parents irradies (Cas particuliers de la sex-ratio). p. 1089-1096 in: 9th International Congress on Radiology, Munich, 1960.

L5 Li, C.C. p. 366 in: Population Genetics. University of Chicago Press, Chicago, 1955.

L6 Lüning, K.G. and A.G. Searle. Estimates of genetic risks from ionizing radiation. Mutat. Res. 12: 291-304 (1971).

L7 Lüning, K.G. Studies of irradiated mouse populations. IV. Effects on productivity in the 7th to 18th generations. Mutat. Res. 14: 331-344 (1972).

L8 Lyon, M.F. Some evidence concerning the "mutational load" in inbred strains of mice. Heredity 13: 341-352 (1959).

L9 Lyon, M.F., R.F.S. Phillips and A.G. Searle. The overall rates of dominant and recessive lethal and visible mutations induced by spermatogonial x-irradiation of mice. Genet. Res. 5: 558-467 (1964).

L10 Lyon, M.F. and R. Renshaw. Induction of congenital malformations in mice by parental irradiation: transmission to later generations. Mutat. Res. 198: 277-283 (1986).

L11 Lyon, M.F. and A.G. Searle (eds.). Genetic Variants and Strains of the Laboratory Mouse. Second edition. Oxford University Press, Oxford, 1989.

M1 Maeda, N. and O. Smithies. The evolution of multigene families: human haptoglobin genes. Annu. Rev. Genet. 20: 81-108 (1986).

M2 Malcolm, S., J. Clayton-Smith, M. Nichols et al. Uniparental paternal disomy in Angelman's syndrome. Lancet 337: 694-697 (1991).

M3 Mange, A.P. and E.J. Mange. p. 286-289 in: Genetics: Human Aspects. Sinauer Associates Inc., Sunderland, MA., 1990.

M4 Martin, R.H., W. Balkan, K. Burns et al. Direct chromosomal analysis of human spermatozoa. Am. J. Hum. Genet. 34: 459-468 (1982).

M5 Martin, R.H., W. Balkan, K. Burns et al. The chromosome constitution of 1000 human spermatozoa. Hum. Genet. 63: 305-309 (1983).

M6 Mathias S.L., A.F. Scott, H.H. Kaazian et al. Reverse transcriptase encoded by a human transposable element. Science 254: 1808-1810 (1991).

M7 McKusick, V.A. Mendelian Inheritance in Man. 4th, 7th and 8th editions. Johns Hopkins University Press, Baltimore, 1975, 1986 and 1988.

M8 McKusick, V.A. Communication to the UNSCEAR Secretariat (1977).

M9 McKusick, V.A. Current trends in mapping human genes. FASEB J. 5: 12-20 (1991).

M10 Modell, B. and A. Kuliev. Changing paternal age distribution and the human mutation rate in Europe. Hum. Genet. 86: 198-202 (1990).

M11 Murphee, A.L. and W.F. Benedict. Retinoblastoma: clues to human oncogenesis. Science 223: 1028-1033 (1984).

M12 Muratani, K., H. Toshikazu, Y. Yoshihiro et al. Inactivation of the cholinesterase gene by Alu insertion. Proc. Natl. Acad. Sci. (USA) 88: 11315-11319 (1991).

N1 Nakamura, Y., M. Leppert, P. O'Connell et al. Variable number of tandem repeat (VNTR) markers for human gene mapping. Science 235: 1616-1622 (1987).

N2 Nance, W.E. Twin Research, Part B: Biology and Epidemiology. Proceedings of the 2nd International Congress on Twin Studies. Alan Liss, New York, 1978.

N3 Neel, J.V. and W.J. Schull. p. xvi and 241 in: The Effect of Exposure to the Atomic Bombs on Pregnancy Termination in Hiroshima and Nagasaki. Publication 461. National Academy of Sciences, National Research Council, Washington, 1956.

N4 Neel, J.V., C. Satoh, K. Goriki et al. Search for mutations altering protein charge and/or function in children of atomic bomb survivors: Final report. Am. J. Hum. Genet. 42: 663-676 (1988).

N5 Neel, J.V., W.J. Schull, A.A. Awa et al. Implications of the Hiroshima-Nagasaki genetic studies for the estimation of the human "doubling dose" of radiation. Proceedings of the 16th International Congress Genetics, Toronto, 1988.

N6 Neel, J.V., W.J. Schull, A.A. Awa et al. The children of parents exposed to atomic bombs: estimates of the genetic doubling dose of radiation for humans. Am. J. Hum. Genet. 46: 1053-1072 (1990).

N7 Neel, J.V. and S.E. Lewis. The comparative radiation genetics of humans and mice. Annu. Rev. Genet. 24: 327-362 (1990).

N8 Neel, J.V. Update on the genetic effects of ionizing radiation. J. Am. Med. Assoc. 266: 698-701 (1991).

N9 Neel, J.V. and W.J. Schull (eds.). p. vi and 518 in: The Children of Atomic Bomb Survivors. National Academy Press, Washington, 1991.

N10 Nuclear Regulatory Commission, United States. Health effects models for nuclear power plant accident consequence analysis. Modifications of models resulting from recent reports on health effects of ionizing radiation. Low-LET radiation. Part II: Scientific bases for health effects models. NUREG/CR-4214, Rev. 1 (1991).

N11 Nelson, K. and L.B. Holmes. Malformations due to presumed spontaneous mutations in newborn infants. N. Engl. J. Med. 320: 19-23 (1989).

N12 Nicholls, R.D., D.R. Higgs, J.B. Clegg et al. Alpha-thalassemia due to recombination between the alpha-1-globin gene and an AluI repeat. Blood 65: 1434-1438 (1985).

N13 Nomura, T. Changed urethane and radiation response of the mouse germ cell to tumor induction. p. 873-891 in: Tumors of Early Life in Man and Animals. (L. Severi, ed.) Perugia University Press, Perugia, 1978.

N14 Nomura, T. Parental exposure to X-rays and chemicals induces heritable tumours and anomalies in mice. Nature 296: 575-577 (1982).

N15 Nomura, T. Further studies on X-ray and chemically induced germ-line alterations causing tumors and malformations in mice. p. 13-20 in: Genetic Toxicology of Environmental Chemicals, Part B: Genetic Effects and Applied Mutagenesis. (C. Ramel, B. Lambert, J. Magnusson, eds.) Alan Liss, New York, 1986.

N16 Nomura, T. X-ray and chemically induced germ-line mutation causing phenotypical anomalies in mice. Mutat. Res. 198: 309-320 (1988).

N17 Nomura, T. Of mice and men? Nature 345: 671 (1990).

O1 Orkin, S.H. and A. Michelson. Partial deletion of the alpha-globin structural gene in human alpha-thalassemia. Nature 266: 538-540 (1980).

O2 Otake, M., W.J. Scull and J.V. Neel. Congenital malformations, stillbirths and early mortality among the children of atomic bomb survivors: a reanalysis. Radiat. Res. 122: 1-11 (1990).

P1 Pacchierotti, F., A. Russo and P. Metalli. Meiotic non-disjunction induced by fission neutrons relative to X-rays observed in mouse secondary spermatocytes. II. Dose-effect relationshipos after treatment of pachytene cells. Mutat. Res. 176: 233-241 (1987).

P2 Peltomäki, P., S. Knuutila, A. Ritvanen et al. Pallister-Killian syndrome: cytogenetic and molecular studies. Clin. Genet. 31: 399-405 (1987).

P3 Preston, D.L. and D.A. Pierce. The effect of changes in dosimetry on cancer mortality, risk estimates in the atomic bomb survivors. Radiat. Res. 114: 437-466 (1988).

P4 Peltomäki, P., L.A. Aaltonen, P. Sistonen et al. Genetic mapping of a locus predisposing to human colorectal cancer. Science 260: 810-812 (1993).

P5 Petrushkina, I., O. Musatova, N. Okladnikova et al. Genetic effects of radiation. Nuclear Society International, Moscow: Scientific Informational and Methodical Bulletin 4: 23-27 (1992). Consequences of Nuclear Tests on South Ural. (1993, in press).

R1 Reichert, W., W. Buselmaier and F. Vogel. Elimination of X-ray-induced chromosomal aberrations in the progeny of femal emice. Mutat. Res. 139: 87-94 (1984).

R2 Richter, C., J.W. Park and B.N. Ames. Normal oxidative damage to mitochondrial and nuclear DNA is extensive. Proc. Natl. Acad. Sci. (USA) 85: 6465-6467 (1988).

R3 Russell, L.B. and E.M. Rinchik. Genetic and molecular characterization of genomic regions surrounding specific loci of the mouse. p. 109-121 in: Mammalian Cell Mutagenesis. Banbury Report 28. (M.M. Moore et al., eds.) Cold Spring Harbor Laboratory Press, New York, 1987.

R4 Russell, L.B. Functional and structural analyses of mouse genomic regions screened by the morphological specific-locus test. Mutat. Res. 212: 23-32 (1989).

R5 Russell, W.L. X-ray-induced mutations in mice. Cold Spring Harbor Symp. Quant. Biol. 16: 327-336 (1951).

R6 Russell, W.L., L.B. Russell and E.M. Kelly. Radiation dose rate and mutation frequency. Science 128: 1546-1550 (1958).

R7 Russell, W.L., L.B. Russell, M.H. Steele et al. Extreme sensitivity of an immature stage of the mouse ovary to sterilization. Science 129: 1228 (1959).

R8 Russell, W.L. Effect of interval between radiation and conception on mutation frequency in female mice. Proc. Natl. Acad. Sci. (USA) 54: 1552-1557 (1965).

R9 Russell, W.L. Studies in mammalian radiation genetics. Nucleonics 23: (1965).

R10 Russell, W.L. The nature of dose-rate effect of radiation on mutation in mice. Jpn. J. Genet. 40 (Suppl.): 128-140 (1965).

R11 Russell, W.L. Mutation frequencies in female mice and the estimation of genetic hazards of radiation in women. Proc. Natl. Acad. Sci. (USA) 74: 3523-3527 (1977).

R12 Russell, W.L. and E.M. Kelly. Mutation frequencies in male mice and the estimation of genetic hazards of radiation in men. Proc. Natl. Acad. Sci. (USA) 79: 542-544 (1982).

R13 Rinchik, E.M., J.P. Stoye, W.N. Frankel et al. Molecular analysis of viable spontaneous and radiation-induced albino (c)-locus mutations in the mouse. Mutat. Res. 286: 199-207 (1993).

S1 Sankaranarayanan, K. Genetic Effects of Ionizing Radiation in Multicellular Eukaryotes and the Assessment of Genetic Radiation Hazards in Man. Elsevier, Amsterdam, 1982.

S2 Sankaranarayanan, K. Invited review: prevalence of genetic and partially genetic diseases in man and the estimation of genetic risks of exposure to ionizing radiation. Am. J. Hum. Genet. 42: 651-662 (1988).

S3 Sankaranarayanan, K. Ionizing radiation and genetic risks. I. Epidemiological, population genetic, biochemical and molecular aspects of Mendelian diseases. Mutat. Res. 258: 3-49 (1991).

S4 Sankaranarayanan, K. Ionizing radiation and genetic risks. II. Nature of radiation-induced mutations in experiemental mammalian in vivo systems. Mutat. Res. 258: 51-73 (1991).

S5 Sankaranarayanan, K. Ionizing radiation and genetic risks. III. Nature of spontaneous and radiation-induced mutations in mammalian in vitro systems and mechanisms of induction of mutations by radiation. Mutat. Res. 258: 75-97 (1991).

S6 Sankaranarayanan, K. Ionizing radiation and genetic risks. IV. Current methods, estimates of risk of Mendelian disease, human data and lessons from biochemical and molecular studies of mutations. Mutat. Res. 258: 99-122 (1991).

S7 Sankaranarayanan, K. Ionizing radiation, genetic risk estimation and molecular biology: impact and inferences. Trends Genet. 9: 79-84 (1993).

S8 Scholte, P.J.L. and F.H. Sobels. Sex ratio shift among progeny from patients having received therapeutic X-radiation. Am. J. Hum. Genet. 16: 26-39 (1964).

S9 Schroeder, W.T., L.Y. Chao, D.D. Dao et al. Non-random loss of maternal chromosome 11 alleles in Wilms' tumour. Am. J. Hum. Genet. 40: 413-420 (1987).

S10 Schull, W.J., J.V. Neel and A. Hashizume. Some further observations on the sex ratio among infants born to the survivors of the atomic bombings at Hiroshima and Nagasaki. Am. J. Hum. Genet. 18: 328-338 (1966).

S11 Scrable, H., W. Cavenee, F. Ghavimi et al. A model for embryonal rhabdomyosarcoma tumorigenesis that involves genome imprinting. Proc. Natl. Acad. Sci. (USA) 86: 7480-7484 (1989).

S12 Searle, A.G. Genetic effects of spermatogonial X-irradiation on productivity of F_1 female mice. Mutat. Res. 1: 99-108 (1964).

S13 Searle, A.G. Mutation induction in mice. Adv. Radiat. Biol. 4: 131-207 (1974).

S14 Searle, A.G. and C.V. Beechey. Complementation studies with mouse translocations. Cytogenet. Cell Genet. 22: 127-146 (1978).

S15 Searle, A.G. and D.G. Papworth. Analysis of pre- and post-natal mortality after spermatogonial irradiation of mice. Communication to the UNSCEAR Secretariat (1986).

S16 Searle, A.G. and J.H. Edwards. The estimation of genetic risks from the induction of recessive mutations after exposure to ionizing radiation. J. Med. Genet. 23: 220-226 (1986).

S17 Searle, A.G., J. Peters, M.F. Lyon et al. Chromosome maps of man and mouse, IV. Ann. Hum. Genet. 53: 89-140 (1989).

S18 Selby, P.B. Radiation-induced dominant skeletal mutations in mice: mutation rate, characteristics, and usefulness in estimating genetic hazard to humans from radiation. p. 537-544 in: Proceedings of the 6th International Congress on Radiation Research, 1979. Toppan Printing Co., Tokyo, 1979.

S19 Selby, P.B. Radiation genetics in the mouse. p. 263-283 in: The Mouse in Biomedical Research: History, Genetics and the Wild Mouse. (H.L. Foster, J.D. Small, J.G. Fox, eds.) Academic Press, New York, 1981.

S20 Selby, P.B. Applications in genetic risk estimation of data on the induction of dominant skeletal mutations in mice. p. 191-210 in: Utilization of Mammalian Specific-locus Studies in Hazard Evaluation and Estimation of Genetic Risk. (F.J. de Serres and W. Sheridan, eds.) Plenum Press, New York, 1983.

S21 Selby, P.B. Experimental induction of dominant mutations in mammals by ionizing radiations and chemicals. p. 181-253 in: Issues and Reviews in Teratology. Volume 5. (H. Kalter, ed.) Plenum Press, New York, 1990.

S22 Selby, P.B. The importance of the direct method of genetic risk estimation and ways to improve it. p. 437-449 in: Biology of Mammalian Germ Cell Mutagenesis. Banbury Report 34. (J.W. Allen et al., eds.) Cold Spring Harbor Laboratory Press, New York, 1990.

S23 Selby, P.B. and P.R. Selby. Gamma-ray-induced dominant mutations that cause skeletal abnormalities in mice. I. Plan, summary of results and discussion. Mutat. Res. 43: 357-375 (1977).

S24 Selby, P.B. and P.R. Selby. Gamma-ray-induced dominant mutations that cause skeletal abnormalities in mice. II. Description of proved mutations. Mutat. Res. 51: 199-236 (1978).

S25 Selby, P.B. and P.R. Selby. Gamma-ray-induced dominant mutations that cause skeletal abnormalities in mice. III. Description of presumed mutations. Mutat. Res. 50: 341-351 (1978).

S26 Selby, P.B. and S.L. Niemann. Non-breeding-test methods for dominant skeletal mutations shown by ethylnitrosourea to be easily applicable to offspring examined in specific-locus experiments. Mutat. Res. 127: 93-105 (1984).

S27 Selby, P.B. and W.L. Russell. First-generation litter-size reduction following irradiation of spermatogonial stem cells in mice and its use in risk estimation. Environ. Mutagen. 7: 451-469 (1985).

S28 Selby, P.B., S.S. Lee, E.M. Kelly et al. Specific-locus experiments show that female mice exposed near the time of birth to low-LET ionizing radiation exhibit both a low mutational response and a dose-rate effect. Mutat. Res. 249: 351-367 (1991).

S29 Selby, P.B., V.S. Mierzejewski, E.M. Garrison et al. Preliminary results in assessment of dominant damage (ADD) experiments and their implications for genetic risk estimation. Communication to the UNSCEAR Secretariat (1993).

S30 Shen D.W., I. Pastan and M.M. Gottesman. In situ hybridization analysis of acquisition and loss of the human multidrug-resistance gene. Cancer Res. 48: 4334-4339 (1988).

S31 Sillence, D.O., H.E. Ritchie and P.B. Selby. Animal model: skeletal anomalies in mice with Cleidocranial dysplasia. Am. J. Med. Genet. 27: 75-85 (1987).

S32 Silverman, L.J., W.N. Kelley and T.D. Palell. Genetic analysis of human hypoxanthine-guanine phosphoribosyltransferase deficiency. Enzyme 38: 36-44 (1987).

S33 Singer, M.F. Highly repeated sequences in mammalian genomes. Int. Rev. Cytol. 76: 67-112 (1982).

S34 Smith, D.W. and J.M. Aase. Polygenic inheritance of certain common malformations: evidence and empiric recurrence risk data. J. Pediatr. 76: 653-659 (1970).

S35 Spranger, J., K. Benirschke, J.G. Hall et al. Errors of morphogenesis: concepts and terms. J. Pediatr. 100: 160-165 (1982).

S36 Stephens, J.C., M.L. Cavanaugh, M.I. Gradie et al. Mapping the human genome: current status. Science 250: 237-234 (1990).

S37 Straume, T. Biological Effectiveness of Neutron Irradiation on Animals and Man. Ph.D. Thesis, University of California, 1982.

S38 Straume, T., T.C. Kwan, L.S. Goldstein et al. Measurement of neutron-induced genetic damage in mouse immature oocytes. Mutat. Res. 248: 123-133 (1991).

S39 Strobel, D. and F. Vogel. Ein statistischer Gesichtspunkt für das Planen von Untersuchungen über Änderungen der Mutationsrate beim Menschen. Acta Genet. Stat. Med. 8: 274-286 (1958).

S40 Sheridan, W. and I. Wardell. The frequency of recessive lethals in an irradiated mouse population. Mutat. Res. 5: 313-321 (1968).

S41 Spotila, L.D., L. Sereda and D.J. Prockop. Partial isodisomy for maternal chromosome 7 and short-stature in an individual with a mutation at the COLIA2 locus. Am. J. Hum. Genet. 51: 1396-1405 (1992).

S42 Schmiady, H., H. Kentenich and M. Stauber. Chromosome studies of human in vitro fertilization (IVF) failures. p. 184-197 in: Cytogenetics, Basic and Applied Aspects. Chapter 9. (G. Obe and A. Basler, eds.) Springer Verlag, Berlin, 1987.

S43 Silver, A. and R. Cox. Telomere-like DNA polymorphisms associated with genetic predisposition to acute myeloid leukaemia in irradiated CB mice. Proc. Natl. Acad. Sci. (USA) 90: 1407-1410 (1993).

S44 Sankaranarayanan, K. Genetic effects of ionizing radiation in man. p. 75-94 in: Risks Associated With Ionizing Radiations. Annals of the ICRP 22(1). Pergamon Press, Oxford, 1991.

T1 Tanaka, K. and K. Ohkura. Evidence for genetic effects of radiation on offspring of radiologic technicians. Jpn. J. Hum. Genet. 3: 135-145 (1958).

T2 Temple, I.K., A. Cockwell, T. Hassold et al. Maternal uniparental disomy for chromosome 14. J. Med. Genet. 28: 511-514 (1991).

T3 Thompson, J.S. and M.W. Thompson. Genetics in Medicine. W.B. Saunders Co., Philadelphia, 1991.

T4 Tiwari, J.L. and P.I. Terasaki. HLA and Disease Associations. Springer Verlag, New York, 1985.

T5 Tretyakov, F.D., Z.I. Voronina, P.F. Voronin et al. Infant mortality rates and structure in a town near a nuclear power enterprise. Med. Radiol. 7: 7-10 (1991).

T6 Trimble, B.K. and J.H. Doughty. The amount of hereditary disease in human populations. Ann. Hum. Genet. 38: 199-223 (1974).

T7 Thibodeau, S.N., G. Bren and D. Schnaid. Microsatellite instability in cancer of the proximal colon. Science 260: 816-819 (1993).

T8 Takahashi, T., H. Watanabe, K. Dohi et al. ^{252}Cf relative biological effectiveness and inheritable effect of fission neutrons in mouse liver tumorigenesis. Cancer Res. 52: 1948-1953 (1992).

T9 Timofeeff-Ressovsky, N.W. Gerichtetes Variieren in der phänotypischen Manifestierung einiger Genovariationen von Drosophila funebris. Naturwissenschaften 19: 493-497 (1931).

U1 United Nations. Sources, Effects and Risks of Ionizing Radiation. United Nations Scientific Committee on the Effects of Atomic Radiation, 1988 Report to the General Assembly, with annexes. United Nations sales publication E.88.IX.7. United Nations, New York, 1988.

U2 United Nations. Genetic and Somatic Effects of Ionizing Radiation. United Nations Scientific Committee on the Effects of Atomic Radiation, 1986 Report to the General Assembly, with annexes. United Nations sales publication E.86.IX.9. United Nations, New York, 1986.

U3 United Nations. Ionizing Radiation: Sources and Biological Effects. United Nations Scientific Committee on the Effects of Atomic Radiation, 1982 Report to the General Assembly, with annexes. United Nations sales publication E.82.IX.8. United Nations, New York, 1982.

U4 United Nations. Sources and Effects of Ionizing Radiation. United Nations Scientific Committee on the Effects of Atomic Radiation, 1977 Report to the General Assembly, with annexes. United Nations sales publication E.77.IX.1. United Nations, New York, 1977.

U5 United Nations. Ionizing Radiation: Levels and Effects. United Nations Scientific Committee on the Effects of Atomic Radiation, 1972 Report to the General Assembly, with annexes. United Nations sales publication E.72.IX.17 and 18. United Nations, New York, 1972.

U11 United States Department of Energy. Understanding our genetic inheritance. p. 17 in: The US Human Genome Project: The First Five Years (1991).

U12 Urabe, K., A. Kimura, F. Harada et al. Gene conversion in steroid 21-hydroxylase genes. Am. J. Hum. Genet. 46: 1178-1186 (1990).

V1 van Buul, P.P.W. X-ray induced translocations in premeiotic germ cells of monkeys. Mutat. Res. 251: 31-39 (1991).

V2 Vanin, E.F., P.S. Henthorn, D. Kioussis et al. Unexpected relationships between four large deletions in the human beta globin gene cluster. Cell 35: 701-709 (1983).

V3 Vnencak-Jones, C.L. and J.A. Phillips III. Hot spots for growth hormone gene deletions in homologous regions outside of Alu repeats. Science 250: 1745-1748 (1990).

V4 Vogel, F. ABO blood groups and disease. Am. J. Hum. Genet. 22: 464-275 (1970).

V5 Vogel, F. Clinical consequences of heterozygosity for autosomal-recessive diseases. Clin. Genet. 25: 381-415 (1984).

V6 Vogel, F. Risk calculations for hereditary effects of ionizing radiation in humans. Hum. Genet. 89: 127-146 (1992).

V7 Vogel, F. and W. Helmbold. Blutgruppen - Populationsgenetik und Statistik. p. 129-557 in: Humangenetik. Ein kurzes Handbuch, Volume 1. (P.E. Becker, ed.) Georg Thieme Verlag, Stuttgart, 1972.

V8 Vogel, F. and R. Rathenberg. Spontaneous mutation in man. Adv. Hum. Genet. 5: 223-318 (1975).

V9 Vogel, F. and K. Altland. Utilization of material from PKU-screening programmes for mutation screening. p. 143-157 in: Proceedings of an International Symposium on Chemical Mutagenesis, Human Population Monitoring and Genetic Risk Assessment. Progress in Mutation Research. Volume 3. (K.C. Bora, ed.) Elsevier, Amsterdam, 1982.

V10 Vogel, F. and A.G. Motulsky. p. 344 in: Human Genetics. Springer Verlag, Berlin, 1986.

V11 Voss, R., E. Ben-Simon, A. Avital et al. Isodisomy of chromosome 7 in a patient with CF: could uniparental disomy be common in humans? Am. J. Hum. Genet. 45: 373-380 (1989).

V12 van Allem, M., D. Kalousek. and G. Chernoff. Evidence for multi-site closure of the neural tube in humans. Am. J. Med. Genet. 47 (1993, in press).

W1 Wang, J.C., M.B. Passage, P.H. Yen et al. Uniparental heterodisomy for chromosome 14 in a phenotypically abnormal familial balanced 13/14 translocation carrier. Am. J. Hum. Genet. 48: 1069-1074 (1991).

W2 Wagstaff, J., J.H. Knoll, J. Fleming et al. Localization of the gene encoding the GABA A receptor beta 3 subunit to the Angelman/Prader-Willi region of human chromosome 15. Am. J. Hum. Genet. 49: 330-337 (1991).

W3 Wahls, W.P., L.J. Wallace and P.D. Moore. Hypervariable minisatellite DNA is a hotspot for homologous recombination in human cells. Cell 60: 95-103 (1990).

W4 Wald, N., J. Sneddon, J. Donsem et al. MRC Vitamin Study Research Group: Prevention of neural tube defects. Lancet 338: 131-137 (1991).

W5 Watson, J.D. and R.M. Cook-Deegan. Origins of the human genome project. FASEB J. 5: 8-11 (1991).

W6 Welch, T.R., L.S. Beischel, E. Choi et al. Uniparental isodisomy 6 associated with deficiency of the fourth component of complement. J. Clin. Invest. 86: 675-678 (1990).

W7 Wilson, G.N. Heterochrony and human malformation. Am. J. Med. Genet. 29: 311 (1988).

W8 World Health Organization. Congenital Malformations Worldwide: A Report from the International Clearinghouse for Birth Defects Monitoring Systems. Elsevier, New York, 1991.

W9 Wright, S. The results of crosses between inbred strains of guinea pigs, differing in number of digits. Genetics 19: 537-551 (1934).

W10 Wallace, M.R., L.B. Andersen, A.M. Saulino et al. A de novo Alu insertion results in neurofibromatosis type 1. Nature 353: 864-866 (1991).

W11 Willman, C.L., C.E. Sever, M.G. Pallavicini et al. Deletion of IRF-1, mapping to chromosome 5q31.1, in human leukaemia and preleukaemia myelodysplasia. Science 259: 968-971 (1993).

W12 Wallace, D. Mitochondrial diseases: genotype versus phenotype. Trends Genet. 9: 128-133 (1993).

Y1 Yoshimoto, Y., J.V. Neel, W.J. Schull et al. Malignant tumours during the first 2 decades of life in the offspring of atomic bomb survivors. Am. J. Hum. Genet. 46: 1041-1052 (1990).

Y2 Yoshimoto, Y., W.J. Schull, H. Kato et al. Mortality among the offspring (F_1) of atomic bomb survivors, 1946-1985. Radiat. Res. 32: 27-35 (1991).

Y3 Yu, S., M. Pritchard, E. Kremer et al. Fragile X genotype characterized by an unstable region of DNA. Science 252: 1179-1181 (1991).

ANNEX H

Radiation effects on the developing human brain

CONTENTS

INTRODUCTION

1. The developing human brain has been shown to be especially sensitive to ionizing radiation. Mental retardation has been observed in the survivors of the atomic bombings in Japan exposed *in utero* during sensitive periods [M2, M3, O1, P1, T1, W1, W2], and clinical studies of pelvically irradiated pregnant women have demonstrated damaging effects on the fetus [G1, I1, M1, Z4]. The sensitivity of the brain undoubtedly reflects its structural complexity, its long developmental (and hence sensitive) period, the vulnerability of the undifferentiated neural cells, the need for cell migration to functional position and the inability of the brain to replace most lost neurons.

2. Previous UNSCEAR reports have considered the general developmental effects of prenatal irradiation. In the UNSCEAR 1977 Report [U4], mainly animal data were considered. In the UNSCEAR 1986 Report [U2], more recent animal data and, to the extent possible, data on effects in humans were considered in order to derive risk estimates. The risks of effects, including mortality and the induction of malformations, leukaemia and other malignancies and mental retardation, were assessed to be 0.4 Gy^{-1} at the time of peak sensitivity and 0.1 Gy^{-1} in less sensitive periods. These values were derived on the assumption that the induction of effects is linear with dose. In the UNSCEAR 1988 Report [U1], these findings were summarized with the further statement that the risk estimates "may need substantial revision downward (particularly in the low-dose ranges)" and that "the Committee intends to review this in the near future". These points are considered in the further study outlined in this Annex.

3. The most significant point to investigate is whether the revised dosimetry system (DS86) [R1] for the survivors of the atomic bombings in Japan alters the interpretation of results previously gained and, therefore, requires the risk estimates to be changed. In particular, it will be necessary to establish whether it should be assumed that there is linearity of the dose-response and whether there may be thresholds of doses for effects at particular stages of fetal development.

4. In this Annex the emphasis is on reviewing the results of the study of the survivors of the atomic bombings in Japan. The results of other human epidemiological investigations and of pertinent experimental studies provide supplementary information, and these have been considered as well.

I. THE HUMAN BRAIN

A. DEVELOPMENT

5. The brain is the culmination of a long and interrelated sequence of molecular, cellular and tissue events. Some of these occur before birth and some after. Those occurring before birth are classifiable on the basis of the time after fertilization at which they occur as either embryonic or fetal. Conventionally, embryogenesis describes the phase of prenatal development from the appearance of the embryonic disk to the end of week 8 after fertilization. After this time, the developing organism is called a fetus. Most of the structural complexity of the brain evolves in the fetal period through a series of interconnected events involving the production of neuronal cells, their migration from the periventricular proliferative zones to the cortex, their further differentiation, their growth in size and complexity of structural and molecular organization, and the establishment of primary neuritic processes that contribute to the emerging fields of

connection. The details of these developmental events have been described elsewhere [C6, C7, I1, M8, M9, O15, R2, R6, R10, R11, S17, U2] and will not be reviewed in depth here. In this Annex, discussion will be limited to certain general principles of brain development that have emerged largely in the last several decades and to recent experimental and epidemiological findings that bear on an understanding of the mechanisms through which prenatal exposure to ionizing radiation can lead to brain dysfunction.

6. One of the first differentiation events in the very early embryo is the appearance of discrete neural precursors, the neuroblasts, which separate from a defined region of the primitive ectoderm. These cells are aggregated around the ventricles of the developing brain, and their descendants will populate the cortex. The mechanisms that operate within this ventricular zone to determine the ultimate fate of immature cortical cells are not well understood. However, evidence accumulates that in early corticogenesis there is a cooperation among the cells in the proliferative zone. For example, recent studies have shown that the neuroblasts in the proliferative zone are physiologically coupled by gap junctions into clusters of 15-90 cells [L4]. This has been demonstrated through the use of a low molecular weight dye, Lucifer yellow, that can be injected into a single cell and can easily pass through gap junctions from one cell to another. To distinguish between coupling through gap junctions and coupling through cytoplasmic bridges, possibly stemming from membrane fusion, the investigators also injected into single cells horseradish peroxidase (HRP), which does not pass through gap junctions because of its molecular size but can pass through cytoplasmic bridges. The injected HRP was invariably restricted to a single cell, indicating that the coupling was not due to cytoplasmic bridges. Similarly, experiments designed to decrease the conductance of gap junction channels and thus increase membrane resistance showed that the membrane resistance of cells within clusters was increased, but there was no increase in membrane resistance among non-coupled neurons in the cortical plate. The coupled cells, identified by the cell to cell diffusion of Lucifer yellow, form columns within the ventricular zone. The clusters themselves allow direct cell-to-cell interaction at the earliest stages of corticogenesis, and these interactions could participate in determining the fates of the developing neurons. This behaviour suggests an interdependency of the fate of these cells such that the death of one, whatever the cause, could lead indirectly to the impairment of the developmental potential of others. Once migration commences, however, the number of cells within the clusters decreases, and apparently the individual immature neurons divorce themselves from the clusters, since they can no longer be shown to be dye-coupled.

7. It is important to note here that experimental studies currently suggest that each cortical neuron has not only a designated date of birth but also a definite functional address (see, e.g. [R16]). Since cerebral neuronal cells proliferate in specific peri- or circumventricular zones, proper function implies migration. The event (or events) that initiates the movement of post-mitotic, undifferentiated neurons from the proliferative zones to their normal sites of function is still unknown. However, once initiated, the movement of cells extends over weeks in aggregate, although an individual cell may reach its destination in a matter of days at the most. The migratory process itself is an active, timed phenomenon dependent to a large degree on an interaction between the surface membranes of the neurons and their guidance cells, on matrix materials such as cytotactin and on the subsequent morphological shaping of the two different families of cells, neurons and neuroglia. Not all of the factors involved in this phenomenon are known; however, there is experimental evidence that a modification of cell surfaces or spaces on or near the glial processes, which guide the neurons during their movement, is involved [F1]. The cells probably advance by making adhesive contacts at their leading edges, or growth cones, and then pulling themselves forward. Edelman [E2], for example, has shown that specific molecules, known as cell adhesion molecules, whose structure and function are apparently under genetic control, play a central role in these movements and that they do so through local alteration of the cell surface. It has also been demonstrated experimentally that within the optic tectum the growth cones are able to read gradients of surface-associated information in the process of axonal path-finding [B15]. Thus, any damage to the surface membranes or impairment of these molecular processes, however transitory, could impair the timing of migration. It is known, for example, that blockade of the cell surface adhesion molecules with appropriate antibodies prevents proper migration of external granule cells in cerebellar slices in culture [C9, H12, L3] and would presumably also do so *in vivo*.

8. Two waves of neuronal migration take place [R15]. The first of these commences at about week 7 after fertilization and appears to involve cells from the inner area of proliferation, the ventricular zone. (Here and elsewhere, unless specifically stated otherwise, time is expressed in weeks following fertilization, estimated from and therefore assumed synonymous with time of ovulation.) The intermediate zone through which they pass is then sparsely structured and contains few impediments to their movement. This wave ceases at about week 10, when numerous nerve fibres appear in the intermediate zone, which thickens markedly. The second wave, numerically much the larger, begins about week 10, normally terminates about week 15 or so and involves cells from a zone

further from the lumen than the zone from which the earlier migrants came. This time the migratory cells must traverse a denser intermediate zone and move past those earlier formed neurons that have already migrated, are positioned and have formed connections. The later-formed neurons are assisted on their way to the cortical plate by the long processes of specialized cells, the radial glia. At a subsequent time, the radial glia will begin to divide anew and become differentiated into astrocytes. However, at this juncture, they seemingly serve two functions: first, to guide the migrating neurons through the densely packed intermediate zone and secondly, to ensure the faithful mapping of the ventricular surface onto the expanding and convoluted cerebral cortex by preventing or minimizing the intermixing of cells generated in different regions of the proliferative zone. While the majority of young neurons do migrate along these radial pathways, some mixing of these clonally related cells occurs. Walsh and Cepko [W8], using a retroviral marking method *in vivo*, have shown that in the rat some labelled cells appear to migrate up different radial glial fibres and even along the ventricular surface, perpendicular to the fibres themselves. The latter form of migration could cause a wide dispersion of related cells and suggests that the pathways for neuronal migration are far more complex than the simple routes offered by radial glia. It is not yet clear how common this occurrence is, whether it is species-dependent or whether all of the labelled cells are indeed clonal or reflect an inhomogeneous distribution of the viral label [K13]. However, these authors, using a new method to identify the functional specification of the progenitors in the cortex, have recently confirmed their earlier findings and argue that this widespread and numerically significant dispersion of neuronal clones implies that the functional specification of cortical areas occurs after neurogenesis [W14]. O'Rourke et al. [O14] have confirmed these observations with time-lapse confocal microscopy.

9. The cellular and molecular mechanisms of cell migration are not yet well understood, and little attention has heretofore been paid to cell membrane properties and changes in ionic concentration during cell movement. Only recently, for example, has it been recognized that migrating neurons in the developing central nervous system express voltage-sensitive ion channels before they reach their final destination. These channels appear to play a transient but specific developmental role in directing the migration of immature neurons. Thus, Komuro and Rakic [K14] have shown, using laser scanning confocal microscopy, that in the mouse cerebellum, granular neurons will not migrate until they have begun to express N-type (conotoxin-sensitive) calcium channels on their plasmalemmal surface. If these specific channels are inhibited by the addition of conotoxin to the tissue culture medium, the neurons will not migrate; however, the inhibition of other calcium channels, as well as those of sodium and potassium, had no effect on the rate of granule cell migration. Accordingly, they speculate that "the early expression of conotoxin-sensitive calcium channels in postmitotic cells may be an essential prerequisite to both the initiation and the execution of their movement".

10. Once migration has ceased, the fate of the migrating cells will ultimately depend on their abilities to connect with other neuronal cells; formation of these axonal pathways is a competitive phenomenon, and those cells that do not form the connections that allow stimuli to be passed from one cell to another will die and disappear. How these growing neurons find their targets has been one of the central problems of neurobiology for the last 40 or so years. It is now generally believed that the answer lies in chemo-affinity, that is to say, that the biochemical specification of growing axons is crucial in leading them to their appropriate targets [S15]. The precise nature of this process is unclear, and competing theories exist. Some speculate that there is a structural or strict chemospecificity in which the ultimate pattern rests on the complementary recognition of mutually specific cell surface markers, but this implies the existence of a very large number of such markers, much larger than has yet been identified. Others argue that the pattern arises through a regulatory or dynamic modulation of a relatively small number of specificities (see, e.g. [E2]). Evidence in support of this latter notion can be found in the fact, as previously stated, that late-formed neurons must migrate past those that have already migrated, are positioned, and have formed connections. Chuong et al. [C9] have shown that modulation of the neural cell adhesion molecule (N-CAM), which is present on all neurons (but not on the glia), or of the neuralglial cell adhesion molecule (Ng-CAM), which binds neurons to glia or glial molecules such as cytotactin, is implicated in the differential adhesiveness and regulation of this passing movement. N-CAM exists in two forms, an adult and an embryonic, which differ in their degree of sialylation. The embryonic form, E-N-CAM, is highly sialylated, whereas the adult form is not. In the cerebellum, E-N-CAM is never expressed in the germinal zone of neuroblasts destined to form or forming the external granular layer. It is, however, expressed by the granule cells during their migration but ceases to be demonstrable when these cells have reached their final position in the internal granular layer. Other cerebellar cell types do express E-N-CAM as histogenesis unfolds, but they, too, cease to do so with the overt cessation of cerebellar histogenesis [H14]. These findings suggest that E-N-CAM is only characteristic of growing and moving cellular structures.

11. Establishment of the proper axonal pathways entails cooperativeness as well as competition. It has been shown that in the developing mammalian telencephalon there exists a special group of early arising neurons, the subplate or transient pioneer neurons, that are instrumental in the laying down of the first axonal pathways and may be essential to the establishment of permanent subcortical projections [K4, M13]. These subplate neurons will disappear in postnatal life after the adult pattern of axonal projections is well established. It is also known that in the development of the central nervous system in some invertebrates, the grasshopper for instance, if the pioneer cells are prevented from differentiating through heat shock, the sensory growth cones that would have migrated along the pathways established by the pioneers are blocked and fail to reach the central nervous system [K4]. While the death or failure of a pioneer cell to differentiate may not always preclude the establishment of a specific pathway, since the function of the pioneer may be assumed by another cell, it is clear that in some instances the pathway will not develop if the pioneer cell is prevented from differentiating. Moreover, at least in some insect species, where the geometry of a specific neuronal pathway may be quite complex and involve sharp angles, it has been shown that other specialized cells contribute to the delineation of the pathway. These cells have been called "landmark" cells, and their presence and proximity apparently signal the pioneer to change course. Finally, as knowledge of the embryology of the brain increases and recognition of the functional specificity and diversity that exists among neurons grows, it becomes more plausible to assume that the loss of relatively small numbers of neuronal cells could have an effect on brain development out of proportion to the actual number of cells that are killed or whose differentiation is impaired.

12. Some cerebral neurons, presently thought to be relatively few in number, do not have their origin in the circumventricular proliferative zones but arise elsewhere and migrate into the cerebrum. It has been shown, for example, that those neurons that secrete the hormone that releases the luteinizing hormone, the one responsible for stimulating production of the sex hormones testosterone and oestrogen, actually have their origin in the olfactory placode. These neurons, known as LHRH cells, begin to migrate from their sites of birth in the placode through the olfactory bulb and into the cerebrum at about gestational day 12 or 13 in the mouse, following the terminal nerve (nervus terminalis). Most of the migration is completed by gestational day 16, and the cells, which are ciliated and morphologically distinguishable from other neurons, are diffusely distributed through the cerebrum [S9, W7]. These events in the human would be occurring at about 12-14 weeks after fertilization.

13. Many areas of the mammalian brain are characterized by repeated ensembles of anatomically and physiologically distinguishable nerve cells. Among such ensembles are those of the barrels and columns seen in the somatosensory cortex, the pattern of glomeruli in the olfactory bulbs and the columns of the visual cortex. Understanding the development of these neuronal assemblages has an important bearing on the nature of critical periods, the manner in which neural information is stored and the age-dependent neuronal response to injury. Progress in this understanding has been slow for lack of suitable study techniques, and it has not been clear whether the initial assemblages persist or whether they are lost or gained as the brain develops. Recently, LaMantia et al. [L2] have been able to show that with regard to the glomerular pattern in the olfactory bulbs, the brain is gradually constructed by the addition of new glomeruli to a persisting population, without apparent losses from the original population. Customarily regressive phenomena (cell death, synaptic loss and axon elimination) are known to play an important role in the development of the brain, but their findings suggest that these regressive events must proceed during the construction of olfactory neural circuits, if they occur at all in this region of the brain. However, LaMantia et al. [L2] note that the olfactory system has several extraordinary features that may lead to an exaggeration in the elaboration of these functional units in the olfactory bulbs. These findings suggest a need to reconcile the observation that some portions of the brain evolve through ongoing construction with the commonly accepted notion of development through the selection of useful circuits from a larger initial repertoire (see, e.g. [E2]).

14. Three general features of the development and organization of the human brain and its adnexa are important to an understanding of the nature of its vulnerability to malformation or maldevelopment, namely:

(a) the brain is one of the most complex organs of the body, with an involved architecture in which different functions are localized in different structures. Differentiation of the latter takes place at different times and for different durations. This is particularly true of the development of the neocortex, which proceeds over a long time;
(b) brain function critically depends on the disposition and interconnection of structures and cells, neuronal and glial, and normal structure and function hinge on an orderly sequence of events (cell division; programmed cell death; migration, including the positioning and selective aggregation of cells of the same kind; differentiation with the acquisition of new membrane proper-

ties; and synaptic inter-connection), each of which must occur correctly in time and space. Both cooperation and competition are involved in many of these events;

(c) the neurons of the cerebrum are not self-renewing. The capacity of neuronal precursors to divide is exhausted during the populating of the cerebral cortex and culminates in differentiated neurons that do not undergo further division.

Proper cortical function depends ultimately not only on the quantity of neuronal cells but their quality as well, and the latter depends, in turn, upon a variety of cellular and molecular processes, some intrinsic to these cells but some not. This has been particularly well illustrated through studies of the genetic disease, ataxia-telangiectasia (see [B17]).

15. ***Summary.*** The majority of neurons in the developing central nervous system migrate from the site of their last cell division to their final, functional position. The processes of acquisition of this position, the endowing of neurons of the six cortical layers of the cerebrum with their laminar identities and the parcellation of the neocortex into over 40 functionally distinct areas remain poorly understood and pose a major problem for neurobiology [S18]. Understanding these phenomena and the plasticity of the brain, i.e. its capacity to continually remodel itself, is also central to understanding how exposure to ionizing radiation impinges on the cytoarchitectonic structure of the central nervous system and its functioning.

B. DEVELOPMENTAL DEFECTS

16. Malformations of the brain may occur either in the course of major organogenesis, or take place during the differentiation and growth of the brain mantle. Among the former defects are malformations such as anencephaly and encephalomeningocele, which represent failures in the normal formation and elevation of the neural folds and the subsequent proper closure of the neural tube [M11, M15, O4], and holoprosencephaly, which reflects the failure of the forebrain to divide into hemispheres or lobes. At this time, the undifferentiated neural cells retain their regenerative capacity, and tissue damage can theoretically be repaired. The closure of the neural tube and the division of the prosencephalic vesicle take place relatively rapidly, probably within a few days [O5]. These events occur early in embryogenesis, 4-6 weeks after fertilization.

17. Disturbances in the production of neurons and their migration to the cerebral cortex give rise to malformations of the brain mantle [S1, S2]. Recent advances in developmental neurobiology have shown that many of these stem from failures in the normal interactions of cells (neural and non-neural) during the development of the primate brain. Normal interactions hinge upon (a) production of a sufficient number of neurons; (b) their appropriate positioning; (c) establishment of the requisite cell shapes; and (d) formation of synaptic connections [R3, R4, R5]. Among such malformations are, for example, an absent corpus callosum or a disorganized cortical architecture, which may later result in abnormal fissuring of the cerebral hemispheres, heterotopic cortical grey matter and microcephaly.

18. The sensitivity of the differentiating neural tissue to damage changes with age, and so does its capacity to replace damaged cells. It is therefore impossible to say whether the intrinsic or apparent sensitivity of the structures changes as a function of time. At any given time in development, the probability of causing abnormalities, and their severity, changes as the dose of the teratogenic agent changes. Moreover, for a given dose, damage can vary as a function of the time in development at which the insult occurs, and therefore defects that arise in the growth and differentiation of the brain mantle, unlike those that arise in the course of organogenesis, can also differ substantially in severity. Broadly stated, the sensitive period for such abnormalities is months instead of days. The longer sensitive period and the limited repair capability must be important reasons why these malformations are much more common than organogenetic ones [D7]. The complexity of the origin of these defects is illustrated by the relationship between brain function and cellular repair that characterizes the human genetic disorder, ataxia-telangiectasia [B17, C13, C14]. In addition to the neurological defects ataxia-telangiectasia is also associated with immunodeficiency, an elevated incidence of lymphoreticular neoplasms and *in vivo/in vitro* cellular radiosensitivity [C13]. Recent molecular studies suggest that the primary defect in ataxia-telangiectasia may center on the misrepair of DNA double strand breaks (see Annex E, "Mechanisms of radiation oncogenesis") and given the dramatic neurological dysfunction that characterizes the disorder it may be concluded that DNA repair is critical for neuronal development and maintenance.

19. The cells of the different structures of the brain are produced at different times. If the proliferating ventricular and subventricular cells are damaged during periods when a certain cell type is being produced, the loss may be permanent. Thus, a brief insult may lead to the preferential damage to a particular region and consequently cause a permanent functional or behavioural abnormality.

20. The period of maximum sensitivity or vulnerability to developmental disorders is understood

as that period in development during which defined teratological effects are most likely to be produced. This does not imply that some malformations can be produced only at certain times but rather that a given dose is more effective at some stages [U4] and that the duration of the period of effectiveness may be broadened by increasing the dose. Table 1, adapted from Williams [W10], sets forth the weeks after fertilization at which major developmental features of the brain evolve. By extension, it would be possible to suggest the damage that could ensue if the normal pattern of orderly differentiation and development did not occur (see also [J2, Z2]).

1. Cerebral and cerebellar abnormalities

21. The critical period for abnormalities in the development of the cerebral cortex occurs when the telencephalic matrix cells undergo their last cellular division, begin to migrate to the cortical plate and differentiate into specific phenotypes (see, e.g. [K8]). The production of neuronal cells accelerates and their migration to the cortical plate commences at about week 8 after fertilization. Cortical neuron production has largely terminated by week 16 after fertilization. Subsequently the laminar cortical structure becomes apparent and dendritic arborization, a process that extends into postnatal life, begins. Migrational errors involving the superficial cortico-cortical cells of the developing brain, or the loss of some of these cells, can lead to convolutional abnormalities [C2, G7], which since neuronal function follows position, may in turn contribute to the origin of functional and behavioural abnormalities.

22. Disorders such as the dyslexias (severe inabilities to read) appear to be due to aberrations in specific cortical areas [G5, K2]. Galaburda et al. [G6], for example, have described a severely dyslexic child with small focal wartlike accumulations of ectopic neurons in layer I and scattered focal cortical dysplasias; these aberrations were confined to the speech region of the left hemisphere. Other cases with comparable structural abnormalities have been described subsequently.

23. Similarly, auditory, olfactory and visual anomalies could be the consequence of damage to the specific cortical areas involved in these sensory functions rather than to the end-organs themselves or to specific sensory fibres in the corpus callosum [G9]. In the case of olfaction, at least, damage can apparently arise through a failure of the LHRH cells to migrate into the cerebrum, since anosmia is a part of the syndrome of hypogonadism and hypergonadotrophism known to be associated with migrational errors in these cells [S9].

24. Hypoplasia with deranged cortical structure stemming from injury to the external granular matrix is the most common abnormality of the cerebellum. Although some cell classes, e.g. the Golgi Type II cells, are generated early in the cerebellar anlage, other and more numerous cells, such as the granular neurons, are generated late. Overall, cerebellar growth starts later, proceeds more slowly and therefore ends later than that of the rest of the brain. This bimodal and protracted growth may account for the differential susceptibility of the cerebellum to growth restriction [R3]. In all major respects, the development of the human cerebellum resembles that in other mammals, when allowance is made for the different timing of birth relative to brain development [D6]. Because of its unique developmental sequence, in which two populations of neurons are generated at opposite sides of the cortical plate and migrate in a subsequent phase to bypass each other, the cerebellum is the most frequent site of genetic abnormalities [C1].

2. Abnormalities of the brain adnexa

25. Abnormalities involving the brain adnexa arise from either maldevelopment of the end-organs themselves, the eyes or ears, for example, (see [O11] for a description of the early normal development of these organs), or in the processing of the signals transmitted from these organs to the brain, or both [O6]. Failures in signal processing could be the consequence of a defect in the optic or auditory nerves or in the various cortical areas involved in auditory, olfactory and visual function.

26. Defects in the optic tract, for instance, could be manifested as aberrations in the field of vision, their nature and extent depending on the severity of the damage. Total destruction of the retina or the optic nerve would result in blindness. Damage to the optic chiasm could give rise to total or unilateral blindness, depending on the location and severity of the lesion. Damage to the iris could culminate in a coloboma or be manifested as heterochromia or other pigmentary disturbance. Neither of these latter defects have been seen, however, among the prenatally exposed survivors of the atomic bombings [K12].

27. Rhinencephalic damage could, if severe, produce anosmia, and if less severe, an inability to perceive specific classes of odours, a selective anosmia. Whether such prenatal damage to the brain adnexa can be subsequently ameliorated is unclear; however, some experimental evidence, based on the exposure of only a portion of the brain, suggests that the undamaged areas can compensate for the loss of function in the damaged regions. If such amelioration is possible, the effects of prenatal irradiation will be more difficult to assess. Special neurons in the nose are capable of

detecting a myriad of odors and communicating these to the brain. These neurons, unlike most others, when they age and die, are replaced with new ones derived from a population of progenitor cells in the nasal epithelium. These new neurons will acquire chemosensitivity and form synaptic connections in the olfactory bulb of the brain. This process occurs continuously, but despite this constant change the sense of smell is normally quite stable. Whether this would be true following exposure to ionizing radiation is not known.

28. *Summary*. The cells of the different structures of the brain are produced at different times, and hence the sensitivity of these structures to damage changes with age at exposure. A brief insult that might at one stage of embryogenesis have little or no effect can, at another stage in development, lead to preferential damage to a particular region and consequently cause a permanent functional or behavioural abnormality. At any given time, the probability of causing abnormalities and their severity change as the dose of the teratogenic agent changes. For a given dose, however, defects that arise in the growth and differentiation of the brain mantle, unlike those arising in the course of organogenesis, can differ substantially in severity, since the sensitive period for such abnormalities is months instead of days. The longer sensitive period and the limited repair capability must be important reasons why these malformations are much more common than organogenetic ones [D7].

II. RADIATION EFFECTS

29. Cells that are actively dividing are more responsive to radiation than those that only divide occasionally, or cannot divide. Given the number of proliferating cell populations in the embryo or fetus, it is to be expected that their tissues would be especially prone to radiation injury. This damage could take a variety of forms, ranging from necrotic to apoptotic death (see, e.g. [G11, H10]) to the impairment of the cell membrane without death. Apoptosis, that is, programmed cell death, is the most common form of cell death in the body and is particularly important in embryo- and fetogenesis in the shaping and reshaping of tissues and organs. It differs from death due to necrosis in a number of ways. Normally the cell dies quickly, within four hours or so, rather than through a process that extends over a much longer period, as in necrosis. Moreover, in apoptosis the cell membrane remains intact as death occurs, whereas in necrosis the integrity of the membrane is rapidly lost. Inoue et al. [I6] have demonstrated that radiation-induced cell death in the external granular layer of the cerebellum of newborn mice is of an apototic nature.

30. Where and how exposure to ionizing radiation at critical developmental junctures acts to impair brain function is unknown at the moment. However, ionizing radiation could interfere in a variety of ways [B3, B4, H1, H2, Y2]:

(a) radiation effects could arise from the death at mitosis of glial or neuronal precursors or both, or the killing of postmitotic, but still immature, neurons;
(b) such effects could result from an intrusion on cell migration either through an alteration of the cell surface phenomena that are involved, through the death of the glial cells that guide the migrating neurons or through infringement on gap-junction-mediated intercellular communication [F1]. It is not clear whether neuronal and glial cells are equally radiosensitive; however, disturbances of myelin formation, a mature glial function, have been described in brain stem fibre tracts in experimental situations following irradiation and appear more severe after exposure to neutrons than to x rays [G7];
(c) abnormality might reflect an impaired capacity of the neurons to connect correctly. The development of neuronal connections, or synaptogenesis, is a multifaceted phenomenon; it involves timing, space, surface-mediated competition and, possibly, diffusible agents;
(d) irradiation could also lead to disoriented dendritic arborization, or a reduced number of dendrites or dendritic spines per cerebral cortical neuron [B5, B6];
(e) programmed cell death, which is essential to the development of the normal brain and its adnexa, could also be accelerated or otherwise altered by ionizing radiation.

If cell death is not the sole mechanism through which irreparable damage occurs and if ionizing radiation can contribute to one or more of the levels or sites at which neuronal variation can arise, then there are numerous possible effects. Edelman [E2], for example, has identified seven major levels of neuronal variation, and within each of these there is commonly more than one site at which variation can be envisaged (see Table 2). Relatively few of these sites or levels of variation have been studied from a radiobiological perspective.

31. Distinguishing between the possible alternative mechanisms of damage and sites of altered variation, although formidable, is essential to more complete

understanding of the nature of the effects of ionizing radiation. How rapidly this understanding will be attained is unknown, but there are promising developments. For example, the study of neuron-specific proteins such as neuron-specific enolase, a cytosolic form of the glycolytic enzyme enolase (phosphopyruvate hydratase), may provide a means to discriminate between cortical dysfunction stemming from radiation-related neuronal death or necrosis, on the one hand, and errors in migration, on the other [I4]. Enolase is a dimeric enzyme composed of various permutations of three immunologically distinct subunits (alpha, beta and gamma). Immunohistochemical studies, using antibodies to the gamma subunit, have localized alpha-gamma and gamma-gamma dimers specifically within neuronal and neuroendocrine tissues. It is this specificity of distribution that makes neuron-specific enolase a useful marker not only for neuronal damage but also for neuroendocrine tumours. Coquerel et al. [C8], for example, have shown that the level of neuron-specific enolase in the cerebrospinal fluid increases as the necrosis volume increases and that at birth, the cerebrospinal fluid level of this enzyme is highly prognostic of infants who will subsequently exhibit confirmed brain damage. It has also been reported that cerebrospinal fluid as well as serum levels of neuron-specific enolase are elevated in non-febrile seizure disorders but not in cases of simple febrile convulsions [K10]. It is, however, not yet clear whether similar elevations occur in well-recognized migrational disorders, such as schizencephaly, a rare abnormality of the brain in which clefts extend across the cerebral hemispheres; if they do not, this enzyme might provide a simple tool for separating cortical functional errors associated with neuronal ectopias from abnormalities stemming from neuronal death.

32. Progress in the understanding of brain organization and function entails not only the use of newer tools but also the formulation of testable propositions [F5, K5]. One such organizational notion is the radial unit hypothesis of Rakic [R12, R13], who argued that the cortex is a collection of ontogenetic columns, each arising from a specific proliferative unit and clonal in nature. Substantial data support this contention. Mountcastle [M12], for example, showed that the neurons within a single column in the somatosensory cortex are responsive to a specific modality and receptive field of stimulation. Other sensory and association areas in the cortex behave similarly. It is thought that those columns innervated by a single thalamic nucleus (subnucleus or cell cluster) serve as a basic processing module. If this perception of cortical organization (and indirectly function) is correct, the loss of a few cells, conceivably even a single cell, could result in the loss, or compromise, of specific somatosensory or association abilities, if the loss occurs in the formative periods for these processing modules.

33. This radial unit thesis can only explain how neurons acquire proper positions; it does not define what initiates or governs their subsequent differentiation, including the course of synaptogenesis, nor does it necessarily establish when the specification of functional areas of the cortex occurs [W14]. Moreover, it does not provide answers to questions such as what prompts the shift from symmetric division of the neuronal stem cell, with one stem cell giving rise to two others, to asymmetric division, with one stem cell producing another stem cell and also an undifferentiated neuron that divides no further? If a single progenitor in the proliferative zone can produce more than one cell phenotype, how does this happen? What mechanism or mechanisms switch on the migratory process? How does the migrating neuron dissociate itself from its guidance mechanism when it nears its functional site? What further clues does it need to position itself properly within its functional domain?

34. The causal relationship between irradiation of the embryo and fetus at specific stages of development and the subsequent morphologic and functional damage to the brain, if not the molecular events involved, are well established in a number of experimental animals. There is abundant information on the biological effects caused by prenatal exposure of mammals to ionizing radiation. Much of this evidence has already been summarized in the UNSCEAR 1986 Report [U2]. These data give, however, little quantitative insight into effects on the brain in humans, although they serve to identify possible effects.

35. The limitations of the human data make studies on other species inevitable, if the risks of exposure are to be understood. There are, of course, differences in the brain development of different species. These are attributable partly to the differing complexity of the adult organ, but especially to the different rates of brain growth and the different time of birth in relation to developmental events in the brain [D1]. In general, the histological structure of the brain is comparable from one species to another, both in composition and function, and the sequence of developmental events in all mammalian species studied is also similar. However, the sizes of the various cytoarchitectonic areas of the cortex devoted to specific functions can and do vary greatly. For example, the primary visual cortex occupies 1/5 of the neocortical surface in monkeys but only 1/30 of it in humans, and Broca's language area exists only in the human species. This suggests that the target zone associated with specific cortical functions differs in different species and that the extrapolation of experimental observations on subhuman forms must take account of these dissimilarities. Finally, although structures in a particular part of the brain are broadly alike in animals of the same and even different species, as previously stated, at the finer level of

axonal and dendritic ramifications and connections there is a considerable degree of diversity among individuals within a species.

36. In order to examine the radiation effects observed in laboratory animals and to relate them to human observations, the timing of an insult, in relation to the developmental events in the brain that dictate the consequences, must be considered [D6, D7]. Experimental procedures must be applied at comparable stages in brain growth rather than at comparable gestational periods. The duration of exposures must also match the different time-scales, but if these factors are taken into account, even the small laboratory species can provide at least some qualitative information of relevance to the human. The complexity of the non-human primate brain obviously makes it valuable for many experimental purposes, and its protracted span of development increases the resolution of temporal sequences in neurogenesis; but the use of rats and mice can much more conveniently and quickly lead to a better understanding of human teratogenesis than has sometimes been supposed. Although extrapolations must be made with care, the use of experimental animals is vital to progress in understanding the effects of ionizing radiation. At the same time, direct evidence, especially that of a quantitative nature, must be continually sought from human studies and will eventually be the most convincing.

37. In this Chapter the primary epidemiological study of the prenatally exposed survivors of the atomic bombings in Japan is reviewed. These results are supplemented by additional but much more limited epidemiological investigations of other exposed individuals. Experimental studies may be particularly important to clarify mechanisms of actions. Some comments on recent findings from this field conclude this Chapter.

A. PRENATAL EXPOSURE TO ATOMIC BOMBINGS

38. Few population-based studies of the effects of prenatal exposure on the developing human embryo and fetus exist. Present knowledge rests mainly on the observation of those survivors exposed prenatally during the bombings of Hiroshima and Nagasaki and, to a lesser degree, on studies carried out on children who were prenatally exposed to radium or x rays in the course of radiotherapeutic treatment of their mothers and on comparative embryological studies. Among these, however, the size, length of study, variability in dose and post-ovulatory age at exposure make the experiences in Hiroshima and Nagasaki the most important source of data.

39. Over the years, the Atomic Bomb Casualty Commission (ABCC) and its successor, the Radiation Effects Research Foundation (RERF), have established several overlapping samples of individuals prenatally exposed to the atomic bombings of Hiroshima and Nagasaki. These samples, the studies and the findings are described in some detail in this Annex because of their inherent importance and to illustrate the breadth and consistency of the effects that have emerged.

40. *Study samples.* The earliest observations, those of Plummer [P1] and Yamazaki et al. [Y3], were based on opportunistic samples and made no systematic attempt to be complete. They were restricted in the method of ascertainment and in structure; often only one city or a limited prenatal age distribution was involved. In 1955, however, the construction of an exhaustive clinical sample of the prenatally exposed survivors was started. This gave rise to what has been termed the PE-86 Sample. Its members were ascertained through a variety of sources but primarily through birth registrations, interviews with women who were enrolled in the genetics programme in 1948-1954 and were possibly pregnant at the time of the bombing, the National Census of 1950, and earlier ad hoc censuses conducted by the city authorities and the ABCC. No attempt was made to match, by sex or prenatal age at the time of the bombing, the more distally exposed or the non-exposed with those survivors exposed within 2,000 meters.

41. In 1959, this sample was revised [B7] according to the following considerations:

(a) the earlier (1955) sample contained a disproportionate number of prenatally exposed survivors who were thought to have received doses of less than 0.01 Gy, and since clinical facilities and personnel were limited, examination of these individuals strained resources and seemed unproductive in view of the probable exposures. In the interests of clinical efficiency, sample size was limited, at the loss, presumably, of little or no information;

(b) special censuses conducted in 1950 and 1951 by the ABCC appeared to offer a better basis for the selection of a comparison group of non-exposed individuals than had previously obtained.

42. This new sample, known as the Revised PE-86 Sample, or the Clinical Sample, differs in several important respects from the unrevised one:

(a) it includes no survivors prenatally exposed at distances between 2,000 and 2,999 meters;

(b) exposed individuals are limited to those survivors prenatally exposed within 2,000 meters (the proximally exposed) or between 3,000 and 5,000 meters (the distally exposed);

(c) non-exposed persons include only those individuals who were beyond 10,000 meters at the time of the bombing and were enumerated in the special censuses;

(d) the survivors within the 3,000-5,000 meter zone, as well as the non-exposed, were matched for sex and age (by trimester of pregnancy) with those exposed within 2,000 meters.

These steps reduced the clinical burden substantially but resulted in little change in the number of persons within 2,000 meters. Both samples include virtually all individuals who received substantial exposures (those with estimated tissue absorbed doses of 0.5 Gy or more) and differ primarily in the number and ascertainment of individuals in the dose range 0-0.01 Gy. It is this group that has been the basis of most subsequent analyses (see, e.g. [M3, W1, W2]).

43. The data on severe mental retardation are restricted to the Clinical Sample, since it involves the only individuals on whom extensive clinical observations are available in both cities. In so far as intelligence tests and school performance data are concerned, attention is focused on the earlier, unrevised sample to bring the largest practicable number of observations to bear on the issue of possible brain damage more subtle than severe mental retardation. The intelligence tests were conducted and the school performance data obtained in 1955, that is, before the definition of the revised sample.

44. ***Dose estimates.*** The analyses of the effects of prenatal exposure to ionizing radiation to be described in the paragraphs to follow all employ the estimated absorbed dose to the mother's uterus based on the DS86 dosimetry ([R1]; see also [H5, K3]), unless otherwise specifically noted. Estimates of the absorbed doses to the fetus itself are not yet available and may not be for some time. Parenthetically, it should be noted that the organ absorbed doses computed under the DS86 system are actually age-specific population averages rather than individual-specific estimates, since the mean dose to an organ depends not only on the energy spectrum of the gamma rays and neutrons involved but also on the size of the organ. This will vary with the size of an individual survivor, which is not known. The organ doses estimated are, therefore, based on a "reference" man or woman, a hypothetical individual whose size approximates that of the average Japanese man or woman at the time of the bombings. The doses are derived from a mathematical phantom that simulates the human body by a series of simple geometric shapes: ellipsoids, elliptical cylinders and cones, or parts of these. The size of the phantom can be adjusted to represent individuals of different ages or genders. Six different phantoms were used: an infant, a juvenile and an adult for each of the two sexes. When one of these phantoms is used in concert with a computer program that models the transport of neutrons or photons through the body by Monte Carlo methods, an estimate of the average absorbed dose in an organ can be calculated.

45. The element of uncertainty introduced by this method of estimating doses is presumably not serious except, possibly, in the case of a pregnant woman. Here the difficulty arises because the reference woman used in the DS86 calculations was assumed not to be pregnant, as was certainly true of the vast majority of women survivors. However, in the pregnant woman the size of the uterus changes dramatically as pregnancy advances, and as the uterus enlarges, the other organs of the abdomen are shifted from their normal position and compressed. Thus the estimated dose to the uterus based on the reference woman describes the actual dose to the uterus more poorly in the later stages of pregnancy than in the early ones, before the uterus has undergone much change in size, and it may therefore be a poorer surrogate later in pregnancy. Although the error in the dose this may introduce is presumably small, given the energy spectrum involved, it should be noted, nonetheless, that to the extent that doses are overestimated, the risk to the embryo or fetus will be underestimated, or conversely if the doses are underestimated.

46. ***Developmental age.*** One of the most important factors, aside from dose, in determining the nature of the insult to the embryo or fetus resulting from exposure to ionizing radiation is the developmental age. Accordingly, since, as previously stated, different functions in the human brain are localized in different structures and since the differentiation of these takes place at different stages of development and over different periods of time, the estimated post-ovulatory ages at exposure (here taken to be synonymous with developmental age) have been grouped so as to reflect these known phases in normal development. Post-ovulatory age has been estimated to be 280 days less the number of days between the bombing and the birth. The average duration of a pregnancy, measured from the onset of the last menstrual period is taken to be 280 days. Fourteen days are subtracted from the days of pregnancy at time of bombing to account for the time between the onset of the last menstrual period and ovulation (and fertilization of the oocyte). Four age periods have been used: 0-7 weeks (0-55 days), 8-15 weeks, 16-25 weeks and 26 or more weeks after ovulation.

47. At the post-ovulatory age of 0-7 weeks (0-55 days), the precursors of the neurons and neuroglia, the two principal types of cells that give rise to the cerebrum, have emerged and are mitotically active. At 8-15 weeks, a rapid increase in the number of neurons occurs; they lose their capacity to divide, becoming perennial cells, and migrate to their functional sites. At 16-25 weeks, differentiation *in situ* accelerates,

synaptogenesis that began about week 8 increases, and the definitive cytoarchitecture of the brain unfolds. At 26 or more weeks, architectural and cellular differentiation and synaptogenesis of the cerebrum continue, with, at the same time, accelerated growth and development of the cerebellum.

48. Experimental studies [H11] have shown that irradiation at about day 16 in the rat (roughly week 28 in the human) will produce gross distortions of the leaf-like gyri, or folia, of the cerebellar cortex, as well as deficiencies in the granular and molecular layers of the cerebellum. The defects in these layers are even more common when exposure occurs shortly after birth, although the folial changes are not. In the rat, when irradiated between day 19 and day 21 (about week 31 to week 35 in the human), disordered cerebellar migration is a common occurrence [C12, H20].

49. ***Effects on brain growth and development.*** So far, only two conspicuous effects on brain growth and development have emerged in the study of prenatally exposed survivors of the atomic bombings of Hiroshima and Nagasaki. These are some cases of severe mental retardation and some of small head size without apparent mental retardation. Additionally, groups within the survivors have shown an increased frequency of unprovoked seizures and significantly reduced intelligence scores and performance in school. The severe mental retardation and the reduced intelligence scores and school performance may be manifestations of the same process, in which all the individuals significantly exposed in the relevant stages of pregnancy suffer some dose-related reduction in cortical function, thus increasing the number of those classified clinically as being severely retarded.

1. Severe mental retardation

50. Individuals classified here as severely mentally retarded are those who cannot form simple sentences, perform simple arithmetic calculations, care for themselves, or have been or are institutionalized or unmanageable. Thirty cases of severe mental retardation were observed in the 1,544 individuals included in the Clinical Sample for whom DS86 doses can be computed (doses were not available for 55 survivors in this sample at the time of this analysis). Details of exposures and clinical findings for the 30 cases of severe mental retardation are given in Table 3.

51. Three of the severely mentally retarded children, all in Hiroshima (estimated uterine absorbed doses 0, 0.29 and 0.56 Gy; post-ovulatory ages 36, 13, and 12 weeks, respectively), are known to have or to have had Down's syndrome (one child died in 1952). A fourth child, also in Hiroshima (estimated uterine absorbed dose 0.03 Gy; post-ovulatory age 20 weeks) had Japanese B encephalitis in infancy, and a fifth, in Hiroshima, had a retarded sibling (dose 0 Gy; post-ovulatory age 20 weeks). It is conceivable that, in these instances, the mental retardation was merely a part of the former syndrome or secondary to the infection, but in either event not radiation-related.

52. When the prenatally exposed survivors, exclusive of the three cases of Down's syndrome, are distributed over the four post-ovulatory age groupings described in paragraph 47 and the frequency of mentally retarded individuals is examined in the light of their estimated doses and the post-ovulatory age at which they were irradiated, the following emerges (see Table 4 and Figure I) [O1]:

(a) the highest risk of severe mental retardation occurred with exposure 8-15 weeks after ovulation. This exceptionally vulnerable period coincides with the most active production of cortical neurons and when all or nearly all of the migration of the immature neurons to the cerebral cortex from the proliferative layers takes place;

(b) within this critical period, damage expressed as the frequency of subsequent severe mental retardation increases as the dose estimated to have been received by the fetal tissues increases. Some 75% (9 of 12) of fetuses exposed to 1 Gy or more in this period are mentally retarded; this is an incidence more than 50 times greater than that in the unexposed comparison group;

(c) a period of lesser vulnerability appears to exist in the interval 16-25 weeks after ovulation. However, no increase in incidence is seen at doses estimated to be less than 0.5 Gy;

(d) there is no apparent increased risk before week 8 or after week 25. Whether the seeming absence of an effect in the first two months after ovulation is real, or merely reflects the fact that embryos exposed at that stage of development commonly fail to survive to an age at which mental retardation can be recognized, is unclear. However, experimental studies (see, e.g. [H11, H13]), have also failed to find effects on the developing mouse or rat nervous system at doses as high as 3 Gy in the first 8 days after fertilization, a period of time corresponding to the first 8 weeks or so in the human.

2. Small head size

53. The small head sizes to which reference has been made were two or more standard deviations below the mean head size of all of the individuals in the revised study sample. About 10% of these individuals with

small head sizes were also mentally retarded. Among the mentally retarded in the 1,598 births in the entire sample [B2, M2, M3, M4, T1], 18 persons (60%) have been previously reported to have or to have had disproportionately small heads [W1, W2]. This value may be spuriously low, since head circumference was not standardized against body size and since mental retardation is often seen in individuals whose head circumferences are disproportionately small for their body sizes. It is commonly thought that the development of the bones forming the vault is closely associated with the development of the brain and dura, and it is known that in fetal life these bones move with the growing brain. It is not clear, therefore, how independent this seeming abnormality may be of severe mental retardation nor what small head size may imply about the nature of the radiation-related damage. It is tempting to believe that the smaller head arises as a result of fewer neurons (because of cell death), but this may not be so. Reyners et al. [R14] have found that in the rat at low doses of x-radiation (0.09-0.45 Gy), the numerical densities of neurons and glial cells are actually increased, although the size of the cells is significantly reduced. The authors suggest that the brain has undergone a "miniaturization" rather than necrosis. However, as previously noted, glial cells retain their proliferative ability and could replace lost tissue mass, as D'Amato et al. [D2] observed experimentally. If so, brain volume could remain the same and head size develop normally, but cortical function would be diminished.

54. Recently, Otake and Schull [O13] re-examined the relationship to radiation exposure of small head size among the prenatally exposed population in Hiroshima and Nagasaki, using the estimated DS86 doses. The study population consisted of the 1,598 individuals (Hiroshima 1,250, Nagasaki 348) used by Otake et al. [O1] in the analysis of severe mental retardation. DS86 doses were available on 1,566 of these persons (1,242 in Hiroshima and 324 in Nagasaki; this represents an addition of 22 cases to the number described in [O1]). Among these subjects, 1,473 had their head circumference measured at least once in the period from 9 to 19 years of age.

55. As stated above, an individual with a small head size is defined as someone with a head circumference less than 2 standard deviations below the mean observed at his or her specific age at measurement. It should be noted that often, in the past, these individuals have been described as microcephalic. This term seems inappropriate, however, for two reasons: first, microcephaly denotes a clinically recognizable smallness of the head, which is often misshapen as well, and secondly, the clinical diagnosis generally is applied to individuals whose head is even smaller in circumference (often 3 standard deviations or more below the mean) than the criteria used here. Accordingly, either of two terms, "atypically small head" or "small head size" would seem to be more appropriate to describe the individuals satisfying the criteria described above.

56. Of the 30 cases with severe mental retardation described elsewhere [O1], 26 were included among the 1,473 study subjects. Three of the four lost cases died before 1954, that is, before they were 9 years of age. The one remaining case, a non-exposed individual, survives, but she did not have a physical examination between 9 and 19 years of age.

57. Among the sample of 1,473 individuals, 62 had small heads according to the criterion previously described. It should be noted that the criteria are different for males and females of the same chronological age; the differences range from -0.98 to 1.34 cm.

58. ***Small head size and trimester of exposure.*** The frequency of individuals with small head sizes, with and without severe mental retardation, is shown in Table 5 by trimester at exposure and estimated DS86 uterine absorbed dose. Figure II gives the proportion of small head sizes by trimester at exposure. As is evident from Figure II, the incidence of individuals with small head sizes in the first trimester unquestionably increases with increasing estimated dose; it also increases in the second trimester, but to a lesser extent. Hardly any increase is observed in the third trimester. Of the 26 mentally retarded individuals, 15 (58%) had small heads (Table 5). About 24% of the 62 individuals with small head size (determined by age-specific criteria) among the 1,473 clinical subjects from both cities were mentally retarded. This rate increases to 29% (13/45) when only those survivors exposed to 0.01 Gy or more are considered. These rates, it will be noted, are greater than that (10%) previously reported by Wood et al. [W1, W2].

59. Almost all of the individuals with small head sizes were exposed in the first or second trimester, 55% in the former and 31% in the latter. The risk of an atypically small head and severe mental retardation observed among individuals exposed in the second trimester to an estimated 0.01 Gy or more is 57% (8/14), but only 19% (5/27) in the first trimester. Alternatively stated, among individuals with an atypically small head and severe mental retardation, the bulk, 62% (8/13), were exposed in the second trimester.

60. ***Small head size and post-ovulatory age (weeks) at exposure.*** The proportion of individuals with small head size for the four post-ovulatory periods, namely, 0-7 weeks, 8-15 weeks, 16-25 weeks and ≥26 weeks, is also shown in Table 5. The proportion of indivi-

duals with small head size increases with increasing estimated dose in only the first two periods, and an especially sharp rising trend is seen in the 8-15 week period (Figure II).

61. In the 17 individuals from both cities with a small head in the 0-7 week period there was no apparent mental retardation. Twelve of these individuals were exposed to an estimated dose of 0.01 Gy or more. One of two (50%) of the individuals exposed to ≥1.00 Gy had small head size and two of four (50%) exposed to 0.50-0.99 Gy had small head size. There were 29 individuals with small head size in the 8-15 week period, 26 of whom received an estimated dose of ≥0.01 Gy; 12 of them (46.2%) were severely mentally retarded. Seven (87.5%) of the eight small head cases who were exposed to ≥1.00 Gy had severe mental retardation. Thus, 12 (80%) of the 15 individuals with an atypically small head and severe mental retardation occurred at the most radiosensitive period, 8-15 weeks after ovulation. In the 16-25 week period, only one (33.3%) of the three individuals with small head in the >0.01 Gy group was mentally retarded, and he had been exposed to a dose of more than 1.00 Gy.

62. The rubric "small head size" may, indeed probably does, cover a variety of different developmental "abnormalities". Among the individuals with small head size and severe mental retardation, for example, some clearly invite the clinical diagnosis of microcephaly, since the head is not only unusually small but misshapen, often pointed or oxycephalic-like. Still others, and they are more common, have a head size that is proportionate in all dimensions, albeit small. Moreover, since head size varies in all populations, it can be assumed that some of the individuals here designated as having small head size merely represent the lower extreme of normal variability. Indeed, based on the criterion for small head size used here, if head sizes are approximately normally distributed, some 2.5% of "normal" individuals would be so classified.

63. Since the mean intelligence quotient (IQ) and its standard deviation among the 47 individuals having small head size without severe mental retardation approximate the values seen in the entire clinical sample, it is conceivable that a significant fraction of these individuals are the "normals" alluded to above. Accordingly, Otake and Schull [O13] attempted to estimate the excess number of individuals with small heads ostensibly attributable to exposure to ionizing radiation (see Table 6). Among the 62 individuals with small head size, some 37 would be expected normally, and the observed and expected numbers agree reasonably well when exposure occurred in the 16th week or later. However, there is a striking excess prior to this time, where 16 are expected but 46 were actually observed, an excess of 30 cases. If it is assumed that the small head size among those 12 individuals with severe mental retardation is secondary to brain damage, this leaves 18 cases that might represent radiation-related instances of growth retardation without accompanying mental impairment. But can these latter individuals be distinguished from those expected by chance? To explore this possibility, the locations of the 47 cases of small head size without mental retardation were determined in a bivariate plot of standing versus sitting height expressed as age- and sex-standardized deviates based upon the full sample of 1,473 individuals. The individuals with a small head size but no apparent mental retardation were found to be disproportionately represented among the lower values defined by either the 95% or 99% probability ellipse (see Figure 4 in [O13]). Three individuals were outside the 99% ellipse, but only one of these three received an estimated dose of known biological consequence. Specifically, the DS86 uterine absorbed doses in the mother were 0, 0.04 and 0.49 Gy. These observations suggest that small head size is not an independent teratogenic effect but is either secondary to mental retardation or to a more generalized growth impairment without clinically recognizable mental retardation (see [O16]).

3. Intelligence test scores

64. Intelligence has been variously described as the ability to manage oneself and one's affairs prudently; to combine the elements of experience; to reason, compare, comprehend, use numerical concepts and combine objects into meaningful wholes; to have the faculty to organize subject-matter experience into new patterns; or to have the aggregate capacity to act purposefully, think rationally and deal effectively with one's environment. Given such differences in definition, it is natural that the bases of measurement should vary.

65. Intelligence tests differ one from another in the importance given to verbal ability, psychomotor reactions, social comprehension and so on. Thus, the score attained by an individual will depend to some degree upon the specific test used; generally, however, individuals scoring high on one test tend to score high on other tests. It is important to note, however, that even with the same test an individual's score is not an immutable value, as retesting has shown. Thus, a change of a few points in a particular child's score may not be clinically significant, but a change of only a few points in the mean score for a population of children can have important public health implications, resulting in a higher proportion of socially dysfunctional individuals. Most intelligence tests are so structured that the distribution of test results follows an

approximately normal curve, with a mean of 100 and a standard deviation of 12-15 points. Thus, normally some 95% of the population will have scores in the range 70-75 to 125-130, that is, will fall within two standard deviations of the mean. Individuals whose scores lie, consistently, two standard deviations or more below the mean would commonly be described as retarded. In the Japanese experience, the mean Koga score of some 1,673 tested children was 107.7 (standard deviation 16.08) [S4], and the highest IQ achieved by any of the clinically diagnosed severely mentally retarded children was 64 [O1].

66. Schull et al. [S4] have described an analysis of the results of intelligence tests of the prenatally exposed survivors of the atomic bombings of Hiroshima and Nagasaki conducted in 1955 by trained psychometrists. This analysis of the Koga test scores [K1, T2], which also used estimates of the DS86 uterine absorbed dose, reveals the following (see Figure III):

(a) there is no evidence of a radiation-related effect on intelligence among those individuals exposed at 0-7 weeks or >26 weeks after ovulation;
(b) for individuals exposed at 8-15 weeks after ovulation, and to a lesser extent those exposed at 16-25 weeks, the mean test scores, but not the variation in scores about the mean, are significantly heterogeneous among the four exposure categories;
(c) the fact that the mean test score declines significantly with increasing estimated dose without a statistically demonstrable change in the variance of the test scores suggests a progressive shift downwards in all individual scores with increasing exposure.

67. While intuitively it is reasonable to assume that achievement on intelligence tests is related to the quality of brain function, and that the diminished performance described above reflects some functional impairment, the biological basis (or bases) of that impairment is far from clear. Performance on intelligence tests can be affected by factors other than ionizing radiation, such as motivation, socialization at home and in school, and physical impairment (defective vision or hearing, for example). Of necessity, since information on these extraneous sources of variability does not exist, they must be assumed to be part of the random error in the analyses of such tests, but the possibility that they change systematically with dose cannot be ignored, although there is no evidence that this is so.

68. Qualitatively, these findings are consistent with the interpretation that there is a dose-related shift in IQ and that this could explain the increase in clinically classified cases of severe mental retardation.

4. School performance

69. As a part of the continuing assessment of the effects on the developing embryonic and fetal brain of exposure to ionizing radiation, the school performances of prenatally exposed survivors of the atomic bombing of Hiroshima and a suitable comparison group have been studied [O2].

70. The Japanese place strong emphasis on school performance and school attendance [B9]. As a consequence, the Japanese child rarely misses school without good cause and places high value upon achievement in school. If a child's attendance record is correlated with illness and performance with innate ability, attendance might be correlated with exposure as a consequence of more (or less) frequent illness, and performance might reflect the nature of the developmental events that took place when exposure occurred. Accordingly, with the approval and assistance of the Municipal Board of Education in Hiroshima and the written consent of the parents of those prenatally exposed, their school records were microfilmed in 1956. At that time these children were 10-11 years old, and most had recently completed their fourth year in elementary school. The records themselves include information on school attendance, performance in various subjects, behaviour and physical status.

71. The attendance records of the public schools of Japan indicate the actual number of days of school and the total number of days of school missed by a specific child, the number of days tardy and the number of days the child left school prematurely. The days missed are further subdivided into absences because of illness and absences for other reasons, such as death or illness of another member of the child's family. The ratio of the days missed through illness to the total days of school affords a crude measure of the health of a given child.

72. With some 250 school days per academic year, the typical child in these years failed to attend school fewer than 5 days a year. On average, school absences for illness tend to increase generally with dose among the four post-ovulatory age groupings, when the clinically recognized mentally retarded cases are included in the sample analysed. Absences also tend to diminish in number as the child advances in school. This continues to be true when the mentally retarded, who are more prone to illness, are excluded, but the overall effect of radiation on attendance becomes more equivocal. When one turns to age-specific categories, it is observed that (a) the number of absences continues to diminish in all age groupings as the child advances in school; and (b) the largest and most consistent effect of radiation, with and without respect to sex, involves the age group exposed 8-15 weeks after ovulation.

73. In the first four years of elementary schooling the Japanese child studies seven subjects: the Japanese language, civics, arithmetic, science, music, drawing and handicrafts, and gymnastics. Every student's performance with respect to these subjects is evaluated routinely, and at the end of every semester (there are three in the academic year) a score is assigned for each. At the end of the academic year, these scores are summarized into a single value for each subject. The latter varies, normally, in unit steps from +2 to -2. The highest and lowest five percentiles of the class are assigned scores of +2 (very good) and -2 (poor), respectively. The next highest and lowest 20 percentiles are given +1 (somewhat above average) and -1 (somewhat below average), and finally, the middle 50% are given zero (average). Otake et al. [O2] have converted these assigned values to a five-point scale (5, 4, ..., 1), giving the highest and lowest scores the values 5 and 1, respectively, and so on. Some scores for some individuals were either missing or illegible in the copies of the original records; all of the information that was available was used in these instances.

74. Before determining what measure of school performance should be fitted to the dose data, given the interdependence of the various school performance scores, the investigators examined the structure of the matrix of correlation coefficients among the seven subjects previously enumerated. The correlations were high, ranging from 0.62 to 0.82, suggesting a strong interdependence of the scores. Accordingly, to determine whether some combination of the scores would provide a more suitable measure of radiation-related damage than the scores individually, summary characteristics of the correlation matrix were computed. These computations revealed that assigning approximately equal weights to the scores and summing the product of the score and its weight would account for 75% of the collective variability. More mathematically stated, the vast majority of the variability was explained by the first eigenvector, which since it weights subjects equally, is tantamount to the mean of the individual subject scores. No other combination of the scores explained more than 6% of the variability, and all were associated primarily with a single subject, the second with music, the third with gymnastics, etc.

75. Achievements in school of the prenatally exposed survivors, as judged by the relationship of the average school performance score in these subjects, can be summarized as follows (see Figure III):

(a) for 8-15 weeks after ovulation, scholastic achievement in school diminishes as the estimated absorbed dose increases;
(b) a similar diminution is seen for 16-25 weeks after ovulation. This trend is stronger, however, in the earliest years of schooling;
(c) in the groups exposed 0-7 weeks after ovulation or 26 or more weeks after ovulation, there is no evidence of a radiation-related effect on academic performance.

Not unexpectedly, given the correlation between average school performance and IQ score (r = 0.54), these results parallel those previously found in prenatally exposed survivors with respect to achievement in standard intelligence tests in childhood.

5. Seizures

76. Seizures are a frequent sequela of impaired brain development and could therefore be expected to affect more children with radiation-related brain damage than children without. Dunn et al. [D3] have described the incidence and type of seizures among the prenatally exposed survivors of the atomic bombings and their association with specific stages of prenatal development at the time of irradiation. Histories of seizures were obtained at biennial routine clinical examinations starting at the age of 2 years.

77. Seizures, as here defined, include all references in the clinical records to "seizure", "epilepsy" or "convulsion". All of the medical records of participants in this programme of examinations who were coded for seizures were reviewed to characterize the nature of the seizure (i.e. its severity, clinical symptomatology, presence of fever, cause of the seizure, duration), the presence of other neurological disease, developmental landmarks, school performance, and any other medical problem. The records were not sufficiently explicit nor were electroencephalographic findings available to permit detailed clinical classification. However, there was enough description to allow a limited categorization of seizures by aetiology for epidemiologic purposes. Starting with all seizures, cases were classified as febrile, acute symptomatic (seizures due to acute central nervous system insult, such as head trauma) and unprovoked.

78. Cases of unprovoked seizures are those seizures without a record of a concomitant acute insult, that is, a known precipitating cause of a seizure, e.g. fever, trauma, post-vaccination reaction, or anoxia during an acute postnatal event. A seizure was so classified if the medical records revealed no clear statement of exposure to an accompanying infectious, traumatic or fever-producing agent. Strictly neonatal seizures (within the first month post-partum) were difficult to ascertain in this study, which did not begin until the children were 2 years old. Since neonatal seizures appear to have a different aetiology and were most likely underascertained, they were routinely excluded.

79. Fever is the most common precipitating cause of seizure in infancy or childhood. In the event of multiple seizures, however, fever might accompany only one seizure, and then not necessarily the first, and scoring these cases was undoubtedly arbitrary. The investigators adopted the following convention: if fever accompanied only one of several seizures, making it doubtful that fever was a generally precipitating cause in an individual, the case was scored as unprovoked.

80. No seizures were recorded among individuals exposed 0-7 weeks after ovulation at estimated doses higher than 0.10 Gy. In the group exposed 8-15 weeks after ovulation, the incidence of seizures was highest among those who received doses exceeding 0.10 Gy and increased with the level of fetal exposure. This was the case for all seizures without regard to the presence of fever or precipitating causes, and for unprovoked seizures. When the 22 cases of severe mental retardation were excluded, the increase in seizures was only slightly significant, and then only for unprovoked seizures. After exposure at later stages of development, there was no increase in recorded seizures.

81. Other data on the occurrence of seizures following *in utero* exposure are sparse, and there is little to which these observations can be compared. However, two case reports suggest that the period between 8 and 15 weeks may be a vulnerable time for exposure of the human fetus to radiation, with subsequent development of seizures [G10]. The first individual was a male exposed in the second to fourth month of gestation in the course of his mother's radiotherapy (dose unknown) for uterine myomatosis. He then developed epilepsy at the age of 3.5 years. The second was a female exposed during months 2 and 3, again in the course of maternal treatment for uterine myomatosis (dose unknown); she developed epilepsy at 2 years of age.

82. ***Summary.*** To summarize paragraphs 50-81, studies of the prenatally exposed survivors of the atomic bombings of Hiroshima and Nagasaki have revealed a statistically demonstrable dose-related increase in the frequency of mental retardation, seizures, individuals with atypically small heads, diminution in intelligence test scores and academic achievement. These effects are most conspicuous in weeks 8-15 following ovulation; however, there is a significant increase in the number of individuals with small heads in the first two months post-ovulation (12 of 81) and some evidence that mental retardation may be more common than expected in post-ovulatory weeks 16-25, particularly at doses estimated to be 0.5 Gy or more, where 3 (12.5%) of 24 children were retarded.

6. Pathologic and other findings of brain abnormalities

83. The biology of mental retardation remains enigmatic, and without a clear understanding of the molecular and cellular events that culminate in this functional defect, the role ionizing radiation may play in its origin is elusive. Despite important recent advances in diagnostic methods, causation is unknown in the great majority of cases of mental retardation. Often (10%-20% of cases) the brain appears normal by all standard methods of neuropathologic examination. Even more frequently the structural changes that are seen are mild and non-specific: the brain may be small, the grey matter may be aggregated abnormally in the subcortical areas, the columnar arrangement of cells may be unusual or the neurons may be more tightly packed than customary. However, two observations are common: a dysgenesis of dendritic spines on the cortical pyramidal neurons and impaired growth of dendritic trees of pyramidal neurons, affecting both basal and apical dendritic branches [H18]. These findings suggest defects in the geometry of the cerebral cortex, which form a plausible, but obviously not established, basis for the mental retardation. They further suggest that the difference between the normal brain and the retarded one may be as much quantitative as qualitative. But the brain is a structure that undergoes major postnatal developmental changes, including the pruning and rearrangement of synapses, and these continue into adolescence. Since this postnatal growth may modify errors that arose prenatally or perinatally, neuropathologic abnormalities seen in the cortex may depend on the age at which the individual was studied. Catch-up growth has been observed in some instances in experimental animals, but the prevalence of this in the human is unknown. Postnatal growth changes may merely lead to mismatched connections and a brain with the normal numbers of synapses, which have not, however, been incorporated into functional units.

84. Whether the cases of mental retardation seen among the prenatally exposed survivors of the atomic bombings of Hiroshima and Nagasaki represent malformations or instances of maldevelopment is not clear. The issue is more than semantic; it strikes at the mechanism of damage. This mechanism can be perceived as involving a dose-related large effect on a small number of individuals, i.e. as a malformation, or as a small effect on a large number of individuals, i.e. as maldevelopment, or, conceivably, as a mixture of the two. In maldevelopment, mental retardation reflects a dose-proportional effect on a variable that is continuously distributed. Otherwise stated, exposure results in a shifting downwards of the distribution of capacities for intelligence and results in some individuals whose capacity falls below that associated

with clinical judgments of retardation. An analogy involves small-statured individuals, some of whom are small because of a single gene effect, such as the achondroplastic dwarfs, and others merely represent the lower end of the normally occurring variation in stature. Other analogies could be drawn, such as spermatogenesis or haematopoiesis.

85. Pathological findings are still too limited to provide an unequivocal answer to the origin of mental retardation following exposure to ionizing radiation. The information available from studies performed is presented here.

86. Four individuals of the Clinical Sample who died have been submitted for autopsy; two were mentally retarded and two were not. Of the two with normal intelligence, a 9-year-old male exposed in week 20 after ovulation to a dose estimated to be less than 0.01 Gy, died from granulocytic leukaemia; autopsy disclosed extensive brain haemorrhages, which were thought to be the final cause of death. His brain had a normal weight of 1,440 g and a normal structure. The death of the other, a 29-year-old female, was ascribed to cardiac insufficiency. She had been exposed in fetal week 24 to an estimated dose of less than 0.01 Gy. The autopsy revealed multiple bilateral pulmonary infarcts and evidence suggestive of autoimmune disease (the clinical data were too scanty, however, to pursue this possibility). Cut sections of the cerebrum, cerebellum, brain stem and spinal cord showed no abnormality on gross or on microscopic examination. The brain had a normal weight of 1,450 g; there was no evidence of edema, which would have increased brain weight.

87. Both of the mentally retarded individuals had brain weights substantially below normal. One of these individuals, a 20-year-old overweight female (MF 400133) exposed in week 31 after ovulation to an estimated dose of less than 0.01 Gy, died of congestive heart failure. Her body mass index (defined as weight in kilograms divided by the square of the height in meters) was 28.6; a body mass index of 27 or greater is commonly used to define obesity. Autopsy disclosed severe edema and congestion of both lungs as well as marked, diffuse fatty infiltration of the liver. Multiple transections of the brain, which weighed 1,000 g, revealed the usual pattern of grey and white matter and no evidence of edema. Her mental retardation was presumably not related to her exposure, given the very low dose involved. The other mentally retarded individual, a male (MF 142623), died of acute meningitis at the age of 16 years [N3, Y1]. If he had been carried to the normal termination of a pregnancy, he would have been exposed 12 weeks after ovulation, but given his birth weight (1,950 g), he was undoubtedly premature. His weight suggests that he was actually exposed at week 8 or 9, since a full-term Japanese infant would weigh about 3,200 g. The estimated absorbed dose to the uterus of his mother was 1.2 Gy, and his brain weighed 840 g. He was bilaterally microphthalmic and had microcorneae and bilateral hypoplasia of the retina, particularly in the macular area. Posterior subcapsular opacities were present in both eyes. Coronal sections of the cerebrum revealed massive heterotopic grey matter around the lateral ventricles. Histologically there was an abortive laminar arrangement of nerve cells within the heterotopic grey areas, imitating the normal laminar arrangement of the cortical neurons. The cerebellum and hippocampi were histologically normal, but both mamillary bodies were missing. These bodies, which can be seen in reconstructions at 6 weeks after conception but are not externally recognizable in their double form until somewhat later, are thought to function as a part of the limbic system, which controls emotions and motivations, and interestingly this boy was not only retarded but severely emotionally disturbed. Heterotopic grey matter was not observed in any of the other three cases, including the second mentally retarded individual.

88. Heterotopic masses are collections of nerve cells in abnormal locations within the brain. They are due to an arrest in the migration of the immature neurons. They may be single, multiple, unilateral, bilateral, periventricular or located deep within the white matter. The most common locations are subependymal and just below the neocortex. They may be isolated or associated with other anomalies in brain development, such as schizencephaly, a rare abnormality of the brain in which clefts extend across the cerebral hemispheres. Individuals with isolated heterotopias can be clinically asymptomatic; when symptomatic, they often present with seizures in infancy or early childhood, but seizures have also been reported associated with other neurological defects, such as homonomous hemianopsia, the loss of vision in one half of the visual field in one or both eyes [O12]. Seizures have also been seen accompanied by the partial or complete absence of the corpus callosum [B13]. Most heterotopias are probably microscopic, but if sufficiently large (0.5 cm or so), they can be readily visualized with either computed tomography or magnetic resonance imaging [B13, O12]. The incidence of isolated heterotopias, either asymptomatic or symptomatic, is not known.

89. Ectopic grey matter is commonly seen in rodents following exposure to ionizing radiation. Hicks et al. [H9] reported such occurrences more than three decades ago and argued that they arose from surviving cells that retained the capacity to divide but did so in an abnormal environment. More recently, Donoso et al. [D8] found that all rats exposed to 1.25 Gy of

x-radiation on gestational day 15 developed ectopic areas beneath the corpus callosum and adjacent to the caudate nucleus. It is presumed that these isolated islands, or rosettes, of neuronal cells arise through faulty repair of radiation-related damage to the ependymal wall of the lateral ventricles, leading to an encirclement of mitotic cells. Subsequent divisions of these cells result in neuroblasts migrating in all directions. Structurally, the rosettes are not laminated but contain neurons with the shapes and sizes characteristic of cortical pyramidal cells. At 4 weeks of age, these cells are immature and seldom seen in the layered cortex above the corpus callosum. At 4 months of age, however, the immature cells are no longer present in the ectopias, and the ectopic pyramidal cells resemble those in the cortical layer. Donoso et al. [D8] found the number and distribution of spines on the ectopic pyramidal cells to be lower than for the layered cortical neurons. They further found that, whereas the number of apical spines decreased with age in the control animals, this did not occur in the ectopic zones. Synapses in the layered and ectopic cortex were morphologically indistinguishable. Since synaptogenesis in the rat is largely a postnatal phenomenon, and synapses were seen in the ectopic areas, these areas may have retained some functional activity.

90. The brains of five of the mentally retarded individuals exposed to the atomic bombings, all during week 8-15 after ovulation, have been examined using magnetic resonance imaging techniques [S8]. Although the number of individuals that have been studied is small, several different anomalies of development have been seen, and these correlate well with the embryological events transpiring at the time the individuals were exposed.

91. Two individuals, both males (MF 404259 and 471693), exposed during weeks 8 and 9 after ovulation, showed ventricles somewhat larger than normal and areas of heterotopic grey matter adjacent to the lateral ventricles. One of these individuals (MF 404259) exhibited an underdeveloped area in the left temporal region, an anterior commissure somewhat wider than normal and a thickened nucleus accumbens sept. Formation of the caudate lenticular bridge also appeared to be poor. It is noteworthy that this is the period when the first wave of neuronal migration develops, the one that proceeds without the support of the radial glial fibres. The findings in these two cases are strikingly similar but not identical to those on the autopsied case described earlier. However in these two instances, unlike the autopsied case, both mamillary bodies are clearly visible in the images. While this fact could be attributable to variation in developmental age, it could also suggest that the estimated ages at exposure are not exact.

92. Ectopic grey matter occurs in other instances of mental retardation not related to exposure to ionizing radiation, but its prevalence among mentally retarded individuals is not reliably known, and it may vary with the type and severity of the retardation. Thus, for example, Rosman and Kakulas [R20] have contrasted the brains of six mentally retarded individuals with muscular dystrophy with those of six dystrophic patients without mental defect. The average brain weight of the deficient group was significantly less than that of the controls. Grossly visible malformations of cerebral development were present in three of the deficient patients, four showed pachygyria and all six had significant microscopic heterotopias. There were no gross lesions in the control subjects, and significant microscopic heterotopias were present in only one of the patients whose intelligence was considered to be normal. A similar comparison of individuals with multiple neurofibromatosis (von Recklinghausen's disease) with and without mental retardation found the cortical architecture to be grossly or microscopically abnormal among the mentally retarded but not among those who were not retarded [R19]. These architectural abnormalities included random orientation of neurons, a disarray of normal cortical lamination and heterotopic neurons within the cortical molecular layer. Among the retarded individuals they also commonly saw (three out of five cases) small heterotopias in the deep cerebral white matter (defined as more than 10 mm from the cortico-white matter junction). These were not seen in the individuals of normal intelligence. However, subcortical heterotopias were present in all instances of the disease.

93. Ectopic grey matter is not invariably associated with mental retardation. The neuro-imaging of individuals with the inherited fragile X syndrome, where varying degrees of mental retardation commonly occur, has not revealed this defect. Of 27 individuals who have been studied, eight were found to be abnormal [W13]. Seven of these individuals exhibited only a mild enlargement of the ventricles, but in one a moderate, generalized dilation was seen. Autopsy studies have, however, disclosed abnormalities in dendritic spine morphology; very thin, long, tortuous spines with prominent heads and irregular dilatations were noted [W13]. This suggests a developmental error occurring after migration was completed.

94. Two individuals, both females (MF 401081 and one unregistered case not included in the clinical sample), exposed at 12-13 weeks after ovulation, that is after completion of the initial wave of migration and late in the second, exhibit no evidence of conspicuous migrational errors but do show a faulty brain structure. There is an enlargement of the prominently rounded elevations of the brain, the gyri. These elevations are separated by furrows or trenches, the sulci, and the

latter are shallower than normal. Both individuals have a mega cisterna magna, that is, an enlargement of the subarachnoid cistern that lies between the under surface of the cerebellum and the posterior surface of the medulla oblongata. One of the cases (the unregistered one) studied at this time exhibited a corpus callosum (the network of nerves that provides communication between the two halves of the brain) markedly smaller than normal and a poorly developed furrow immediately above the corpus, suggesting an aberration in the development of the band of association fibres, the cingulum, that passes over the corpus callosum. Interestingly, animal experiments suggest the cingulum to be particularly radiosensitive [R14, R17]. Indirectly, these findings suggest errors in migration.

95. Still later in development, a male exposed to an estimated dose of 1.5 Gy at week 15 exhibited neither migrational errors nor conspicuous changes in brain structure (MF 143818). It is therefore presumed that the functional impairment that exists must be related to the degree of connectedness between neurons. There is experimental evidence to show that exposure at this time in the development of the brain in primates leads to a diminished number of connections between neuronal cells [B6]. If all of the connections can be presumed to have functional significance, then the diminution must compromise performance in some manner.

96. Are the developmental errors described in the preceding paragraphs causally related to prenatal exposure to ionizing radiation, or are they merely fortuitous, characteristics of mental retardation generally? Two lines of evidence suggest causation. First, although the data are limited, similar findings have been reported in other individuals who were exposed to ionizing radiation prenatally. For example, Driscoll et al. [D5] have described the acute damage to two fetuses, one a male exposed at 16 or 17 weeks of pregnancy and the other a female exposed at 22 weeks to radium therapy in the course of treatment of maternal squamous cell carcinoma of the cervix uteri. Both were alive at the time of hysterectomy, a day following the cessation of treatment in the first instance and six days later in the second. The doses were large, estimated to be about 4.3 Gy at the centre of the fetal head and 7.7 Gy at the nearest point inside the cranium in the 16-17 week fetus, and about 16 Gy in the second fetus. In both cases, the brain incurred the greatest damage, but then it was also closest to the source of ionizing radiation. Neuronal cell loss was shown to be selective. The primitive post-mitotic migratory cells were promptly killed by the radiation, and in this respect the findings parallel those seen in experimental animals. Damage to the cerebellum was less extensive but still noticeable, particularly in the older fetus exposed to 16 Gy. Extensive changes were seen in other organs, notably the bone marrow and lymph nodes.

97. Thus the findings of Driscoll et al. as well as those of other investigators (see, e.g. [M19]), clearly indicate that if the dose is sufficiently high, severe damage to the brain can occur at stages in gestation consistent with those seen in the survivors of the atomic bombings in Japan. Unfortunately, the ages at exposure are described in terms of weeks of pregnancy, but if it is assumed that this implies time from the onset of the last menstrual period, as is commonly the case, then, measured from the moment of ovulation, these fetuses were 14-15 and 20 weeks of development at the time of exposure. However, dose-response extrapolations to the situation among the prenatally exposed survivors of the atomic bombings must be guarded. The doses were three to eight times higher than the highest received by any one of the survivors of the atomic bombings, and well above the presumed whole body fetal LD_{50}. Moreover, the Japanese studies are based upon live-born children surviving at least to an age where a clinical diagnosis of mental retardation could be made. Given the extensiveness of the damage in the cases described by Driscoll et al., it is questionable whether these fetuses would have survived gestation and parturition.

98. Second, although migrational errors are often seen associated with well-recognized, often inherited, syndromes in which mental retardation occurs (for specific instances, see [D9, H19, M20], and for a review [B16]), they appear relatively uncommon in idiopathic (unclassified) mental retardation. Crome [C10], for example, describes the findings at autopsy on 282 institutionalized mentally defective individuals. He points out rather carefully the limitations of the sample of individuals he studied and does not argue that his findings are representative of "the large number of mentally retarded individuals in the community or special hospitals". Among 191 individuals with unclassified mental retardation, he identified about 500 main abnormalities (each individual was counted as many times as main diagnoses occurred). About half of these abnormalities involved either dilation of the ventricles or a small brain (based on weight). However, smallness was defined as anything under 90% of the average, which implies that some 40% or so of a random sample of individuals would be diagnosed as having an abnormally small brain. Of more immediate interest and relevance to the prenatally exposed is the frequency of macrogyria (or pachygyria) and ectopic grey matter, since these are the primary findings reported in the Japanese studies. Crome identified only two cases (among 500-odd diagnoses) of pachygyria and two of "ectopic nodules of grey matter". Another, smaller series of autopsies of mentally retarded individuals in Finland revealed three cases of pachygyria or agyria among 80 individuals [P3]. Finally, a study of retarded individuals in Denmark reported 34 cases of microgyria or pachy-

gyria among 175 autopsies [C11]. Thus, the abnormalities seen among the prenatally exposed survivors of the atomic bombings of Hiroshima and Nagasaki would not appear to be common findings among the mentally retarded.

99. ***Summary.*** A variety of anatomical abnormalities of the brain have been seen among the prenatally exposed, mentally retarded survivors of the atomic bombings of Hiroshima and Nagasaki and in other embryos or fetuses also exposed to ionizing radiation. Although the data are limited, these gross anatomical effects have thus far been seen only at doses in excess of 0.5 Gy. Some of these abnormalities have been observed among mentally retarded individuals who were not exposed to radiation, but they appear to be less common. The abnormalities commonly correlate well with the embryological events occurring at the time of exposure, suggesting a causal relationship. However, the observations are essentially descriptive and subject to different interpretations; they suggest but cannot establish the nature of the cellular or molecular events that are impaired. Further similar studies are obviously needed.

B. OTHER HUMAN STUDIES

1. Prenatal exposure

100. Numerous studies and a variety of case reports (see, e.g. [B1, D5], and [M19] for a review) have been published that further the understanding of the possible role of ionizing radiation in the origin of brain abnormalities [G1, M1]. However, few of these studies or reports provide a reliable basis for risk estimation. Generally, there is little information on the exposures or on the developmental ages after fertilization at the time of exposure, and the sample sizes are often small. An exception to this is the study of some 998 children born at the Chicago Lying-In Hospital to women who had pelvimetry during the course of their pregnancy [O3, O8, O9]. The pelvimetric procedure was standard and resulted in an estimated dose of 0.005 Gy to the fetus. Since the date at which pelvimetry occurred was recorded, the age of the fetus at exposure could be estimated. While the bulk (87%) were exposed in the second half of pregnancy, 120 or so were exposed prior to the day 140 after the onset of the last menstrual cycle. A variety of end-points were examined in this group of children, relative to two control groups (born before or after the pelvimetry series was completed), including the occurrence of malignant neoplasms and congenital malformations, and the presence of mental deficiency. Only one statistically significant difference between the exposed and the comparison groups was observed: the frequency of haemangiomas was increased in the pelvimetry group, particularly when exposure occurred in the second or third trimester [G8]. Subsequent studies have indicated that this increase was due primarily to flame nevi, and the investigators are inclined to attribute no biological significance to their finding [O8]. Although the sample ascertained by Oppenheim et al. [O3, O8, O9] is relatively large (about 1,000 first-born children) and the irradiation occurred routinely rather than for medically indicated diagnostic purposes, the doses are generally small, 0.01-0.03 Gy, and as previously indicated, the bulk of the children were exposed in the third trimester. Unlike those studies of individuals where irradiation had occurred on a selective basis (e.g. [D4]), these authors find no evidence of a radiation-related effect on morbidity or mortality, save the one described above, but the analyses usually pooled all ages at exposure, and the power of the tests, in the statistical sense, is small in light of the expected effect at these doses, based on the Japanese studies.

101. Granroth [G2] has examined the association of diagnostic x-ray examinations in Finland with the occurrence of defects of the central nervous system. The data, drawn from the Finnish Registry of Congenital Malformations, reveal a significant increase in abnormalities of the brain, primarily anencephaly, hydrocephaly and microcephaly, among newborn infants prenatally exposed, when contrasted with control subjects matched by time and area. No estimate is given of the fetal absorbed dose. Moreover, as the author notes, the majority of these infants were exposed because of the clinical suspicion of either maternal pelvic anomaly or fetal anomaly, so the exposures were unlikely to have occurred at a time when abnormalities such as anencephaly are induced [M11]. Accordingly, it seems unlikely that the results reflect a teratogenic effect of radiation.

102. Neumeister [N1] has described the findings on 19 children prenatally exposed to doses estimated to be between 0.015 and 0.1 Gy. No instances of severe mental retardation are recorded, but post-ovulatory age at the time of exposure was not taken into consideration and no suitable comparison group was found. A subsequent report, on 73 children, merely states that mental development followed a normal course [N7]. Meyer et al. [M5] failed to find evidence of an increased frequency of severe mental retardation among 1,455 women who were prenatally exposed to small doses of radiation as a result of diagnostic pelvic examinations of their mothers. It seems uncertain, however, whether their case-finding mechanism would have identified women who were severely mentally retarded. An increased probability of premature death among such individuals leads to underrepresentation of the mentally retarded later in life. In addition, exposure must commonly have occurred late in pregnancy, after the most vulnerable period.

103. Other studies, such as those of Nokkentved [N2], are similarly inappropriate for the estimation of radiation effects. Nokkentved examined 152 children exposed in the first four months after fertilization to doses ranging from 0.002 to 0.07 Gy. The findings among these children were compared with the findings among their unirradiated siblings. Only one child, in the exposed group, was found to be microcephalic. There were no cases of microcephaly among the siblings. Two children in each group were reported to be retarded. Given the purported doses and sample sizes, these findings are not inconsistent with the experience in Hiroshima and Nagasaki.

104. Recently, Chinese investigators [H8, H17] published the results of a study of the long-term effects of prenatal exposure to diagnostic x-radiation on childhood physical and mental development that addresses some of the limitations, previously cited, of other studies. The exposed group consisted of 1,026 children who had been born in hospitals in Beijing, Shanghai and Changchun and were between the ages of 4 and 7 years when recruited. The absorbed dose to the fetus ranged from about 0.012-0.043 Gy; these doses were estimated using a thermoluminescent dosimeter in a human fetus phantom exposed to x rays from the posterior-anterior, lateral and axial views with typical exposure factors. Only one child, however, was exposed before week 8 following ovulation; 13 were exposed in weeks 8-15, 41 in weeks 16-25 and the remainder in week 26 or subsequently (most of them in week 37 or thereafter). The comparison group was comprised of 1,191 children matched to the exposed group by sex, age and hospital of birth. Height, weight and head circumference measurements were obtained, and intelligence was assessed using a 50-item intelligence and ability scale developed by the Capital Institute of Pediatrics of the Chinese Academy of Medical Sciences and standardized nationally. No significant difference between exposed and controls emerged in the measurements of physical development. The mean intelligence test score was reduced to a modest but statistically significant extent among the exposed group as compared to the non-exposed group (mean IQ: 100.35 and 101.71, respectively), and the distribution of individual scores was slightly shifted towards lower values. However, when possible confounding factors were taken into account, this difference was no longer statistically significant, nor was a significant difference found when attention was focused on those cases exposed between 8 and 15 weeks after conception. Given the small doses and the small sample size in the critical period, it is not surprising that these authors found no significant effects.

105. Ragozzino et al. [R21] have described the outcome of 9,970 pregnancies recorded for 2,980 women in the Rochester, Minnesota, metropolitan area in the United States in the years 1935-1960. The health status of the children was followed for more than 20 years in 70% of the entire cohort. This was possible because of the linkage system for medical records, which facilitated the retrospective determination of radiation absorbed dose and the comprehensive, long-term follow-up of mothers and offspring. Absorbed dose to the fetus for examinations in which the uterus was in the primary radiation beam was estimated for five intervals of gestation by multiplying calculated fetal dose at conception by a scale factor based on average maternal anterior-posterior dimension at different gestational ages. Fetal absorbed dose was expressed as the total absorbed dose in the first trimester, as the total dose absorbed by mid-gestation and as the absorbed dose accumulated throughout gestation. For purposes of analysis, the doses were classified into three categories, namely, 0 Gy, 0-3 mGy, and >3 mGy. Among the 8,014 children where the data were complete, 63 cases of mental retardation were recorded. The relative risk in the highest dose group, based on the mid-gestation total absorbed dose, was not statistically significant; the value was 1.1 (95% CI: 0.06-5.39). Data were not reported on the occurrence of seizures.

106. Results are also now available from a 5-year clinical-physiological study of children who were born after the Chernobyl accident whose mothers lived in contaminated areas at the time of pregnancy [T6, T7]. The critical periods for cerebro- and corticogenesis (8-15 and 16-25 weeks) for 370 of these children occurred in May, June and July of 1986, but the doses accumulated in these periods are not clear. However, the findings of Ilyin et al. [I5] suggest that they were probably a few tens of milligray at most.

107. Some delay in myelination, accompanied by slight psychomotor disorders, was seen in 14.5% of children exposed in the critical period of cerebrogenesis, but in only 7.5% of children born in the first half of 1988. EEG studies of these children showed a delay in normal alpha rhythm formation, with significant input of slow waves and later formation of zone differentiation. This was found in 16%-18% of children examined at 2 and 5 years of age. For the critical group of children, symptoms associated with an increase in intracranial pressure were seen, as revealed by special function studies. This was found in 18%-35% of cases, more frequently among children 2-3 years old.

108. The occurrence of seizures, confirmed by repeated EEG examinations, was observed in 14 of 342 children [T6, T7]. However, seven of these children were excluded since they had other proved causes of symptomatic seizures. For the other seven there were no other apparent causes than radiation exposure.

Seizures were observed more frequently in the group exposed at 8-15 weeks (13.4%) than in the group exposed at 16-25 weeks (8.2%); in the comparison group, the frequency of seizures was only 3.0%-3.2%. Insofar as the developmental period of vulnerability is concerned, these findings are consistent with those that have been reported for the prenatally exposed survivors in Hiroshima and Nagasaki. No cases of microencephaly, Down's syndrome or any gross CNS defect were observed in the study group.

109. ***Summary***. Aside from the observations on the prenatally exposed survivors of the atomic bombings of Hiroshima and Nagasaki, there are few other population-based studies of the effects of prenatal exposure on the developing human embryo and fetus. Those that have been published often provide no information on the doses received by the embryo or fetus or on the developmental ages after fertilization at which exposure occurred. Moreover, the sample sizes are often small and the power of the statistical tests inadequate in the light of the expected effect based on the Japanese experience. These caveats notwithstanding, the information provided by those studies that are available is broadly consistent with the Japanese data and not clearly contradictory.

2. Exposure of the infantile and juvenile brain

110. Because maturation of the human brain continues beyond birth, possible late-stage effects of prenatal exposure of the brain to ionizing radiation (especially in the later weeks of gestation) may be similar to effects from exposures of the infantile and juvenile brain. It is clear that ionizing radiation used therapeutically in the treatment of brain tumours or acute leukaemia at these ages can have deleterious effects, as measured by conventional intelligence testing (e.g. [E1, H3, M10, R7, S3]). Meadows et al. [M10] stated that "significant reductions were found in overall intelligence score for the majority of children, younger patients being most affected". The exposures involved in these instances were high, tens of gray, and most of the individuals involved were also receiving chemotherapy. It is also important to bear in mind that protracted hospitalization of the young often denies them the opportunity to socialize with their contemporaries and the intellectual interactions this affords. Neuropsychologic and other effects of therapeutic irradiations of children are discussed in Annex I, "Late deterministic radiation effects in children".

111. X-ray induced epilation was extensively used between 1910 and 1959 for the treatment of tinea capitis. It has been estimated that more than 200,000 children worldwide received this form of treatment. Albert et al. [A1], in their study of one group of children treated for tinea capitis, reported a higher incidence of mental illness, including psychosis, personality disorders and psychoneurosis, among 1,905 children treated for this disease by x rays than among 1,501 children with tinea capitis treated by other means. It has been estimated that, in the Adamson-Kienbock treatment regimen used in these instances, the brain received 1.5-1.75 Gy at its surface, decreasing to 0.7 Gy at the base.

112. Subsequently, Omran et al. [O7] described the results of psychiatric and psychometric evaluations of 109 children with tinea capitis treated by x-ray therapy and 65 treated with chemotherapy. They found more patients with deviant Minnesota Multiphasic Personality Inventory scores among those who had been irradiated than in those chemotherapeutically treated, and the former were judged more maladjusted by their MMPI profiles. Hence, there is evidence that exposure to ionizing radiation can modify personality traits, but interpretation of these data is difficult, because x-ray treatment and chemotherapy treatment differ in aspects other than radiation exposure and because a variety of emotional disturbances are associated with protracted hospitalization of the young. However, Ron et al. [R8] (see also [A1, O7, S5]) have reported a similar finding among individuals treated for tinea capitis who were not on adjuvant therapy nor hospitalized and who received similar radiation doses, possibly 1.3 Gy, on the average. Ron et al. [R8] have stated that "the irradiated children had lower examination scores on scholastic aptitude, intelligence quotient (IQ) and psychologic tests, completed fewer school grades, and had an increased risk for mental hospital admissions for certain disease categories". Apparently no estimate was made of the diminution in intelligence test score per unit exposure. The increased frequency of cases of cortical dysfunction reported by these authors and in the studies described in the preceding paragraph are not known to be associated with demonstrable anatomic changes in the brain.

113. Studies of children exposed during the first few months of life to absorbed doses in the brain of 1.0-5.2 Gy as a result of therapy for haemangiomas of the head, face and neck also reveal impaired subsequent brain development (see, e.g. [T3, T4, T5]). These investigators assessed brain function using not only conventional clinical and neurological examinations but also electroencephalography, electromyography, rheoencephalography and a variety of psychological tests. More than half of the children exposed to doses ranging from 0.46 to 1.3 Gy exhibited functional central nervous system changes. These were commonly manifested as memory and emotional defects. At somewhat higher doses (2.3-3.4 Gy), damage was more pronounced and included structural-functional asymmetries that could be demonstrated electroencephalographically. Long-term follow-up has re-

vealed some amelioration of these effects in some instances. At doses of 4.2-5.2 Gy, arrested physical and endocrinological growth was seen, accompanied by a reduction in head size with deformity. Mental retardation combined with epileptoid phenomena was also seen. No amelioration occurred with time in these cases. Generally, it was found that the older the child at the time of exposure, the higher the dose required to produce a specific effect.

114. Studies have been made in the former Soviet Union of the late consequences of radiation therapy for brain tumours, using concentrated beams in fractionated exposures [M25]. Observations after 5-10 years disclosed a number of asthenoneurotic cerebrasthenic syndromes, combined with hypertension, vestibular and atactic insufficiency, and residual hemiparesis in some children. Psychological studies have revealed passive attention instability, active attention exhausti-bility, rapid loss of interest due to fatigue and memory and intellect reduction; some children exhibited overt emotional disorders. In nearly half of the cases studied, however, some amelioration of these effects occurred, and after 5-7 years there was an apparently satisfactory social and school adaptation. Seven individuals developed an epileptoid syndrome after 10 years, and nine had a lowered convulsion preparedness threshold, based on electroencephalogram (EEG) tests.

115. Long-term observations have also been made on 89 Soviet children treated with ^{60}Co gamma rays for haemangiomas of the skin in the first 6 months and the first 2 years after birth [T4, T5]. Local doses were estimated to be 15-28 Gy, but exposure of the brain was non-uniform, varying from 1 to 3 Gy. A retardation in the development of motor and motorstatic functions, as evidenced by psychomotor performance or partial-speech, was seen in 11 children. By 5-6 years of age, almost a quarter of the children (22 per cent) exhibited an encephalopathy syndrome, often with evidence of minor organic damage to the central nervous system. Among the symptoms they exhibited were headache, difficulty in falling asleep, increased fatiguability of the neuromuscular system, vegetative-vestibular disorders (vegetative as used here and subsequently implies the autonomic nervous system) and a reduction in memory and associative abilities. Eight children had psychovegetative disorders and lowered IQ. After puberty, during adolescence and youth, satisfactory or good social adaptation occurred in some instances, but neuropsychic dysadaptational periods were seen. EEG tests disclosed an epileptoid syndrome, as well as a lowering of the convulsion preparedness threshold in seven individuals, including two with epileptiform seizures (radiation dose 22-26 Gy). These neuropsychic organic and functional changes were most pronounced in children exposed at 1-6 months and 1-3 years of age.

C. EXPERIMENTAL STUDIES

116. As noted in paragraph 2, previous UNSCEAR reports (see, in particular, [U2, U4]) have considered the general developmental effects of prenatal irradiation as revealed by experimental studies. It is not the intent of this Annex to re-examine the voluminous literature, but to comment on certain recent findings that deal specifically with the development of the brain. Mole [M19] reviewed this literature and the basis it affords for predicting malformations after irradiation of the developing human.

117. Experimental studies have demonstrated that the relative sensitivity of different components of the brain to ionizing radiation differs, and possibly substantially so. Reyners et al. [R17, R18], for example, have shown that the cingulum bundle, a myelinated substructure of the corpus callosum, is an especially sensitive indicator of exposure to x-radiation. Changes in this structure occur at doses as low as 0.1 Gy, that is, at doses too low for the effects to be readily explicable in terms of mitotic cell death, and suggest a disordered sequence of morphogenetic events. More recently, using 600 keV neutrons from a Van de Graaff accelerator, Reyners et al. [R22] have shown a significant effect on brain weight at doses as low as 10 mGy. This diminished brain weight is accompanied by a significant reduction in the size of the cingulum bundle. Reyners et al. concluded from their studies that "the threshold dose for detectable effects to a developing brain may be lower than 35 mSv, in particular for acute exposure to high energy transfer particles during the period of corticogenesis." Lent et al. [L1] have shown that mice exposed to 2 or 3 Gy of gamma radiation on gestational day 16 are invariably acallosal. It is not clear, however, whether these changes in the cingulum and the corpus callosum are conspicuously detrimental to the animal nor is it known why the cingulum appears to be so radiosensitive, more so than the entire corpus callosum.

118. Until relatively recently, most experimental studies have focused on changes in brain morphology or weight (e.g. [A3, H7, S13]) following exposure to ionizing radiation rather than changes in brain function. There are exceptions to this statement. Studies conducted almost three decades ago have revealed that seizures occur in rodents following prenatal exposure. Sikov et al. [S12, W11], for example, reported an increased frequency of seizures among the offspring of albino rats exposed at 15 days of gestation to a dose of 0.5 or 1.9 Gy. These seizures were described as focal in onset, with rapid progression from face to forelimb and hind limbs, and then quickly becoming generalized. They were said to be equivalent to the typical Jacksonian seizure in man, in which the attack usually proceeds from the distal to the proximal limb

musculature. No increase in seizures was seen when exposure occurred on day 10 of gestation, and no effort was made to define a dose-response relationship at 15 days of age. Other neurological deficits were noted, such as gait defects, forced circling and hypersensitivity to some sensory stimuli, which manifested itself as exaggerated myoclonic jerks. Although some of these effects were seen in rats exposed on day 10, they were more common among the rats exposed on day 15 and at the higher dose.

119. However, behavioural studies of rodents following prenatal irradiation have now revealed that a variety of behaviours are correlated with cortical morphology. Norton [N5, N6], for example, has reported that cortical thinning is associated with changes in an animal's angle of stride, negative geotaxis and continuous corridor activity, as well as with other behavioural measures. She has further shown that some behavioural tests exhibit a clear dose-response relationship to doses as low as 0.25 Gy (the lowest dose used in her experiment), although several behavioural parameters were not altered by radiation. Jensh et al. [J4, J5] have described similar findings in the Wistar rat at doses of 0.2 Gy and higher, but they concluded that all of the parameters they had studied had thresholds at or above 0.2 Gy. Kimler et al. [K6] have shown that the organ most sensitive to radiation-induced alterations changes: it is the pituitary gland at gestational day 11 and the primitive cortex of the brain at days 13-17, with a peak of sensitivity at day 15. They further noted that a spectrum of related functional and morphological deficits can be produced even by low-dose *in utero* irradiation (0.25 Gy), with the specific end-point showing the greatest change being determined by the day on which exposure occurs. Finally, Minamisawa et al. demonstrated an effect of aggressive behaviour in adult male mice following fetal exposure to gammarays [M24]. These anatomical and behavioural experi-mental results accord surprisingly well with what has been seen in the human (for a comparison see [S24]).

120. Still other neurophysiologic effects, with different critical periods, have been identified. Recently, for example, it has been shown that mice irradiated prenatally on day 18 (corresponding, roughly, to week 33 in the human) suffer a significant loss in spatial memory [S16]. The integrity of spatial memory appears to depend on the proper development of the hippocampus, a primitive, anatomically distinct part of the cortex lying beneath the cerebral hemispheres. This structure arises relatively late in the development of the human brain, but damage to it results in a recognized cognitive defect characterized by severe amnesia and includes deficits in learning mazes. Moreover, there is evidence that associates a reduction in the pyramidal cells within the hippocampus with memory impairment.

121. Analogous behavioural changes have been seen in primates following prenatal exposure [O10]. Brizzee et al. [B12], for example, have reported that the exposure of squirrel monkeys on days 89 and 90 of gestation to ^{60}Co gamma-radiation at doses of 0.5 or 1.0 Gy results in less accurate and poorly coordinated reflexes and neuromuscular coordination. The percentage of correct responses in tests on visual orientation, discrimination and reversal learning were significantly lower in the exposed animals than in the controls. At doses of 0.1 Gy, no structural or behavioural alterations were seen; however, the authors conjecture that more sensitive behavioural testing and the use of computerized microscopic techniques (and, possibly, the computer-aided mapping of specific neuronal populations [K9]) will reveal changes.

122. It is difficult to put these observations into a perspective suitable to the purposes of this Annex: the tests used to measure cortical dysfunction have no obvious human counterparts, the nature of the dose-response relationship is often clouded by the large inherent variability in the end-points measured, and so forth. Moreover, abscopal effects either in the experimental animal, the human or both cannot be excluded. Sloviter et al. [S11], for example, have shown that adrenalectomy of adult male rats results in a nearly complete loss of hippocampal granule cells 3-4 months after surgery. The hippocampus, as previously stated, is involved in learning, memory and a variety of other behaviours and is known to be the target of adrenal steroids. How widespread this phenomenon may be is not known, nor is it clear that radiation-related damage to the adrenals would effect similar changes. However, damage to the adrenals from prenatal exposure has been seen in the human [D5, Y1].

123. ***Summary.*** Three general conclusions seem warranted from the experimental evidence. First, it appears clear that low doses (that is, doses in the range of 0.2 Gy or so) produce measurable behavioural and anatomic effects. Secondly, behavioural changes have their structural counterparts in the architecture of the brain. Thirdly, there is a high degree of functional specificity in the information transmitted over neural systems.

III. RISK ESTIMATES

124. Quantitative risk estimates for radiation damage to the brain after prenatal exposure of human beings are of importance because they have practical implications for radiation protection. However, the human data on which to base such estimates are limited and imperfect. The data on the survivors of the atomic bombings of Hiroshima and Nagasaki provide the primary basis for the risk evaluation. As described in Chapter II, four types of observation are available from these data:

(a) the frequency of severe mental retardation recognized clinically;
(b) the diminution of intelligence, as measured by conventional tests;
(c) scholastic achievement in school;
(d) the occurrence of unprovoked seizures.

Each has its limitations, and there must be an awareness, when interpreting the available information, of these limitations and other difficulties. However, until more direct measures of brain damage, such as cell death or impaired cell migration, are available, these observations are the only ones on which risk estimates can be based. Unquantified clinical descriptions are of little assistance, and experimental data, though important qualitatively, provide an uncertain basis for quantitative estimates of prenatal risks in humans.

125. One of the most important problems in estimating the risk to the developing brain from exposure to ionizing radiation is the shape of the dose-response relationship. As stated, much of the data that have helped to identify the teratogenic effects of radiation have limited applicability, for either the doses are too poorly known or too invariant to permit discrimination between different plausible models. The information on the atomic bomb survivors represents one of a very few sets of data that may be relevant. But even here, the multiplicity of ways in which radiation could affect the normal development of the brain and culminate in cortical dysfunction makes it hard to assess the reasonableness of an observed dose-response relationship. This limitation will remain until the different causes of a neurological deficit of an organic nature can be distinguished one from another.

126. As stated in paragraph 84, it is presently unclear whether the cases of mental retardation seen among the prenatally exposed survivors of the atomic bombings of Hiroshima and Nagasaki represent malformations or instances of maldevelopment. Their origin can be perceived either as involving a dose-related large effect on a small number of individuals or as a small effect on a large number or, conceivably, a mixture of the two. Since the suggested shift of the IQ curve towards lower values must increase the frequency of mentally retarded individuals with increasing dose, the fall in IQ and the increase in severely mentally retarded individuals with dose may be interrelated. Indeed, the observed increase in mental retardation in the critical 8-15 week period and the shift in mean IQ in this same interval of time can be shown to be mathematically compatible. This fact has led the International Commission on Radiological Protection (ICRP) to conclude that the shift in IQ "appears to be a deterministic effect, probably with a threshold determined only by the minimum shift in IQ that can be clinically recognized" and to assert further that "the observed shift of 30 IQ units per Sv is best suited to describe the risk" of radiation-related mental impairment [I2]. The Commission also concluded that "if both observations (alluded to above) are correct, the most likely interpretation is that the dose required to cause an IQ change large enough to make an otherwise normal individual mentally retarded would be high, while the dose that would bring an individual with potentially low IQ over the borderline may be a few tenths of a Sv".

127. It should be noted that ICRP interpretation of the data stemming from the studies in Japan has not gone unchallenged, most notably by Mole [M23]. He argues that the neuroembryology and plasticity of the brain do not support this interpretation, that the correlation between the shift in IQ and the occurrence of severe mental retardation reflects the way in which IQ tests are constructed and is not indicative of a common underlying biologic process, and that the data are actually better described by a threshold model, with the threshold being in the neighborhood of 0.5 Gy.

128. Mole contends that the interpretation of the damage to the developing brain depends upon the choice between two competing proposals about the mechanism of construction of the primitive cerebral cortex. One of these hypotheses, the radial column hypothesis, argues that the development of the cerebral cortex arises through the radial migration of neurons from their sites of birth to predetermined destinations in the cortex, forming, as they move, radial columns with specific functions (see, in particular, [R12, R13]). The other hypothesis (see [W8, W14]) asserts that the migration of neurons is not limited to outward radial movement but can occur in other directions and over longer distances than envisaged by the radial column hypthesis. He argues that ICRP in favoring the radial column hypothesis has erred in denying the plasticity of the human brain. This argument is specious for at least two reasons. First, the hypotheses stated briefly above are not competitive but supplemental; it is not a matter of the choice of one and the rejection of the other. Evidence

clearly exists for both mechanisms of migration. This should not be unexpected, since collectively they afford an explanation for both the known plasticity of the human brain and the necessity that some cortical functions be rigidly encoded. This does not deny plasticity, but asserts that cortical function is a complex process some portion of which is conservative. Secondly, ICRP, while favoring the radial column hypothesis, does not assert that all migration of neuronal cells must conform to this hypothesis. They do note, however, that the radial column hypothesis provides a basis for presuming that some small local lesions could have lasting effects on mental function.

A. RISK FROM ACUTE EXPOSURE

129. Re-evaluation of the data on the survivors of the atomic bombings of Hiroshima and Nagasaki has provided a new perspective on the periods of sensitivity of the developing brain to radiation-related damage and the possible nature of the dose-response relationship. These findings have been described in some detail previously. The main points that specifically concern risk estimation are the following:

(a) the period of maximum vulnerability to radiation appears to be the time between 8-15 weeks after ovulation, that is, the interval when neurons are produced in greatest number and when they migrate to the cerebral cortex;

(b) a period of lesser vulnerability occurs in the succeeding period, 16-25 weeks after ovulation. This period accounts for about a quarter of the apparently radiation-related cases of severe mental retardation;

(c) the least vulnerable period is 0-7 weeks after ovulation, during which no radiation-related cases of severe mental retardation occur.

However, as previously stated, within the 0-7 week period, a higher proportion of exposed embryos fail to survive gestation, and it may be that brain-damaged embryos are less likely to survive to an age where their handicap can be recognized clinically. Moreover, a significant increase in the incidence of individuals with an atypically small head, presumably due to generalized growth retardation, does occur in these weeks.

1. Mental retardation

130. In fetuses exposed to radiation in the period 8-15 weeks after ovulation, the prevalence of severe mental retardation at estimated mean doses to the mother's uterus of 0, 0.05, 0.23, 0.64 and 1.38 Gy, was 0.8%, 4.5%, 1.8%, 20% and 75% (Table 4). Within this period of maximum vulnerability, it is difficult to know, a priori, what the appropriate dose-response model should be, since mental retardation could arise through a variety of different biological or genetic events, ranging from cell killing to mismanaged neuronal migration to errors in synaptogenesis or to some combination of these events. Each of these processes could have its own unique, but currently unknown dose-response relationship. Accordingly the Committee has elected not to fit a specific model or models but to cite the risks as they have been observed empirically.

131. Although the Committee does not believe that a linear dose-response model has much, if any, biological credence, prudence suggests the need to examine such a model, since presumably it would maximize the estimated risk at low doses. Within the most vulnerable age group (irradiation at 8-15 weeks after ovulation), the incidence of severe mental retardation at 1 Gy is 0.39, with a standard error of about 0.09 Gy^{-1}.

132. In fetuses exposed to radiation in the period 16-25 weeks after ovulation, the prevalence of severe mental retardation at estimated mean doses to the mother's uterus of 0, 0.05, 0.23, 0.64 and 1.38 Gy was 0.6%, 1.8%, 0%, 0% and 37.5% (Table 4). Thus, the only demonstrably increased risk occurs at doses estimated to be 1 Gy or more.

2. Small head size

133. A variety of dose-response relationships, with and without a threshold, have been fitted to the data on head size grouped by trimester and post-ovulatory age (weeks) at exposure. A significant radiation-related effect on the incidence of individuals with a small head was noted only in the first and second trimesters and for the 0-7 week and 8-15 week periods after ovulation. It is worth noting that these findings are similar to those of Miller and Blot [M3], when allowance is made for the difference in dosimetry (they used the T65 maternal kerma) and some subsequent small changes in the data. They observed "a progressive increase with dose in the frequency of the abnormality (small head circumference) among persons whose mothers were exposed before the 18th week of pregnancy". When exposure occurred in the first trimester, the risk of an atypically small head suggests a possible linear-quadratic dose-response relationship. Both linear and quadratic terms are significant, but the quadratic term is negative. The results of fitting a linear-quadratic model to the 0-15 week period after ovulation suggest a linear dose-response relationship (Figure II). No excess risk for small head size is seen in the third trimester or among individuals exposed at 16 weeks or more after ovula-

tion. The estimated threshold, based on either a linear or a linear-quadratic dose-response relationship, is zero or nearly so. This apparent absence of a threshold and the somewhat different periods of developmental vulnerability suggest an embryological difference in the events culminating in small head size, on the one hand, and severe mental retardation, on the other.

134. The relationship of small head size to exposure to ionizing radiation and gestational weeks was evaluated using four physical measurements of growth and development: standing height, weight, sitting height and chest circumference. These variables are highly correlated. Accordingly, the four measurements were evaluated as a set, using a multivariate analysis with estimated DS86 dose and gestational week as covariates and sex and small head size as categorical factors. A retardation in growth is observed among individuals with a small head, with or without severe mental retardation, when their physical measurements are compared with those of individuals with a "normal" head size.

135. In order to investigate the possibility of growth retardation using the four physical measurements simultaneously, a multivariate analysis of covariance was attempted, using data for individuals 10-12 and 16-18 years old, for whom comparatively large numbers of observations were available. The retardation of growth with increasing radiation dose is observed at almost all ages, as judged by the negative estimates of the dose parameters associated with the four measurements. However, a statistically significant retardation of growth and development, after adjusting for confounding factors based on sex, small head and gestational age, is noted only at 17 years of age with or without inclusion of severe mental retardation and at 18 years of age with the severe mental retardation cases included. At 16 years of age there is a suggestive retardation of growth among individuals with small head size and severe mental retardation ($p < 0.10$). At all other ages, no statistically significant retardation of growth is observed; however, as previously noted, at these ages too, growth seems to diminish as the radiation dose increases. It must be borne in mind that where a statistically significant effect of radiation on growth is not seen, the pubertal growth spurt and its variability in age of onset could increase the generalized variance of the measurements, diminishing the sensitivity of the statistical tests. This conjecture is not supported, however, by a test of the homogeneity of the generalized variances, since these cannot be shown to be significantly heterogeneous.

136. Post-ovulatory age is statistically significant and negative for all coefficients associated with the four physical measurements, except for chest circumference at 10 years of age, with or without the inclusion of individuals with severe mental retardation in the analysis. Individuals with small heads, with or without the inclusion of the cases with severe mental retardation, exhibit a highly significant retardation of growth and development with gestational age at exposure, as judged by the four physical measurements. Why this should be true is not obvious. But since the measurements decline as gestational age increases, it suggests that there may have been some selection for body size in the earlier gestational ages. Expressed in another way, individuals who survived exposure in the early stages of gestation may have represented healthier pregnancies, on average, that were therefore destined to give rise to larger children and young adults. If this were true, it would be reasonable to assume that no gestational age effect would be observed if the comparisons were restricted to those sample members who were either not exposed or exposed to estimated doses of less than 0.01 Gy. When the data are so restricted, however, the effect of gestational age remains, and its origin is unclear.

3. Diminution in intelligence and academic performance

137. The observations on intelligence tests and school performance suggest the same two post-ovulatory age periods of vulnerability to radiation. The period 8-15 weeks again shows the greatest sensitivity, although with the data available so far, it has not been possible to establish the form of the dose-response relationship unequivocally. However, within the post-ovulatory age group most sensitive to the occurrence of clinically recognizable severe mental retardation (exposure 8-15 weeks after ovulation) the diminution in IQ under the linear model is 21-33 points at 1 Gy, based on the new dosimetry and the specific set of observations used.

138. A linear-quadratic model does not generally provide a better fit to the intelligence test data (see Table 7), nor does it reveal persuasive evidence of curvilinearity in the dose response in the most critical post-ovulatory age group. However, the significance of the effect at 16-25 weeks after ovulation is more equivocal with a linear-quadratic model than with a linear one. Regression coefficients obtained in fitting linear and linear-quadratic models to school performance results are shown in Table 8.

139. The effects of diminished mental capacity considered here result from damage to the cerebrum in prenatally exposed individuals. Although experimental studies [A2, C12, H20] and case reports [B1, D5] have established that the cerebellum is sensitive to radiation damage, no evidence has emerged from the studies of the prenatally exposed survivors in Hiro-

shima and Nagasaki of such damage, and for several reasons it may be difficult to identify. First, Purkinje cells, the only efferent neurons in the cerebellum, are proliferating and migrating in the same developmental period as the neuronal cells that populate the cerebral cortex, so damage to precursors or differentiated Purkinje cells would occur at the same time and might be inseparable from damage to those cells that give rise to the cerebral cortex [Z1]. Secondly, the granular neurons, the most numerous nerve cells in the cerebellum, retain their proliferative abilities after birth and could, in theory, repopulate areas of the developing cerebellum that were damaged by radiation. To the extent that this occurs, granular cell damage might be mitigated. Estimates of the risk of damage to the cerebellum following prenatal exposure, based on fixed or progressive neurologic deficit, are presently not possible. No evidence of damage to the mid-brain or the brain stem following prenatal exposure has been reported; accordingly, radiation risks to these parts of the central nervous system cannot be estimated.

4. Seizures

140. The risk ratios for unprovoked seizures, following exposure at weeks 8-15 after ovulation are as follows: after doses of 0.1-0.49 Gy, 4.4 (90% CI: 0.5-40.9); after doses of ≥0.5 Gy, 24.9 (90% CI: 4.1-192, mentally retarded included); 14.5 (90% CI: 0.4-200, mentally retarded excluded). Table 9 gives the results of fitting a linear response model to the grouped dose data including and excluding the severely mentally retarded.

141. It is not clear which of these sets of risk ratios, that based on the inclusion or that based on the exclusion of the mentally retarded, should be given the greater weight. The answer hinges ultimately on the mechanisms underlying the occurrence of seizures and mental retardation following prenatal exposure to ionizing radiation, and these are presently unknown. If seizures can arise by two independent mechanisms, both possibly dose-related, one of which causes seizures and the other of which causes mental retardation in some individuals who are then predisposed to develop seizures, the mentally retarded must necessarily be excluded if one is to explore the dose-response relationship associated with the first mechanism. If, however, mental retardation and seizures arise from a common brain defect, which manifests itself in some instances as mental retardation and in other instances as seizures, then the mentally retarded should not be excluded.

142. At present the only evidence suggesting a common radiation-related developmental defect is the occurrence of ectopic grey matter in some instances of both disorders. However, even this evidence is difficult to put into perspective, because while it is known that ectopic grey matter occurs among some of the radiation-related instances of mental retardation, the observation of ectopia in individuals with seizures is based on other studies. As yet, there has been no investigation of the incidence of ectopic grey matter among the prenatally exposed survivors of the atomic bombings of Hiroshima and Nagasaki who have seizures but no mental retardation.

143. A search for a threshold in the occurrence of seizures (see Table 10) discloses the following: the central values of the threshold for all seizures range between 0.11 and 0.15 Gy in the most critical period, that is, 8-15 weeks after ovulation, and the estimates are even lower for unprovoked seizures (0.04-0.08 Gy). In all of these instances, however, the lower 95% bound on the threshold includes zero, so the data provide no compelling evidence for a threshold.

B. RISK FROM FRACTIONATED OR CHRONIC EXPOSURE TO NEUROTOXINS

1. Ionizing radiation

144. Little is known about the effects on the developing human embryo and fetus of fractionated or chronic exposures to ionizing radiation. Given the complexity of brain development and the differing durations of specific developmental phenomena, it is reasonable, however, to assume that reducing the dose rate or dose fractionation will have some effect. The hippocampus, for example, and the cerebellum continue to have limited neuronal multiplication, and migration does occur in both organs. Changes continue in the hippocampus and cerebellum into the first and second years of life. Continuing events such as these may show dose-rate effects differing from those associated with the multiplication of the cells of the ventricular and subventricular areas of the cerebrum, or the migration of neurons to the cerebral cortex.

145. Most of the information available on the effects of dose rate involves the experimental exposure of rodents. Since these findings have been summarized in previous reviews (see, e.g. [K11, M19, U2, U4]), attention here is restricted to only one or two representative observations. Brizzee et al. [B10] (see also [J1]) have examined cell recovery in the fetal brain of rats. Pregnant rats were exposed to ^{60}Co radiation on gestation day 13 in single doses, ranging from 0.25 to 2 Gy in increments of 0.25 Gy, and in split doses of 1 Gy, followed 9 hours later by a second dose of 0.25 to 1.5 Gy, again in increments of 0.25 Gy. The animals were disected and examined on the day 19 of gestation. The incidence and severity of

tissue alterations generally varied directly with dose and were clearly greater in single dose than in split dose groups with the same total exposure. The authors observed that "the presence of a threshold (shoulder) zone on the dose-response curve in the split-dose animals suggests that cell recovery occurred in some degree in the interval between the two exposures". This reduction in damage with the protraction of dose seems greater for continuous gamma-ray exposure than for serial, brief x-ray exposures, and it has been argued that this may indicate a further sparing when the protracted dose is evenly distributed over time [M19]. If true, this obviously has important regulatory implications.

146. Recently, Vidal-Pergola et al. [V1] reported results of fractionated prenatal doses on postnatal development in Sprague-Dawley derived rats. Their experiment consisted of exposing pregnant females to single doses of 0.5 or 1.0 Gy, or to two doses of 0.5 Gy 6 hours apart. Offspring were subjected to four behavioural tests (negative geotaxis, reflex suspension, continuous corridor activity and gait) on postnatal days 7-28. The rats were then sacrificed, and the brains were removed and processed for histology. For all four behavioural end-points, the fractionated dose produced an effect that was intermediate between the 0.5 and 1.0 Gy doses and that, by linear interpolation, could be expressed as equivalent to a single dose of about 0.7 Gy. Measurements of the upper four layers, the lower two layers and the total thickness of the sensorimotor cortex in the dose-fractionated group revealed significantly less damage than was seen at a single dose of 1.0 Gy but more than that seen at a single dose of 0.5 Gy. Reyners et al. [R22] have examined the effects of protracted exposures to low doses of gamma rays on Wistar rats from day 12 to 16 post conception and found a significant reduction in brain weight at an accumulated dose as low as 160 mGy.

147. Newly developed techniques for the culturing of neuronal cells *in vitro* make such cell studies more practical now than in the past. For example, the means exist to culture cells from a snippet of the embryonic forebrain of the mouse (see, e.g. [F2, H15, H16]). These cells, when dissociated and plated in a monolayer, will form structures with a well-defined lumen and dispose themselves radially around the latter much like the proliferative zones seen in the fetal brain. The cells will divide, become post-mitotic, as evidenced by the presence of neural filament protein, and actually migrate to the periphery of the globular aggregate. At about 5-7 days after the formation of the aggregates, they collapse, presumably for want of a supporting structure, and although the cells will continue to divide and migrate, they no longer have a well-defined architecture. No studies have been published describing the effect of exposure to ionizing radiation on this sequence of events in these cultures. However, even a week could be long enough to determine whether radiation does alter, even transitorily, the surface properties of these neuronal cells, much as Feinendegen et al. reported for haematopoietic stem cells [F3, F4]. The measurements on the haematopoietic stem cells are essentially indirect, but given the existence of specific monoclonal antibodies to a variety of the neuronal cell adhesion molecules and cytoskeletal proteins, a more direct test of alterations in the neuronal or glial cell membrane or the cytoskeleton of the neuronal cell is possible. If such studies are to be informative, however, it will be necessary to demonstrate that the changes seen *in vitro* parallel changes *in vivo* and are not merely the consequence of the experimental manipulations.

2. Neurotoxic chemicals

148. Some insight into the nature of the developmental effects to be anticipated from chronic radiation exposure may come from toxicological effects in embryos and fetuses exposed to toxic chemicals [W3, W4, W5]. In Minamata, Japan, where the bay and its marine life were contaminated by methylmercury, 23 of 359 children born between 1955 and 1959 showed symptoms of cerebral palsy, a proportion 10 to 60 times higher than normally expected. Fetal exposure reduced brain weight in severely poisoned children to one half or less of normal, and abnormal cells could be seen distributed throughout the brain. Severe, permanent central nervous system damage leading to behavioural and other neurological disorders was also seen in Iraq, where seed grain contaminated with methylmercury was used as food. These incapacitating consequences were often observed in children of mothers whose most common symptom of methylmercury poisoning during pregnancy was a mild, transient paraesthesia. Such observations suggest that the embryo and fetus are much more sensitive to methylmercury than the mother, but it should also be noted that methylmercury accumulates to higher concentrations in the blood and tissues of the embryo and fetus than in those of the mother [I3, W6].

149. The fetal alcohol syndrome offers another possible paradigm. Abnormalities of the central nervous system, particularly mental retardation and small head size, are also the most pronounced effects of heavy intra-uterine exposure to alcohol [S6]. The average IQ of individuals with fetal alcohol syndrome is about 65, although scores may vary from 16 to 105 [S7]; also, the severity of the mental retardation correlates with the severity of the dysmorphic features in the individual. Clarren et al. [C3, C4] (see also

[H4]) have noted that areas of ectopic grey matter in the frontal and temporal white regions of the cerebral hemispheres and leptomeningeal neuroglial heterotopias, both evidences of abnormal cell migration, are common among infants with fetal alcohol syndrome. This appears true not only among those infants born to chronically alcoholic mothers, but also those born to women who describe themselves as infrequent drinkers who have occasional episodes of intensive drinking.

150. It is generally assumed that the teratogenic effect of alcohol, insofar as abnormalities of the central nervous system are concerned, is initiated during the first trimester, but this has not been well established. Given the commonly chronic nature of the exposure, it is not surprising that the sensitive period is imperfectly known. Renwick et al. [R9], using an argument based upon seasonality in the prevalence of fetal alcohol syndrome, on the one hand, and ethanol use, on the other, suggested that the damage may occur as late as weeks 18-20 of gestation. Since they apparently measured gestation from the last menstrual period [R9], this corresponds to 16-18 weeks after ovulation and suggests that the vulnerable periods for alcohol use and exposure to ionizing radiation may be similar. It should be noted, however, that leptomeningeal heterotopias of the kind observed in fetal alcohol syndrome have not been reported in either humans or other primates exposed to ionizing radiation, although heterotopic grey matter has been seen, as previously described. These leptomeningeal neuroglial heterotopias are seen as a sheet of neural and glial tissue that covers a part of the brain surface and may partially incorporate the pia mater. They are apparently continuous with the molecular layer of the cortex and may represent a persistence of its subpial granular layer [B8]. If so, they arise somewhat later, probably after week 24 [B8, Z2]. The aberration in migration that occurs appears less a failure of the neurons to move from the periventricular proliferative areas than an inability to recognize when to stop; the cells commonly migrate beyond their normal sites of final differentiation.

151. Further insight into the effects of ionizing radiation on the developing human brain is to be found in the neurotoxic effects of prenatal exposure to lead (see, e.g. [M22, S19, S20]). Although the toxic effects of this metal are many and varied, four findings appear especially pertinent to this Annex. First, the effects of prenatal exposure to lead on the development of the central nervous system appear to be linear over a wide range of doses. For example, the decline in performance on the Bayley Mental Development Index, which has a mean of 100 and a standard deviation of 16, is 2-8 points per 10 μg of lead per deciliter of blood [M22]. But the epidemiological data do not allow a threshold to be established with confidence. Linearity does not seem to be true for all neurotoxic effects, however. The lead-related impairment of peripheral nerve conductance, for example, appears to follow a quadratic dose-response curve, suggesting that a threshold may exist for this effect [S21]. In this instance neurotoxicity apparently requires the recruitment of several nerve fibers if a dysfunctional state is to obtain. This suggests that the shape of the dose-response relationship is intimately related to the developmental biology of the end effect measured. Secondly, since there are no absolutely lead-free societies, it is not possible to compare lead-free situations with those involving very low levels of lead exposure in order to determine whether there are non-monotonic regions in the empirical dose-response relationship. This situation is similar to that involving exposure to ionizing radiation. Thirdly, there is substantial evidence supporting the notion that lead toxicity involves molecular interactions of this metal with calcium and sodium [S19]. Given the ubiquity of exposure to lead, its effect on the transmembranal influx of calcium and the possible role of N-type calcium channels in neuronal migration, this suggests the need, in the case of ionizing radiation, to explore carefully the molecular and cellular mechanisms that may subtend radiation damage. Finally, in so far as lead provides a paradigm for the potentiation of radiation-related effects on the central nervous system through other toxic exposures, it is important to recognize that evaluation of the mother at the time of pregnancy may not predict the actual exposure of the embryo or fetus to a neurotoxin. In the case of lead, there is evidence that bone stores of this metal can be mobilized during pregnancy and cause rapid changes in internal exposure.

152. Brock et al. [B11], as well as others, have shown that chemically induced injury to the postnatal mammalian brain is often manifested by alterations in the cytoarchitecture of specific neuroanatomical regions. More importantly, they have shown that these anatomic changes are accompanied by quantitative changes in the proteins associated with specific cell types. Thus, for example, the organometallic compound trimethyltin, which preferentially destroys the neurons of the limbic system, depresses the concentration of the synaptic vesicle proteins synapsin I and p38 but increases that of glial fibrillary acid protein (GFAP) in a dose-related manner. This suggests a widespread astrocytic response to the chemical, since GFAP is the major protein of intermediate filaments in astrocytes. Presumably trimethyltin stimulates astrocyte division and, possibly, other glial elements as well. Whether this also occurs in the prenatal brain is not clear; however, it is known that the radial glial cells that provide guidance during migration of the immature neurons to the cortex will ultimately develop into astrocytes and, possibly, oligodendroglial cells [C5]

once their guidance function ceases. Astrocytes have many neuronal characteristics, such as neurotransmitter receptors, ion channels and neurotransmitter uptake systems. Moreover, it has been shown that cultured astrocytes express certain neuropeptide genes preferentially and specifically for the brain region from which the cultured cells were derived, suggesting that the peptides synthesized in astrocytes may play a role in the development of the central nervous system [S10].

153. ***Summary.*** The information available on exposure of the developing human brain to protracted doses of ionizing radiation is still too limited to permit estimates of risk at low dose rates; however, the animal data that are available suggest that the risk is lower but the degree of attenuation is uncertain. Moreover, it is difficult to extrapolate this information to the human case because of the differences in duration of the relevant neuroembryologic events. Data on exposure to neurotoxic chemicals have provided some insight into the molecular and cellular events associated with such exposures, which may be pertinent to radiation-related brain damage.

C. UNCERTAINTIES

154. Estimates of risks from prenatal radiation exposure of the developing human brain have been derived only from the high-dose-rate, acute exposures of survivors of the atomic bombings of Hiroshima and Nagasaki. Many uncertainties are associated with these risk estimates. They include the limited nature of the data, especially on mental retardation and seizures, the appropriateness of the comparison group, errors in the estimates of the tissue absorbed doses and in the estimates of prenatal ages at exposure. Moreover, there are other confounding factors that would play a role. Socio-economic circumstances in the final year of the war and immediately thereafter were stringent, affecting both the availability of food and the resources to treat disease. Thus, maternal nutrition and health status and the possibility of intercurrent disease could contribute to higher risks than might be seen otherwise.

155. ***Sample size and comparison group.*** Only 21 of the 30 severely mentally retarded individuals in the Clinical Sample received fetal absorbed doses estimated to be 0.01 Gy or more, and three of these had health problems that could account for their retardation, making it unrelated to radiation (two cases of Down's syndrome and one case of Japanese encephalitis in infancy). With their removal, there are only 18 cases in the critical period without known cause and might be attributable to exposure to ionizing radiation or other factors.

156. As to the comparison group, the atomic bombings resulted in exceptional circumstances that could have altered the normal frequency of severe mental retardation or have interacted non-additively with exposure. However, comparison of the frequency of mental retardation among children whose mothers were present in the city at the time of the bombing but received an estimated dose of less than 0.01 Gy with the frequency of severe mental retardation among children whose mothers migrated into these cities after the bombing reveals no difference.

157. ***Estimation of prenatal age.*** The apparent timing of vulnerable events in development can be affected by errors in the determination of prenatal age, possibly seriously so in specific cases. Gestational age is usually estimated from the onset of the last menstrual period, assuming that 280 days, on average, intervene between the beginning of menstruation and parturition. Post-ovulatory age is then calculated by subtracting two weeks. This method is sensitive to at least two types of errors, namely, misestimation of the onset of menstruation and that associated with the tacit assumption that all pregnancies proceed to term. If any terminated prematurely, as must surely have been true for some of the sample of prenatally exposed survivors in Hiroshima and Nagasaki, the estimated age of the child at exposure would be incorrect. Prematurity is generally determined by an infant's size and weight at birth, but these measurements were not routinely made and recorded in the months immediately following the bombings. At the initial physical examination of these survivors the mother was asked about the child's weight at birth. The trustworthiness of her recollections is uncertain, however, since a subsequent mail survey often revealed large discrepancies between the weight obtained at interview and that given in the survey. Women with irregular menstrual cycles or who miss a menstrual period for any of several reasons, notably lactational amenorrhea, illness or malnutrition, could erroneously identify the onset of their last cycle. Japanese women formerly nursed their infants longer, so lactational amenorrhea may have been more common. Some were undernourished due to the economic stringencies that obtained during and following the war, and infectious diseases were more frequent in the surviving populations. Another possible source of error may arise from variations between individuals in the prenatal age at which specific developmental events occur [M7, N4, S17]. This does not seem likely to be a major limitation of the data, but little or no information is available on the probable magnitude of this source of variability.

158. ***Dosimetry.*** All estimates of doses in the study of survivors of the atomic bombings in Japan are subject to at least three sources of error: (a) determinations of dose in air with distance from the epicentre,

(b) the attenuation factors for building materials and tissues and (c) the locations and positions of the survivors. Some of these, notably (c), can never be evaluated rigorously for all of the individuals concerned. Errors of this nature can affect inferences on the overall shape of the dose-response relationship as well as parameter values defining that shape [G3, G4, J3, P2]. Pierce et al. [P2] have shown that random dosimetric errors can lead to a 10%-15% underestimation of the cancer risk among the survivors, and presumably a similar error could obtain in the estimates described here. Nevertheless, there remain troublesome inconsistencies in the DS86 system, notably with regard to neutrons in Hiroshima. Straume et al. [S22], for example, using all of the available measurement data on thermal neutron activation including new measurements for ^{36}Cl, suggest that thermal neutron activation at about 1 km in Hiroshima was 2 to 10 or more times higher than that calculated based on DS86. The implications of this discrepancy with regard to risk estimates is not wholly clear, since it must be noted that low-energy neutron activation contributed little to the dose in Hiroshima. It is not presently known whether the fast neutrons, those with energies in the range ~0.1 to 1 MeV, which comprised the bulk of the neutron dose in Hiroshima, have been similarly underestimated. However, Preston et al. [P5] and Sasaki et al. [S23] have attempted to determine the possible impact of this discrepancy on risk estimates. Preston et al., based on several different assumptions regarding the neutron RBE, found that the cancer risk estimates might be in error by 2% to 20%; whereas Sasaki and his colleagues, using a series of *in vitro* experiments, found that the difference in chromosome aberration frequencies between the two cities is explicable if the neutron dose in Hiroshima was as large as 5% of the total dose in Gy rather than the estimate of 2% or less provided by the DS86 dosimetry.

159. ***Dose-response function.*** Within the period of maximum vulnerability, all the data on the prenatally exposed survivors of the atomic bombings of Hiroshima and Nagasaki can be satisfactorily approximated by more than one dose-response function. Given that neuronal death, mismanaged migration and faulty synaptogenesis could all play a role in the occurrence of mental retardation or other cortical dysfunction and that each could have its own different dose-response relationship, there is little or no prior basis for presuming that one or the other of these models better describes the fundamental biological events involved. The most appropriate model, therefore, remains a matter of conjecture, and it seems unlikely that epidemiological studies will ever be able to determine this. This means necessarily that the estimation of risk must rest on a series of considerations not all of which are biological.

160. First, the experimental data are often contradictory. Some of the disparity in results may reflect the choice of experimental animal; some investigators have used inbred strains of mice or rats and others outbred lines. Some may reflect the choice of the end-point measured. However, Hoshino et al. [H6] have reported the frequency of pycnotic cells to be linear with dose, even at doses below 0.24 Gy, and Wanner et al. [W9] reported a measurable, but not statistically significant, diminution in brain weight in guinea pigs at exposures as low as 0.04 Gy. More recently, Wagner et al. [W12] demonstrated a statistically significant diminution in the brain weight of guinea pigs exposed to 0.075 Gy on day 21 following conception (this corresponds to approximately week 5 or 6 following ovulation in the human). The loss in brain weight was approximately 1 mg mGy^{-1}. Studies of beagles exposed on the day 26 post-ovulation have shown a similar linear decrease in brain weight over a range of doses extending from 0.16 Gy to 3.6 Gy [H7]. Konermann [K7] has argued that the lowest dose in animals causing overt brain damage is generally 0.1 Gy or higher. This is consonant with other experimental studies. However, he noted that more subtle changes, such as the alignment of the small and medium-sized pyramidal neurons in the inner pyramidal cell layer of the mouse cortex, can be seen at doses as low as 0.025 Gy and that errors in alignment are marginally significant at 0.05 Gy ($p < 0.10$). It is not obvious what the occurrence of pycnotic cells or malaligned neurons is measuring in so far as functional brain damage is concerned. Nor is it clear what a loss in brain weight implies if the numerical densities of brain cells are increased, as has been reported [R14]. An increased cell density can, of course, mean less neuropil (fewer axons, dendrites and glial processes between the nerve cells), and it is reasonable to assume that fewer intercellular connections could reduce the quality of brain function.

161. Secondly, Müller et al. [M14], in a study of x-ray irradiation of preimplantation stages in the mouse, have shown that exposure at the single-cell stage can produce malformed fetuses, although the risk of death of the fetus is greater. They not only noted that the single-cell stage is characterized by a high radiation sensitivity but also asserted that their observations are best described by a linear-quadratic dose-response function without a threshold in this (their) special case. This conclusion, they contended, is consistent with theoretical considerations, since the exposure of a single cell differs from the exposure of polycytic stages in development, where the high capacity of embryonic cells to replace damaged cells and the need for a number of cells to be affected if a malformation is to ensue argues for a threshold. However, the fact that they found teratogenic effects following the exposure of a single cell, whereas most

other experimental studies have focused on later critical stages in development and have commonly found no evidence of a radiation-related effect, suggests that the mechanisms involved in their findings may be quite different from those of others. Indeed, Pampfer and Streffer [P4], in a study of female mice irradiated with neutrons (7 MeV) or x rays when the embryos were at an early zygote stage, interpreted their results as suggesting that the reactions of preimplantation embryos to irradiation could be more complex than the simple all-or-none response generally considered. In these experiments, the most commonly encountered malformation was gastroschisis, but omphaloceles and anencephalies were also observed [M21]. The proportion of malformed fetuses increased with dose in a linear-quadratic manner for both radiation qualities. These investigators estimated the relative biological effectiveness of neutrons in the induction of external malformations to lie between 2 and 3, increasing somewhat as the reference x-ray dose increased.

162. ***Extraneous variations.*** Alternative, non-radiation-related explanations can be found to cause or confound the effects to the developing human brain observed in the study of survivors of the atomic bombings in Japan. These include (a) genetic variation, (b) nutritional deprivation, (c) bacterial and viral infections in the course of pregnancy, and (d) embryonic or fetal hypoxemia, since there is substantial evidence to suggest that the cerebrum and its adnexa are especially sensitive to oxygen deprivation. There were also exposures to other potentially noxious physical or chemical agents, including the blast wave, the fumes associated with the extensive conflagration that followed the bombing, and the volatilization of chemicals, such as lead, the fires produced. The possible roles some of these may play in the present context have been explored elsewhere [M6, M16, O1], but the roles of others can only be a source of speculation, since no relevant data are available.

163. Mole [M18], in particular, has contended that the radiation-related depression of fetal haematopoiesis may have played an important role in the occurrence of severe mental retardation among the prenatally exposed survivors in Hiroshima and Nagasaki by reducing oxygen transport to the fetal brain. While the abscopal effect to which he alludes cannot be established unequivocally, it remains a contention to bear in mind in interpreting the human data. However, the issue of the oxygenation of the developing embryonic and fetal brain is a complex one, involving not only blood volume and concentration of haemoglobin, as Mole suggests, but also the specific haemoglobin present, since this affects the binding and unloading of oxygen. The earliest haemoglobins present in the developing individual, the embryonic ones, are produced in the yolk sac, but from about week 8 through week 28 after fertilization, the major site of erythropoiesis in the fetus is the liver and not the bone marrow [B14]. If a depression in erythropoiesis occurred at this time, it would have to entail damage to the haematopoietic cells in the liver or, to a lesser extent, perhaps, the spleen. The single case of fetal marrow irradiation at 21 weeks to which Mole alluded has little relevance, therefore, despite the fact that the marrow was apparently normal. The site of erythropoiesis does gradually shift from the liver and spleen to the bone marrow in the last half of gestation, making bone marrow depression a more important threat to the fetus at this later stage of development. This is not the time when the brain appears especially vulnerable. It is, of course, not known whether significant damage to the liver does or does not occur at the doses and times of relevance in the human case; however, studies of prenatal exposure of rats at comparable stages of development, 10 and 15 days of gestation, failed to show an alteration in liver weight as a percentage of body weight, although spleen weight did decrease [S13]. It would be reasonable to presume, nonetheless, that haematopoietic cells in the liver have the same sensitivity to radiation as those in the marrow itself and that a diminution in their number might not be reflected in liver weight. At about 9 weeks of gestation, the bulk (90%) of the haemoglobin to be found in fetal red cells is fetal haemoglobin, and even at birth this haemoglobin still accounts for 80% of the haemoglobin present. Fetal haemoglobin has a substantially enhanced alkaline Bohr effect, which in concert with the fall in pH of maternal blood as it passes through the placenta facilitating maternal oxygen unloading, maximizes oxygen transport to the fetus. Finally, the incidence of hypoxia-producing complications of late pregnancy does not appear to be significantly different among pregnancies terminating in a mentally handicapped child from that seen in general [D10].

164. No fully satisfactory assessment of the contribution of the sources of variation alluded to above can be made so many years after the event. It is only possible to speculate on their importance. Given the present uncertainties (since most of these extraneous sources of variation would have a greater impact at high than at low doses, and thus produce a concave upwards dose-response function), the careful course would be to assume that the dose-response relationship is not materially altered other than additively by these potential confounders. This would have the effect of overestimating the risk at low doses, which are of greatest concern in radiation protection.

IV. FUTURE PERSPECTIVES

165. Numerous events are involved in the processes that bring forth a functional brain, any one of which is potentially susceptible to radiation damage. There is clearly a need to confirm and extend the findings on cerebral cortical impairment following prenatal exposure to ionizing radiation described in the earlier paragraphs. To do so, however, will entail not only more neurologically focused clinical examinations, including the various non-invasive techniques now available to image the living brain, but a concerted effort, national and international, to identify groups of individuals prenatally exposed to ionizing radiation that might be able to contribute information. Such studies will have value well beyond the immediate assessment of the risk of prenatal exposure to radiation; they can contribute to a deeper understanding of human embryonic and fetal development, to a clearer appreciation of the diversity among individuals in the age at which specific embryonic or fetal landmarks are achieved, and to a sharper definition of the developmental ages most vulnerable to exposure to chemical or physical teratogens. Some methods of investigation which might be profitably exploited in future research studies are considered in this Chapter.

166. ***Epidemiological studies.*** The prenatally exposed survivors of the atomic bombing of Hiroshima and Nagasaki are unusual in many respects, not the least of which is the fact that they are the only group of survivors whose life experience subsequent to exposure can be followed literally from birth to death and who can thus provide unique insights into the effect of the exposure on central nervous system aging. As yet, however, there have been no studies directed at determining the effect of radiation on specific cortical functions. Nevertheless, many of these functions can be investigated with a surprising degree of precision, and the time at which cortical neurogenesis is initiated and its duration, are often reasonably well known. Particularly appealing as subjects of study are the various aspects of visual function. Some 30% or so of the human cortex appears to be involved in the processing of visual stimuli, and the mechanisms through which this processing occurs are better understood than for any other cortical area. Similarly, it has long been known that the brain exhibits weak electrical activity, which can be measured. Its recording is not painful or invasive, and other studies have revealed measurable radiation-related alterations in the normal record of these electrical potentials.

167. Future investigations of central nervous system impairment should look for damage not only to the cerebrum but also to the cerebellum and brain stem, to the extent that effects on the latter can be dissociated from effects on the former. Methods of visualizing the living brain such as magnetic resonance imaging (MRI) or positron emission tomography (PET) might give subclinical evidence of radiation-related central nervous system damage. If there are metabolic differences between neuronal and non-neuronal cells, PET scans, since they can measure some metabolic functions, could give evidence of impaired migration or of sites in the brain that are non-functional but seem to be histologically normal. Individuals with intractable seizures, for example, often have regions of the brain that show no functional activity yet appear grossly normal. Similarly, recent advances in MRI, which does not involve exposure to ionizing radiation, have made possible some functional measurements of brain activity, and further developments can be anticipated. Singly and collectively, these techniques hold great promise for furthering the understanding of the function and physiology of the brain in the healthy as well as the diseased state.

168. Of particular import have been the recent developments in MRI that allow functional parameters to be added to the information content of the images themselves (see, e.g. [M17]). Although these newer uses of MRI have not been applied to the study of functional damage to the brain following prenatal exposure to ionizing radiation, their promise seems great. High-resolution MRI, together with neurological findings has demonstrated, for example, that selective bilateral damage to the hippocampal formation is sufficient to cause significant, permanent memory impairment [S14]. Also, neuropsychological studies of patients with confirmed hippocampal damage suggest that the hippocampus is essential in the establishment of long-term memory. This role of the hippocampus appears to be a time-limited one, however, and ultimately the role is transferred to the neocortex [Z3]. Where practical, the use of these non-invasive but highly informative techniques should be encouraged in clinical as well as experimental studies. They could be the means not only of determining the functional impairment associated with grossly visible changes in the brain but also of identifying damage that cannot be related to gross morphological changes.

169. Radiation-related damage to the brain could also be evaluated by simpler means. Cognitive tests, such as those measuring word association, learning ability, memory and intelligence, could be informative. Moreover, in the light of experimental findings on other primates, careful studies of auditory and visual acuity and olfaction and taste should be useful. These might include the audiometric assessment of the left and right ears and the conventional appraisal of visual acuity. Smell and taste could be evaluated through exposure to a battery of tastes or aromas at different

concentrations. Evidence of premature loss of hearing or vision should be sought, since a lesser initial number of neuronal cells could lead to earlier manifestation of an aging central nervous system.

170. Still other neurophysiologic effects, with different critical periods, can be envisaged. Recently, for example, it has been shown that mice irradiated prenatally on day 18 (corresponding to about week 35 in the human) suffer a significant loss in spatial memory. The integrity of spatial memory appears to depend on the proper development of the hippocampus. This structure arises relatively late in the development of the human brain, but damage to it results in a recognized cognitive defect characterized by severe amnesia and evidenced by deficits in learning mazes. There is evidence that associates a reduction in the pyramidal cells within the hippocampus with memory impairment. Here even simple pencil-and-paper mazes might be informative.

171. Prenatal exposure to a nuclear accident might give rise to a dysfunctional child, either because of organic damage to the developing brain or because of the disturbed psychosocial milieu into which the child is born. The frequency, severity and pathogenesis of these psychosocial disorders have been poorly studied. If their origins are to be understood, the children found to be abnormal need to be studied to ascertain ways in which the children, families, and community and culture interact to cause psychosocial dysfunction and to form perceptions of risk. A child's perception of risk is not independently formed, but is inculcated, at least in part, by the attitudes of his or her age peers and family, and their attitudes are shaped, in turn, by community and culture. Thus, to understand the origin of psychosocial disorders arising out of a nuclear accident, it is essential to understand the workings of the larger milieu. Without this understanding, purely pragmatic ameliorative or preventive efforts are likely to be unproductive and ultimately self-defeating because they arouse expectations than cannot be fulfilled.

172. ***Experimental studies.*** Although no animal species is an ideal model for human brain development, experimental studies will and must continue to play an important role in understanding the effects of prenatal exposure on the developing human brain. Such studies can serve to confirm epidemiological findings in humans, to provide data on possible dose-response relationships and to afford insight into molecular and cellular mechanisms that is not easily available from human investigations. It warrants noting, as well, that extrapolations to the human being of molecular and cellular mechanisms revealed by animal experimentation are likely to be better than extrapolations based upon gross, phenotypic end-points, although the latter are often a necessary first step in the detection of radiation-related effects. Numerous questions of a mechanistic nature exist for which answers are not now available. For example, what initiates migration? How does the migrating neuron know that it has reached its destination, which is the point at which it disengages from its radial glial pathway? Recent advances in neuromolecular biology and the ability to culture specific neuronal cells *in vitro* hold promise for providing answers to these fundamental questions.

CONCLUSIONS

173. The human brain is relatively sensitive to ionizing radiation at certain stages in its prenatal development. Data from Hiroshima and Nagasaki, as well as from a few other studies, indicate that there can be consequences to the central nervous system from exposure to radiation at these stages. The abnormalities that have been observed correlate well with animal experiments and with current knowledge of the developmental embryology of the brain. It should be noted, however, that these findings do not represent a major public health problem. There were about 100,000 deaths at Hiroshima and Nagasaki, and somewhat more than 285,000 survivors. Among these survivors there were possibly as many as 10,000 pregnant women whose greatest immediate risk was the loss of their pregnancy. Although the observations on loss of pregnancy are limited, this risk appears to have been markedly elevated among those women in the first eight weeks of pregnancy, but it was also greater than normal among women in the 8-15 week interval [C15]. Nonetheless, the epidemiological data do indicate substantial risk of abnormalities in the central nervous system following high doses at certain periods of pregnancy. The risk is highest for exposures occurring during post-ovulatory weeks 8-15, that is, when the greatest number of neurons are produced and when they migrate to their functional sites in the cerebral cortex. During weeks 16-25 after ovulation, a lesser vulnerability is observed, with little apparent risk for exposures before week 8 or after week 25.

174. Among the prenatally exposed survivors of the atomic bombings of Hiroshima and Nagasaki who have been under clinical scrutiny, there are 30 cases of

severe mental retardation, some of which are probably not radiation-related, 30 with small head size without apparent mental retardation, 52 with seizures, of which 24 appear to be unprovoked (those with no clinically identifiable precipitating cause) and some with reduced intelligence quotient scores or with lower scholastic achievement in school.

175. Both severe mental retardation and lower intelligence test scores are observed to occur following prenatal exposures during the two sensitive periods of development previously described. These effects are mutually consistent if radiation is seen as operating on a continuum of qualities of brain function. The damage caused by exposure to 1 Gy within the most vulnerable period, namely 8-15 weeks after ovulation, increases the frequency of mental retardation to about 40% (background frequency: 0.8%), and lowers IQ by 25-30 points, which is consistent with the observed increase in mental retardation. The specific value of the IQ decrement depends on the sample used to estimate the risk and on whether the mentally retarded individuals are included in that sample. Prenatal exposure to 1 Gy in the most critical period appears to cause a decrement in average school performance score equivalent to the shifting of an average individual from the 50th percentile to the lower 10th percentile and increases the risk of unprovoked seizures by a factor of approximately 25. For the period 16-25 weeks, no cases of severe mental retardation were observed at exposures of less than 0.5 Gy. Thus, albeit with some uncertainty, a threshold could be assumed for that period. As to unprovoked seizures, at estimated doses in the range of 0.1 to 0.49 Gy the relative risk is 4.4; whereas at doses of 0.5 Gy or greater the relative risk is 14.5 when the cases of mental retardation are excluded from the data.

176. The risks cited in the preceding paragraphs assume the dose to have been an acute one. It is reasonable to assume, however, that these risks would be smaller for chronic exposure over the same critical periods, and this assumption is supported by the experimental animal information that is available. However, there are numerous potential confounding factors, and the human data are still far too limited to provide quantitative estimates of the possible reduction in risk at low doses.

177. The limitations in the data presently available and the uncertainties in the risk estimates have been pointed out. Definite risk estimates cannot be obtained at doses lower than 0.5 Gy or at low dose rates. The above estimates are therefore obviously provisional until additional evidence from further investigations can be obtained.

Table 1
Temporal pattern of brain development
[W10]

Post-ovulatory age	*Important developmental events*
3 weeks	Neural folds close to form neural tube Cervical region begins to form Cranial and cervical flexures appear Cranial and spinal motor nuclei develop
4 weeks	Paired optic vesicles evert; cranial and spinal nerves emerge Spinal ganglia develop and axons enter central nervous system Closure of neural tube
5 weeks	Diencephalic nuclei develop Pineal and hypophysis evert Eversion of cerebral vesicles Orbit and lens induced by the optic primordia Choroid plexus develops and cerebrospinal fluid fills neural tube Basal ganglia and amygdala develop Major cerebral arteries form Canalization and development of caudal spinal cord; posterior commissure develops Beginnings of the cerebellum and cerebellar nuclei appear Thinning of the roof of the 4th ventricle allows cerebrospinal fluid to flow out
6 weeks	Neural retina develops Olfactory nerves grow to base of brain; secretory vesicles appear in choroid plexus Beginnings of hippocampus and olfactory apparatus appear
7 weeks	Neocortical primordia appears Olfactory bulb everts Formation of pigmented retinal epithelium and ciliary body
8-11 weeks	Cortical plate appears in neocortex First synapses in the molecular and subplate regions of the neocortex Neurons migrate from the proliferative zones; optic nerve pathways form Proliferative zone of 3rd ventricle is exhausted Cortical plate of cerebellum appears Anterior commissure develops Cortical plate of the hippocampus appears Sylvan and hippocampal fissures form Skeletal muscle innervated and joint cavities appear Basal foramina and subarachnoid spaces open
12-15 weeks	Corpus callosum forms Cavum septum pellicidum formed Migration of neurons to neocortex in full swing Cortical wall triples in thickness Corticospinal fibers dessucate Purkinje cell migration complete, inward migration of external granule cells begins
16-20 weeks	Germinal zones of lateral ventricles are depleted Last wave of neocortical migration Prominence of subventricular germinal zone and first wave of glial migration Thalamocortical afferents invade the depths of the cortical plate, synapses appear and large pyramidal neurons begin to differentiate Cerebral subarachnoid spaces are open to the sagittal sinus Active phase of natural nerve cell death
20-24 weeks	Neuronal migration to neocortex complete Granule cells of cerebellum and dentate gyrus of hippocampus continue to proliferate and migrate Radial glial cells release ventricular attachments and migrate into cortex as protoplasmic astrocytes Primary gyri and sulci form Myelination begins Retinogeniculate, brain stem auditory and visual motor, and sensory lemniscal pathways are among the first to develop
25 weeks to end of term	Granule cell migration continues Glial proliferation continues Appearance of glial fibrils and acidic glial fibrillary protein signal increasing capacity for glial response to injury Secondary gyri and sulci form Maturation of supragranular neocortical layers begins Myelination of internal capsule begins Robust growth of dendrites and axons, and synaptogenesis

Table 2
Sites and levels of neuronal variation
[E2]

Genetic traits and developmental primary processes	*Variations in cell division, migration, adhesion, differentiation, death*
Cell morphology	Variation in cell shape and size; variation in dendritic and axonal arborizations (spatial distribution, branching order, length of branches, number of spines)
Connection patterns	Variations in number of inputs and outputs; connection order with other neurons; local versus long-range connections; degree of overlap of arbors
Cytoarchitectonics	Variation in number or density of cells; thickness of individual cortical layers; relative thickness of supragranular, infragranular and granular layers; position of somata; variation in columns; variation in strips or patches of terminations; variation in anisotropy of fibers
Transmitters	Variations between cells in a population; between cells at different times
Dynamic response	Variations in synaptic chemistry and size of synapse; in electrical properties; in excitatory/inhibitory ratios and locations of synapses; in short- and long-term synaptic alteration; in metabolic state
Neuronal transport	
Interactions with glia	

Table 3
Severely mentally retarded individuals exposed *in utero* to the atomic bombings in Japan
[O1]

File number	*Date of birth*	*Date of death*	*Cause of death*	Sex	Post-ovulatory age at exposure (weeks)	Absorbed dose in uterus (Gy)		Koga IQ score 1955-1956	Small head size	Significant clinical findings
						Total	Neutron			
Hiroshima										
245977	5.3.1946	14.1.1953	Malignant neoplasm of liver	F	8	1.4	0.01		Yes	Neo-natal jaundice
404239	1.3.1946			M	8	0.14	0		Yes	
246116	28.2.1946			M	8	0.87	0	64	Yes	
400590	25.2.1946			M	9	1.36	0.01		Yes	
471693	24.2.1946			M	9	0.69	0		Yes	
401141	12.2.1946			M	10	1.02	0		Yes	
400210	15.2.1946	21.1.1952	Ill-defined, unkown	F	11	2.22	0.01		Yes	
857279	11.2.1946			M	11	0.05	0		No	
401023	6.2.1946	28.6.1952	Accidental drowning	F	12	0.56	0		Yes	Down's syndrome
444522	4.2.1946			F	12	1.39	0.01		Yes	
401081	27.1.1946			F	13	1.64	0.01	56	Yes	
404032	23.1.1946			F	13	0.29	0		Yes	Down's syndrome
245763	15.1.1946	30.8.1958	Tuberculosis	M	15	0.61	0		Yes	
241728	11.1.1946			F	15	0.06	0		Yes	
312021	5.1.1946			F	16	0	0		Yes	
400716	12.12.1945	18.2.1970	Renal failure	M	19	1.23	0.01	64	No	
226683	12.12.1945	19.9.1956	Heart failure, epilepsy	M	20	0	0		No	Retarded sibling
433800	8.12.1945			F	20	0.03	0		No	Encephalitis at age 4
440463	22.11.1945			M	22	1.0	0	59	Yes	
440056	29.10.1945			M	26	0	0	60	No	
400133	22.9.1945	26.3.1966	Heart failure, epilepsy	F	31	0	0		No	
403929	18.8.1945			M	36	0	0		Yes	Down's syndrome
Nagasaki										
050968	22.4.1946			F	1	0	0		No	Possible birth trauma
078487	27.2.1946			M	9	1.16	0	62	No	Neurofibromatosis
142623	6.2.1946	14.3.1962	General symptoms, meningitis	M	12	1.18	0		Yes	
152396	26.1.1946			M	13	0	0		No	
143818	15.1.1946			M	15	1.46	0		Yes	
151845	15.1.1946			F	15	0	0	56	No	
078481	2.11.1945			F	25	1.79	0	60	No	
257021	25.9.1945			F	31	0	0		No	Congenital lues

Table 4
Severe mental retardation in individuals exposed *in utero* to the atomic bombings in Japan [a] [O1]

Post-ovulatory age	*Evaluation categories*	*Dose categories (Gy) [b]*					
		< 0.01	*0.01-0.09*	*0.10-0.49*	*0.50-0.99*	*≥ 1.0*	*Total*
Hiroshima							
0-7 weeks	Number of subjects Number retarded	145 0 (0%)	35 0 (0%)	24 0 (0%)	5 0 (0%)	1 0 (0%)	210 0 (0%)
8-15 weeks	Number of subjects Number retarded	209 0 (0%)	41 2 (4.9%)	50 1 (2.0%)	13 3 (23.1%)	9 6 (66.7%)	322 12 (3.7%)
16-25 weeks	Number of subjects Number retarded	243 2 (0.8%)	47 1 (2.1%)	46 0 (0%)	14 0 (0%)	7 2 (28.6%)	357 5 (14.0%)
≥ 26 weeks	Number of subjects Number retarded	227 2 (0.9%)	57 0 (0%)	47 0 (0%)	4 0 (0%)	2 0 (0%)	337 2 (0.6%)
All ages	Number of subjects Number retarded	824 4 (0.5%)	180 3 (1.7%)	167 1 (0.6%)	36 3 (8.3%)	19 8 (42.1%)	1226 19 (1.5%)
Nagasaki							
0-7 weeks	Number of subjects Number retarded	60 1 (1.7%)	6 0 (0%)	7 0 (0%)	0 0 (0%)	1 0 (0%)	74 1 (1.4%)
8-15 weeks	Number of subjects Number retarded	46 2 (4.3%)	3 0 (0%)	7 0 (0%)	2 0 (0%)	3 3 (100%)	61 5 (8.2%)
16-25 weeks	Number of subjects Number retarded	65 0 (0%)	8 0 (0%)	11 0 (0%)	2 0 (0%)	1 1 (100%)	87 1 (1.1%)
≥ 26 weeks	Number of subjects Number retarded	72 1 (1.4%)	4 0 (0%)	14 0 (0%)	1 0 (0%)	2 0 (0%)	93 1 (1.1%)
All ages	Number of subjects Number retarded	243 4 (1.6%)	21 0 (0%)	39 0 (0%)	5 0 (0%)	7 4 (57.1%)	315 8 (2.5%)
Both cities							
0-7 weeks	Number of subjects Number retarded	205 1 (0.5%)	41 0 (0%)	31 0 (0%)	5 0 (0%)	2 0 (0%)	284 1 (0.4%)
8-15 weeks	Number of subjects Number retarded	255 2 (0.8%)	44 2 (4.5%)	57 1 (1.8%)	15 3 (20.0%)	12 9 (75.0%)	383 17 (4.4%)
16-25 weeks	Number of subjects Number retarded	308 2 (0.6%)	55 1 (1.8%)	57 0 (0%)	16 0 (0%)	8 3 (37.5%)	444 6 (1.4%)
≥ 26 weeks	Number of subjects Number retarded	299 3 (1.0%)	61 0 (0%)	61 0 (0%)	5 0 (0%)	4 0 (0%)	430 3 (0.7%)
All ages	Number of subjects Number retarded	1067 8 (0.7%)	201 3 (1.5%)	206 1 (0.5%)	41 3 (7.3%)	26 12 (46.2%)	1541 27 (1.8%)

[a] Three cases of Down's syndrome have been excluded.
[b] DS86 uterine absorbed dose; mean doses within dose categories for total sample are 0, 0.05, 0.23, 0.64 and 1.38 Gy, respectively.

Table 5
Small head size in children exposed *in utero* to the atomic bombings in Japan
[O13]

Post-ovulatory age	*Evaluation categories*	*Dose categories (Gy)* [a]					
		< 0.01	*0.01-0.09*	*0.10-0.49*	*0.50-0.99*	*≥ 1.0*	*Total*
		Hiroshima					
First trimester	Number of subjects	222	57	52	9	3	343
	Number with small head size	7 (3.2%)	3 (5.3%)	12 (23.1%)	5 (55.7%)	2 (66.7%)	29 (8.5%)
	Number mentally retarded [b]	0, 0	0, 1	0, 1	2, 0	2, 0	4, 2
Second trimester	Number of subjects	317	62	57	17	10	463
	Number with small head size	3 (0.95%)	3 (4.8%)	4 (7.0%)	2 (11.8%)	3 (30.0%)	15 (3.2%)
	Number mentally retarded [b]	0, 1	1, 1	1, 0	1, 0	3, 1	6, 3
Third trimester	Number of subjects	229	61	46	7	2	345
	Number with small head size	5 (2.2%)	2 (3.3%)	1 (2.2%)	0 (0.0%)	0 (0.0%)	8 (2.3%)
	Number mentally retarded [b]	2, 1	0, 0	0, 0	0, 0	0, 0	2, 1
		Nagasaki					
First trimester	Number of subjects	88	9	15	1	3	116
	Number with small head size	0 (0.0%)	0 (0.0%)	1 (6.7%)	1 (100%)	3 (100%)	5 (4.3%)
	Number mentally retarded [b]	0, 1	0, 0	0, 0	0, 0	1, 0	1, 1
Second trimester	Number of subjects	80	9	12	3	2	106
	Number with small head size	2 (2.5%)	0 (0.0%)	0 (0.0%)	0 (0.0%)	2 (100%)	4 (3.8%)
	Number mentally retarded [b]	0, 2	0, 0	0, 0	0, 0	2, 0	2, 2
Third trimester	Number of subjects	74	7	15	1	3	100
	Number with small head size	0 (0.0%)	0 (0.0%)	1 (6.7%)	0 (0.0%)	0 (0.0%)	1 (1.0%)
	Number mentally retarded [b]	0, 1	0, 0	0, 0	0, 0	0, 1	0, 2
		Both cities					
First trimester	Number of subjects	310	66	67	10	6	459
	Number with small head size	7 (2.3%)	3 (4.6%)	13 (19.4%)	6 (60.0%)	5 (83.3%)	34 (7.4%)
	Number mentally retarded [b]	0, 1	0, 1	0, 1	2, 0	3, 0	5, 3
Second trimester	Number of subjects	397	71	69	20	12	569
	Number with small head size	5 (1.3%)	3 (4.2%)	4 (5.8%)	2 (10.0%)	5 (41.7%)	19 (3.3%)
	Number mentally retarded [b]	0, 3	1, 1	1, 0	1, 0	5, 1	8, 5
Third trimester	Number of subjects	303	68	61	8	5	445
	Number with small head size	5 (1.7%)	2 (2.9%)	2 (3.3%)	0 (0.0%)	0 (0.0%)	9 (2.0%)
	Number mentally retarded [b]	2, 2	0, 0	0, 0	0, 0	0, 1	2, 3
		Hiroshima					
0-7 weeks	Number of subjects	135	36	25	4	1	201
	Number with small head size	5 (3.7%)	3 (8.3%)	5 (20.0%)	2 (50.0%)	0 (0.0%)	15 (7.5%)
	Number mentally retarded [b]	0, 0	0, 0	0, 0	0, 0	0, 0	0, 0
8-15 weeks	Number of subjects	187	41	48	12	7	295
	Number with small head size	3 (1.6%)	1 (2.4%)	11 (22.9%)	5 (41.7%)	4 (57.1%)	24 (8.1%)
	Number mentally retarded [b]	0, 0	1, 1	1, 1	3, 0	4, 0	9, 2
16-25 weeks	Number of subjects	232	45	38	13	5	333
	Number with small head size	2 (0.9%)	2 (4.4%)	0 (0.0%)	0 (0.0%)	1 (20.0%)	5 (1.5%)
	Number mentally retarded [b]	0, 1	0, 1	0, 0	0, 0	1, 1	1, 3
≥ 26 weeks	Number of subjects	214	58	44	4	2	322
	Number with small head size	5 (2.3%)	2 (3.5%)	1 (2.3%)	0 (0.0%)	0 (0.0%)	8 (2.5%)
	Number mentally retarded [b]	2, 1	0, 0	0, 0	0, 0	0, 0	2, 1
		Nagasaki					
0-7 weeks	Number of subjects	60	7	7	0	1	75
	Number with small head size	0 (0.0%)	0 (0.0%)	1 (14.3%)	0 (0.0%)	1 (100%)	2 (2.7%)
	Number mentally retarded [b]	0, 1	0, 0	0, 0	0, 0	0, 0	0, 1
8-15 weeks	Number of subjects	46	4	9	2	4	65
	Number with small head size	0 (0.0%)	0 (0.0%)	0 (0.0%)	1 (50.0%)	4 (100%)	5 (7.7%)
	Number mentally retarded [b]	0, 2	0, 0	0, 0	0, 0	3, 0	3, 2

Table 5 (continued)

Post-ovulatory age	*Evaluation categories*	*Dose categories (Gy)* [a]					
		< 0.01	*0.01-0.09*	*0.10-0.49*	*0.50-0.99*	*≥ 1.0*	*Total*
16-25 weeks	Number of subjects	65	8	12	2	1	88
	Number with small head size	2 (3.1%)	0 (0.0%)	0 (0.0%)	0 (0.0%)	0 (0.0%)	2 (2.3%)
	Number mentally retarded [b]	0, 0	0, 0	0, 0	0, 0	0, 1	0, 1
≥ 26 weeks	Number of subjects	71	6	14	1	2	94
	Number with small head size	0 (0.0%)	0 (0.0%)	1 (7.1%)	0 (0.0%)	0 (0.0%)	1 (1.1%)
	Number mentally retarded [b]	0, 1	0, 0	0, 0	0, 0	0, 0	0, 1
Both cities							
0-7 weeks	Number of subjects	195	43	32	4	2	276
	Number with small head size	5 (2.6%)	3 (7.0%)	6 (18.8%)	2 (50.0%)	1 (50.0%)	17 (6.2%)
	Number mentally retarded [b]	0, 1	0, 0	0, 0	0, 0	0, 0	0, 1
8-15 weeks	Number of subjects	233	45	57	14	11	360
	Number with small head size	3 (1.3%)	1 (2.2%)	11 (19.3%)	6 (42.9%)	8 (72.7%)	29 (8.1%)
	Number mentally retarded [b]	0, 2	1, 1	1, 1	3, 0	7, 0	12, 4
16-25 weeks	Number of subjects	297	53	50	15	6	421
	Number with small head size	4 (1.4%)	2 (3.8%)	0 (0.0%)	0 (0.0%)	1 (16.7%)	7 (1.7%)
	Number mentally retarded [b]	0, 1	0, 1	0, 0	0, 0	1, 2	1, 4
≥ 26 weeks	Number of subjects	285	64	58	5	4	416
	Number with small head size	5 (1.8%)	2 (3.1%)	2 (3.5%)	0 (0.0%)	0 (0.0%)	9 (2.2%)
	Number mentally retarded [b]	2, 2	0, 0	0, 0	0, 0	0, 0	2, 2
Al ages	Number of subjects	1010	205	197	38	23	1473
	Number with small head size	17 (1.7%)	8 (3.9%)	19 (9.6%)	8 (21.1%)	10 (43.5%)	62 (4.2%)
	Number mentally retarded [b]	2, 6	1, 2	1, 1	3, 0	8, 2	15, 11

[a] DS86 uterine absorbed dose; mean doses within dose categories for total sample are 0, 0.05, 0.23, 0.63 and 1.30 Gy, respectively.
[b] Number of mentally retarded with small head size followed by number of mentally retarded with normal head size.

Table 6
Expected and observed incidence of small head size in individuals exposed *in utero* to the atomic bombings in Japan
[O13]

Post-ovulatory age	*Number of subjects*	*Number with small head size*	
		Expected [a]	*Observed* [b]
0-7 weeks	276	7	17 (0, 17)
8-15 weeks	360	9	29 (12, 17)
16-25 weeks	421	11	7 (1, 6)
≥ 26 weeks	416	10	9 (2, 7)
All ages	1473	37	62 (15, 47)

[a] Estimated from assumed 2.5% deviance in the normal distribution.
[b] Number with and without severe mental retardation given in parentheses.

Table 7
Regression coefficients obtained in fitting models to intelligence test scores and uterine absorbed dose for individuals exposed *in utero* to the atomic bombings in Japan
[S4]

Post-ovulatory age	*Regression model*	*Regression coefficient* [a]			*Significance level of*	
		a	*b*	*c*	*b*	*c*
Clinical subsample, all cases included						
0-7 weeks	Linear	106 ± 1.2	-2.7 ± 5.3			
8-15 weeks		108 ± 0.99	-29.0 ± 4.2		p < 0.01	
16-25 weeks		111 ± 0.89	-20.4 ± 4.4		p < 0.01	
≥ 26 weeks		107 ± 0.80	-4.2 ± 5.0			
All ages		108 ± 0.47	-15.8 ± 2.4		p < 0.01	
0-7 weeks	Linear-quadratic	107 ± 1.2	-34.0 ± 13.5	16.4 ± 6.5	p < 0.05	p < 0.05
8-15 weeks		108 ± 1.0	-25.8 ± 11.1	-2.9 ± 9.2	p < 0.05	
16-25 weeks		111 ± 0.91	-3.6 ± 9.3	-16.8 ± 8.2		p < 0.05
≥ 26 weeks		107 ± 0.82	-10.1 ± 12.8	7.1 ± 14.2		
All ages		109 ± 0.48	-20.7 ± 4.8	4.2 ± 3.6	p < 0.01	
PE-86 subsample, all cases included						
0-7 weeks	Linear	106 ± 0.94	-1.7 ± 5.1			
8-15 weeks		110 ± 0.92	-25.3 ± 4.0		p < 0.01	
16-25 weeks		110 ± 0.76	-21.4 ± 4.2		p < 0.01	
≥ 26 weeks		108 ± 0.68	-4.7 ± 5.0			
All ages		109 ± 0.40	-15.7 ± 2.2		p < 0.01	
0-7 weeks	Linear-quadratic	107 ± 0.97	-24.1 ± 12.5	12.1 ± 6.1	p < 0.10	p < 0.05
8-15 weeks		110 ± 0.97	-33.6 ± 9.7	6.1 ± 6.6	p < 0.01	
16-25 weeks		110 ± 0.77	-6.9 ± 8.8	-14.9 ± 8.0		p < 0.10
≥ 26 weeks		108 ± 0.71	-11.9 ± 12.5	8.8 ± 14.0		
All ages		109 ± 0.42	-20.2 ± 4.6	3.7 ± 3.3	p < 0.01	
Clinical subsample, retardation cases excluded						
0-7 weeks	Linear	106 ± 1.2	-2.7 ± 5.3			
8-15 weeks		108 ± 0.98	-25.0 ± 5.1		p < 0.01	
16-25 weeks		111 ± 0.89	-9.8 ± 5.7		p < 0.10	
≥ 26 weeks		107 ± 0.79	-4.4 ± 5.0			
All ages		108 ± 0.47	-10.2 ± 2.6		p < 0.01	
0-7 weeks	Linear-quadratic	107 ± 1.2	-34.0 ± 13.5	16.4 ± 6.5	p < 0.05	p < 0.05
8-15 weeks		108 ± 1.0	-26.1 ± 12.2	1.2 ± 11.7	p < 0.05	
16-25 weeks		111 ± 0.92	-5.9 ± 15.6	-6.2 ± 23.3		
≥ 26 weeks		108 ± 0.82	-10.8 ± 12.7	7.7 ± 14.0		
All ages		109 ± 0.48	-19.0 ± 4.8	8.1 ± 3.8	p < 0.01	p < 0.05
PE-86 subsample, retardation cases excluded						
0-7 weeks	Linear	106 ± 0.94	-1.7 ± 5.1			
8-15 weeks		110 ± 0.91	-21.0 ± 4.5		p < 0.01	
16-25 weeks		110 ± 0.76	-13.3 ± 5.2		p < 0.01	
≥ 26 weeks		108 ± 0.68	-4.9 ± 5.0			
All ages		108 ± 0.40	-11.0 ± 2.5		p < 0.01	
0-7 weeks	Linear-quadratic	107 ± 0.97	-24.1 ± 12.5	12.1 ± 6.1	p < 0.10	p < 0.05
8-15 weeks		110 ± 0.94	-29.3 ± 9.9	6.3 ± 6.7	p < 0.01	
16-25 weeks		110 ± 0.79	-5.1 ± 15.0	-12.8 ± 22.0		
≥ 26 weeks		108 ± 0.70	-12.5 ± 12.4	9.3 ± 13.9		
All ages		109 ± 0.41	-17.8 ± 4.6	5.9 ± 3.4	p < 0.01	p < 0.10

[a] The regression coefficient a is the estimated IQ score at zero dose (intercept); b is the increase in IQ score per unit dose (Gy^{-1}); c is the increase in IQ score per unit dose squared (Gy^{-2}).

Table 8
Regression coefficients obtained in fitting models to average school performance and uterine absorbed dose for individuals exposed *in utero* to the atomic bombings in Japan
[O2]

Post-ovulatory age	*Regression model*	*Regression coefficient* [a]			*Significance level of*	
		a	*b*	*c*	*b*	*c*
			First grade			
0-7 weeks	Linear	3.09 ± 0.08	0.23 ± 0.32			
8-15 weeks		2.86 ± 0.06	-1.15 ± 0.22		p < 0.01	
16-25 weeks		3.03 ± 0.05	-0.97 ± 0.24		p < 0.01	
≥ 26 weeks		3.11 ± 0.05	0.23 ± 0.36			
All ages		3.03 ± 0.03	-0.70 ± 0.14		p < 0.01	
0-7 weeks	Linear-quadratic	3.18 ± 0.08	-2.68 ± 0.89	1.38 ± 0.40	p < 0.01	p < 0.01
8-15 weeks		2.87 ± 0.06	-1.21 ± 0.58	0.06 ± 0.48	p < 0.05	
16-25 weeks		3.05 ± 0.05	-1.53 ± 0.72	0.67 ± 0.80	p < 0.05	
≥ 26 weeks		3.10 ± 0.05	0.84 ± 0.79	-0.82 ± 0.95		
All ages		3.05 ± 0.03	-1.51 ± 0.27	0.70 ± 0.20	p < 0.01	p < 0.01
			Second grade			
0-7 weeks	Linear	3.09 ± 0.09	0.36 ± 0.34			
8-15 weeks		2.86 ± 0.06	-1.27 ± 0.22		p < 0.01	
16-25 weeks		3.05 ± 0.05	-0.96 ± 0.24		p < 0.01	
≥ 26 weeks		3.16 ± 0.05	0.01 ± 0.36			
All ages		3.05 ± 0.03	-0.76 ± 0.14		p < 0.01	
0-7 weeks	Linear-quadratic	3.17 ± 0.09	-2.14 ± 0.98	1.19 ± 0.44	p < 0.05	p < 0.01
8-15 weeks		2.86 ± 0.06	-1.14 ± 0.57	-0.12 ± 0.48	p < 0.05	
16-25 weeks		3.06 ± 0.05	-1.79 ± 0.72	0.97 ± 0.80	p < 0.05	
≥ 26 weeks		3.15 ± 0.05	0.21 ± 0.80	-0.28 ± 0.97		
All ages		3.07 ± 0.03	-1.64 ± 0.27	0.76 ± 0.20	p < 0.01	p < 0.01
			Third grade			
0-7 weeks	Linear	3.11 ± 0.10	0.12 ± 0.38			
8-15 weeks		2.86 ± 0.06	-1.17 ± 0.25		p < 0.01	
16-25 weeks		3.02 ± 0.06	-1.01 ± 0.25		p < 0.01	
≥ 26 weeks		3.10 ± 0.05	-0.06 ± 0.37			
All ages		3.02 ± 0.03	-0.74 ± 0.15		p < 0.01	
0-7 weeks	Linear-quadratic	3.21 ± 0.10	-3.04 ± 1.08	1.50 ± 0.48	p < 0.01	p < 0.01
8-15 weeks		2.86 ± 0.06	-0.90 ± 0.62	-0.25 ± 0.54		
16-25 weeks		3.02 ± 0.06	-1.17 ± 0.77	0.19 ± 0.85		
≥ 26 weeks		3.10 ± 0.05	-0.13 ± 0.81	0.10 ± 0.98		
All ages		3.05 ± 0.03	-1.57 ± 0.29	0.73 ± 0.21	p < 0.01	p < 0.01
			Fourth grade			
0-7 weeks	Linear	2.78 ± 0.11	-1.72 ± 0.84		p < 0.05	
8-15 weeks		2.88 ± 0.06	-0.95 ± 0.42		p < 0.05	
16-25 weeks		3.03 ± 0.05	-1.09 ± 0.26		p < 0.01	
≥ 26 weeks		3.13 ± 0.05	-0.35 ± 0.32			
All ages		3.02 ± 0.03	-0.89 ± 0.18		p < 0.01	
0-7 weeks	Linear-quadratic	2.82 ± 0.11	-4.42 ± 2.88	5.66 ± 5.78		
8-15 weeks		2.89 ± 0.07	-1.52 ± 0.98	0.90 ± 1.39		
16-25 weeks		3.05 ± 0.06	-1.88 ± 0.75	0.95 ± 0.84	p < 0.05	
≥ 26 weeks		3.13 ± 0.05	-0.44 ± 0.78	0.11 ± 0.88		
All ages		3.03 ± 0.03	-1.52 ± 0.45	0.82 ± 0.54	p < 0.01	

[a] The regression coefficient a is the mean school score at zero dose (intercept); b is the increase in mean school score per unit dose (Gy^{-1}); c is the increase in mean school score per unit dose squared (Gy^{-2}).

Table 9
Regression coefficients obtained in fitting a linear model to seizures and uterine absorbed dose for individuals exposed *in utero* to the atomic bombings in Japan
[O3]

Post-ovulatory age	*Regression model*	*Regression coefficient* [a]		*Significance level of b*
		a	*b*	
All seizures				
0-7 weeks [b]	Linear	4.55	-0.046 ± 0.34	
8-15 weeks [b]		2.51	0.18 ± 0.087	$p < 0.05$
8-15 weeks [b, c]		3.87	0.15 ± 0.084	$p < 0.10$
16-25 weeks [b]		4.73	0.001 ± 0.052	
≥ 26 weeks [b]		3.89	0.024 ± 0.064	
All ages [b]		3.97	0.054 ± 0.037	$p < 0.10$
0-7 weeks [d]	Linear	4.62	-0.058 ± 0.12	
8-15 weeks [d]		2.61	0.11 ± 0.11	
8-15 weeks [c, d]		3.70	0.083 ± 0.10	
16-25 weeks [d]		4.39	0.016 ± 0.067	
≥ 26 weeks [d]		3.62	0.029 ± 0.071	
All ages [d]		3.88	0.026 ± 0.040	
Febrile seizures				
0-7 weeks [b]	Linear	4.06	-0.041 ± 0.34	
8-15 weeks [b]		1.80	-0.018 ± 0.071	
8-15 weeks [b, c]		2.21	-0.023 ± 0.073	
16-25 weeks [b]		2.79	-0.030 ± 0.048	
≥ 26 weeks [b]		1.81	0.033 ± 0.052	
All ages [b]		2.46	-0.012 ± 0.015	
0-7 weeks [d]	Linear	4.10	-0.050 ± 0.30	
8-15 weeks [d]		1.96	-0.018 ± 0.081	
8-15 weeks [c, d]		2.21	-0.028 ± 0.017	$p < 0.10$
16-25 weeks [d]		2.83	-0.036 ± 0.11	
≥ 26 weeks [d]		1.84	0.033 ± 0.056	
All ages [d]		2.61	-0.013 ± 0.021	
Unprovoked seizures				
0-7 weeks [b]	Linear	-	-	
8-15 weeks [b]		0.89	0.20 ± 0.084	$p < 0.01$
8-15 weeks [b, c]		1.71	0.18 ± 0.083	$p < 0.05$
16-25 weeks [b]		1.98	0.042 ± 0.054	
≥ 26 weeks [b]		1.89	-0.019 ± 0.070	
All ages [b]		1.45	0.074 ± 0.033	$p < 0.05$
0-7 weeks [d]	Linear	-	-	
8-15 weeks [d]		0.921	0.15 ± 0.10	$p < 0.10$
8-15 weeks [c, d]		1.50	0.13 ± 0.099	
16-25 weeks [d]		1.58	0.067 ± 0.065	
≥ 26 weeks [d]		1.69	-0.018 ± 0.065	
All ages [d]		1.30	0.052 ± 0.035	$p < 0.10$

[a] The regression coefficient a is the number of seizures per 100 individuals at zero dose (intercept); b is the increase in frequency of seizures per unit dose (Gy^{-1}).
[b] Cases of severe mental retardation included in sample.
[c] Pooled controls. Data for controls (> 0.01 Gy) over all gestational ages were used.
[d] Cases of severe mental retardation excluded from sample.

Table 10
Regression coefficients and estimated thresholds obtained in fitting a linear model to seizures and uterine absorbed dose for individuals exposed *in utero* to the atomic bombings in Japan
[O1]

Post-ovulatory age	*Regression model*	*Regression coefficient* [a]		*Significance level of b*	*Threshold* [b] *(Gy)*
		a	*b*		
All seizures					
8-15 weeks [c] 8-15 weeks [c, d] All ages [c]	Linear with threshold	2.71 3.94 4.08	0.26 ± 0.13 0.25 ± 0.14 0.10 ± 0.06	$p < 0.05$ $p < 0.10$ $p < 0.10$	0.15 0.20 0.23
8-15 weeks [e] 8-15 weeks [d, e] All ages [e]	Linear with threshold	2.70 3.72 3.93	0.17 ± 0.16 0.17 ± 0.20 0.06 ± 0.07		0.11 0.17 0.23
Unprovoked seizures					
8-15 weeks [c] 8-15 weeks [c, d] All ages [c]	Linear with threshold	0.90 1.72 1.44	0.26 ± 0.11 0.25 ± 0.11 0.09 ± 0.04	$p < 0.01$ $p < 0.05$ $p < 0.05$	0.08 0.11 0.04
8-15 weeks [e] 8-15 weeks [d, e] All ages [e]	Linear with threshold	0.91 1.49 1.28	0.19 ± 0.13 0.17 ± 0.12 0.07 ± 0.04	$p < 0.10$ $p < 0.10$	0.04 0.04 0.04

[a] The regression coefficient a is the number of seizures per 100 individuals at zero dose (intercept); b is the increase in frequency of seizures per unit dose (Gy^{-1}).
[b] 95% CI in parentheses.
[c] Cases of severe mental retardation included in sample.
[d] Pooled controls.
[e] Cases of severe mental retardation excluded from sample.

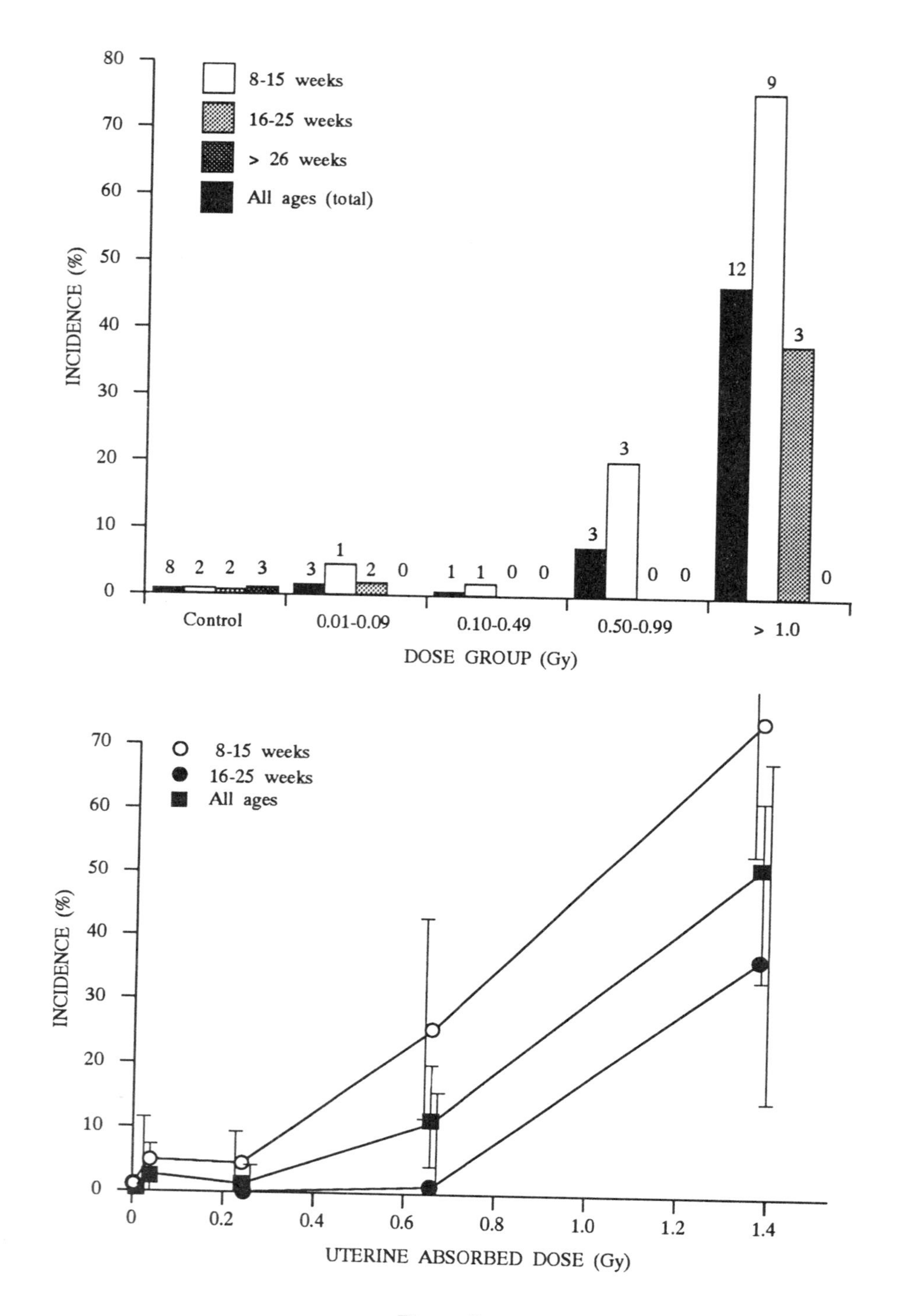

Figure I.
Incidence of severe mental retardation in individuals exposed *in utero* to the atomic bombings in Japan. Number of cases indicated in upper figure. Total number of cases is 27; one case in controls exposed at 0-7 weeks not shown; three cases of Down's syndrome excluded.
[O1]

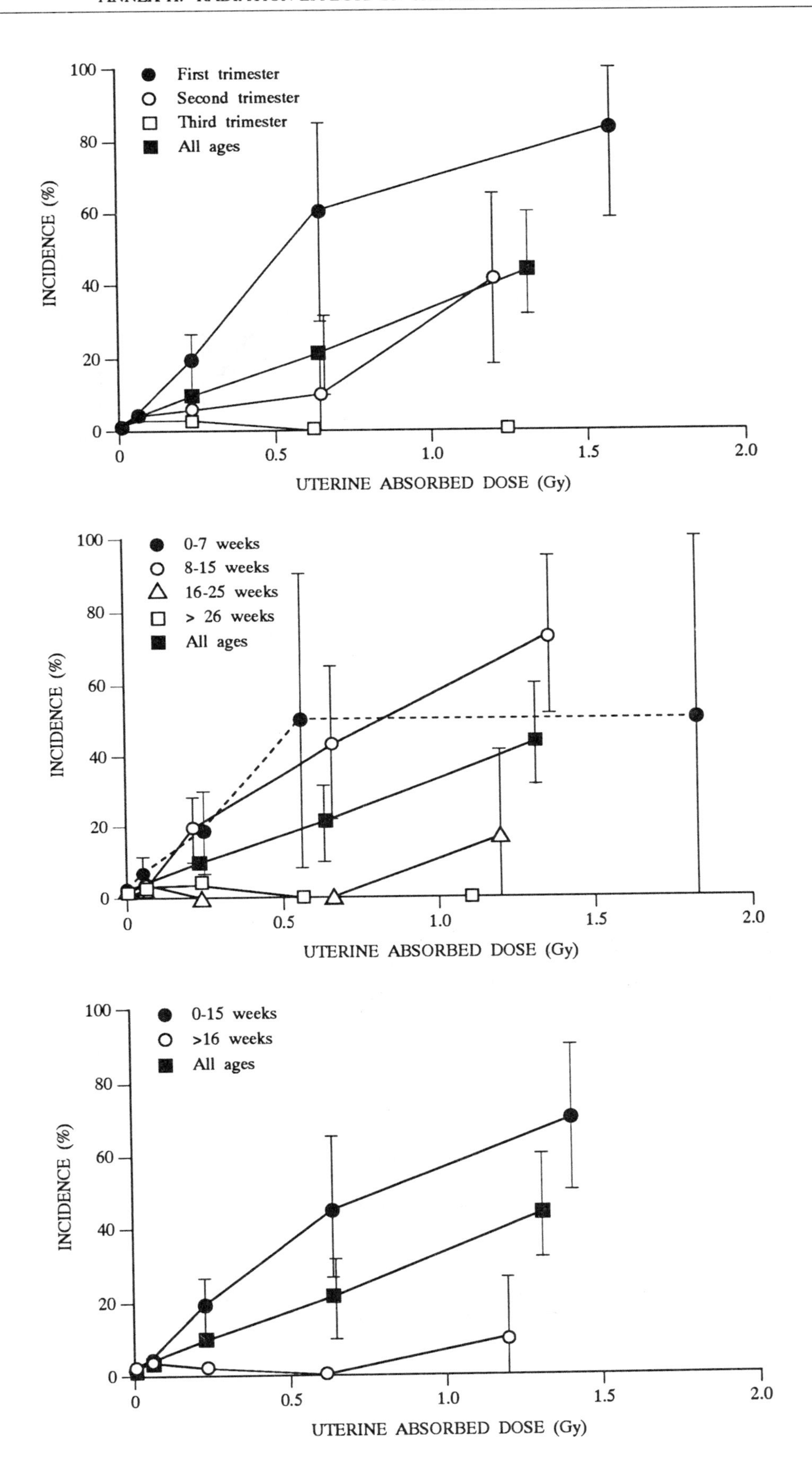

Figure II.
Incidence of small head size in individuals exposed *in utero* to the atomic bombings in Japan [O13]

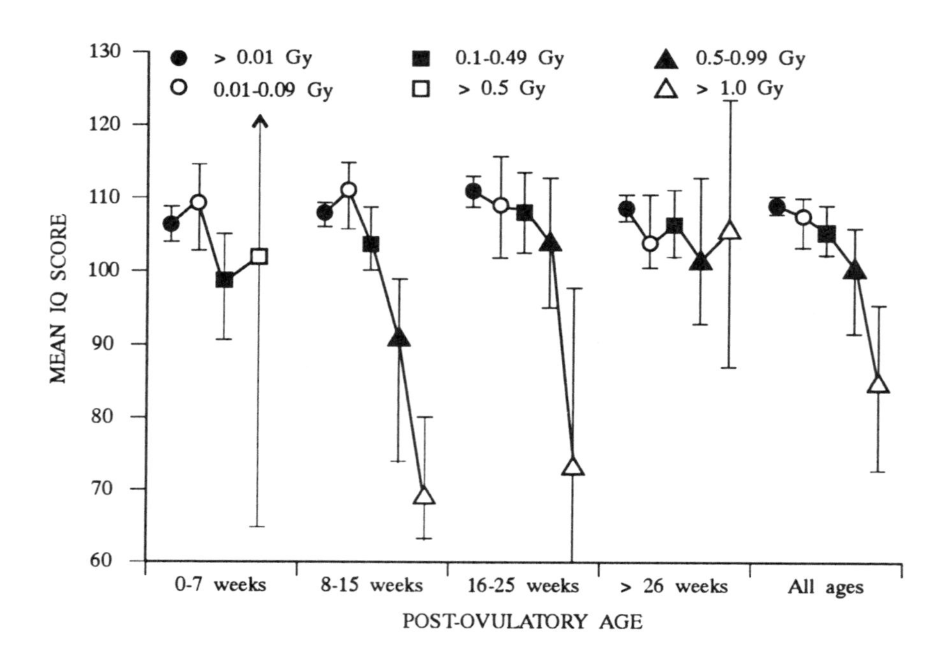

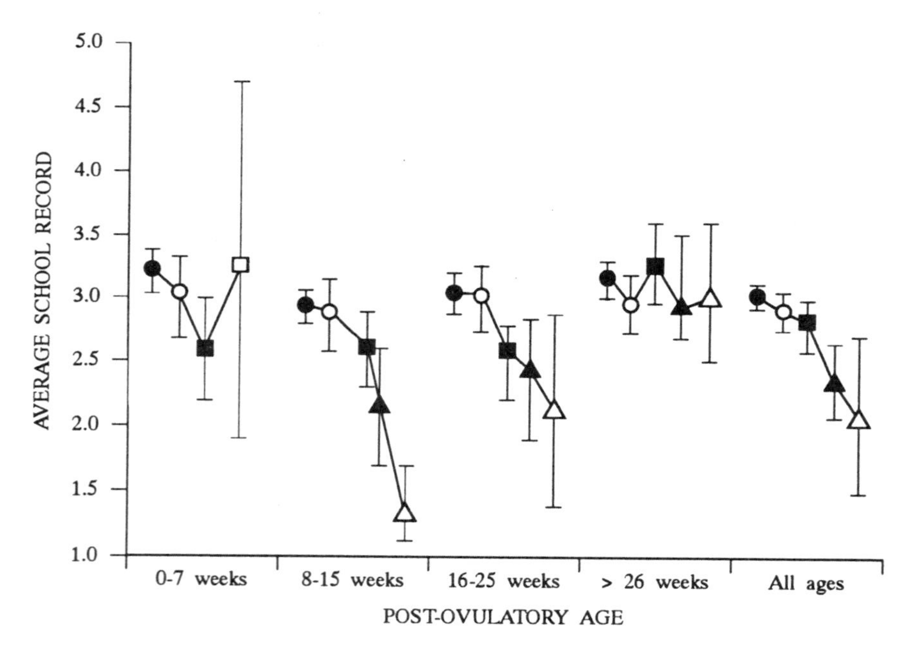

Figure III.
Change in intelligence scores and school performance in individuals exposed *in utero* to the atomic bombings in Japan [O2, S4]

Glossary

abscopal	the effect on non-irradiated tissue of the irradiation of other tissues of an organism
acallosal	in the context used here, implying without a corpus callosum
anencephaly	a congenital anomaly of the brain with the absence of the bones of the cranial vault; usually the cerebral and cerebellar hemispheres are lacking and the brain stem is rudimentary.
anosmia	the inability to smell
apoptosis	a particular form of cell death, apparently programmed, in which death occurs relatively rapidly without conspicuous damage to the cell membrane
arborization, dendritic	development of the tree-like network of nerve processes
astrocyte	a star-shaped neuroglia cell; the final differentiated form of the radial glial cells that provide guidance to the neurons as they migrate from the proliferative zones surrounding the ventricles to the cortex
axon	a nerve fibre that is continuous with the body of a nerve cell and is the essential stimulus conducting portion of the cell. It consists of a series of neurofibrils surrounded by a well-defined sheath, known as the axolemma; the latter is in turn encased in myelin, a mixture of lipids, and a final sheath, the neurolemma.
brain	the mass of nervous matter that lies within the cranium or skull and consists of a number of discrete parts, such as the brain stem, the cerebrum and the cerebellum
brain mantle	the distinctively laminated layering of grey matter covering the cerebral hemispheres
brain stem	the portion of the brain that connects the cerebrum with the spinal column
Broca's area	the region in the left hemisphere involved in language. It lies in the frontal lobe above the lateral sulcus (the Sylvian fissure) between the two anterior limbs of this fissure. It is also known as the parolfactory area or the area subcallosa.
bulb, olfactory	the greyish expanded forward extremity of the olfactory tract, lying on a sieve-like plate above the ethmoid bone and receiving the olfactory nerves
CAM	an abbreviation of the words cell adhesion molecule; a number of surface molecules are known, such as N-CAM, a molecule that allows one neuron to recognize another, or Ng-CAM, that is involved in neuron-glial recognition. N-CAM exists in at least two forms, an embryonic (E-N-CAM) and an adult, which differ in the degree of sialylation.
caudate nucleus	a long horse shoe-shaped mass of grey matter that is closely related to the lateral ventricle throughout its entire length. It consists of a head, a body and a tail.
cerebellum	the posterior portion of the brain, consisting of two hemispheres connected by a narrow mass of tissue known as the vermis
cerebrum	the largest portion of the brain including the cerebral hemispheres. In its earlier stages of development, the cerebrum is characterized by four major layers, namely, the mantle, the outermost margin of the brain; the cortical plate; the intermediate or migratory zone; and the matrix or proliferative zone.
cingulum	a well-marked band of nerve fibres lying immediately above the corpus callosum that relate the cingulate to the hippocampal gyri
cisterna magna	the largest of the cisterns lying in the space between the pia mater and the arachnoid membrane of the brain; it lies between the under surface of the cerebellum and the posterior surface of the medulla oblongata. The term mega cisterna magna implies an abnormal enlargement of this cistern.
coloboma	a mutilation of a structure, generally of the eye. For example, coloboma iridis is a congenital cleft of the iris.
commissure	a bundle of nerve fibres passing from one side to the other of the brain
corpus callosum	the great transverse commissure between the two cerebral hemispheres; it lies beneath the longitudinal fissure and is covered on each side by the cingulate gyrus.

cortex	the outer layers of the cerebral hemispheres and the cerebellum where most of the neurons in the brain are located. The cells of the cortex are arranged in extensive, stacked layers that are distinguishable histologically. Six layers are recognized, namely, the molecular or plexiform layer (Layer I), the outer granule cell layer (II), the outer pyramidal cell layer (III), the inner granule cell layer (IV), the inner pyramidal cell layer (V) and the polymorphous layer (VI). Layer V, the inner pyramidal cell layer, is often further subdivided into two sublayers, known as V_a and V_b. V_a consists of small and medium-sized pyramidal neurons, whereas V_b is made up of large pyramidal neurons. The spheres of projection of these two sublayers are also different.
cortico-cortical cells	the most superficial of the cells of the cortex
cytoarchitectonics	the cytoarchitecture of a structure, particularly the cerebral cortex, where different areas may be mapped according to the manner in which various cells are distributed in the cell layers
dendrite	one of the branching protoplasmic processes of the nerve cell
diencephalon	the part of the brain that includes the thalamus and related structures. It is derived from the posterior part of the prosencephalon.
DS86	the revised system of computing the gamma and neutron doses received by the survivors of the atomic bombing of Hiroshima and Nagasaki; this system was introduced in 1986, hence the acronym DS86 (dosimetry system 1986).
dyslexia (severe)	an uncorrectable inability to read understandably, now attributed to a specific lesion in the language centre of the brain located in the left temporal lobe
ectopia	as used in the present context, the displacement or malpositioning of neuronal cells; synonymous with heterotopia
encephalomeningocele	a protrusion of the brain and its membranes through a bony defect in the skull
enolase, neuron-specific	a form of the glycolytic enzyme enolase, or phosphopyruvate hydratase, which appears to be restricted to neuronal and neuroendocrine tissues and can be a useful marker for neuronal damage
ependymal layer	the layer of cells that line the ventricles; the term subependymal implies the region beneath the ependymal layer.
folia cerebelli	the narrow, leaf-like gyri of the cerebellar cortex
fragile X syndrome	an inherited, X-linked form of mental retardation associated with a characteristic secondary constriction (often called a fragile site) of the X-chromosome. The extent of the mental retardation can vary substantially.
ganglia (ganglion)	a term generally used to describe a knot or knot-like collection of nerve cell bodies outside the central nervous system
gap junction	the cells of a multicellular organism are able to influence the activities of one another through a variety of processes. Collectively, these processes are referred to as inter-cellular communication. Adjacent cells, for example, can transport small molecules back and forth through their cell walls by means of a specific channel, known as the gap junction. Their capacity to do this, however, is influenced or modulated by a number of factors, such as the calcium levels within the cells. Regulation of this communication through gap junctions is presumed to play a role in the occurrence of cancer and in the development of the brain.
gastroschisis	a congenital defect in the abdominal wall, usually with protrusion of the viscera
GFAP	glial fibrillary acid protein, a biochemical marker of glial cells
glomerulus, olfactory	a rounded body in the olfactory bulb formed by the synapses of dendrites of one class of olfactory cells, known as mitral cells, with the axons of the olfactory cells of the nasal mucous membrane
granular neurons	one of the five discrete types of neuronal cells found in the cerebellum; these cells arise in the outer granular layer of the cerebellar cortex and migrate inwards to their sites of function. They make synaptic connections with the spiny processes on the Purkinje cell.
growth cone	the specialized end of a growing axon (or dendrite) that provides the motive force for its elongation

gyrus	one of the prominent rounded elevations of the surface of the hemispheres of the brain; the cingulate gyrus or the callosal gyrus, a synonym, is a long, curved convolution that arches over the corpus callosum.
hemianopsia, homonomous	defective vision or blindness affecting the right halves or the left halves of the visual fields of the two eyes
heterochromia iridis	a difference in coloration of the iris of the two eyes, or different parts of the iris of the same eye
heterotopia	see ectopia
hippocampus	a deeply infolded portion of the cerebral cortex, lying on the floor of the inferior horn of the lateral ventricle. It is a submerged elevation that forms the largest part of the olfactory cortex. It is now thought to be involved in learning and memory since damage to it results in a recognized cognitive defect characterized by severe amnesia and includes deficits in learning mazes.
holoprosencephaly	a failure of the forebrain to divide into hemispheres
horseradish peroxidase	an enzyme derived from horseradish that catalyzes the oxidation of certain compounds by peroxide
hydrocephaly	a condition marked by the excessive accumulation of fluid in the cerebral ventricles, resulting in a thinning of the brain and causing a separation of the cranial bones
hypergonadotrophism	the overproduction or excretion of the gonadotrophic hormones, the hormones of pituitary origin
hypogonadism	inadequate gonadal function, represented either by deficiencies in gametogenesis or the secretion of gonadal hormones
leptomeninges	the combined pia mater and the middle layer of membranes covering the brain and spinal cord known as the arachnoid
LHRH cells (luteinizing hormone releasing hormone cells)	these are specialized ciliated neurons that arise in the olfactory placode and migrate into the cerebrum. Their function is to release the hormone that stimulates the production of the luteinizing hormone, which in turn is involved in the elaboration of the sex hormones.
limbic system	a group of subcortical structures of the brain (the hippocampus, hypothalamus, amygdala) that are concerned with emotions and motivations
macrogyria (also called pachygyria)	a developmental abnormality of the brain in which the gyri are fewer in number than expected and relatively broad, and the sulci are short, shallow and straighter than normal. In its most extreme form, known as argyria or lissencephaly, there may be a total or almost total absence of gyri. Macrogyria is an abnormality in neuronal migration.
mamillary bodies	two protuberances on the under surface of the brain beneath the corpus callosum; they are a part of the brain known as the hypothalamus.
medulla oblongata	the portion of the brain that is continuous above with the pons and below with the spinal cord
mesencephalon (or midbrain)	the part of the central nervous system that arises from the middle portion of the initial divisions of the embryonic neural tube
micrencephaly (microencephaly)	abnormal smallness of the brain
motoneuron (motor neuron)	a neuron that enervates muscle fibres
motor cortex	the region of the cortex lying in front of the central furrow, or sulcus, that divides the cerebral hemispheres into anterior and posterior portions. It is the site of the processing of motor impulses.
myelin	a mixture of lipids arranged around the axons of nerve fibres. Myelination refers to the development or formation of the myelin sheath around a nerve fibre.
neocortex	the laminated, evolutionarily younger portion of the cerebral cortex in humans and higher vertebrates
neurite	see axon

neuroblasts — embryonic cells that develop into neurons

neurofibromatosis, multiple (von Recklinghausen's disease) — an inherited neurological disorder characterized generally by the appearance early in childhood of discrete, small, pigmented lesions in the skin, followed by the development of multiple subcutaneous neurofibroma. The latter can develop along almost any nerve trunk. Two different types of this disorder have been identified, each associated with a different genetic locus.

neuroglia (or often just, glia) — the non-nervous cellular components of the nervous system; they provide support to the developing structures of the nervous system and perform important metabolic functions. There are a variety of different glial cells, distinguishable by their morphology and function. One especially important group is the transitory set, known as radial glia cells, that provide guidance to the neurons as they migrate from the proliferative zones to their sites of function.

neuron — a nerve cell, consisting of the cell body and its various processes, the dendrites, axons and ending. Neurons do not normally divide.

neuropil — a collective term describing the network of neuroglia, axons and dendrites and their synapses in the brain

nucleus accumbens septi — an area of the brain immediately beneath the head of the caudate nucleus and medial to the putamen

oligodendroglia — a class of neuroglial cells having few processes that form a sheath around nerve fibres or a capsule around nerve cell bodies

olfactory bulb — a specialized area on the ventral aspect of the cerebral hemispheres, distinguishable about mid-gestation; related to the development of olfaction

omphalocele — congenital protrusion of the abdominal viscera at the umbilicus

optic tectum — the first central station in the visual pathway of many vertebrates. It is located in the midbrain and is analogous in mammals to the superior colliculus, a rounded eminence on the dorsal aspect of the mesencephalon concerned with visual reflexes.

oxycephaly — a condition in which the top of the head is pointed

pachygyria — see macrogyria

paleocortex — the cortex of the primate brain is often divided on the basis of the antiquity of origin of specific segments; the paleocortex is the evolutionarily older part (the neocortex in the younger) and includes the olfactory cortex.

parahippocampal gyrus — a convolution of the interior surface of each cerebral hemisphere, lying between the hippocampal and collateral sulci (or furrows)

PE-86 sample — the sample of prenatally exposed survivors in Hiroshima and Nagasaki. It was constructed, beginning in 1955, based upon birth registrations, ad hoc censuses by the city authorities and the Atomic Bomb Casualty Commission, and interviews of women who were enrolled in the genetics programme in these cities in 1948-1954 and were possibly pregnant at the time of the bombing.

periventricular (or circumventricular) — meaning around the ventricles of the brain

pia mater — the innermost of the three membranes (or meninges) that cover the brain spinal cord. The other two membranes are known as the dura mater, the outermost of the three, and the arachnoid that lies between the pia and dura maters. The arachnoid membrane is separated from the pia mater by the subarachnoid space.

placode, olfactory — a thickening of embryonic cells lying in the bottom of the olfactory pit as the pits are deepened by the growth of the surrounding nasal processes

plasmalemma — the plasma membrane

premotor cortex — the region of the cortex of the brain lying just before the motor cortex, where complex motor movements are organized

prosencephalon (or forebrain) — the most forward part of the three primary division of the neural tube; it gives rise to the diencephalon and telencephalon.

Purkinje cell — a large nerve cell of the cerebellar cortex; these cells are the only ones in the cerebellum that carry nerve impulses out of the cerebellum itself.

pyknosis (also spelled pycnosis)	a degeneration of a cell in which the nucleus shrinks in size and the chromatin condenses into a solid, structureless mass
radial glia	a specialized group of neuroglia cells that assist immature neurons in their migration to the cortical plate; later in the development of the brain these cells will differentiate into astrocytes.
Rathke's pouch	a pouch of embryonic ectoderm that gives rise to the anterior lobe of the pituitary body
rhinencephalon	one of the portions of the telencephalon, specifically that part comprising the structures toward the centre of the furrow separating the forward part of the parahippocampal gyrus from the remainder of the temporal lobe of the brain
rhombencephalon (or hindbrain)	the most posterior of the three initial divisions of the neural tube; it subsequently gives rise to the metencephalon and the mylencephalon.
schizencephaly	an abnormality of the development of the brain in which there are abnormal divisions or clefts of the brain substance
somatosensory cortex	that portion of the cortex of the brain that is involved in the processing of sensory stimuli that arise in the body outside of the brain
subarachnoid	implying beneath the arachnoidea, a delicate membrane interposed between the dura and pia maters; the subarachnoid space lies between the arachnoidea and the pia mater.
subplate neurons	a special group of early arising neurons that appear to be instrumental in the laying down of the first axonal pathways; also known as transient pioneer neurons
sulcus	one of the grooves or furrows on the surface of the brain that bounds or delimits the convolutions, the gyri. The sulcus that separates the corpus callosum from the gyrus cinguli is called the sulcus corporis callosi.
syncytium	a multinucleated protoplasmic mass formed by the secondary union of originally separate cells
synaptogenesis	the process or processes that culminate in the formation of synapses, that is, the places where a nerve impulse is transmitted from one neuron to another
telencephalon	the part of the brain that includes the cerebral hemispheres and is derived from the foremost part of the neural tube
tinea capitis	infection of the skin of the scalp with one or several different genera of fungi
uterine myomatosis	the occurrence of benign neoplasms in the musculature of the uterus
ventricles	as used here, the cavities within the brain derived from the lumen, or open canal, of the primitive neural tube. The term ventricular is used to describe the layer in the brain immediately adjacent to the ventricles.
von Recklinghausen's disease	see neurofibromatosis, multiple

References

A1 Albert, R.E., A.R. Omran, E.W. Brauer et al. Follow-up study of patients treated by x ray for tinea capitis. Am. J. Public Health 56: 2114-2120 (1966).

A2 Altman, J. and J.W. Anderson. Experimental reorganization of the cerebellar cortex. Morphological effects of elimination of all microneurons with prolonged X-irradiation started at birth. Volume 1. J. Comp. Neurol. 146: 355-406 (1972).

A3 Antal, S., A. Fonagy, Z. Fulop et al. Decreased weight, DNA, RNA and protein content of the brain after neutron irradiation of the 18-day mouse embryo. Int. J. Radiat. Biol. 46: 425-433 (1984).

B1 Bogaert, L. van and M.A Radermecker. Une dysgenesie cerebelleuse chez un enfant du radium. Rev. Neurol. 93: 65-82 (1955).

B2 Blot, W.J. and R.W Miller. Small head size following in utero exposure to atomic radiation, Hiroshima and Nagasaki. ABCC TR/35-72 (1972).

B3 Brent, R.L. Radiation teratogenesis. Teratology 21: 281-298 (1980).

B4 Brent, R.L. Effects of ionizing radiation on growth and development. Contr. Epidemiol. Biostat. 1: 147-183 (1979).

B5 Brizzee, K.R., J.M. Ordy, M.B. Kaack et al. Effect of prenatal ionizing radiation on the visual cortex and hippocampus of newborn squirrel monkeys. J. Neuropathol. Exp. Neurol. 39: 523-540 (1980).

B6 Brizzee, K.R., J.M. Ordy and A.N. D'Agostino. Morphological changes of the central nervous system after radiation exposure in utero. p. 145-173 in: Developmental Effects of Prenatal Irradiation. Gustav Fischer Verlag, Stuttgart, 1982.

B7 Beebe, G.W. and M. Usagawa. The major ABCC samples. ABCC TR/12-68 (1968).

B8 Brun, A. The subpial granular layer of the foetal cerebral cortex in man: its ontogeny and significance in congenital cortical malformations. Acta Pathol. Microbiol. Scand. 179 (Suppl.): 7-98 (1965).

B9 Beardsley, R.K., J.W. Hall and R.E. Ward. p. 498 in: Village Japan: A Study Based on Niiike Buraku. University of Chicago Press, Chicago, 1959.

B10 Brizzee, K.R. and R.B Brannon. Cell recovery in foetal brain after ionizing radiation. Int. J. Radiat. Biol. 21: 375-388 (1972).

B11 Brock, T.O. and J.P. O'Callahan. Quantitative changes in the synaptic vesicle proteins synapsin I and p38 and the astrocyte-specific protein glial fibrillary acidic protein are associated with chemical-injury to the rat central nervous system. J. Neurosci. 7: 931-942 (1987).

B12 Brizzee, K.R. and J.M. Ordy. Effects of prenatal ionizing irradiation on neural function and behavior. p. 255-282 in: Radiation Risks to the Developing Nervous System. (H. Kriegel et al., eds.) Gustav Fischer Verlag, Stuttgart, New York, 1986.

B13 Byrd, S.E., R.E. Osborn and T.P. Bohan. Computed tomography in the evaluation of the migration disorders of the brain. Part II: Schizencephaly, heterotopia, and polymicrogyria. J. Med. Imaging 2: 232-239 (1988).

B14 Bunn, H.F. and B.G. Foreyt. Hemoglobin: Molecular, Genetic and Clinical Aspects. Chapter 4. p. vii and 690. W.B. Saunders, Philadelphia, 1986.

B15 Baier, H. and F. Bonhoeffer. Axon guidance by gradients of a target-derived component. Science 255: 472-475 (1992).

B16 Barth, P.G. Disorders of neuronal migration. Can. J. Neurol. Sci. 14: 1-16 (1987).

B17 Bridges, B.A. and D.G. Harnden (eds.). Ataxia-Telangiectasia. John Wiley and Sons, Chichester, 1982.

C1 Caviness, V.S. and P. Rakic. Mechanisms of cortical development: a view from mutations in mice. Annu. Rev. Neurosci. 1: 297-326 (1978).

C2 Chi, J.G., E.C. Dooling and F.H. Gilles. Gyral development of the human brain. Ann. Neurol. 1: 86-93 (1977).

C3 Clarren, S.K., E.C. Alvord, M.S. Sumi et al. Brain malformations related to prenatal exposure to ethanol. J. Pediatr. 92: 64-67 (1978).

C4 Clarren, S.K. and D.M. Bowden. Fetal alcohol syndrome: a new primate model for binge drinking and its relevance to human ethanol teratogenesis. J. Pediatr. 101: 819-824 (1982).

C5 Choi, B.H., R.C. Kim and L.W. Lapham. Do radial glia give rise to both astroglial and oligodendroglial cells? Dev. Brain Res. 8: 119-130 (1983).

C6 Caviness, V.S. Jr. Normal development of cerebral neocortex. Dev. Neurobiol. 12: 1-10 (1989).

C7 Commission on Radiological Protection of the Federal Republic of Germany. Effects of Pre-natal Irradiation. Gustav Fischer Verlag, Stuttgart, 1989.

C8 Coquerel, C., E. Jeannot, A. Loeb et al. A brain damage marker with prognostic value in newborns: neuron-specific enolase in cerebrospinal fluid. Eur. J. Nucl. Med. 16 (Suppl.): S131 (1990).

C9 Chuong, C.-M., K.L. Crossin and G.M. Edelman. Sequential expression and differential function of multiple adhesion molecules during the formation of cerebellar cortical layers. J. Cell Biol. 104: 331-342 (1987).

C10 Crome, L. and J.F. Stern. Pathology of Mental Retardation (2nd edition). The Williams and Wilkins Company, Baltimore, 1972.

C11 Christiansen, E., J.C. Melchior and G.V. Bredmose. A survey of neuropathological findings in 175 mentally retarded patients. in: Proceedings of the International Copenhagen Congress on the Scientific Study of Mental Retardation. Volume 1. Copenhagen, 1964.

C12 Cowen, D. and L.M. Geller. Long-term pathological effects of prenatal X-irradiation on the central nervous system of the rat. J. Neuropathol. Exp. Neurol. 19: 488-527 (1960).

C13 Cox, R., P.G. Debenham, W.K. Masson et al. Ataxia-telangiectasia: a human mutation giving high frequency misrepair of DNA double strand scissions. Mol. Biol. Med. 3: 229-244 (1986).

C14 Cox, R. A cellular description of the repair defect ataxia-telangiectasia. p. 141-153 in: Ataxia-telangiectasia. (B.A. Bridges and D.G. Harnden, eds.) John Wiley and Sons, Chichester, 1982.

C15 Committee for the Compilation of Materials on Damage Caused by the Atomic Bombs in Hiroshima and Nagasaki. p. xiv and 706 in: Hiroshima and Nagasaki: The Physical, Medical, and Social Effects of the Atomic Bombings. Iwanami Shoten, Tokyo, 1981.

D1 Dobbing, J. The developing brain: a plea for more critical interspecies extrapolation. Nutr. Rep. Int. 7: 401-406 (1973).

D2 D'Amato, C.J. and S.P. Hicks. Effects of low levels of ionizing radiation on the developing cerebral cortex of the rat. Neurology 15: 1104-1116 (1965).

D3 Dunn, K., H. Yoshimaru, M. Otake et al. Prenatal exposure to ionizing radiation and subsequent development of seizures. Am. J. Epidemiol. 131: 114-123 (1990). See also RERF TR/5-88 (1988).

D4 Diamond, E.L., H. Schmerler and A.M. Lilienfeld. The relationship of intra-uterine radiation to subsequent mortality and development of leukemia in children. Am. J. Epidemiol. 97: 283-313 (1973).

D5 Driscoll, S.G., S.P. Hicks, E.H. Copenhaver et al. Acute radiation injury in two human fetuses. Arch. Pathol. 76: 125-131 (1963).

D6 Dobbing, J. and J. Sands. Comparative aspects of the brain growth spurt. Early Hum. Dev. 3: 109-126 (1979).

D7 Dobbing, J. The later development of the brain and its vulnerability. in: Scientific Foundations of Pediatrics (2nd edition). (J.A. Davis and J. Dobbing, eds.) William Heineman, London, 1981.

D8 Donoso, J.A. and S. Norton. The pyramidal neuron in cerebral cortex following prenatal X-irradiation. Neurotoxicology 3: 72-84 (1982).

D9 De Bleecker, J., J. de Reuck, J.J. Martin et al. Autosomal recessive inheritance of polymicrogyria and dermatomyositis with paracrystalline inclusions. Clin. Neuropath. 9: 299-304 (1990).

D10 Drillien, C.M. Studies in mental handicap. II: Some obstetric factors of possible aetiological significance. Arch. Dis. Childhood 43: 283-294 (1968).

E1 Eiser, C. Intellectual abilities among survivors of childhood leukemia as a function of CNS irradiation. Arch. Dis. Childhood 53: 391-395 (1978).

E2 Edelman, G.M. Neural Darwinism: The Theory of Neuronal Group Selection. Basic Books, New York, 1987.

F1 Fushiki, S. Cell-to-cell interactions during development of the neocortex, with special reference to neuronal migration. Congenit. Anom. 28: 111-125 (1988).

F2 Fushiki, S., A. Soshiki, M. Kusakabe et al. Analyses on the cellular mechanisms of histogenesis in the mouse cerebrum with scanning electron microscope fractography, cultures and chimeras. Proceedings of the International Symposium on Growth and Aging of the Brain: Clinical, Cellular and Molecular Aspects. J. Kyoto Prefectural Medical University 101 (Suppl.): 14-30 (1983).

F3 Feinendegen, L.E., H. Mühlensiepen, W. Proschen et al. Acute non-stochastic effect of very low dose whole-body exposure, a thymidine equivalent serum factor. Int. J. Radiat. Biol. 41: 139-150 (1982).

F4 Feinendegen, L.E., H. Mühlensiepen, C. Lindberg et al. Acute and temporary inhibition of thymidine kinase in mouse bone marrow cells after low-dose exposure. Int. J. Radiat. Biol. 45: 205-215 (1984).

F5 Filjushkin, I.V. On the mechanism of induction of congenital nervous and immune deficiencies in newborns resulting from in utero exposure to radiation and other risk factors. Radiobiology 5: (1993, in press).

G1 Goldstein, L. and D.P. Murphy. Etiology of the ill-health in children born after maternal pelvic irradiation. Part 2. Defective children born after post-conception pelvic irradiation. Am. J. Roentgenol. 22: 322-331 (1929).

G2 Granroth, G. Defects of the central nervous system in Finland. IV. Associations with diagnostic X-ray examinations. Am. J. Obstet. Gynecol. 133: 191-194 (1979).

G3 Gilbert, E.S. Some effects of random dose measurement errors on analysis of atomic bomb survivor data. Radiat. Res. 98: 591-605 (1984).

G4 Gilbert, E.S. and J.L. Ohara. An analysis of various aspects of atomic bomb dose estimation at RERF using data on acute radiation symptoms. Radiat. Res. 100: 124-138 (1984).

G5 Geschwind, N. and A.M. Galaburda. Anatomical asymmetries. p. 11-25 in: Cerebral Dominance: The Biological Foundations. Harvard University Press, Cambridge, Massachussetts, 1984.

G6 Galaburda, A.M. and T.L. Kemper. Cytoarchitectonic abnormalities in developmental dyslexia: a case study. Ann. Neurol. 6: 94-100 (1979).

G7 Goldman-Rakic, P.S. and P. Rakic. Experimental modification of gyral patterns. p. 179-194 in: Cerebral Dominance: The Biological Foundations. (N. Geschwind and A.M. Galaburda, eds.) Harvard University Press, Cambridge, Massachussetts, 1984.

G8 Griem, M.L., P. Meier and G.D. Dobben. Analysis of the morbidity and mortality of children irradiated in fetal life. Radiology 88: 347-349 (1967).

G9 Gazzaniga, M.S. Organization of the human brain. Science 245: 947-952 (1989).

G10 Guerke, W. and W. Goetze. EEG changes, psychomotor epilepsy and intracranial calcification occurring as late results of radiation therapy. Clin. Elec. 2: 146-153 (1971).

G11 Gobe, G.C., R.A. Axelsen, B.V. Harmon et al. Cell death by apoptosis following X-irradiation of the foetal and neonatal rat kidney. Int. J. Radiat. Biol. 54: 567-576 (1988).

H1 Hicks, S.P. and C.J. D'Amato. Effects of radiation on development, especially of the nervous system. Am. J. Forensic Med. Pathol. 1: 309-317 (1980).

H2 Hicks, S.P. and C.J. D'Amato. Effects of ionizing radiation on mammalian development. p. 196-250 in: Advances in Teratology. Volume 1. (D.H.M. Woollum, ed.) Logos Press, London, 1966.

H3 Hochberg, F.H. and B. Slotnick. Neurospsychologic impairment in astrocytoma survivors. Neurology 30: 172-177 (1980).

H4 Hammer, R.P. et al. Morphologic evidence for a delay of neuronal migration in fetal alcohol syndrome. Exp. Neurol. 74: 587-596 (1981).

H5 Hashizume, T., T. Maruyama, K. Nishizawa et al. Dose estimation of human fetus exposed in utero to radiations from atomic bombs in Hiroshima and Nagasaki. J. Radiat. Res. 14: 346-362 (1973).

H6 Hoshino, K. and Y. Kameyama. Developmental-stage-dependent radiosensitivity of neural cells in the ventricular zone of telencephalon in mouse and rat fetuses. Teratology 37: 257-262 (1988).

H7 Hamilton, B.F., S.A. Benjamin, G.M. Angleton et al. The effect of prenatal ^{60}Co-gamma radiation on brain weight in beagles. Radiat. Res. 119: 366-379 (1989).

H8 Hu, Y.M. and J.X. Yao. Effect of prenatalexposure to diagnostic radiation on childhood physical and intellectual development. Chin. J. Radiol. Med. Prot. 12: 2-6 (1992). (in Chinese)

H9 Hicks, S.P., C.J. D'Amato and M.J. Lowe. The development of the mammalian nervous system. I. Malformations of the brain, especially of the cerebral cortex, induced in rats by ionizing radiation. II. Some mechanisms of the malformations of the cortex. J. Comp. Neurol. 113: 435-469 (1959).

H10 Harmon, B.V. and D.J. Allan. X-ray induced cell death by apoptosis in immature rat cerebellum. Scanning Microsc. 2: 561-568 (1988).

H11 Hicks, S.P., C.A. Schaufus, A.A. Williams et al. Some effects of ionizing radiation and metabolic inhibition of the developing mammalian nervous system. J. Pediatr. 40: 489-513 (1952).

H12 Hoffman, S., D.R. Friedlander, C.-M. Chuong et al. Differential contributions of Ng-CAM and N-CAM to cell adhesion in different neural regions. J. Cell Biol. 103: 145-158 (1986).

H13 Hicks, S.P. and C.J. D'Amato. Malformation and regeneration of the mammalian retina following experimental radiation. p. 45-51 in: Les Phakomatoses Cerebrales, Deuxieme Colloque Internationale, Malformations Congenitales de L'Encephale. (L. Michaux and M. Feld, eds.) S.P.E.I., Paris, 1963.

H14 Hekmat, A., D. Bitter-Suermann and M. Schachner. Immunocytological localization of the highly polysialylated form of the neural cell adhesion molecule during development of the murine cerebellar cortex. J. Comp. Neurol. 291: 457-467 (1990).

H15 Hatten, M.A. and R.H.K. Liem. Astroglia provide a template for the positioning of cerebellar neurons in vitro. J. Cell Biol. 90: 622-630 (1981).

H16 Hatten, M.A., R.H.K. Liem and C.A. Mason. Defects in specific associations between astroglia and neurons occur in microcultures of weaver mouse cerebellar cells. J. Neurosci. 4: 1163-1172 (1984).

H17 Hu, Y.M. and J.X. Yao. Long-term effects of prenatal diagnostic X-rays on childhood physical and intellectual development. J. Radiat. Res. (1993, in press).

H18 Huttenlocher, P.R. Dendritic and synaptic pathology in mental retardation. Pediatr. Neurol. 7: 79-85 (1991).

H19 Harbord, M.G., S. Boyd, M.A. Hall-Crags et al. Ataxia, developmental delay and an extensive neuronal migration abnormality in 2 siblings. Neuropediatrics 21: 218-221 (1990).

H20 Hicks, S.P. Developmental malformations produced by radiation. A time table of their development. Am. J. Roentgenol. 69: 272-293 (1953).

I1 International Commission on Radiological Protection. Developmental effects of irradiation on the brain of the embryo and fetus. ICRP Publication 49. Pergamon Press, Oxford, 1986.

I2 International Commission on Radiological Protection. 1990 Recommendations of the International Commission on Radiological Protection. ICRP Publication 60. Annals of the ICRP 21 (1-3). Pergamon Press, Oxford, 1991.

I3 Inskip, M.J. and J.K. Piotrowski. Review of health effects of methyl-mercury. J. Appl. Toxicol. 5: 113-133 (1985).

I4 Iwanaga, T., Y. Takahashi and T. Fujita. Immunohistochemistry of neuron-specific and glia-specific protenis. Arch. Histol. Cyto. 52 (Suppl.): 13-24 (1989).

I5 Ilyin, L.A., M.I. Balonov, L.A. Buldakov et al. Radiocontamination patterns and possible health consequences of the accident at the Chernobyl nuclear power station. J. Radiol. Prot. 10: 3-29 (1990).

I6 Inoue, M., M. Tamaru and Y. Kameyama. Effects of cycloheximide and actinomycin D on radiation-induced apototic cell death in the developing mouse cerebellum. Int. J. Radiat. Biol. 61: 669-674 (1992).

J1 Jacobs, L.A. and K.R. Brizzee. Effects of total-body X-irradiation in single and fractionated doses on developing cerebral cortex in rat foetus. Nature 210: 31-33 (1966).

J2 Jordaan, H.V. Development of the central nervous system in prenatal life. Obstet. Gynecol. 53: 146-150 (1979).

J3 Jablon, S. Atomic bomb radiation dose estimation at ABCC. ABCC TR/23-71 (1971).

J4 Jensh, R.P. and R.L. Brent. Effects of 0.6 Gy prenatal irradiation on postnatal neurophysiologic development in the Wistar rat. Proc. Soc. Exp. Biol. Med. 181: 611-619 (1986).

J5 Jensh, R.P. and R.L. Brent. The effect of low-level prenatal X-irradiation on postnatal development in the Wistar rat. Proc. Soc. Exp. Biol. Med. 184: 256-263 (1987).

K1 Koga, Y. Two intelligence test methods viewed in relation to evaluated intelligence. p. 923-988 in: Collection of Reports in Commemoration of Dr. Matsumoto, Studies in Psychology and Arts, Tokyo, 1937. (in Japanese.)

K2 Kemper, T.L. Asymmetrical lesions in dyslexia. p. 75-92 in: Cerebral Dominance: The Biological Foundations. (N. Geschwind and A.M. Galaburda, eds.) Harvard University Press, Cambridge, Massachussetts, 1984.

K3 Kerr, G.D. Organ dose estimates for the Japanese atomic bomb survivors. Health Phys. 37: 487-508 (1979).

K4 Klose, M. and D. Bentley. Transient pioneer neurons are essential for formation of an embryonic peripheral nerve. Science 245: 982-983 (1989).

K5 Kurnit, D.M., W.M. Layton and S. Matthysse. Genetics, chance and morphogenesis. Am. J. Hum. Genet. 41: 979-995 (1987).

K6 Kimler, B.F. and S. Norton. Behavioral changes and structural defects in rats irradiated in utero. Int. J. Radiat. Oncol. Biol. Phys 15: 1171-1177 (1988).

K7 Konermann, G. Postnatal brain maturation damage induced by prenatal irradiation: modes of effect manifestation and dose-response relations. p. 364-376 in: Low Dose Radiation: Biological Bases of Risk Estimation. (K.F. Baverstock and J.W. Stather, eds.) Taylor and Francis, London, 1989.

K8 Kameyama, K. and K. Hoshino. Sensitive phases of CNS development. p. 75-92 in: Radiation Risks to the Developing Nervous System. (H. Kriegel et al., eds.) Gustav Fischer Verlag, Stuttgart, New York, 1986.

K9 Koh, E.T., E.G. Stopa, J.C. King et al. Computer-aided mapping of specific neuronal populations in the human brain. Biocomputing 7: 596-602 (1989).

K10 Ko, F.J., C.H. Chiang, C.C. Wu et al. Studies of neuron-specific enolase levels in serum and cerebrospinal fluid of children with neurological diseases. Kao-Hsiung (Taiwan) Journal of Medical Science 6: 137-143 (1990).

K11 Konermann, G. Postimplantation defects in development following ionizing radiation. Adv. Radiat. Biol. 13: 91-167 (1987).

K12 Kawamoto, S., T. Fujino and H. Fujisawa. Ophthalmological status in children exposed in utero. ABCC/TR 23-64 (1964).

K13 Kirkwood, T.B.L., J. Price and E.A. Grove. The dispersion of neuronal clones across the cerebral cortex. Science 258: 317 (1992).

K14 Komuro, H. and P. Rakic. Selective role of N-type calcium channels in neuronal migration. Science 257: 806-809 (1992).

L1 Lent, R. and S.L. Schmidt. Dose-dependent occurrence of the aberrant longitudinal bundle in the brains of mice born acallosal after prenatal gamma irradiation. Dev. Brain Res. 25: 127-132 (1986).

L2 LaMantia, A.-S. and D. Purves. Development of glomerular pattern visualized in the olfactory bulbs of living mice. Nature 341: 646-649 (1989).

L3 Lindner, J., F.G. Rathjen and M. Schachner. Monoclonal and polyclonal antibodies modify cell-migration in early postnatal mouse cerebellum. Nature 305: 427-430 (1983).

L4 Lo Turco, J.J. and A.R. Kriegstein. Clusters of coupled neuroblasts in embryonic neocortex. Science 252: 563-566 (1991).

M1 Murphy, D.P. Maternal pelvic irradiation. in: Congenital Malformations (2nd edition). (D.P. Murphy, ed.) Lippincott, Philadelphia, 1947.

M2 Miller, R.W. Delayed effects occurring within the first decade after exposure of young individuals to the Hiroshima atomic bomb. Pediatrics 18: 1-18 (1956).

M3 Miller, R.W. and W.J. Blot. Small head size after in-utero exposure to atomic radiation. Lancet II: 784-787 (1972).

M4 Miller, R.W. and J.J. Mulvihill. Small head size after atomic irradiation. Teratology 14: 355-358 (1976).

M5 Meyer, M.B., J.A. Tonascia and T. Merz. Long-term effects of prenatal X ray on development and fertility of human females. p. 273-284 in: Biological and Environmental Effects of Low-level Radiation. Volume II. STI/PUB/409. IAEA, Vienna, 1976.

M6 Mole, R.H. Consequences of pre-natal radiation exposure for post-natal development: a review. Int. J. Radiat. Biol. 42: 1-12 (1982).

M7 Moore, G.W., G.M. Hutchins and R. O'Rahilly. The estimated age of staged human embryos and early fetuses. Am. J. Obstet. Gynecol. 139: 500-506 (1981).

M8 Martinez, P.F.A. Neuroanatomy: Development and Structure of the Central Nervous System. W.B. Saunders Co., Philadelphia, 1982.

M9 Müller, F. and R. O'Rahilly. The first appearance of the major divisions of the human brain at stage 9. Anat. Embryol. 168: 419-432 (1983).

M10 Meadows, A.T., J. Gordon, D.J. Massari et al. Declines in IQ scores and cognitive dysfunctions in children with acute lymphocytic leukaemia treated with cranial irradiation. Lancet II: 1015-1018 (1981).

M11 Müller, F. and R. O'Rahilly. Cerebral dysraphia (future anencephaly) in a human twin embryo at stage 13. Teratology 30: 167-177 (1984).

M12 Mountcastle, V.B. An organizing principle for cerebral function: the unit module and the distributed system. p. 21-42 in: The Neurosciences: Fourth Study Program. (F.O. Schmitt and F.G. Worden, eds.) MIT Press, Cambridge, Massachussetts, 1979.

M13 McConnell, S.K., A. Ghosh and C.J. Shatz. Subplate neurons pioneer the first axon pathway from the cerebral cortex. Science 245: 978-982 (1989).

M14 Müller, W.-U., C. Streffer and S. Pampfer. Teratogenic effects of ionizing radiation after exposure of preimplantation stages of mouse embryos. p. 377-381 in: Low Dose Radiation: Biological Bases of Risk Estimation. (K.F. Baverstock and J.W. Stather, eds.) Taylor and Francis, London, 1989.

M15 Marin-Padilla, M. The closure of the neural tube in the golden hamster. Teratology 3: 39-45 (1970).

M16 Mole, R.H. The effect of prenatal radiation exposure on the developing human brain. Int. J. Radiat. Biol. 57: 647-663 (1990).

M17 Moonen, C.T.W., P.C.M. van Zijl, J.A. Frank et al. Functional magnetic resonance imaging in medicine and physiology. Science 250: 53-62 (1990).

M18 Mole, R.H. Severe mental retardation after large prenatal exposure to bomb radiation. Reduction in oxygen transport to fetal brain: a possible abscopal mechanism. Int. J. Radiat. Biol. 58: 705-711 (1990).

M19 Mole, R.H. Expectation of malformations after irradiation of the developing human in utero: the experimental basis for predictions. Adv. Radiat. Biol. 15: 217-301 (1992).

M20 Marion, R.W., L.A. Alvarez, Z.S. Marans et al. Computed tomography of the brain in the Smith-Lemli-Optiz syndrome. J. Child Neurol. 2: 198-200 (1987).

M21 Müller, W.-U. and C. Streffer. Lethal and teratogenic effects after exposure to X-rays at various stages in early murine gestation. Teratology 42: 643-650 (1990).

M22 Mushak, P., J.M. Davis, A.F. Crocetti et al. Prenatal and postnatal effects of low level lead exposure: integrated summary of a report to the U.S. Congress on childhood lead poisoning. Environ. Res. 50: 11-36 (1989).

M23 Mole, R.H. ICRP and impairment of mental function following prenatal irradiation. J. Radiol. Prot. 12: 93-105 (1992).

M24 Minamisawa, T., K. Hirokaga, S. Sasaki et al. Effects of fetal exposure to gamma-rays on aggressive behavior in adult male mice. J. Radiat. Res. 33: 243-249 (1992).

M25 Mirimova, T.D. Delayed Effects of Radiation Therapy in Children. Medicina, Moscow, 1968.

N1 Neumeister, K. Findings in children after radiation exposure in utero from X-ray examination of mothers. p. 119-134 in: Late Biological Effects of Ionizing Radiation. Volume I. STI/PUB/489. IAEA, Vienna, 1978.

N2 Nokkentved, K. Effects of Diagnostic Radiation Upon the Human Fetus. Munksgaard, Copenhagen, 1968.

N3 Neriishi, S. and H. Matsumura. Morphological observations of the central nervous system in an in-utero exposed autopsied case. J. Radiat. Res. 24: 18 (1983).

N4 Nishimura, H. Introduction. Atlas of Human Perinatal Histology. Igaku-Shoin, Tokyo, 1983.

N5 Norton, S. Correlation of cerebral cortical morphologys with behavior. Toxicol. Ind. Health 5: 247-255 (1989).

N6 Norton, S. Behavioral changes in preweaning and adult rats exposed prenatally to low ionizing radiation. Toxicol. Appl. Pharmacol. 83: 240-249 (1986).

N7 Neumeister, K. and S. Wässer. Findings in children after radiation exposure in utero from x-ray examination of mothers: results from children studied after one to ten years. p. 229-242 in: Effects of Prenatal Irradiation with Special Emphasis on Late Effects. CEC EUR 8067 (1984).

O1 Otake, M., H. Yoshimaru and W.J. Schull. Severe mental retardation among the prenatally exposed survivors of the atomic bombing of Hiroshima and Nagasaki: a comparison of the T65DR and DS86 dosimetry systems. RERF TR/16-87 (1987).

O2 Otake, M., W.J. Schull, Y. Fujikoshi et al. Effect on school performance of prenatal exposure to ionizing radiation in Hiroshima: a comparison of the T65DR and DS86 dosimetry systems. RERF TR/2-88 (1988).

O3 Oppenheim, B.E., M.L. Griem and P. Meier. An investigation of effects of prenatal exposure to diagnostic X rays. p. 249-260 in: Biological and Environmental Effects of Low-level Radiation. Volume II. IAEA, Vienna, 1976.

O4 O'Rahilly, R. and F. Müller. The first appearance of the human nervous system at stage 8. Anat. Embryol. 163: 1-13 (1981).

O5 O'Rahilly, R. and E. Gardner. The developmental anatomy and histology of the human central nervous system. p. 17-40 in: Handbook of Clinical Neurology. Volume 30. (P.J. Vinken and G.W. Bruyn, eds.) North-Holland Publication Co., New York, 1977.

O6 Ordy, J.M., K.R. Brizzee and R. Young. Prenatal cobalt-60 irradiation effects on visual acuity, maturation of the fovea in the retina, and the striate cortex of squirrel monkey offspring. p. 205-217 in: Developmental Effects of Prenatal Irradiation. Gustav Fischer Verlag, Stuttgart, 1982.

O7 Omran, A.R., R.E. Shore, R.A. Markoff et al. Follow-up study of patients treated by x-ray epilation for tinea capitis: psychiatric and psychometric evaluation. Am. J. Public Health 68: 561-567 (1978).

O8 Oppenheim, B.E., M.L. Griem and P. Meier. Effects of low-dose prenatal irradiation in humans: analysis of Chicago Lying-in data and comparison with other studies. Radiat. Res. 57: 508-544 (1974).

O9 Oppenheim, B.E., M.L. Griem and P. Meier. The effects of diagnostic x-ray exposure on the human fetus: an examination of the evidence. Radiology 114: 529-534 (1975).

O10 Ordy, J.M., K.R. Brizzee, W.P. Dunlap et al. Effects of prenatal Co-60 irradiation on the post-natal neural, learning and hormonal development of the squirrel monkey. Radiat. Res. 89: 309-324 (1982).

O11 O'Rahilly, R. The timing and sequence of events in the development of the human eye and ear during the embryonic period proper. Anat. Embryol. 168: 87-99 (1983).

O12 Osborn, R.E., S.E. Byrd, T.P. Naidich et al. MR imaging of neuronal migrational disorders. AJNR, Am. J. Neuroradiol. 9: 1101-1106 (1988).

O13 Otake, M. and W.J. Schull. Radiation-related small head sizes among prenatally exposed A-bomb survivors. Int. J. Radiat. Biol. 63: 255-270 (1993).

O14 O'Rourke, N.A., M.E. Dailey, S.J. Smith et al. Diverse migratory pathways in the developing cerebral cortex. Science 258: 299-302 (1992).

O15 O'Rahilly, R. and F. Müller. Human Embryology and Teratology. John Wiley and Sons, New York, 1992.

O16 Otake, M., Y. Fujikoshi, W.J. Schull et al. A longitudinal study of growth and development of stature among prenatally exposed atomic bomb survivors. Radiat. Res. 134: 94-101 (1993).

P1 Plummer, G. Anomalies occurring in children in utero, Hiroshima. ABCC TR/29-C-59 (1952).

P2 Pierce, D.A. and M. Vaeth. Cancer risk estimation from the A-bomb survivors: extrapolation to low doses, use of relative risk models and other uncertainties. p. 54-69 in: Low Dose Radiation: Biological Bases of Risk Estimation. (K.F. Baverstock and J.W. Stather, eds.) Taylor and Francis, London, 1989.

P3 Palo, J., K. Lydecken and E. Kivalo. Etiological aspects of mental deficiency in autopsied patients. Am. J. Ment. Defic. 71: 401-405 (1966).

P4 Pampfer, S. and C. Streffer. Prenatal death and malformations after irradiation of mouse zygotes with neutrons or X-rays. Teratology 37: 599-607 (1988).

P5 Preston, D.L., D. Pierce and M. Vaeth. Neutrons and radiation risk: a commentary. p. 5 in: RERF Update (1993).

R1 Roesch, W.C. (ed.). US-Japan Joint Reassessment of Atomic Bomb Radiation Dosimetry in Hiroshima and Nagasaki: Final Report. RERF (1987).

R2 Rakic, P. Neuronal migration and contact guidance in the primate telencephalon. Postgrad. Med. J. 54: 25-40 (1978).

R3 Rakic, P. and R.L. Sidman. Histogenesis of cortical layer in human cerebellum, particularly the lamina dissecans. J. Comp. Neurol. 139: 473-500 (1970).

R4 Rakic, P. Timing of major ontogenetic events in the visual cortex of the Rhesus monkey. p. 3-40 in: Brain Mechanisms in Mental Retardation. Academic Press, New York, 1975.

R5 Rakic, P. Prenatal genesis of connections subserving ocular dominance in the rhesus monkey. Nature 261: 467-471 (1976).

R6 Rakic, P. Limits of neurogenesis in primates. Science 227: 1054-1055 (1985).

R7 Raimondi, A.J. and T. Tomita. The advantages of total resection of medulloblastoma and disadvantages of full head post-operative radiation therapy. Child's Brain 5: 550 (1979).

R8 Ron, E., B. Modan, S. Floro et al. Mental function following scalp irradiation during childhood. Am. J. Epidemiol. 116: 149-160 (1982).

R9 Renwick, J.H. and R.L. Asker. Ethanol-sensitive times for the human conceptus. Early Hum. Dev. 8: 99-111 (1983).

R10 Rakic, P. Mechanisms of neuronal migration in developing cerebellar cortex. p. 139-160 in: Molecular Bases of Neural Development. (G.M. Edelman et al., eds.) John Wiley and Sons, New York, 1985.

R11 Rakic, P. Neuronal-glial interaction during brain development. Trends Neurosci. 4: 184-187 (1981).

R12 Rakic, P. Specification of cerebral cortical areas. Science 241: 170-241 (1988).

R13 Rakic, P. Defects of neuronal migration and the pathogenesis of cortical malformations. Prog. Brain Res. 73: 15-37 (1988).

R14 Reyners, H., E. Gianfelici de Reyners and J.R. Maisin. Brain lesions caused by low dose levels of X-rays administered during fetogenesis. Biol. Cell. 51: 28a (1984).

R15 Rakic, P. Mode of cell migration to the superficial layers of fetal monkey neocortex. J. Comp. Neurol. 145: 61-83 (1972).

R16 Rakic, P. Neurons in Rhesus monkey visual cortex: systematic relation between time of origin and eventual disposition. Science 183: 425-427 (1974).

R17 Reyners, H., E. Gianfelici de Reyners, R. Hooghe et al. Irradiation prenatal du Rat a tres faible dose de rayons X: lesions de la substance blanche. C.R. Seances Soc. Biol. Fil. 180: 224-228 (1986).

R18 Reyners, H., E. Gianfelici de Reyners and J.R. Maisin. The role of the GLIA in late damage after prenatal irradiation. p. 118-131 in: Radiation Risks to the Developing Nervous System. (H. Kriegel et al., eds.) Gustav Fischer Verlag, Stuttgart, New York, 1986.

R19 Rosman, N.P. and J. Pearce. The brain in multiple neurofibromatosis (von Recklinghausen's disease): a suggested neuropathological basis for the associated mental defect. Brain 90: 829-838 (1967).

R20 Rosman, N.P. and B.A. Kakulas. Mental deficiency associated with muscular dystrophy: a neuropathological study. Brain 89: 769-787 (1966).

R21 Ragozzino, M.W., J.E. Gray, P.C. O'Brien et al. Risk of malignancy in offspring from preconception and in utero fetal medical ionizing radiation. (1993, in press).

R22 Reyners, H., E. Gianfelici de Reyners, F. Poortman et al. Brain atrophy after foetal exposure to very low doses of ionizing radiation. Int. J. Radiat. Biol. 62: 619-626 (1992).

S1 Sidman, R.L. and P. Rakic. Neuronal migration, with special reference to developing human brain: a review. Brain Res. 62: 1-35 (1973).

S2 Sidman, R.L. and P. Rakic. Development of the human central nervous system. p. 3-145 in: Histology and Histopathology of the Nervous System. (W. Haymaker and R.D. Adams, eds.) C.C. Thomas, Springfield, 1982.

S3 Soni, S.S., G.W. Marten, S.E. Pitner et al. Effects of central nervous system irradiation on neuropsychologic functioning of children with acute lymphocytic leukemia. N. Engl. J. Med. 293: 113-118 (1975).

S4 Schull, W.J., M. Otake and H. Yoshimaru. Effect on intelligence test score of prenatal exposure to ionizing radiation in Hiroshima and Nagasaki: a comparison of the T65DR and DS86 dosimetry systems. RERF TR/3-88 (1988).

S5 Shore, R.E., R.E. Albert and B.S. Pasternack. Follow-up study of patients treated by x-ray for tinea capitis: resurvey of post-treatment illness and mortality experience. Arch. Environ. Health 31: 21-28 (1976).

S6 Streissguth, A.P., S. Landesman-Dwyer, J.C. Martin et al. Teratogenic effects of alcohol in humans and laboratory animals. Science 209: 353-361 (1980).

S7 Streissguth, A.P., C.S. Herman and D.W. Smith. Intelligence, behavior and dysmorphogenesis in the fetal alcohol syndrome. J. Pediatr. 92: 363-367 (1978).

S8 Schull, W.J., H. Nishitani, K. Hasuo et al. Brain abnormalities among the mentally retarded prenatally exposed survivors of the atomic bombing of Hiroshima and Nagasaki. RERF TR/13-91 (1991).

S9 Schwanzel-Fukuda, M. and D.W. Pfaff. Origin of luteinizing hormone-releasing hormone neurons. Nature 338: 161-164 (1989).

S10 Shinoda, H., A.M. Marini, C. Costi et al. Brain region and gene specificity of neuropeptide gene expression in cultured astrocytes. Science 245: 415-417 (1989).

S11 Sloviter, R.S., G. Valiquette, G.M. Abrams et al. Selective loss of hippocampal granule cells in the mature rat brain after adrenalectomy. Science 243: 535-538 (1989).

S12 Sikov, M.R., C.F. Resta, J.E. Lofstrom et al. Neurological deficits in the rat resulting from x-irradiation in utero. Exp. Neurol. 5: 131-138 (1962).

S13 Sikov, M.R., C.F. Resta and J.E. Lofstrom. The effects of prenatal x-irradiation of the rat on postnatal growth and mortality. Radiat. Res. 40: 133-148 (1969).

S14 Squire, L.R., D.G. Amaral and G.A. Press. Magnetic resonance imaging of the hippocampal formation and mammillary nuclei distinguish medial temporal lobe and diencephalic amnesia. J. Neurosci. 10: 3106-3117 (1990).

S15 Sperry, R.W. Chemoaffinity in the orderly growth of nerve fiber patterns and connections. Proc. Natl. Acad. Sci. (USA) 50: 703-710 (1963).

S16 Sienkiewicz, Z.J., R.D. Saunders and B.K. Rutland. Prenatal irradiation and spatial memory in mice: investigation of critical period. Int. J. Radiat. Biol. 62: 211-219 (1992).

S17 Shiota, K., D. Fisher and D. Neubert. Variability of development in the human embryo. in: Non-Human Primates: Developmental Biology and Toxicology. (D. Neubert et al., eds.) Ueberreuter Wissenschaft, Wien, Berlin, 1988.

S18 Shatz, C.J. Dividing up the neocortex. Science 258: 237-239 (1992).

S19 Silbergeld, E.K. Toward the twenty-first century: lessons from lead and lessons yet to be learned. Environ. Health Perspect. 86: 191-196 (1990).

S20 Schwartz, J., P.J. Landrigan, R.G. Feldman et al. Threshold effect in lead-induced peripheral neuropathy. J. Pediatr. 112: 12-17 (1988).

S21 Schell, L.M. Effects of pollutants on human prenatal and postnatal growth: noise, lead, polychlorobiphenyl compounds and toxic wastes. Yearb. Phys. Anthropol. 34: 157-188 (1991).

S22 Straume, T., S.D. Egbert, W.A. Woolson et al. Neutron discrepancies in the DS86 Hiroshima dosimetry system. Health Phys. 63: 421-426 (1992).

S23 Sasaki, M.S., S. Saigusa, I. Kimura et al. Biological effectiveness of fission neutrons: energy dependency and its implication for risk assessment. p. 31-35 in: Proceedings of the International Conference on Radiation Effects and Protection, Mito, Japan. JAERI, Japan, 1992.

S24 Schull, W.J., S. Norton and R.P. Jensh. Ionizing radiation and the developing brain. Neurotoxicol. Teratol. 12: 249-260 (1990).

T1 Tabuchi, A., T. Hirai, S. Nakagawa et al. Clinical findings on in utero exposed microcephalic children. ABCC TR/28-67 (1967).

T2 Tanebashi, M. Intelligence and intelligence tests. p. 128-158 in: Outline of Educational Psychology (20th edition). (Y. Koga, ed.) Kyodo Shuppansha, Tokyo, 1972. (in Japanese)

T3 Tereschenko, N.Y. Study of child nervous system damage at long-term period of postnatal irradiation. p. 31-33 in: Proceedings of the Symposium on Central Nervous System Exposure to Low Doses of Ionizing Radiation. Minsk, 1968.

T4 Tereschenko, N.Y., L.I. Burtseva and A.V. Gezin. Results of dynamic clinico-physiological study of the child nervous system exposed during the first months after birth. p. 273-283 in: Problems of General Radiobiology. (M.P. Domshlak, ed.) Atomizdat, Moscow, 1971.

T5 Tereschenko, N.Y., L.I. Burtseva and V.M. Abdullaeva. Delayed clinical effects of applicational gamma-therapy for angioma cutis among the children of early age. Med. Radiol. 11: 49-53 (1982).

T6 Tereschenko, N.Y., A.M. Lyaginskaya and L.I. Burtseva. Stochastic, non-stochastic effects and some population-genetic characteristics in critical groups of children who were born and lived on zones of radiation control in BSSR. p. 73-74 in: Abstracts of Republic Conference on Scientific and Practical Issues of Safe Health of People Exposed to Radiation Resulting from the Chernobyl Accident. Minsk, 1991.

T7 Tereschenko, N.Y., L.I. Burtseva and A.M. Lyaginskaya. Features of CNS development and some population-genetic characteristics of children in case of pre-natal brain exposure in the critical periods of cerebro- and corticogenesis. p. 140-143 in: Chernobyl Disaster and Medico-psychological Rehabilitation of Victims (Proceedings). Minsk, 1992.

U1 United Nations. Sources, Effects and Risks of Ionizing Radiation. United Nations Scientific Committee on the Effects of Atomic Radiation, 1988 Report to the General Assembly, with annexes. United Nations sales publication E.88.IX.7. United Nations, New York, 1988.

U2 United Nations. Genetic and Somatic Effects of Ionizing Radiation. United Nations Scientific Committee on the Effects of Atomic Radiation, 1986 Report to the General Assembly, with annexes. United Nations sales publication E.86.IX.9. United Nations, New York, 1986.

U4 United Nations. Sources and Effects of Ionizing Radiation. United Nations Scientific Committee on the Effects of Atomic Radiation, 1977 report to the General Assembly, with annexes. United Nations sales publication E.77.IX.1. United Nations, New York, 1977.

V1 Vidal-Pergola, G.M., B.F. Kimler and S. Norton. Effect of in utero radiation dose fractionation on rat postnatal development, behavior, and brain structure: 6 hour interval. Radiat. Res. 134: 369-374 (1993).

W1 Wood, J.W., K.G. Johnson and Y. Omori. In utero exposure to the Hiroshima atomic bomb: follow-up at twenty years. ABCC TR/9-65 (1965).

W2 Wood, J.W., K.G. Johnson, Y. Omori et al. Mental retardation in children exposed in utero, Hiroshima-Nagasaki. ABCC TR/10-66 (1966).

W3 Weiss, B. Behavior as a measure of adverse responses to environmental contaminants. p. 1-57 in: Handbook of Psychopharmacology. Volume 18. (L.L. Iversen et al., eds.) Plenum Publishing Corp., New York, 1984.

W4 Weiss, B. Behavioral toxicology of heavy metals. p. 1-50 in: Neurobiology of the Trace Elements. (I. Droesti and R. Smith, eds.) The Humana Press, New Jersey, 1983.

W5 Weiss, B. Behavioral toxicology and environmental health science. Am. J. Psychol. 38: 1174-1187 (1983).

W6 Wannag, A. The importance of organ blood mercury when comparing foetal and maternal rat organ distribution of mercury after methylmercury exposure. Acta Pharmacol. Toxicol. 38: 289-298 (1976).

W7 Wray, S., A. Nieburgs and S. Elkabes. Spatiotemporal cell expression of luteinizing hormone-releasing hormone in the prenatal mouse: evidence for an embryonic origin in the olfactory placode. Dev. Brain Res. 46: 309-318 (1989).

W8 Walsh, C. and C.L. Cepko. Clonally related cortical cells show several migration patterns. Science 241: 1342-1345 (1988).

W9 Wanner, R.A. and M.J. Edwards. Comparison of the effects of radiation and hyperthermia on prenatal retardation of brain growth of guinea-pigs. Br. J. Radiol. 56: 33-39 (1983).

W10 Williams, R.S. Cerebral malformations arising in the first half of gestation. Dev. Neurobiol. 12: 11-20 (1989).

W11 Werboff, J., J. Havlena and M.R. Sikov. Behavioral effects of small doses of acute x-irradiation administered prenatally. Atompraxis 9: 103-105 (1963).

W12 Wagner, L.K., D.A. Johnston and D.J. Felleman. Radiation induced microencephaly in guinea pigs. Radiat. Res. 132: 54-60 (1992).

W13 Wisniewski, K.E., S.M. Segan, C.M. Miezejeski et al. The FRA(X) syndrome: neurological, electrophysiological, and neuropathological abnormalities. Am. J. Med. Genet. 38: 476-480 (1991).

W14 Walsh, C. and C.L. Cepko. Widespread dispersion of neuronal clones across functional regions of the cerebral cortex. Science 255: 434-440 (1992).

Y1 Yokota, S., D. Tagawa, S. Otsuru et al. Dissection examination of an individual with Down's syndrome exposed in utero to the atomic bombing. Med. J. 38: 92-95 (1963). (in Japanese)

Y2 Yamazaki, J.N. A review of the literature on the radiation dosage required to cause manifest central nervous system disturbances from in utero and postnatal exposure. Pediatrics 37: 877-903 (1966).

Y3 Yamazaki, J.N., S.W. Wright and P.M. Wright. Out-come of pregnancy in women exposed to the atomic bomb in Nagasaki. Am. J. Dis. Child. 87: 448-455 (1954).

Z1 Zecevic, N. and P. Rakic. Differentiation of Purkinje cells and their relationship to other components of developing cerebellar cortex in man. J. Comp. Neurol. 167: 27-47 (1976).

Z2 Zamorano, L. and B. Chuaqui. Teratogenic periods for the principal malformations of the central nervous system. Virchows Arch., Abt. A Pathol. Anat. 384: 1-18 (1979).

Z3 Zola-Morgan, S.M. and L.R. Squire. The primate hippocampal formation: evidence for a time-limited role in memory storage. Science 250: 288-290 (1990).

Z4 Zappert, J. Über röntgenogene fötale Mikrozephalie. Arch. Kinderheilkd. 80: 34-50 (1926).

ANNEX I

Late deterministic effects in children

CONTENTS

INTRODUCTION

1. Deterministic effects of ionizing radiation in humans are the result of whole-body or local exposures that cause sufficient cell damage or cell killing to impair function in the irradiated tissue or organ. The damage is the result of collective injury to substantial numbers or proportions of cells. For any given deterministic effect, a given number or proportion of cells must be affected, so that there will be a threshold dose below which the number or proportion of cells affected is insufficient for the defined injury or clinical manifestation of the effect to occur [F1, I1]. With increasing radiation dose fewer cells survive intact, and therefore the deterministic effects increase in severity and frequency with the dose [U3]. If the radiation exposure is severe enough, death may result as a consequence of the exposure. Death is generally the result of severe cell depletion in one or more critical organ systems of the body.

2. Ionizing radiation can impair function in all tissues and organs in the body because of cell killing; however, tissues vary in their sensitivity to ionizing radiation [F1, I1]. The ovary, testis, bone marrow, lymphatic tissue and the lens of the eye belong to the most radiosensitive tissues. In general, the dose-response function for these tissues, i.e. the plot on linear axes of the probability of harm against dose, is sigmoid in shape. Above the appropriate threshold, the effect becomes more severe as the radiation dose increases, reflecting the number of cells damaged. The effect will usually also increase with dose rate, because a more protracted dose causes the cell damage to be spread out in time, allowing for more effective repair or repopulation [I2]. This type of effect, which is characterized by a severity that increases with dose above some clinical threshold, was previously called "non-stochastic". The initial changes on the cellular level occur essentially at random, but the large number of cells required to result in a clinically observable, non-stochastic effect gives the effect a deterministic character. For this reason such effects are now called "deterministic" effects. The dose levels that result in the clinical appearance of pathological effects are generally of the order of a few gray to some tens of gray. This clinical threshold or critical dose is based on clinical examination and laboratory tests. The time of appearance of tissue damage ranges from a few hours to many years after the exposure, depending on the type of effect and the characteristics of the particular tissue.

3. Radiation-induced deterministic damage in a tissue or organ will often have a more severe impact on the individual during childhood, when tissues are actively growing, than during adulthood. Examples of deterministic sequelae after radiation exposure in childhood include effects on growth and development, hormonal deficiencies, organ dysfunctions and effects on intellectual and cognitive functions. In this Annex, a review is made of late, deterministic damage to normal tissues in children caused by ionizing radiation. Life shortening is not discussed due to the paucity of data. Other effects of radiation exposure, such as cancer induction, hereditary effects and early radiation effects, are not considered. One objective of this review is to try to determine the critical dose levels for the appearance of clinical deterministic effects. Such dose levels will depend on the end-points considered and on the sensitivity of the techniques for measuring the effects. Permanent rather than transient biochemical changes are emphasized in the attempts to define the threshold doses.

4. The Committee reviewed the deterministic effects of radiation in Annex J of the UNSCEAR 1982 Report [U3]. The basic concepts of cell survival were reviewed, including the factors influencing tissue response to fractionated or continuous exposures to radiation. That review of effects was based mainly on results of animal experiments and clinical observations of adults who had received radiotherapy. Its main objective was to identify the nature of effects in various tissues and the doses and modalities of irradiation that cause the effects. It was the Committee's opinion that better quantitative results in man would be required, although it was recognized that such data were difficult to obtain. For effects in children, the need for data and the difficulties were considered to be even greater.

5. The information in this Annex on the possible deterministic effects specific to the exposure of children comes from the application of new methods to derive data and the continued monitoring of patients who received radiotherapy and other individuals exposed to doses high enough to cause deterministic damage to specific tissues or to the whole body. For practical applications it is important that attempts should be made to quantify this damage in terms of the degree of detriment. Owing to the paucity of data, it is not really possible to quantify effects by age in most situations.

I. DETERMINISTIC EFFECTS OF RADIATION EXPOSURES

6. Although the pathobiology of radiation-induced late deterministic effects is poorly understood, it is reasonable to believe that late damage can result from a combination of loss of parenchymal cells, injury to the fine vasculature and/or dysfunction of the fibrocytes and other cells [C1]. Radiation-induced late tissue injury of a deterministic nature appears to have its origin in the sterilization of a large proportion of the stem-like cells of the tissue or organ in question, although these cells may be only a small proportion of the total number of cells in that tissue/organ. The consequent injury results from the natural loss of post-mitotic cells that are not replaced or from the loss of cells that are stimulated into mitosis. The timing of tissue injury depends on the natural proliferation characteristics of cells and also on kinetic changes resulting from the radiation exposure that are characteristic of the tissue [U3]. In addition to the loss of functional cells, supporting blood vessels may be damaged, resulting in secondary tissue damage. Damage to the capillary network has been implicated in the degenerative changes that are accompanied by a progressive reduction of functional capacity [F1]. Other mechanisms for late effects include increased vascular permeability, which causes plasma proteins to leak into interstitial spaces, resulting in the deposition of collagen and leading to atrophy of parenchymal cells. There may also be some replacement of functional cells by fibrous tissue, reducing organ function. The clinical effect that ensues depends on the specific function of the tissue in question.

7. Various processes of repair and repopulation will increase the threshold level of dose when radiation is given over a long period or when a second period of irradiation is encountered sometime after an earlier exposure. The exact role of repopulation, recruitment and intracellular repair of radiation injury over long periods is not clear [C1]. Another aspect that is not well understood is the effect of prior radiation therapy on late injuries following a second course of radiotherapy. There is repair of sublethal damage related to fraction size and fraction number, as well as to dose rate. There appears to be a wide range in the amount of repair that can occur between radiation doses or at decreasing dose rates, which seems to be a tissue-specific phenomenon [C1]. Increasing tolerance occurs as a function of time (days to weeks between fractions) in organs expressing late damage and is thought to be based on slow cell renewal.

8. Late radiation effects often occur in tissues with little or very little proliferation. The radiation effects have been attributed to parenchymal depletion secondary to endothelial changes in small blood vessels or to the direct depletion of parenchymal or stromal cells [R1, R2, R3, T1, W1]. The dose-survival relationship for late effects differs from that of acute responses. Injury to slowly responding tissues is more dependent on fraction size. When conventional radiotherapy fractionation schedules have been altered to fewer fractions of larger doses, an increase in late complications has ensued, with little or no difference in the severity of acute effects [T2]. Studies in animals indicate that the dose-survival characteristics of target cells for late injuries are different from those of target cells of acutely responding tissues. The slopes of the isoeffect curves as a function of dose per fraction are greater for late effects, indicating a greater influence on sparing from dose fractionation for late effects [T2, W2]. The data for low-LET radiation in adults show a wide range of sensitivities of different tissues [I1, R1]. Few tissues show clinically significant effects after acute exposures of less than a few gray, with the exception of the gonads, lens and the bone marrow, which show higher sensitivities.

9. There is little direct correlation between acute reactions and late effects of radiation [B1, R2, R3]. It is, therefore, the late radiation effects that are the dose-limiting factors in curative radiotherapy. Interactions with other treatment modalities may also limit the radiation dose. For example, chemotherapy administered during, before or after irradiation may reduce the tolerance of the tissues exposed to ionizing radiation [R3, W1]. In radiotherapy, normal tissues are unavoidably included in the target volume, and it is the effects in these tissues that limit the dose that can be tolerated. There is still poor understanding of the exact tolerance of a given organ or tissue and of changes in tolerance caused by variations in fraction size, target volume, duration of treatment, dose rate and the presence of various chemical compounds. For a variety of tissues or organs, a critical radiation dose for a limited volume of this tissue has been established empirically, mainly in adults. This dose is usually defined as the dose that will produce a small but detectable incidence of serious complications resulting from the radiation effect on the normal tissue, and often 5% of serious complications is considered reasonable in radiotherapy [C1, R1]. This critical dose or dose range is different from the term "tolerance dose", historically used in radiation protection. Most clinical practice involves daily fractionation with approximately 1.5-2 Gy four or five days per week. In the following paragraphs this will be referred to as conventionally fractionated radiotherapy. Rubin et al. [R1] and Molls and Stuschke [M41] have published data on acceptable doses in radiotherapy and have presented estimates of radiation doses for deterministic effects in organs and tissues of adults and children. There are wide variations in the critical dose from one tissue to another (Tables 1-2).

10. There is great variability in the latent intervals between radiation exposure and the clinical manifestation of late deterministic effects, which may develop at times varying from months to 10 or more years after treatment. The latent interval depends on the tissue or organ affected and is, for example, up to 2 years for myelitis, one to several years for nephritis, 1-5 years for eye effects and 6 months to many years for fibrosis in subcutaneous and connective tissues [T2]. The rate at which radiation injury becomes manifest in a tissue reflects the rate of turnover of target cells and their progeny [F1].

11. Only a few large epidemiological studies of deterministic effects in children exposed to ionizing radiation have been published. Most data are obtained from clinical follow-up of small groups of patients successfully treated for paediatric tumours. In the 1950s and early 1960s the prognosis for a child with a malignant tumour disease was grave, and for many types of tumours death would follow in a matter of months. With the introduction of modern surgery, high-voltage radiotherapy and chemotherapy, the prognosis has improved considerably, and today a large proportion of children with paediatric tumours are cured. The proportion of two-year survivors, which implies the cured fraction, in 1980 ranged from approximately 40% for patients with neuroblastoma or brain tumours to 80%-90% for patients with Wilms' tumour or Hodgkin's disease [S1]. Consequently, many children are now surviving into adulthood, making it possible to study the late effects of their treatment. Increasing reports of late effects have led to systematic investigations by groups of paediatric cancer treatment institutions, such as the Childrens Cancer Study Group in the United States and Canada and the International Late Effects Study Group.

12. In this review of deterministic effects in children, the various observed effects have been grouped according to the organ or tissue affected. It is generally difficult to single out the specific effect of radiation in children with paediatric tumours, as most have also been treated with other modalities, e.g. surgery, cytostatic drugs and/or hormones. Most clinical evaluations are, moreover, based on small numbers of patients, and often appropriate control groups are lacking. Furthermore, the long duration of the illness, the need for hospitalization, the lack of school attendance and other social factors may have had an impact on certain effects measured, such as neuropsychologic functioning. The fact that most data are obtained from studies of patients with paediatric tumours makes it even more difficult to draw conclusions that can be generalized to the general paediatric population. One reason for this is that groups of children treated for malignant disease may include individuals with a genetic predisposition to cancer, some of whom can perhaps have a higher sensitivity to other radiation-induced effects as well. In general, there is a great variability in the ages of the patients studied, and many studies have also assessed patients at widely different ages. A sizeable portion of eligible patients are often not assessed: the children may not be available for evaluation, owing to, for example, their refusal or that of their parents, the disease itself or geographical factors. These selection criteria obviously also affect the interpretation of data.

13. Radiation therapy has been claimed to account for about 80% of the long-term sequelae in surviving children with neoplasms [M1]. Severe disabilities were noted in 41% of 200 children treated for cancer who had no sign of disease for at least five years after therapy [M2]. The disabilities included severe cosmetic changes (16%), severe growth retardation (10%), the need for special education (8%), gonadal failure (7%) and other apparent organ dysfunctions (12%). Hypothyroidism (3%), minimal scoliosis and hypoplasia (22%) were some of the mild to moderate disabilities. Li and Stone [L1] studied late effects in 142 patients treated for childhood cancer and observed major defects in treated organs in 52% of the patients. Despite this, a large proportion of the patients had fully active lives, 61% had attended college, 53% were married and 32% had progeny.

II. RADIATION EFFECTS IN TISSUES AND ORGANS

A. BRAIN

1. Organic effects

14. The developing human brain is especially sensitive to ionizing radiation. Previous UNSCEAR Reports have considered the general developmental effects of prenatal irradiation [U2, U4]. A review of the results of the study of survivors of the atomic bombings in Japan, as well as reviews of other epidemiological investigations relating to prenatal exposure to ionizing radiation and effects on the brain, are presented in Annex H, "Radiation effects on the developing human brain". The mechanisms of observed effects from exposure in fetal life are different from the mechanisms in a nearly fully developed brain. This Section reviews data on late effects following exposure of the brain of infants and children.

15. The response of the normal brain to radiation depends on the total and fractional doses of radiation, the duration of exposure, the exposed tissue volume and the age of the exposed subject. The outcome of iatrogenic radiation damage to the normal brain depends on the magnitude of the damage and the brain's lack of cellular repopulation. Although partial recovery takes place between fractionated exposures, the brain has very little repair function [K1, M3]. After birth, the period of greatest radiosensitivity of the human brain is during the first two years of life, before maturation is completed. Treatment involving the whole brain is more likely to have an adverse effect on younger children by interfering with neural development before maturation of the brain is complete.

16. There is a large body of evidence indicating that radiotherapy to the central nervous system is associated with adverse late effects [B2, B3, D1, D26, F2, K2, K3, O1, P2]. This delayed type of damage is believed to be the effect of injury to the fine vasculature and/or loss of parenchymal cells, resulting in ischaemic necrosis and loss of parenchymal function [A1, C1, C2, S2]. Vascular changes may occur after relatively low radiation doses. Glial cells proliferate during the first years after birth and are therefore sensitive to ionizing radiation. A decrease in the replacement of glial cells and the associated interference with myelination have also been postulated as causes of delayed radiation injury [M4].

17. Treatment-related sequelae of the central nervous system have been documented in children with brain tumours and acute leukaemia, as well as in children having other tumours that require treatment of the central nervous system. The concept of treating the central nervous system of children with acute lymphoblastic leukaemia was developed in the 1960s in order to avoid leukaemic relapse of the central nervous system [A2, A3]. Most patients with leukaemia or solid tumours other than of the brain do not have primary disease of the central nervous system, and the effects of treatment can therefore be better distinguished from the effects of disease. In addition, the radiotherapy in these patients generally involves relatively low radiation doses in the brain. Analysis of radiation effects in brain tumour patients is more difficult because of the much higher radiation doses and the possible effect of the tumour on brain function. In a follow-up study of 102 subjects treated for brain tumour in childhood [L2], 40% of the subjects had mild to moderate disabilities but were living independently, 9% were capable of self-care and 4% required institutionalization. Moderate or severe disabilities were reported in 13 of 30 (43%) irradiated patients and in 11 of 72 (15%) who did not receive radiotherapy. Functional deficits were more common among those treated before two years of age.

18. Five distinctive forms of late effects in the central nervous system have been described: necrotizing leukomyelopathy, leukoencephalopathy, mineralizing microangiopathy, cortical atrophy and necrosis. Necrotizing leukomyelopathy is a spinal cord lesion that does not appear to be related to radiotherapy, since the majority of cases have been observed in non-irradiated patients [P2]. Leukoencephalopathy is a syndrome caused by demyelination; it develops in patients who have received cranial irradiation with intrathecal and/or systemic methotrexate treatment [P1, P2, R4]. Histopathologically, leukoencephalopathy is characterized by demyelination, beginning with axonal swelling and fragmentation and progressing to necrosis and gliosis [B4]. Leukoencephalopathy presents as multifocal coalescing areas of necrosis in the deep white matter, and in the late stage white matter is reduced to a relatively thin gliotic calcified layer. Cortical grey matter and basal ganglia are not affected. Clinical findings range from poor school performance and mild confusion to lethargy, dysarthria, ataxia, spasticity, progressive dementia and even death.

19. Both intrathecal methotrexate and cranial radiotherapy affect endothelial pinocytosis, and damage to the endothelial barrier could be involved in late effects following such treatments [L3]. The interactions between methotrexate and radiation within the central nervous system may be due to the overlapping neurocytotoxicity of the two treatment modalities or to methotrexate acting as a radiosensitizer. Irradiation of the central nervous system may also increase the permeability of the blood-brain barrier or may slow the turnover of cerebrospinal fluid and clearance of methotrexate from the central nervous system. This would alter the distribution of methotrexate in the central nervous system so that some areas accumulate higher amounts of the agent [B4]. Significant levels of methotrexate can also be found in the spinal fluid after it has been administered systemically. The risk and severity of leukoencephalopathy are directly proportional to the total radiation dose, the cumulative dose of systemic methotrexate and the number of therapeutic modalities used (Figure I) [B2, B4]. The highest incidence of leukoencephalopathy is found in patients receiving radiotherapy and methotrexate administered both intravenously and intrathecally. The least neurotoxic combination appears to be intrathecal plus intravenous methotrexate. If radiotherapy to the central nervous system must be combined with methotrexate therapy, the least neurotoxic approach appears to be to administer these modalities in sequence [B2].

20. Leukoencephalopathy has been reported after 20 Gy or more in combination with intrathecal methotrexate [M6, P3, R4]. No evidence of leukoencephalopathy has been found in children for whom intra-

venous or intrathecal methotrexate was discontinued before radiotherapy. Leukoencephalopathy has not been reported after fractionated radiotherapy of the central nervous system with 18-24 Gy alone and rarely with intrathecal methotrexate alone [B4, K4]. Leukoencephalopathy can also occur after a single dose of 10 Gy whole-body irradiation prior to bone marrow transplantation [A4, D2, J1]. Almost all such reported cases have occurred in children, suggesting that the maturing brain is more susceptible. These patients were usually given intensive chemotherapy and cranial radiotherapy with 20-24 Gy over a few weeks prior to the whole-body irradiation. Leukoencephalopathy occurred within a few years of whole-body irradiation in these patients and has usually resulted in severe neurologic deterioration.

21. Mineralizing microangiopathy affects predominantly cerebral grey matter and sometimes cerebellar grey matter and is characterized by focal calcifications in the central nervous system. This degenerative and mineralizing disorder is believed to result from radiation-induced damage to the small vessels [B4, P2, P4]. Histopathologically, calcifications are found in small blood vessels occluding the lumen with mineralized necrotic brain tissue around the vessels. Neurological abnormalities, such as poor muscular control, ataxia, headaches and seizures, have been observed in patients with this complication. Mineralizing microangiopathy is not fatal, and its effect on neuropsychologic functioning may be minimal, although permanent destruction of specific regions of the brain may occur. Mineralizing microangiopathy has not been found in children who did not receive cranial radiotherapy [P4]. It occurs predominantly in children who received 20 Gy or more. Between 25% and 30% of patients who survive more than nine months after intrathecal methotrexate and cranial irradiation with 24 Gy have evidence of mineralizing microangiopathy. The lesion occurs more often in young children [B4, D5]. When mineralizing microangiopathy and leukoencephalopathy coexist, the clinical manifestations of the leukoencephalopathy will predominate.

22. Cortical atrophy is perhaps the most common manifestation after treatment of the central nervous system. It is the result of multiple areas of radiation-induced focal necrosis causing loss of cortical tissue and production of ventricular and subarachnoid space dilatation [C3, D3, D4, D5]. The cortex of atrophic brains is microscopically characterized by an irregular, neuronal loss from all six layers. Astroglial proliferation is sometimes present, usually confined to the marginal layer. Cerebral atrophy occurs after fractionated cranial radiotherapy in nearly half of the patients receiving >30 Gy to the entire brain. The latent period between radiotherapy and the onset of atrophic changes detectable with computed tomography is 1-4 years or even longer [D3].

23. After cranial radiotherapy with 25-65 Gy to the whole brain (delivered at ≤2 Gy per day) to treat brain tumours, cortical atrophy has been found in half of the children [D5], abnormalities of the white matter in 26% and calcifications in 8% of the patients. Cortical atrophy has also been demonstrated in one third of children with acute lymphoblastic leukaemia receiving 24 Gy prophylactic cranial irradiation and intrathecal methotrexate [K2]. Crosley et al. [C3] found evidence of abnormality of the central nervous system at autopsy in 93% of 91 children treated for acute leukaemia. Moderate to severe atrophy was observed in 13% of patients receiving no prophylactic treatment of the central nervous system, in 19% of patients receiving radiotherapy given in 1-2 Gy fractions over 2-15 days (the total brain dose was not stated), in 43% of patients given intrathecal methotrexate and in 47% of patients who received both chemotherapy and radiotherapy. Atrophy did not correlate with leukaemic infiltrations or vascular or infectious processes. Children with the most severe atrophy were the ones who were youngest at onset (mean age: 2.5 years).

24. Cerebral necrosis is a serious sequelae and is usually diagnosed 1-5 years after treatment but may develop more than a decade later. It is characterized by an insidious onset of clinical features [K2]. Post-irradiation myelopathy occurs with rapidly increasing incidence at doses above 45-50 Gy with conventional fractionation. The dose per fraction is critical, and almost all cases of necrosis following total doses of <60 Gy had fractions of >2.5-3.0 Gy [K1, M7, S2]. An interaction between chemotherapy and radiotherapy has been observed for methotrexate in children but has been difficult to show for other agents. A total dose of 50 Gy with 2 Gy per fraction or 55 Gy in 1.8 Gy fractions over six weeks, five daily fractions per week, is considered to be tolerable in adults [A5, K2, S56]. A more recent estimate has been given by Bloom [B35], who assumed that the maximum tolerable radiation dose for children up to 3 years old is 33% lower than in adults, and for children 3-5 years old the dose has to be reduced by 20%.

25. Very few data are available on the effects of hyperfractionated radiotherapy. Freeman et al. [F3] studied 34 patients 3-18 years old (mean: 7 years) who were irradiated for brain stem tumours with 1.1 Gy twice daily with a minimum interval of 4-6 hours, to a total dose of 66 Gy given in 60 fractions over 6 weeks. In the 16 patients who were alive at one year (only 7 were free of progressive disease), there was no clinical suspicion of radiation-related injury. Microscopical examination of the brain in 8 patients failed to show any injury attributable to the radiotherapy.

26. Abnormalities are frequently observed by computed tomographic scanning in long-term survivors of childhood acute leukaemia treated with cranial radiotherapy and intrathecal methotrexate [B5, B6, C14, D24, E1, M5, O2, O3, O13, O14, P5, P7, R5, S55]. Abnormal brain scan findings may not become apparent until many years have elapsed since therapy. The type of brain abnormalities detected include intracerebral calcifications, white matter hypodensity and cortical atrophy (Table 3). Patients who received 24 Gy in 2 Gy fractions with intrathecal chemotherapy appear to have a higher incidence of each of the various abnormalities detected by computed tomography than those who did not receive radiotherapy. On average, there is a 40% incidence of brain abnormalities after 24 Gy in 12 fractions over 2.5 weeks combined with intrathecal methotrexate, although the incidence varies from study to study, depending on the number of patients and length of follow-up. At brain doses of 18-20 Gy combined with intrathecal methotrexate or after intrathecal plus intravenous methotrexate, the average prevalence of brain abnormalities detected is 10%-15%.

27. Magnetic resonance imaging appears to be more sensitive than computed tomography in demonstrating treatment-related neurologic damage in irradiated children. The types of changes observed by magnetic resonance correlate well with the type and severity of the neurologic dysfunctions [A6, C4, K5, P6]. Constine et al. [C4] observed radiation-induced changes in the white matter in 90% of the patients by magnetic resonance imaging, and 68% of these changes were not visible by computed tomography. Enlargement of the sulci was demonstrated in 76% by magnetic resonance imaging and in 52% by computed tomography. Patients treated on a hyperfractionated schedule (1.2 Gy per fraction) had less severe changes, despite the fact that some received over 70 Gy.

28. *Summary*. The available clinical data on deterministic radiation effects on the brain in children are based on small and often heterogenous groups of patients with varying age at exposure and varying lengths of follow-up. Well-designed epidemiological studies of late effects are lacking, and it is therefore not possible to draw any firm conclusions about the radiation effects on the brain and the exact critical dose levels for the appearance of various clinical pathological entities. There is evidence that the incidence of late brain effects will increase as the number of fractions is decreased and the fraction size is increased. The most important effects in the brain following radiotherapy to the central nervous system are leukoencephalopathy, mineralizing microangiopathy, cortical atrophy and cerebral necrosis. Radiotherapy involving the whole brain is more likely to have more severe adverse effects in young children by interfering with neural development before maturation of the brain is complete. Brain changes have been demonstrated with computed tomography and magnetic resonance imaging after 18 Gy of fractionated radiotherapy to the brain. Leukoencephalopathy has been observed after >20 Gy in 1.8-2 Gy daily fractions to the whole brain together with systemic methotrexate and has rarely been reported after 18-24 Gy without methotrexate (Table 4). Leukoencephalopathy has been found in children who were given a single dose of 9-10 Gy whole-body irradiation, but they had generally received cranial radiotherapy prior to the whole-body treatment. Mineralizing microangiopathy has rarely been reported following radiation doses below 20 Gy in 1.8-2 Gy fractions in combination with methotrexate. Cortical atrophy has been observed after 18 Gy in 1.8-2 Gy daily fractions combined with intrathecal methotrexate. A whole-brain dose of 50 Gy in 2 Gy fractions over 6 weeks is generally considered to be a critical dose in adults for radiation-induced necrosis. For children up to 3 years old, the dose should be reduced by 33% and for children 3-5 years old the dose has to be reduced by 20%.

2. Neuropsychologic effects

29. Individuals vary in personality characteristics and mental abilities, and tests have been designed to measure such differences. Ability tests are among the most widely used tools in psychology. They can be divided into achievement tests (designed to measure accomplished skills and indicate what the person can do at present) and aptitude tests (designed to predict what the person can accomplish with training), although the distinction between these two types of tests is not clear-cut. The intelligence quotient (IQ) is an index of mental development and expresses intelligence as a ratio of mental age to chronological age. Heredity plays a role in intelligence, and environmental factors such as nutrition, intellectual stimulation and the emotional climate of the home will influence where within the reaction range determined by heredity a person's IQ will fall. Ability tests are, despite their limitations, still the most objective method available for assessing individual capabilities [A7].

30. Intelligence and academic achievement testings of long-term survivors of childhood cancer reveal a high incidence of memory deficits, visual-spatial skill impairment and attentional deficit disorders. Available data identify radiotherapy to the central nervous system and the synergism with intrathecal chemotherapy as primary etiologic factors in the neuropsychologic sequelae of survivors of childhood cancer [G1, M8]. The brain is particularly sensitive to biologic insults during periods of rapid growth and development, which after birth comprise the first four years

when glial cells proliferate and myelination occurs. Therefore the age at which the child receives cranial irradiation is of importance, and the younger the age of the child at the time of exposure the more serious the intellectual deficit will be. The effect of age at which brain damage occurs depends heavily on the type of psychological ability measured and the instruments for that measurement as on well as the location, extent and permanence of the damage. Multiple factors may be involved in the causation of intellectual deterioration, and the interpretation of IQ may be confounded by the type, location, extent and permanence of lesion, hydrocephalus, age of the child at the time of diagnosis, the aggressiveness of the surgery, radiotherapy and chemotherapy, lack of school attendance, and by anxieties and fears experienced by the child at the time [D1, E3, M8]. Parental social class or parental education level have in some studies been found to be strong predictors of IQ in the survivors of acute childhood leukaemia [T7, W3]. This emphasizes the importance of controlling for social class differences.

31. Neuropsychologic dysfunction with behaviourial or intellectual impairment may occur in up to 50% of children with brain tumours [B6, B7, B8, D6, D7, D8, D9, D10, D11, E2, H2, K6, L2, M9, M10, R6, S3, S4]. These children have received high radiation doses to the brain, and the direct effects of tumour and/or increased intracranial pressure may have contributed to the development of the intellectual problems. Radiotherapy is the most important factor for cognitive sequelae in long-term survivors of paediatric brain tumours who received brain doses of 40 Gy or more in 1.8-2 Gy daily fractions [D8, D9, E2, J2, K6, L4, S3]. In some studies a strong correlation has been observed between IQ and radiotherapy, and young children have generally shown the greatest IQ losses.

32. Radiotherapy to the central nervous system in acute childhood leukaemia (usually 24 Gy fractionated over 2.5 weeks) has been associated with subsequent adverse neuropsychologic effects [C4, C5, C7, E3, E4, E5, H3, I3, K5, L22, M2, M5, M6, M11, M12, O3, O17, P5, R7, R8, R9, S5, T4, T14]. The most common finding is decrements in general intelligence. Other documented effects include general memory impairment, difficulties with short-term memory, distractibility, deficits in abstract reasoning, quantitative skills, visual-motor and visual-spatial skills [C6, D9, E3, E4, J3, M4, M6, M11, M13]. Neuropsychological dysfunction has been reported in up to 30% in children with acute leukaemia, although the deficiencies have been mild, and the children have usually functioned well within the wide normal range. Some studies suggest that adverse effects on intellect are not noted until 2-5 years after treatment. Prophylactic radiotherapy with 24 Gy is associated with poorer intellectual function than is intrathecal chemotherapy (Figure II). Mean overall intelligence scores in irradiated children are, in general, 10-15 points lower than mean scores in non-irradiated children. Performance skills are usually more affected than verbal skills, irradiated patients scoring an average of 15-25 points lower than the mean performance IQ of non-irradiated children [B2, B7]. The younger the child is at the time of irradiation, the greater the neuropsychologic deficit [C7, H4, J3]. Children treated with 24 Gy plus cytotoxic agents for acute leukaemia generally display greater neuropsychological disabilities in a variety of neuropsychologic tests [B9, C5, E3, E5, L5, M11, M12, R8, R9], although some studies have failed to detect such deficits [H4, M8, S6, V2]. Overall, data show that radiotherapy in conjunction with methotrexate has a deleterious effect on later cognitive development. Intrathecal methotrexate as the only prophylactic therapy does not appear to be associated with any global or specific neuropsychologic impairment [P5, T5]. There is some evidence that chemotherapy combined with radiotherapy impairs intellectual functions to a greater extent in children with acute leukaemia who are less than 5 years of age than in older ones [E3, E4, E5, J3, M12].

33. Neuropsychologic late effects can also be seen after doses to the brain of 18 Gy from fractionated radiotherapy [M13, O1, O4, O17, R7, T4, T6]. Studies by Tamaroff et al. [T4, T6] suggest that a dose to the brain of 18 Gy or 24 Gy in children with acute leukaemia in combination with intrathecal methotrexate may have similar deleterious sequelae for neuropsychologic functions. Patients receiving radiotherapy had significantly lower mean full-scale IQ scores and performance IQ scores than non-irradiated children. Ochs et al. [O1, O4, O17], on the other hand, did not observe any significant difference in initial or final full-scale IQ scores between long-term survivors of acute leukaemia having received 18 Gy cranial fractionated radiotherapy plus intrathecal methotrexate and those having received methotrexate only. However, statistically significant decreases in overall and verbal IQ and arithmetic achievement were found in both groups. Thus, 18 Gy of cranial radiotherapy and intrathecal methotrexate may be associated with comparable decreases in neuropsychologic function.

34. A clear dose-response relationship for impaired neuropsychologic functions has, however, not yet been established. Ron et al. [R10, R30] studied a cohort of 10,842 Israeli children who were irradiated for tinea capitis at a mean age of 7 years, receiving a mean brain dose of 1.5 Gy (range: 1.0-6.0 Gy), a control group of ethnicity-, sex- and age-matched subjects from the general population and another control group of siblings. For a subgroup taking scholastic aptitude tests between 1966 and 1970, the irradiated children

achieved lower examination scores. For males born between 1949 and 1955, irradiated subjects achieved lower examination scores on IQ and psychologic tests, completed fewer school grades and had a slight excess of mental hospital admissions. Males with multiple irradiations had twice the mental hospital admission rate of males with a single irradiation (34.0 versus 17.4 per 1,000); there was no such difference among females. The standardized risk ratio for mental hospital admissions was 1.0 for non-irradiated males, 1.1 for males having one treatment, 2.4 for two treatments and 4.8 for ≥3 treatments (test for linear trend, $p < 0.01$). There were also changes in the electroencephalogram among the irradiated subjects and significant differences between the irradiated and control subjects in visual-evoke-response averages, providing further evidence of impaired brain function following the radiotherapy. Children irradiated at less than six years had a relative risk of 1.7 (95% CI: 1.1-2.8) for mental hospital admissions, whereas for older children that relative risk did not differ significantly from 1 [R10].

35. An indication of an excess of admissions to mental institutions was also observed in a survey of American children with tinea capitis after similar radiation doses [O5, S7]. Shore et al. [S7] studied 2,215 patients given radiotherapy for tinea capitis in childhood. The brain received 1.5-1.8 Gy at the surface and 0.7 Gy at the base. There was a 30% excess of psychiatric disorders in the irradiated group overall when controlling for race, sex, socio-economic status, age at therapy and interval from treatment to disease. Omran et al. [O5] made a psychometric and psychiatric evaluation of 177 subjects treated 10-29 years earlier for ringworm of the scalp. Radiotherapy was given to 109 subjects, and 68 received topical medications. Average age at treatment was eight years in both groups. The irradiated group manifested more psychiatric problems and were judged more maladjusted in the testings when controlling for educational level and family psychiatric disorders. However, the psychiatrist's overall rating of current psychiatric status showed only a borderline difference between the two groups.

36. The Israeli and American studies of children irradiated for tinea capitis suggest that doses to the brain of 1-2 Gy would be associated with late neuropsychologic effects. The dose given to these patients is the lowest that has been reported to lead to functional neuropsychologic disturbances after radiotherapy in childhood. However, it is difficult to identify mechanisms that could explain these functional changes after such relatively low radiation doses. Furthermore, the observations are not supported by clinical follow-up of patients treated for childhood tumours, and the possibility that confounding factors are responsible for this observed association cannot be ruled out. The trauma of baldness and of having had treatment for tinea capitis may have caused some of the psychological problems. Also, at least in the Israeli cohort, parts of the brain received higher doses than the mean doses of 1-2 Gy.

37. *Summary*. The incidence and extent of neuropsychologic dysfunction among children given radiotherapy to the central nervous system are difficult to define. A variety of factors complicate the study of a possible association between effect and dose, including the underlying disease and associated clinical findings, other treatment modalities, the impact of illness on body image and school attendance, and perhaps also parental social class. Most studies contain a small number of patients of varying ages, who received a variety of treatment modalities and had varying follow-ups. Several studies, however, indicate that radiotherapy increases the risk of adverse neuropsychologic effects. Younger children, particularly those less than five years of age at time of treatment, are more severely affected. Clinical follow-ups of survivors of paediatric cancers have demonstrated a decline in IQ after doses to the brain of 18 Gy with conventional fractionation. In general, performance skills are more affected than verbal skills. It is difficult to distinguish the impact of radiotherapy from that of methotrexate. It is possible that intrathecal methotrexate administered prior to radiotherapy in children with acute leukaemia may be associated with less intellectual impairment than its administration during and after radiotherapy. Two epidemiological studies of children irradiated for tinea capitis of the scalp suggest adverse neuropsychologic effects after 1-2 Gy to the brain, with parts of the brain having received more than the mean doses in at least one of the studies. It is likely that these observations can be at least partially explained by confounding factors. The available data on neuropsychologic effects after radiotherapy in childhood do not allow an analysis of the possible effect of the fraction size on neuropsychologic functions, since most studies deal with conventional fractionation schedules.

3. Neuroendocrine effects

38. Growth depends on a delicate interplay of endocrine and metabolic factors, and secretion of growth hormone from the pituitary gland is necessary for normal growth [S31, W4]. Growth hormone deficiency is usually defined as an impaired response of serum growth hormone to various provocative tests. The commonly used tests include stimulation with arginine, ornithine, insulin-induced hypoglycemia, L-dopa, growth-hormone-releasing hormone or exercise. Neuroendocrine abnormalities have been observed in

children with tumours who received cranial radiotherapy. The abnormalities primarily involve the hypothalamus and/or the pituitary gland and range from impaired growth hormone response to complete panhypopituitarism [A8, A10, D8, D11, D12, D13, O6, P8, R11, S8, S9]. Radiation-induced damage to the hypothalamic-pituitary axis is the dominant cause of the observed abnormalities and the major site of radiation-induced damage causing hypothalamic-pituitary dysfunction appears to be the hypothalamus, although the pituitary gland itself may also be damaged. The most sensitive endocrinological target is the cells producing the growth hormone releasing hormone in the hypothalamus, and impaired growth hormone secretion is the most commonly finding [S10, S11]. Growth hormone is always the first and often the only anterior pituitary hormone to be affected by radiation damage, and panhypopituitarism occurs only after doses above 50 Gy. Radiotherapy appears to have an almost immediate suppressive effect on the hypothalamic-pituitary axis [D25]. Younger patients seem to be at greater risk for neuroendocrine damage [B8, D9, O7, S12]. Chemotherapy may contribute to growth impairment, but the effect is usually temporary when it is given alone. In this Section it is mainly the effects on growth hormone production that are discussed; the effects on thyroid-stimulating hormone are discussed in Section II.B, and the effects on gonadotropins, in Sections II.C and II.D.

39. Cranial radiotherapy and growth hormone deficiency are not the only causes of impaired growth in children treated for intracranial tumours. Other possible contributing factors to the impaired growth of these children include impaired spinal growth following spinal irradiation (see Section II.E), chemotherapy, poor nutrition and tumour relapse. The different results in various studies of growth hormone production in children receiving similar radiation doses to the central nervous system may be due to the use of different methods for studying growth hormone and/or to variation in time intervals between exposure and growth hormone determination. After 24 Gy of cranial radiotherapy, there are normal growth hormone responses to arginine but not to insulin stimulation, higher doses are associated with abnormal growth hormone responses to both [D14]. Since insulin-induced hypoglycemia is believed to affect receptors in the hypothalamus and arginine causing them to stimulate the pituitary gland, lower radiation doses affect the hypothalamus and higher doses also destroy pituicytes involved in growth hormone secretion [D1]. There is a correlation between the radiation dose to the hypothalamic-pituitary axis and the growth hormone response to stimulation, but a dose threshold below which no pituitary dysfunction follows has not yet been defined [C10, S10]. Although children treated for acute leukaemia may have biochemical growth hormone deficiency, they usually have a normal longitudinal growth pattern. Children with brain tumours, on the other hand, are more likely to have clinically significant endocrine dysfunction because they receive higher radiation doses. Growth hormone deficiency becomes apparent within a few months after the completion of radiotherapy for brain tumours, and after 30 Gy or more to the hypothalamus or pituitary gland using conventional fractionation, severe growth retardation has been observed in more than 50% of the survivors of childhood brain tumours [A9, C9, D1, D9, H5, O6, O8, P8, R12, R23, S4, S10, S11, S13, S14, S15, S16].

40. Absorbed doses to the brain of 30 Gy or more fractionated over several weeks result in significant long-term reduction in growth hormone secretion and impaired growth. Stunted growth has been most frequently observed among children irradiated for brain tumours at an age of 6-10 years, and it occurs in about 50% of those who have received >30 Gy to the hypothalamic-pituitary region fractionated over several weeks [A9, A11, D6, D9, O4, O6, O8, S11]. After a hypothalamic-pituitary dose of 37 Gy or more delivered in 2 Gy fractions five times per week, the 24-hour growth hormone profile is disturbed, with low overall secretion and few peaks of low amplitude but with a discernable diurnal rhythm [L6]. The normal diurnal rhythm of growth hormone secretion may be blunted but is not completely lost. There is a prompt rise in growth hormone after stimulation with growth-hormone-releasing hormone, and this response decreases with time after radiotherapy (Figure III). Patients with brain tumours who have received radiation doses of 50 Gy or more exhibit the most severe abnormalities, and multiple pituitary hormonal deficiencies may occur [B10, P8, R8, S17, S18].

41. Clayton [C12] assessed growth hormone secretion in 82 children who received cranial or craniospinal radiotherapy with up to 48 Gy (estimated by a schedule of 16 fractions over three weeks) to the hypothalamic-pituitary region. Stepwise multiple regression analysis showed that dose ($p < 0.01$) and time from radiotherapy ($p < 0.05$), but not age at therapy, had a significant influence on growth hormone response. Growth hormone deficiency developed more rapidly in those who received higher radiation doses. Shalet et al. [S14] noted a significant inverse correlation between dose and growth hormone response in 56 children with brain tumours or acute leukaemia and evaluated two years or more after radiotherapy. Thirty-seven patients (66%) had impaired growth hormone response, and all but one received >29 Gy to the hypothalamic-pituitary axis. Only five patients who received such a dose had normal growth hormone response, and four of them were older than 13 years at the time of treatment. In another study,

Shalet et al. [S11] found normal growth hormone response to hypoglycaemia in 14 children with brain tumours prior to treatment, and growth hormone deficiency occurred after a brain dose of 25-29 Gy in 7 patients within two years of radiotherapy. Of 13 children in whom growth could be assessed, 12 had poor growth.

42. Cranial irradiation with 24 Gy in 12-16 fractions over 2-2.5 weeks for acute leukaemia has also been associated with a measurable reduction in growth hormone response, although growth remains relatively unaffected at this dose [M14, M15, M16, M17, O9, P2, S19, S20]. Others have claimed whole-brain irradiation to be an important cause of short stature in survivors of childhood acute leukaemia [D15, K7, O7, P8, W5]. Some data suggest that a significant number of children less than 4 years of age with acute lymphoblastic leukaemia are short before the onset of therapy [B11]. Some data suggest that the effect of radiation on growth hormone secretion can be reduced by decreasing the dose per fraction. Shalet et al. [S19, S21] studied growth hormone levels and growth in 17 leukaemic children who received 25 Gy in 10 fractions over 2.5 weeks and in 9 children who received 24 Gy in 20 fractions over 4 weeks. Of the 17 children who received 25 Gy in 10 fractions, 14 had subnormal growth hormone response to insulin, compared to 1 of 9 patients who received 24 Gy in 20 fractions ($p < 0.002$). Arginine stimulation test was carried out in 16 children given 25 Gy and in 7 children receiving 24 Gy, and impaired response was seen in 6 and 1 patients, respectively. The greater impairment of growth hormone response to insulin hypoglycaemia following irradiation with 25 Gy in 10 fractions to the hypothalamic-pituitary axis suggests that the hypothalamus rather than the pituitary gland was the site of damage. There was no difference in mean standing height standard deviation score between the two irradiated groups, but they both differed significantly in this respect from normal children.

43. Griffin and Wadsworth [G2] compared the growth of 66 children with acute leukaemia to the growth of normal children matched for age and sex by calculation of the standard deviation score. All patients had cranial radiotherapy with 24-25 Gy in 15-20 fractions over 21-28 days, and 24 of them also had spinal radiotherapy with 10-24 Gy in 5-20 fractions over 7-28 days. The standard deviation score for height [calculated as $(\bar{x}-x)/SD$ where $\bar{x}$ = mean of the normal population; x = the measurement; SD = standard deviation] of the patients fell significantly in the first year of treatment (Figure IV). This was specifically related to craniospinal radiotherapy but not to age or chemotherapy. Robison et al. [R13] studied 187 children (mean age: 5 years) with acute leukaemia who received either cranial irradiation with a median of 24 Gy (range: 14-28 Gy) in 1.2-2 Gy fractions five times a week plus intrathecal methotrexate; craniospinal irradiation alone (24 Gy); or craniospinal irradiation plus abdominal irradiation (12 Gy). At diagnosis no significant difference was observed in the height distribution compared to expected population standards. After treatment, an excess was observed in the proportion of patients in the lower percentiles in conjunction with a decrease in the proportion of patients in the highest percentiles. The only factor found to have a significant impact on attained height percentile was radiotherapy.

44. Children with acute leukaemia have a high frequency of biochemically abnormal growth hormone response to stimuli, but growth hormone deficiency is uncommon. Impaired response to stimuli, suggesting abnormality in the hypothalamic-pituitary axis, does not necessarily indicate absolute growth hormone deficiency. The presence of growth hormone abnormalities is not necessarily correlated with clinical findings of short stature [O7, S19]. Most of the adverse central nervous system sequelae in patients with acute leukaemia have been observed among those who received 24 Gy of cranial radiation and intrathecal chemotherapy.

45. The dose required to prevent leukaemic infiltration into the central nervous system can now be safely lowered from 24 Gy to 18 Gy [N1]. Few data exist on the effect on growth of radiation doses below 24 Gy. In some studies, growth impairment has been similar after 24 Gy and after 18 Gy [R13, S22, W5]. Others have observed that growth impairment in children with acute leukaemia has been less frequent and generally milder below 24 Gy [B12, C11, C23, G2, S19, V1, V2]. Cicognani et al. [C23] found that children who had received 18 Gy in 10 fractions had complete growth recovery and normal growth hormone responses to pharmacological tests. Children who had received 24 Gy in 12 fractions showed significantly lower standard deviation scores for height than at diagnosis and had impaired growth hormone response.

46. After a single whole-body dose of 10 Gy, severe growth retardation appear in most children [D2, S23]. Many if not most of these children also received cranial radiotherapy prior to the whole-body irradiation. The majority of paediatric patients treated with whole-body irradiation have decreased growth rates on longitudinal growth velocity curves, and growth hormone levels have been subnormal in about one third of the patients [D14, S24, S25]. Sanders [S24] reported subnormal levels of growth hormone in 87% of children who received both cranial radiotherapy and whole-body irradiation, compared to 42% of those who received whole-body irradiation only. Deeg et al. [D2] observed normal growth velocity curves in

transplant-treated children who did not receive whole-body irradiation, whereas irradiated children had impaired growth and decreased growth velocity. Growth hormone levels were subnormal in about one third of the irradiated patients.

47. Some data suggest that fractionation will reduce the adverse effects of whole-body irradiation. Barrett et al. [B13] reported growth hormone deficiency in 6 of 8 children after a single whole-body dose of 10 Gy and in 3 of 8 children who had a fractionated whole-body dose of 12-14 Gy in 6 fractions given twice daily for 3 days. Sanders et al. [S23] evaluated growth in 144 patients following marrow transplantation for childhood leukaemia at a median age of 10 years. All children had received multiagent chemotherapy, and 55 had received a median of 24 Gy (range: 18-29 Gy) to the central nervous system, 5 of whom had also received a median of 12 Gy to the spine. A whole-body dose of 9.2-10 Gy in a single exposure was given to 79 patients, and 63 patients had a fractionated regimen of 2.0-2.3 Gy per day for 6-7 days for cumulative doses of 12-16 Gy. Growth hormone levels were measured in 43 patients 1-8 years after transplant, and growth hormone deficiency was present in 27 subjects (63%). Of these, 21 patients had received pre-transplant cranial irradiation. By three or more years after transplant, boys who received single whole-body exposure were 8.0 ± 2.3 cm shorter than boys who received fractionated whole-body exposure ($p < 0.03$). Among boys who had not received cranial irradiation, those given single whole-body exposure were 15.2 ± 3.2 cm shorter than those given fractionated whole-body exposure ($p < 0.04$). Girls showed similar trends that were not statistically significant.

48. Hiroshima survivors exposed to >1 Gy at ages 0-19 years were shorter and weighed less than the overall population. Those who were less than 6 years old and who also received >1 Gy [B14] at the time of the bombings were shorter still, on average. The analyses were based on the T65 dosimetry. Exposure to high radiation doses markedly reduced mean height for those who were very young at the time of the bombings, but this effect diminished with increasing age. Average height for those aged 0-5 years at the time of the bombings was significantly smaller for the >1.0 Gy dose group than for the groups 0 Gy (not in city), 0-0.09 Gy and 0.10-0.99 Gy for both males and females: smaller by 4.4 cm or more for males and by 2.5 cm or more for females (Table 5). For those aged 6-11 years at the time of the bombings, smaller heights were again found for the >1 Gy dose group, although to a lesser degree. For subjects aged 12-17 years at the time of the bombings, no apparent differences between the four dose groups were found. When the high dose group was further divided into 1.00-2.49 Gy and ≥2.50 Gy groups, the mean heights were less for both males and females aged 0-5 years at the time of the bombings in the ≥2.50 Gy group. The difference from the 1.00-2.49 Gy group was statistically significant for males. Average heights of females aged 6-11 years at the time of the bombings and for males and females aged 12-17 years at the time of the bombings were approximately the same for the two dose groups (Table 6). In Nagasaki, the effect of dose on height was not statistically significant, although the mean height of Nagasaki females aged 0-5 years at the time of the bombings was least for those who were exposed to >1 Gy (Table 5). Among males, those exposed to 0-0.09 Gy at ages 0-5 years at the time of the bombings showed the smallest mean height. For both the 6-11 year and 12-17 year groups, however, the mean height for boys in the high dose exposure group was the smallest. A reanalysis based on the same T65 dosimetry was undertaken of the relationship between attained adult height and radiation dose of 628 survivors of the atomic bombings in Hiroshima and Nagasaki aged less than 10 years at the time of the bombings [I4]. Average height tended to be lower as exposure increased, except among Nagasaki males (Table 7). Two-way analysis of variance of height in relation to sex and dose by city showed that height was significantly different by sex and total kerma in Hiroshima. In Nagasaki, however, it was significantly different by sex but not kerma total dose. Growth and development of stature depends on nutrition, socio-economic conditions, the quality and quantity of radiation received and, possibly, other factors. Contrary to the report by Belsky and Blot [B14], the results of Ishimaru et al. [I4] suggested that diminished stature was not significantly related to age at the time of the bombings for individuals exposed before the adolescent growth spurt, something which was probably due to the small sample size. The observed difference between the two cities may change with new analyses based on the new DS86 dosimetry.

49. Children on the Marshall Islands exposed to radioactive fallout in 1954 were also found to have a significant reduction in height, which was probably mainly due to radiation-induced hypothyroidism [R14, S26] (see Section II.B).

50. Children with radiation-induced growth hormone deficiency can now be treated with growth hormone, although there are as yet no long-term studies of the effects of such a therapy in a large number of children. Some data suggest a significant growth response to therapy in children who received cranial irradiation alone, whereas the response in patients receiving cranio-spinal irradiation has been less satisfactory [G3, S20].

51. *Summary*. Irradiation of the central nervous system may produce damage to the hypothalamic-pituitary axis, resulting most commonly in impaired

growth hormone secretion. The hypothalamic cells producing the growth-hormone-releasing hormone are the most sensitive endocrinological target. Growth hormone deficiency can be expected in approximately 75% of children treated for brain tumours, and a growth velocity or height below the 10th percentile can be expected in 70%. The growth hormone deficiency is permanent. Patients with acute leukaemia have in general received lower doses to the central nervous system but growth hormone secretion is still affected. After 25-30 Gy, the growth hormone response to insulin-induced hypoglycaemia is impaired within two years of irradiation. After 24 Gy in 12-16 fractions, there is also a measurable reduction in growth hormone response to stimuli. Growth has been less affected after 24 Gy than after higher radiation doses in the brain, suggesting that the normal physiologic requirements of growth hormone secretion have been met. No effect on growth hormone secretion has been observed below 18 Gy. A 10 Gy whole-body dose in a single fraction results in severe growth retardation in the majority of children, who generally have been pretreated with chemotherapy and cranial radiotherapy. Fractionation appears to be of importance for the effect on growth hormone secretion and growth, and increasing fraction size will result in a higher proportion of patients with subnormal growth hormone response. Growth impairment is seen more often after a single-dose whole-body irradiation with 10 Gy than after a fractionated regimen of 12-16 Gy in 2 Gy fractions over a week. It is not possible to define the lowest dose capable of impairing growth hormone secretion, since available data are obtained from small studies with varying ages at exposure and lengths of follow-up, as well as different methods for assessing the growth hormone level. Such a dose appears to be lower than 18 Gy from fractionated exposure. Growth has been affected in the survivors of the atomic bombings in Japan at acute doses of >1 Gy, especially among children less than 6 years of age. This effect may be due to a combination of brain damage, damage to the spine, nutritional factors etc.

B. THYROID GLAND

52. Hypothyroidism is the most common late deterministic effect of the thyroid gland following exposure to ionizing radiation. Thyroid nodularity is considered to be a stochastic phenomenon and is therefore not discussed in this Section. Clinical damage to the pituitary and thyroid glands is usually manifested several years after exposure and is preceded by a subclinical phase [F4]. Direct damage to the thyroid gland by radiation can cause primary hypothyroidism, whereas damage to the hypothalamic-pituitary axis may produce secondary hypothyroidism. Primary hypothyroidism has been demonstrated in 40%-90% of patients with paediatric tumours given 15-70 Gy to the thyroid gland and followed for up to six years [B10, C5, C13, D16, F4, G4, K8, O8, P9, S9, S23, S27, S28]. The onset of hypothyroidism may be several months to years following the radiotherapy. Administration of oral thyroxine during radiotherapy does not appear to prevent later thyroid hypofunction [B15]. Radiotherapy alone and with chemotherapy have been associated with similar high incidences of hypothyroidism. Patients treated with chemotherapy only have generally not had any significant thyroid hypofunction, although transient thyroid dysfunction has been reported [G4, G5, H7, L7, S27, S28, S29].

53. The incidence of overt [low serum T4 and elevated thyroid-stimulating hormone (TSH)] and compensated (normal serum T4 and elevated TSH) hypothyroidism varies with the radiation dose in the thyroid gland, the length of follow-up and the way in which the thyroid function was determined. Thyroid surgery, iodine-containing contrast material and age of the patient at the time of radiotherapy may contribute to the development of hypothyroidism. The effect of age at the time of radiotherapy on the development of hypothyroidism is a matter of controversy. In one study, 48% of patients with Hodgkin's disease who were younger than 20 years of age at the time of treatment had elevated TSH levels compared to 33% of older patients [G4]. Green et al. [G5], observed that 7 of 15 children with Hodgkin's disease and irradiated at the age of less than 13 years developed hypothyroidism, compared to 3 of 12 among those who had been older than 13 years. In a study by Tarbell et al. [T9] of patients irradiated for Hodgkin's disease, the 15-year actuarial risk for hypothyroidism was 64% among patients aged 16 years or less, as compared to 29% among those older than 16 years. Others have not identified age as a contributory factor [D16, K8, N2, S28, S29]. The possibility that the thyroid is more sensitive in childhood is also supported by the high incidence of increased TSH levels in children irradiated for Hodgkin's disease [D16, S27].

54. Elevated TSH levels have been observed in children who received radiotherapy for brain tumours after 25-30 Gy to the hypothalamic-pituitary axis or 24 Gy to the thyroid gland [C26, D6, H6, O6, S15]. Various studies show that hypothyroidism is dose-dependent. In a study by Glatstein et al. [G4], no patient had an elevated TSH level after 15 Gy to the thyroid, as compared to 44% of the patients receiving 40 Gy or more. Kaplan et al. [K8] found elevated TSH levels in 15% of patients who received <30 Gy and in 68% of those who received higher doses. Logistic regression analysis showed that both higher radiation dose (≥30 Gy) and lymphangiography increased the risk of having an elevated serum TSH level. Constine et al. [C15] measured thyroid function

in 119 children irradiated for Hodgkin's disease. Radiotherapy was delivered over 4-5 weeks: 24 children received a neck dose of 26 Gy or less (mean: 22 Gy) and 95 received >26 Gy (mean: 44 Gy). More than 75% of the children receiving >26 Gy had elevated TSH levels, compared to 17% of those treated with lower doses. A weak correlation with age ($p < 0.05$) was found, and the doubling dose for the mean peak TSH value was 11 Gy (Figure V).

55. Most of the experience in radiation-related late effects in the thyroid has been gained from the treatment of Hodgkin's disease. Compensated hypothyroidism occurs in up to 75% of the treated children, and uncompensated hypothyroidism has been observed in less than 30% of the children [C14, D16, D17, F4, F5, G4, G5, M18, S17, S27, S28, S29, T8]. Patients irradiated for lymphomas or head and neck cancers have generally received 24-60 Gy fractionated over several weeks. In some studies lymphangiography prior to radiotherapy has been shown to increase the risk of hypothyroidism [G4, G5, K8, S27, S28, S29]; in others, it has not [C14, G5, N2, T8]. Lymphangiography may increase thyroid damage from subsequent irradiation for the following reason: the iodine released from the contrast material could inhibit thyroid hormone synthesis and secretion within a few days, thereby causing increased thyrotropin secretion and consequent stimulation of thyroid cells at the time of irradiation [K8]. An expanded extrathyroidal pool of iodine may increase susceptibility to hypothyroidism in irradiated subjects.

56. Lower radiation doses may also increase the risk of hypothyroidism. In children with acute leukaemia receiving cranial irradiation with 18 Gy, the thyroid dose is 3%-8% of the cranial dose [R15]. Hypothyroidism has been observed in up to 20% of long-term survivors of childhood acute leukaemia after 18-25 Gy of cranial or craniospinal radiotherapy with conventional fractionation [N3, R16, R18, S12]; others have failed to observe such an effect after cranial doses of 8.5-24 Gy in 2 Gy fractions [O7, V1]. Mean thyroid doses of 4-10 Gy in infancy or childhood from fractionated radiotherapy for benign disease has not been associated with clinical hypothyroidism, although follow-up lasted as long as 25 years [H8, R19]. In contrast, hypothyroidism has been reported in 7 of 9 Russian children after radiotherapy for skin angioma with thyroid doses of >1.1 Gy [T15].

57. Thyroid hypofunction can occur after whole-body irradiation. Children who received a regimen of chemotherapy in preparation for a transplant have an incidence of thyroid dysfunction that is not greater than normally observed among non-transplant children [S24, S25]. Radiotherapy appears to be the major, if not the sole, cause of subsequent thyroid hypofunction in these patients. In terms of its effects on thyroid hypofunction [T17], single-dose radiotherapy has been claimed to be equivalent to a total radiation dose 4-5 times larger when it is delivered in conventional fractions. Sanders et al. [S23, S24] studied 142 patients 1-17 years old after bone marrow transplantation to treat haematological malignancies. All patients had received multiagent chemotherapy, 55 had been pretreated with 24 Gy fractionated cranial radiotherapy and 12 had received 12 Gy spinal irradiation. Whole-body irradiation was delivered as a single dose of 9.2-10 Gy ($n = 79$) or 2-2.2 Gy daily for 6-7 days to 12.0-15.8 Gy ($n = 63$). Among children who received 10 Gy single whole-body exposure, 56% had compensated hypothyroidism and 13% had overt hypothyroidism, and the figures for children who received fractionated whole-body irradiation were 21% and 3%, respectively. These differences most likely reflect the shorter observation times after fractionated exposure (median nine years versus five years). Longer follow-up is needed to determine whether there is any real difference between the two types of whole-body exposure. Katsanis et al. [K9] evaluated thyroid function in 80 patients after bone marrow transplantation for aplastic anaemia or acute leukaemia. Median age at the time of transplantation was 10 years (range: 2-21 years). Patients with aplastic anaemia received high-dose chemotherapy and total lymphoid irradiation with a single dose of 7.5 Gy, and leukaemia patients received either whole-body irradiation as a single fraction of 7.5-8.5 Gy ($n = 33$) or fractionated whole-body irradiation with 13.2 Gy ($n = 20$) in 1.7 Gy fractions twice daily for four days. Of 27 patients with aplastic anaemia plus total lymphoid irradiation, 11 showed thyroid hypofunction, as compared with 9 of 53 patients with acute leukaemia plus whole-body irradiation. The five-year actuarial risk estimate of hypothyroidism after total lymphoid irradiation was 42% (95% CI: 23%-61%), which was significantly different from 10% after fractionated whole-body irradiation (95% CI: 0%-23%) ($p < 0.05$), but not different from 21% after single-dose whole-body irradiation (95% CI: 7%-35%).

58. The thyroid gland has the capacity to actively concentrate iodine, and radioiodine can therefore deliver considerable radiation doses to the gland, a fact that has been and is still used in diagnostic and therapeutic medical procedures [D18, G6]. The most commonly used radioiodine is ^{131}I, which has a half-life of eight days. Most data on hypothyroidism after ^{131}I exposure emanate from studies on patients with hyperthyroidism, and their experience may not be directly transferable to a normal euthyroid population. In patients with hyperthyroidism, hypothyroidism is common even after surgery or treatment with anti-thyroid drugs [B17, H10]. The thyroid uptake of ^{131}I is higher in hyperthyroid patients, but the turnover of

the nuclide is more rapid. It may therefore be possible to approximate the experience of hyperthyroid patients to that of euthyroid subjects [M19, M20, N4]. In adult hyperthyroid patients treated with a single dose of ^{131}I, the cumulative probability of hypothyroidism is related to the ^{131}I activity administered per unit thyroid weight [B16]. Holm et al. [H9] observed an annual hypothyroidism of 3% the first 24 years after ^{131}I therapy for hyperthyroidism. There are only very limited data on the effects of thyroid absorbed doses from ^{131}I of <25 Gy and the effects in children. NCRP Report No. 55 [N4] cited unpublished data from Hamilton and Tompkins, who observed that 8 of 443 subjects (2%) less than 16 years old and judged to have normal thyroids became hypothyroid after diagnostic ^{131}I tests. The incidence of hypothyroidism was 0% per year in 146 subjects who received <0.3 Gy in the thyroid, 0.15% per year in 146 subjects who received 0.3-0.8 Gy and 0.23% per year in 151 subjects after thyroid doses of >0.8 Gy. A linear model with a threshold was postulated for hypothyroidism; owing to the large functional capacity of the thyroid gland, a large number of cells would have to be affected to result in hypothyroidism. Hayek et al. [H11] observed hypothyroidism in 8 of 30 (26%) patients between the ages of 8 and 18 years who received ^{131}I therapy for hyperthyroidism. The mean amount of ^{131}I administered was 240 MBq, and the mean follow-up was nine years. Freitas et al. [F6] found a 92% prevalence of hypothyroidism in 51 patients aged 6-18 years after ^{131}I therapy for hyperthyroidism (mean ^{131}I activity, 520 MBq).

59. In 1954, following detonation of a megatonne nuclear device at Bikini, 250 inhabitants of the Rongelap, Ailingnae and Utirik atolls of the Marshall Islands were exposed to radioactive fallout [C16, L8, R14]. This consisted of whole-body gamma-irradiation, beta-irradiation of the skin from fallout deposited on the skin, and internal absorption of radionuclides from the ingestion of contaminated food and water. The most serious internal exposure was that to the thyroid gland, from radioiodines in the fallout. The estimated thyroid dose varied from 0.3 to 3.4 Gy among those aged 18 years or more to 0.6-20 Gy among those less than 10 years of age. Many uncertainties were involved in the dose calculations, and particularly in the thyroid dosimetry. The most widespread late effects of fallout exposure among the Marshallese have been related to radiation injury to the thyroid gland. The growth status of children exposed to fallout radiation has been studied in 67 unexposed and 38 exposed children, 4 children exposed *in utero*, 39 children born to exposed parents and 53 children born to unexposed parents [S26]. Retardation in both statural growth and skeletal maturation has been observed among exposed boys, as compared with unexposed children. The retardation was noted among boys who were under 5 years of age when exposed to the fallout, being most prominent among those aged 12-18 months at the time of exposure. No significant differences were noted in the growth patterns between exposed and unexposed girls and between children born to exposed or unexposed parents.

60. The incidence of subclinical hypothyroidism was 31% among children less than 10 years of age at exposure after an estimated thyroid dose of >2 Gy. No case of hypothyroidism occurred in this age group at lower doses (Table 8). Among subjects 10 years or older, one case (1%) of hypothyroidism was observed at an estimated thyroid dose of <1 Gy, one case (8%) at 1-2 Gy and four cases (9%) at doses higher than 2 Gy. Only two of the subjects exposed at less than 10 years of age had clinical hypothyroidism. The incidence of hypothyroidism began to increase approximately one decade after exposure. A thorough re-evaluation of the absorbed dose in the thyroid was done by Lessard et al. [L9]. The recalculated cumulative external doses of gamma rays were close to the initial estimates, but doses from internally deposited radionuclides were much higher. Most of the thyroid dose resulted from short-lived radionuclides. The re-evaluation of the thyroid absorbed dose makes the observed results compatible with those of other studies with similar doses [R20].

61. Rallison et al. [R21, R22] observed two cases of hypothyroidism in 1,378 children exposed to ^{131}I fallout from nuclear weapons tests, compared to four cases in 3,801 non-irradiated control subjects. The follow-up time was, on average, 16 years, and the mean thyroid dose was estimated to be <0.5 Gy. The difference in the incidence of hypothyroidism between the two groups was not statistically significant. Clinical examinations were performed in 1990, and levels of free T4 and thyroid stimulating hormone were measured in children living in Russia, Belarus and Ukraine at the time of the nuclear plant accident in Chernobyl in 1986 and in children born in 1989 [I8]. There was no evidence that thyroid function had been affected in a way that could be detected either clinically or by laboratory testing at that time.

62. Thyroid disorders were studied 30 years after exposure in 978 individuals under 20 years of age at the time of the bombings in Hiroshima and Nagasaki [M21, M22]. The estimated doses from the atomic bomb fallout radiation were based on T65 dosimetry. There were 200 males and 277 females in the >1.0 Gy exposed group and 219 males and 282 females in the unexposed (0 Gy) group. Of these, 128 were aged 0-9 years and 349 were 10-19 years at the time of the bombings in the >1.0 Gy group; and 139 subjects were aged 0-9 years and 362 were 10-19 years at the time of the bombings in the unexposed group. There were

no significant differences in mean serum TSH levels or mean serum thyroglobulin levels between the 0 Gy (unexposed) group and the >1 Gy (exposed) group. In a recent analysis [N7] of 2,774 subjects of the Nagasaki Adult Health Study cohort, the prevalence of hypothyroidism was 5% in exposed subjects and 2% in controls. Inoue et al. [I7] studied nearly 2,600 individuals from the same cohort and observed hypothyroidism in 3% of the subjects. The fitted relative risk increased from 1 for those less than 5 years at the time of the bombings to 3 for those 30 years at the time of the bombings.

63. ***Summary***. Thyroid dysfunction may result from irradiation of the thyroid gland or the hypothalamic-pituitary axis. A substantial proportion of patients receiving radiotherapy for various paediatric tumours have impaired thyroid function. The incidence of hypothyroidism varies with the definition used and is highest when elevated TSH levels are used to define the impairment. Young children seem to be more sensitive to radiation-induced hypothyroidism. Various studies show that hypothyroidism is dose-dependent. The prevalence of hypothyroidism is increased in leukaemic children who have received cranial radiotherapy of 18-24 Gy over 2-2.5 weeks. The thyroid doses in these cases have been calculated to be 3%-8% of the brain dose, i.e. 1-2 Gy. However, the children also received associated chemotherapy, which may affect the risk for hypothyroidism. No epidemiologic study has demonstrated hypothyroidism in children after a thyroid dose from external irradiation <1 Gy. There is limited evidence that dose rate may be of importance and that the risk of hypothyroidism is reduced when fraction size is reduced. There are insufficient data on the effects of ^{131}I to determine a possible threshold dose for the induction of hypothyroidism.

C. OVARY

64. The ovary is a highly radiosensitive organ, and single doses of 0.6-4 Gy have caused temporary sterility in adults, with higher doses required to produce the same effect when fractionated. Permanent sterility results from 2.5-10 Gy in a single dose and from 6 Gy with protracted exposure [F1, I1, U3]. The radiosensitivity of the ovary depends on the degree of maturity, and the threshold for permanent sterility decreases with age, although the age-related differences are hard to estimate [A12, F1]. The fact that the ovary of a young woman is more resistant is explained by the reduction, over time, in the fixed pool of oocytes, since these cells are not replaced. The radiation dose required to destroy all the oocytes is therefore larger in younger than in older women. Ovarian dysfunction has been observed in more than 50% of adolescents and young women after doses of 2.5-4.0 Gy. Recovery has been age-related. After 4 Gy, permanent amenorrhea and infertility have occurred in approximately one third of younger women and in all women older than 40 years of age [A12, H12].

65. The most common cause of ovarian dysfunction in patients treated for paediatric tumours is direct damage to the gonads by radiation and/or cytotoxic agents. The observed ovarian effects have basically been fibrosis and follicle destruction with elevated levels of luteinizing hormone and follicle stimulating hormone. Irradiation of the hypothalamic-pituitary area can also result in gonadotropin deficiency or hyperprolactinaemia, which may impair subsequent reproductive function [A13, R23]. Quiescent ovaries have been found in children after radiotherapy with 20-30 Gy to the abdomen over 21-30 days, either alone or combined with chemotherapy [H13]. Chemotherapy used for a short time has been reported to be without effect on the small follicles, whereas prolonged treatment destroys them [M23].

66. Pelvic or abdominal irradiation has been associated with ovarian failure, resulting in elevated levels of follicle-stimulating hormone, amenorrhea and failure to develop secondary sexual characteristics [G7, O9, S32, S33, W6]. In a study by Wallace et al. [W6], ovarian failure occurred before 16 years of age in 19 patients irradiated in childhood for abdominal tumours with 30 Gy in 16-26 fractions over 21-38 days. An upper limit for the LD50 of the human oocyte was estimated at 4 Gy. Stillman et al. [S33] observed signs of ovarian failure in 12% of 182 long-term survivors of childhood cancer. Of 25 patients (68%) with both ovaries within the treatment fields (mean ovarian dose: 32 Gy), 17 showed ovarian failure, as compared with 5 of 35 patients (14%) whose ovaries were on the border of the treatment field (mean: 2.9 Gy), none of 34 patients with one or both ovaries outside the treatment field (mean: 0.5 Gy) and none of 88 patients receiving no radiation to the ovaries. The likelihood of ovarian failure in patients with both ovaries in the field was 19.7 (95% CI: 5.3-72.8), higher than those for other irradiated patients. Subsequent fertility has been observed in prepubertal girls after pelvic doses of 10-30 Gy, despite follicular depletion and elevated follicle-stimulating hormone levels [H13, L11, S32].

67. Horning et al. [H12] studied 103 women aged 13-38 years (median age: 19 years) with Hodgkin's disease treated by chemotherapy alone (n = 34), total-lymphoid irradiation alone (n = 19) or irradiation plus chemotherapy (n = 50). The pelvic dose was 30-40 Gy, delivered with conventional fractionation. Menses were present in 94% after total-lymphoid irradiation alone, 85% after chemotherapy alone and in 48% after total-lymphoid irradiation plus chemo-

therapy, of which 47%, 56% and 20%, respectively, were regular. Chemotherapy was associated with the highest and combination therapy with the lowest probability of regular menses. The probability of regular menses decreased with age at treatment (Figure VI). When age at treatment, interval after completion of treatment, stage of disease, number of cycles of chemotherapy and pelvic radiation dose were included in a multivariate analysis to determine factors predicting regular menses, only age was significant for any of the three treatment modalities.

68. Irradiation of the central nervous system and chemotherapy can destroy gonadal function by causing damage to the hypothalamus or direct damage to the gonads themselves [B18]. Various hormonal effects have been observed after cranial or craniospinal radiotherapy with 25-50 Gy fractionated over 3-4 weeks, e.g. elevated, normal or reduced levels of gonadotropins, secondary amenorrhea and lack of pubertal progression [A13, B10, C17, L10, R23, S15]. Leiper et al. [L12] observed early puberty in 10% of 233 children given cranial radiotherapy with 18-24 Gy in 10-15 fractions over 2-3 weeks for acute leukaemia at a mean age of 4 years. Three girls had precocious puberty, i.e. signs of sexual maturation occurring before 8 years. Early onset of menarche after cranial radiotherapy has also been observed by others [B19, M15, Q1, R23, S15]. Others have reported normal levels of gonadotropins and oestrogens after 24 Gy cranial radiotherapy in 2 Gy fractions over 2.5 weeks [D5, O7, V1].

69. Hamre et al. [H14] assessed gonadal function in 163 children treated for acute leukaemia at an average age of 6 years and who were randomized to receive 18 or 24 Gy to one of three fields: cranial, craniospinal or craniospinal plus 12 Gy abdominal, including the ovaries or testes. Gonadal evaluation 4 years later showed elevated levels of follicle-stimulating hormone and/or luteinizing hormone in 36% of the patients. There was an association between elevated gonadotropins and the radiotherapy field: 9% of patients who had cranial fields had elevated levels, as compared to 49% for craniospinal fields and 93% for craniospinal plus abdominal fields ($p < 0.001$). Girls receiving 24 Gy had a relative risk of 14 for elevated follicle-stimulating hormone and 8.7 for elevated luteinizing hormone compared with girls receiving 18 Gy. Craniospinal plus abdominal radiotherapy was significantly associated with abnormal gonadotropin levels and lack of pubertal development.

70. Patients who receive only chemotherapy prior to bone marrow transplantation have normal pubertal development and normal levels of gonadotropins and sex hormones. The majority of children receiving 10 Gy single whole-body exposure experience a delayed onset of puberty, and their gonadotropin levels reflect primary gonadal failure. Nearly half of children receiving fractionated whole-body irradiation have normal pubertal development and normal gonadotropin levels [B13, D2, S24, S34]. Ovarian failure appears to develop in almost all females of postpubertal age after whole-body irradiation with 10-12 Gy. Normal gonadotropin levels have been observed in the majority of girls who were prepubertal at the time of transplantation.

71. Sanders et al. [S23] studied ovarian function in 142 children (52 girls) treated with bone marrow transplantation at the median age of 10 years. All patients had received chemotherapy, and one third of the patients also had received radiotherapy to the central nervous system. Patients were given chemotherapy and whole-body irradiation, as a single dose of 9.2-10 Gy ($n = 79$) or as fractionated doses of 2-2.3 Gy daily for 6-7 days to a cumulative dose of 12-15.8 Gy ($n = 63$). Of 35 girls who were prepubertal at transplant, 10 had delayed development of secondary sexual characteristics at evaluation 4 years later. Gonadotropin and oestradiol levels were determined for 11 of 16 girls older than 12 years of age, and 7 had elevated levels of follicle-stimulating hormone, low levels of oestradiol and delayed onset of puberty. Gonadal failure occurred in nearly all who were post-pubertal at transplant, with amenorrhea and elevated levels of luteinizing hormone and follicle-stimulating hormone. It was not possible to determine how many of these endocrine abnormalities occurred as a result of treatment administered prior to transplantation. No information was provided on the effect of fractionation on gonadal function.

72. Sarkar et al. [S35] studied fertility in 33 subjects after ^{131}I therapy for thyroid cancer in childhood or adolescence. They received a mean ^{131}I amount of 7,250 MBq, with a range of 2,960-25,560 MBq, and the estimated cumulative gonadal dose ranged from 0.08 to 0.69 Gy. The incidence of infertility and miscarriage did not differ significantly from that in the general population.

73. ***Summary***. The effects of radiation on the ovary are age- and dose-dependent. The ovary of young women is less sensitive to radiation-induced deterministic effects because of their higher number of oocytes, although it is difficult to define the magnitude of these differences. A variety of factors complicate the study of a possible association between radiation dose and the effects on the ovary, including the underlying disease for which treatment was given. Unfortunately, most studies have been performed on a limited number of patients of varying ages at exposure, who received a variety of treatment modalities and had varying lengths of follow-up. The available data therefore do not allow an analysis of the dose-effect

patterns to define a critical dose for different gonadal parameters, nor can the impact of the fraction size be determined, since most studies have used fractionation schedules with about 2 Gy per day. An ovarian dose of 20 Gy or more causes microscopically evident damage and results in increased levels of gonadotropins and follicle-stimulating hormone. Amenorrhea has been observed in more than 10% of patients exposed in childhood with ovarian doses of 0.5 Gy on average and in two thirds of girls who received 3 Gy, on average, to both ovaries. Infertility occurs in approximately one third of girls receiving 4 Gy, as compared to almost all women over 40 years of age. The radiation dose required to ablate ovarian function seems to be around 20 Gy for girls, and the greater number of oocytes explains the higher doses needed for castration. Amenorrhea and the failure to develop secondary sexual characteristics have been documented in prepubertal girls following 10 Gy of whole-body irradiation, and ovarian failure has been seen in all pubertal women, of whom 50% had menopausal symptoms. Cranial radiotherapy may disturb sexual maturation by damaging the hypothalamus or the pituitary gland. Evidence of hypogonadism and of precocious puberty has been reported. Since chemotherapy may also cause ovarian dysfunction, the age of the patient, the amount of chemotherapy and the combined use of radiotherapy are all important factors in assessing ovarian injury.

D. TESTIS

74. The germ cells of the testis are the cells of the male reproductive system that are the most sensitive to exposure to ionizing radiation. Their depletion results in impaired fertility, the degree of which is dose-dependent. In adults, few stem cells survive a dose of 3-5 Gy, and sterility may be permanent. The lowest single acute dose that will impair fertility in adults is of the order of 0.15 Gy [R24]. Fractionated treatment may have more effect than single doses, e.g. 20 doses of 0.25 Gy each cause more rapid depletion and a slower recovery than a single dose of 5 Gy [L13, U3]. Blot et al. [B40] observed no clear evidence of sterility in 14 men exposed to the atomic bombings *in utero* with maternal doses ranging from 1 Gy to more than 6 Gy, nor among 66 men exposed to similar doses before 15 years of age. Data suggest that fractionated irradiation of 20 Gy is required to produce an incidence of more than 50% sterilization for more than five years [L14]. As little as 0.2 Gy can cause germinal epithelial damage with decreased sperm count and an elevated level of follicle-stimulating hormone [R24]. The damaged epithelium may recover with time, which related to the total dose received. A threshold dose required to damage the germinal epithelium in childhood has not been established, and doses as low as 0.1 Gy have been reported to cause temporary sterility, although >2 Gy and possibly about 6 Gy are needed to produce permanent aspermia [I1, U3]. Assessments of the effects of conventionally fractionated irradiation on testicular function indicate that gonadal function is compromised at doses as low as 0.5 Gy and that a cumulative dose of 2 Gy results in testicular dysfunction persisting at least three years [S36, S37]. There are no substantive studies of the effects of low-dose radiation on testicular function in boys, and it is generally not possible to distinguish between gonadal toxicity from chemotherapy and from radiotherapy.

75. The ability of the Leydig cells to produce testosterone appears to be appreciably reduced after testicular irradiation with high doses (24 Gy), resulting in androgen deficiency, testicular atrophy and clinical hypogonadism with elevated levels of follicle-stimulating hormone in the majority of boys [B20, L15, S20, S40]. The prepubertal boy appears more sensitive to radiation-induced Leydig cell damage than the adult male after testicular radiotherapy with 27-30 Gy in 20-28 fractions over 27-38 days [S38]. Normal Leydig cell function has been observed after testicular irradiation for childhood leukaemia with 12-15 Gy in 2 Gy fractions, although high gonadotropin levels suggest subclinical Leydig cell damage [C19]. According to Shalet [S20, S39], a fractionated testicular dose of <10 Gy in 20 fractions over 4 weeks does not appear to impair Leydig cell function in boys, whereas 24 Gy over 2.5-3 weeks causes Leydig cell failure.

76. The testicular germinal epithelium is more susceptible than Leydig cells to chemotherapy-induced damage and appears to be more sensitive to moderate doses of alkylating agents after puberty than before [S36]. In contrast to that given to prepubertal boys, chemotherapy given during puberty may result in injury to both Leydig cells and the seminiferous epithelium and may thus have profound effects on both endocrine function and germ cell production [A13, C18]. The use of alkylating agents has been associated with testicular dysfunction that may be related to age and the total dose of the agent used. Recovery of spermatogenesis is variable. Others have found that chemotherapy for acute leukaemia may be compatible with normal gonadal development [B21, B22].

77. Of 10 men who had radiotherapy for Wilms' tumour in childhood with estimated testicular doses of 2.7-9.8 Gy, eight had oligo- or azoospermia and seven had elevated follicle-stimulating hormone levels [S39]. Only one man had evidence of Leydig cell dysfunction. Shalet et al. [S39] also studied a second group of eight prepubertal males who had received testicular doses of 1-30 Gy. Despite these substantial doses, which are higher than those required to cause tubular

in the postpubertal male, plasma testosterone and gonadotropin levels were normal. Only one boy had an elevated follicle-stimulating hormone level. The radiation-induced damage to the germinal epithelium thus resulted in raised levels of follicle-stimulating hormone after puberty but not before. In respect of pelvic radiotherapy and/or chemotherapy for Hodgkin's disease in childhood, Green et al. [G7] did not observe any difference in gonadal function between nine boys and male adolescents who received a gonadal dose of 1 Gy and seven patients who received only chemotherapy. Six and five men, respectively, had elevated levels of follicle-stimulating hormone up to eight years after completion of treatment.

78. Abnormal puberty and gonadotropin deficiency have been observed in about 10% of children irradiated to the hypothalamic-pituitary region with 25-50 Gy over 3-4 weeks [L10, R23]. After cranial radiotherapy for leukaemia in childhood, varying results have been observed. Quigley et al. [Q1] found evidence of germ-cell damage in 25 boys who received chemotherapy and 24 Gy in 15 fractions over three weeks. Germ-cell damage was confirmed by the absence of germ cells in testicular biopsy specimens and by the small size of the testes in all boys. Boys reached puberty at a mean age of 12 years. Plasma sex steroids were normal, but the level of luteinizing hormone after stimulation with gonadotropin-releasing hormone was elevated in pubertal children, suggesting compensation for decreased gonadal function. Sklar et al. [S41] evaluated testicular function in 60 long-term survivors of childhood acute leukaemia who had been randomized to cranial radiotherapy with 18 or 24 Gy (n = 26), 18 or 24 Gy plus intrathecal methotrexate (n = 23) or 24 Gy craniospinal radiotherapy plus 12 Gy to the abdomen including gonads (n = 11). Treatment was delivered in 1.2-2 Gy daily fractions, and the scattered dose in the testes was 0.4-3.6 Gy after craniospinal radiotherapy. Primary germ-cell dysfunction on average five years after cessation of therapy was significantly associated with type of radiotherapy field: 55% after craniospinal plus abdominal field, 17% after craniospinal and 0% after cranial radiotherapy ($p < 0.01$). Leydig cell function was unaffected in the majority of patients regardless of type of radiotherapy. Leiper et al. [L12] observed early puberty in five boys treated with 18-24 Gy in 10-15 fractions over 2-3 weeks. The mean age for onset of puberty in these children was 9 years, which was greater than two standard deviations from the mean. Precocious puberty, i.e. signs of sexual maturation occurring before 9 years, has also been reported [B19, L12]. Von Muehlendahl et al. [V1] noted normal levels of luteinizing hormone and follicle-stimulating hormone in 17 boys after 8-18 Gy of cranial radiotherapy. Jaffe et al. [J4] evaluated reproductive function in 27 male long-term survivors of childhood cancer treated during prepuberty and puberty with a mean testicular dose of 1.9 Gy (range: 0-25 Gy). Sperm samples were obtained from 23 subjects, and the 4 who refused had fathered healthy children. Four patients were oligospermic and 14 were azoospermic. The four sterile men had received at least 1.4 Gy to the testes without chemotherapy and as low as 0.08 Gy in combination with alkylating agents. Sterility was mainly associated with alkylating agents.

79. After chemotherapy and whole-body irradiation with a single exposure of 10 Gy, delayed pubertal development occurred in one of 12 boys (he also received testicular irradiation); four were still prepubertal at evaluation and seven boys had normal pubertal development [B13]. Four of the boys with normal pubertal development had elevated levels of follicle-stimulating hormone with normal luteinizing hormone and testosterone. Another seven boys received fractionated whole-body irradiation with 12-14 Gy in 6 fractions over three days, and five of them were still prepubertal and two had achieved puberty, one after testosterone administration. Deeg et al. [D2] observed that 5 of 16 boys subjected to whole-body irradiation developed secondary sex characteristics appropriate for their age and 11 had delayed onset of puberty. Forty-one male patients who were past puberty at the time of transplantation developed primary gonadal failure and azoospermia. Two had recovery of spermatogenesis approximately six years after transplantation, and one of them had two normal children. Gonadal failure therefore appeared to be nearly universal after whole-body irradiation with 10-12 Gy in patients of post-pubertal age. Sanders et al. [S23] studied gonadal function in 90 boys 1-17 years old who had bone marrow transplantation after prior chemotherapy and radiotherapy to the central nervous system (n = 55). Whole-body irradiation was given as a single dose of 9.2-10 Gy or fractionated doses of 2-2.3 Gy daily for 6-7 days to a cumulative dose of 12-15.8 Gy. At evaluation on average four years later, 21 of the 63 boys who were prepubertal at transplant had delayed development of secondary sexual characteristics. Gonadal failure occurred in nearly all who were postpubertal at transplant.

80. *Summary*. The effects of radiation on the testis are age- and dose-dependent. Radiation appears to have its greatest effect on the germ cells rather than on Leydig cells. It is difficult to draw any certain conclusions regarding the effect of ionizing radiation on the gonadal function in boys and male adolescents. The data have been obtained from studies based on heterogeneous materials, with great variation in age at exposure and treatment modalities. Furthermore, gonadal function has been assessed in many different ways. The threshold radiation dose that will damage the germinal epithelium in childhood cannot therefore

be clearly defined at present. Testicular function may be compromised at doses as low as 0.5 Gy. Leydig cell function appears more resistant to ionizing radiation, and impaired function occurs after 10 Gy or more. Testicular function is also impaired by chemotherapy and may also be abnormal prior to therapy for malignancy that does not involve the testis. Irradiation to the prepubertal gonads may not always result in irreversible damage. Whole-body irradiation has been shown to produce primary gonadal failure of various degrees in the majority of boys receiving 10 Gy, regardless of pubertal status. In most of these patients, Leydig cell function appeared adequate.

E. MUSCULOSKELETAL SYSTEM

81. Two processes of bone formation occur within the human skeleton: membranous bone formation and enchondral bone formation [P10]. Flat bones and the cortices of long bones are formed by membranous bone formation, in which there is no pre-existing cartilage template, and osteoid tissue is laid down adjacent to existing collagen, cartilage or bone. In enchondral bone formation, which is responsible for longitudinal bone growth, new bone is formed at the epiphyseal growth plate. Chondroblast proliferation is responsible for widening of the epiphyseal growth plate and lengthening of the bone, and osteoid is formed by osteoblasts. External irradiation affects, in particular, dividing chondroblasts and small blood vessels. Membraneous bone formation is disturbed to a lesser extent than enchondral bone growth. Epiphyseal irradiation causes arrest of chondrosis due to direct effects on the chondrocytes and secondary vascular effects. Radiotherapy also disrupts the normal processes of resorption of bone at the epiphysis. Actinomycin D and adriamycin enhance the effects of radiotherapy [E6]. Bone absorbs less radiation in the megavoltage range than in the orthovoltage range, and it has been believed that there is less growth disturbance in bone after megavoltage therapy. However, the major radiation changes occur in the chondroblasts and the fine blood vessels of the physis. Since both are materials of unit density, it is reasonable to expect growth disturbances to be largely independent of radiation voltage quality.

82. The first evidence of growth disturbances following x-ray treatment in patients under 20 years of age was reported in 1929 by Hueck et al. [H15]. In adults, cartilage tolerates 40 Gy over 4 weeks or >70 Gy over 10-12 weeks, and bone tolerates 65 Gy over 6-8 weeks. Higher doses cause necrosis [C24]. These tissues are more sensitive in children, and some growth retardation may occur after 1 Gy, depending on the age at irradiation and the conditions of exposure [I1, T10]. The maximum growth depression has been observed in children treated up to the age of 6 years and in young puberty [G9, P10, R25, R26]. Roentgenographic changes of the bone in children less than 1 year of age occur after conventionally fractionated radiotherapy of >4 Gy, while a dose of >18 Gy with similar fractionation is required to produce significant changes in children 1-2 years of age and >26 Gy is required in older children [N5, T10]. Other skeletal changes occur in children at doses >20 Gy, including scoliosis, kyphosis and slipped capital femoral epiphysis.

83. Growth in children can be adversely affected by direct radiation damage to long bones and spine, malnutrition, steroid therapy, cytotoxic drugs, the presence of residual tumour and endocrine complications [B3, B23, B24, B25, D17, G8, P11, P12, S20, S42, T10, W7]. The effects of radiotherapy on the skeleton are related to the anatomical site, the target volume, the radiation dose, the source and pattern of the radiation used, the age of the patient and chemotherapy. These effects may be seen in any bone but are most often observed in the spine after fractionated radiotherapy with cumulative doses of 20 Gy or more [P13]. The severity increases with increasing radiation dose and with decreasing age at time of treatment. Mature bone and cartilage may also be devitalized by ionizing radiation without showing clinical consequences until stressed by, for example, infection or trauma. Prednisone and doxorubicin depress cartilage responsiveness to somatomedin and also growth-hormone-stimulated somatomedin production [P12]. It is difficult to quantify the effects of ionizing radiation on growing bones for several reasons:

(a) there is a lack of large groups of patients of various ages in whom the same epiphyseal cartilage has been irradiated with a range of doses;
(b) the tumour itself and other treatment modalities can contribute to the growth disturbance;
(c) patients must be followed until growth is completed;
(d) often patients with growth disturbances have deformities corrected surgically, making it impossible to quantify the damage [G8].

84. Children less than 6 years old and at the time of the adolescent growth spurt, i.e. during periods of rapid bone growth, are especially sensitive to irradiation of the vertebral column. Impaired growth has been observed after total doses of 25 Gy, and higher doses to the entire spine result in suppression of spinal growth and decreased sitting height [D17, P10, P11, S25]. Probert et al. [P10] observed changes in both the sitting and standing heights of 44 children treated with megavoltage radiation, particularly among those receiving >35 Gy in 2-2.5 Gy fractions, whereas only slight changes were observed among those receiving <25 Gy with similar fractionation (Figure VII). Shalet

et al. [S43] measured growth after radiotherapy for brain tumour in 37 children who had received cranio-spinal irradiation with 27-35 Gy to the vertebrae in 17-20 fractions over 3-4 weeks and in 42 children who received cranial radiotherapy. The cranial dose was not stated. All had completed their growth at the time of evaluation, and at that time there were significant differences between the two groups on standard deviation scores for standing height and sitting height, but not for leg length. The younger the child was at the time of treatment the greater the subsequent skeletal disproportion; the estimated eventual loss in height was 9 cm when spinal irradiation was given at 1 year, 7 cm when given at 5 years, and 6 cm when given at 10 years.

85. Growth retardation has also been observed in children injected with ^{224}Ra for intended treatment of tuberculosis of bone and soft tissue [M24, S44]. Spiess et al. [S44] obtained the adult heights of 133 patients injected as juveniles. Radium-224-induced growth retardation was greatest in young children, who had the greatest amount of potential growth after exposure. The growth retardation increased with radiation dose, and there was a 2% decrease in potential growth post-irradiation per gray for average skeletal doses up to 20-25 Gy.

86. Functional and cosmetic disabilities involving bone, teeth, muscle and other soft tissues have been reported to occur after radiotherapy in up to 38% of survivors of paediatric cancers, in particular after treatment for solid tumours [D19, L16, M2, M25, S43]. The clinically significant problems often involve bone abnormalities, such as scoliosis, atrophy or hypoplasia, avascular necrosis and osteoporosis. Scoliosis may occur following radiotherapy to segments of the spinal column in patients with solid tumours [H16, J5, S42, S45, W8]. Scoliosis has been most apparent in children treated with orthovoltage radiation to fields extending to the midline, resulting in asymmetric radiation of the vertebrae. The degree of scoliosis has increased with dose and has been mild after 20-32 Gy and significant after higher doses [O10, P10, R27]. Vertebral abnormalities have been less pronounced with high voltage radiotherapy and with radiation fields encompassing the entire vertebrae, and significant scoliosis below 35 Gy is uncommon [H16, P10, T11]. The cases of scoliosis that occur at present are usually not so severe that orthopaedic intervention is required.

87. Slipped epiphyses can develop in patients who have received radiotherapy to the proximal femoral epiphysis, combined with chemotherapy, in childhood [B26, L17, R1, S46, W9, W10]. Silverman et al. [S46] studied 50 patients under 15 years of age who had radiotherapy that included the non-fused capital femoral epiphyseal plate in the treatment field. Mean dose to the epiphyseal plates was 23 Gy (range: 1.5-53 Gy), and 10% of the 83 plates at risk showed epiphyseal slippage or other severe radiographical abnormalities. Children under the age of 4 years at the time of irradiation were at higher risk (47%) than older children (5%). No complications occurred below 25 Gy and no dose-response curve was obtained. A mean difference of up to 12 cm in clinical length between unirradiated and irradiated extremities has been observed after ≥6 Gy to the epiphyseal plates [G8]. Figure VIII shows the relationship between age at irradiation, dose and shortening for 20 patients who had epiphyseal plate irradiation. Damage increased dramatically at doses up to 40 Gy but levelled off beyond that. Shortening was strongly age-dependent, amounting to 9-12 cm in several patients who were less than 1 year old. When growth expected to remain after irradiation was taken into account, age at irradiation did not influence the final effect, and the radiation dose was the most important factor. Radiation-induced aseptic necrosis of the femoral heads have been observed in children after doses of 30-40 Gy [L17]. Chemotherapy may be a contributing factor, since aseptic osteonecrosis has been reported in children after chemotherapy alone [P14]. Slipped proximal humeral epiphysis has also been reported after slightly higher radiation doses than those received by children with slipped capital femoral epiphysis [E6]. That the shoulder is not as stressed as the hip may be the reason why slipped proximal humeral epiphysis is less frequent than slipped femoral epiphysis.

88. Bony hypoplasia of the orbit with facial asymmetry was reported in half of 50 children with orbital rhabdomyosarcoma after 50-60 Gy in 5-6 weeks [H17]. The degree of hypoplasia appeared to be higher the younger the child was at the time of treatment. Other common findings were asymmetry of the face and/or neck and the presence of dental problems, both of which occurred in 58% of the patients. Evidence of muscle atrophy or fibrosis of the subcutaneous tissues was evident in 40% of the patients in the head or face and 33% in the neck. Hypoplasia of bones in treated sites was documented in one third of the patients and judged to be largely due to radiotherapy. Similar late effects have been observed by others [E7, G10].

89. Radiotherapy may also have adverse effects on developing dentition, including root abnormalities, incomplete calcification, delayed or arrested tooth development and caries [B27, D19, H18, J6, M26]. These and other maxillofacial abnormalities, such as trismus, abnormal occlusal relationships and facial deformities are more severe in patients irradiated at an earlier age and at higher doses. Jaffe et al. [J6] observed dental and maxillofacial abnormalities in 82% of 45 long-term survivors of childhood cancer

after maxillofacial radiotherapy. Younger patients and those treated with higher doses, i.e. rhabdomyosarcoma patients (median dose: 55 Gy) as opposed to Hodgkin's disease and leukaemia patients (median dose: 35 Gy, $p < 0.001$) had more severe abnormalities. In a study by Sonis et al. [S47], abnormal dental development occurred five or more years later in 94% of 97 children with acute leukaemia treated before 10 years of age with intrathecal methotrexate alone (n = 19) or in combination with 18-24 Gy cranial radiotherapy (n = 78). All children who received treatment before 5 years of age and those who received radiotherapy had the most severe abnormalities. Tooth breakage due to tooth resorption has been common among patients injected with ^{224}Ra, especially those injected as teenagers [S48]. The incidence of tooth breakage increased significantly with dose. The tooth fractures resembled those observed in radium dial painters in the United States [R25]. Children given a single whole-body exposure of 10 Gy for marrow transplantation have developed similar disturbances in dental development and facial growth similar to those seen after 18-65 Gy fractionated radiotherapy to the maxillofacial region for leukaemia or solid tumours [D20, S25]. The most severe effects have been seen in children irradiated when they were less than 6 years of age.

90. Anthropometric analyses were performed in 1990 on children living in Russia, Belarus and Ukraine at the time of the nuclear plant accident in Chernobyl in 1986, and in children born in 1989 [I8]. The main conclusion from these studies was that there were no significant differences in height or weight between the control and contaminated regions.

91. ***Summary***. Growth in children can be adversely affected by direct radiation damage and by malnutrition, other treatment modalities, the presence of residual tumour, and endocrine late radiation effects. Most clinical data are based on small and heterogeneous groups of patients treated in different ways at varying ages. The skeletal effects have also been assessed in a variety of ways, and it is not possible to give any estimates of late deterministic effects based on large-scale epidemiologic data. Skeletal changes in children generally occur at doses exceeding 20 Gy and include scoliosis, kyphosis, slipped femoral epiphyses, hypoplasia, growth retardation, dental problems etc. Absolute shortening of the long bone depends on the absorbed radiation dose and the age at the time of irradiation. Exposure at ages less than 6 years and during puberty appears to have the greatest effect on growth retardation. However, other studies have observed that when growth expected to occur after irradiation was taken into account, the age at irradiation did not influence the final effect, and the radiation dose was then the most important factor. Scoliosis and kyphosis are common after spinal or flank irradiation following doses of >20 Gy. Slipped femoral capital epiphysis does not occur below 20 Gy, and this late effect is more common in children under 4 years of age at the time of irradiation. A dose exceeding 20 Gy is required to arrest encondral bone formation, and doses of 10-20 Gy cause the partial arrest of bone growth. There is little alteration in bone growth below 10 Gy of fractionated exposure directly to the bone. No radiation-related effect on height has been observed in children living in Russia, Belarus or Ukraine at the time of the Chernobyl accident.

F. EYE

92. Ionizing radiation, chemotherapy and corticosteroids have all been found to increase the risk of cataract formation [C20, H19, I1, O11, P15, S49, U3]. Different components of the eye have different sensitivity to ionizing radiation, and the lens is especially sensitive when uniformly irradiated. There are different forms of cataract, and radiation-induced cataract is in its early stages a characteristic lesion, which is defined as a posterior subcapsular opacity. The threshold dose for cataract in adults is about 2 Gy of x rays from a single exposure and 4-6 Gy when fractionated over 3-13 weeks [F1, M27]. Minimal stationary opacities have been observed after single doses of 1-2 Gy, and with 5 Gy more serious progressive cataracts occur [U3]. The threshold dose for cataract formation is increased by non-uniform irradiation [B28]. Higher radiation doses yield more progressive cataracts with a greater loss of vision. The average latent period is 2 years but may be up to 35 years. The combination of radiotherapy and chemotherapy enhances the risk for cataract formation [F7]. Other late radiation effects in the eye include retinopathy, optic neuropathy and lacrimal gland atrophy. These types of injuries rarely occur below 45 Gy.

93. Decreased vision due to cataract formation in the treated eye is common in children treated for orbital rhabdomyosarcoma after doses to the tumour of 50-60 Gy in 2 Gy fractions over 5-6 weeks [H17]. The time to first reported evidence of cataract varied from one to four years after radiotherapy. Other reported structural late effects include changes in the cornea or retina, enophthalmos, and stenosis of the lacrimal duct.

94. Qvist and Zachau-Christiansen [Q2] estimated the minimum lenticular dose to produce cataract in children to be 13.8 Gy from radium moulds; the maximum non-cataract dose for infants was 9.9 Gy and for school-aged children, 11.4 Gy. Notter et al. [N8] observed cataracts after considerably lower doses in 234 patients who had been irradiated with ^{226}Ra-containing applicators for skin haemangioma between

1920 and the mid-1950s. An ophthalmologic examination was conducted in 1961-1965. Of 468 eyes examined, cataract was observed in 51 (11%). No cataract was observed in the 246 eyes receiving <2.5 Gy in the lens. The prevalence of cataract was 8% (100 eyes) after a lenticular dose of 2.5-3.5 Gy and 54% (122 eyes) after higher doses.

95. Stefani et al. [S37, C25] reported on the development of cataract in 899 patients receiving multiple injections of ^{224}Ra for the intended treatment of tuberculosis or ankylosing spondylitis. Cataracts were found in 6% of the 218 juvenile patients and in 5% of the 681 adult patients. In those with known injected activities, juveniles receiving >1 MBq kg^{-1} of ^{224}Ra had a cataract incidence of 14% (11 of 80) compared to 0.8% (1 of 131) receiving less than that amount. The cataract incidence increased significantly with dosage in both juveniles and adults.

96. The dose received by the lens in cranial radiotherapy for acute leukaemia is of importance for the induction of cataract [K10]. The dose to the lens is approximately 15%-30% of the midline dose, depending on the type of treatment fields. Nesbit et al. [N3] found one case of posterior subcapsular cataracts in 50 survivors of childhood acute leukaemia. In contrast, Inati et al. [I3] observed a 50% incidence of cataract formation in 69 children with acute leukaemia given 24 Gy cranial radiotherapy in 13 fractions over 2.5 weeks, intrathecal methotrexate and high doses of steroids. All cataracts were small and did not impair vision. In another study of 34 long-term survivors of acute leukaemia, all 18 patients in the non-irradiated group had normal results in eye examinations, while 4 of 16 of those receiving 24 Gy to the whole brain in 12 fractions over 2.5 weeks had ocular abnormalities [W11]. None of the ocular findings could, however, be definitely attributed to radiation, and all patients had normal visual acuity.

97. Posterior subcapsular cataracts occur in the great majority of patients after 10 Gy of single whole-body exposure but in only about 20% after 12-15.8 Gy of fractionated exposure [A14, B13, C8, D21, L23, S24, V7]. Among 105 patients given 10 Gy single-dose whole-body irradiation, 80% developed cataracts by six years compared to 19% of 76 patients given fractionated whole-body irradiation (12-15 Gy in 2-5 Gy fractions over 6-7 days) and 18% in patients who did not receive radiotherapy [D2]. This last figure indicates that factors other than irradiation, e.g. steroids or previous treatments may have contributed to the development of cataracts. Nearly all cataracts developed after a single exposure need to be removed, whereas a smaller fraction of those developed after fractionated exposure require removal.

98. In a study conducted among subjects of the Adult Health Study of Hiroshima and Nagasaki, a significant excess risk for posterior subcapsular changes was observed for all ages in the group receiving >3 Sv in comparison with those in the control group among residents in Hiroshima but not in Nagasaki [C21]. The study was based on the T65 dosimetry and the examination was conducted on 2,385 persons. The relative risk of cataract for persons in Hiroshima exposed to >3 Sv was 4.8 in persons under age 15 years at the time of the bombings, 2.3 in persons 15-24 years at the time of the bombings and 1.4 in persons more than 25 years at the time of the bombings. The relative risk for posterior subcapsular changes in Hiroshima for persons under age 15 years at the time of the bombings was 2.8 in the 1-1.9 Sv group, 4.3 in the group receiving 2-2.9 Sv and 5.3 in the group receiving >3 Sv. A comparison of relative risks in the different age groups suggested a stronger effect in Hiroshima for persons under age 15 years at the time of the bombings. These results support the hypothesis that younger individuals are more sensitive to radiation-induced cataract than older individuals. A more recent assessment of the dose-effect relationship for cataract induction has been made using the DS86 dosimetry system [O15, O16]. This new study confirms the previous findings of a higher sensitivity in young persons. The magnitude of log relative risks for cataracts in persons aged 40, 50, 60 and 70 years at the time of examination was 8.2, 6.4, 4.6 and 2.8-fold higher, respectively, than in persons aged 80 years at the time of examination. The best-fitting relationship for posterior postcapsular changes suggested a linear-quadratic dose-response.

99. *Summary.* The available data on radiation-induced cataract formation in adults suggest a sigmoid dose-response relationship with an apparent threshold. This threshold varies from 2 to 5 Gy after x rays and gamma rays given as single exposure and is about 10 Gy for doses fractionated over a period of months. Data on radiation-induced cataracts in children are scarce and are based on small groups of patients receiving different treatment modalities. Cataracts have been reported after 24 Gy cranial radiotherapy for childhood leukaemia resulting in 5-7 Gy in the lens. Cataracts have been observed after 2.5 Gy or more in the lens, and in one study the prevalence of cataract was 8% (100 eyes) after a lenticular dose of 2.5-3.5 Gy. Whole-body exposure of 10 Gy in childhood has also been associated with cataract formation in the majority of cases, whereas fractionated whole-body irradiation with 12-15.8 Gy is associated with cataract in about 20% of the patients. Cataracts were observed in the survivors of the atomic bombings in Japan exposed to >3 Gy, and the risk for cataract was higher in persons less than age 15 years at the time of the bombings than in persons older than that.

G. CARDIOVASCULAR SYSTEM

100. Ionizing radiation affects small and large vessels within the treatment field, and changes may develop within months and up to two decades after radiotherapy [K2]. The main changes that occur consist of premature atherosclerosis with vascular occlusion. The heart was formerly thought to be relatively resistant to ionizing radiation. The increasing use of radiotherapy to the mediastinum, however, has been associated with well-documented instances of cardiac abnormalities. Late effects following radiotherapy have been reported in both adults and children and usually occur as cardiomyopathy, coronary artery disease, pericardial effusions or constrictive pericarditis [A15, B29, B30, D17, G11, G12, K11, L1, P9, R28, T9]. Interstitial myocardial fibrosis and coronary artery changes have been reported after 30 Gy, and pericarditis has been reported after 15 Gy [B29, G12, K12, M28, M29]. In children as well as in adults, a dose of 40 Gy to the heart appears to be the critical dose for clinical cardiomyopathy.

101. The incidence of post-irradiation pericarditis increases with dose and fraction size [S50]. In patients irradiated for Hodgkin's disease, the frequency of radiation-related pericarditis correlates with the pericardial dose [C22]. Carmel and Kaplan [C22] found a 7% incidence of pericarditis after doses <6 Gy, 12% after 6-15 Gy, 19% after 15-30 Gy and 50% after >30 Gy. Symptomatic pericarditis may first appear as late as 45 years after therapy [B29, G13, H20, K12, S51]. Kadota et al. [K12] evaluated cardiopulmonary function in 11 children who received radiotherapy for Hodgkin's disease with a mean dose of 36 Gy (range: 20-55 Gy) with conventional fractionation. Mean age at radiotherapy was 11 years, and evaluation was performed, on average, nine years later. Ten patients had no clinical evidence of cardiopulmonary dysfunction, and one had constrictive pericarditis. Four had thickened cardiac valves on echocardiography, without significant stenosis or insufficiency. Only three had normal cardiopulmonary function, and the others had one or more abnormal tests.

102. Mäkinen et al. [M30] evaluated cardiac sequelae in 41 individuals who had received chest radiotherapy or doxorubicin for childhood cancer at a median of 17 years earlier. Radiotherapy had been used in 21 patients, and in 13 of them irradiation was directed at the heart with doses of 12-60 Gy in 8-30 fractions over 12-47 days. Of the 41 patients, 20 (49%) showed some abnormality in cardiac tests (e.g. abnormal ECG or echocardiogram, reduced exercise capacity), and each additional year of follow-up was associated with a 1.3-fold increase in pathologic cardiac findings. The risk of an abnormal cardiac test result in the 13 patients who had received radiotherapy to the heart was 12.8 times the risk for other patients (95% CI: 1.8-90.8). No detailed analysis of the effect of radiotherapy was presented.

103. The anthracyclines doxorubicin and daunomycin are cardiotoxic and may cause electrocardiographic changes and congestive heart failure. There is a dose-response relationship between the total dose of anthracyclines and cardiomyopathy, and children appear to be more susceptible to drug-induced cardiomyopathy [P16, P17, S52, V3, V4]. Several studies have shown that mediastinal irradiation enhances the myocardial toxicity of anthracyclines [B31, G14, M31, P16, P18]. Gilladoga et al. [G14] observed severe cardiomyopathy with congestive heart failure in 16% of 50 children receiving adriamycin and in 3% of 60 children receiving daunomycin. Four of 8 children who also had incidental cardiac irradiation prior to or during adriamycin administration had severe cardiomyopathy. In contrast, Von Hoff et al. [V5] observed a lower risk of cardiomyopathy for children than for adults at any given cumulative doxorubicin dosage.

104. *Summary*. Radiation exposures cause occlusion of both small and large blood vessels. Cardiac abnormalities have been observed particularly following irradiation of the mediastinum. Patients may have abnormal cardiac function without clinical evidence of such dysfunction. Myocardial fibrosis has occurred after 30 Gy. The few data available suggest that 40 Gy with conventional fractionation can be considered as a critical dose for clinical cardiomyopathy in both children and adults. The anthracyclines are cardiotoxic and enhance the effects of mediastinal irradiation.

H. LUNG

105. The lung is the most radiosensitive organ in the thorax. The mechanism for respiratory damage in young children may be different from that in adults or in adolescents. Specific radiation effects in children can include the impaired formation of new alveoli or failures in the development of the thoracic skeleton and thus a reduced size of the lung [B32, R17]. Interstitial fibrosis of the lung, resulting in decreased total lung capacity, vital capacity and diffusion, is a late effect that has been observed in adults after doses of >30 Gy and above [D22, H21, L1, L18, M18, M32, S54]. The effect in children appears to be similar for the same dose and fractionation schedules [D17, S53, T9, W12]. Children younger than 3 years at the time of treatment may be at higher risk for lung dysfunction [M32]. The effects depend on the target volume and on the concurrent use of chemotherapy [W13]. Interstitial pneumonitis and pulmonary fibrosis have also been reported after chemotherapy in children and adults [A16].

106. Restrictive lung volume with total lung capacity between 62% and 80% of normal capacity was recorded after treatment for Hodgkin's disease in 5 of 11 patients (mean age: 11 years) who received mantle field radiotherapy with 20-55 Gy [K12]. Six children had reduced exercise tolerance, manifested by reduced maximum oxygen uptake (<65% of predicted) and exercise duration (<75% of predicted). Miller et al. [M32] observed reduced forced vital capacity and/or total lung capacity in half of 29 children with childhood cancer. The incidence of pulmonary dysfunction was high in both irradiated children and in individuals who did not receive radiotherapy to the thorax.

107. After fractionated pulmonary radiotherapy for Wilms' tumour at age 2-4 years with a lung dose of 20 Gy, children may develop dyspnoea and evidence of interstitial and pleural thickening on chest x-ray examination up to 14 years after treatment [W14]. Mean total lung volumes may be reduced by approximately 40% after such radiotherapy owing to effects on lung growth and on chest wall growth. Restrictive lung changes after fractionated radiotherapy with 11-14 Gy to the whole lung have been reported in other studies of children with paediatric tumours [B32, L19]. Benoist et al. [B32] studied the effects of whole-lung irradiation on lung function in 48 children treated for Wilms' tumour with pulmonary metastases. The mean age was 3 years, and all patients received fractionated radiotherapy with 20 Gy bilateral pulmonary irradiation over three weeks plus actinomycin D. Greatly reduced sagittal and frontal thoracic diameters were observed in nearly all of the cases 3-4 years after radiotherapy. Lung volumes and dynamic lung compliance and functional residual capacity decreased with time. Static pressure volume curves, blood gases and carbon monoxide transfer were normal, making it unlikely that post-radiation pulmonary fibrosis was involved.

108. Littman et al. [L19] evaluated pulmonary function in 33 patients treated for Wilms' tumour and followed for up to 20 years after diagnosis. All but five children received at least one course of actinomycin D. Eighteen children who did not receive lung irradiation had normal pulmonary function. Radiotherapy was given to 10 children for pulmonary metastases and to 5 children as prophylaxis with a lung dose of 12-14 Gy and varying fractionations. Patients treated for metastases had findings suggestive of moderately reduced lung volumes, whereas patients receiving prophylactic treatment had essentially normal lung volumes. Vital capacity and functional residual capacity were significantly lower in the irradiated group of patients than in the non-irradiated patients. Residual volume was lower in the irradiated group as was forced expiratory volume. The fact that patients who were treated for metastatic disease had greater abnormalities in pulmonary function than those irradiated for prophylaxis suggests that the presence of metastatic nodules and additional lung treatment could have aggravated the effects.

109. Two studies did not observe any impairment of lung function in patients 15 years old or less after whole lung irradiation with 20 Gy in 1.5-2 Gy fractions five times per week [B39, Z1]. According to Margolis et al. [M34], the maximum safe dose to the whole lung for patients receiving actinomycin D is 15 Gy in 1.5 Gy fractions. However, doses lower than that may affect pulmonary function. Wohl et al. [W14] reported that total lung capacity averaged 71% of the expected value in six children treated with fractionated and bilateral pulmonary irradiation for Wilms' tumour and evaluated more than seven years later. The exposures at the midplane of the chest ranged from 8-12 Gy delivered over an average of 11 days. The total lung capacity for eight children receiving no radiotherapy was 94% of the expected value. Springmeyer et al. [S53] found restrictive ventilatory changes in 79 patients with haematologic malignancies or aplastic anaemia one year or more after bone marrow transplantation. There was a mean loss in total lung capacity of 0.8 and in vital capacity of 0.5, but these changes were not significantly associated with whole-body irradiation.

110. *Summary*. The lung is a radiosensitive organ, and radiotherapy during a period of lung growth and chest wall growth primarily results in a reduction of the subsequent size of both lungs and chest wall. Respiratory damage in young children is more severe than in adults at the same doses. The effects depend on the target volume and concurrent use of chemotherapy. Interstitial fibrosis may occur 6-12 months after absorbed doses to the lung of 30 Gy or more. A lung dose of 15 Gy in 1.5 Gy fractions is generally considered as the maximum safe dose in children receiving radiotherapy to the whole lung and simultaneous treatment with actinomycin D. However, restrictive lung changes have been reported after doses of 11 Gy or more in children treated for paediatric tumours, and reduced total lung capacity has been found after 8 Gy or more to the whole lung with similar fractionation.

I. BREAST

111. Breast development is readily inhibited by radiotherapy in infancy, and severe hypoplasia of breast tissue has been reported in women having a history of breast irradiation in childhood [D19, F8, F9, G15, H22, K13, U11]. Breast hypoplasia or aplasia have also been noted as sequelae after radiotherapy for paediatric tumours in childhood [F8]. The knowledge

of dose-effect patterns is scarce [I1, I5]. Moss [M35] stated that an exposure giving a skin dose of 15-20 Gy over eight days would impair breast development. According to Rubin et al. [R2], a dose exceeding 10 Gy to the prepubertal female breast of conventionally fractionated x-ray therapy may result in the absence of breast development in 1%-5% of the patients.

112. Fürst et al. [F9] studied the prevalence and degree of breast hypoplasia in 129 women irradiated in infancy or childhood for haemangioma in the breast region. The patients were treated in 1934-1943 at an age of 4 years or less. Radiotherapy was mainly given with applicators containing ^{226}Ra, with flat applicators or needles and/or tubes having been used. Mean absorbed dose to the breast anlage for the whole cohort was 2.3 Gy (range: 0.01-18.3 Gy). Breast asymmetry was estimated by responses to a mail questionnaire to all patients and by the clinical examination of 53 patients living in Stockholm county. Breast hypoplasia on the treated side was reported by 57% of the patients and on the contralateral side by 8%. Among women reporting a smaller breast on the untreated side, the mean dose to the treated breast was 0.5 Gy (range: 0.01-1.0 Gy). In 28 of the 53 clinically examined patients, breast hypoplasia exceeding 10% was found on the treated side, and five patients had hypoplasia of more than 10% on the contralateral side (Figure IX). The frequency and the severity of impaired breast development increased with the radiation dose. In this study, the possibility of a threshold dose for radiation-induced breast hypoplasia could neither be established nor ruled out, and the results suggested that the available risk estimates for breast hypoplasia underestimate the effect [I1, R2]. At lower doses, the dose-effect relationship may be confounded by normal variations in breast size. At higher doses and with larger fields than were used in the Swedish study, there may also be a radiation effect on the chest wall with subsequent growth impairment.

113. ***Summary***. The sensitivity of breast tissue in the irradiated child is recognized, with low threshold doses for the occurrence of clinical effects. One study has reported that hypoplasia occurs in more than 50% of children treated with radiotherapy at less than 4 years of age with doses to the breast of the order of 2 Gy. Higher doses cause increased incidence and severity of impaired breast development.

J. DIGESTIVE SYSTEM

114. Late radiation effects of the gastro-intestinal tract develop months or years after exposure and include fibrosis, stricture, intestinal perforation and fistula formation [R1]. The liver appears to have a low threshold for late injury, and in adults veno-occlusive disease has been observed after single doses of 10 Gy or 18-30 Gy with conventional fractionation [F10]. The damage is due to changes that interfere with mitosis in the irradiated hepatocytes and to vascular changes [I1]. Radiation-induced liver disease is characterized structurally by progressive fibrosis and obliteration of central veins, possibly by injuring preferentially the endothelial cells of central veins [F10, L20]. Veno-occlusive disease may also be caused by antineoplastic drugs, and hepatic fibrosis has been observed in children receiving chemotherapy [M36, N6].

115. The risk for radiation-induced liver damage increases when large volumes of the liver are irradiated or when the liver is irradiated after resection. A larger dose can be tolerated if only part of the liver is exposed [F1, I6, K14]. In children, Tefft et al. [T13] noted liver abnormalities after radiotherapy to the liver with doses of 12-30 Gy. This could be related to the greater sensitivity of the younger child, who generally also received the lower doses. Thomas et al. [T11] observed liver fibrosis in 3 of 26 long-term survivors of Wilms' tumour who had received at least 30 Gy to the liver in 1.5-2 Gy fractions. Hepatic disease, ranging from abnormal liver enzymes and thrombocytopenia to death, has also been reported by others [S45, T12].

116. Hepatitis following irradiation and chemotherapy at doses and volumes of irradiation ordinarily considered within the tolerance of hepatic function has been reported [K15]. Fatal liver damage occurred in a 13-year-old boy who had received adriamycin before and during radiotherapy of 24 Gy in 17 fractions over 28 days to the upper abdomen including the entire liver. A 13-year-old girl had moderate clinical liver changes following 25 Gy in 23 fractions over 32 days with adriamycin administered before and during irradiation. In this case much of the right lobe was shielded during radiotherapy. About 20 patients have been reported to have developed liver disease after fractionated radiotherapy with 12-40 Gy to the liver in childhood together with chemotherapy [J7]. Most patients were asymptomatic, and their condition was discovered because of hepatomegaly or abnormalities shown in a routine liver scintigram. When hepatitis is observed following radiation exposure, especially if exposure is received in conjunction with chemotherapy, it is important to note that not only post-irradiation effects but also toxic and infectious complications requiring appropriate therapeutic and prophylactic measures will occur.

117. The small intestine has a high radiosensitivity but is somewhat spared by its mobility. Thus, repeated exposure of a particular segment is avoided. This is not the case for the rectum, which is fixed to adjacent

tissues and consequently experiences the effects of radiation more frequently [H1]. In adults, the risk of small bowel complications depends on radiation dose, volume of bowel irradiated and fractionation schedule. Surgery increases the risk of developing radiation enteropathy. The manifestations of late radiation enteropathy are considered to be due mainly to vascular and connective tissue damage. Mage et al. [M37] reported late gastro-intestinal effects in 17 children receiving abdominal fractionated radiotherapy with 30-55 Gy. Stenosis, submucous infiltrations and mesenteritis were observed 2-13 months after radiotherapy. No details of the radiotherapeutic regimens were given. The combined effects of radiation damage to the mucous membrane and exacerbation of already existing gastro-intestinal infections can cause perforation and ulceration.

118. Donaldson et al. [D23] reviewed late radiation effects in the gastro-intestinal tract of 44 children receiving whole abdominal radiotherapy for lymphoma, Wilms' tumour or teratoma. Of 14 long-term survivors, 5 developed severe radiation injury with small bowel obstruction within two months after completion of radiotherapy. Their mean age at the time of therapy was 6 years, and the abdominal dose was 31 Gy (range: 10-40 Gy) delivered in 7-20 fractions over 11-39 days. Surgery contributed to the presence of abdominal adhesions and fibrosis.

119. ***Summary***. The risk of radiation-induced liver damage increases with increasing volume of the liver irradiated and after liver resection with regenerating liver tissue. Some data suggest that children are more sensitive to such late effects than are adults. Liver abnormalities have been observed after 12 Gy with conventional fractionation and often in combination with chemotherapy. Clinical radiation-induced hepatitis has rarely been reported at doses below 30 Gy in 0.9-1.0 Gy fractions five times per week. Case-reports have presented data on liver damage in children after 24-25 Gy in 1.1-1.4 Gy fractions with concomitant use of anthracyclines. Radiation effects in the gastro-intestinal tract include fibrosis, stricture, perforation and formation of fistulae. There are hardly any data available on such effects in children.

K. KIDNEY

120. The urinary system shows a wide range in radiosensitivity, with the kidney being the most sensitive organ, the bladder having an intermediate sensitivity and the ureter being more resistant, although the full length is seldom irradiated [U1]. Late radiation sequelae of the kidney are directly related to the total dose to the tissue and are characterized by tissue necrosis and fibrosis, which may occur a few months to several years after exposure [F1, K16, L21, M38, M39, U1]. The critical dose for the kidneys in adults is usually set at about 23 Gy over five weeks. Rubin [R3] suggested the critical dose for 5% chronic nephrosclerosis to be 20 Gy with conventional fractionation. Radiation nephritis results from lesions of the tubules and microvasculature of the kidney. Radiation injury to large and medium-sized arteries can also result in stenosis or occlusion [M38]. The severity of radiation injury seems to be a function of the radiation dose and the size of the vessel. Larger doses and smaller vessels are more likely to end in total occlusion, whereas larger vessels or smaller doses result in stenosis or hypoplasia of the vessel. Children are more susceptible to vascular injury, because of their small, growing arteries and relative sensitivity to a given dose of radiation. Radiation injury to the renal artery may produce a renovascular hypertension, which can be distinguished from the more common radiation nephritis.

121. Renal injury is more severe in children, and they have limited tolerance for combined chemotherapy and radiotherapy. A normal creatinine clearance and glomerular filtration rate may be anticipated below a fractionated dose of 15 Gy when actinomycin D is used concurrently, but progressive renal insufficiency occurs after doses of 20 Gy and more [J5]. However, radiation nephritis has been reported 20 years after 14 Gy to the kidney in childhood [O12]. Reduced creatinine clearance has been found in 18% of 108 children who underwent nephrectomy for malignant disease and received <12 Gy to the remaining kidney and in 33% among those receiving 12-24 Gy [M33]. In another study, Levitt et al. [L24] observed that children with Wilms' tumour and less than 2 years old who received chemotherapy with >12 Gy to the remaining kidney had a worse renal prognosis than other children. In children exposed *in utero* in Hiroshima and Nagasaki, urinary examination revealed transient proteinuria, which was not found in adults [F11].

122. Radiotherapy for Wilms' tumour has also been associated with late effects in the kidney [A17, K16, M40, V6]. McGill et al. [M40] reported post-irradiation renovascular hypertension in a boy who received chemotherapy and fractionated radiotherapy with 30 Gy to the abdomen at the age of 9 months and in another boy 14 months of age who received 51 Gy to the abdomen. Severe hypertension developed 6-8 years later. Koskimies [K16] reported three patients aged 1-2 years with Wilms' tumour who developed hypertension more than 10 years after receiving >36 Gy postoperatively to the tumour area. The hypertension was considered to be of renal origin for three reasons: the likelihood of renal damage was supported by gross macroscopic changes in the nearby organs; two patients had proteinuria indicating renal damage; and

other causes known to cause secondary hypertension had been excluded. In another study of 14 patients with Wilms' tumour evaluated at a median of 17 years later, four had elevated diastolic blood pressure and two had mild proteinuria [B33]. That study provided no data on the radiotherapy. Arneil et al. [A17] reported nephritis four months after surgery in two children aged 2 and 5 years who received actinomycin D and vincristine followed by 15-20 Gy to the remaining kidney fractionated over 2-3 weeks.

123. Radiation nephropathy is common after whole-body irradiation for bone marrow transplantation [T3, V8]. After 12-14 Gy in 6-8 fractions over 3-4 days, the child may develop anaemia, haematuria and elevated creatinine. This renal insufficiency is due both to the radiotherapy and to the chemotherapeutic regimens employed.

124. ***Summary***. Late effects following irradiation of the kidney include nephritis, tissue necrosis and fibrosis, renal dysfunction and hypertension. Available data do not indicate that children are more susceptible to radiation-induced renal injury than adults. Radiation nephritis has been reported after fractionated doses of 14 Gy, and decreased creatine clearance has occurred after doses around 12 Gy. The seemingly higher sensitivity among children can probably be explained by the combination of radiotherapy and chemotherapy, which can enhance the side-effects in the kidney [R3].

L. BONE MARROW

125. Few studies have been performed to determine the long-term deterministic effects on bone marrow function after exposure to ionizing radiation in childhood, and most available data refer to exposure in adulthood. Rubin et al. [R29] studied the repopulation and redistribution of bone marrow in 27 adults irradiated for Hodgkin's disease with 40-45 Gy of fractionated radiotherapy to large segments of their bone marrow (mantle and inverted fields). Bone marrow scanning techniques using ^{99m}Tc-sulphur colloid, which parallels ^{59}Fe activity and can be used to reflect haematopoietic activity, indicated that prolonged suppression of bone marrow occurs immediately following completion of radiotherapy and persists for 2-3 years. Partial to complete bone marrow regeneration after fractionated radiotherapy with 40 Gy occurs in 85% of the exposed bone marrow sites at two years. Mechanisms of this recovery may include increased haematopoietic production in shielded marrow sites, expansion of bone marrow space and infield regeneration of bone marrow. The study suggested that the dose-response data for bone marrow suppression following localized and segmental exposure need to be revised upwards for fractionated radiotherapy. At the 40 Gy level there was evidence of prolonged suppression of bone marrow activity starting in the immediate post-irradiation period and continuing for one year. Regeneration of bone marrow activity and expansion of bone marrow occurred after one year following the 40 Gy treatment and continued to improve with time from the first to the third post-irradiation year. Baisogolov and Shiskin [B36, B37, B38] observed bone marrow hypoplasia in 8% of examined bone marrow from exposed parts in 200 patients irradiated for Hodgkin's disease, and in 89% the marrow was aplastic.

126. Magnetic resonance imaging can detect radiation-induced marrow changes. There are at least two distinct types of late marrow patterns [S57]: homogeneous fatty replacement and another pattern possibly representing haematopoietic marrow surrounding the central marrow fat. These changes have been observed in the lumbar vertebral bone marrow of adults after 15-50 Gy delivered over 3-6 weeks. No similar studies have been performed in paediatric patients.

127. No evidence exists of a late radiation effect of primary disturbance of haematopoiesis in the absence of malignant disease in the populations of Hiroshima and Nagasaki [F12]. There is no evidence for radiation-induced disturbance of granulocyte function, but the age-related accelerated decline in the immunological functions of T-lymphocytes and age-related alteration in the number of certain subsets of circulating T- and B-lymphocytes appear to be radiation-related.

128. The Chernobyl accident does not appear to have caused statistically significant effects on the major haematological parameters of children living in Russia, Belarus or Ukraine at the time of the accident, or who were born later [A18, I8, K17, K18, L25, L29, V9]. There were no differences between control and contaminated settlements. From the calculated and measured radiation dose levels, no changes should have been expected as a direct result of radiation exposure.

129. In children having an intact thymus, immune function recovers more rapidly and does not necessarily have permanent effects. Blomgren et al. [B34] analysed peripheral lymphocyte populations and serum immunoglobulin levels in 10 long-term survivors of Wilms' tumour (age: 0.5-6 years) and 6 long-term survivors of non-Hodgkin lymphoma (age: 3-13 years). All received chemotherapy, and the tumour dose was 7-32 Gy and 2-21 Gy, respectively. Lymphocyte counts, as well as frequencies of E, EA and EAC rosette-forming cells, did not differ from those of healthy controls. Serum levels of immunoglobin E were somewhat lower in patients treated for lymphoma, but for other immunoglobulins there was no difference between patients and controls. The treatment did not have any long-lasting effects on the lym-

phatic system. In comparison, adults receiving radiotherapy for breast cancer developed T-cell lymphopenia that persisted for a decade. Studies on more than 900 children from contaminated areas in Russia and Ukraine have not demonstrated any radiation-related effect on T-cells [L26, L27, L28].

130. ***Summary***. Studies of bone marrow suppression, recovery, late marrow changes and effects on the immune system pertain only to adults. Too few data exist on the effects of ionizing radiation on bone marrow and on immune function to determine or even suggest critical levels for clinical effects to appear.

CONCLUSIONS

131. Deterministic effects of ionizing radiation in humans depend on the dose and can be expected to have thresholds below which the radiation effects are too small to impair function of the irradiated tissue or organ. In children, tissues are actively growing, and a radiation-induced deterministic damage in a tissue or organ will often be more severe than in adults. Examples of such deterministic sequelae include effects on growth and development, hormonal deficiencies, organ dysfunctions and effects on intellectual and cognitive functions.

132. Well-designed epidemiological studies of late deterministic effects are generally lacking, and it is therefore not possible to draw any firm conclusions about the exact critical dose levels at which various late deterministic effects appear. Most data concerning such effects are obtained from the clinical follow-up of groups of patients treated for paediatric tumours. These groups generally comprise small numbers of patients of different ages and who were followed for different lengths of time. The treatment modalities have usually included surgery, radiotherapy and chemotherapy, and it is not always possible to single out the effect of radiation alone. A variety of factors complicate the study of a possible association between effect and dose, including the underlying disease and associated clinical findings, other treatment modalities, the impact of illness on body image and lack of school attendance.

133. The methods for assessing a given deterministic effect vary greatly, and this makes comparisons between different studies difficult. Based on the available findings, some general conclusions can be drawn. Children appear to be more sensitive to radiation than adults, and, in general, younger children are more sensitive than older children. Radiation doses indicated in this Annex are usually given with fractionation over a period of several weeks. The deterministic effects following radiation exposures in childhood are summarized in Table 9.

134. ***Brain***. Leukoencephalopathy, microangiopathy and cortical atrophy have been reported after cumulative brain doses of 18 Gy or more given in 1.8-2 Gy fractions or after 10 Gy given as a single whole-body exposure. Necrosis occurs after considerably higher doses, and a whole-brain dose of 54 Gy in 2 Gy fractions over six weeks is generally considered to be a critical dose for radiation-induced necrosis in children older than 5 years. For children 3-5 years old the dose should be reduced by about 20%, and for children less than 3 years old the dose should be reduced by about 30%. Brain doses of 18 Gy or more of fractionated radiotherapy have been associated with neuropsychologic effects and decline in IQ.

135. ***Endocrine system***. The most important endocrine effects of radiation exposure are impaired secretions of growth hormone, thyroid-stimulating hormone, gonadotropins, thyroid hormones and oestrogens/testosterone. Impaired growth has been observed after fractionated radiotherapy to the brain with cumulative doses of more than 24 Gy and after >1 Gy in a single exposure among the survivors of the atomic bombings in Japan, whereas impaired growth hormone secretion has been observed in patients after 18 Gy of fractionated radiotherapy. Hypothyroidism has been reported in leukaemic children receiving thyroid doses of 1-2 Gy over 2-2.5 weeks from cranial radiotherapy and chemotherapy. In subjects under 20 years at the time of the bombings in Hiroshima and Nagasaki, those exposed to greater than 1 Gy had a significantly higher incidence of thyroid disorders than those in the unexposed control group. No study has so far demonstrated hypothyroidism in children after a thyroid dose <1 Gy. There are insufficient data on the effects of ^{131}I to determine a possible threshold dose for the induction of hypothyroidism.

136. ***Gonads***. The effects of radiation on the testis and ovary are age- and dose-dependent. The radiation dose required to ablate ovarian function seems to be around 20 Gy for girls; because of the greater number of oocytes in young girls, higher doses are tolerated before castration. Infertility occurs in approximately one third of girls receiving 4 Gy and in almost all women over 40 years of age. Ovarian failure has been documented in prepubertal girls following 10 Gy of whole-body irradiation and occurs in all pubertal girls. Amenorrhea has been observed in two thirds of girls

who have received 3 Gy on average to both ovaries and in more than 10% of patients exposed in childhood with ovarian doses of 0.5 Gy on average. Ionizing radiation appears to have its greatest effect on the germ cells in the testes rather than on the Leydig cells. Testicular function may be compromised at doses as low as 0.5 Gy. Leydig cell function appears more resistant to ionizing radiation, and impaired function occurs only after 10 Gy or more. Whole-body irradiation has been shown to produce primary gonadal failure of various degrees in the majority of boys receiving 10 Gy, regardless of pubertal status. In most of these patients, Leydig cell function appeared adequate.

137. ***Skeleton.*** Skeletal changes generally occur at doses >20 Gy from fractionated radiotherapy and include scoliosis, kyphosis, slipped femoral epiphyses, hypoplasia, growth retardation and dental problems. A dose exceeding 20 Gy is required to arrest encondral bone formation, and doses of 10-20 Gy cause partial arrest of bone growth. There is little alteration in bone growth below 10 Gy of fractionated exposure.

138. ***Eye.*** Data on cataracts from radiation exposure in childhood are scarce. Cataracts have been observed after a lenticular dose of 2 Gy. Whole-body exposure of 10 Gy in childhood has been associated with cataract formation.

139. ***Cardiovascular system.*** The few data available on cardiovascular effects suggest that 40 Gy can be considered as a threshold for clinical cardiomyopathy in children. A considerable proportion of patients have abnormal cardiac function without clinical evidence of such dysfunction, and the critical dose for cardiovascular effects is therefore probably lower than 40 Gy. The anthracyclines are cardiotoxic and enhance the effects of mediastinal irradiation.

140. ***Lung.*** The lung is a radiosensitive organ, and a lung dose of 15 Gy in 1.5 Gy fractions has generally been considered as the maximum safe dose in children receiving radiotherapy to the whole lung and simultaneous treatment with actinomycin D. However, restrictive lung changes have been reported after doses of 11 Gy or more in children treated for paediatric tumours, and reduced total lung capacity has been found after 8 Gy or more to the whole lung with similar fraction size.

141. ***Breast.*** Breast hypoplasia has been reported in more than 50% of children less than 4 years of age receiving breast irradiation with doses of about 2 Gy. Higher doses cause increased frequency and severity of impaired breast development.

142. ***Liver and gastro-intestinal tract.*** Clinical radiation-induced hepatitis has rarely been reported at doses below 30 Gy at 0.9-1.0 Gy fractions in five fractions per week. However, case-reports have presented data on sometimes fatal radiation-induced liver damage in children after fractionated radiotherapy with 24-25 Gy in 1.1-1.4 Gy fractions with concomitant use of anthracyclines. Non-fatal liver disease has been reported after of 12 Gy or more in children who also received chemotherapy. Radiation effects in the gastro-intestinal tract include fibrosis, stricture, perforation and formation of fistulae. There are hardly any data available on such effects in children.

143. ***Kidney.*** Late effects following irradiation of the kidney include nephritis, tissue necrosis and fibrosis, renal dysfunction and hypertension. The threshold dose for effects in children has been estimated to be 16-18 Gy of fractionated radiotherapy to the entire kidney in combination with chemotherapy, but it may be even lower since radiation nephritis has been reported after fractionated doses of 14 Gy and reduced creatine clearance after 12 Gy.

144. ***Bone marrow.*** There are insufficient data on the effects of ionizing radiation on bone marrow and on immune function in children to determine or even suggest critical dose levels for the appearance of clinical deterministic effects.

Table 1
Estimates of doses for 1%-5% and 25%-50% incidences of clinically detrimental deterministic effects in adults at five years after radiation exposure [a]
[I1, R2]

Organ	*Treatment field*	*Injury at five years*	*Approximate dose (Gy)*	
			Effect in 1%-5% of patients	*Effect in 25%-50% of patients*
Bone marrow	Whole	Hypoplasia	2	5
Ovary	Whole	Permanent sterility	2-3	6-12
Testis	Whole	Permanent sterility	5-15	20
Lens	Whole	Cataract	5	12
Kidney	Whole	Nephrosclerosis	23	28
Liver	Whole	Liver failure	35	45
Lung	lobe	Pneumonitis, fibrosis	40	60
Heart	Whole	Pericarditis, pancarditis	40	>100
Thyroid	Whole	Hypothyroidism	45	150
Pituitary	Whole	Hypopituitarism	45	200-300
Brain	Whole	Necrosis	50	>60
Spinal cord	5 cm^2	Necrosis	50	>60
Breast	Whole	Atrophy, necrosis	>50	>100
Skin	100 cm^2	Ulcer, severe fibrosis	55	70
Eye	Whole	Panophthalmitis	55	100
Oesophagus	75 cm^2	Ulcer, stricture	60	75
Bladder	Whole	Ulcer, contracture	60	80
Bone	10 cm^2	Necrosis, fracture	60	150
Ureter	5-10 cm	Stricture	75	100
Muscle	Whole	Atrophy	>100	

[a] Based on responses of patients conventionally treated with fractionated therapeutic x- or gamma-irradiation.

Table 2
Estimates of doses for 1%-5% and 25%-50% incidences of clinically detrimental deterministic effects in children at five years after radiation exposure [a]
[I1, R2]

Organ	*Treatment field*	*Injury at five years*	*Approximate dose (Gy)*	
			Effect in 1%-5% of patients	*Effect in 25%-50% of patients*
Breast	5 cm^2	No development	10	15
Cartilage		Arrested growth	10	30
Bone	10 cm^2	Arrested growth	20	30
Muscle		Hypoplasia	20-30	40-50

[a] Based on responses of patients conventionally treated with fractionated therapeutic x- or gamma-irradiation.

Table 3
Effects on the brain in children treated for acute leukaemia detected by computed tomography scans

Treatment		*Number of patients*	*Abnormalities*		*Type of brain abnormalities detected*	*Ref.*
Radiotherapy dose to the brain (Gy)	*Chemotherapy* [a]		*Number*	*Per cent*		
24	IT	23	13	56	Intracerebral califications, cortical atrophy	[B6]
24	IT	19	11	56	Intracerebral califications, cortical atrophy	[P5]
24	IT	24	13	54	Intracerebral califications, cortical atrophy	[R5]
24	IT	32	17	53	Intracerebral califications, cortical atrophy	[P7]
24	IT	72	35	49	Intracerebral califications, cortical atrophy	[C14]
24	IT	14	6	43	Intracerebral califications, cortical atrophy	[E1]
24	IT	25	10	40	Intracerebral califications	[M5]
24	IT	30	12	40	Cortical atrophy	[B5]
24	IT	45	11	24	Intracerebral califications, cortical atrophy	[S55]
24	IT	19	3	16	Cortical atrophy	[O3]
24	IT	44	5	11	Intracerebral califications	[O13]
20	IT	27	1	4	Cortical atrophy	[D24]
18	IT	55	5	9	White matter hypodensity, cortical atrophy	[O2]
0	IV+IT	12	3	25	Cortical atrophy	[E1]
0	IV+IT	43	8	19	Cortical atrophy	[O14]
0	IV+IT	23	1	4	Cortical atrophy	[P5]

[a] IT = intrathecal methotrexate and IT + IV = intrathecal and intravenous methotrexate.

Table 4
Effects on the brain of radiotherapy to the central nervous system in children

Effect	*CNS therapy*	*Comments*	*Ref.*
Leukoencephalopathy	>20 Gy in 1.5-2.0 Gy fractions plus systemic methotrexate 10 Gy whole-body irradiation	Young children more sensitive	[M6, P3, R4]
Mineralizing microangiopathy	>15 Gy in 1.5-2.0 Gy fractions	Young children more sensitive	[B4, D5]
Cortical atrophy	>18 Gy in 1.5-2.0 Gy fractions and intrathecal methotrexate	Severest atrophy in young children	[C3, D3, D5, K2]
Cerebral necrosis	>54 Gy in 1.8 Gy fractions		[B35, K2]

Table 5
Average adult heights of individuals exposed in the lower dose groups in Hiroshima and Nagasaki and under 18 years old at the time of bombing
[B14]

Sex	*Age at time of bombing (years)*	*Average adult height (cm) in dose group*			
		0 Gy	*0-0.09 Gy*	*0.10-0.99 Gy*	*> 1.00 Gy*
Hiroshima					
Male	0-5 6-11 12-17	166.4 [a] 162.3 164.3	166.1 [a] 164.2 163.6	165.9 [a] 166.3 164.3	161.5 162.2 163.4
Female	0-5 6-11 12-17	153.3 [b] 152.5 152.1	153.6 [a] 153.6 [b] 152.3	152.9 [b] 153.6 [b] 152.2	150.4 150.5 151.9
Nagasaki					
Male	0-5 6-11 12-17	166.2 164.0 163.2	166.2 164.1 163.9		166.2 162.7 161.8
Female	0-5 6-11 12-17	152.8 152.4 151.8	152.9 151.3 151.6		150.8 151.5 151.2

[a] Significantly different ($p < 0.01$) compared with the average of group exposed to > 1.00 Gy.
[b] Significantly different ($p < 0.05$) compared with the average of group exposed to > 1.00 Gy.

Table 6
Average adult heights of children exposed in the higher dose group in Hiroshima and under 18 years old at the time of bombing
[B14]

Sex	*Age at time of bombing (years)*	*Average adult height (cm)* [a]	
		In dose group 1.0-2.49 Gy	*In dose group > 2.5 Gy*
Male	0-5 6-11 12-17	164.2 (12) 162.7 (13) 163.2 (43)	159.8 (18) 161.5 (10) 163.5 (46)
Female	0-5 6-11 12-17	151.8 (11) 150.4 (17) 152.1 (58)	149.8 (23) 150.5 (11) 151.7 (59)

[a] Number of individuals in parentheses.

Table 7
Average height of individuals followed in the Adult Health Study and under age 10 years at the time of bombing [I4]

Sex	*Dose range (Gy)*	*Average adult height (cm) ± standard deviation* [a]	
		Hiroshima	*Nagasaki*
Male	< 0.01	164.9 ± 6.02 (52)	163.3 ± 5.72 (53)
	0.01-0.99	166.4 ± 6.18 (91)	164.4 ± 5.43 (31)
	1.00-2.99	164.4 ± 5.55 (20)	165.1 ± 5.04 (31)
	3.00-6.00	161.0 ± 5.18 (20)	164.3 ± 6.64 (18)
Total		164.9 ± 6.11 (148)	164.1 ± 5.61 (128)
χ^2 statistical test [b]		1.04 ($p > 0.05$)	1.90 ($p > 0.05$)
Female	< 0.01	153.0 ± 5.54 (74)	152.8 ± 4.81 (53)
	0.01-0.99	153.6 ± 5.84 (91)	152.1 ± 4.25 (38)
	1.00-2.99	151.1 ± 5.34 (25)	151.5 ± 5.26 (32)
	3.00-6.00	149.9 ± 6.90 (20)	149.8 ± 5.33 (19)
Total		152.7 ± 5.87 (210)	151.9 ± 4.89 (142)
χ^2 statistical test [b]		2.00 ($p > 0.05$)	2.00 ($p > 0.05$)

[a] Number of individuals in parentheses.
[b] Homogeneity test of variance for four dose groups; df = 3.

Table 8
Thyroid hypofunction in individuals exposed to fallout radiation in the Marshall Islands [C16]

Age at exposure (years)	*Incidence of thyroid hypofunction for various estimated doses to the thyroid*			
	0 Gy	*< 1.00 Gy*	*1.00-2.00 Gy*	*≥ 2.00 Gy*
<10	1/229 (0.4%)	0/64 (0%)	-	9/29 (31%)
≥10	1/371 (0.3%)	1/100 (1%)	1/12 (8%)	4/45 (9%)

Table 9
Estimates of lowest radiation doses associated with late deterministic effects from exposure in childhood to ionizing radiation, usually in the form of fractionated radiotherapy

Organ	*Effect*	*Dose (Gy)*
Testis	Germ cell depletion Leydig cell dysfunction	0.5 10
Ovary	Amenorrhea Infertility Ablation	> 0.5 4 20
Thyroid gland	Hypothyroidism	> 1
Brain	Cognitive functions Histopathologic changes Neuroendocrine effects	18 18, (10 [a]) > 18, (> 1 [a])
Breast	Hypoplasia	2
Eye	Cataract	2
Lung	Fibrosis	8-11
Liver	Fibrosis	12
Kidney	Reduced creatinine clearance	12
Skeleton	Skeletal changes	10
Cardiovascular system	Cardiomyopathy	40
Bone marrow	Hypofunction	Insufficient data available

[a] Single whole-body exposure.

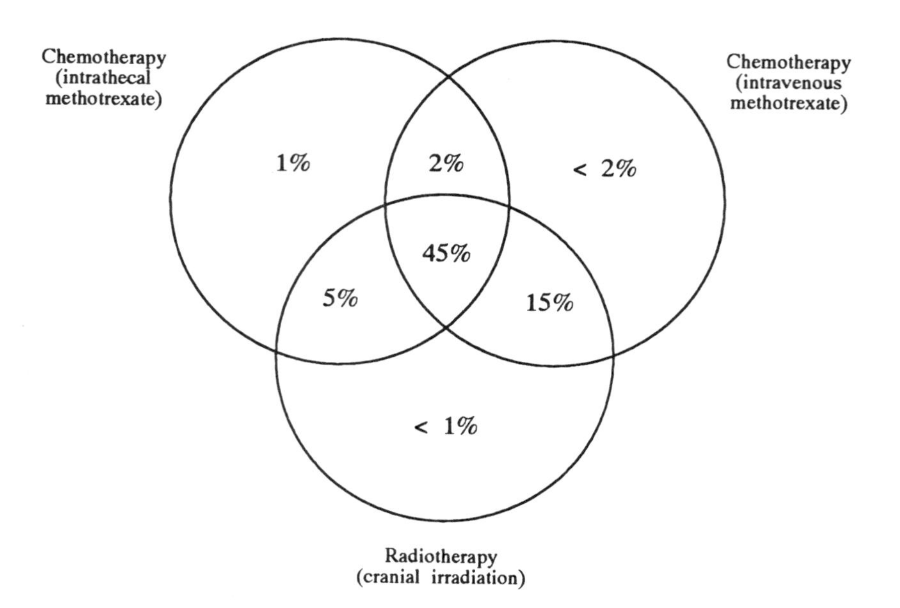

Figure I.
Approximate incidence rates of clinical leukoencephalopathy in patients treated by cranial irradiation, chemotherapy or combination therapies.
[B4]

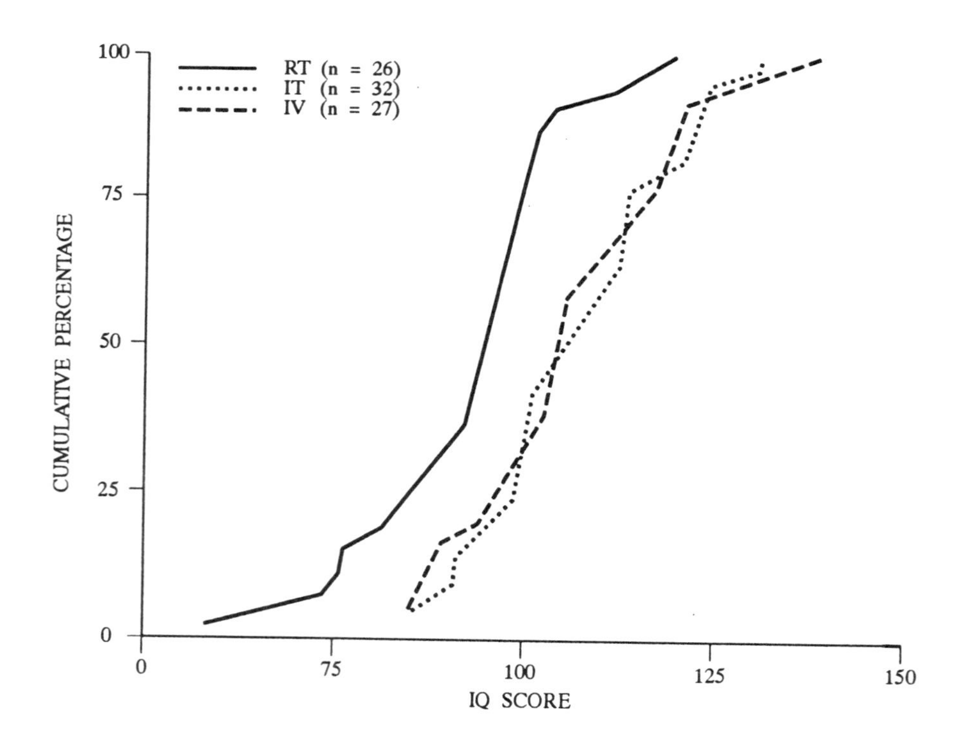

Figure II.
IQ score distribution in children treated for acute lymphocytic leukaemia by cranial radiotherapy (RT), intrathecal methotrexate (IT) or intravenous methotrexate (IV).
[B2]

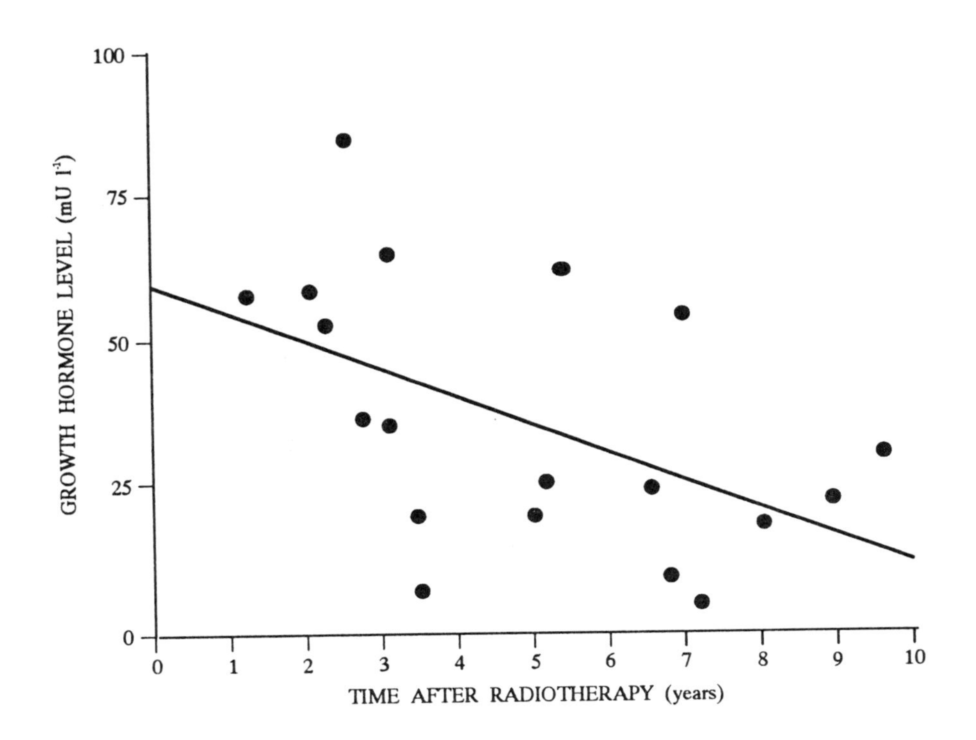

Figure III.
Maximum growth hormone response to growth-hormone-releasing hormone in children treated for brain tumours by radiotherapy.
[L6]

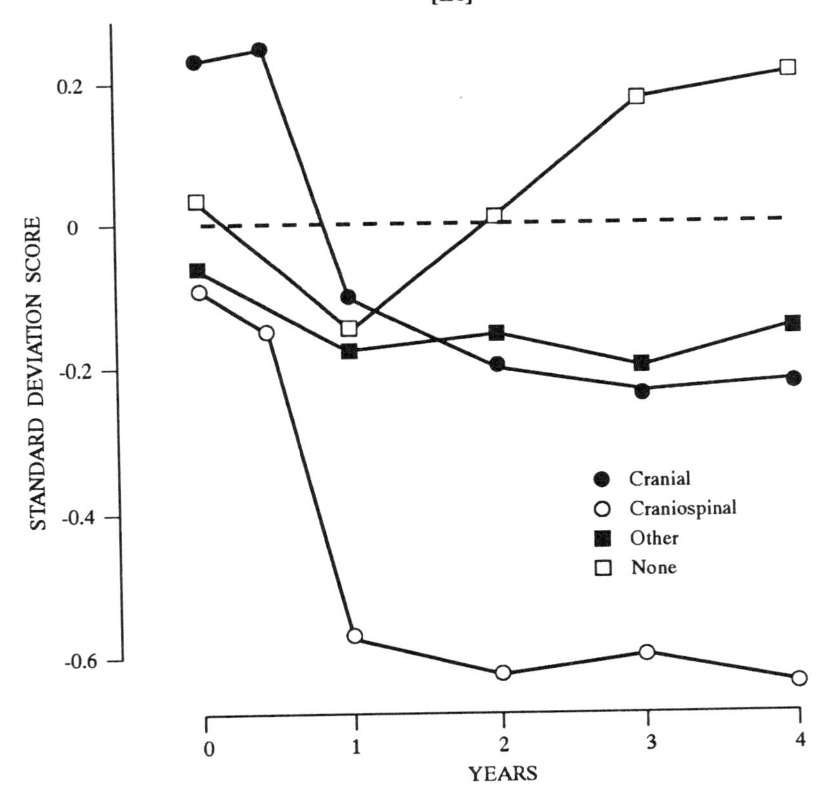

Figure IV.
Mean standard deviation score of height in children treated for malignant disease by radiotherapy to various sites. Results for those receiving cranial and craniospinal treatment were significantly lower ($p < 0.001$) at 1-4 years than at the time of initial treatment.
[G2]

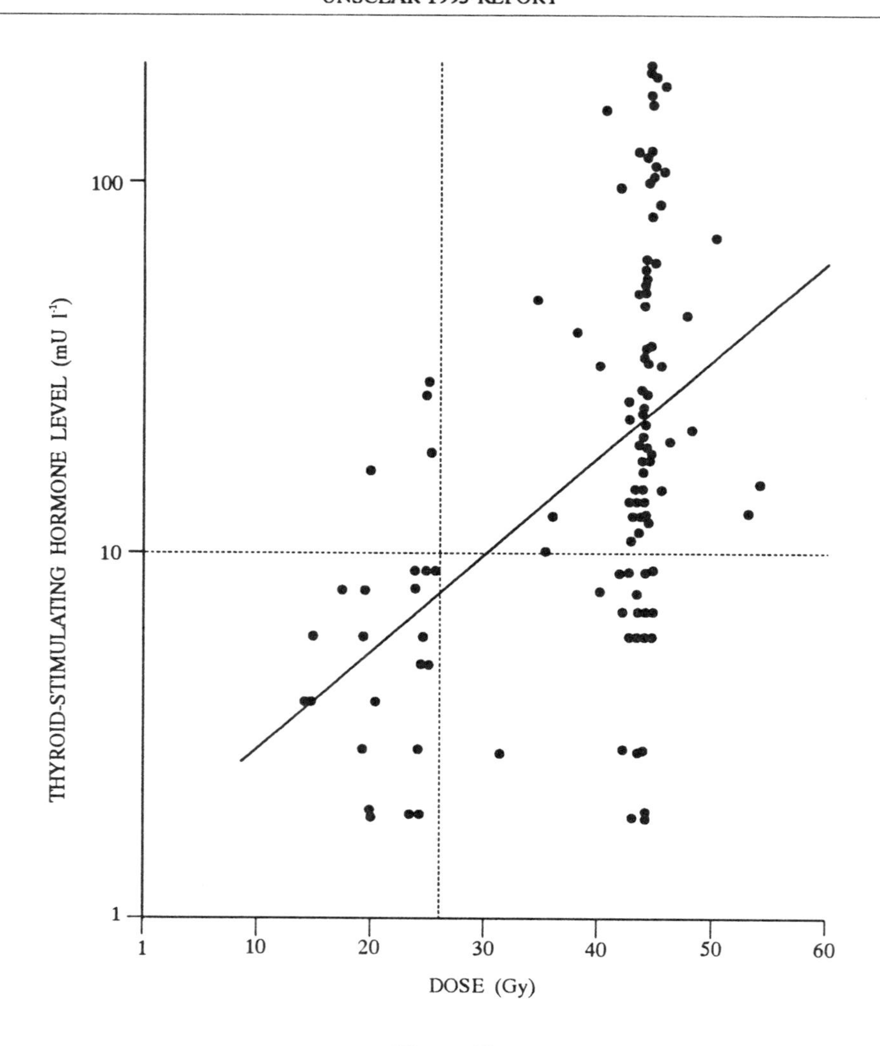

Figure V.
Thyroid-stimulating hormone levels in 116 patients aged 16 years or less treated for Hodgkin's disease by radiotherapy.
[C15]

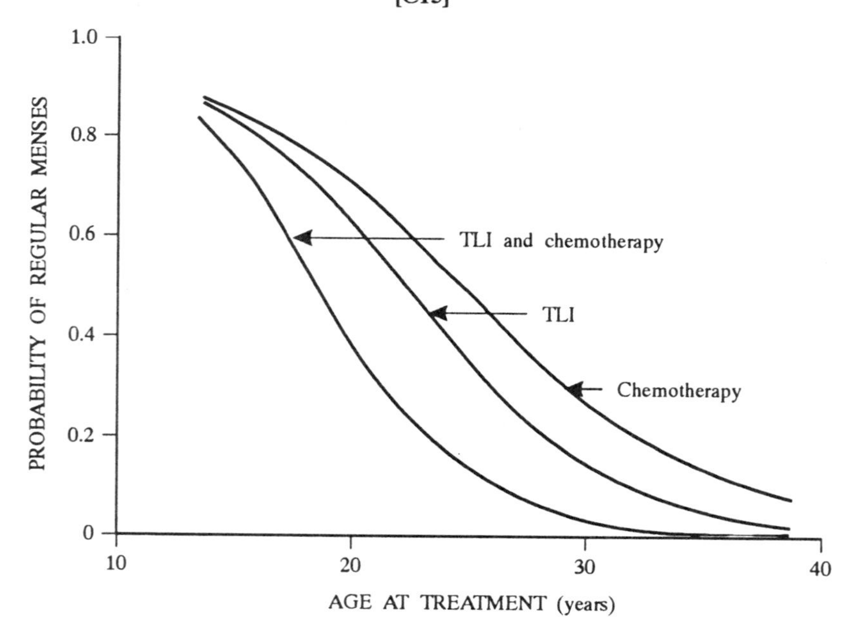

Figure VI.
Probability of regular menses in women treated for Hodgkin's disease by total lymph irradiation (TLI) and/or chemotherapy.
[H12]

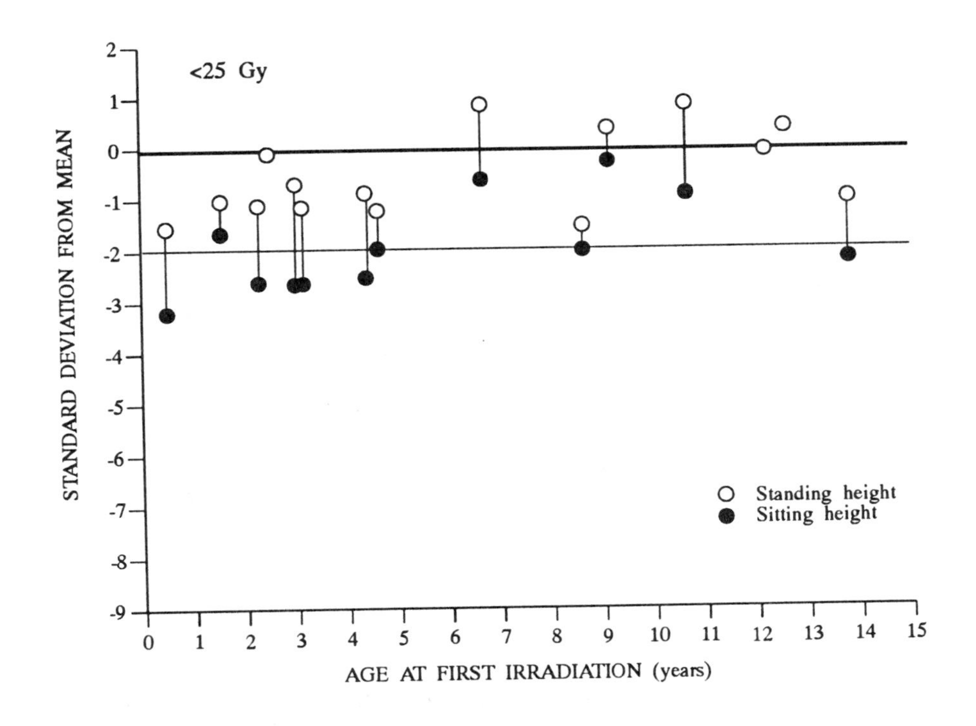

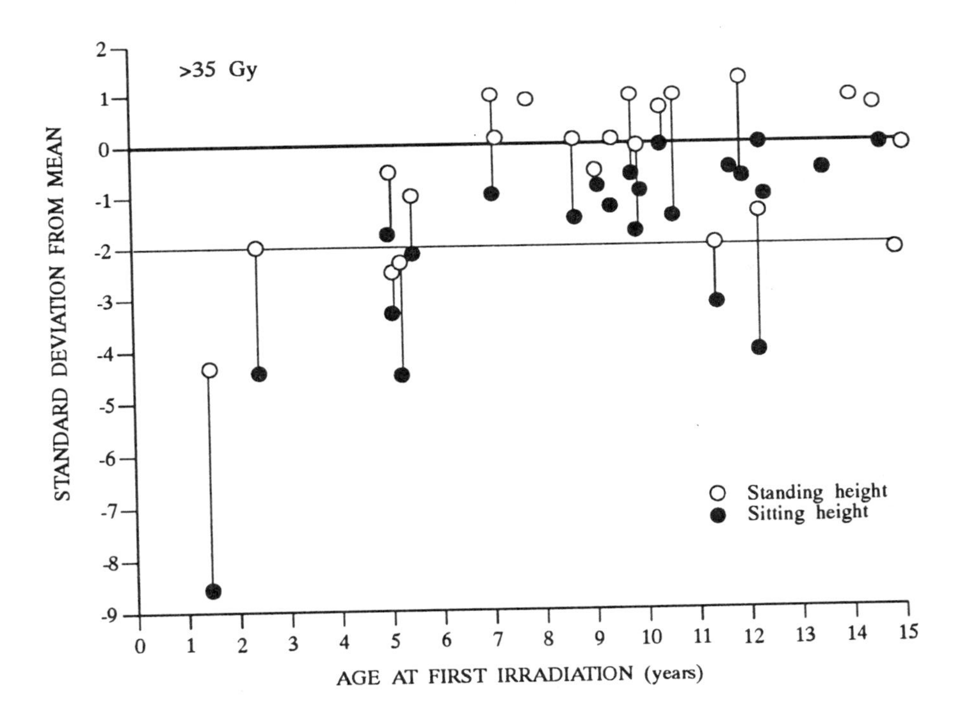

Figure VII.
Deviation from mean standing and sitting heights in children treated by radiotherapy with <25 Gy or >35 Gy.
[P10]

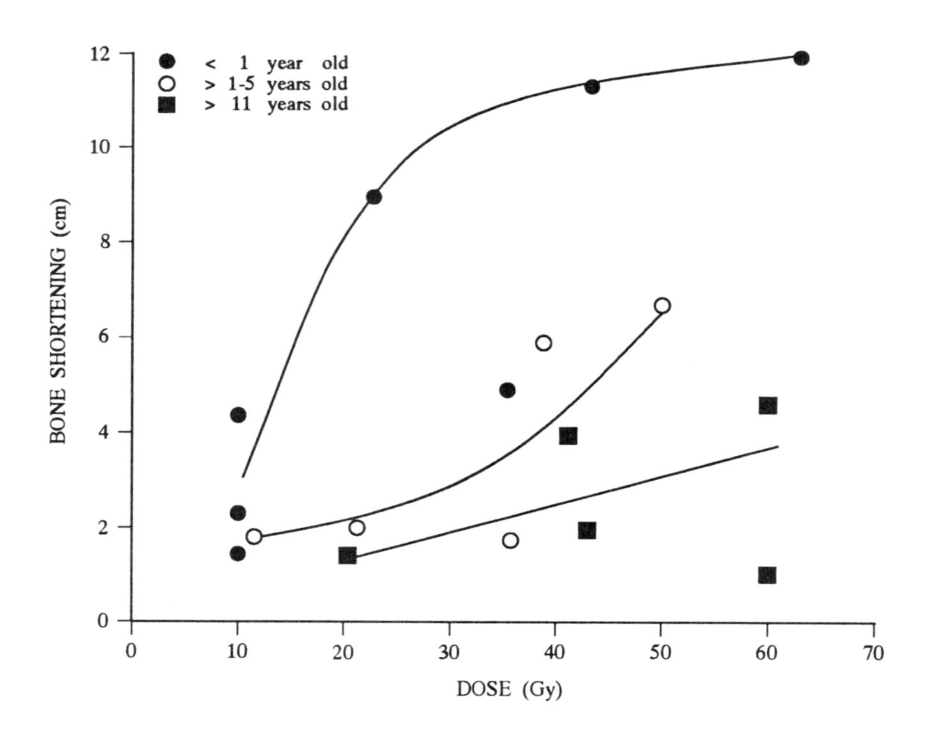

Figure VIII.
Dose-effect relationship for bone shortening in children treated by radiotherapy that included epiphysial plate irradiation.
[G8]

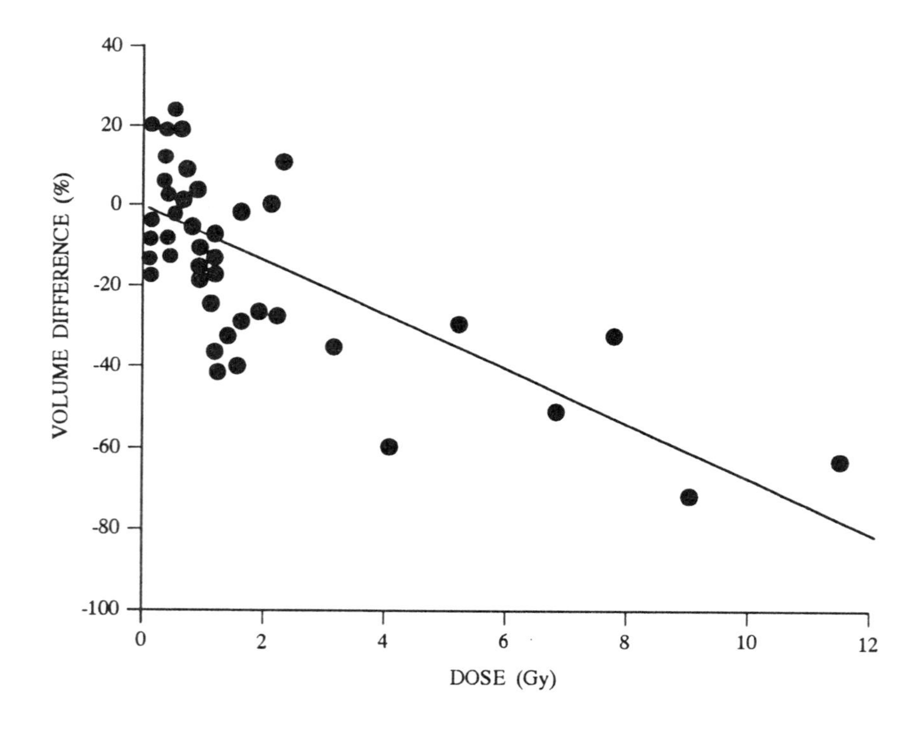

Figure IX.
Difference in breast volume in 53 women treated in childhood for haemangioma by radiotherapy of the breast region.
[F9]

References

A1 Allen, J.C. The effects of cancer therapy on the nervous system. J. Pediatr. 93: 903-909 (1978).

A2 Aur, R.J.A., J.V. Simone, H.O. Hustu et al. Central nervous system therapy and combination chemotherapy of childhood lymphocytic leukemia. Blood 37: 272-281 (1971).

A3 Aur, R.J.A., J.V. Simone, H.O. Hustu et al. A comparative study of central nervous system irradiation and intensive chemotherapy early in remission of childhood acute lymphocytic leukemia. Cancer 29: 381-391 (1972).

A4 Atkinson, K., H. Clink, S. Lawler et al. Encephalopathy following bone marrow transplantation. Eur. J. Cancer 13: 623-625 (1977).

A5 Abbatucci, J.S., T. Delozier, R. Quint et al. Radiation myelopathy of the cervical spinal cord: time, dose and volume factors. Int. J. Radiat. Oncol. Biol. Phys. 4: 239-248 (1978).

A6 Atlas, S.W., R.I. Grossman, R.J. Packer et al. Magnetic resonance imaging diagnosis of disseminated necrotizing leukoencephalopathy. J. Comput. Assist. Tomogr. 11: 39-43 (1987).

A7 Atkinson, R.L., R.C. Atkinson and E.R. Hilgard. (eds.). Mental abilities and their measurement. p. 349-381 in: Introduction to Psychology, Eighth Edition. Harcout Brace Jovanovich, Inc., New York, 1983.

A8 Ahmed, S.R. and S.M. Shalet. Hypothalamic growth hormone releasing factor deficiency following cranial irradiation. Clin. Endocrinol. 21: 483-488 (1984).

A9 Abayomi, O.K. and A. Sadeghi-Nejad. The incidence of late endocrine dysfunction following irradiation for childhood medulloblastoma. Int. J. Radiat. Oncol. Biol. Phys. 12: 945-948 (1986).

A10 Ahmed, S.R., S.M. Shalet and C.G. Beardwell. The effects of cranial irradiation on growth hormone secretion. Acta Paediatr. Scand. 75: 255-260 (1986).

A11 Albertsson-Wikland, K., B. Lannering, I. Márky et al. A longitudinal study on growth and spontaneous growth hormone (GH) secretion in children with irradiated brain tumors. Acta Paediatr. Scand. 76: 966-973 (1987).

A12 Ash, P. The influence of radiation on fertility in man. Br. J. Radiol. 53: 271-278 (1980).

A13 Ahmed, S.R., S.M. Shalet, R.H.A. Campbell et al. Primary gonadal damage following treatment of brain tumors in childhood. J. Pediatr. 103: 562-565 (1983).

A14 Applebaum, F.R. and E.D. Thomas. Treatment of acute leukemia in adults with chemoradiotherapy and bone marrow transplantation. Cancer 55: 2202-2209 (1985).

A15 Applefeld, M.M. and P.H. Wiernik. Cardiac disease after radiation therapy for Hodgkin's disease: analysis of 48 patients. Am. J. Cardiol. 51: 1679-1681 (1983).

A16 Alvarado, C.S., T.F. Boat and A.J. Newman. Late-onset pulmonary fibrosis and chest deformity in two children treated with cyclophosphamide. J. Pediatr. 92: 443-446 (1978).

A17 Arneil, G.C., F. Harris, I.G. Emmanuel et al. Nephritis in two children after irradiation and chemotherapy for nephroblastoma. Lancet 1: 960-963 (1974).

A18 Andreeva, A.P., E.G. Kazanets, N.A. Karamjan et al. Erythropoiesis of children exposed to low radiation doses in the contaminated areas. Sov. Med. Rev. Hematol. (1993). (in Russian)

B1 Bloomer, W.D. and S. Hellman. Normal tissue responses to radiation therapy. N. Engl. J. Med. 293: 80-83 (1975).

B2 Bleyer, W.A. and D.G. Poplack. Prophylaxis and treatment of leukemia in the central nervous system and other sanctuaries. Semin. Oncol. 12: 131-148 (1985).

B3 Bloom, H.J.G., E.N.K. Wallace and J.M. Henk. The treatment and prognosis of medulloblastoma in children. Am. J. Roentgenol. 105: 43-62 (1969).

B4 Bleyer, W.A. and T.W. Griffin. White matter necrosis, mineralizing microangiopathy, and intellectual abilities in survivors of childhood leukemia: associations with central nervous system irradiation and methotrexate therapy. p. 155-174 in: Radiation Damage to the Nervous System. (H.A. Gilbert and A.R. Kagan, eds.) Raven Press, New York, 1980.

B5 Brecher, M.L., P. Berger, A.I. Freeman et al. Computerized tomography scan findings in children with acute lymphocytic leukemia treated with three different methods of central nervous system prophylaxis. Cancer 56: 2439-2433 (1985).

B6 Brouwers, P., R. Riccardi, P. Fedio et al. Long-term neuropsychological sequelae of childhood leukemia: correlation with CT brain scan abnormalities. J. Pediatr. 106: 723-728 (1985).

B7 Bordeaux, J., R. Dowell, D. Copeland et al. Intellectual functioning of children who survive brain tumors. Abstract. p. 2 in: Childhood Cancer Survivors: Living Beyond Cure. Tenth Annual Mental Health Conference, Houston, Texas, 1985.

B8 Bamford, F.N., P.H. Morris Jones, D. Pearson et al. Residual disabilities in children treated for intracranial space-occupying lesions. Cancer 37: 1149-1151 (1976).

B9 Bleyer, W.A. Neurologic sequelae of methotrexate and ionizing radiation: a new classification. Cancer Treat. Rep. 65 (Suppl. 1): 89-98 (1981).

B10 Bajorunas, D.R., F. Ghavimi, B. Jereb et al. Endocrine sequelae of antineoplastic therapy in childhood head and neck malignancies. J. Clin. Endocrinol. Metab. 50: 329-335 (1980).

B11 Berry, D.H., M.J. Elders, W. Crist et al. Growth in children with acute lymphocytic leukemia: a Pediatric Oncology Group study. Med. Pediatr. Oncol. 11: 39-45 (1983).

B12 Bode, U., A. Oliff, B.B. Bercu et al. Absence of CT brain scan and endocrine abnormalities with less intensive CNS prophylaxis. Am. J. Pediatr. Hematol./ Oncol. 2: 21-24 (1980).

B13 Barrett, A., J. Nicholls and B. Gibson. Late effects of total body irradiation. Radiother. Oncol. 9: 131-135 (1987).

B14 Belsky, J.L. and W.J. Blot. Adults stature in relation to childhood exposure to the atomic bombs of Hiroshima and Nagasaki. Am. J. Public Health 65: 489-494 (1975).

B15 Bantle, J.P., C.K.K. Lee and S.H. Levitt. Thyroxine administration during radiation therapy to the neck does not prevent subsequent thyroid dysfunction. Int. J. Radiat. Oncol. Biol. Phys. 11: 1999-2002 (1985).

B16 Becker, D.V., W.M. McConahey, B.M. Dobyns et al. The results of radioiodine treatment of hyperthyroidism. A preliminary report of the thyrotoxicosis therapy follow-up study. p. 603-609 in: Further Advances in Thyroid Research. Vol. 1. (K. Fellinger and R. Höfer, eds.) Verlag der Wiener Medizinischen Akademie, Wien, 1971.

B17 Becker, D.V. Medical radiation: comparison of iodine-131 therapy and alternative treatments of hyperthyroidism. p. 57-67 in: Radiation and the Thyroid. (S. Nagataki, ed.) Excerpta Medica, Amsterdam, 1989.

B18 Brauner, R., R. Rappaport, P. Czernichow et al. Effects of hypothalamic and gonadal irradiation on pubertal development in children with cranial, cervical and abdominal tumors and acute leukemia. p. 163-173 in: Pathophysiology of Puberty. (E. Cacciari and A. Prader, eds.) Academic Press, London, 1980.

B19 Brauner, R., P. Czernichow and R. Rappaport. Precocious puberty after hypothalamic and pituitary irradiation in young children. N. Engl. J. Med. 310: 920 (1984).

B20 Brauner, R., P. Czernichow, P. Cramer et al. Leydig-cell function in children after direct testicular irradiation for acute lymphoblastic leukemia. N. Engl. J. Med. 309: 25-28 (1983).

B21 Blatt, J., D.G. Poplack and R.J. Sherins. Testicular function in boys after chemotherapy for acute lymphoblastic leukemia. N. Engl. J. Med. 304: 1121-1124 (1981).

B22 Blatt, J., R.J. Sherins, D. Niebrugge et al. Leydig cell function in boys following treatment for testicular relapse of acute lymphoblastic leukemia. J. Clin. Oncol. 3: 1227-1231 (1985).

B23 Butler, M.S., W.W. Robertson, W. Rate et al. Skeletal sequelae of radiation therapy for malignant childhood tumors. Clin. Orthop. 251: 235-240 (1990).

B24 Broadbent, V.A., N.D. Barnes and T.K. Wheeler. Medulloblastoma in childhood: long-term results of treatment. Cancer 48: 26-30 (1981).

B25 Bleher, E.A. and H. Tschäppeler. Spätveränderungen an der Wirbelsäule nach Strahlentherapie und kombinierter Behandlung bei Morbus Hodgkin im Kindes- und Adoleszentenalter. Strahlentherapie 155: 817-828 (1979).

B26 Barrett, I.R. Slipped capital femoral epiphysis following radiotherapy. J. Pediatr. Orthop. 5: 268-273 (1985).

B27 Burke, F.J.T. and J.W. Frame. The effect of irradiation on developing teeth. Oral Surg., Oral Med., Oral Pathol. 47: 11-13 (1979).

B28 Britten, M.J.A., K.E. Halnan and W.J. Meredith. Radiation cataract: new evidence on radiation damage to the lens. Br. J. Radiol. 39: 612-617 (1966).

B29 Brosius, F.C., B.F. Waller and W.C. Roberts. Radiation heart disease. Analysis of 16 young (aged 15 to 33 years) necropsy patients who received over 3,500 rads to the heart. Am. J. Med. 70: 519-530 (1981).

B30 Burns, R.J., B.-Z. Bar-Schlomo, M.N. Druck et al. Detection of radiation cardiomyopathy by gated radionuclide angiography. Am. J. Med. 74: 297-302 (1983).

B31 Billinghamn, M.E., J.W. Mason, M.R. Bristow et al. Anthracycline carciomyopathy monitored by morphologic changes. Cancer Treat. Rep. 62: 865-872 (1978).

B32 Benoist, M.R., J. Lemerle, R. Jean et al. Effects on pulmonary function of whole lung irradiation for Wilms' tumor in children. Thorax 37: 175-180 (1982).

B33 Barrera, M., L.P. Roy and M. Stevens. Long-term follow-up after unilateral nephrectomy and radio-therapy for Wilms' tumour. Pediatr. Nephrol. 3: 430-432 (1989).

B34 Blomgren, H., S. Hayder, I. Lax et al. Studies on the lymphatic system in long-term survivors treated for Wilms' tumour or non-Hodgkin's lymphoma during childhood. Clin. Oncol. 6: 3-13 (1980).

B35 Bloom, H.J.G. Intracranial tumors: response and resistance to therapeutic endeavors, 1970-1980. Int. J. Radiat. Oncol. Biol. Phys. 8: 1083-1113 (1982).

B36 Baisogolov, G.D. and I.P. Shiskin. Spätfolgen nach Bestrahlung (a) Fellzusammensetzung in bestrahlten Knochenmarkabschnitten. Radiobiol. Radiother. 22 (4): 377-381 (1981).

B37 Baisogolov, G.D. and I.P. Shiskin. Zustand des Strohmas in bestrahlten und intakten Abschnitten des menschlichen Knochenmarks. Radiobiol. Radiother. 23 (1): 31-35 (1982).

B38 Baisogolov, G.D. and I.P. Shiskin. Blutbildung in bestrahlten und unbestrahlten Knochenmarksbereichen. Radiobiol. Radiother. 24 (N1): (1983).

B39 Breur, K., P. Cohen, O. Schweisguth et al. Irradiation of the lungs as an adjuvant therapy in the treatment of osteosarcoma of the limbs. Eur. J. Cancer 14: 461-471 (1978).

B40 Blot, W.J., I.M. Moriyama and R.W. Miller. Reproductive potential of males exposed in utero or prepubertally to atomic radiation. ABCC TR/39-72 (1972).

C1 Committee for Radiation Oncology Studies. Normal tissue tolerance and damage. Cancer 37 (Suppl.): 2046-2055 (1976).

C2 Casarett, G. Basic mechanisms for permanent and delayed radiation pathology. Cancer 37 (Suppl. 2): 1002-1010 (1976).

C3 Crosley, C.J., L.B. Rorke, A. Evans et al. Central nervous system lesions in childhood leukemia. Neurology 28: 678-685 (1978).

C4 Constine, L., A. Konski, S. Ekholm et al. Adverse effects of brain irradiation correlated with MR and CT imaging. Abstract. Int. J. Radiat. Oncol. Biol. Phys. 13 (Suppl. 1): 88 (1987).

C5 Cap, J., Z. Misikova, A. Foltinova et al. Consequences of intensive therapy of acute lymphoblastic leukemia in children in initial complete remission lasting more than five years. Czech. Med. 8: 35-44 (1985).

C6 Copeland, D.R., J.M. Fletcher, B. Pfefferbaum-Levine et al. Neuropsychological sequelae of childhood cancer in long-term survivors. Pediatrics 75: 745-753 (1985).

C7 Copeland, D.R., R.E. Dowell, J.M. Fletcher et al. Neuropsychological effects of childhood cancer treatment. J. Child Neurol. 3: 53-62 (1988).

C8 Calissendorff, B., P. Bolme and M. el-Azazi. The development of cataract in children as a late side-effect of bone marrow transplantation. Bone Marrow Transplant. 7: 427-429 (1991).

C9 Chin, H.W. and Y. Maruyama. Age at treatment and long-term performance results in medulloblastoma. Cancer 53: 1952-1958 (1984).

C10 Czernichow, P., O. Cachin, R. Rappaport et al. Sequelles endocriniennes des irradiations de la tete et du cou pour tumeurs extracraniennes. Arch. Fr. Pédiatr. 34 (Suppl. 7): 154-164 (1977).

C11 Clayton, P.E., S.M. Shalet, P.H. Morris-Jones et al. Growth in children treated for acute lymphoblastic leukemia. Lancet 1: 460-462 (1988).

C12 Clayton, P.E. and S.M. Shalet. Dose dependency of time of onset of radiation-induced growth hormone deficiency. J. Pediatr. 118: 226-228 (1991).

C13 Cramer, P., G. Schaison and J.M. Andrieu. Maladie de Hodgkin de l'enfant résultants à long terme du traitement. Bull. Cancer (FR) 68: 456-464 (1981).

C14 Carli, M., G. Perilongo, A.M. Lavarda et al. Risk factors for cerebral calcifications in patients treated with conventional CNS prophylaxis. in: Third International Symposium on Therapy of Acute Leukemias, Rome, 1982.

C15 Constine, L.S., S.S. Donaldson, I.R. McDougall et al. Thyroid dysfunction after radiotherapy in children with Hodgkin's disease. Cancer 53: 878-883 (1984).

C16 Conard, R.A. Late radiation effects in Marshall Islanders exposed to fallout 28 years ago. p. 57-71 in: Radiation Carcinogenesis: Epidemiology and Biological Significance. (J.D. Boice Jr. and J.F. Fraumeni Jr., eds.) Raven Press, New York, 1984.

C17 Clayton, P.E., S.M. Shalet, D.A. Price et al. Ovarian function following chemotherapy for childhood brain tumours. Med. Pediatr. Oncol. 17: 92-96 (1989).

C18 Clayton, P.E., S.M. Shalet, D.A. Price et al. Testicular damage after chemotherapy for childhood brain tumors. J. Pediatr. 112: 922-926 (1988).

C19 Castillo, L.A., A.W. Craft, J. Kernahan et al. Gonadal function after 12 Gy testicular irradiation in childhood acute lymphoblastic leukemia. Med. Pediatr. Oncol. 18: 185-189 (1990).

C20 Committee on Biological Effects of Ionizing Radiations (BEIR III). The Effects on Populations of Exposure to Low Levels of Ionizing Radiation: 1980. United States National Academy of Sciences, National Research Council. National Academy Press, Washington, 1980.

C21 Choshi, K., I. Takaku, H. Mishima et al. Ophtalmologic changes related to radiation exposure and age in the adult health study sample, Hiroshima and Nagasaki. Radiat. Res. 96: 560-579 (1983).

C22 Carmel, R.J. and H.S. Kaplan. Mantle irradiation in Hodgkin's disease. An analysis of technique, tumor eradication and complications. Cancer 37: 2813-2825 (1976).

C23 Cicognani, A., E. Cacciari, V. Vecci et al. Differential effects of 18- and 24-Gy cranial irradiation on growth rate and growth hormone release in children with prolonged survival after acute lymphocytic leukemia. Am. J. Dis. Child. 142: 1199-1202 (1988).

C24 Caceres, E. and M. Zaharia. Massive preoperative radiation therapy in the treatment of osteogenic sarcoma. Cancer 30 (3): 634-638 (1972).

C25 Chmelevsky, D., C.W. Mays, H. Spiess et al. An epidemiological assessment of lens opacifications that impaired vision in patients injected with radium-224. Radiat. Res. 115: 238-257 (1988).

C26 Constine, L.S., P.D. Woolf, D. Cann et al. Hypothalamic-pituitary dysfunction after radiation for brain tumors. N. Engl. J. Med. 328: 87-94 (1993).

D1 Duffner, P.K., M.E. Cohen, P.R.M. Thomas et al. The long-term effects of cranial irradiation on the central nervous system. Cancer 56 (Suppl.): 1841-1846 (1985).

D2 Deeg, H.J., R. Storb and E.D. Thomas. Bone marrow transplantation: a review of delayed complications. Br. J. Haematol. 57: 185-208 (1984).

D3 Deck, M.D.F. Imaging techniques in the diagnosis of radiation damage to the central nervous system. p. 107-127 in: Radiation Damage to the Nervous System. (H.A. Gilbert and A.R. Kagan, eds.) Raven Press, New York, 1980.

D4 Di Chiro, G., E. Oldfield, D.C. Wright et al. Cerebral necrosis after radiotherapy and/or intraarterial chemotherapy for brain tumors: PET and neuro-pathologic studies. Am. J. Roentgenol. 150: 189-197 (1988).

D5 Davis, P.C., J.C. Hoffman, G.S. Pearl et al. CT evaluation of effects of cranial radiation therapy in children. Am. J. Roentgenol. 147: 587-592 (1986).

D6 Duffner, P.K., M.E. Cohen, S.W. Anderson et al. Long-term effects of treatment on endocrine function in children with brain tumors. Ann. Neurol. 14: 528-532 (1983).

D7 Deutsch, M. Radiotherapy for primary brain tumors in very young children. Cancer 50: 2785-2789 (1982).

D8 Duffner, P.K., M.E. Cohen and P. Thomas. Late effects of treatment in the intelligence of children with posterior fossa tumors. Cancer 51: 233-237 (1983).

D9 Danoff, B.F., F.S. Cowchock, C. Marquette et al. Assessment of the long-term effects of primary radiation therapy for brain tumors in children. Cancer 49: 1580-1586 (1982).

D10 Danoff, B.F., F.S. Cowchock and S. Kramer. Childhood craniopharyngioma: survival, local control, endocrine and neurologic function following radiotherapy. Int. J. Radiat. Oncol. Biol. Phys. 9: 171-175 (1983).

D11 Duffner, P.K., M.E. Cohen, P.R.M. Thomas et al. The long-term effects of cranial irradiation on the central nervous system. Cancer 56: 1841-1846 (1985).

D12 Duffner, P.K., M.E. Cohen, M.L. Voorhess et al. Long-term effects of cranial irradiation on endocrine function in children with brain tumors. Cancer 56: 2189-2193 (1985).

D13 Duffner, P.K. and M.E. Cohen. Recent developments in pediatric neuro-oncology. Cancer 58: 561-568 (1986).

D14 Dickinson, W.P., D.H. Berry, L. Dickinson et al. Differential effects of cranial radiation on growth hormone response to arginine and insulin infusion. J. Pediatr. 92: 754-757 (1978).

D15 Drinnan, C.R., J.D. Miller, H.J. Guyda et al. Growth and development of long-term survivors of childhood acute lymphoblastic leukemia treated with and without prophylactic radiation of the central nervous system. Clin. Invest. Med. 8: 307-314 (1985).

D16 Devney, R.B., C.A. Sklar, M.E. Nesbit et al. Serial thyroid function measurements in children with Hodgkin's disease. J. Pediatr. 105: 223-227 (1984).

D17 Donaldson, S.S. and H.S. Kaplan. Complications of treatment of Hodgkin's disease in children. Cancer Treat. Rep. 66: 977-989 (1982).

D18 Danowski, T.S. Thyroid. p. 255-256 in: Clinical Endocrinology. Volume II. The Williams & Wilkins Company, Baltimore, 1962.

D19 Dawson, W.B. Growth impairment following radiotherapy in childhood. Clin. Radiol. 19: 241-256 (1968).

D20 Dahllöf, G., M. Barr, P. Bolme et al. Disturbances in dental development after total body irradiation in bone marrow transplant recipients. Oral Surg. Oral Med. Oral Pathol. 65: 41-44 (1988).

D21 Deeg, H.J., N. Flournoy, K.M. Sullivan et al. Cataracts after total body irradiation and marrow transplantation: a sparing effect of dose fractionation. Int. J. Radiat. Oncol. Biol. Phys. 10: 957-964 (1984).

D22 do Pico, G.A., A.L. Wiley, P. Rao et al. Pulmonary reaction to upper mantle radiation therapy for Hodgkin's disease. Chest 75: 688-692 (1979).

D23 Donaldson, S.S., S. Jundt, C. Ricour et al. Radiation enteritis in children. Cancer 35: 1167-1178 (1975).

D24 Day, R.E., J. Kingston, J.A. Bullimore et al. CAT brain scans after central nervous system prophylaxis for acute lymphoblastic leukaemia. Br. Med. J. 2: 1752-1753 (1978).

D25 Dacou-Voutetakis, C., A. Xypolyta, S. Haidas et al. Irradiation of the head. Immediate effect on growth hormone secretion in children. J. Clin. Endocrinol. Metab. 44: 791-794 (1977).

D26 DeAngelis, L.M. and W.R. Shapiro. Drug/radiation interactions and central nervous system injury. p. 361-381 in: Radiation Injury to the Nervous System. (P.H. Gutin, S.A. Leibel and G.E. Sheline, eds.) Raven Press Ltd., New York, 1991.

E1 Esseltine, D.W., C.R. Freeman, L.M. Chevalier et al. Computed tomography brain scans in long-term survivors of childhood acute lymphoblastic leukemia. Med. Pediatr. Oncol. 9: 429-438 (1981).

E2 Ellenberg, L., J.G. McComb, S.E. Siegel et al. Factors affecting intellectual outcome in pediatric brain tumor patients. Neurosurgery 21: 638-644 (1987).

E3 Eiser, C. Intellectual abilities among survivors of childhood leukaemia as a function of CNS irradiation. Arch. Dis. Childhood 53: 391-395 (1978).

E4 Eiser, C. and R. Lansdown. Retrospective study of intellectual development in children treated for acute lymphoblastic leukemia. Arch. Dis. Childhood 52: 525-529 (1977).

E5 Eiser, C. Effects of chronic illness on intellectual development. Arch. Dis. Childhood 55: 766-770 (1980).

E6 Edeiken, B.S., H.I. Libshitz and M.A. Cohen. Slipped proximal humoral epiphysis: a complication of radiotherapy to the shoulder in children. Skelet. Radiol. 9: 123-125 (1982).

E7 Egawa S., I. Tsukiyama, Y. Akine et al. Suppression of bony growth of the orbit after radiotherapy for retinoblastoma. Radiat. Med. 5: 207-211 (1987).

F1 Field, S.B. and A.C. Upton. Non-stochastic effects: compatibility with present ICRP recommendations. Int. J. Radiat. Oncol. Biol. Phys. 48: 81-94 (1985).

F2 Fusner, J.E., D.G. Poplack, P.A. Pizzo et al. Leukoencephalopathy following chemotherapy for rhabdomyosarcoma: reversibility of cerebral changes demonstrated by computed tomography. J. Pediatr. 91: 77-79 (1977).

F3 Freeman, C.R., J. Krischer, R.A. Sanford et al. Hyperfractionated radiotherapy in brain stem tumors: results of a pediatric oncology group study. Int. J. Radiat. Oncol. Biol. Phys. 15: 311-318 (1988).

F4 Fuks, Z., E. Glatstein, G.W. Marsa et al. Long-term effects of external radiation on the pituitary and thyroid glands. Cancer 37: 1152-1161 (1976).

F5 Fleming, I.D., T.L. Black, E.I. Thompson et al. Thyroid dysfunction and neoplasia in children receiving neck irradiation for cancer. Cancer 55: 1190-1194 (1985).

F6 Freitas, J.E., D.P. Swanson, M.D. Gross et al. Iodine-131: optimal therapy for hyperthyroidism in children and adolescents? J. Nucl. Med. 20: 847-850 (1979).

F7 Fromm, M., P. Littman, R.B. Raney et al. Late effects after treatment of twenty children with soft tissue sarcomas of the head and neck. Experience at a single institution with a review of the literature. Cancer 57: 2070-2076 (1986).

F8 François, P. Etude dosimetrique retrospective chez des enfants ayant fait une seconde tumeur après radiotherapie. Thèse N.D.'ordre: 132. L'Université Paul Sabatier de Toulouse, 1987.

F9 Fürst, C.J., M. Lundell, S.-O. Ahlbäck et al. Breast hypoplasia following irradiation of the female breast in infancy and early childhood. Acta Oncol. 28: 519-523 (1989).

F10 Fajardo, L.F. and T.V. Colby. Pathogenesis of veno-occlusive liver disease after radiation. Arch. Pathol. Lab. Med. 104: 584-588 (1980).

F11 Freedman, L.R. and R.K. Keehen. Urinary findings of children who were in utero during the atomic bombings of Hiroshima and Nagasaki. Yale J. Biol. Med. 39: 196-206 (1966).

F12 Finch, S.C. and C.A. Finch. Summary of the studies at ABCC-RERF concerning the late hematologic effects of atomic bomb exposure in Hiroshima and Nagasaki. RERF TR/23-88 (1988).

G1 Gamis, A.S. and M.E. Nesbit. Neuropsychologic (cognitive) disabilities in long-term survivors of childhood cancer. Pediatrics 18: 11-19 (1991).

G2 Griffin, N.K. and J. Wadsworth. Effect of treatment of malignant disease on growth in children. Arch. Dis. Childhood 55: 600-603 (1980).

G3 Growth Hormone Treatment of Short Stature. State-of-the-Art in 1989. Acta Paediatr. Scand. (Suppl.) 362: 1-75 (1989).

G4 Glatstein, E., S. McHardy-Young, N. Brast et al. Alternation in serum thyrotropin (TSH) and thyroid function following radiotherapy in patients with malignant lymphoma. J. Clin. Endocrinol. 32: 833-841 (1971).

G5 Green, D.M., M.L. Brecher, D. Yakar et al. Thyroid function in pediatric patients after neck irradiation for Hodgkin's disease. Med. Pediatr. Oncol. 8: 127-136 (1980).

G6 Goolden, A.W. and J.B. Davey. The ablation of normal thyroid tissue with iodine-131. Br. J. Radiol. 36: 340-345 (1963).

G7 Green, D.M., M.L. Brecher, A.N. Lindsay et al. Gonadal function in pediatric patients following treatment for Hodgkin's disease. Med. Pediatr. Oncol. 9: 235-244 (1981).

G8 Gonzalez, D.G. and K. Breur. Clinical data from irradiated growing long bones in children. Int. J. Radiat. Oncol. Biol. Phys. 9: 841-846 (1983).

G9 Gauverky, F. Über die Strahlenschädigung des wachsenden Knochens. Strahlentherapie 113: 325-350 (1960).

G10 Guyuron, B., A.P. Dagys and I.R. Munro. Long-term effects of orbital irradiation. Head Neck Surg. 10: 85-87 (1987).

G11 Gottdiener, J.S., M.J. Katin, J.S. Borer et al. Late cardiac effects of therapeutic mediastinal irradiation. Assessment by echocardiography and radionuclide angiography. N. Engl. J. Med. 308: 569-572 (1983).

G12 Greenwood, R.D., A. Rosenthal, R. Cassady et al. Constrictive pericarditis in childhood due to mediastinal irradiation. Circulation 50: 1033-1039 (1974).

G13 Green, D.M., R.L. Gingell, J. Pearce et al. The effect of mediastinal irradiation on cardiac function of patients treated during childhood and adolescence for Hodgkin's disease. J. Clin. Oncol. 5: 239-245 (1987).

G14 Gilladoga, A.C., C. Manuel, C.T.C. Tan et al. The cardiotoxicity of adriamycin and daunomycin in children. Cancer 37: 1070-1078 (1976).

G15 Gregl, A. and J.W. Weiss. Mammohypoplasie nach Röntgenbestrahlung von Hämangiomen im Säuglingsalter. Fortschr. Geb. Röntgenstr. Nuklearmed. 96: 272-277 (1962).

H1 Hauer-Jensen, M. Late radiation injury of the small intestine. Clinical, pathophysiologic and radiobiologic aspects. A review. Acta Oncol. 29: 401-415 (1989).

H2 Hirsch, J.F., D. Renier, A. Pierre-Kahn et al. Les médulloblastomes de l'enfant. Survie et résultats fonctionnels. Neurochirurgie 24: 391-397 (1978).

H3 Harten, G., U. Stephani, G. Henze et al. Slight impairment of psychomotor skills in children after treatment of acute lymphoblastic leukemia. Eur. J. Pediatr. 142: 189-197 (1984).

H4 Hanefeld, F. and H. Riehm. Therapy of acute lymphoblastic leukemia in childhood: effects on the nervous system. Neuropediatrics 11: 3-16 (1980).

H5 Herber, S.M., R. Kay, R. May et al. Growth of long-term survivors of childhood malignancy. Acta Paediatr. Scand. 74: 438-441 (1985).

H6 Hirsch, J.F., D. Renier, P. Czernichow et al. Medulloblastoma in childhood. Survival and functional results. Acta Neurochir. 48: 1-15 (1979).

H7 Heidemann, P.H., P. Stubbe and W. Beck. Transient secondary hypothyroidism and thyroxine binding globulin deficiency in leukemic children during polychemotherapy: an effect of L-asparaginase. Eur. J. Pediatr. 136: 291-295 (1981).

H8 Hempelmann, L.H. Neoplasms in youthful populations following X-ray treatment in infancy. Environ. Res. 1: 338-358 (1967).

H9 Holm, L.-E., G. Lundell, A. Israelsson et al. Incidence of hypothyroidism occurring long after iodine-131 therapy for hyperthyroidism. J. Nucl. Med. 23: 103-107 (1982).

H10 Holm, L.-E. and I. Ålinder. Relapses after thionamide therapy for Graves' disease. Acta Med. Scand. 211: 489-492 (1982).

H11 Hayek, A., F.M. Chapman and J.D. Crawford. Long-term results of treatment of thyrotoxicosis in children and adolescents with radioactive iodine. N. Engl. J. Med. 283: 949-953 (1970).

H12 Horning, S.J., R.T. Hoppe, H.S. Kaplan et al. Female reproductive potential after treatment for Hodgkin's disease. N. Engl. J. Med. 304: 1377-1382 (1981).

H13 Himmelstein-Braw, R., H. Peters and M. Faber. Influence of irradiation and chemotherapy on the ovaries of children with abdominal tumours. Br. J. Cancer 36: 269-275 (1977).

H14 Hamre, M.R., L.L. Robison, M.E. Nesbit et al. Gonadal function in survivors of childhood acute lymphoblastic leukemia (ALL). Abstract. Proc. Am. Soc. Clin. Oncol. 4: 166 (1985).

H15 Hueck, H. and W. Spiebs. Zur Frage der Wachstumsstörungen bei Röntgen bestrahlten Knochen und Gelenktuberculosen. Strahlentherapie 32: 322-342 (1929).

H16 Heaston, D.K., H.I. Libshitz and R.C. Cahn. Skeletal effects of H2. megavoltage irradiation in survivors of Wilms' tumor. Am. J. Roentgenol. 133: 398-395 (1979).

H17 Heyn, R., A. Ragab, R.B. Raney et al. Late effects of therapy in orbital rhabdomyosarcoma in children. A report from the Intergroup Rhabdomyosarcoma Study. Cancer 57: 1738-1743 (1986).

H18 Hazra, T.A. and B. Shipman. Dental problems in pediatric patients with head and neck tumors undergoing multiple modality therapy. Med. Pediatr. Oncol. 10: 91-95 (1982).

H19 Holbeck, S. and N. Ehlers. Long-term visual results in eyes cured for retinoblastoma by radiation. Acta Ophthalmol. 67: 560-566 (1989).

H20 Haas, J.M. Symptomatic constrictive pericarditis developing 45 years after radiation therapy to the mediastinum. A review of radiation pericarditis. Am. Heart J. 77: 89-95 (1969).

H21 Höst, H. and J.R. Vale. Lung function after mantle field irradiation in Hodgkin's disease. Cancer 32: 328-332 (1973).

H22 Harms, C. Entwicklungshemmung der weiblichen Brustdrüse durch Röntgenbestrahlung. Strahlentherapie 19: 586-588 (1925).

I1 International Commission on Radiological Protection. Non-stochastic Effects of Ionizing Radiation. ICRP Publication 41. Annals of the ICRP 14(3). Pergamon Press, Oxford, 1984.

I2 International Commission on Radiological Protection. 1990 Recommendations of the International Commission on Radiological Protection. ICRP Publication 60. Annals of the ICRP 21(1-3). Pergamon Press, Oxford, 1991.

I3 Inati, A., S.E. Sallan, J.R. Cassady et al. Efficacy and morbidity of central nervous system "prophylaxis" in childhood acute lymphoblastic leukemia: eight years' experience with cranial irradiation and intrathecal methotrexate. Blood 61: 297-303 (1983).

I4 Ishimaru, T., T. Amano and S. Kawamoto. Relationship of stature to gamma and neutron exposure among atomic bomb survivors aged less than 10 at the time of the bomb, Hiroshima and Nagasaki. RERF TR/18-81 (1981).

I5 International Commission on Radiological Protection. Recommendations of the International Commission on Radiological Protection. ICRP Publication 26. Annals of the ICRP 1(3). Pergamon Press, Oxford, 1977.

I6 Ingold, J.A., G.B. Reed, H.S. Kaplan et al. Radiation hepatitis. Am. J. Roentgenol. 93: 200-208 (1965).

I7 Inoue, S., Y. Shibata, H. Hirayu et al. Thyroid diseases among A-bomb survivor in Nagasaki. RERF TR/12-92 (1992).

I8 International Chernobyl Project. Assessment of radiological consequences and evaluation of protective measures. Technical Report. International Advisory Committee, IAEA (1991).

J1 Johnson, F.L., E.D. Thomas, B.S. Clark et al. A comparison of marrow transplantation with chemotherapy for children with acute lymphoblastic leukemia in second or subsequent remission. N. Engl. J. Med. 305: 846-851 (1981).

J2 Jannoun, L. and H.J.G. Bloom. Long-term psychological effects in children treated for intracranial tumors. Int. J. Radiat. Oncol. Biol. Phys. 18: 747-753 (1990).

J3 Jannoun, L. Are cognitive and educational development affected by age at which prophylactic therapy is given in acute lymphoblastic leukaemia? Arch. Dis. Childhood 58: 953-958 (1983).

J4 Jaffe, N., M.P. Sullivan, H. Ried et al. Male reproductive function in long-term survivors of childhood cancer. Med. Pediatr. Oncol. 16: 241-247 (1988).

J5 Jaffe, N., M. McNeese, J.K. Mayfield et al. Childhood urologic cancer therapy related sequelae and their impact on management. Cancer 45: 1815-1822 (1980).

J6 Jaffe, N., B.B. Toth, R.E. Hoar et al. Dental and maxillofacial abnormalities in long-term survivors of childhood cancer: effects of treatment with chemotherapy and radiation to the head and neck. Pediatrics 73: 816-823 (1984).

J7 Johnson, F.L. and F.M. Balis. Hepatopathy following irradiation and chemotherapy for Wilms' tumor. Am. J. Pediatr. Hematol./Oncol. 4: 271-221 (1983).

K1 Kramer, S., M.E. Southard and C.M. Mansfield. Radiation effect and tolerance of the central nervous system. p. 332-345 in: Frontiers of Radiation Therapy and Oncology. Volume 6. (J.M. Vaeth, ed.) Karger, Basel and University Park Press, Baltimore, 1972.

K2 Kingsley, D.P. and B.E. Kendall. CT of the adverse effects of therapeutic radiation of the central nervous system. Am. J. Neuroradiol. 2: 453-460 (1981).

K3 Kramer, J. and M. Moore. Late effects of cancer therapy on the central nervous system. Semin. Oncol. Nurs. 5: 22-28 (1989).

K4 Kay, H.E.M., P.J. Knapton, J.P. O'Sullivan et al. Encephalopathy in acute leukaemia associated with methotrexate therapy. Arch. Dis. Childhood 47: 344-354 (1972).

K5 Kramer, J.H., D. Norman, M. Brant-Zawadzki et al. Absence of white matter changes on magnetic resonance imaging in children treated with CNS prophylaxis therapy for leukemia. Cancer 61: 928-930 (1988).

K6 Kun, L.E., R.K. Mulhern and J.J. Crisco. Quality of life in children treated for brain tumors. Intellectual, emotional, and academic function. J. Neurosurg. 58: 1-6 (1983).

K7 Kirk, J.A., P. Raghupathy, M.M. Stevens et al. Growth failure and growth-hormone deficiency after treatment for acute lymphoblastic leukaemia. Lancet 1: 190-193 (1987).

K8 Kaplan, M.M., M.B. Garnick, R. Gelber et al. Risk factors for thyroid abnormalities after neck irradiation for childhood cancer. Am. J. Med. 74: 272-280 (1983).

K9 Katsanis, E., R.S. Shapiro, L.L. Robison et al. Thyroid dysfunction following bone marrow transplantation: long-term follow-up of 80 pediatric patients. Bone Marrow Transpl. 5: 335-340 (1990).

K10 Kline, R.W., M.T. Gillin and L.E. Kun. Cranial irradiation in acute leukemia: dose estimate in the lens. Int. J. Radiat. Oncol. Biol. Phys. 5: 117-121 (1979).

K11 Kopelson, G. and K.J. Herwig. The etiologies of coronary artery disease in cancer patients. Int. J. Radiat. Oncol. Biol. Phys. 4: 895-906 (1978).

K12 Kadota, R.P., E.O. Burgert, D.J. Driscoll et al. Cardiopulmonary function in long term survivors of childhood Hodgkin's lymphoma: a pilot study. Abstract. Proc. Am. Soc. Clin. Oncol. 5: 198 (1986).

K13 Kolár, J., V. Bek and R. Vrabec. Hypoplasia of the growing breast after contact x-ray therapy for cutaneous angiomas. Arch. Dermatol. 96: 427-430 (1967).

K14 Kraut, J.E., M.A. Bagshaw and E. Glatstein. Hepatic effects of irradiation. p. 182-195 in: Frontiers of Radiation Therapy and Oncology. Volume 6. (J.M. Vaeth, ed.) Karger, Basel and University Park Press, Baltimore, 1972.

K15 Kun, L.E. and B.M. Camita. Hepatopathy following irradiation and adriamycin. Cancer 42: 81-84 (1978).

K16 Koskimies, O. Arterial hypertension developing 10 years after radiotherapy for Wilms' tumour. Br. Med. J. 285: 996-998 (1982).

K17 Kazanets, E.G., A.P. Andreeva, N.A. Karamjan et al. Pathogenesis of anemia in children of the Brjansk region. in: Molecular and Genetic Mechanisms of Influence of Low Radiation Doses. Moscow, 1993. (in Russian)

K18 Karamjan, N.A., S.S. Loria, S.G. Pobpova et al. Hypochronic erythrocytes and secondary erythrocytosis in children from contaminated areas exposed to low radiation doses. in: Molecular and Genetic Mechanisms of Influence of Low Radiation Doses. Moscow, 1993. (in Russian)

L1 Li, F.P. and R. Stone. Survivors of cancer in childhood. Ann. Intern. Med. 84: 551-553 (1976).

L2 Li, F.P., K.R. Winston and K. Gimbrere. Follow-up of children with brain tumors. Cancer 54: 135-138 (1984).

L3 Livrea, P., I.L. Simone, G.B. Zimatore et al. Acute changes in blood-CSF barrier permselectivity to serum proteins after intrathecal methotrexate and CNS irradiation. J. Neurol. 231: 336-339 (1985).

L4 Lannering, B., I. Márky, A. Lundberg et al. Long-term sequelae after pediatric brain tumors: their effect on disability and quality of life. Med. Pediatr. Oncol. 18: 304-310 (1990).

L5 Longeway, K., R. Mulhern, J. Crisco et al. Treatment of meningeal relapse in childhood acute lymphoblastic leukemia: II. A prospective study of intellectual loss specific to CNS relapse and therapy. Am. J. Pediatr. Hematol./Oncol. 12: 45-50 (1990).

L6 Lannering, B. and K. Albertsson-Wikland. Growth hormone release in children after cranial irradiation. Horm. Res. 27: 13-22 (1987).

L7 Livesey, E.A. and C.G.D. Brook. Thyroid dysfunction after radiotherapy and chemotherapy of brain tumours. Arch. Dis. Childhood 64: 593-595 (1989).

L8 Larsen, P.R., R.A. Conard, K.D. Knudsen et al. Thyroid hypofunction after exposure to fallout from a hydrogen bomb explosion. J. Am. Med. Assoc. 247: 1571-1575 (1982).

L9 Lessard, E., R. Miltenberger, R. Conard et al. Thyroid absorbed dose for people at Rongelap, Utirik and Sifo on March 1, 1954. BNL-51882 (1985).

L10 Livesey, E.A. and C.G.D. Brook. Gonadal dysfunction after treatment of intracranial tumours. Arch. Dis. Childhood 63: 495-500 (1988).

L11 Li, F.P., K. Gimbrere, R.D. Gelber et al. Adverse pregnancy outcome after radiotherapy for childhood Wilms' tumor. Abstract. Proc. Am. Soc. Clin. Oncol. 5: 202 (1986).

L12 Leiper, A.D., R. Stanhope, P. Kitching et al. Precocious and premature puberty associated with treatment of acute lymphoblastic leukemia. Arch. Dis. Childhood 62: 1107-1112 (1987).

L13 Lushbaugh, C.C. and R.C. Ricks. Some cytokinetic and histopathologic considerations of irradiated male and female gonadal tissues. p. 228-248 in: Frontiers of Radiation Therapy and Oncology. Volume 6. (J.M. Vaeth, ed.) Karger, Basel and University Park Press, Baltimore, 1972.

L14 Lushbaugh, C.C. and G.W. Casarett. The effects of gonadal irradiation in clinical radiation therapy: a review. Cancer 37: 1111-1120 (1976).

L15 Leiper, A.D., D.B. Grant and J.M. Chessells. The effect of testicular irradiation on Leydig cell function in prepubertal boys with acute lymphoblastic leukaemia. Arch. Dis. Childhood 58: 906-910 (1983).

L16 Larson, D.L., S. Kroll, N. Jaffe et al. Long-term effects of radiotherapy in childhood and adolescence. Am. J. Surg. 160: 348-351 (1990).

L17 Libshitz, H.I. and B.S. Edeiken. Radiotherapy changes of the pediatric hip. Am. J. Roentgenol. 137: 585-588 (1981).

L18 Lockich, J.J., H. Bass, F.E. Eberly et al. The pulmonary effect of mantle irradiation in patients with Hodgkin's disease. Radiology 108: 397-402 (1973).

L19 Littman, P., A.T. Meadows, G. Polgar et al. Pulmonary function in survivors of Wilms' tumor. Patterns of impairment. Cancer 37: 2773-2776 (1976).

L20 Lewin, K. and R.R. Millis. Human radiation hepatitis. A morphologic study with emphasis on the late changes. Arch. Pathol. 96: 21-26 (1973).

L21 Luxton, R.W. Radiation nephritis. Q. J. Med. 22: 215-242 (1953).

L22 Ladavas, E., G. Missiroli, P. Rosito et al. Intellectual function in long-term survivors of childhood acute lymphoblastic leukaemia. Int. J. Neurol. Sci. 6: 451-455 (1985).

L23 Lappi, M., J. Rajantie and R.J. Uusitalo. Irradiation cataract in children after bone marrow transplantation. Graefes Arch. Klin. Exp. Ophthalmol. 228: 218-221 (1990).

L24 Levitt, G.A., E. Yeomans, C. Dicks Mireaux et al. Renal size and function after cure of Wilms' tumour. Br. J. Cancer 66: 877-882 (1992).

L25 Lenskaya, R.V., E.V. Samotsatova, V.M. Bujankin et al. Leukopoiesis in children from Krasnogorsk district of the Brjansk region. p. 95-97 in: Medical Aspects on the Influence of Small Radiation Doses. Obninsk, 1992. (in Russian)

L26 Lenskaya, R.V., O.A. Ikonnikova, A.M. Dzerschinskaja et al. Non-specific esterase of lymphocytes in 101 children from Polesskoje, Ukraine. J. Clin. Lab. Diagn. 11-12: (1992). (in Russian)

L27 Lenskaya, R.V., V.M. Bujankin, O.A. Ikonnikova et al. Cytochemical markers of lymphocytes for the screening of children from radiation contaminated areas. Hematol. Transfusiol. 8: 31-33 (1993). (in Russian)

L28 Lenskaya, R.V., V.M. Bujankin, V.N. Blindar et al. Cytochemical criteria for the screening of children in the radiation contaminated Brjansk region. in: Molecular and Genetic Mechanisms of Influence of Low Radiation Doses. Moscow, 1993. (in Russian)

L29 Lenskaya, R.V., A.G. Rumjantsev, V.M. Bujankin et al. Blood and bone marrow data for 28 children one year after the Chernobyl accident. Hematol. Transfusiol. 4: 25-28 (1991). (in Russian)

M1 Meadows, A.T. The concept of care for life. J. Assoc. Pediatr. Oncol. Nurses 5: 7-9 (1988).

M2 Meadows, A.T., W. Hobbie, P. Jarrett et al. Disabilities in long-term survivors of childhood cancer: results of a systematic follow-up program. Abstract. Proc. Am. Soc. Clin. Oncol. 5: 211 (1986).

M3 Mikhael, M.A. Dosimetric considerations in the diagnosis of radiation necrosis of the brain. p. 59-91 in: Radiation Damage to the Nervous System. (H.A. Gilbert and A.R. Kagan, eds.) Raven Press, New York, 1980.

M4 Moore, I.M., J. Kramer and A. Ablin. Late effects of central nervous system prophylactic leukemia therapy on cognitive functioning. Oncol. Nurs. Forum 13: 45-51 (1986).

M5 McIntosh, S., E.H. Klatskin, R.T. O'Brien et al. Chronic neurologic disturbance in childhood leukemia. Cancer 37: 853-857 (1976).

M6 Meadows, A.T. and A.E. Evans. Effects of chemotherapy on the central nervous system. A study of parenteral methotrexate in long-term survivors of leukemia and lymphoma in childhood. Cancer 37: 1079-1085 (1976).

M7 Marks, J.E., R.J. Baglan, S.C. Prassad et al. Cerebral radionecrosis: incidence and risk in relation to dose, time, fractionation and volume. Int. J. Radiat. Oncol. Biol. Phys. 7: 243-252 (1981).

M8 Mulhern, R.K., J.J. Crisco and L.E. Kun. Neuropsychological sequelae of childhood brain tumors: a review. J. Clin. Child Psychol. 12: 66-73 (1983).

M9 Mulhern, R.K., M.E. Horowitz, E.H. Kovnar et al. Neurodevelopment status of infants and young children treated for brain tumors with pre-irradiation chemotherapy. J. Clin. Oncol. 7: 1660-1666 (1989).

M10 Mulhern, R.K. and L.E. Kun. Neuropsychologic function in children with brain tumors. III. Interval changes in the six months following treatment. Med. Pediatr. Oncol. 13: 318-324 (1985).

M11 Meadows, A.T., J. Gordon, D.J. Massari et al. Declines in IQ scores and cognitive dysfunctions in children with acute lymphocytic leukaemia treated with cranial irradiation. Lancet 2: 1015-1018 (1981).

M12 Moss, H.A., E.D. Nannis and D.G. Poplack. The effects of prophylactic treatment of the central nervous system on the intellectual functioning of children with acute lymphocytic leukemia. Am. J. Med. 71: 47-52 (1981).

M13 Muchi, H., T. Satoh, K. Yamamoto et al. Studies on the assessment of neurotoxicity in children with acute lymphoblastic leukemia. Cancer 59: 891-895 (1987).

M14 Mauras, N., H. Sabio and A.D. Rogol. Neuro-endocrine function in survivors of childhood acute lymphocytic leukemia and non-Hodgkins lymphoma: a study of pulsatile growth hormone and gonadotropin secre-tions. Am. J. Pediatr. Hematol./Oncol. 10: 9-17 (1988).

M15 Moëll, C. Disturbed pubertal growth in girls after acute leukaemia: a relative growth hormone insufficiency with late presentation. Acta Paediatr. Scand. (Suppl.) 343: 162-166 (1988).

M16 Moëll, C., S. Garwicz, U. Westgren et al. Disturbed pubertal growth in girls treated for acute lymphoblastic leukemia. Am. J. Pediatr. Hematol./Oncol. 4: 1-5 (1987).

M17 Moëll, C., S. Garwicz, U. Westgren et al. Suppressed spontaneous secretion of growth hormone in girls after treatment for acute lymphoblastic leukaemia. Arch. Dis. Childhood 64: 252-258 (1989).

M18 Mefferd, J.M., S.S. Donaldson and M.P. Link. Pediatric Hodgkin's disease: pulmonary, cardiac, and thyroid function following combined modality therapy. Int. J. Radiat. Oncol. Biol. Phys. 16: 679-685 (1989).

M19 Maxon, H.R., S.R. Thomas, E.L. Saenger et al. Ionizing irradiation and the induction of clinically significant disease in the human thyroid gland. Am. J. Med. 63: 967-978 (1977).

M20 Maxon, H.R. Radiation-induced thyroid disease. Med. Clin. North Am. 69: 1049-1061 (1985).

M21 Morimoto, I., Y. Yoshimoto, K. Sato et al. Serum TSH, thyroglobulin, and thyroid disorders in atomic bomb survivors exposed in youth: a study 30 years after exposure. RERF TR/20-85 (1985).

M22 Morimoto, I., Y. Yoshimoto, K. Sato et al. Serum TSH, thyroglobulin, and thyroidal disorders in atomic bomb survivors exposed in youth: 30-year follow-up study. J. Nucl. Med. 28: 1115-1122 (1987).

M23 Miller, J.J., G.F. Williams and J.C. Leissring. Multiple late complications of therapy with cycholophosphamide, including ovarian destruction. Am. J. Med. 50: 530-535 (1971).

M24 Mays, C.W., H. Speiss and A. Gerspach. Skeletal effects following 224-Ra injections into humans. Health Phys. 35: 83-90 (1978).

M25 Meadows, A.T., N.L. Krejmas and J.B. Belasco. The medical cost of cure: sequelae in survivors of childhood cancer. p. 263-276 in: Status of the Curability of Childhood Cancers. (J. van Eys and M.P. Sullivan, eds.) Raven Press, New York, 1980.

M26 McGinnis, J.P., K.P. Hopkins, E.I. Thompson et al. Mandibular third molar development after mantle radiation in long-term survivors of childhood Hodgkin's disease. Oral Surg. Oral Med. Oral Pathol. 63: 630-633 (1987).

M27 Merriam, G.R., A. Szechter and E.F. Focht. The effects of ionizing radiations on the eye. p. 346-385 in: Frontiers of Radiation Therapy and Oncology. Volume 6. (J.M. Vaeth, ed.) Karger, Basel and University Park Press, Baltimore, 1972.

M28 Marks, R.D., S.K. Agarwal and W.C. Constable. Radiation induced pericarditis in Hodgkin's disease. Acta Radiol. Ther. Phys. Biol. 12: 305-312 (1973).

M29 Martin, R.G., J.C. Rukdeschel, P. Chang et al. Radiation-related pericarditis. Am. J. Cardiol. 35: 216-220 (1975).

M30 Mäkinen, L., A. Mäkipernaa, J. Rautonen et al. Long-term cardiac sequelae after treatment of malignant tumors with radiotherapy or cytostatics in childhood. Cancer 65: 1913-1917 (1990).

M31 Minow, R.A., R.S. Benjamin and J.A. Gottlieb. Adriamycin (NSC-123127) cardiomyopathy - an overview with determination of risk factors. Cancer Chemother. Rep. 6: 195-200 (1975).

M32 Miller, R.W., J.E. Fusner, R.J. Fink et al. Pulmonary function abnormalities in long-term survivors of childhood cancer. Med. Pediatr. Oncol. 14: 202-207 (1986).

M33 Mitus, A., M. Tefft, F.X. Fellers. Long-term follow-up of renal functions in 108 children who underwent nephrectomy for malignant disease. Pediatrics 44: 912-921 (1969).

M34 Margolis, L. and T.L. Phillips. Whole-lung irradiation for metastatic tumor. Radiology 93: 1173-1179 (1969).

M35 Moss, W.T. Therapeutic Radiology. Mosby, St. Louis, 1959.

M36 McIntosh, S., D.L. Davidson, R.T. O'Brien et al. Methotrexate hepatotoxicity in children with leukemia. J. Pediatr. 90: 1019-1021 (1977).

M37 Mage, K., J.F. Duhamel, J. Sauvegrain et al. Lesions radiques du tube digestif de l'enfant apres irradiation de l'abdomen. Aspects radiologiques. J. Radiol. Electrol. Med. Nucl. 61: 763-768 (1980).

M38 Maher, J.F. Toxic and irradiation nephropathies. p. 1431-1472 in: Strauss and Welt's Diseases of the Kidney. 3rd edition. (L.E. Earley and C.W. Gottschalk, eds.) Little Brown, Boston, 1979.

M39 Maier, J.G. Effects of radiations on kidney, bladder and prostate. p. 196-227 in: Frontiers of Radiation Therapy and Oncology. Volume 6. (J.M. Vaeth, ed.) Karger, Basel and University Park Press, Baltimore, 1972.

M40 McGill, C.W., T.M. Holder, T.H. Smith et al. Post-radiation renovascular hypertension. J. Pediatr. Surg. 14: 831-833 (1979).

M41 Molls, M. and M. Stuschke. Radiotherapy in childhood: normal tissue injuries and carcinogenesis. p. 461-481 in: Medical Radiology, Radiopathology of Organs and Tissues. (E. Scherer, Ch. Streffer and K.-R. Trott, eds.) Springer Verlag, Berlin, 1991.

N1 Nesbit, M.E., H.N. Sather, L.L. Robison et al. Presymptomatic central nervous system therapy in previously untreated childhood acute lymphoblastic leukaemia: comparison of 1800 rad and 2400 rad. A report for Childrens Cancer Study Group. Lancet 1: 461-466 (1981).

N2 Nelson, D.F., K.V. Reddy, R.E. O'Mara et al. Thyroid abnormalities following neck irradiation for Hodgkin's disease. Cancer 42: 2553-2562 (1978).

N3 Nesbit, M.E., L.L. Robison, H.N. Sather et al. Evaluation of long-term survivors of childhood acute lymphoblastic leukemia (ALL). Abstract. Proc. Am. Assoc. Cancer Res. 23: 107 (1982).

N4 National Council on Radiation Protection and Measurements. Protection of the thyroid gland in the event of releases of radioiodine. NCRP Report No. 55 (1977).

N5 Neuhauser, E.B.D., M.H. Wittenborg, C.Z. Berman et al. Irradiation effects of roentgen therapy on the growing spine. Radiology 59: 637-650 (1952).

N6 Nesbit, M.E., W. Krivit, R. Heyn et al. Acute and chronic effects of methotrexate on hepatic, pulmonary, and skeletal systems. Cancer 37: 1048-1054 (1976).

N7 Nagataki, S. Delayed effects of atomic bomb radiation on the thyroid. p. 1-10 in: Radiation and the Thyroid. (S. Nagataki, ed.) Excerpta Medica, Amsterdam, 1989.

N8 Notter, G., R. Walstam and L. Wikholm. Radiation induced cataracts after radium therapy in children. A preliminary report. Acta Radiol. 254 (Suppl.): 87-92 (1966).

O1 Ochs, J., R. Mulhern, D. Fairclough et al. Prospective evaluation of central nervous system (CNS) changes in children with acute lymphoblastic leukemia (ALL) treated with prophylactic cranial irradiation (RT) or iv methothrexate (MTX). Abstract. Proc. Annu. Meet. Am. Soc. Clin. Oncol. 8: A824 (1989).

O2 Ochs, J.J., L.S. Parvey, J.N. Whitaker et al. Serial cranial computed tomography scans in children with leukemia given two different forms of central nervous system therapy. J. Clin. Oncol. 1: 793-798 (1983).

O3 Obetz, S.W., R.J. Ivnik, W.A. Smithson et al. Neuropsychologic follow-up study of children with acute lymphocytic leukemia. A preliminary report. Am. J. Pediatr. Hematol./Oncol. 1: 207-213 (1979).

O4 Ochs, J., R. Mulhern, D. Fairclough et al. Comparison of neuropsychologic functioning and clinical indicators of neurotoxicity in long-term survivors of childhood leukemia given cranial radiation or parenteral methotrexate: a prospective study. J. Clin. Oncol. 9: 145-151 (1991).

O5 Omran, A.R., R.E. Shore, R.A. Markoff et al. Follow-up study of patients treated by X-ray epilation for tinea capitis: psychiatric and psychometric evaluation. Am. J. Public Health 68: 561-567 (1978).

O6 Oberfield, S.E., J.C. Allen, J. Pollack et al. Long-term endocrine sequelae after treatment of medulloblastoma: prospective study of growth and thyroid function. J. Pediatr. 108: 219-223 (1986).

O7 Oliff, A., U. Bode, B.B. Bercu et al. Hypothalamic-pituitary dysfunction following CNS prophylaxis in acute lymphocytic leukemia: correlation with CT scan abnormalities. Med. Pediatr. Oncol. 7: 141-151 (1979).

O8 Onoyama, Y., M. Abe, M. Takahashi et al. Radiation therapy of brain tumors in children. Radiology 115: 687-693 (1975).

O9 Olive, D., B.P. LeHeup and M. Pierson. Ovarian function in 12 long term surviving patients (PTS) with Wilms' tumor. Abstract. Proc. Annu. Meet. Am. Soc. Clin. Oncol. 6: A875 (1987).

O10 Oliver, J.H., G. Gluck, R.B. Gledhill et al. Musculoskeletal deformities following treatment of Wilms' tumour. Can. Med. Assoc. J. 119: 459-464 (1978).

O11 Oglesby, R.B., R.L. Black, L. von Sallmann et al. Cataracts in patients with rheumatic diseases treated with corticosteroids. Further observations. Arch. Ophthalmol. 66: 41-46 (1961).

O12 O'Malley, B., G.J. D'Angio and G.F. Vawter. Late effects of roentgen therapy given in infancy. Am. J. Roentgenol. 89: 1067 (1963).

O13 Ochs, J.J., R. Berg, L. Ch'ien et al. Structural and functional central nervous system (CNS) changes in long-term acute lymphocytic leukemia (ALL) survivors. Proc. Am. Soc. Clin. Oncol. 1: 27 (1982).

O14 Ochs, J.J., P. Berger, M.L. Brecher et al. Computed tomography brain scans in children with acute lymphocytic leukemia receiving methotrexate alone as central nervous system prophylaxis. Cancer 45: 2274-2278 (1980).

O15 Otake, M. and W.J. Schull. Radiation-related posterior lenticular opacities in Hiroshima and Nagasaki atomic bomb survivors based on the DS86 dosimetry system. Radiat. Res. 121: 3-13 (1990).

O16 Otake, M., S.C. Finch, K. Choshi et al. Radiation-related optalmologic changes and aging among a-bomb survivors: a reanalysis. RERF TR/18-91 (1991).

O17 Ochs, J. and R.K. Mulhern. Prospective evaluation of neuropsychological function following cranial irradiation or intermediate dose methotrexate. p. 23-30 in: Late Effects of Treatment for Childhood Cancer. (D.M. Green and G.J. D'Angio, eds.) Wiley-Liss Inc., New York, 1992.

P1 Pizzo, P.A., D.G. Poplack and W.A. Bleyer. Neurotoxicities of current leukemia therapy. Am. J. Pediatr. Hematol./Oncol. 1: 127-140 (1979).

P2 Poplack, D.G. and P. Brouwers. Adverse sequalae of central nervous system therapy. Clin. Oncol. 4: 263-285 (1985).

P3 Price, R.A. and P.A. Jamieson. The central nervous system in childhood leukemia. II. Subacute leukoencephalopathy. Cancer 35: 306-318 (1975).

P4 Price, R.A. and D.A. Birdwell. The central nervous system in childhood leukemia. III. Mineralizing microangiopathy and dystrophic calcification. Cancer 42: 717-728 (1978).

P5 Pavlovsky, S., J. Castano, R. Leiguarda et al. Neuropsychological study in patients with ALL. Am. J. Pediatr. Hematol./Oncol. 5: 79-86 (1983).

P6 Packer, R.J., R.A. Zimmerman and L.T. Bilaniuk. Magnetic resonance imaging in the evaluation of treatment-related central nervous system damage. Cancer 58: 635-640 (1986).

P7 Peylan-Ramu, N., D.G. Poplack, P.A. Pizzo et al. Abnormal CT scans of the brain in asymptomatic children with acute lymphocytic leukemia after prophylactic treatment of the central nervous system with radiation and intrathecal chemotherapy. N. Engl. J. Med. 298: 815-818 (1978).

P8 Perry-Keene, D.A., J.F. Connelly, R.A. Young et al. Hypothalamic hypopituitarism following external radiotherapy for tumours distant from the adenohypophysis. Clin. Endocrinol. 5: 373-380 (1976).

P9 Poussin-Rosillo, H., L.Z. Nisce and B.J. Lee. Complications of total nodal irradiation of Hodgkin's disease stages III and IV. Cancer 42: 437-441 (1978).

P10 Probert, J.C. and B.R. Parker. The effects of radiation therapy on bone growth. Radiology 114: 155-162 (1975).

P11 Probert, J.C., B.R. Parker and H.S. Kaplan. Growth retardation in children after megavoltage irradiation of the spine. Cancer 32: 634-639 (1973).

P12 Price, D.A., M.J. Morris, K.V. Rowsell et al. The effects of anti-leukaemic drugs on somatomedin production and cartilage responsiveness to somatomedin in vitro. Abstract. Pediatr. Res. 15: 1553 (1981).

P13 Parker, R.G. and H.C. Berry. Late effects of therapeutic irradiation on the skeleton and bone marrow. Cancer 37: 1162-1171 (1976).

P14 Prindull, G., W. Weigel, E. Jentsch et al. Aseptic oestonecrosis in children treated for acute lymphoblastic leukemia and aplastic anemia. Eur. J. Pediatr. 139: 48-51 (1982).

P15 Parsons, J.T., C.R. Fitzgerald, C.I. Hood et al. The effects of irradiation on the eye and optic nerve. Int. J. Radiat. Oncol. Biol. Phys. 9: 609-622 (1983).

P16 Prout, M.N., M.J.S. Richards, K.J. Chung et al. Adriamycin cardiotoxicity in children. Case reports, literature review, and risk factors. Cancer 39: 62-65 (1977).

P17 Pratt, C.B., J.L. Ransom and W.E. Evans. Age-related adriamycin cardiotoxicity in children. Cancer Treat. Rep. 62: 1381-1385 (1978).

P18 Pinkel, D., B. Camitta, L. Kun et al. Doxorubicin cardiomyopathy in children with left-sided Wilms' tumor. Med. Pediatr. Oncol. 10: 483-488 (1982).

Q1 Quigley, C., C. Cowell, M. Jimenez et al. Normal or early development of puberty despite gonadal damage in children treated for acute lymphoblastic leukemia. N. Engl. J. Med. 321: 143-151 (1989).

Q2 Qvist, C.F. and B. Zachau-Christiansen. Radiation cataract following fractionated radium therapy in childhood. Acta Radiol. 51: 207-216 (1959).

R1 Rubin, P. and G.W. Casarett. Clinical Radiation Pathology. Volume 1. Saunders, Philadelphia, 1968.

R2 Rubin, P. and G.W. Casarett. A direction for clinical radiation pathology. The tolerance dose. p. 1-16 in: Frontiers of Radiation Therapy and Oncology. Volume 6. (J.M. Vaeth, ed.) Karger, Basel and University Park Press, Baltimore, 1972.

R3 Rubin, P. The Franz Buschke lecture: Late effects of chemotherapy and radiation therapy: a new hypothesis. Int. J. Radiat. Oncol. Biol. Phys. 10: 5-34 (1984).

R4 Rubinstein, L.J., M.M. Herman, T.F. Long et al. Disseminated necrotizing leukoencephalopathy: a complication of treated central nervous system leukemia and lymphoma. Cancer 35: 291-305 (1975).

R5 Riccardi, R., P. Brouwers, G. Di Chiro et al. Abnormal computed tomography brain scans in children with acute lymphoblastic leukemia: serial long-term follow-up. J. Clin. Oncol. 3: 12-18 (1985).

R6 Raimondi, A.J. and T. Tomita. The disadvantages of prophylactic whole CNS post-operative radiation therapy for medulloblastoma. p. 209-218 in: Multidisciplinary Aspects of Brain Tumor Therapy. (P. Paoletti, M.D. Walker, G. Butti et al., eds.) Elsevier/North Holland Biomedical Press, New York, 1979.

R7 Rubinstein, C.L., J.W. Varni and E.R. Katz. Cognitive functioning in long-term survivors of childhood leukemia; a prospective analysis. J. Dev. Behav. Pediatr. 11: 301-305 (1990).

R8 Rowland, J.H., O.J. Glidewell, R.F. Sibley et al. Effects of different forms of central nervous system prophylaxis on neuropsychologic function in childhood leukemia. J. Clin. Oncol. 2: 1327-1335 (1984).

R9 Robison, L.L., A.T. Meadows, M.E. Nesbit et al. Factors associated with IQ scores in long-term survivors of childhood acute lymphoblastic leukemia. Am. J. Pediatr. Hematol./Oncol. 6: 115-120 (1984).

R10 Ron, E., B. Modan, S. Floro et al. Mental function following scalp irradiation during childhood. Am. J. Epidemiol. 116: 149-160 (1982).

R11 Richards, G.E., W.M. Wara, M.M. Grumbach et al. Delayed onset of hypopituitarism: sequelae of therapeutic irradiation of central nervous system, eye, and middle ear tumors. J. Pediatr. 89: 553-559 (1976).

R12 Romshe, C.A., W.B. Zipf and A. Miser. Evaluation of growth hormone release and human growth hormone treatment in children with cranial irradiation - associated short stature. J. Pediatr. 104: 177-181 (1984).

R13 Robison, L.L., M.E. Nesbit, H.N. Sather et al. Height of children successfully treated for acute lymphoblastic leukemia: a report from the late effects study committee of Childrens Cancer Study Group. Med. Pediatr. Oncol. 13: 14-21 (1985).

R14 Robbins, J., J.E. Rall and R.A. Conard. Late effects of radioactive iodine in fallout. Ann. Intern. Med. 66: 1214-1242 (1967).

R15 Rogers, P.C.J., C.J.H. Fryer and S. Hussein. Radiation dose to the thyroid in the treatment of acute lymphoblastic leukemia (ALL). Med. Pediatr. Oncol. 10: 385-388 (1982).

R16 Robison, L.L., M.E. Nesbit, H.N. Sather et al. Thyroid abnormalities in long-term survivors of childhood acute lymphoblastic leukemia. Pediatr. Res. 19: 226A (1985).

R17 Rubin, P., P. van Houtte and L. Constine. Radiation sensitivity and organ tolerances in pediatric oncology: a new hypothesis. Front. Radiat. Ther. Oncol. 16: 62-82 (1982).

R18 Robison, L.L. Delayed consequences of therapy in childhood acute lymphoblastic leukaemia. Clin. Oncol. 4: 321-332 (1985).

R19 Refetoff, S., J. Harrison, B.T. Karanfilski et al. Continuing occurrence of thyroid carcinoma after irradiation to the neck in infancy and childhood. N. Engl. J. Med. 292: 171-175 (1975).

R20 Robbins, J. and W.H. Adams. Radiation effects in the Marshall Islands. p. 11-24 in: Radiation and the Thyroid. (S. Nagataki, ed.) Excerpta Medica, Amsterdam, 1989.

R21 Rallison, M.L., B.M. Dobyns, F.R. Keating et al. Thyroid disease in children. A survey of subjects potentially exposed to fallout radiation. Am. J. Med. 56: 457-463 (1974).

R22 Rallison, M.L., B.M. Dobyns, F.R. Keating et al. Thyroid nodularity in children. J. Am. Med. Assoc. 233: 1069-1072 (1975).

R23 Rappaport, R., R. Brauner, P. Czernichow et al. Effect of hypothalamic and pituitary irradiation on pubertal development in children with cranial tumors. J. Clin. Endocrinol. Metab. 54: 1164-1168 (1982).

R24 Rowley, M.J., D.R. Leach, G.A. Warner et al. Effect of graded doses of ionizing radiation on the human testis. Radiat. Res. 59: 665-678 (1974).

R25 Rubin, P., R.B. Duthie and L.W. Young. Significance of scoliosis in post-irradiated Wilms' tumor and neuroblastoma. Radiology 79: 539-559 (1962).

R26 Rausch, L., W. Koch and G. Hagemann. Klinische und dosimetrische Untersuchungen zur Frage der kritischen Dosis und typischer Strahlenschäden am Skelett bestrahlter Angiom-Patienten. Strahlentherapie (Sonderbände) 55: 198-514 (1964).

R27 Riseborough, E.J., S.L. Grabias, R.I. Burton et al. Skeletal alternations following irradiation for Wilms' tumor with particular reference to scoliosis and kyphosis. J. Bone Jt. Surg. 58A: 526-536 (1976).

R28 Ruckdeschel, J.C., P. Chang, R.G. Martin et al. Radiation-related pericardial effusions in patients with Hodgkin's disease. Medicine 54: 245-259 (1975).

R29 Rubin, P., S. Landman, E. Mayer et al. Bone marrow regeneration and extension after extended field irradiation in Hodgkin's disease. Cancer 32: 699-711 (1973).

R30 Ron, E., B. Modan, J.D. Boice et al. Tumors of the brain and nervous system after radiotherapy in childhood. N. Engl. J. Med. 319: 1033-1039 (1988).

S1 Sposto, R. and G.D. Hammond. Survival in childhood cancer. Clin. Oncol. 4: 195-204 (1985).

S2 Sheline, G.E., W.M. Wara and V. Smith. Therapeutic irradiation and brain injury. Int. J. Radiat. Oncol. Biol. Phys. 6: 1215-1228 (1980).

S3 Silverman, C.L., H. Palkes, B. Talent et al. Late effects of radiotherapy on patients with cerebellar medulloblastoma. Cancer 54: 825-829 (1984).

S4 Suc, E., C. Kalifa, R. Brauner et al. Brain tumours under the age of three. The price of survival. A retrospective study of 20 long-term survivors. Acta Neurochir. 106: 93-98 (1990).

S5 Sawyer, M.G., I. Toogood, M. Rice et al. School performance and psychological adjustment of children treated for leukemia. A long-term follow-up. Am. J. Pediatr. Hematol./Oncol. 11: 146-152 (1989).

S6 Soni, S.S., G.W. Marten, S.E. Pitner et al. Effects of central-nervous-system irradiation on neuropsychologic functioning of children with acute lymphocytic leukemia. N. Engl. J. Med. 293: 113-118 (1975).

S7 Shore, R.E., R.E. Albert and B.S. Pasternack. Follow-up study of patients treated by x-ray epilation for tinea capitis. Resurvey of post-treatment illness and mortality experience. Arch. Environ. Health 31: 21-28 (1976).

S8 Spunberg, J.J., C.H. Chang, M. Goldman et al. Quality of long-term survival following irradiation for intracranial tumors in children under the age of two. Int. J. Radiat. Oncol. Biol. Phys. 7: 727-736 (1981).

S9 Samaan, N.A., P.N. Schultz, K.-P.P. Yang et al. Endocrine complications after radiotherapy for tumors of the head and neck. J. Lab. Clin. Med. 109: 364-372 (1987).

S10 Shalet, S.M. Growth and hormonal status of children treated for brain tumours. Child's Brain 9: 284-293 (1982).

S11 Shalet, S.M., C.G. Beardwell, B.M. Aarons et al. Growth impairment in children treated for brain tumours. Arch. Dis. Childhood 53: 491-494 (1978).

S12 Shalet, S.M., C.G. Beardwell, J.A. Twomey et al. Endocrine function following the treatment of acute leukemia in childhood. J. Pediatr. 90: 920-923 (1977).

S13 Shalet, S.M., C.G. Beardwell, P.H. Morris-Jones et al. Growth hormone deficiency in children with brain tumors. Cancer 37: 1144-1148 (1976).

S14 Shalet, S.M., C.G. Beardwell, D. Pearson et al. The effect of varying doses of cerebral irradiation on growth hormone production in childhood. Clin. Endocrinol. 5: 287-290 (1976).

S15 Shalet, S.M., C.G. Beardwell, I.A. MacFarlane et al. Endocrine morbidity in adults treated with cerebral irradiation for brain tumors during childhood. Acta Endocrinol. 84: 673-680 (1977).

S16 Shalet, S.M., C.G. Beardwell, P.H. Morris-Jones et al. Pituitary function after treatment of intracranial tumours in children. Lancet 2: 104-107 (1975).

S17 Samaan, N.A., R. Vieto, P.N. Schultz et al. Hypothalamic pituitary and thyroid dysfunction after radiotherapy to the head and neck. Int. J. Radiat. Oncol. Biol. Phys. 8: 1857-1867 (1982).

S18 Samaan, N.A., M.M. Bakdash, J.B. Caderao et al. Hypopituitarism after external irradiation. Evidence for both hypothalamic and pituitary origin. Ann. Intern. Med. 83: 771-777 (1975).

S19 Shalet, S.M., D.A. Price, C.G. Beardwell et al. Normal growth despite abnormalities of growth hormone secretion in children treated for acute leukemia. J. Pediatr. 94: 719-722 (1979).

S20 Shalet, S.M. The effects of cancer treatment on growth and sexual development. Clin. Oncol. 4: 223-238 (1985).

S21 Shalet, S.M., C.G. Beardwell, P.H. Morris-Jones et al. Growth hormone deficiency after treatment of acute leukaemia in children. Arch. Dis. Childhood 51: 489-493 (1976).

S22 Starceski, P.J., P.A. Lee, J. Blatt et al. Comparable effects of 1800- and 2400-rad (18- and 24-Gy) cranial irradiation on height and weight in children treated for acute lymphocytic leukemia. Am. J. Dis. Child. 141: 550-552 (1987).

S23 Sanders, J.E., S. Pritchard, P. Mahoney et al. Growth and development following marrow transplantation for leukemia. Blood 68: 1129-1135 (1986).

S24 Sanders, J.E. Late effects in children receiving total body irradiation for bone marrow transplantation. Radiother. Oncol. 18 (Suppl. 1): 82-87 (1990).

S25 Sanders, J.E. Implications of cancer therapy to the head and neck on growth and development and other delayed effects. Natl. Cancer Inst. Monogr. 9: 163-167 (1990).

S26 Sutow, W.W., R.A. Conard and K.M. Griffith. Growth status of children exposed to fallout radiation on the Marshall Islands. Pediatrics 36: 721-31 (1965).

S27 Shalet, S.M., J.D. Rosenstock, C.G. Beardwell et al. Thyroid dysfunction following external irradiation to the neck for Hodgkin's disease in childhood. Clin. Radiol. 28: 511-515 (1977).

S28 Schimpff, S.C., C.H. Diggs, J.G. Wiswell et al. Radiation-related thyroid dysfunction: implications for the treatment of Hodgkin's disease. Ann. Intern. Med. 92: 91-98 (1980).

S29 Smith, R.E., R.A. Adler, P. Clark et al. Thyroid function after mantle irradiation in Hodgkin's disease. J. Am. Med. Assoc. 245: 46-49 (1981).

S30 Sklar, C.A., T.H. Kim and M.K.C. Ramsay. Thyroid dysfunction among long-term survivors of bone marrow transplantation. Am. J. Med. 73: 688-694 (1982).

S31 Sklar, C.A. Physiology of growth hormone production and release. p. 49-54 in: Late Effects of Treatment for Childhood Cancer. (D.M. Green and G.J. D'Angio, eds.) Wiley-Liss Inc., New York, 1992.

S32 Shalet, S.M., C.G. Beardwell, P.H. Morris-Jones et al. Ovarian failure following abdominal irradiation in childhood. Br. J. Cancer 33: 655-658 (1976).

S33 Stillman, R.J., J.S. Schinfeld, I. Schiff et al. Ovarian failure in long-term survivors of childhood malignancy. Am. J. Obstet. Gynecol. 139: 62-66 (1981).

S34 Sanders, J.E., C.D. Buckner, K.M. Sullivan et al. Growth and development after bone marrow transplantation. p. 375-382 in: Advances and Controversies in Thalassemia Therapy: Bone Marrow Transplantation and Other Approaches. (C.D. Buckner, R.P. Galce and G. Lucarelli, eds.) Alan R. Liss Inc., New York, 1989.

S35 Sarkar, S.D., W.H. Beierwaltes, S.P. Gill et al. Subsequent fertility and birth histories of children and adolescents treated with ^{131}I for thyroid cancer. J. Nucl. Med. 17: 460-464 (1976).

S36 Sherins, R.J. and J.J. Mulvihill. Gonadal dysfunction. p. 2170-2180 in: Cancer. Principles & Practice of Oncology. (V.T. Devita, S. Hellman and S.A. Rosenberg, eds.) J.B. Lippincott Company, Philadelphia, 1989.

S37 Stefani, F.H., H. Spiess and C.W. Mays. Cataracts in patients injected with 224-Ra. p. 51-59 in: The Radiobiology of Radium and Thorotrast. (W. Gössner, G.B. Gerber, U. Hagen et al., eds.) Urban & Schwarzenberg, München, 1986.

S38 Shalet, S.M., A. Tsatsoulis, E. Whitehead et al. Vulnerability of the human Leydig cell to radiation damage is dependent upon age. J. Endocrinol. 120: 161-165 (1989).

S39 Shalet, S.M., C.G. Beardwell, H.S. Jacobs et al. Testicular function following irradiation of the human prepubertal testis. Clin. Endocrinol. 9: 483-490 (1978).

S40 Shalet, S.M., A. Horner, S.R. Ahmed et al. Leydig cell damage after testicular irradiation for lymphoblastic leukaemia. Med. Pediatr. Oncol. 13: 65-68 (1985).

S41 Sklar, C.A., L.L. Robison, M.E. Nesbit et al. Effects of radiation on testicular function in long-term survivors of childhood acute lymphoblastic leukemia. A report from the Childrens Cancer Study Group. J. Clin. Oncol. 8: 1981-1987 (1990).

S42 Smith, R., J.K. Davidson and G.E. Flatman. Skeletal effects of orthovoltage and megavoltage therapy following treatment of nephroblastoma. Clin. Radiol. 33: 601-613 (1982).

S43 Shalet, S.M., B. Gibson, R. Swindell et al. Effect of spinal irradiation on growth. Arch. Dis. Childhood 62: 461-464 (1987).

S44 Spiess, H., C.W. Mays and E. Spiess-Paulus. Growth retardation in children injected with 224-Ra. p. 45-50. in: The Radiobiology of Radium and Thorotrast. (W. Gössner, G.B. Gerber, U. Hagen et al., eds.) Urban & Schwarzenberg, München, 1986.

S45 Schultz, H., B. Jacobsen, K. Bjørn Jensen et al. Nephroblastoma. Results and complications of treatment. Acta Radiol. Oncol. 18: 449-459 (1979).

S46 Silverman, C.L., P.R.M. Thomas, W.H. McAlister et al. Slipped femoral capital epiphyses in irradiated children: dose, volume and age relationships. Int. J. Radiat. Oncol. Biol. Phys. 7: 1357-1363 (1981).

S47 Sonis, A.L., N. Tarbell, R.W. Valachovic et al. Dentofacial development in long-term survivors of acute lymphoblastic leukemia. A comparison of three treatment modalities. Cancer 66: 2645-2652 (1990).

S48 Sonnabend, E., H. Spiess and C.W. Mays. Tooth breakage in patients injected with 224-Ra. p. 60-64 in: The Radiobiology of Radium and Thorotrast. (W. Gössner, G.B. Gerber, U. Hagen et al., eds.) Urban & Schwarzenberg, München, 1986.

S49 Spaeth, G.L. and L. von Sallmann. Corticosteroids and cataracts. Int. Ophthalmol. Clin. 6: 915-928 (1966).

S50 Stewart, J.R. and L.F. Fajardo. Dose response in human and experimental radiation-induced heart disease. Application of the nominal standard dose (NSD) concept. Radiology 99: 403-408 (1971).

S51 Scott, D.L. and R.D. Thomas. Late onset constrictive pericarditis after thoracic radiotherapy. Br. Med. J. 1: 341-342 (1978).

S52 Smith, P.J., H. Ekert, K.D. Waters et al. High incidence of cardiomyopathy in children treated with adriamycin and DTIC in combination chemotherapy. Cancer Treat. Rep. 61: 1736-1738 (1977).

S53 Springmeyer, S.C., N. Flournoy, K.M. Sullivan et al. Pulmonary function changes in long-term survivors of allogeneic marrow transplantation. p. 343-353 in: Recent Advances in Bone Marrow Transplantation. (R.P. Gale, ed.) Alan R. Liss Inc., New York, 1983.

S54 Shapiro, S.J., S.D. Shapiro, W.B. Mill et al. Prospective study of long-term pulmonary manifestations of mantle irradiation. Int. J. Radiat. Oncol. Biol. Phys. 19: 707-714 (1990).

S55 Scotti, G., M. Bracchi, G. Masera et al. Prophylactic treatment of the central nervous system in acute lymphoblastic leukemia. CT findings in 45 children of therapy. J. Neurol. Sci. 2(4): 361-365 (1981).

S56 Sheline, G.E., W.M. Wara and V. Smith. Therapeutic irradiation and brain injury. Int. J. Radiat. Oncol. Biol. Phys. 6: 1215-1218 (1980).

S57 Stevens, S.K., S.G. Moore and I.D. Kaplan. Early and late bone-marrow changes after irradiation: MR evaluation. AJR, Am. J. Roentgenol. 154: 745-750 (1990).

T1 Trott, K.-R. Chronic damage after radiation therapy: challenge to radiation biology. Int. J. Radiat. Oncol. Biol. Phys. 10: 907-913 (1984).

T2 Thames, H.D., H.R. Withers, L.J. Peters et al. Changes in early and late radiation responses with altered dose fractionation: implications for dose-survival relationships. Int. J. Radiat. Oncol. Biol. Phys. 8: 219-226 (1982).

T3 Tarbell, T.J., E.C. Guinan, L. Chin et al. Renal insufficiency after total body irradiation for pediatric bone marrow transplantation. Radiother. Oncol. 18 (Suppl. 1): 139-142 (1990).

T4 Tamaroff, M., R. Salwen, D.R. Miller et al. Comparison of neuropsychologic performance in children treated for acute lymphoblastic leukemia (ALL) with 1800 rads cranial radiation plus intrathecal methotrexate or intrathecal methotrexate alone. Abstract. Proc. Am. Soc. Oncol. 3: 198 (1984).

T5 Tamaroff, M., D.R. Miller, M.L. Murphy et al. Immediate and long-term post-therapy neuropsychologic performance in children with acute lymphoblastic leukemia treated without central nervous system radiation. J. Pediatr. 101: 524-529 (1982).

T6 Tamaroff, M., R. Salwen, D.R. Miller et al. Neuropsychologic sequelae in irradiated (1800 rads (r) & 2400r) and non-irradiated children with acute lymphoblastic leukemia (ALL). Abstract. Proc. Am. Soc. Clin. Oncol. 4: 165 (1985).

T7 Trautman, P.D., C. Erickson, D. Shaffer et al. Prediction of intellectual deficits in children with acute lymphoblastic leukemia. J. Dev. Behav. Pediatr. 9: 122-128 (1988).

T8 Tamura, K., K. Shimaoka and M. Friedman. Thyroid abnormalities associated with treatment of malignant lymphoma. Cancer 47: 2704-2711 (1981).

T9 Tarbell, N.J., L. Thompson and P. Mauch. Thoracic irradiation in Hodgkin's disease: disease control and long-term complications. Int. J. Radiat. Oncol. Biol. Phys. 18: 275-281 (1990).

T10 Tefft, M., P.B. Lattin, B. Jereb et al. Acute and late effects on normal tissues following combined chemo- and radiotherapy for childhood rhabdomyosarcoma and Ewing's sarcoma. Cancer 37: 1201-1213 (1976).

T11 Thomas, P.R.M., K.D. Griffith, B.B. Fineberg et al. Late effects of treatment for Wilms' tumor. Int. J. Radiat. Oncol. Biol. Phys. 9: 651-657 (1983).

T12 Thomas, P.R.M., M. Tefft, G.J. D'Angio et al. Radiation associated toxicities in the Second National Wilms' Tumor Study (NWTS-2). Abstract. Int. J. Radiat. Oncol. Biol. Phys. 10 (Suppl. 2): 88 (1984).

T13 Tefft, M., A. Mitus, L. Das et al. Irradiation of the liver in children: review of experience in the acute and chronic phases, and in the intact normal and partially resected. Am. J. Roentgenol. 108: 365-385 (1970).

T14 Twaddle, V., P.G. Britton, A.C. Craft et al. Intellectual function after treatment for leukaemia or solid tumours. Arch. Dis. Childhood 58: 949-952 (1983).

T15 Tereshenko, N.Ya., L.I. Burtseva and V.M. Abdulaeva. Delayed clinical effects of contact gamma-irradiation therapy for angioma cutis in young children. Med. Radiol. 11: 49-53 (1988). (in Russian)

T16 Tarbell, N.J., E.C. Guinan, C. Niemeyer et al. Late onset of renal dysfunction in survivors of bone marrow transplantation. Int. J. Radiat. Oncol. Biol. Phys. 15: 99-104 (1988).

T17 Tichelli, A., A. Gratwohl, M. Uhr et al. Gesundheitszustand und Spätkomplikationen nach allogener Knochenmarktransplantation. Eine Übersicht. Schweiz. Med. Wochenschr. 121: 1473-1481 (1991).

U1 United Nations. Sources, Effects and Risks of Ionizing Radiation. United Nations Scientific Committee on the Effects of Atomic Radiation, 1988 Report to the General Assembly, with annexes. United Nations sales publication E.88.IX.7. United Nations, New York, 1988.

U2 United Nations. Genetic and Somatic Effects of Ionizing Radiation. United Nations Scientific Committee on the Effects of Atomic Radiation, 1986 Report to the General Assembly, with annexes. United Nations sales publication E.86.IX.9. United Nations, New York, 1986.

U3 United Nations. Ionizing Radiation: Sources and Biological Effects. United Nations Scientific Committee on the Effects of Atomic Radiation, 1982 Report to the General Assembly, with annexes. United Nations sales publication E.82.IX.8. United Nations, New York, 1982.

U4 United Nations. Sources and Effects of Ionizing Radiation. United Nations Scientific Committee on the Effects of Atomic Radiation, 1977 report to the General Assembly, with annexes. United Nations sales publication E.77.IX.1. United Nations, New York, 1977.

U11 Underwood, G.B. and L.E. Gaul. Disfiguring sequelae from radium therapy. Results of treatment of a birthmark adjacent to the breast in a female infant. Arch. Dermatol. Syphilology 57: 918-919 (1948).

V1 Von Muehlendahl, K.E., H. Gadner, H. Riehm et al. Endocrine function after antineoplastic therapy in 22 children with acute lymphoblastic leukaemia. Helv. Paediatr. Acta 31: 463-471 (1976).

V2 Verzosa, M.S., R.J.A. Aur, J.V. Simone et al. Five years after central nervous system irradiation of children with leukemia. Int. J. Radiat. Oncol. Biol. Phys. 1: 209-215 (1976).

V3 Von Hoff, D.D., M. Rozencweig and M. Piccart. The cardiotoxicity of anticancer agents. Semin. Oncol. 9: 23-33 (1982).

V4 Von Hoff, D.D., M. Rozencweig, M. Layard et al. Daunomycin-induced cardiotoxicity in children and adults. A review of 110 cases. Am. J. Med. 62: 200-208 (1977).

V5 Von Hoff, D.D., M.W. Layard, P. Basa et al. Risk factors for doxorubicin-induced congestive heart failure. Ann. Intern. Med. 91: 710-717 (1979).

V6 Van Slyck, E.J. and G.A. Bermudez. Radiation nephritis. Yale J. Biol. Med. 41: 243-256 (1968).

V7 Van Weel-Sipman, M.H., E.T. van't Veer-Korthof, H. van den Berg et al. Late effects of total body irradiation and cytostatic preparative regimen for bone marrow transplantation in children with hematological malignancies. Radiother. Oncol. 18 (Suppl. 1): 155-157 (1990).

V8 Van Why, S.K., A.L. Friedman, L.J. Wei et al. Renal insufficiency after bone marrow transplantation in children. Bone Marrow Transplant. 7: 383-388 (1991).

V9 Vladimirskaja, E.B., I.V. Zamaraeva, E.U. Osipova et al. Granulocytopoiesis in children from the radio-contaminated areas. in: Molecular and Genetic Mechanisms of Influence of Low Radiation Doses. Moscow, 1993. (in Russian)

W1 Withers, H.R. Predicting late normal tissue responses. Int. J. Radiat. Oncol. Biol. Phys. 12: 693-698 (1986).

W2 Withers, H.R., L.J. Peters, H.D. Thames et al. Hyperfractionation. Int. J. Radiat. Oncol. Biol. Phys. 8: 1807-1809 (1982).

W3 Whitt, J.K., R.J. Wells, M.M. Lauria et al. Cranial radiation in childhood acute lymphocytic leukemia. Neuropsychological sequelae. Am. J. Dis. Child. 138: 730-736 (1984).

W4 Westergren, U. Is growth hormone secretion related to growth? Acta Paediatr. Scand. 362(S): 32-35 (1989).

W5 Wells, R.J., M.B. Foster, A.J. D'Ercole et al. The impact of cranial irradiation on the growth of children with acute lymphocytic leukemia. Am. J. Dis. Child. 137: 37-39 (1983).

W6 Wallace, W.H.B., S.M. Shalet, J.H. Hendry et al. Ovarian failure following abdominal irradiation in childhood: the radiosensitivity of the human oocyte. Br. J. Radiol. 62: 995-998 (1989).

W7 Wilimas, J., E. Thompson and K.L. Smith. Long-term results of treatment of children and adolescents with Hodgkin's disease. Cancer 46: 2123-2125 (1989).

W8 Willich, E., H. Kuttig, G. Pfeil et al. Wirbelsäulenveränderungen nach Bestrahlung wegen Wilms' tumor im Kleinkindersalter. Strahlenther. Onkol. 166: 815-821 (1990).

W9 Walker, S.J., L.A. Whiteside, W.H. McAlister et al. Slipped capital femoral epiphysis following radiation and chemotherapy. Clin. Orthop. 159: 186-193 (1981).

W10 Wolf, E.L., W.E. Berdon, J.R. Cassady et al. Slipped femoral capital epiphysis as a sequela to childhood irradiation for malignant tumors. Radiology 125: 781-784 (1977).

W11 Weaver, R.G., A.R. Chauvenet, T.J. Smith et al. Ophtalmic evaluation of long-term survivors of childhood, acute lymphoblastic leukemia. Cancer 58: 963-968 (1986).

W12 Wara, W.M., T.L. Phillips, L.W. Margolis et al. Radiation pneumonitis: a new approach to the derivation of time-dose factors. Cancer 32: 547-552 (1973).

W13 Watchie, J., C.N. Coleman, T.A. Raffin et al. Minimal long-term cardiopulmonary dysfunction following treatment for Hodgkin's disease. Int. J. Radiat. Oncol. Biol. Phys. 13: 517-524 (1987).

W14 Wohl, M.E., N.T. Griscom, D.G. Traggis et al. Effects of therapeutic irradiation delivered in early childhood upon subsequent lung function. Pediatrics 55: 507-514 (1975).

Z1 Zaharia, M., E. Caceres, S. Valdivia et al. Postoperative whole lung irradiation with or without adriamycin in osteogenic sarcoma. Int. J. Radiat. Oncol. Biol. Phys. 12: 907-910 (1986).